fifth edition

Family
Health Care
Nursing

Theory, Practice, and Research

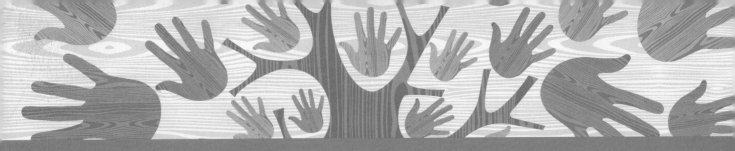
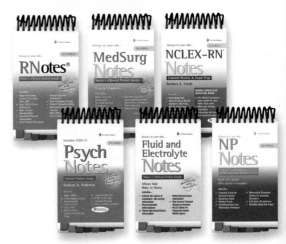
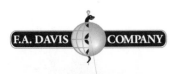

fifth edition

Family Health Care Nursing

Theory, Practice, and Research

Joanna Rowe Kaakinen, PhD, RN
Professor, School of Nursing
Linfield College
Portland, Oregon

Deborah Padgett Coehlo, PhD, C-PNP, PMHS, CFLE
Developmental and Behavioral Specialist
Juniper Ridge Clinic
Bend, Oregon

Rose Steele, PhD, RN
Professor, School of Nursing, Faculty of Health
York University
Toronto, Ontario, Canada

Aaron Tabacco, RN, BSN
Doctoral Candidate, School of Nursing
Oregon Health and Science University
Portland, Oregon

Shirley May Harmon Hanson, RN, PhD, PMHNP/ARNP, FAAN, CFLE, LMFT
Professor Emeritus, School of Nursing
Oregon Health and Science University
Portland, Oregon
Adjunct Faculty, College of Nursing
Washington State University
Spokane, Washington

 F.A. Davis Company • Philadelphia

F. A. Davis Company
1915 Arch Street
Philadelphia, PA 19103
www.fadavis.com

Copyright © 2015 by F. A. Davis Company

Printed in the United States of America

Last digit indicates print number: 10 9 8 7 6 5 4 3 2

Publisher, Nursing: Joanne P. DaCunha
Director of Content Development: Darlene D. Pedersen
Content Project Manager: Jacalyn C. Clay
Electronic Project Editor: Katherine E. Crowley
Cover Design: Carolyn O'Brien

As new scientific information becomes available through basic and clinical research, recommended treatments and drug therapies undergo changes. The author(s) and publisher have done everything possible to make this book accurate, up to date, and in accord with accepted standards at the time of publication. The author(s), editors, and publisher are not responsible for errors or omissions or for consequences from application of the book, and make no warranty, expressed or implied, in regard to the contents of the book. Any practice described in this book should be applied by the reader in accordance with professional standards of care used in regard to the unique circumstances that may apply in each situation. The reader is advised always to check product information (package inserts) for changes and new information regarding dose and contraindications before administering any drug. Caution is especially urged when using new or infrequently ordered drugs.

Library of Congress Cataloging-in-Publication Data

Family health care nursing : theory, practice, and research / [edited by] Joanna Rowe Kaakinen, Deborah Padgett Coehlo, Rose Steele, Aaron Tabacco, Shirley May Harmon Hanson. — 5th edition.
    p. ; cm.
Includes bibliographical references and index.
ISBN 978-0-8036-3921-8
I. Kaakinen, Joanna Rowe, 1951- editor. II. Coehlo, Deborah Padgett, editor. III. Steele, Rose, editor. IV. Tabacco, Aaron, editor. V. Hanson, Shirley M. H., 1938- editor.
[DNLM: 1. Family Nursing. 2. Family. WY 159.5]
RT120.F34
610.73—dc23

2014015448

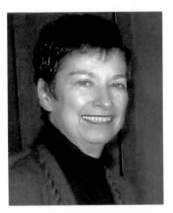

Vivian Rose Gedaly-Duff, RN, DNS

Family nursing lost an exemplary family nurse and nursing scholar in September 2012: Vivian Rose Gedaly-Duff, our esteemed colleague and friend. As one of the editors of Family Health Care Nursing: Theory, Practice, and Research *for the third and fourth editions, Vivian worked tirelessly to elevate our collective thoughts and work. Even as Vivian courageously battled breast cancer, she always asked about this edition of this textbook, offering her wisdom and insight to us. Our work in family nursing, and family nursing itself, is infinitely better because of Vivian.*

We dedicate this fifth edition of Family Health Care Nursing: Theory, Practice, and Research *to Vivian Rose Gedaly-Duff. Vivian, we miss you and think of you often.*

—Editorial Team
   Joanna, Deborah, Rose, Aaron, and Shirley

I am proud to have been the founder of *Family Health Care Nursing: Theory, Practice, and Research* with the first edition published in 1996. I am honored to be asked to write this particular foreword, as this fifth edition of this textbook attests and gives credence to the ongoing evolution and development in the field of family nursing. This edition also marks the end of my long nursing, academic, and writing career. It is time to retire and step aside for the younger generation of family nurses to take over. It is exciting to think about what family nursing will look like in the future.

Family Health Care Nursing: Theory, Practice, and Research (I–V) is an ever changing and comprehensive textbook originally developed to reflect and promote the art and science of family nursing. This all-inclusive far-reaching compendium of integrating theory, practice, and research continues in this fifth edition of this textbook.

All editions of this distinctive textbook were published by F. A. Davis. I am grateful for their faith, trust, and support in carrying the legacy of family nursing forward. This book originated when I was teaching family nursing at Oregon Health and Science University (OHSU) School of Nursing in Portland, Oregon. At that time there was no comprehensive or authoritative textbook on the nursing care of families that matched our program of study. This was the impetus I needed to write and edit the first edition of *Family Health Care Nursing: Theory, Practice, and Research* (Hanson and Boyd, 1996). The first edition met a need of nursing educators in many other nursing schools around the world, so F. A. Davis invited me to revise, update, and publish the second edition, which came out in 2001. For the third edition, I asked two additional scholars to join me in writing and editing this edition: the late Dr. Vivian Rose Gedaly-Duff from OHSU (see Dedication) and Dr. Joanna Rowe Kaakinen, then from the University of Portland and now from Linfield College Portland campus. A separate *Instructors' Manual*, a new feature of the third edition, was developed by Dr. Deborah Padgett Coehlo when she was on faculty at Oregon State University (Bend, OR). This wonderful infusion of nursing colleagues and scholars elevated this textbook to a whole other level.

After my retirement from active full-time teaching and professional practice, the capable Dr. Joanna Rowe Kaakinen assumed the leadership for the fourth edition (2010). Along with Drs. Vivian Gedaly-Duff, Deborah Padgett Coehlo, and myself, we produced the fourth edition of this cutting-edge family nursing textbook that included some Canadian-specific family content. For the fourth edition Dr. Deborah Padgett Coehlo wrote the first online teachers' manual that accompanied this edition; two other online chapters were added to this fourth edition: research in families/family nursing and international family nursing. Dr. Joanna Rowe Kaakinen is the lead editor of this fifth edition. In thinking about the sixth edition and the future of the text, a younger family nursing scholar Aaron Tabacco (PhC) was added to the editorial team. Dr. Rose Steele, our Canadian colleague from Toronto, joined our writing team. Dr. Deborah Coehlo continues as editor and now brings the perspective of family nursing from her pediatric practice as a PNP in Bend, Oregon. My last contribution to this book is as editor on this fifth edition. This edition has taken on a much more international flair, especially for North America, as Canadian authors were added to many of the writing teams.

The first three editions of this textbook received the following awards: the American Journal of Nursing Book of the Year Award and the Nursing Outlook Brandon Selected Nursing Books Award. Every new edition has been well received around the world and every edition has brought forth new converts to family nursing. Previous editions of the text were translated or published in Japan, Portugal, India, Pakistan, Bangladesh, Burma, Bhutan, and

Nepal. I anticipate even more international interest for this fifth edition as the message of family nursing continues to spread across the globe. It is also interesting to note that online sales of the book come from many countries.

Contributors to this edition were selected from distinguished practitioners, researchers, theorists, scholars, and teachers from nursing and family social scientists across the United States and Canada. Like any good up-to-date textbook, some subject matter stayed foundational and other subject matter changed based on current evidence. As family nursing evolved, different authors and editors were added to the writing team. This textbook is a massive undertaking involving 30 committed nurses and family scholars, not to mention the staff of F. A. Davis. The five editors of this fifth edition are grateful for this national and international dedication to family nursing. Together we all continue to increase nursing knowledge pertaining to the nursing care of families across the globe.

This fifth edition builds on the previous editions. The primary shift in the direction of this edition is to make family nursing practice meaningful and realistic for nursing students. The first unit of the book addresses critical foundational knowledge pertaining to families and nursing. The second unit concentrates on theory-guided, evidence-based practice of the nursing care of families across the life span and in a variety of specialties. In addition to the large increase of Canadian contributors, substantial updates took place in all chapters. A new chapter, Trauma and Family Nursing, was added. Other new or updated features of this edition include the following:

- A strong emphasis on evidence-based practice in each chapter.
- Five selected family nursing theories interwoven throughout the book.
- Family case studies that demonstrate the practice of family nursing.
- Content that addresses family nursing in both Canada and the United States (North America).

Family nursing, as an art and science, has transformed in response to paradigm shifts in the profession and in society over time. As a nursing student in the United States during the 1950s, the focus of care was on individuals and centered in hospitals. As time passed and the profession matured, nursing education and practice expanded and shifted to more family-centered care and community-based nursing. The codified version of family nursing really emerged and peaked during the 1980s and 1990s in the United States and Canada, where the movement was headquartered. Even though this initial impetus for family nursing came from North America, the concept spread quickly around the world. Asian countries, in particular, have embraced family nursing, and though they initially translated books coming from the United States or Canada, they have matured to creating their own books and theories for family nursing. The Scandinavian countries have expanded their own scholarship and tailored family nursing to their own unique countries and populations. Today, it could be said that family nursing is without borders and that no one country owns family nursing.

The International Family Nursing Association (IFNA) was established in 2009 for the purpose of advancing family nursing and creating a global community of nurses who practice with families. The 11th International Family Nursing Conference (and the first official conference of IFNA) took place June 19–22, 2013, in Minneapolis, Minnesota, USA. This new professional body (IFNA) is assuming the leadership for keeping family nursing at the forefront of theory development, practice, research, education, and social policy across the globe.

Family nursing has become more than just a "buzzword" but rather an actual reality. Family nursing is being taught in many educational institutions, practiced in multiple health care settings, and globally actualized by many nurses. Nursing care to individuals, regardless of place, occurs within the context of families and communities— all of which can be called "family nursing." Most everyone in the nursing profession agrees that a profound, reciprocal relationship exists between families, health, and nursing.

This book and current edition recognizes that nursing as a profession has a close alignment with families. Nurses share many of the responsibilities with families for the care and protection of their family members. Nurses have an obligation to help families promote and advance the care and growth of both individual family members and families as a unit. This textbook provides nursing students the knowledge base and the processes to become effective in their nursing care with families. Additionally, families benefit when already practicing registered nurses use this knowledge to reorganize their nursing care to be more family centered and develop working partnerships with families to strengthen family systems. *Family Health Care Nursing: Theory, Practice, and Research* was written by nurses for nurses who practice nursing care of families. Students will learn how to tailor their assessment and interventions with families in health and illness, in physical as well as mental health, across the life span, and in all the settings in which nurses and families interface. I firmly believe that this fifth edition of this textbook is at the cutting edge of this practice challenge for the next decade, and will help to marshal the nursing profession toward improving nursing care of families.

—SHIRLEY MAY HARMON HANSON, RN, PhD,
PMHNP/ARNP, FAAN, CFLE, LMFT
Professor Emeritus, School of Nursing
Oregon Health and Science University
Portland, Oregon
Adjunct Faculty, College of Nursing
Washington State University
Spokane, WA

Overview of the Fifth Edition

Ask anyone about a time they were affected by something that happened to one of their family members, and you will be overwhelmed with the intensity of the emotions and the exhaustive details. Every individual is influenced significantly by their families and the structure, function, and processes within their families. Even individuals who do not interact with their families have been shaped by their families. The importance and connection between individuals and their families have been studied expansively in a variety of disciplines, including nursing.

As such, the importance of working in partnerships with families in the health care system is evident. Yet many health care providers view dealing with patients' families as an extra burden that is too demanding. Some nurses are baffled when a family acts or reacts in certain ways that are foreign to their own professional and personal family experiences. Some nurses avoid the tensions and anxiety that exist in families during a crisis situation. But it is in just such situations that families most need nurses' understanding, knowledge, and guidance. The purpose of this book is to provide nursing students, as well as practicing nurses, with the understanding, knowledge, and guidance to practice family nursing. This fifth edition of the textbook focuses on theory-guided, evidence-based practice of the nursing care of families throughout the family life cycle and across a variety of clinical specialties.

Use of the Book

Family Health Care Nursing: Theory, Practice, and Research, fifth edition, is organized so that it can be used on its own and in its entirety to structure a course in family nursing. An alternative approach for the use of this text is for students to purchase the book at the beginning of their program of study so that specific chapters can be assigned for specialty courses throughout the curriculum. The fifth edition complements a concept-based curriculum design. For example, Chapter 16, Family Mental Health Nursing, could be assigned when students take their mental health nursing course, and Chapter 13, Family Child Health Nursing, could be studied during a pediatric course or in conjunction with life-span–concept curriculum for chronic illness and acute care courses. Thus, this textbook could be integrated throughout the undergraduate or graduate nursing curriculum.

Canadian Content

Moreover, this fifth edition builds on successes of the past editions and responds to recommendations from readers/users of past editions. Because of the ever-evolving nature of families and the changing dynamics of the health care system, the editors added new chapters, consolidated chapters, and deleted some old chapters. Importantly, this fifth edition incorporates additional Canadian-specific content. Though it is true that the United States and Canada have different health care systems, so many of the stressors and challenges for families overlap. One of the editors for this fifth edition, Rose Steele, is from Toronto and helped expand our concepts about Canadian nursing. Moreover, a number of chapters in the text have a combined author team of scholars from both Canada and the United States: Chapter 5, Family Social Policy and Health Disparities; Chapter 12, Family Nursing With Childbearing Families; and Chapter 17, Families and Community/Public Health Nursing. Two chapters in this edition were written by an all-Canadian team: Chapter 6, Relational

Nursing and Family Nursing in Canada and Chapter 10, Families in Palliative and End-of-Life Care. All of the chapters in this edition include information, statistics, programs, and interventions that address the individual needs of families and family nurses from both Canada and the United States.

Additions and Deletions

This edition contains one new chapter: Chapter 11, Trauma and Family Nursing. Between the advanced understanding of brain function and general physiology; the mind and body response to severe and/or prolonged stress; and the increase in trauma experienced by families through war, natural disasters, and family violence, the need to understand, prevent, treat, and monitor the effects of trauma on individuals and families has never been more vital. Therefore, we felt it was essential to include ways family nurses could work with these families. All chapters have been changed and updated significantly to reflect the present state of "family," current evidence-based practice, research, and interventions. Many of the chapters now include a second family case study to illustrate further the evidence discussed throughout that specific chapter. We deleted the chapter on the future of families and family nursing because changes in health care reform, social policy, and families are occurring at such a rate that it is impossible to predict what the future will hold.

Structure of the Book

Each chapter begins with the critical concepts to be addressed within that chapter. The purpose of placing the critical concepts at the beginning of the chapter is to focus the reader's thinking and learning and offer a preview and outline of what is to come. Another organizing framework for the book is presented in Chapter 3, Theoretical Foundations for the Nursing of Families. This chapter covers the importance of using theory to guide the nursing of families and presents five theoretical perspectives, with a case study demonstrating how to apply these five theoretical approaches in practice. These five theories are threaded throughout the book and are applied in many of the chapter case studies. As stated earlier, most of the chapters include two case studies; all of the case studies contain family genograms and ecomaps.

The main body of the book is divided into three units: Unit 1: Foundations in Family Health Care Nursing, which includes Chapters 1 to 5; Unit 2: Families Across the Health Continuum, which includes Chapters 6 to 11; and Unit 3: Nursing Care of Families in Clinical Areas, which includes Chapters 12 to 17. The *Family Health Care Nursing Instructors' Guide* is an online faculty guide that provides assistance to faculty using/teaching family nursing or the nursing care of families in a variety of settings. Each chapter also includes a Power-Point presentation, Case Study Learning Activities, and other online assets, which can be found at www.DavisPlus.com.

UNIT 1

Foundations in Family Health Care Nursing

Chapter 1: Family Health Care Nursing: An Introduction provides foundational materials essential to understanding families and nursing. Two nursing scholars have worked on this chapter now for three editions: Joanna Rowe Kaakinen, PhD, RN, Professor at the Linfield College School of Nursing and Shirley May Harmon Hanson, RN, PhD, PMHNP/ARNP, FAAN, CFLE, LMFT, Professor Emeritus at Oregon Health and Science University School of Nursing. The chapter lays down crucial foundational knowledge about families and family nursing.

The first half of the chapter discusses dimensions of family nursing and defines family, family health, and healthy families. The chapter follows with an explanation of family health care nursing and the nature of interventions in the nursing care of families, along with the four approaches to family nursing (context, client, system, and component of society). The chapter then presents the concepts or variables that influence family nursing, family nursing roles, obstacles to family nursing practice, and the history of family nursing. The second half of the chapter elaborates on theoretical ideas involved with understanding family structure, family functions, and family processes.

Chapter 2: Family Demography: Continuity and Change in North American Families provides nurses with a basic contextual orientation to the demographics of families and health. All three authors are experts in statistics and family demography. Three sociologists joined to update and write this chapter: Lynne M. Casper, PhD, Professor of Sociology and Director of the South California Population Research Center, University of Southern California (USC); Sandra M. Florian, MA, PhD Candidate, who is a graduate student/research assistant, Population Research Center at USC Department of Sociology; and Peter D. Brandon, PhD, Professor, Department of Sociology, The University at Albany (SUNY), New York. This chapter examines changes and variations in North American families in order to understand what these changes portend for family health care nursing during the first half of this century. The subject matter of the chapter is structured to provide family nurses with background on changes in the North American family so that they can understand their patient populations. The chapter briefly touches on the implications of these demographic patterns on practicing family nursing.

Chapter 3: Theoretical Foundations for the Nursing of Families is co-authored by two of the editors of this textbook: Joanna Rowe Kaakinen and Shirley May Harmon Hanson. This chapter lays the theoretical groundwork needed to practice family nursing. The introduction builds a case for why nurses need to understand the interactive relationship among theory, practice, and research. It also makes the point that no single theory adequately describes the complex relationships of family structure, function, and processes. The chapter then continues by delineating and explaining relevant theories, concepts, propositions, hypotheses, and conceptual models. Selected for this textbook, and explained in this chapter, are five theoretical/conceptual models: Family Systems Theory, Developmental and Family Life Cycle Theory, Bioecological Theory, Rowland's Chronic Illness Framework, and the Family Assessment and Intervention Model. Using basic family case studies, the chapter explores how each of the five theories could be used to assess and plan interventions for a family. This approach enables learners to see how different interventions are derived from different theoretical perspectives.

Chapter 4: Family Nursing Assessment and Intervention is co-authored by Joanna Rowe Kaakinen and Aaron Tabacco, BSN, RN, Doctoral Candidate, who is a Student Instructor, Undergraduate Nursing Programs at Oregon Health Sciences University, Portland, Oregon. The purpose of this chapter is to present a systematic approach to develop a plan of action for the family, *with* the family, to address its most pressing needs. These authors built on the traditional nursing process model to create a dynamic systematic family nursing assessment approach. Assessment strategies include selecting assessment instruments, determining the need for interpreters, assessing for health literacy, and learning how to diagram family genograms and ecomaps. The chapter also explores ways to involve families in shared decision making, and explores analysis, a critical step in the family nursing process that helps focus the nurse and the family on identification of the family's primary concern(s). The chapter uses a family case study as an exemplar to demonstrate the family nursing assessment and intervention.

Chapter 5: Family Social Policy and Health Disparities exposes nurses to social issues that affect the health of families and strongly challenge nurses to become more involved in the political aspects of health policy. This chapter is co-authored by two experienced nurses in the social policy arena and a sociology professor: Isolde Daiski, RN, BScN, EdD, Associate Professor, School of Nursing, from York University, Toronto, Ontario, Canada; Casey R. Shillam, PhD, RN-BC, Director of the BSN program at Western Washington State University, Bellingham, Washington; Lynne M. Casper, PhD, Professor Sociology at the University of Southern California; and Sandra Florian, MA, a graduate student at the University of Southern California. These authors discuss the practice of family nursing within the social and political structure of society. They encourage the readers to understand their own biases and how these contribute to health disparities. In this chapter, students learn about the complex components that contribute to health disparities. Nurses are called to become politically active, advocate for vulnerable families, and assist in the development of creative alternatives to social policies that limit access to quality care and resources. These authors present the difficulties families face in the current political climate in both the United States and Canada, as the legal definition of family is being challenged and family life evolves. The chapter touches on social policies, or lack of them, specifically policies that affect education, socioeconomic status, and health insurance. The chapter also explores determinants of health disparities, which include infant mortality rates, obesity, asthma, HIV/AIDS, aging, women's issues, and health literacy.

UNIT 2

Families Across the Health Continuum

Chapter 6: Relational Nursing and Family Nursing in Canada is co-authored by Canadian nursing scholars Colleen Varcoe, PhD, RN, Associate Professor and Associate Research Director at the University of British Columbia, School of Nursing in Vancouver, British Columbia, Canada; and Gweneth Hartrick Doane, PhD, RN, Professor, School of Nursing, University of Victoria, British Columbia, Canada. Relational inquiry family nursing practice is oriented toward enhancing the capacity and power of people/families to live a meaningful life (meaningful from their own perspective). Understanding and working directly with context provides a key resource and strategy for responsive, health-promoting family nursing practice. Grounded in a relational inquiry approach, this chapter focuses specifically on the significance of context in family nursing practice in Canada. The chapter highlights the interface of sociopolitical, historical, geographical, and economic elements in shaping the health and illness experiences of families in Canada and the implications for family nursing practice. The chapter covers some of the key characteristics of Canadian society, and how those characteristics shape health, families, health care, and family nursing. Informed by a relational inquiry approach to family nursing, the chapter turns to the ways nurses might practice more responsively and effectively based on this understanding.

Chapter 7: Genomics and Family Nursing Across the Life Span is authored by a nursing expert in nursing genomics, Dale Halsey Lea, MPH, RN, CGC, FAAN, Consultant, Public Health Genomics and Adjunct Lecturer for University of Maine School of Nursing. The ability to apply an understanding of genetics in the care of families is a priority for nurses and for all health care providers. As a result of genomic research and the rapidly changing body of knowledge regarding genetic influences on health and illness, more emphasis has been placed on involving all health care providers in this field, including family nursing. This chapter describes nursing responsibilities for families of persons who have, or are at risk for having, genetic conditions. These responsibilities are described for families before conception, with neonates, teens in families, and families with

members in the middle to elder years. The goal of the chapter is to describe the relevance of genetic information within families when there is a question about genetic aspects of health or disease for members of the family. The chapter begins with a brief introduction to genomics and genetics. The chapter then explains how families react to finding out they are at risk for genetic conditions, and decide how and with whom to disclose genetic information, and the critical aspect of confidentiality. The chapter outlines the components of conducting a genetic assessment and history, and offers interventions that include education and resources. Several specific case examples and a detailed case study illustrate nurses working with families who have a genetic condition.

Chapter 8: Family Health Promotion is written by Yeoun Soo Kim-Godwin, PhD, MPH, RN, Professor of Nursing; and Perri J. Bomar, PhD, RN, Professor Emeritus, who are both from the School of Nursing at the University of North Carolina, Wilmington. Fostering the health of the family as a unit and encouraging families to value and incorporate health promotion into their lifestyles are essential components of family nursing practice. The purpose of this chapter is to introduce the concepts of family health and family health promotion. The chapter presents models to illuminate these concepts, including the Model of Family Health, Family Health Model, McMaster Model of Family Functioning, Developmental Model of Health and Nursing, Family Health Promotion Model, and Model of the Health-Promoting Family. The chapter also examines internal and external factors through a lens of the bioecological systems theory that influence family health promotion. It covers family nursing intervention strategies for health promotion, and presents two family case studies demonstrating how different theoretical approaches can be used for assessing and intervening in the family for health promotion. The chapter also discusses the role of nurses and intervention strategies in maintaining and regaining the highest level of family health. Specific interventions presented include family empowerment, anticipatory guidance, offering information, and encouraging family rituals, routines, and time together.

Chapter 9: Families Living With Chronic Illness is co-authored by Joanna Rowe Kaakinen and Sharon A. Denham, DSN, RN, Professor, Houston J. and Florence A. Doswell Endowed

Chair in Nursing for Teaching Excellence, Texas Woman's University, Dallas, Texas. The purpose and focus of this chapter is to describe ways for nurses to think about the impact of chronic illness on families and to consider strategies for helping families manage chronic illness. The first part of this chapter briefly outlines the global statistics of chronic illness, the economic burden of chronic diseases, and three theoretical perspectives for working with families living with chronic illness. The majority of the chapter describes how families and individuals are challenged to live a quality life in the presence of chronic illness and how nurses assist these families. Specific attention is drawn to families with children who have a chronic illness and families with an adult member living with a chronic illness. The chapter addresses adolescents who live with a chronic illness as they transition from pediatric to adult medical care, siblings of children with a chronic illness and their specific needs, and the needs of young caregivers who provide care for a parent who has a chronic illness. The chapter presents two case studies: one a family who has an adolescent with diabetes and one a family helping its elderly parent and grandparent manage living with Parkinson's disease.

Chapter 10: Families in Palliative and End-of-Life Care is written by Rose Steele, PhD, RN, Professor, York University School of Nursing, Toronto, Ontario, Canada; Carole A. Robinson, PhD, RN, Associate Professor, University of British Columbia, Okanagan School of Nursing, British Columbia, Canada; and Kimberley A. Widger, PhD, RN, Assistant Professor, Lawrence S. Bloomberg Faculty of Nursing, University of Toronto, Ontario, Canada. This chapter details the key components to consider in providing palliative and end-of-life care, as well as families' most important concerns and needs when a family member experiences a life-threatening illness or is dying. It also presents some concrete strategies to assist nurses in providing optimal palliative and end-of-life care to all family members. More specifically, the chapter begins with a brief definition of palliative and end-of-life care, including its focus on improving quality of life for patients and their families. The chapter then outlines principles of palliative care and ways to apply these principles across all settings and regardless of whether death results from chronic illness or a sudden or traumatic event. Two evidence-based, palliative care and end-of-life case studies conclude the chapter.

Chapter 11: Trauma and Family Nursing is written by Deborah Padgett Coehlo, PhD, C-PNP, PMHS, CFLE, Developmental and Behavioral Specialist, Juniper Ridge Clinic, Bend, Oregon, and adjunct faculty at Oregon State University. Dr. Coehlo has been on the editorial team for two editions of this text. Using theory-guided practice, this chapter helps nurses develop knowledge about trauma and family nurses' key role in the field of trauma. It emphasizes the importance of prevention, early treatment, encouraging family resilience, and helping the family to make meaning out of negative events. This chapter also stresses an understanding of secondary trauma, or the negative effects of witnessing trauma of others. This discussion is particularly salient for family nurses, because they are some of the most likely professionals to encounter traumatized victims in their everyday practice. Two case studies explicate family nursing when working with families who are experiencing the effects of traumatic life events.

UNIT 3

Nursing Care of Families in Clinical Areas

Chapter 12: Family Nursing With Childbearing Families is written by Linda Veltri, PhD, RN, Clinical Assistant Professor, Oregon Health Science University, School of Nursing, Ashland, Oregon, Campus; Karline Wilson-Mitchell, RM, CNM, RN, MSN, Assistant Professor, Midwifery Education Program, Ryerson University, Ontario, Canada; and Kathleen Bell, MSN, CNM, AHN-BC, Clinical Associate, School of Nursing, Linfield College, Portland, Oregon. The focus of childbearing family nurses is family relationships and the health of all family members. Therefore, nurses involved with childbearing families use family concepts and theories as part of developing the plan of nursing care. A review of literature provides current evidence about the processes families experience when deciding on and adapting to childbearing, including theory and clinical application of nursing care for families planning pregnancy, experiencing pregnancy, adopting and fostering children, struggling with infertility, and coping with illness during the early postpartum period. This chapter starts by presenting theoretical perspectives that guide nursing practice with childbearing families. It continues with an exploration of family nursing with childbearing families before conception through the postpartum period. The chapter covers specific issues childbearing families may experience, including postpartum depression, attachment concerns, and postpartum illness. Nursing interventions are integrated throughout this chapter to demonstrate how family nurses can help childbearing families prevent complications, increase coping strategies, and adapt to their expanded family structure, development, and function. The chapter concludes with two case studies that explore family adaptations to stressors and changing roles related to childbearing.

Chapter 13: Family Child Health Nursing is written by Deborah Padgett Coehlo. A major task of families is to nurture children to become healthy, responsible, and creative adults who can develop meaningful relationships across the life span. Families experience the stress of normative transitions with the addition of each child and situational transitions when children are ill. Knowledge of the family life cycle, child development, and illness trajectory provides a foundation for offering anticipatory guidance and coaching at stressful times. Family life influences the promotion of health and the experience of illness in children, and is influenced by children's health and illness. This chapter provides a brief history of family-centered care of children and then presents foundational concepts that will guide nursing practice with families with children. The chapter goes on to describe nursing care of well children and families with an emphasis on health promotion, nursing care of children and families in acute care settings, nursing care of children with chronic illness and their families, and nursing care of children and their families during end of life. Case studies illustrate the application of family-centered care across settings.

Chapter 14: Family Nursing in Acute Care Adult Settings is written by Vivian Tong, PhD, RN, and Joanna Rowe Kaakinen, PhD, RN, both professors of nursing at Linfield College-Good Samaritan School of Nursing, Portland, Oregon. Hospitalization for an acute illness, injury, or exacerbation of a chronic illness is stressful for patients and their families. The ill adult enters the hospital usually in a physiological crisis, and the family most often accompanies the ill or injured family members into the hospital; both the patient and the family are usually in an emotional crisis. Families with members who are acutely or critically ill are seen in adult medical-surgical units, intensive care or cardiac care units, or emergency departments. This chapter covers the major stressors that families experience during hospitalization of adult family members, the transfer of patients from one unit to another, visiting policies, family waiting rooms, home discharge, family presence during cardiopulmonary resuscitation, withdrawal or withholding of life-sustaining therapies, end-of-life family care in the hospital, and organ donation. The content emphasizes family needs during these critical events. This chapter also presents a family case study in a medical-surgical setting that demonstrates how the Family Assessment and Intervention Model and the FS^{3}I can be used as the framework to assess and intervene with a particular family.

Chapter 15: Family Health in Mid and Later Life is co-authored by Diana L. White, PhD, Senior Research Associate in Human Development and Family Studies, Institute of Aging at Portland State University, Portland, Oregon, and Jeannette O'Brien, PhD, RN, Assistant Professor at Linfield College–Good Samaritan School of Nursing, Portland, Oregon. The chapter employs the life course perspective, family systems models, and developmental theories as the guiding organizational structure. The chapter presents evidence-based practice on working with adults in mid and later life, including a review of living choices for older adults with chronic illness, and the importance of peer relationships and intergenerational relationships to quality of life. This chapter includes extensive information about family caregiving for and by older adults, including spouses, adult children, and grandparents. Two case studies conclude the chapter. One family case study illustrates the integrated generational challenges facing older adults today. The second case study addresses care of an elderly family member who never married and has no children. This case presents options for caregiving and the complexity of living healthy.

Chapter 16: Family Mental Health Nursing has been completely revised for this edition. It is written by Laura Rodgers, PhD, RN, PMHNP, Professor of Nursing at Linfield College–Good Samaritan School of Nursing, Portland, Oregon. Dr. Rodgers brings to her writing both her scholarly perspective and clinical practice as a psychiatric nurse practitioner in private practice. The chapter begins with a brief demographic overview of the pervasiveness of mental health conditions (MHCs) in both Canada and the United States. The remainder of the chapter focuses on the impact a specific MHC can have on the individual with the MHC, individual family members, and the family as a unit. Although the chapter does not go into specific diagnostic criteria for various conditions, it does offer nursing interventions to assist families. One case study explores the impact and treatment of substance abuse. The second presents how a family nurse can work with a family to improve the health of all family members when one family member lives with paranoid schizophrenia.

Chapter 17: Families and Community/Public Health Nursing is co-authored by a North American writing team: Linda L. Eddy, PhD, RN, CPNP, Associate Professor, Washington State University Intercollegiate College of Nursing, Vancouver, Washington; Annette Bailey, PhD, RN, Assistant Professor, Daphne Cockwell School of Nursing, Ryerson University, Toronto, Ontario, Canada; and Dawn Doutrich, PhD, RN, CNS, Associate Professor, Washington State University Intercollegiate College of Nursing, Vancouver, Washington. Healthy communities are comprised of healthy families. Community/public health nurses understand the effects that communities can have on individuals and families, and recognize that a community's health is reflected in the health experiences of its members and their families. This chapter offers a description of community health nursing promoting the health of families in communities. It begins with a definition of community health nursing, and follows with a discussion of concepts and principles that guide the work of these nurses, the roles they enact in working with families and communities, and the various settings where they work. This discussion is organized around a visual representation of community health nursing. The chapter ends with discussion of current trends in community/public health nursing and a family case study that demonstrates working with families in the community.

ANNETTE BAILEY, PhD, RN
Assistant Professor, Daphne Cockwell School of
   Nursing
Ryerson University
Toronto, Ontario, Canada

KATHLEEN BELL, RN, MSN, CNM,
   AHN-BC
Clinical Associate, School of Nursing
Linfield College
Portland, Oregon

PERRI J. BOMAR, PhD, RN
Professor Emeritus, School of Nursing
University of North Carolina at Wilmington
Wilmington, North Carolina

PETER D. BRANDON, PhD
Professor, Department of Sciology
The University at Albany - SUNY
Albany, New York

LYNNE, M. CASPER, PhD
Professor of Sociology and Director, Southern
   California Population Research Center
University of Southern California
Los Angeles, California

DEBORAH PADGETT COEHLO, PhD,
   C-PNP, PMHS, CFLE
Developmental and Behavioral Specialist
Juniper Ridge Clinic
Bend, Oregon
Adjunct Professor
Oregon State University
Bend, Oregon

ISOLDE DAISKI, RN, BScN, EdD
Associate Professor, School of Nursing
York University
Toronto, Ontario, Canada

SHARON A. DENHAM, DSN, RN
*Professor and Houston J. and Florence A. Doswell
   Endowed Chair in Nursing for Teaching Excellence*,
   College of Nursing
Texas Woman's University, Dallas
Dallas, Texas

GWENETH HARTRICK DOANE, PhD, RN
Professor, School of Nursing
University of Victoria
Victoria, British Columbia, Canada

DAWN DOUTRICH, PhD, RN, CNS
Associate Professor, Intercollegiate College of
   Nursing
Washington State University
Vancouver, Washington

LINDA L. EDDY, PhD, RN, CPNP
Associate Professor, Intercollegiate College of Nursing
Washington State University
Vancouver, Washington

SANDRA M. FLORIAN, MA
PhD Candidate, Department of Sociology
University of Southern California
Los Angeles, California

DALE HALSEY LEA, MPH, RN, CGC, FAAN
Adjunct Lecturer, School of Nursing
University of Maine
Cumberland Foreside, Maine

SHIRLEY MAY HARMON HANSON, RN, PhD,
   PMHNP/ARNP, FAAN, CFLE, LMFT
Professor Emeritus, School of Nursing
Oregon Health and Science University
Portland, Oregon
Adjunct Faculty, College of Nursing
Washington State University
Spokane, Washington

JOANNA ROWE KAAKINEN, PhD, RN
Professor, School of Nursing
Linfield College
Portland, Oregon

YEOUN SOO KIM-GODWIN,
  PhD, MPH, RN
Professor, School of Nursing
University of North Carolina, Wilmington
Wilmington, North Carolina

JEANNETTE O'BRIEN, PhD, RN
Assistant Professor, School of Nursing
Linfield College
Portland, Oregon

CAROLE A. ROBINSON, PhD, RN
Associate Professor, School of Nursing
University of British Columbia, Okanagan
Kelowna, British Columbia, Canada

LAURA RODGERS, PhD, PMHNP
Professor, School of Nursing
Linfield College
Portland, Oregon

CASEY R. SHILLAM, PhD, RN-BC
Director, School of Nursing
Western Washington University
Bellingham, Washington

ROSE STEELE, PhD, RN
Professor, School of Nursing, Faculty of Health
York University
Toronto, Ontario, Canada

AARON TABACCO, BSN, RN
Doctoral Candidate, School of Nursing
Oregon Health and Science University
Portland, Oregon

VIVIAN TONG, PhD, RN
Professor, School of Nursing
Linfield College
Portland, Oregon

COLLEEN VARCOE, PhD, RN
Associate Professor, School of Nursing
University of British Columbia
Vancouver, British Columbia, Canada

LINDA VELTRI, PhD, RN
Clinical Assistant Professor, School of Nursing
Oregon Health Science University, Ashland
Ashland, Oregon

DIANA L. WHITE, PhD
Senior Research Associate, Institute on Aging
Portland State University
Portland, Oregon

KIMBERLEY A. WIDGER, PhD, RN
Assistant Professor, Lawrence S. Bloomberg School of
  Nursing
University of Toronto
Toronto, Ontario, Canada

KARLINE WILSON-MITCHELL, RM, CNM,
  RN, MSN
Assistant Professor, Midwifery Education Program
Ryerson University
Toronto, Ontario, Canada

ELLEN J. ARGUST, MS, RN
Lecturer
State University of New York
New Paltz, New York

AMANDA J. BARTON, DNP, FNP, RN
Assistant Professor
Hope College
Holland, Michigan

LAURA J. BLANK, RN, MSN, CNE
Assistant Clinical Professor
Northern Arizona University
Flagstaff, Arizona

BARBARA S. BROOME, PhD, RN
Associate Dean and Chair
University of South Alabama
Mobile, Alabama

SHARON L. CARLSON, PhD, RN
Professor
Otterbein College
Westerville, Ohio

BARBARA CHEYNEY, BSN, MS, RN-BC
Adjunct Faculty
Seattle Pacific University
Seattle, Washington

MICHELE D'ARCY-EVANS, PhD, CNM
Professor
Lewis-Clark State College
Lewiston, Idaho

MARGARET C. DELANEY, MS, CPNP, RN
Faculty Instructor
Benedictine University
Lisle, Illinois

SANDRA K. EGGENBERGER, PhD, RN
Professor
Minnesota State University Mankato
Mankato, Minnesota

ANNELIA EPIE, RN, MN(c)
Public Health Nurse
City of Toronto Public Health
Toronto, Ontario, Canada

BRIAN FONNESBECK, RN
Associate Professor
Lewis Clark State College
Lewiston, Idaho

MARY ANN GLENDON, PhD, MSN, RN
Associate Professor
Southern Connecticut State University
New Haven, Connecticut

RACHEL E. GRANT, RN, MN
Research Associate
University of Toronto
Toronto, Ontario, Canada

SHEILA GROSSMAN, PhD, FNP-BC
Professor and FNP Specialty Track Director
Fairfield University
Fairfield, Connecticut

AAFREEN HASSAN, RN
Registered Nurse
Scarborough Hospital
Toronto, Ontario, Canada

ANNA JAJIC, MN-NP, MSc, RPN, BSsN
Faculty and Nurse Practitioner
Douglas College
New West Minster, British Columbia, Canada

MOLLY JOHNSON, MSN, CPNP, RN
Nursing Instructor
Ohio University
Ironton, Ohio

KATHY KOLLOWA, MSN, RN
Nurse Educator
Platt College
Aurora, Colorado

KEN KUSTIAK, RN, RPN, BScN, MHS(c)
Nursing Instructor
Grant MacEwan College
Ponoka, Alberta, Canada

MAUREEN LEEN, PhD, RN, CNE
Professor
Madonna University
Livonia, Michigan

KAREN ELIZABETH LEIF, BA, RN, MA
Nurse Educator
Globe University, Minnesota School of Business
Richfield, Minnesota

BARBARA MCCLASKEY, PhD, MN, RNC, ARNP
Professor
Pittsburg State University
Pittsburg, Kansas

VICKI A. MOSS, DNSc, RN
Associate Professor
University of Wisconsin, Oshkosh
Oshkosh, Wisconsin

VERNA C. PANGMAN, MEd, MN, RN
Senior Instructor
University of Manitoba
Winnipeg, Manitoba, Canada

CINDY PARSONS, DNP, PMHNP-BC, FAANP
Assistant Professor
University of Tampa
Tampa, Florida

SUSAN PERKINS, MSN, RN
Lead Faculty and Instructor
Washington State University
Spokane, Washington

CINDY PETERNELJ-TAYLOR, RN, BScN, MSc, PhD(c)
Professor
University of Saskatchewan
Saskatoon, Saskatchewan, Canada

THELMA PHILLIPS, MSN, RN, NRP
Instructor
University of Detroit, Mercy
Detroit, Michigan

TREVA V. REED, BScN, MSN, PhD
Professor
Canadore College/Nipissing University
North Bay, Ontario, Canada

NANCY ROSS, PhD, ARNP
Professor
University of Tampa
Tampa, Florida

CARMEN A. STOKES, PhD(c), RN, MSN, FNP-BC, CNE
Assistant Professor
University of Detroit, Mercy
Detroit, Michigan

JILL STRAWN, EdD, APRN
Associate Professor
Southern Connecticut State University
New Haven, Connecticut

SARA STURGIS, MSN, CRNP
Manager, Pediatric Clinical Research
Hershey Medical Center
Hershey, Pennsylvania

BARBARA THOMPSON, RN, BScN, MScN
Professor
Sault College
Sault Ste. Marie, Ontario, Canada

SHARON E. THOMPSON, MSN, RN
Assistant Clinical Professor
Northern Arizona University
Flagstaff, Arizona

MARYANN TROIANO, MSN, RN, APN
Assistant Professor and Family Nurse Practitioner
Monmouth University
West Long Branch, New Jersey

LOIS TSCHETTER, EdD, RN, IBCLC
Associate Professor
South Dakota State University
Brookings, South Dakota

WENDY M. WHEELER, RN, MN
Instructor
Red Deer College
Red Deer, Alberta, Canada

MARIA WHEELOCK, MSN, NP
Clinical Assistant Professor and Nurse Practitioner
State University of New York, Upstate Medical University
Syracuse, New York

UNIT 1 Foundations in Family Health Care Nursing 1

chapter 1 Family Health Care Nursing 3
An Introduction
Joanna Rowe Kaakinen, PhD, RN
Shirley May Harmon Hanson, RN, PhD, PMHNP/ARNP, FAAN, CFLE, LMFT

chapter 2 Family Demography 33
Continuity and Change in North American Families
Lynne M. Casper, PhD
Sandra M. Florian, MA, PhD Candidate
Peter D. Brandon, PhD

chapter 3 Theoretical Foundations for the Nursing of Families 67
Joanna Rowe Kaakinen, PhD, RN
Shirley May Harmon Hanson, RN, PhD, PMHNP/ARNP, FAAN, CFLE, LMFT

chapter 4 Family Nursing Assessment and Intervention 105
Joanna Rowe Kaakinen, PhD, RN
Aaron Tabacco, BSN, RN, Doctoral Candidate

chapter 5 Family Social Policy and Health Disparities 137
Isolde Daiski, RN, BScN, EdD
Casey R. Shillam, PhD, RN-BC
Lynne M. Casper, PhD
Sandra M. Florian, MA, PhD Candidate

UNIT 2 Families Across the Health Continuum 165

chapter 6 Relational Nursing and Family Nursing in Canada 167
Colleen Varcoe, PhD, RN
Gweneth Hartrick Doane, PhD, RN

chapter 7 Genomics and Family Nursing Across the Life Span 187
Dale Halsey Lea, MPH, RN, CGC, FAAN

chapter 8 Family Health Promotion 205
Yeoun Soo Kim-Godwin, PhD, MPH, RN
Perri J. Bomar, PhD, RN

chapter 9 Families Living With Chronic Illness 237
Joanna Rowe Kaakinen, PhD, RN
Sharon A. Denham, DSN, RN

chapter 10 Families in Palliative and End-of-Life Care 277
Rose Steele, PhD, RN
Carole A. Robinson, PhD, RN
Kimberley A. Widger, PhD, RN

chapter 11 Trauma and Family Nursing 321
Deborah Padgett Coehlo, PhD, C-PNP, PMHS, CFLE

UNIT 3 **Nursing Care of Families in Clinical Areas** 351

chapter 12 Family Nursing With Childbearing Families 353
Linda Veltri, PhD, RN
Karline Wilson-Mitchell, RM, CNM, RN, MSN
Kathleen Bell, RN, MSN, CNM, AHN-BC

chapter 13 Family Child Health Nursing 387
Deborah Padgett Coehlo, PhD, C-PNP, PMHS, CFLE

chapter 14 Family Nursing in Acute Care Adult Settings 433
Vivian Tong, PhD, RN
Joanna Rowe Kaakinen, PhD, RN

chapter 15 Family Health in Mid and Later Life 477
Diana L. White, PhD
Jeannette O'Brien, PhD, RN

chapter 16 Family Mental Health Nursing 521
Laura Rodgers, PhD, PMHNP

chapter 17 Families and Community/Public Health Nursing 559
Linda L. Eddy, PhD, RN, CPNP
Annette Bailey, PhD, RN
Dawn Doutrich, PhD, RN, CNS

APPENDICES

appendix A Family Systems Stressor-Strength Inventory (FS³I) 583
appendix B The Friedman Family Assessment Model (Short Form) 599

INDEX 603

Foundations in Family Health Care Nursing

chapter 1

Family Health Care Nursing
An Introduction

Joanna Rowe Kaakinen, PhD, RN

Shirley May Harmon Hanson, PhD, PMHNP/ARNP, FAAN, CFLE, LMFT

Critical Concepts

- Family health care nursing is an art and a science that has evolved as a way of thinking about and working with families.
- Family nursing is a scientific discipline based in theory.
- Health and illness are family events.
- The term *family* is defined in many ways, but the most salient definition is, *The family is who the members say it is.*
- An individual's health (on the wellness-to-illness continuum) affects the entire family's functioning, and in turn, the family's ability to function affects each individual member's health.
- Family health care nursing knowledge and skills are important for nurses who practice in generalized and in specialized settings.
- The structure, function, and processes of families have changed, but the family as a unit of analysis and service continues to survive over time.
- Nurses should intervene in ways that promote health and wellness, as well as prevent illness risks, treat disease conditions, and manage rehabilitative care needs.
- Knowledge about each family's structure, function, and process informs the nurse in how to optimize nursing care in families and provide individualized nursing care, tailored to the uniqueness of every family system.

Family health care nursing is an art and a science, a philosophy and a way of interacting with families about health care. It has evolved since the early 1980s as a way of thinking about, and working with, families when a member experiences a health problem. This philosophy and practice incorporates the following assumptions:

- Health and illness affect all members of families.
- Health and illness are family events.
- Families influence the process and outcome of health care.

All health care practices, attitudes, beliefs, behaviors, and decisions are made within the context of larger family and societal systems.

Families vary in structure, function, and processes. The structure, functions, and processes of the family influence and are influenced by individual family member's health status and the overall health status of the whole family. Families even vary within given cultures because every family has its own unique culture. People who come from the same family of origin create different families over time. Nurses need to be knowledgeable in the theories of families, as well as the structure, function, and processes of families to assist them in achieving or maintaining a state of health.

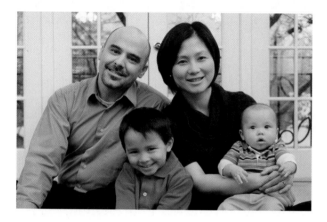

When families are considered the unit of care—as opposed to individuals—nurses have much broader perspectives for approaching health care needs of both individual family members and the family unit as a whole (Kaakinen, Hanson, & Denham, 2010). Understanding families enables nurses to assess the family health status, ascertain the effects of the family on individual family members' health status, predict the influence of alterations in the health status of the family system, and work with members as they plan and implement action plans customized for improved health for each individual family member and the family as a whole.

Recent advances in health care, such as changing health care policies and health care economics, ever-changing technology, shorter hospital stays, and health care moving from the hospital to the community/family home, are prompting changes from an individual person paradigm to the nursing care of families as a whole. This paradigm shift is affecting the development of family theory, practice, research, social policy, and education, and it is critical for nurses to be knowledgeable about and at the forefront of this shift. The centrality of family-centered care in health care delivery is emphasized by the American Nurses Association (ANA) in its publication, *Nursing's Social Policy Statement* (ANA,

2010a). In addition, *ANA's Nursing: Scope and Standards of Practice* mandates that nurses provide family care (ANA, 2010b). "Nurses have an ethical and moral obligation to involve families in their health-care practices" (Wright & Leahey, 2013, p. 1).

The overall goal of this book is to enhance nurses' knowledge and skills in the theory, practice, research, and social policy surrounding nursing care of families. This chapter provides a broad overview of family health care nursing. It begins with an exploration of the definitions of family and family health care nursing, and the concept of healthy families. This chapter goes on to describe four approaches to working with families: family as context, family as client, family as system, and family as a component of society. The chapter presents the varied, but ever-changing, family structures and explores family functions relative to reproduction, socialization, affective function, economic issues, and health care. Finally, the chapter discusses family processes, so that nurses know how their practice makes a difference when families experience stress because of the illness of individual family members.

THE FAMILY AND FAMILY HEALTH

Three foundational components of family nursing are: (1) determining how family is defined, (2) understanding the concepts of family health, and (3) knowing the current evidence about the elements of a healthy family.

What Is the Family?

There is no universally agreed-upon definition of family. Now more than ever, the traditional definition of family is being challenged, with Canadian recognition of same-sex marriages and with several states in the United States giving same-sex families the freedom to marry. Family is a word that conjures up different images for each individual and group, and the word has evolved in its meaning over time. Definitions differ by discipline, for example:

- *Legal:* relationships through blood ties, adoption, guardianship, or marriage
- *Biological:* genetic biological networks among and between people
- *Sociological:* groups of people living together with or without legal or biological ties
- *Psychological:* groups with strong emotional ties

Historically, early family social science theorists (Burgess & Locke, 1953, pp. 7–8) adopted the following traditional definition in their writing:

The family is a group of persons united by ties of marriage, blood, or adoption, constituting a single household; interacting and communicating with each other in their respective social roles of husband and wife, mother and father, son and daughter, brother and sister; and creating and maintaining a common culture.

Currently, the U.S. Census Bureau defines *family* as two or more people living together who are related by birth, marriage, or adoption (U.S. Census Bureau, 2011). This traditional definition continues to be the basis for the implementation of many social programs and policies. Yet, this definition excludes many diverse groups who consider themselves to be families and who perform family functions, such as economic, reproductive, and affective functions, as well as child socialization. Depending on the social norms, all of the following examples could be viewed as "family": married or remarried couples with biological or adoptive children, cohabitating same-sex couples (gay and lesbian families), single-parent families with children, kinship care families such as two sisters living together, or grandparents raising grandchildren without the parents.

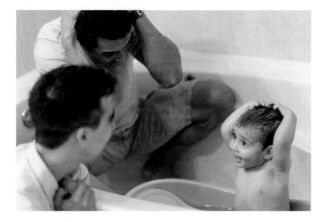

The definition of *family* adopted by this textbook and that applies from the previous edition (Kaakinen et al., 2010) is as follows: *Family refers to two or more individuals who depend on one another for emotional, physical, and economic support. The members of the family are self-defined.* Nurses who work with families should ask clients who they consider to be members of their family and should include those persons in health care planning with the patient's permission.

What Is Family Health?

The World Health Organization (2008) defined *health* to include a person's characteristics, behaviors, and physical, social, and economic environment. This definition applies to individuals and to families. Anderson and Tomlinson (1992) suggested that the analysis of family health must include, simultaneously, health and illness, the individual and the collective. They underscored evidence that the stress of a family member's serious illness exerts a powerful influence on family function and health, and that familial behavioral patterns or reactions to illness influence the individual family members. The term *family health* is often used interchangeably with the terms *family functioning*, *healthy families*, or *familial health*. To some, family health is the composite of individual family members' physical health, because it is impossible to make a single statement about the family's physical health as a single entity.

The definition of *family health* adopted in this textbook and that applies from the previous edition (Kaakinen et al., 2010) is as follows: *Family health is a dynamic, changing state of well-being, which includes the biological, psychological, spiritual, sociological, and culture factors of individual members and the whole family system.* This definition and approach combines all aspects of life for individual members, as well as for the whole family. An individual's health (on the wellness-to-illness continuum) affects the entire family's functioning, and in turn, the family's ability to function affects each individual member's health. Assessment of family health involves simultaneous data collection on individual family members and the whole family system (Craft-Rosenberg & Pehler, 2011).

What Is a Healthy Family?

While it is possible to define family health, it is more difficult to describe a healthy family. Characteristics used to describe healthy families or family strengths have varied throughout time in the literature. Krysan, Moore, and Zill (1990) described "healthy families" as "successful families" in a report prepared by the U.S. Department of Health and Human Services. They identified some of the ideas put forward by many family scholars over time. For example, Otto (1963) was the first scholar to develop psychosocial criteria for assessing family strengths, and he emphasized the need to focus on positive family attributes instead of the pathological approach that accentuated family problems and weaknesses. Pratt (1976) introduced the idea of the "energized family" as one whose structure encourages and supports individuals to develop their capacities for full functioning and independent action, thus contributing to family health. Curran (1985) investigated not only family stressors but also traits of healthy families, incorporating moral and task focus into traditional family functioning. These traits are listed in Box 1-1.

For more than three decades, Driver, Tabares, Shapiro, Nahm, and Gottman (2011) have studied the interactional patterns of marital success or failure. The success of a marriage does not depend on the presence or the amount of conflict. Success of a marriage depends primarily on how the couple handles conflict. The presence of four characteristics of couple interaction was found to predict divorce with 94% accuracy (Carrere, Buehlman, Coan, Gottman, & Ruckstuhl, 2000):

1. *Criticism:* These are personal attacks that consist of negative comments, to and about

each other, that occur over time and that erode the relationship.
2. *Contempt:* This is the most corrosive of the four characteristics between the couple. Contempt includes comments that convey disgust and disrespect.
3. *Defensiveness:* Each partner blames the other in an attempt to deflect a verbal attack.
4. *Stonewalling:* One or both of the partners refuse to interact or engage in interaction, both verbally and nonverbally.

In contrast, conflict is addressed in three ways in positive, healthy marriages. *Validators* talk their problems out, expressing emotions and opinions, and are skilled at reaching a compromise. *Volatiles* are two partners who view each other as equals, as they engage in loud, passionate, explosive interactions that are balanced by a caring, loving relationship. Their conflicts do not include the four negative characteristics identified earlier. The last type of couple is the *Avoiders.* Avoiders simply agree not to engage in conflicts, thus minimizing the corrosive effects of negative conflict resolution. The crucial point in all three styles of healthy conflict is that both partners engage in a similar style. Thus how conflict is used and resolved in the parental or couple dyad relationship suggests the health and longevity of the family unit.

The described positive interactions occur far more often than the negative interactions in happily married couples. These healthy family couples find ways to work out their differences and problems, are willing to yield to each other during their arguments, and make purposeful attempts to repair their relationship.

Olson and Gorall (2005) conducted a longitudinal study on families, in which they merged the concepts of marital and family dynamics in the Circumplex Model of Marital and Family Systems. They found that the ability of the family to demonstrate flexibility is related to its ability to alter family leadership roles, relationships, and rules, including control, discipline, and role sharing. Functional, healthy families have the ability to change these factors in response to situations. Dysfunctional families, or unhealthy families, have less ability to adapt and flex in response to changes. See Figures 1-1 and 1-2, which depict the differences in functional and dysfunctional families in the Circumplex Model. Balanced families will function more adequately across the family life cycle and

---

BOX 1-1
Traits of a Healthy Family

- Communicates and listens
- Fosters table time and conversation
- Affirms and supports each member
- Teaches respect for others
- Develops a sense of trust
- Has a sense of play and humor
- Has a balance of interaction among members
- Shares leisure time
- Exhibits a sense of shared responsibility
- Teaches a sense of right and wrong
- Abounds in rituals and traditions
- Shares a religious core
- Respects the privacy of each member
- Values service to others
- Admits to problems and seeks help

Source: From Kaakinen, J. R., Hanson, S. M. H., & Denham, S. (2010). Family health care nursing: An introduction. In J. W. Kaakinen, V. Gedaly-Duff, D. P. Coehlo, & S. M. H. Hanson (Eds.), *Family health care nursing: Theory, practice and research* (4th ed.). Philadelphia, PA: F. A. Davis, with permission.

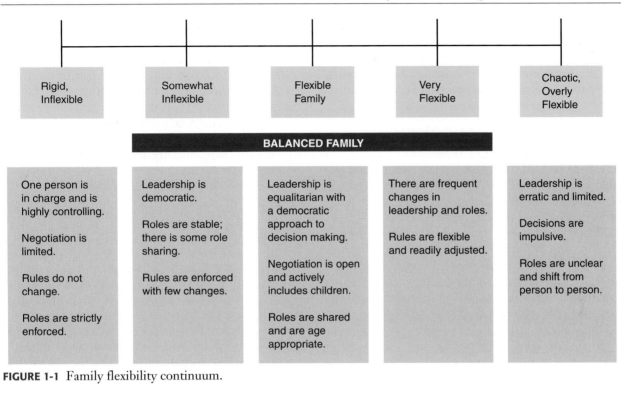

FIGURE 1-1 Family flexibility continuum.

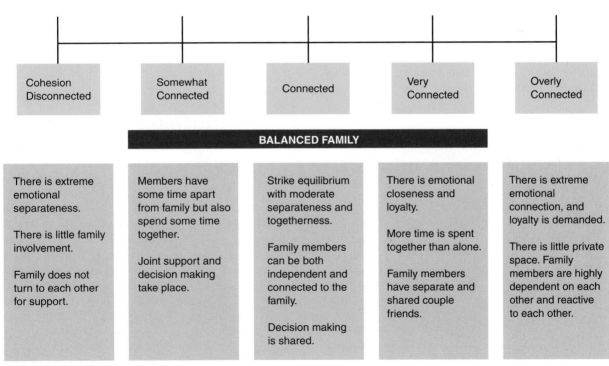

FIGURE 1-2 Family cohesion continuum.

tend to be healthier families. The family communication skills enable balance and help families to adjust and adapt to situations. Couples and families modify their levels of flexibility and cohesion to adapt to stressors, thus promoting family health.

FAMILY HEALTH CARE NURSING

The specialty area of family health care nursing has been evolving since the early 1980s. Some question how family health care nursing is distinct from other specialties that involve families, such as maternal-child health nursing, community health nursing, and mental health nursing. The definition and framework for *family health care nursing* adopted by this textbook and that applies from the previous edition (Kaakinen et al., 2010) is as follows:

> *The process of providing for the health care needs of families that are within the scope of nursing practice. This nursing care can be aimed toward the family as context, the family as a whole, the family as a system, or the family as a component of society.*

Family nursing takes into consideration all four approaches to viewing families. At the same time, it cuts across the individual, family, and community for the purpose of promoting, maintaining, and restoring the health of families. This framework illustrates the intersecting concepts of the individual, the family, nursing, and society (Fig. 1-3).

Another way to view family nursing practice is conceptually, as a confluence of theories and strategies from nursing, family therapy, and family social science as depicted in Figure 1-4. Over time, family nursing continues to incorporate ideas from family therapy and family social science into the practice of family nursing. See Chapter 3 for discussion about how theories from family social science, family therapy, and nursing converge to inform the nursing of families.

Several family scholars have written about levels of family health care nursing practice. For example, Wright and Leahey (2013) differentiated among several levels of knowledge and skills that family nurses need for a generalist versus specialist practice, and they defined the role of higher education for the two different levels of practice. They propose that nurses receive a generalist or basic level of knowledge and skills in family nursing during their undergraduate work, and advanced specialization in family nursing or family therapy at the graduate level. They recognize that advanced specialists in family nursing have a narrower focus than generalists. They purport, however, that family assessment is an important skill for all nurses practicing with families. Bomar (2004) further delineated five levels of family health care nursing practice using Benner's levels of practice: expert, proficient, competent, advanced beginner, and novice. See Table 1-1, which describes how the two levels of generalist and advanced practice have been delineated further with levels of education and types of clients (Benner, 2001).

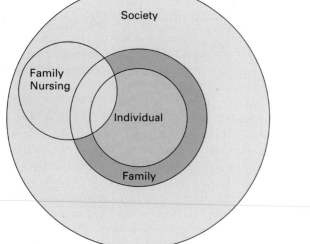

FIGURE 1-3 Family nursing conceptual framework.

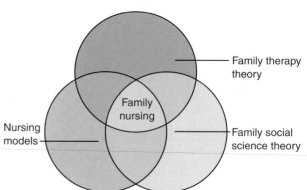

FIGURE 1-4 Family nursing practice.

Table 1-1	**Levels of Family Nursing Practice**		
Level of Practice	**Generalist/Specialist**	**Education**	**Client**
Expert	Advanced specialist	Doctoral degree	All levels
			Family nursing theory development
			Family nursing research
Proficient	Advanced specialist	Master's degree with added experience	All levels
			Beginning family nursing research
Competent	Beginning specialist	Master's degree	Individual in the family context
			Interpersonal family nursing
			Family unit
			Family aggregates
Advanced beginner	Generalist	Bachelor's degree with added experience	Individual in the family context
			Interpersonal family nursing (family systems nursing)
			Family unit
Novice	Generalist	Bachelor's degree	Individual in the family context

Source: Bomar, P. J. (Ed.). (2004). *Promoting health in families: Applying family research and theory to nursing practice* (3rd ed.). Philadelphia, PA: Saunders/Elsevier, with permission.

NATURE OF INTERVENTIONS IN FAMILY NURSING

The following 10 interventions family nurses use provide structure to working with families regardless of the theoretical underpinning of the nursing approach. These are enduring ideas that support the practice of family nursing (Gilliss, Roberts, Highley, & Martinson, 1989; Kaakinen et al., 2010):

1. Family care is concerned with the experience of the family over time. It considers both the history and the future of the family group.
2. Family nursing considers the community and cultural context of the group. The family is encouraged to receive from, and give to, community resources.
3. Family nursing considers the relationships between and among family members, and recognizes that, in some instances, all individual members and the family group will not achieve maximum health simultaneously.
4. Family nursing is directed at families whose members are both healthy and ill regardless of the severity of the illness in the family member.

5. Family nursing is often offered in settings where individuals have physiological or psychological problems. Together with competency in treatment of individual health problems, family nurses must recognize the reciprocity between individual family members' health and collective health within the family.
6. The family system is influenced by any change in its members. Therefore, when caring for individuals in health and illness, the nurse must elect whether to attend to the family. Individual health and collective health are intertwined and will be influenced by any nursing care given.
7. Family nursing requires the nurse to manipulate the environment to increase the likelihood of family interaction. The physical absence of family members, however, does not preclude the nurse from offering family care.
8. The family nurse recognizes that the person in a family who is most symptomatic may change over time; this means that the focus of the nurse's attention will also change over time.

9. Family nursing focuses on the strengths of individual family members and the family group to promote their mutual support and growth.

10. Family nurses must define with the family which persons constitute the family and where they will place their therapeutic energies.

These are the distinctive intervention statements specific to family nursing that appear continuously in the care and study of families in nursing, regardless of the theoretical model in use.

APPROACHES TO FAMILY NURSING

Four different approaches to care are inherent in family nursing: (1) family as the context for individual development, (2) family as a client, (3) family as a system, and (4) family as a component of society (Kaakinen et al., 2010). Figure 1-5 illustrates these approaches to the nursing of families. Each approach derived its foundations from different nursing specialties: maternal-child nursing, primary care nursing, psychiatric/mental health nursing, and community health nursing, respectively. All four approaches have legitimate implications for nursing assessment and intervention. The approach that nurses use is determined by many factors, including the health care setting, family circumstances, and nurse resources. Figure 1-6 shows how a nurse can view all four approaches to families through just one set of eyes. It is important to keep all four perspectives in mind when working with any given family.

Family as Context

The first approach to family nursing care focuses on the assessment and care of an individual client in which the family is the context. Alternate labels for this approach are *family centered* or *family focused*. This is the traditional nursing focus, in which the individual is foreground and the family is background. The family serves as context for the individual as either a resource or a stressor to the individual's health and illness. Most existing nursing theories or models were originally conceptualized using the individual as a focus. This approach is rooted in the specialty of maternal-child nursing and underlies the philosophy of many maternity

and pediatric health care settings. A nurse using this focus might say to an individual client: "Who in your family will help you with your nightly medication?" "How will you provide for child care when you have your back surgery?" or "It is wonderful for you that your wife takes such an interest in your diabetes and has changed all the food preparation to fit your dietary needs."

Family as Client

The second approach to family nursing care centers on the assessment of all family members. The family nurse is interested in the way all the family members are individually affected by the health event of one family member. In this approach, all members of the family are in the foreground. The family is seen as the sum of individual family members, and the focus concentrates on each individual. The nurse assesses and provides health care for each person in the family. This approach is seen typically in primary care clinics in the communities where primary care physicians (PCPs) or nurse practitioners (NPs) provide care over time to all individuals in a given family. From this perspective, a nurse might ask a family member who has just become ill: "How has your diagnosis of juvenile diabetes affected the other individuals in your family?" "Will your nightly need for medication be a problem for other members of your family?" "Who in your family is having the most difficult time with your diagnosis?" or "How are the members of your family adjusting to your new medication regimen?"

Family as System

The third approach to care views the family as a system. The focus in this approach is on the family as a whole as the client; here, the family is viewed as an interactional system in which the whole is more than the sum of its parts. In other words, the interactions between family members become the target for the nursing interventions. The interventions flow from the assessment of the family as a whole. The family nursing system approach focuses on the individual and family simultaneously. The emphasis is on the interactions between family members, for example, the direct interactions between the parental dyad or the indirect interaction between the parental dyad and the child. The more children there are in a family, the more complex these interactions become.

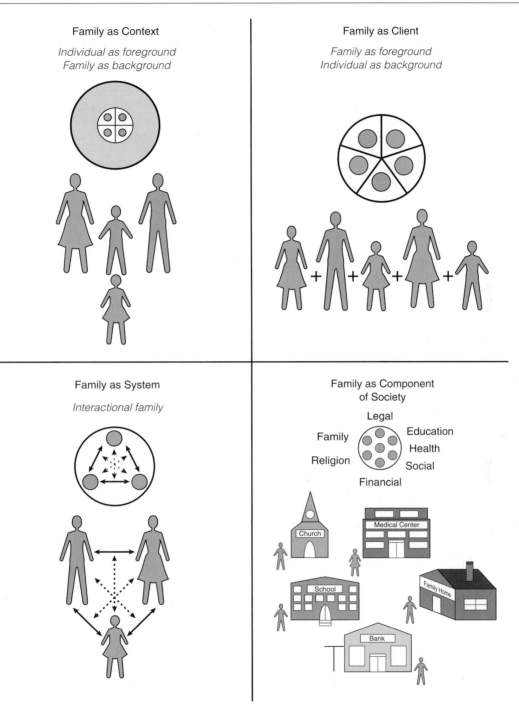

FIGURE 1-5 Approaches to family nursing.

This interactional model had its start with the specialty of psychiatric and mental health nursing. The systems approach always implies that when something happens to one part of the system, the other parts of the system are affected. Therefore, if one family member becomes ill, it affects all other members of the family. Examples of questions that nurses may ask in a systems approach include the following: "What has changed between you and your spouse since your child was diagnosed with juvenile

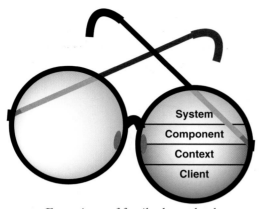

FIGURE 1-6 Four views of family through a lens.

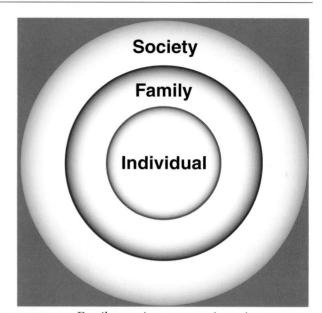

FIGURE 1-7 Family as primary group in society.

diabetes?" or "How has the diagnosis of juvenile diabetes affected the ways in which your family is functioning and getting along with each other?"

Family as Component of Society

The fourth approach to care looks at the family as a component of society, in which the family is viewed as one of many institutions in society, similar to health, educational, religious, or economic institutions. The family is a basic or primary unit of society, and it is a part of the larger system of society (Fig. 1-7). The family as a whole interacts with other institutions to receive, exchange, or give communication and services. Family social scientists first used this approach in their study of families in society. Community health nursing has drawn many of its tenets from this perspective as it focuses on the interface between families and community agencies. Questions nurses may ask in this approach include the following: "What issues has the family been experiencing since you made the school aware of your son's diagnosis of HIV?" or "Have you considered joining a support group for families with mothers who have breast cancer? Other families have found this to be an excellent resource and a way to reduce stress."

VARIABLES THAT INFLUENCE FAMILY NURSING

Family health care nursing has been influenced by many variables that are derived from both historical and current events within society and the profession of nursing. Examples include changing nursing

theory, practice, education, and research; new knowledge derived from family social sciences and the health sciences; national and state health care policies; changing health care behavior and attitudes; and national and international political events. Chapters 3 and 5 provide detailed discussions of these areas.

Figure 1-8 illustrates how many variables influence contemporary family health nursing, making the point that the status of family nursing is dependent on what is occurring in the wider society—family as community. A recent example of this point is that health practices and policy changes are under way because of the recognition that current costs of health care are escalating and, at the same time, greater numbers of people are underinsured or uninsured and have lost access to health care. The goal of this health care reform is to make access and treatment available for everyone at an affordable cost. That will require a major shift in priorities, funding, and services. A major movement toward health promotion and family care in the community will greatly affect the evolution of family nursing.

FAMILY NURSING ROLES

Families are the basic unit of every society, but it is also true that families are complex, varied, dynamic,

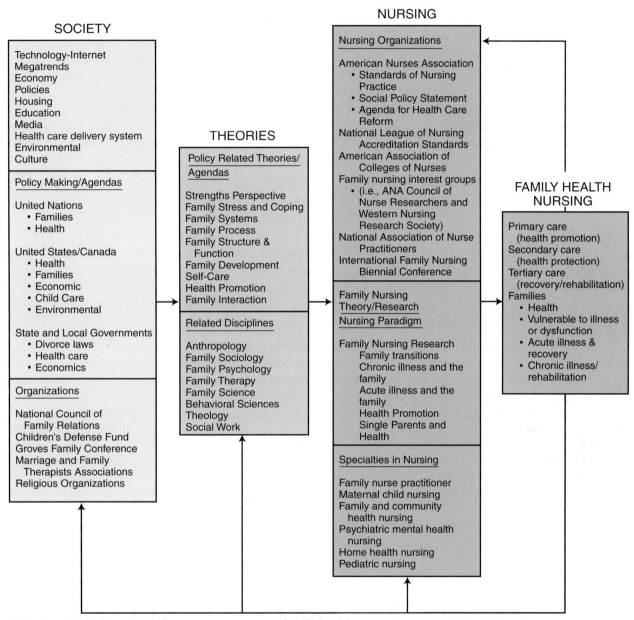

SOCIETY

Technology-Internet
Megatrends
Economy
Policies
Housing
Education
Media
Health care delivery system
Environmental
Culture

Policy Making/Agendas

United Nations
- Families
- Health

United States/Canada
- Health
- Families
- Economic
- Child Care
- Environmental

State and Local Governments
- Divorce laws
- Health care
- Economics

Organizations

National Council of
   Family Relations
Children's Defense Fund
Groves Family Conference
Marriage and Family
   Therapists Associations
Religious Organizations

THEORIES

Policy Related Theories/
Agendas

Strengths Perspective
Family Stress and Coping
Family Systems
Family Process
Family Structure &
   Function
Family Development
Self-Care
Health Promotion
Family Interaction

Related Disciplines

Anthropology
Family Sociology
Family Psychology
Family Therapy
Family Science
Behavioral Sciences
Theology
Social Work

NURSING

Nursing Organizations

American Nurses Association
- Standards of Nursing
   Practice
- Social Policy Statement
- Agenda for Health Care
   Reform
National League of Nursing
   Accreditation Standards
American Association of
   Colleges of Nurses
Family nursing interest groups
- (i.e., ANA Council of
   Nurse Researchers and
   Western Nursing
   Research Society)
National Association of Nurse
   Practitioners
International Family Nursing
   Biennial Conference

Family Nursing
Theory/Research
Nursing Paradigm

Family Nursing Research
   Family transitions
   Chronic illness and the
   family
   Acute illness and the
   family
   Health Promotion
   Single Parents and
   Health

Specialties in Nursing

Family nurse practitioner
Maternal child nursing
Family and community
   health nursing
Psychiatric mental health
   nursing
Home health nursing
Pediatric nursing

FAMILY HEALTH NURSING

Primary care
   (health promotion)
Secondary care
   (health protection)
Tertiary care
   (recovery/rehabilitation)
Families
- Health
- Vulnerable to illness
   or dysfunction
- Acute illness &
   recovery
- Chronic illness/
   rehabilitation

FIGURE 1-8 Variables that influence contemporary family health care. (From Bomar, P. J. [Ed.]. [2004]. *Promoting health in families: Applying family research and theory to nursing practice [3rd ed., p. 17]. Philadelphia, PA: Saunders/Elsevier, with permission.)*

and adaptive, which is why it is crucial for all nurses to be knowledgeable about the scientific discipline of family nursing, and the variety of ways nurses may interact with families (Kaakinen et al., 2010). The roles of family health care nurses are evolving along with the specialty. Figure 1-9 lists the many roles that nurses can assume with families as the focus. This figure was constructed from some of the first family nursing literature that appeared, and

it is a composite of what various scholars believe to be some of the current roles of nurses. Keep in mind that the health care setting affects roles that nurses assume with families.

Health teacher: The family nurse teaches about family wellness, illness, relations, and parenting, to name a few topics. The teacher-educator function is ongoing in all settings in both formal and informal

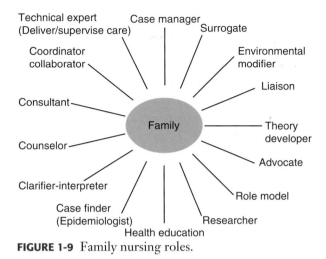

FIGURE 1-9 Family nursing roles.

ways. Examples include teaching new parents how to care for their infant and giving instructions about diabetes to a newly diagnosed adolescent boy and his family members.

Coordinator, collaborator, and liaison:
The family nurse coordinates the care that families receive, collaborating with the family to plan care. For example, if a family member has been in a traumatic accident, the nurse would be a key person in helping families to access resources—from inpatient care, outpatient care, home health care, and social services to rehabilitation. The nurse may serve as the liaison among these services.

"Deliverer" and supervisor of care and technical expert:
The family nurse either delivers or supervises the care that families receive in various settings. To do this, the nurse must be a technical expert both in terms of knowledge and skill. For example, the nurse may be the person going into the family home on a daily basis to consult with the family and help take care of a child on a respirator.

Family advocate:
The family nurse advocates for families with whom he works; the nurse empowers family members to speak with their own voice, or the nurse speaks out for the family. An example is a school nurse advocating for special education services for a child with attention-deficit hyperactivity disorder.

Consultant:
The family nurse serves as a consultant to families whenever asked or whenever necessary. In some instances, she consults with agencies to facilitate family-centered care. For example, a clinical nurse specialist in a hospital may be asked to assist the family in finding the appropriate long-term care setting for their sick grandmother. The nurse comes into the family system by request for a short period and for a specific purpose.

Counselor:
The family nurse plays a therapeutic role in helping individuals and families solve problems or change behavior. An example from the mental health arena is a family that requires help with coping with a long-term chronic condition, such as when a family member has been diagnosed with schizophrenia.

"Case-finder" and epidemiologist:
The family nurse gets involved in case-finding and becomes a tracker of disease. For example, consider the situation in which a family member has been recently diagnosed with a sexually transmitted disease. The nurse would engage in sleuthing out the sources of the transmission and in helping other sexual contacts to seek treatment. Screening families and subsequent referral of the family members may be a part of this role.

Environmental specialist:
The family nurse consults with families and other health care professionals to modify the environment. For example, if a man with paraplegia is about to be discharged from the hospital to home, the nurse assists the family in modifying the home environment so that the patient can move around in a wheelchair and engage in self-care.

Clarify and interpret:
The nurse clarifies and interprets data to families in all settings. For example, if a child in the family has a complex disease, such as leukemia, the nurse clarifies and interprets information pertaining to diagnosis, treatment, and prognosis of the condition to parents and extended family members.

Surrogate:
The family nurse serves as a surrogate by substituting for another person. For example, the nurse may stand in temporarily as a loving parent to an adolescent who is giving birth to a child by herself in the labor and delivery room.

Researcher:
The family nurse should identify practice problems and find the best solution for dealing with these problems through the process of scientific investigation. An example might be

collaborating with a colleague to find a better intervention for helping families cope with incontinent elders living in the home.

Role model: The family nurse is continually serving as a role model to other people. A school nurse who demonstrates the right kind of health in personal self-care serves as a role model to parents and children alike.

Case manager: Although case manager is a contemporary name for this role, it involves coordination and collaboration between a family and the health care system. The case manager has been empowered formally to be in charge of a case. For example, a family nurse working with seniors in the community may become assigned to be the case manager for a patient with Alzheimer's disease.

OBSTACLES TO FAMILY NURSING PRACTICE

There are several obstacles to practicing family nursing. A vast amount of literature is available about families, but there has been little taught about families in the nursing curricula until the past three decades. Most practicing nurses have not had exposure to family theory or concepts during their undergraduate education and continue to practice using the individualist paradigm. Even though there are several family assessment models and approaches, families are complex, so no one assessment approach fits all family situations. There is a paucity of valid and reliable psychometrically tested family evaluation instruments.

Furthermore, some students and nurses may believe that the study of family and family nursing is "common sense," and therefore does not belong formally in nursing curricula, either in theory or practice. Nursing also has strong historical ties with the medical model, which has traditionally focused on the individual as client, rather than the family. At best, families have been viewed in context, and many times families were considered a nuisance in health care settings—an obstacle to overcome to provide care to the individual.

Another obstacle is the fact that the traditional charting system in health care has been oriented to the individual. For example, charting by exception focuses on the physical care of the individual and does not address the whole family or members of families. Likewise, the medical and nursing diagnostic systems used in health care are disease centered, and diseases are focused on individuals and have limited diagnostic codes that pertain to the family as a whole. To complicate matters further, most insurance companies require that there be one identified patient, with a diagnostic code drawn from an individual disease perspective. Thus, even if health care providers are intervening with entire families, companies require providers to choose one person in the family group as the identified patient and to give that person a physical or mental diagnosis, even though the client is the whole family. Although there are family diagnostic codes that address care with families, insurance companies may not pay for care for those codes, especially if the care is more psychological or educational in nature. See Chapter 4 for a detailed discussion on diagnostic codes.

The established hours during which health care systems provide services pose another obstacle to focusing on families. Traditionally, office hours take place during the day, when family members cannot accompany other family members. Recently, some urgent care centers and other outpatient settings have incorporated evening and weekend hours into their schedules, making it possible for family members to come in together. But many clinics and physician offices still operate on traditional Monday through Friday, 9:00 a.m. to 5:00 p.m. schedules, thus making it difficult for all family members to attend together. These obstacles to family-focused nursing practice are slowly changing; nurses should continue to lobby for changes that are more conducive to caring for the family as a whole.

HISTORICAL PERSPECTIVES

A brief historical outline of the development of the specialty of family nursing will help nurses understand how nurses have actually always provided care for the family from several different viewpoints. An outline of the history of families in North America is presented to provide an overview of the family development up until present time.

History of Family Nursing

Family health nursing has roots in society from prehistoric times. The historical role of women has been inextricably interwoven with the family, for it was the responsibility of women to care for family members who fell ill and to seek herbs or remedies to treat the illness. Women have been the primary child care providers throughout history. In addition, through "proper" housekeeping, women made efforts to provide clean and safe environments for the maintenance of health and wellness for their families (Bomar, 2004; Ham & Chamings, 1983; Whall, 1993).

During the Nightingale era in the late 1800s, the development of nursing families became more explicit. Florence Nightingale influenced both the establishment of district nursing of the sick and poor, and the work of "health missionaries" through "health-at-home" teaching. She believed that cleanliness in the home could eradicate high infant mortality and morbidity rates. She encouraged family members of the fighting troops to come into the hospitals during the Crimean War to take care of their loved ones. Nightingale supported helping women and children achieve good health by promoting both nurse midwifery and home-based health services. In 1876, in a document titled "Training Nurses for the Sick Poor," Nightingale encouraged nurses to serve in nursing both sick and healthy families in the home environment. She gave both home-health nurses and maternal-child nurses the mandate to carry out nursing practice with the whole family as the unit of service (Nightingale, 1979).

In colonial America, women continued the centuries-old traditions of nurturing and sustaining the wellness of their families and caring for the ill. During the industrial revolution of the late 18th century, family members began to work outside the home. Immigrants, in particular, were in need of income, so they went to work for the early hospitals. This was the real beginning of public health and school nursing. The nurses involved in the beginning of the labor movement were concerned with the health of workers, immigrants, and their families. Concepts of maternal-child and family care were incorporated into basic curriculums of nursing schools. In fact, maternity nursing, nurse midwifery, and community nursing historically focused on the quality of family health. Margaret Sanger fought for family planning. Mary Breckenridge formed the famous Frontier Nursing Service (midwifery) to provide training for nurses to meet the health needs of mountain families.

A concerted expansion of public health nursing occurred during the Great Depression to work with families as a whole. Nevertheless, before and during World War II, nursing became more focused on the individual, and care became centralized in institutional and hospital settings, where it remained until recently.

Since the 1950s, at least 19 disciplines have studied the family and, through research, produced family assessment techniques, conceptual frameworks, theories, and other family material. Recently, this interdisciplinary work has become known as family social science. Family social science has greatly influenced family nursing in the United States, largely because of the professional interdisciplinary group called National Council of Family Relations and its large number of family publications. Many family nurses have become active in this organization. In addition, some nurses are now receiving advanced degrees in family social science departments around the country.

Nursing theorists started in the 1960s to systematize nursing practice. Scholars began to articulate the philosophy and goals of nursing care. Initially, theorists were concerned only with individuals, but gradually, individuals became viewed as part of a larger social system. Also in the 1960s, the NP movement began espousing the family as a primary unit of care in practice, although the grand theories of nursing focused primarily on the individual and not families.

The 1980s saw a shift in focus to families as a unit of care in America and Canada. Small numbers of people across these countries gathered together to discuss and share family nursing concepts. Family nurses started defining the scope of practice, family concepts, and how to teach this information to the next generation of nurses. Family nursing has both old and new traditions and definitions. The discipline and science of family nursing is now beyond youth, more like a young adult, but still in a state of growing up and maturing. The first national family nursing conferences were held in the United States (Portland, Oregon) in 1986–1989. The International Family Nursing Conferences (IFNC) began in the late 1980s and has been held around the world every 2 or 3 years since that time. The 11th International Family Nursing Conference was held in June 2013 in Minneapolis, Minnesota. The International Family Nursing Association (IFNA) grew out of IFNC and became active in 2009–2010. See Table 1-2 for a composite of historical factors that contributed to the development of family health as a focus in nursing.

Table 1-2	**Historical Factors Contributing to the Development of Family Health as a Focus in Nursing**
Time Period	**Events**
Pre-Nightingale era	Revolutionary War "camp followers" were an example of family health focus before Florence Nightingale's influence.
Mid-1800s	Nightingale influences district nurses and health missionaries to maintain clean environment for patients' homes and families.
	Family members provided for soldiers' needs during Civil War through Ladies Aid Societies and Women's Central Association for Relief.
Late 1800s	Industrial Revolution and immigration influence focus of public health nursing on prevention of illness, health education, and care of the sick for both families and communities.
	Lillian Wald establishes Henry Street Visiting Nurse Service (1893).
	Focus on family during childbearing by maternal-child nurses and midwives.
Early 1900s	School of nursing established in New York City (1903).
	First White House Conference on Children occurs (1909).
	Red Cross Town and Country Nursing Service was founded (1912).
	Margaret Sanger opens first birth control clinic (1916).
	Family planning and quality care become available for families.
	Mary Breckinridge forms Frontier Nursing Service (1925).
	Nurses are assigned to families.
	Red Cross Public Health Nursing Service meets rural health needs after stock market crash (1929).
	Federal Emergency Relief Act passed (1933).
	Social Security Act passed (1935).
	Psychiatry and mental health disciplines begin family therapy focus (late 1930s).
1960s	Concept of family as a unit of care is introduced into basic nursing curriculum.
	National League for Nursing (NLN) requires emphasis on families and communities in nursing curriculum.
	Family-centered approach in maternal-child nursing and midwifery programs is begun.
	Nurse-practitioner movement, programs to provide primary care to children begin (1965).
	Shift from public health nursing to community health nursing occurs.
	Family studies and research produce family theories.
1970s	Changing health care system focuses on maintaining health and returning emphasis to family health.
	Development and refinement of nursing conceptual models that consider the family as a unit of analysis or care occur (e.g., King, Newman, Orem, Rogers, and Roy).
	Many specialties focus on the family (e.g., hospice, oncology, geriatrics, school health, psychiatry, mental health, occupational health, and home health).
	Master's and doctoral programs focus on the family (e.g., family health nursing, community health nursing, psychiatry, mental health, and family counseling and therapy).
	ANA Standards of Nursing Practice are implemented (1973).
	Surgeon General's Report focuses on healthy people, health promotion, and disease prevention (1979).
1980s	ANA Social Policy Statement (1980).
	White House Conference on Families.
	Greater emphasis is put on health from very young to very old.
	Increasing emphasis is placed on obesity, stress, chemical dependency, and parenting skills.
	Graduate level specialization begins, with emphasis on primary care outside of acute care settings, health teaching, and client self-care.

(continued)

Table 1-2	Historical Factors Contributing to the Development of Family Health as a Focus in Nursing—cont'd
Time Period	**Events**
	Use of wellness and nursing models in providing care increases.
	Promoting Health/Preventing Disease: Objective for the Nation (1980) is released by U.S. Department of Health and Human Services.
	Family science develops as a discipline.
	Family nursing research increases.
	National Center for Nursing Research is founded, with a Health Promotion and Prevention Research section.
	First International Nursing Conference occurs in Calgary, Canada (1988).
1990s	*Healthy People 2000: National Health Promotion and Disease Prevention Objective* (1990) is released by U.S. Department of Health and Human Services.
	Nursing's Agenda for Health Care Reform is developed (ANA, 1991).
	Family leave legislation is passed (1991).
	Journal of Family Nursing is created (1995).
2000s	*Nursing's Agenda for the Future* is written (ANA, 2002).
	Healthy People 2010 and *Healthy People 2020* are released from U.S. Department of Health and Human Services.
	The quality and quantity of family nursing research continue to increase, especially in the international sector.
	Family-related research is clearly a goal of the *National Institute of Nursing Research Themes for the Future* (NINR, 2003).
	World Health Organization document *Health for All in the 21st Century* calls for support of families.
	The National Council on Family Relations prepared the *NCFR Presidential Report 2001: Preparing Families for the Future.*
	International Family Nursing Conferences start meeting every 2 years instead of every 3 years.

Adapted from Bomar, P. J. (Ed.). (2004). *Promoting health in families: Applying family research and theory to nursing practice* (3rd ed.). Philadelphia, PA: Saunders/Elsevier.

History of Families

A brief macro-analytical history of families is important to an understanding of family nursing. The past helps to make the present realities of family life more understandable, because the influence of the past is evident in the present. This historical approach provides a means of conceptualizing family over time and within all of society. History helps to dispel preferences for family forms that are only personally familiar and broaden nurses' views of the world of families.

Prehistoric Family Life

Archaeologists and anthropologists have found evidence of prehistoric family life, existing before the time of written historical sources. These family forms varied from present-day forms, but the functions of the family have been assumed to have remained somewhat constant over time. Families were then and are now a part of the larger community and constitute the basic unit of society.

It is postulated that the family structure, process, and function were a response to everyday needs in prehistoric times, just as they are in modern times. As communities grew, families and communities became more institutionalized and homogeneous as civilization progressed. Family culture was that aspect of life derived from membership in a particular group and shared by others. Family culture was composed of values and attitudes that allowed early families to behave in a predictable fashion.

Man and woman dyads are the oldest and most tenacious unit in history. Biologically, human children need care and protection longer than other animals' offspring. These needs led humans to form long-term relationships. Economic pairing was not always the same as reproductive pairing, but it was a by-product of reproductive pairing. Moreover, a variety of skills were required for living, and no single person possessed all skills; therefore, male and female roles began to differ and become defined. Early in history, children were part of the economic unit. As small groups of conjugal families formed communities, the complexity of the social order increased.

European History

Many Americans are of European ancestry and stem from the family structure that was present there. Social organizations called families emphasized consanguineous (genetic) bonds. The tendency toward authority was concentrated in a few individuals at the top of the hierarchical structure (kings, lords, fathers). Men were the heads of families.

Property of family transferred through the male line. Women left home to join their husbands' families. Mothers did not establish strong bonds with their daughters because the daughters eventually left their homes of origin to join their husbands' families of origin. Women and children were property to be transferred. Marriage was a contract between families, not individuals. Extended patriarchal family characteristics prevailed until the advent of industrialism.

Industrialization

Great stability existed within family systems until the Industrial Revolution. The revolution first appeared in England around 1750 and spread to Western Europe and North America. Some believe that the nuclear family idea started with the Industrial Revolution. Extended families had always been the norm until families left farms and moved into the cities, or until men left their families in order to work in the factories. Some women stayed at home, maintaining the house and caring for the children, while other women and children took up labor in the city factories.

When factories of the Industrial Revolution started to be built, people began moving about. The state had begun to provide services that families previously had performed for their members. Informal contractual arrangements between public and state power and nuclear families took place, in which the state gave fathers the power and authority over their families in exchange for male individuals giving the state their loyalty and service. Women were not expected to love husbands but to obey them.

Society today is still living with bequests of patriarchal family life. Women are still struggling to get out from under the rules and expectations of the state and of men. The women's movement and the National Organization for Women (NOW) are two of the forces that have improved the level of equality of women in modern society. A lot more work needs to be done on the issues of equality for all Americans, including gender differences.

In recent years, men have also begun identifying the bondage they experience. They cannot meet all of the needs of families and feel inadequate for failing to do so. This is especially true of men who cannot access the resources of money, occupation, and occupational status through education. A men's movement is afoot that is promoting male causes, although this movement is not as dynamic as it may be in the future. One of the organizations supporting this work is the National Congress for Men.

North American Families

North American society and families were molded from the beginning by economic logic rather than consanguineous logic. America does not have the history of Europe's preindustrial age. English patriarchy was not transplanted in its pure form to America. Both women and men had to labor in the New World. This gave women new power. Also, the United States had an ethic of achieved status rather than status inherited through familial lines.

Children were also experiencing a changing status in American families. Originally, they were part of the economic unit and worked on farms. Then with the great immigration of the early 1900s, the expectation shifted to parents creating a better world for their children than they themselves had. To do this, children had to become more educated to deal with the developing society. Each generation of children has generally obtained more education and income than their parents; they left the family farms and moved to distant cities. As a result of this change, parents lost assurance that their children would take care of them during their old age.

In addition, the functions of families were changing greatly. The traditional roles that families played were being displaced by the growing numbers and kinds of social institutions. Families began increasingly surrendering to public agencies many of the socialization functions they previously performed, such as child education, health care, and child care.

Families Today

Today, families cannot be separated from the larger system of which they are a part, nor can they be separated from their historical past. Some people argue that families are in terrible condition, like a rudderless ship in the dark. Other people hail the changes that continue to occur in families, and approve the diversity and options that address modern needs. Idealizing past family arrangements and decrying change has become commonplace in the media. Just as some families of both the past and present engage in behaviors that are destructive to individuals and other social institutions, there are families of the past and present that provide healthy environments. The structure, function, and processes of families have changed, but the family will continue to survive and thrive. It is, in fact, the most tenacious unit in society (Kaakinen et al., 2010).

FAMILY STRUCTURE, FUNCTION, AND PROCESS

Knowledge about family structure, functions, and processes is essential for understanding the complex family interactions that affect health, illness, and well-being (Kaakinen et al., 2010). Knowledge emerging from the study of family structure, function, and process suggests concepts and a framework that nurses can use to provide effective assessment and intervention with families. Many internal and external family variables affect individual family members and the family as a whole. Internal family variables include unique individual characteristics, communication, and interactions, whereas external family variables include location of family household, social policy, and economic trends. Family members generally have complicated responses to all of these factors. Although some external factors may not be easily modifiable, nurses can assist family members to manage change, conflict, and care needs. For instance, a sudden downturn in the economy could result in the family breadwinner becoming unemployed. Although nurses are unable to alter this situation directly, understanding the implications on the family situation provides a basis for planning more effective interventions that may include financial support programs for families. Nurses can assist members with coping skills, communication patterns, location of needed resources, effective use of information, or creation of family rituals or routines (Kaakinen et al., 2010).

Nurses who understand the concepts of family structure, function, and process can use this knowledge to educate, counsel, and implement changes that enable families to cope with illness, family crisis, chronic health conditions, and mental illness. Nurses prepared to work with families can assist them with needed life transitions (Kaakinen et al., 2010). For example, when a family member experiences a chronic condition such as diabetes, family roles, routines, and power hierarchies may be challenged. Nurses must be prepared to address the complex and holistic family problems resulting from illness, as well as to care for the individual's medical needs.

Family Structure

Family structure is the ordered set of relationships within the family, and between the family and other social systems (Denham, 2005). There are many tools available for nurses to use in conducting assessments of family structure. The most fundamental tools are family genograms and ecomaps, which will be introduced later in this chapter. These tools are not new in nursing, but their popularity among nurses and other providers is growing due to the clearly perceived value of the knowledge they generate. Genograms and ecomaps are beginning to make their way out of more obscure settings such as specialty genetics clinics and into mainstream home health, public health, and even acute care settings (Svarvardoittir, 2008).

In terms of family nursing assessment and intervention, it is logical to begin with the "who" of families before moving to the "how" or "why." In determining the family structure, the nurse needs to identify the following:

- The individuals who comprise the family
- The relationships between them
- The interactions between the family members
- The interactions with other social systems

Family patterns of organization tend to be relatively stable over time, but they are modified gradually throughout the family life cycle and often change radically when divorce, separation, or death occurs.

In today's information age and global society, several ideas about the "best family" coexist simultaneously. Different family types have their strengths and limitations, which directly or indirectly affect individuals and family health. Many families still adhere to more customary forms and patterns, but many of today's families fall into categories more clearly labeled nontraditional (Table 1-3). Nurses will confront families structured differently from their own families of origin and will encounter family types that conflict with personal value systems. For nurses to work effectively with families, they must maintain open and inquiring minds.

Table 1-3	Variations of Family and Household Structures
Family Type	**Composition**
Nuclear dyad	Married couple, no children
Nuclear	Husband, wife, children (may or may not be legally married)
Binuclear	Two postdivorce families with children as members of both
Extended	Nuclear family plus blood relatives
Blended	Husband, wife, and children of previous relationships
Single parent	One parent and child(ren)
Commune	Group of men, women, and children
Cohabitation (domestic partners)	Unmarried man and woman sharing a household
Homosexual	Same-gender couple
Single person (adult)	One person in a household

Families in the past were more homogeneous than they are today. Whereas the past norm in predominately Caucasian families was a two-parent family (traditional nuclear family) living together with their biological children, many other family forms are acknowledged and recognized today. It is important to note that the average person born today will experience many family forms during his or her lifetime. Figure 1-10 depicts the many familial forms that the average person can live through today. Nurses are not only experiencing this proliferation of variation in their own personal lives but also with the patients with whom they work in health care settings (Kaakinen & Birenbaum, 2012).

Understanding family structure enables nurses assisting families to identify effective coping strategies for daily life disturbances, health care crises, wellness promotion, and disease prevention (Denham, 2005). In addition, nurses are central in advocating and developing social policies relevant to family health care needs. For example, taking political action to increase the availability of appropriate care for children could reduce the financial and emotional burden of many working and single-parent families when faced with providing care for sick children. Similarly, caregiving responsibilities and health care costs for acutely and chronically ill family members place increasing demands on family members. Nurses well informed about different family structures can

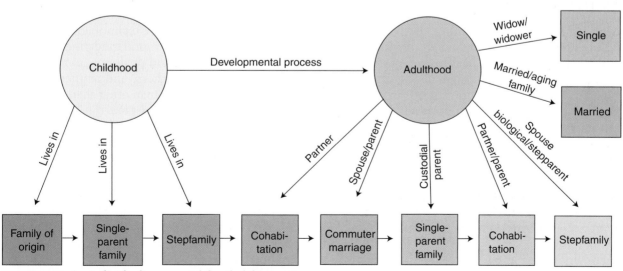

FIGURE 1-10 An individual's potential family life experiences.

identify specific needs of unique families, provide appropriate clinical care to enhance family resilience, and act as change agents to enact social policies that reduce family burdens.

Family Functions

A functional perspective has to do with the ways families serve their members. One way to describe the functional aspect of family is to see the unit as made up of intimate, interactive, and interdependent persons who share some values, goals, resources, responsibilities, decisions, and commitment over time (Steinmetz, Clavan, & Stein, 1990). Family function relates to the larger purposes or roles of families in society at large. It is important to be clear that there is a distinction between the concepts of family function (the prescribed social and cultural obligations and roles of family in society) and family functioning (the processes of family life). Family functioning has been described as "the individual and cooperative processes used by developing persons as to dynamically engage one another and their diverse environments over the life course" (Denham, 2003a, p. 277). Family function includes the ways a family reproduces offspring, interacts to socialize its young, cooperates to meet economic needs, and relates to the larger society. Nurses should ask about specific characteristics that factor into achieving family or societal goals, or both. Families' functional processes such as socialization, reproduction, economics, and health care provision are areas nurses can readily assess and address during health care encounters. Nursing interventions can enhance the family's protective health function when teaching and counseling is tailored to explicit learning needs. Family cultural context and individual health literacy needs are closely related to functional needs of families. Nurses become therapeutic agents as they assist families to identify social supports and locate community resources during times of family transitions and health crisis. Five specific family functions are worth deeper investigation here: reproductive, socialization, affective, economic, and health care.

Reproductive Functions of the Family

The survival of a society is linked to patterns of reproduction. Sexuality serves the purposes of pleasure and reproduction, but associated values differ from one society to another. Traditionally, the family has been organized around the biological function of reproduction. Reproduction was viewed as a major concern for thousands of years when populating the earth was continually threatened by famine, disease, war, and other life uncertainties. Norms about sexual intercourse affect the fertility rate. Fertility rate is "the average number of children that would be born per woman if all women lived to the end of their childbearing years and bore children according to a given fertility rate at each age" (World Factbook, 2013). In general, global fertility rates are in decline, with the most pronounced decline being in industrialized countries, especially Western Europe (World Factbook, 2013). Global concerns about overpopulation and environmental threats, as well as personal views of morality and financial well-being, have been reasons for limiting numbers of family births.

Since the 1980s, the reproductive function has become increasingly separated from the family (Kaakinen et al., 2010). As mores and norms change over time, it is not deemed "unacceptable" in many industrialized countries for birth to occur outside of marriage. Abstinence, various forms of contraception, tubal ligation, vasectomy, family planning, artificial insemination, and abortion have various degrees of social acceptance as means to control reproduction. Many aspects of reproduction continue to be the subject of social and ethical controversy. Nurses working with families find themselves at the forefront of practical issues related to providing care in this complex context.

The ethical dilemmas surrounding abortion, for example, seem compounded by technological advances that affect reproduction and problems of infertility. Reproductive technologies are guided by few legal, ethical, or moral guidelines. Artificial insemination by husband or donor, in vitro fertilization, surrogate mothers, and artificial embryonization, in which a woman other than the woman who will give birth to and raise the child donates an egg for fertilization, create financial and moral dilemmas. Although assistive reproductive technologies can provide a biological link to the child, some families are choosing to adopt children. Many are wrangling over the issues implicit in cross-racial and cross-cultural adoptions. Reproductive technologies and adoption are being considered by all family types to add children to the family unit. Religious, legal, moral, economic, and technological challenges will continue to cause debates in the years ahead about family control over reproduction, such as gender selection of child.

Socialization Functions of the Family

A major function for families is to raise and socialize their children to fit into society. Families have great variability in the ways they address the physical and emotional needs, moral values, and economic needs of children, and these patterns are influenced specifically by the role of parenting and somewhat by the larger society (Grusec, 2011). Children are born into families without knowledge of the values, language, norms, morals, communication, or roles of the society in which they live. A major function of the family continues to be to socialize them about family life and ground them in the societal identity of which they are a part. The function of the family relative to socialization includes protection, mutual reciprocity or interdependence between family members, control, guided learning, and group participation, and all these functions are assumed to be operative in all cultures (Grusec, 2011).

Although the family is not the only institution of society that participates in socialization of children, it is generally viewed as having primary responsibility for this function. When children fail to meet societal standards, it is common to blame this on family deficits and parental inadequacies; however, it is important to keep in mind that the issues are more complex than simple finger pointing.

Today, patterns of socialization require appropriate developmental care that fosters dependence and leads to independence (Denham, 2005). Socialization is the primary way children acquire the social and psychological skills needed to take their place in the adult world. Parents combine social support and social control as they equip children to meet future life tasks. Parental figures interact in multiple roles such as friends, lovers, child care providers, housekeepers, financial providers, recreation specialists, and counselors. Children growing up within families learn the values and norms of their parents and extended families.

Another role of families in the socialization process is to guide children through various rites of passage. Rites of passage are ceremonies that announce a change in status in the ways members are viewed. Examples include events such as a baptism, communion, circumcision, puberty ritual, graduation, wedding, and death. These occasions signal to others changes in role relationships and new expectations. Understandings about families' unique rites of passage can assist nurses working with diverse health care needs.

Affective Functions of the Family

Affective function has to do with the ways family members relate to one another and those outside the immediate family boundaries. Healthy families are able to maintain a consistent level of involvement with one another, yet at the same time, not become too involved in each other's lives (Peterson & Green, 2009). The healthiest families have empathetic interaction where family members care deeply about each other's feeling and activities, and are emotionally invested in each other. Families with a strong affective function are the most effective type of families (Peterson & Green, 2009). All families have boundaries that help to buffer stresses and pressure of systems outside the family on its members. Healthy families protect their boundaries, but at the same time, give members room to negotiate their independence. Achieving this balance is often difficult in our fast-paced culture. And it is particularly difficult in families with adolescents (Peterson & Green, 2009). Emotional involvement is a key to successful family functioning. Researchers have identified several characteristics of strong families. Among these are expressions of appreciation, spending time together, strong commitment to the family, good communication, and positive conflict resolution (Peterson & Green, 2009). When family members feel that they are supported and encouraged and that their personal interests are valued, family interaction becomes more effective.

Families provide a sense of belonging and identity to their members. This identity often proves to be vitally important throughout the entire life cycle. Within the confines of families, members learn dependent roles that later serve to launch them into independent ones. Families serve as a place to learn about intimate relationships and establish the foundation for future personal interactions. Families provide the initial experience of self-awareness, which includes a sense of knowing one's own gender, ethnicity, race, religion, and personal characteristics. Families help members become acquainted with who they are and experience themselves in relationships with others. Families provide the substance for self-identity, as well as a foundation for other-identity. Within the confines of families, individual members learn about love, care, nurturance, dependence, and support of the dying.

Resilience implies an ability to rebound from stress and crisis, the capacity to be optimistic, solve problems, be resourceful, and develop caring support systems. Although unique traits alter potential for emotional and psychological health, individuals exposed to resilient family environments tend to have greater potential to achieve normative developmental patterns and positive sibling and parental relationships (Denham, 2005).

Research on parent-child interactions needs to consider the quantity and quality of time spent together, the kinds of activities engaged in, and patterns of interaction to understand member feelings toward each other. More needs to be known about relationships with nonresidential parents as well as families characterized by polyamory, families in which there is more than one loving sexual relationship at the same time with the consent and knowledge of all partners (Pallotta-Chiarolli, 2006). Variables such as the quality of couples' relationships, the ways families' conflicts are handled, whether abuse or violence has previously occurred in the households or members' lives, frequency of children's contact with nonresidential parents, shared custody arrangements, and emotional relationships between parents and children appear to be important predictors of family affective functions.

Affective functions can best be understood by gathering information from all of the various members involved within a household; lack of access to all points of view within families should not prevent nurses from gaining knowledge from those to whom they have access. It is quite reasonable to inquire about the perceptions and experiences of some individuals through key family informants, but nurses must always remember that more certain knowledge should come from the specific individuals themselves, particularly as family members are known to have diverse viewpoints on issues that affect health and family life. Shared or discrepant views among family members have an important influence on the overall functioning of families' management of illness (Knafl, Breitmayer, Gallo, & Zoeller, 1996 Knafl, Deatrick, & Gallo, 2008).

Economic Functions of the Family

Families have an important function in keeping both local and national economies viable. Economic conditions significantly affect families. When economies become turbulent so become families' structures, functions, and processes. People make decisions about when to enter the labor force, when to marry, when to have children, and when to retire or come out of retirement based on economic factors (Bianchi, Casper, & King, 2005). For a detailed discussion on family and economics, see Chapter 2.

Family income provides a substantial part of family economics, but an equally important aspect has to do with economic interactions and consumerism related to household consumption and finance. Money management, housing decisions, consumer spending, insurance choices, retirement planning, and savings are some of the issues that affect family capacity to care for the economic needs of its members (Lamanna & Reidmann, 2011. These values and skills are passed down to children within the family structure. Financial vulnerability and bankruptcy have increased for middle-class families (Denham, 2005). The ability of the family to earn a sufficient income and to manage its finances wisely is a critical factor related to economic well-being.

In order to meet their own economic needs and maintain family life and health, family members take upon themselves a number of contributory roles for obtaining and utilizing the wages. Family nurses should explore the types of resources available or lacking as families engage in providing health care functions to their members.

Health Care Functions of the Family

Family members often serve as the primary health care providers to their families. Individuals regularly seek services from a variety of health care professionals, but it is within the family that health instructions are followed or ignored. Family members tend to be the primary caregivers and sources of support for individuals during health and illness. Families influence well-being, prevention, illness care, maintenance care associated with chronic illness, and rehabilitative care. Family members often care for one another's health conditions from the cradle to the grave. Families can become particularly vulnerable when they encounter health threats, and family-focused nurses are in a position where they can provide education, counseling, and assistance with locating resources. Family-focused care implies that when a single individual is the target of care, the entire family is still viewed as the unit of care (Denham, 2003a).

Health care functions of the family include many aspects of family life. Family members have different ideas about health and illness, and often these ideas are not discussed within families until problems arise. Availability and cost of health care insurance is a concern for many families, but many families lack clarity about what is and is not covered until they encounter a problem. Lifestyle behaviors, such as healthy diet, regular exercise, and alcohol and tobacco use, are areas that family members may not associate with health and illness outcomes. Risk reduction, health maintenance, rehabilitation, and caregiving are areas where families often need information and assistance. Family members spend far more time taking care of health issues of family members than professionals do.

Family Processes

Family process is the ongoing interaction between family members through which they accomplish their instrumental and expressive tasks (Denham, 2005). Family process indicators describe the interactions between members of a family, including their relationships, communication patterns, time spent together, and satisfaction with family life (World Family Map, 2013). In part, family process makes every family unique within its own particular culture. Families with similar structures and functions may interact differently. Family process, at least in the short term, appears to have a greater effect on the family's health status than family structure and function, and in turn, processes within families are more affected by alterations in health status. Family process certainly appears to have the greatest implications for nursing actions. For example, for the chronically ill, an important determinant for successful rehabilitation is the ability to assume one's familial roles. For rehabilitation to occur, family members have to communicate effectively, make decisions about atypical situations, and use a variety of coping strategies. The usual familial power structure may be threatened or need to change to address unique individual needs. Ultimately, the success or failure of the adaptation processes will affect individual and family well-being.

Alterations in family processes most likely occur when the family faces a transition brought about by developmental changes, adding or subtracting family members, an illness or accident, or other potential crisis situations, such as natural disasters, wars, or personal crises. The family's current modes of operation may become ineffective, and members are confronted with learning new ways of coping with change. For example, when coping with the stress of a chronic illness, families experience alterations in role performance and in power. When individuals are unable to perform usual roles, other members are expected to assume them. A shift in family roles may result in the loss of individual power. During times of change, family nurses can assist family members to communicate, make decisions, identify ways to cope with multiple stressors, reduce role strain, and locate needed resources.

Family communication patterns, member interactions, and interaction with social networks are several areas related to family processes that nurses need to assess systematically. Nursing interventions that promote resiliency in family processes vary with the degree of strain faced by the family. Families have complex needs related to adaptation, goal attainment, integration, pattern, and tension management. When family processes are ineffective or disrupted, the families and their members may be at risk for problems pertinent to health outcomes, and the family itself could be in danger of disintegrating.

Following is a discussion of a few family processes that nurses can influence through their relationships with families in caregiving situations. The family processes covered here include family coping, family roles, family communication, family decision making, and family rituals and routines.

Family Coping

Every family has its own repertoire of coping strategies, which may or may not be adequate in times of stress, such as when a family member experiences an altered health event such as the diagnosis of diabetes, a stroke, or a fractured leg in a biking accident. Coping consists of "constantly changing cognitive and behavioral efforts to manage specific external and/or internal demands that are appraised as taxing or exceeding the resources of the person" (Lazarus & Folkman, 1984, p. 141). Families with support can withstand and rebound from difficult stressors or crises (Walsh, 2011b), which is referred to as *family resilience*. "Family resilience is the successful coping of family members under adversity that enables them to flourish with warmth, support, and cohesion" (Black & Lobo, 2008, p. 33).

Not all families have the same ability to cope because of multiple reasons. There is no universal list of key effective factors that contribute to family resiliency, but a review of research and literature by Black and Lobo (2008) found the following similarities across studies for those families that cope well: a positive outlook, spirituality, family member accord, flexibility, communication, financial management, time together, mutual recreational interests, routines and rituals, and social support (Black & Lobo, 2008). According to Walsh (2011b) some key processes in family resiliency include belief system, organizational patterns, and family communication. The family's belief system involves making meaning of adversity, maintaining a positive outlook, and being able to transcend adversity through a spiritual/faith system (Walsh, 2011b). The families' organization patterns, which speak to their flexibility, connectedness, and social and economic resources, help the family maintain resilience. Finally, families who communicate with clarity, allow open emotional expression, and have a collaborative problem-solving approach facilitate family resiliency (Walsh, 2011b).

Nurses have the ability to support families in times of stress and crisis through empowering processes that work well and are familiar to the family. Using a strengths-based approach, family nurses help families to adjust and adapt to stressors (Black & Lobo, 2008; Walsh, 2011c). Nurses can help families in establishing priorities and responding to everyday needs when a health event occurs that threatens family stability. For example, when an unexpected death in the family occurs, family members are called on to make multiple decisions. At the same time, they may not be able to remember phone numbers, think of whom to call in what order, decide who should pick up the kids, determine which funeral home to use, or decide how or what to tell children or aging parents. Helping families to work through steps and set priorities during this situation is an important aspect of family nursing.

Even families who function at optimal levels may experience difficulties when stressful events pile up. Even families that cope well may still feel stressed (Black & Lobo, 2008). Today's families encounter many challenges that leave them vulnerable to a myriad of stressors. Vulnerability can result from poverty, illness, abuse, and violence. Coping capacities are enhanced whenever families demonstrate resilience or the capacity to survive in the midst of struggle, adversity, and long-term conflict. Families who recover from crisis tend to be more cohesive, value unique member attributes, support one another without criticism, and focus on strengths (Black & Lobo, 2008).

Family Roles

Understanding family roles is crucial in family nursing as it is one area in which nurses can help families to adapt, negotiate, give up expectations, or find additional resources to help decrease family stress during times when a family member is ill. Within the family, regardless of structure, each family position has a number of attached roles, and each role is accompanied by expectations. After a review of the family literature, Nye (1976) identified eight roles associated with the position of spouse/partner:

- Provider
- Housekeeper
- Child care
- Socialization
- Sexual
- Therapeutic
- Recreational
- Kinship

With the rates of divorce and cohabitation in North America, traditional roles such as provider and child care role are stressed and unfold differently. In addition, other roles are added relative to relationship, such as father who lives apart from children, stepparent, and/or half-sibling.

Traditionally, the provider role has been assigned to husbands, whereas wives assumed the housekeeper, child care, and other caregiving roles. With societal changes and variations in family structure, however, the traditional enactment of these roles is not viable for some families anymore (Gaunt, 2013). In two-parent heterosexual families, the roles are still primarily organized by gender, with men as breadwinners and women as primary caregivers (Scott & Braun, 2009). Other family roles form based on generation or location in the family (Haddock, Zimmerman, & Lyness, 2005), such as, for example, middle child, mother, father, stepsister, niece, and grandfather. Attitudes have changed somewhat in regard to rigid gender role enactment (who does what), but the research shows that, in reality, little change has occurred, and most families remain gender based (Haddock et al., 2005; Scott & Braun, 2009).

What has changed relative to family roles is the number of mothers who work outside of the home and the role of the father. The rate of mothers with infants under 1 year old working outside of the home is 55.8% (Bureau of Labor Statistics, 2011). Even though more women work outside of the home and men are participating and doing more in the home and with child care in the family than ever before, the responsibility for child care still remains largely with women (Kaakinen et al., 2010). The role of the father has changed, but the degree of change is unsure. A 2011 Pew Research Center report indicates that one in four children under the age of 18 years lives apart from their father (Livingston & Parker, 2011). Many fathers who live with their children are active in their day-to-day activities. Fathers who live apart from their children are often involved in e-mail and phone conversations and visitation in varying amounts of time. But 27% of the fathers who do not live with their children indicate that they have not been in communication with their children in the last year. In general, the Pew report found no consensus on whether or not today's fathers are more involved in the family life of their children than previous generations of fathers (Livingston & Parker, 2011).

In every household, members have to decide the ways work and responsibilities will be divided and shared. Roles are negotiated, assigned, delegated, or assumed. Division of labor within the family household occurs as various members assume roles, and as families change over time and over the family life cycle. For example, family members need to reconfigure role allocation after the birth or death of family members.

Provider role: The provider role has undergone significant change in the past few decades. Whereas American men were once viewed as the sole primary family breadwinner, this has changed significantly. In today's world, many families need more than one income to meet basic needs. Work conditions have become increasingly stressful for men and women, and external work obligations impinge on members' abilities to meet familial role obligations. For example, working mothers in Canada were found to rely on processed and fast convenience foods in the majority of meal preparations, thus increasing the risk of poor health outcomes for the family members, such as obesity (Slater, Sevenhuysen, Edginton, & O'Neil, 2012).

Housekeeper and child care roles: Today, many women experience significant role strain in balancing provider and other familial roles. Women who work continue to be responsible for most housekeeping and child care responsibilities (Haddock et al., 2005). Women who work outside the home still perform 80% of the child care and household duties (Walsh, 2011a). In a survey by Hewlett and Luce (2006), 77% of women and 66% of men who worked over 60 hours a week said they were unable to maintain their household, 66% of the sample reported they did not get sufficient sleep, and half reported not getting enough exercise. Although husbands' roles in child care are increasing, their focus is often on playing with the children rather than meeting basic needs. Women still are primary in meeting health care needs of all family members, including children and men.

Sick role: Individuals learn health and illness behaviors in their family of origin. Health behaviors are related to the primary prevention of disease, and include health promotion activities to reduce susceptibility to disease and actions to reduce the effects of chronic disease. Kasl and Cobb (1966) identified three types of health behaviors in families:

- Health behavior is any activity undertaken by a person believing himself to be healthy for the purpose of preventing disease or detecting it at an asymptomatic stage.
- Illness behavior is any activity, undertaken by a person who feels ill, to define the state of his health and to discover a suitable remedy.
- Sick-role behavior is any activity undertaken for the purpose of getting well, by those who consider themselves ill.

Once a family member becomes ill, she demonstrates various illness behaviors or enacts the "sick role." Parsons (1951) defines four characteristics of a person who is sick:

- While sick, the person is temporarily exempt from carrying out normal social and family roles. The more severe the illness, the freer one is from role obligations.
- In general, the sick person is not held responsible for being ill.

- The sick person is expected to take actions to get well, and therefore has an obligation to "get well."
- The sick person is expected to seek competent professional medical care and to comply with medical advice on how to "get well."

Voluminous research has been conducted on the theoretical concepts of the sick role. Some criticisms of the Parsons perspective the sick role are as follows: (1) some individuals reject the sick role; (2) some individuals are blamed for their illness, such as alcoholics or individuals with AIDS; and (3) sometimes independence is encouraged in persons who have a chronic illness as a way to "get well."

Regardless of the theoretical debates about the sick role, individuals in families experience acute and chronic illness. Each family, depending on its family processes, defines the sick role differently. Most "sick" people require some level of care; someone needs to assume the family caregiver role. The caregiving role may be as simple as a stop at the store on the way home to buy chicken soup or pick up medicines, or as involved as providing around-the-clock care for someone. The female individuals in our society still provide the majority of the care required when family members become sick or injured.

Role strain, conflict, and overload: Family roles are affected, some more than others, when a family member becomes ill. Usually the women in the family add the role of family caregiver to their other roles. Nurses have a crucial role in helping families adjust to illness by discussing and exploring role strain, role conflict, and role overload. Nurses can facilitate family adaptation by helping to problem-solve role negotiations and helping families access outside resources.

Lack of competence in role performance may be a result of role strain. Some researchers have found that sources of role strain are cultural and interactional. Interactional sources of role strain are related to difficulties in the delineation and enactment of familial roles. Heiss (1981) identifies five sources of difficulties in the interaction process that place strain on a family system:

- Inability to define the situation
- Lack of role knowledge
- Lack of role consensus
- Role conflict
- Role overload

The inability to define the situation creates ambiguity about what one should do in a given scenario. Continual changes in family structures and gender roles means that members increasingly encounter situations in which guidelines for action are unclear. Single parents, stepparents, nonresident fathers, and cohabiting partners deal daily with situations for which there are no norms. What right does a stepparent have to discipline the new spouse's child? Is a nonresident father expected to teach his child about AIDS? What name or names go on the mailbox of cohabiting partners? Who can sign for consent when divorced parents share custody?

Regardless of whether the issues are substantive, they present daily challenges to the people involved. Some choose to withdraw from the situation, and others choose to redefine the situation when they are uncertain how to act. For instance, a blended family might want to operate in the same way as a traditional family but may experience conflict when thinking about which members to include in family decision making. When a solution cannot be found, family members suffer the consequences of role strain.

Role strain sometimes results when family members lack role knowledge, or they have no basis for choosing between several roles that might seem appropriate. In America, most people are not taught how to be parents, and much learning is observational and experiential. Socialization related to caregiving of a chronically ill family member seldom occurs, and many individuals are unfamiliar with and unprepared to assume the roles necessary for providing care. When an individual is learning how to be a parent or a caregiver, role training may be required. Knowledge may be acquired by peer observation, trial and error, or explicit instruction. Parents may have limited opportunities to observe peers, and other family members may not have the knowledge necessary to help. Thus, the family may need to seek external resources or obtain needed information using other means such as child care classes, self-help groups, or instruction from health professionals. When individuals are unable to figure out their roles in a situation, it limits their problem-solving abilities.

Family members may lack role consensus, or be unable to agree about the expectations attached to a role. One family role that is often the source of family disagreement is the housekeeping role, especially for dual-career couples. Men who have been socialized into more traditional male roles are less inclined to accept responsibility for household tasks readily and may limit the amount of time they are willing to spend on these activities. When active participation does not meet the wife's expectations, she tends to assume responsibility for the greater number of household tasks. If she has been socialized into thinking that women are accountable for traditional housekeeping roles, she may feel guilty or neglectful if she asks for help. Lack of agreement about the role sometimes results in familial discord and impedes satisfaction with the partner. Negotiation is likely the most effective way to reach consensus about things that can be done.

Role conflict occurs when expectations about familial roles are incompatible. For example, the therapeutic role might involve becoming a caregiver to an elderly parent, but expectations of this new role may be incompatible with that of provider, housekeeper, sexual partner, and child care provider. Does one go to the child's baseball game or to the doctor with the elderly parent? Role conflict may occur when roles present conflicting demands. Individuals and families often have to set priorities. Demands of caregiver and provider roles may be conflicting and may conflict with other therapeutic familial tasks. The caregiver may withdraw from activities that, in the short term, seem superfluous, but in the long term are sources of much-needed energy. Family nurses are likely to encounter members facing many strains because of role conflict, and may need to assist by providing information and suggesting ways the family could negotiate roles to discover meaningful solutions.

A source of role strain closely related to role conflict is role overload. In role overload, the individual lacks resources, time, and energy to meet role demands. As with role conflict, the first option usually considered is to withdraw from one of the roles. Maintaining a balance between energy-enhancing and energy-depleting roles reduces role strain. An alternative to withdrawing from a role might be to seek time away from some role responsibilities. For example, a friend of the family member could relieve the primary caregiver for several hours. Nurses could arrange for a home-health aide to assist with personal care hygiene.

The dependent family member can be temporarily cared for in a residential facility while the other family members go on a vacation, which is called respite care.

It is the role of the nurse to help families who experience role strain, conflict, and overload. Using anticipatory guidance, nurses work closely with families to discuss and define the family flow of energy and resources when confronted with a family caregiving situation. See Chapter 4 for ways to work with families who experience stress related to caregiving and caregiving roles.

Family Communication

Communication is an ongoing, complex, changing activity and is the means through which people create, share, and regulate meaning in a transactional process to make sense of their world (Dance, 1967). In all families, communication is continuous in that it defines their present reality and constructs family relationships (Dance, 1967). It is through communication that families find ways to adapt to changes as they seek family stability. Families that are highly adaptive change more easily in response to demands. Families with low adaptability have a fixed or more rigid style of interacting (Olson & Gorall, 2005). "Family adaptability is manifested in how assertive family members are with each other, the amount of control in the family, family discipline practices, negotiation, how rigid family roles are adhered to, and the nature and enforcement of rules in the family" (Segrin & Flora, 2011, p. 17).

Family communication affects family physical and mental health. Most programs and intervention strategies for improving family communication are beyond the role and experience of nurses with undergraduate education. The role of the nurse is to facilitate family communication at times when families are stressed by changes that occur with its members, such as birth of an infant, growth and development issues of children, when family members become ill, or the death of family members. It is the role of the nurse to assist family communication to achieve healthful outcomes.

Family Decision Making

Communication and power are family processes that influence decision making. Family decision making is not an individual effort but a joint one. Most health care decisions should be made from a family perspective. Each decision has at least five features: the person raising the issue, what is being said about the issue, supporting action to what is being said, the importance of what is being said, and the responses of the individuals (Friedman, Bowden, & Jones, 2003).

Decision making provides opportunity for various family members to make a contribution to the process, support one another, and jointly set and strive to achieve goals. Disagreements within a family are natural, because members often have different points of view. It is important for members to share their various viewpoints with one another. Problem solving is part of the decision-making process, and frequently means that differences in opinion and emotions need consideration.

Family communication processes influence decision-making outcomes. In the Pew Research Center (2006) report on family communication, 46% of the 3,014 subjects indicated that they turned to their families for help and advice when they had problems. Keep in mind that in family conflicts, the expression of anger is not necessarily destructive, but contempt, belligerence, and defensiveness are counterproductive (Gottman, Coan, Carrere, & Swanson, 1998). Nurses working with families can facilitate family communication skills to help families find an effective way for resolving differences and making decisions.

Families want to be involved in varying degrees with health care decisions. Families are often asked to help make end-of-life decisions, not to resuscitate a loved one or to withdraw/withhold life-sustaining therapies. See Chapter 4 for information on shared decision making.

Family Rituals and Routines

Family rituals and routines have been studied for decades, beginning with Bossard and Boll (1950). Rituals are associated with formal celebrations, traditions, and religious observances with symbolic meaning, such as bar mitzvahs, weddings, funerals. Routines are patterned behaviors or interactions that closely link to daily or regular activities, such as bedtime procedure, mealtimes, greetings, and treatment of guests (Buchbinder, Longhofer, & McCue, 2009). Families have unique rituals and routines that provide organization and give meaning to family life. When family rituals and routines are disrupted by illness, the family system as a whole is affected; therefore, it can affect the health

of each family member and the family as a whole (Buchbinder et al., 2009). The importance and value of rituals in everyday life has been clearly explored in anthropological and sociological literature, but the significance of rituals is largely ignored by nurses (Denham, 2003b).

Assessing rituals and routines related to specific health or illness needs provides a basis to envision distinct family interventions and to devise specific plans for health promotion and disease management, especially when adherence to medical regimens is critical or caregiving demands are burdensome to the families (Fiese, 2007). For example, when a family member develops type 2 diabetes, the whole family may adapt its cooking, eating, and shopping habits to accommodate the needs of this family member (Denham, Manoogian, & Schuster, 2007). It enhances compliance with chronic illness treatment when the family incorporates illness regimens into the basic family tasks and practices (Buchbinder et al., 2009).

SUMMARY

This chapter provides an introduction and broad overview to family health care nursing. The following major concepts were discussed in this chapter:

- Family health care nursing is an art and a science that has evolved as a way of thinking about and working with families.
- Family nursing is a scientific discipline based in theory.
- Health and illness are family events.
- The term *family* is defined in many ways, but the most salient definition is, *The family is who the members say it is.*
- An individual's health (on the wellness-to-illness continuum) affects the entire family's functioning, and in turn, the family's ability to function affects each individual member's health.
- Family health care nursing knowledge and skills are important for nurses who practice in generalized and in specialized settings.
- The structure, function, and processes of families have changed, but the family as a unit of analysis and service continues to survive over time.
- Nurses should intervene in ways that promote health and wellness, as well as prevent

illness risks, treat disease conditions, and manage rehabilitative care needs.

■ Knowledge about each family's structure, function, and process informs the nurse in how to optimize nursing care in families and provide individualized nursing care, tailored to the uniqueness of every family system.

REFERENCES

American Nurses Association. (2010a). *Nursing's social policy statement* (2nd ed.). Washington, DC: American Nurses Association.

American Nurses Association. (2010b). *Nursing: Scope and standards of practice.* Washington, DC: American Nurses Association.

Anderson, K. H., & Tomlinson, P. S. (1992). The family health system as an emerging paradigmatic view for nursing. *Image: Journal of Nursing Scholarship, 24,* 57–63.

Benner, P. (2001). *Novice to expert: Excellence and power in clinical nursing practice.* Menlo Park, CA: Prentice Hall.

Bianchi, S. M., Casper, L. M., & King, R. B. (2005). *Work, family, health, and well-being.* Mahwah, NJ: Lawrence Erlbaum Associates.

Black, K., & Lobo, M. (2008). A conceptual review of family resiliency factors. *Journal of Family Nursing, 14,* 33–55.

Bomar, P. J. (Ed.). (2004). *Promoting health in families: Applying family research and theory to nursing practice* (3rd ed.). Philadelphia, PA: Saunders/Elsevier.

Bossard, J., & Boll, E. (1950). *Ritual in family living.* Philadelphia, PA: University of Pennsylvania Press.

Buchbinder, M., Longhofer, J., & McCue, K. (2009). Family routines and rituals when a parent has cancer. *Families, systems and Health, 27*(3), 213-227.

Bureau of Labor Statistics. (2011). Employment characteristics of families. Retrieved from http://www.bls.gov/news.release/famee.nr0.htm

Burgess, E. W., & Locke, H. J. (1953). *The family: From institution to companionship.* New York, NY: American Book Company.

Carrere, S., Buehlman, K. T., Coan, J., Gottman, J. M., & Ruckstuhl, L. (2000). Predicting marital stability and divorce in newlywed couples. *Journal of Family Psychology, 14*(1), 42–58.

Craft-Rosenberg, M., & Pehler, S. R. (Eds.). (2011). *Encyclopedia of family health.* Los Angeles, CA: Sage.

Curran, D. (1985). *Stress and the healthy family.* Minneapolis, MN: Winston Press (Harper & Row).

Dance, F. E. X. (1967). *Toward a theory of human communication.* In F. E. X. Dance (Ed.), Human communication theory (pp. 288–309). New York, NY: Holt.

Denham, S. A. (2003a). *Family health: A framework for nursing.* Philadelphia, PA: F. A. Davis.

Denham, S. A. (2003b). Relationships between family rituals, family routines, and health. *Journal of Family Nursing, 9*(30), 305–330.

Denham, S. A. (2005). Family structure, function and process. In S. M. H. Hanson, V. Gedaly-Duff, & J. R. Kaakinen (Eds.), *Family health care nursing: Theory, practice and research* (3rd ed., pp. 119–157). Philadelphia, PA: F. A. Davis.

Denham, S., Manoogian, M., & Schuster, L. (2007). Managing family support and dietary routines: Type 2 diabetes in rural Appalachian families. *Families, Systems, & Health, 25,* 36–52.

Driver, H., Tabares, A., Shapiro, A., Nahm, E. Y., & Gottman, J. M. (2011). Couple interaction in happy and unhappy marriages. In F. Walsh (Ed.), *Normal family processes: Growing diversity and complexity* (4th ed., pp. 57–77. New York, NY: Guilford Press.

Fiese, R. (2007). Routines and rituals: Opportunities for participation in family health [Supplemental material]. *OJRT Occupation, Participation and Health, 27,* 41S–49S.

Friedman, M. H., Bowden, V. R., & Jones, E. G. (2003). *Family nursing: Research, theory and practice* (5th ed.). Norwalk, CT: Appleton & Lange.

Gaunt, R. (2013). Breadwinning moms, caregiving dads: Double standard in social judgments of gender norm violators. *Journal of Family Issues, 34*(1), 3–24. Published online before print, April 4, 2012, doi:10.1177/0192513X12438686

Gilliss, C. L., Roberts, B. M., Highley, B. L., & Martinson, I. M. (1989). What is family nursing? In C. L. Gilliss, B. L. Highley, B. M. Roberts, & I. M. Martinson (Eds.), *Toward a science of family nursing* (pp. 64–73). Menlo Park, CA: Addison-Wesley.

Gottman, J. M., Coan, J., Carrere, S., & Swanson, C. (1998). Predicting marital happiness and stability from newlywed interactions. *Journal of Marriage and the Family, 60,* 5–22.

Grusec, J. (2011). Socialization processes in the family: Social and emotional development. *Annual Review of Psychology, 62,* 243-269.

Haddock, S. A., Zimmerman, T. S., & Lyness, K. P. (2005). Changing gender norms: Transitional dilemmas. In F. Walsh (Ed.), *Normal family processes: Growing diversity and complexity* (3rd ed., pp. 301–336). New York, NY: Guilford Press.

Ham, L. M., & Chamings, P. A. (1983). Family nursing: Historical perspectives. In I. Clements & F. B. Roberts (Eds.), *Family health care: Vol. 1. A theoretical approach to nursing care* (pp. 88–109). San Francisco, CA: McGraw-Hill.

Heiss, J. (1981). Family theory 20 years later. *Contemporary Sociology, 9*(2), 201-205.

Hewlett, S. A., & Luce, C. B. (2006). Extreme jobs: The dangerous allure of the 70-hour workweek. *Harvard Business Review, 12,* 49–59.

Kaakinen, J. R., & Birenbaum, L. K. (2012). Family development and family nursing assessment. In M. Stanhope & J. Lancaster (Eds.), *Public health nursing: Population centered health care in the community* (8th ed., pp. 599–623). St. Louis, MO: Mosby.

Kaakinen, J. R., & Hanson, S. M. H. (2008). Family development and family nursing assessment. In M. Stanhope & J. Lancaster (Eds.), *Public Health Nursing* (7th ed.). St. Louis, MO: Mosby.

Kaakinen, J. R., Hanson, S. M. H., & Denham, S. (2010). Family health care nursing: An introduction. In J. W. Kaakinen, V. Gedaly-Duff, D. P. Coehlo, & S. M. H. Hanson (Eds.), *Family health care nursing: Theory, practice and research* (4th ed., pp. 3–33). Philadelphia, PA: F. A. Davis.

Kasl, S. V., & Cobb, S. (1966) Health behavior, illness behavior and sick-role behavior. *Archives of Environmental Health, 12,* 531–541.

Knafl, K., Breitmayer, B., Gallo, A., & Zoeller, L. (1996). Family response to childhood chronic illness: Description of management styles. *Journal of Pediatric Nursing, 11,* 315-326.

Knafl, K., Deatrick, J.A., & Gallo, A. M. (2008). The interplay of concepts, data and methods in the development of the family management style framework. *Journal of Family Nursing, 14*(4), 412-428.

Krysan, M., Moore, K. A., & Zill, N. (1990). Identifying successful families: An overview of constructs and selected measures.

U.S. Department of Health and Human Services. Retrieved December 20, 2012, from http://aspe.hhs.gov/deltcp/reports/idsucfam.htm

Lamanna, M., & Reidmann, A. (2011). *Marriages, families, and relationships: Making choice in a diverse society.* Belmont, CA: Wadsworth Cengage Learning.

Lazarus, R. S., & Folkman, S. (1984). *Stress, appraisal, and coping.* New York, NY: Springer.

Livingston, G., & Parker, P. (2011). A tale of two fathers: More are active but more are absent. Pew Research Center: Social and Demographic Trends. Retrieved from http://www.pewsocialtrends.org/files/2011/06/fathers-FINAL-report.pdf

Nightingale, F. (1979). *Cassandra.* Westbury, NY: Feminist Press.

Nye, F. I. (1976). *Role structure and analysis of the family.* Beverly Hills, CA: Sage.

Olson, D. H., & Gorall, D. N. (2005). Circumplex model of marital and family systems. In F. Walsh (Ed.), *Normal family processes: Growing diversity and complexity* (3rd ed., pp. 514–548). New York, NY: Guilford Press.

Otto, H. (1963). Criteria for assessing family strengths. *Family Process, 2,* 329–338.

Pallotta-Chiarolli, M. (2006). Polyparents having children, raising children, schooling children. *Lesbian and Gay Psychology Review, 7*(1), 48–53.

Parsons, T. (1951). *The social system.* Glencoe, IL: Free Press.

Peterson, R., & Green S., (2009). Families first-keys to successful family functioning: Communication. Retrieved from http://pubs.ext.vt.edu/350/350-092/350-092.htmPew Research Center. (2006). Families drawn together by communication revolution: A social trends report. Retrieved April 24, 2009, from http://pewresearch.org/assets/social/pdf/FamilyBonds.pdf

Pratt, L. (1976). *Family structure and effective health behavior: The energized family.* Boston, MA: Houghton Mifflin.

Scott, J., & Braun, M. (2009). Changing public views of gender roles in seven nations: 1988–2002. In M. Haller, R. Jowell, & T. Smith (Eds.), *Charting the globe* (pp. 358–377). Oxford, England: Routledge.

Segrin, C., & Flora, J. (2011). *Family communication* (2nd ed.). New York: Routledge.

Slater, J., Sevenhuysen, B., Edginton, G., & O'Neil, J. (2012). "Trying to make it all come together": Structuration and employed mothers' experience of family food provisioning in Canada. *Health Promotion International, 27*(3), 405–415.

Steinmetz, S. K., Clavan, S., & Stein, K. F. (1990). *Marriage and family realities: Historical and contemporary perspectives.* New York, NY: Harper & Row.

Svavarsdottir, E.K. (2008). Excellence in nursing: A model for implementing family systems nursing in nursing practice at an institutional level in Iceland. *Journal of Family Nursing, 14*(4), 456-468.

U.S. Census Bureau. (2011). Frequently asked questions. Retrieved from http://www.census.gov/hhes/www/income/about/faqs.html

U.S. Department of Health and Human Services. (2009). *Healthy people 2020* (Vol. 1). Washington, DC: U.S. Government Printing Office. Retrieved December 18, 2012, from http://www.cdc.gov/nchs/healthy_people/hp2020.htm

Walsh, F. (2011a). The new normal: Diversity and complexity. In F. Walsh (Ed.), *Normal family processes: Growing diversity and complexity* (4th ed., pp. 3–27). New York, NY: Guilford Press.

Walsh, F. (2011b). Family resilience: Strengths forged through adversity. In F. Walsh (Ed.), *Normal family processes: Growing diversity and complexity* (4th ed., pp. 399–429). New York, NY: Guilford Press.

Walsh, F. (2011c). *Clinical views of family normality, health and dysfunction: From a deficits to a strengths perspective* (4th ed., pp. 28–56). New York, NY: Guilford Press.

Whall, A. L. (1993). The family as the unit of care in nursing: A historical review. In G. D. Wegner & R. J. Alexander (Eds.), *Readings in family nursing* (pp. 3–12). Philadelphia, PA: J. B. Lippincott.

World Factbook, (2013). Total fertility rates. Retrieved from https://www.cia.gov/library/publications/the-world-factbook/fields/2127.html

World Family Map. (2013). Family processes. Mapping family change and child well-being outcomes. An International Report from Child Trends. Retrieved from http://worldfamilymap.org/2013/wp-content/uploads/2013/01/WFM-2013-Final-lores-11513.pdf

World Health Organization. (2008). The determinants of health. Retrieved July 9, 2008, from http://www.who.int/hia/evidence/doh/en/index.html

Wright, L. M., & Leahey, M. (2013). *Nurses and families: A guide to family assessment and intervention* (6th ed.). Philadelphia, PA: F. A. Davis.

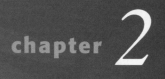
Family Demography
Continuity and Change in North American Families

Lynne M. Casper, PhD

Sandra M. Florian, MA, PhD Candidate

Peter D. Brandon, PhD

Critical Concepts

- Economic, social, and cultural changes have increased family diversity in North America. More families are maintained by single mothers, single fathers, cohabiting couples, and grandparents than in the past.

- Increases in women's labor force participation, especially among mothers, have reduced the amount of nonwork time that families have to attend to health care needs.

- North Americans are more likely to live alone than they were a few decades ago. Thus, people are less likely to have family members living with them who can assist them when they become ill or injured.

- The Great Recession has increased the likelihood that young adults will remain in or return to their parents' homes after graduating from school. Many of them cannot find a stable job that pays enough for them to live on their own. In the United States, many young adults do not have health insurance and, thus, do not seek health care regularly.

- More North Americans are immigrants than was the case a few decades ago. Family nurses provide care for an increasingly ethnically, culturally, and linguistically diverse population.

- Single-mother families are particularly vulnerable. They are more likely to live in poverty than are other families. These mothers are usually the sole wage earners and care providers in their families. Thus, these families are more likely than other families both to be monetarily poor and to face stringent time constraints.

- Single-father families have been increasing in recent decades and fathers are spending more time caring for their children. Nurses will be increasingly likely to encounter fathers who bring their children in for checkups or medical treatments.

- Cohabitation among opposite- and same-sex couples continues to rise in North America. In the United States, because cohabiting relationships are not legally sanctioned in many states and localities, partners may not have the right to make health care decisions on behalf of each other or for the other partner's children.

(continued)

33

■ Couples who are having trouble conceiving are increasingly turning to the medical profession for help. Births resulting from assisted reproductive technologies (ARTs) are on the rise in North America. The ART process is expensive, time consuming, and often increases health risks for the women and children involved.

■ Many children in North America are adopted. These children need time to adjust to their new circumstances and are more likely than other children to have special health care needs.

■ Stepfamilies are common among North American families. Legal arrangements in these families can be complicated; it is not always clear who has the right to make health care decisions for children in these families.

■ Many children are raised by or receive regular care from their grandparents. These grandparents may or may not have legal responsibility for their grandchildren, but may seek medical care for them.

■ The aging of the population, as well as the impending retirement of the baby-boom generation, presents significant challenges for both informal caregivers and the health care system. The need for nurses who specialize in caring for elderly persons will continue to increase.

If there is one "mantra" about family life in the last half century, it is that the family has undergone tremendous change. No other institution elicits as contentious debate as the North American family. Many argue that the movement away from marriage and traditional gender roles has seriously degraded family life. Others view family life as amazingly diverse, resilient, and adaptive to new circumstances (Cherlin, 2009; Popenoe, 1993; Stacey, 1993).

Any assessment of the general "health" of family life in North America, and the health and well-being of family members, especially children, requires a look at what is known about demographic and socioeconomic trends that affect families. A pragmatic approach to family nursing requires an understanding of the broader changes in family within the population. The latter half of the 20th century was characterized by tumultuous change in the economy, civil rights, and sexual freedom and by dramatic improvements in health and longevity. Marriage and family life felt the reverberations of these societal changes.

In the first decades of the 21st century, as North Americans reassess where they have come from and where they are going, one thing stands out—rhetoric about the dramatically changing family may be a step behind the reality. Recent trends suggest a quieting of changes in the family in Canada, as well as the United States, or at least of the pace of change. Little change occurred in the proportions of two-parent or single-parent families since the mid-1990s (U.S. Census Bureau, 2011d). After a significant increase in the proportion of children living with unmarried parents, the living arrangements of children

stabilized, as did the living arrangements of young adults and elderly persons. The divorce rate increased substantially in the mid-1960s and 1970s, reached its peak in 1980, slightly declined during the 1990s, and has remained relatively constant since then. In the United States, between 43% and 46% of marriages contracted today are expected to end in divorce (Schoen & Canudas-Romo, 2006). The rapid growth in cohabitation among unmarried adults has also slowed. In Canada, divorce rates also increased during the 1970s and 1980s, peaked slightly later in 1987, but have slightly declined since then. In 2008, 41% of marriages were expected to end in divorce within the first 30 years (Statistics Canada, 2012b).

Yet, family life is still evolving. Young adults have often postponed marriage and children to complete higher education before attempting to enter labor markets that have become inhospitable to poorly educated workers. Accompanying this delay in marriage was the continued increase in births to unmarried women. By 2010, 41% of all births in the United States were to unmarried women (Martin et al., 2012).

Within marriage or marriage-like relationships, the appropriate roles for each partner are shifting as North American societies accept and value more equal roles for men and women. The widening role of fathers has become a major agent of change in the family. More father-only families exist than in the past, and after divorce, fathers are more likely to share custody of children with the mother. Within two-parent families, fathers are also more likely to be involved in the children's care than in the past (Hernandez & Brandon, 2002). In addition, the number of same-sex couples has been increasing, and a larger proportion of them are now raising children. Family roles in same-sex couples are more likely to be negotiated than in opposite-sex families.

Whether the slowing, and in some cases, cessation, of change in family living arrangements is a temporary lull or part of a new, more sustained equilibrium will only be revealed in the next decades of the 21st century. New norms may be emerging about the desirability of marriage, the optimal timing of children, and the involvement of fathers in child rearing and mothers in breadwinning. Understanding the evolution of North American families and the implications these changes have for family nursing requires taking the pulse of contemporary family life.

This chapter examines changes and variations in North American families in order to understand what these changes portend for family health care nursing during the first half of this century. This chapter draws on information pertaining to family demography from a variety of data sources (Box 2-1). The reader should note that family nursing is not the major focus of this chapter. The subject matter of the chapter is structured to provide family nurses with background on changes in the North American family so that they can understand their patient populations. The chapter does briefly touch upon the implications of these demographic patterns for practicing family nursing.

Where possible, statistics have been reported for both the United States and Canada, but comparable data for Canada were not always readily accessible for the topics covered in this chapter. Readers should note that data are not always collected in the

---

BOX 2-1

Sources of Information on Demography and Public Health

Many of the statistics discussed in this chapter draw on information from the Current Population Surveys (CPS) collected by the U.S. Census Bureau. This is a continuous survey of about 60,000 households, selected at random to be representative of the national population. Each household is interviewed monthly for two 4-month periods. During February through April of each year, the CPS collects additional demographic and economic data, including data on health insurance coverage, from each household. This Annual Demographic Supplement is the most frequently used source of data on demographic and economic trends in the United States and is the data source for the majority of statistics presented in this chapter regarding changes in the family.

For estimates for small areas or subgroups of the population, demographers often used data from the "long form" of the decennial census, which collected data from one-sixth of all households. The census collects a range of economic and demographic information, including incomes and occupations, housing, disability status, and grandparent responsibility for children. The census cannot match the detail found in more specialized surveys. For example, only four short questions measure disability for children; surveys designed for precise and complete estimates of disabilities will usually have dozens of such questions. Since 2004, the American Community Survey replaced the sample data from the census and now provides a more continuous flow of estimates for states, cities, counties, and even towns and rural areas, for which estimates were made only once a decade.

Moreover, several large health-related surveys are conducted by the National Center for Health Statistics. The National Health Interview Survey (NHIS) is a large, continuous survey of about 43,000 households per year, covering the civilian, noninstitutionalized population of the United States. The NHIS is the major source of information on health status and disability, health-related behaviors, and health care utilization for all age groups. The National Health and Nutrition Examination Survey (NHANES) includes physical examinations, mental health questionnaires, dietary data, analyses of urine and blood, and immunization status from a random sample of Americans (about 10,000 in each 2-year cycle). NHANES also collects some basic demographic and income data. It is the major source of information on trends in obesity, cholesterol status, and a host of other conditions in the national population, and in particular age groups and racial/ethnic groups. The National Survey of Family Growth (NSFG) is the primary source of information on marriage and divorce trends, pregnancy, contraceptive use, and fertility behaviors, and the ways in which they vary among different groups and over time. Birth and death certificates, sent by hospitals and funeral homes to state offices of vital events registration, provide the raw material for calculating fertility and mortality rates and life expectancy. The data are collected from the states and analyzed by the National Center for Health Statistics.

In Canada, the National Population Health Survey has interviewed a panel of respondents every 2 years since 1994 to track changes in health-related behaviors, risk factors, and health outcomes.

same year and that some family indicators are defined and measured differently across the two countries.

A CHANGING ECONOMY AND SOCIETY

Consider the life of a North American young woman reaching adulthood in the 1950s or early 1960s. Such a woman was likely to marry straight out of high school or to take a clerical or retail sales job until she married. She would have moved out of her parents' home only after she married to form a new household with her husband. This young woman was likely to marry by about age 20 in the United States (U.S. Census Bureau, 2008), age 22 in Canada, and begin a family soon thereafter. If she were working when she became pregnant, she would probably have quit her job and stayed home to care for her children and husband while her husband had a steady job that paid enough to support the entire family. Thus, usually someone was at home who had the time to care for the health needs of family members, to schedule routine checkups with doctors and dentists, and to take family members to these appointments.

Fast-forward to the first decades of the 21st century. A young woman reaching adulthood in the first decades of the 21st century is not likely to marry before her 26th birthday. She will probably attend higher education and is likely to live by herself, with a boyfriend, or with roommates before marrying. She may move in and out of her parents' house several times before she gets married. Like her counterpart reaching adulthood in the 1950s, she is likely to marry and have at least one child, but the sequence of those events may well be reversed. She probably will not drop out of the labor force after she has children, although she may curtail the number of hours she is employed. She is much more likely to divorce, and possibly even to remarry, compared with a young woman in the 1950s or 1960s. Because she is more likely to be a single mother and to be working outside of the home, she is also not as likely to have the time necessary to devote to caring for the health of family members.

A dramatic change in women's participation in the labor market occurred after 1970, as mothers with young children began entering the labor force

in greater numbers. Historically, unmarried mothers (either never married or formerly married) of young children had higher labor force participation rates than married mothers. These women often were the only earners in their families. One notable change has been the increase in the combination of paid work and mothering among married mothers. In 1960, for example, in the United States, only 19% of married mothers with children younger than age 6 were in the labor force. By 2011, the proportion increased to 62% (U.S. Census Bureau, 2011e). In Canada, 28% of women with children under the age of 3 were employed in 1976 compared with 64% in 2009. Among mothers with children under the age of 16 living at home, the proportion is even higher at 73% (Statistics Canada, 2010). Another truly remarkable change has been the increase in the labor force participation of single mothers from 44% to 77% between 1980 and 2011 (U.S. Census Bureau, 2011j). In Canada, the proportion of single mothers who were employed in 1976 was 28% and increased to 69% in 2009 (Statistics Canada, 2010). What does this trend imply for family nursing? The majority of North American families with young children in the mid-20th century had mothers who were home full-time to care for the health needs of family members, whereas at the beginning of the 21st century such families were in the minority.

Changes in the Economy

Economic conditions have an influence on young people's decisions about when to enter the labor force, when to marry, and when to have children (and how many children to have). After World War II, the United States and Canada enjoyed an economic boom characterized by rapid economic growth, full employment, rising productivity, higher wages, low inflation, and increasing earnings. A man with a high-school education in the 1950s and 1960s could secure a job that paid enough to allow him to purchase a house, support a family on one income, and join the swelling ranks of the middle class.

The economic realities of the 1970s and 1980s were quite different. The two decades after the oil crisis, which began in 1973, were decades of economic change and uncertainty marked by a shift away from manufacturing and toward services, stagnating or declining wages (especially for less-educated workers), high inflation, and a slowdown in productivity growth. The 1990s were just as remarkable for the turnaround: sustained prosperity, low unemployment, and economic growth that seems to have reached many in the poorest segments of society (Farley, 1996; Levy, 1998). The Great Recession, which began in 2008, reversed this trend, and many men and women joined the ranks of the unemployed.

When the economy is on such a roller coaster, family life often takes a similar ride. Marriage occurred early and was nearly universal in the decades after World War II; mothers remained in the home to rear children as the baby-boom generation was born and nurtured. When baby boomers hit working age in the 1970s, the economy was not as hospitable as it had been for their parents. They postponed marriage, delayed having children, and found it difficult to establish themselves in the labor market.

Many of the baby boomers' own children began reaching working age in the 1990s and 2000s, when individuals' economic fortunes were increasingly dependent on their educational attainment. Those who attended higher education were much more likely to become self-sufficient and to live independently from their parents (Rosenfeld, 2007). High-school graduates who did not go to higher education discovered that jobs with high pay and benefits were in relatively short supply. In the United States, a high-school graduate in full-time work earned about 25% (allowing for inflation) less than a comparable new worker would have earned 20 years earlier (Farley, 1996). The increasing relative benefits of further education encouraged more young men and women to delay marriage and attend higher education.

Partly because of these changes in the economy, both men and women are remaining single longer and are more likely to leave home to pursue higher education, to live with a partner, and to launch a career before taking on the responsibility of a family of their own. The traditional gender-based organization of home life (in which mothers have primary responsibility for care of the home and children and fathers provide financial support) has not disappeared, but young women today can expect to be employed while raising children, and young men are more likely to share in some child-rearing and household tasks. Thus, in the first decades of this century,

men are more likely to play a role in looking after the health of family members than they were in previous decades.

Before World War II, most men worked nearly to the end of their lives. Retirement was a privilege for the wealthy or the fortunate workers whose companies provided pensions. Currently, with increases in life expectancy and healthier lives, the passage of the Social Security Acts in 1936 and 1938 in the United States, and the institution of provincial (in the 1920s) and federal (since 1952) pensions in Canada, most workers can look forward to at least a modest guaranteed income for themselves and their spouses and minor children. Social Security benefits constitute more than half of the household income for two-thirds of Americans older than 65. The increased availability of public pensions made possible a growing period of retirement for most workers, a steady decrease in poverty rates for older people, and an increase in the proportion of older people maintaining their own households separately from their adult children.

Changing Family Norms

In 1950, in North America, there was one dominant and socially acceptable way for adults to live their lives. Those who deviated could expect to be censured and stigmatized. The "ideal" family was composed of a homemaker-wife, a breadwinner-father, and two or more children. Americans shared a common image of what a family should look like and how mothers, fathers, and children should behave. These shared values reinforced the importance of the family and the institution of marriage (McLanahan & Casper, 1995). This vision of family life showed amazing staying power, even as its economic underpinnings were eroding. For this 1950s-style family to exist, North Americans had to support distinct gender roles, and the economy had to be vibrant enough for an average man to support a family financially on his own.

Government policies and business practices perpetuated this family type by reserving the best jobs for men and discriminating against working women when they married or had a baby. Beginning in the 1960s, though, women and people from minority backgrounds gained legal protections in the workplace and discriminatory practices began to recede.

A transformation in attitudes toward family behaviors also took place. People became more accepting of divorce, cohabitation, and sex outside marriage; less sure about the universality and permanence of marriage; and more tolerant of blurred gender roles and of mothers working outside the home (Bianchi, Raley, & Casper, 2012; Cherlin, 2009). Society became more open-minded about a variety of living arrangements, family configurations, and lifestyles.

Although the transformation of many of these attitudes occurred throughout the 20th century, the pace of change accelerated in the 1960s and 1970s. These years brought many political, social, and medical upheavals affecting gender issues and views of the family. The women's liberation movement included a highly publicized, although unsuccessful, attempt to pass the Equal Rights Amendment (ERA) to the Constitution of the United States. New and effective methods of contraception were introduced in the 1950s and 1960s. In 1973, the U.S. Supreme Court ruled that state laws banning abortion were unconstitutional. In Canada, abortion was illegal until 1969 when the law was changed to allow abortions for health reasons. Popular literature and music heralded the sexual revolution and an era of "free love." In all industrialized countries, a new ideology was emerging during these years that stressed personal freedom, self-fulfillment, and individual choice in living arrangements and family commitments (Bianchi et al., 2012; Cherlin, 2009). People began to expect more out of marriage and to leave marriages that failed to fulfill their expectations. Certainly not all Americans approved of all these changes in beliefs and behaviors. The general North American culture changed, though, as divorce and single parenting became more widespread realities.

An Aging Society

For Americans born in 1900, the average life expectancy was less than 50 years. But the early decades of the 20th century brought such tremendous advances in the control of communicable diseases of childhood that life expectancy at birth increased to 70 years by 1960. Rapid declines in mortality from heart disease—the leading cause of death—significantly lengthened life expectancy for those aged 65 or older after 1960 (Treas & Torrecilha, 1995). By 2009, life expectancy at birth

was nearly 79 years for Americans (National Center for Health Statistics, 2008) and 81 years for Canadians (World Health Organization, 2011). An American woman who reached age 60 in 2009 could expect to live an additional 25 years, on average, and a 60-year-old American man would live another 22 years. For Canadians, life expectancy at age 60 is even higher—26 years for women and 23 years for men. Women continue to outlive men in North America, though the gender gap in recent years has shrunk somewhat, primarily because of the delayed effects of smoking trends (men have always been more likely to smoke than women, but they have reduced smoking much more than women in recent decades). The gap in life expectancy between men and women means that women tend to outlive their husbands and women predominate in the older age groups. About 60% of the population 75 years and older in the United States and Canada are women (Statistics Canada, 2012d).

Partly because more North Americans are surviving until older ages, and partly because of a long-term decline in fertility rates, the proportion of the population aged 65 or older has grown. In 1900, only 1 of every 25 Americans was aged 65 or older (nearly 3% of the total population). By 2011, the proportion was more than 3 in 25 (13% of the total population). In 2011, the first of some 78 million baby boomers reached their 65th birthdays, and the rate of increase of the population of elderly persons began to accelerate. By 2030, it is expected that one in five Americans will be aged 65 or older. The scenario for Canada is similar, although Canada has a slightly higher proportion of the population aged 65 and older; in 2011, 14.8% of Canada's population was 65 years and older compared with 13.3% of U.S. residents (Statistics Canada, 2011a; U.S. Census Bureau, 2011d).

People do not suddenly become old on their 65th birthday, of course. Together with improvements in life expectancy have come improvements in the disability rates at older ages, so that North Americans are not only living longer than in the past but also enjoying more years of life without chronic illness or disabilities. In the United States, 65 is still a convenient marker for "old age" in health policy terms, because it is the age at which most Americans become eligible for medical and hospital insurance funded mainly by the federal government through Medicare. By 65, as well, most workers (both men and women) have left full-time work, though many continue to work part-time, or for part of the year, often at different jobs than those they pursued during most of their careers. Given the growing number of elderly persons, the Canadian government will raise the eligible age for Old Age Security (OAS) from 65 to 67 between 2023 and 2029 to ease pressures on the OAS budget and to ensure the program's sustainability (Service Canada, 2012).

The aging of the population is often considered a major cause of increasing demand for medical services and of the growth in medical expenditures. Population aging is, indeed, one factor, because older people in every country consume more medical care than younger adults. The major causes of increased health expenditures in industrialized countries, however, have been changes in medical technology, including increased use of pharmaceuticals, rather than the simple growth of the population of elderly persons (Reinhardt, 2003).

Increased life expectancy translates into extended years spent in family relationships. A couple who marry in their twenties could spend the next 50 years together, assuming they remain married. Couples in the past were much more likely to experience the death of one spouse earlier in their adult years. Longer lives (together with lower birth rates) also mean that people spend a smaller portion of their lives parenting young children. More parents live long enough to be part of their grandchildren's and even great-grandchildren's lives (Bengtson, 2001). Many adults are faced with the demands of caring for extremely elderly parents about the time they reach retirement age and begin to experience health limitations of older age themselves.

Immigration and Ethnic Diversity

In 1965, the U.S. Congress amended the Immigration and Naturalization Act to create a fundamental change in the nation's policy on immigration. Visas for legal immigrants were no longer to be based on quotas for each country of origin; instead, preference would be given to immigrants joining family members in the United States. The legislation also removed limitations on immigration from Latin America and Asia. The numbers of legal immigrants to the United States increased, to an average of 900,000 persons per year in the 1990s and to

1.1 million in 2011. Immigration has likewise increased in Canada from about 140,000 in 1980 to 249,000 in 2011. In 2011, 66% of legal immigrants were admitted to the United States because family members already living there petitioned the government to grant them entry (U.S. Department of Homeland Security, 2012). For Canada, the corresponding figure is 61% (Citizenship and Immigration Canada, 2011). Immigrant visas were also granted for economic reasons, usually after employers petitioned the government for admission of persons with special skills or for humanitarian reasons, including asylum granted to refugees because of well-founded fear of persecution in their home countries. In the United States and Canada, immigration laws provide refugees with resettlement assistance including temporary health care services. The goal of these programs is to promote and improve the health of refugees, as well as to control the potential spread of any contagious diseases brought into the country by these immigrants. The benefits of these health programs are restricted to the prevention and treatment of disease that poses a risk to the public health and safety (Citizenship and Immigration Canada, 2012; U.S. Centers for Disease Control and Prevention, 2010).

In addition to legal immigrants, an estimated 10.8 million illegal immigrants lived in the United States in 2010, either because they entered without detection or because they stayed longer than allowed by a temporary visa (Hoefer, Rytina, & Baker, 2011). In 2010, the U.S. Census Bureau estimated that there were 40 million U.S. residents born outside the country, nearly 13% of the total population (Grieco et al., 2012). Because immigrants tend to arrive in the United States early in their working careers, they are younger, on average, than the overall U.S. population and account for a larger share of young families. In 2010, for example, 20% of all births in the United States were to mothers born outside the country (U.S. Census Bureau, 2010e). Illegal immigrants are ineligible for any type of federal public benefits including welfare, Social Security, and health services such as Medicaid and Medicare (U.S. Department of Health and Human Services, 2009).

Estimates based on 2007 U.S. American Community Survey data reveal that 55 million people older than age 5 speak a language other than English at home, the most common being Spanish

(34.5 million) and Chinese (2.5 million). In the United States, half of adults 18 to 40 years old who speak Spanish at home reported that they could not speak English well (Shin & Kominski, 2010). Keep in mind, however, that the overwhelming majority of those who do not speak English well are recent immigrants. More than 96% of the native-born who speak Spanish at home report that they can speak English well (Saenz, 2004). In Canada, although English and French are still dominant, more than 200 languages are now spoken in the country. In 2011, 6.6 million people, representing nearly 20% of the Canadian population, reported speaking a language other than English or French at home. Of them, a third, or 2.1 million, reported speaking *only* a language other than English or French at home, primarily Asian languages. The 10 most common foreign languages spoken in 2011 in Canada were Punjabi, Chinese (not specified), Cantonese, Spanish, Tagalog, Arabic, Mandarin, Italian, Urdu, and German (Statistics Canada, 2012h).

The majority of foreign-born U.S. residents live in states that are the traditional "gateways" to immigrant populations: California, New York, Florida, Texas, and Illinois. In recent decades, however, significant increases have occurred in the immigrant populations of most parts of the country, including the rural South and the Upper Midwest, which had seen few immigrants for most of the 20th century (Singer, 2004).

Implications for Health Care Providers

The aging and the growing diversity of the American and Canadian populations, combined with shifts in the economy and changing norms, values, and laws, have altered the context for the nursing care of families. As the population ages, the demand will increase for nurses who specialize in caring for elderly persons, and even those who do not choose a geriatric specialty will find that older people constitute an increasing portion of the patient population. Improvements in health and physical functioning among those aged 60 to 70 reduce the need for care among this group. Yet rates of population growth are greatest for those aged 80 and older, implying an increased demand for care among the "oldest old" who are likely to suffer from poorer health and require substantial care. Because women continue to outlive men, on average, nurses are more likely to be dealing with the health care needs of older women than of men. Extended lives and delayed childbearing have increased the chances that adults will experience the double whammy of having to provide care and financial support for their children and their parents. Families in these situations can face considerable time and money pressures.

At the same time that changing gender roles point to more men in families taking on caregiving duties, more women are in the labor force and unavailable to care for family members, and it is doubtful that the increase in men's time in caregiving will fully compensate for the decrease in women's time. Individuals and families are increasingly turning to extended kin and informal care providers to meet their health needs. Societal changes also influence individuals' life-course trajectories. All these changes in individual lives and family relationships are transforming North American households and families and, in turn, changing the context in which health needs are defined and both formal and informal health care are provided. Nurses are more likely to encounter fathers seeking health care for their children, and individuals whose health needs are met by informal extended kin or untrained caretakers, especially among the fragile and older populations.

The growth of the immigrant population, and its spread throughout both the United States and Canada, has meant that patient populations in many regions are more racially and ethnically diverse than in the past. Working with a diverse pool of immigrant and refugee populations, health care providers may encounter health conditions and diseases unusual in North America. Nurses in North America work with families whose cultural backgrounds, perceptions of sickness, and expectations of healers may be different from those with which they are familiar. Everyone providing health care can expect to face both the challenges and the professional rewards of adapting to a diverse patient population.

LIVING ARRANGEMENTS

The demographic changes for individuals discussed earlier in this chapter are reflected in changes in living arrangements, which have become more diverse over time. For most statistical purposes, a family is defined as two or more people living together who are related by blood, marriage, or adoption (Casper & Bianchi, 2002). Most households (defined by the U.S. Census Bureau as one or more people who occupy a house, apartment, or other residential unit, as opposed to "group quarters" such as nursing homes or student dormitories) are maintained by families. Demographic trends, including late marriage, divorce, and single parenting, have resulted in a decrease in the "family share" of U.S. and Canadian households. In 1960, in the United States, 85% of households were family households; by 2012, just 66% were family households (U.S. Census Bureau, 2012). Married-couple family households with children under 18 constituted 44% of all households in 1960, but only 20% of all households in 2012 (authors' calculations from U.S. Census Bureau, 2012). Nonfamily households, which consist primarily of people who live alone or who share a residence with roommates or with a partner, have been on the rise. The fastest growth was among persons living alone, although much of this growth occurred during the 1960s and 1970s. The proportion of households with just one person more than doubled from 13% to 27% between 1960 and 2012 (authors' calculations from U.S. Census Bureau, 2012). Thus, fewer Americans live with family members who can help care for them when they are ill or injured.

In Canada, in 1981, two-thirds of households were single-family households maintained by married or cohabiting couples, but by 2011 the percentage declined to 56% (Statistics Canada, 2011c). As in the United States, the percentage of households that contained two parents with children declined from 36% in 1981 to 26% in 2011. The proportion of Canadian households that contained one person grew from 20% in 1981 to 28% in 2011. Single-person households were the fastest growing type of household (Casper & Bianchi, 2002). With the diversity of family forms that have emerged, nurses are increasingly likely to encounter patients who are living alone and have no one to help them in the home should they become seriously ill. Nurses will come into contact with more single-mother families who are more likely than other types of families to be time poor and cash strapped. In fact, most families with children today do not conform to the traditional notion of a breadwinner/homemaker family.

Living Arrangements of Elderly Persons

Improvements in the health and financial status of older Americans helped generate a revolution in lifestyles and living arrangements among elderly persons. Older North Americans now are more likely to spend their later years with their spouse or live alone, rather than with adult children as in the past. The options and choices differ between elderly women and elderly men, however, in large part because women live longer than men, yet have fewer financial resources.

At the beginning of the 20th century, more than 70% of Americans aged 65 or older resided with kin (Ruggles, 1994). In part because of increased incomes of elderly persons but also because of declining numbers of children and increased divorce rates, the proportion of elderly adults living alone has increased dramatically. Just 15% of widows aged 65 or older lived alone in 1900, whereas 66% lived alone in 2011 (Ruggles, 1996; U.S. Census Bureau, 2011b). In 2011, 44% of the population aged 65 and older lived alone (U.S. Census Bureau, 2011l).

A woman is likely to spend more years living alone after a spouse dies than will a man because life expectancy is about 3 years longer for an elderly woman than for an elderly man, and because women usually marry men older than themselves. As a result, older American women are nearly twice as likely as men to be living alone (37% vs. 19%) (U.S. Census Bureau, 2011b). This pattern is similar in Canada; for example, in 2011 among Canadians aged 65 and older, 32% of women lived alone compared with only 16% of men (Statistics Canada, 2011b). Just under half of all American women aged 75 and older live by themselves (U.S. Census Bureau, 2011b). Living alone can mean delays in getting attention for illness or injury and can complicate arrangements for informal care or transportation to formal care when needed.

Elderly American women are also more than twice as likely as men to be living with someone other than their spouse (19% vs. 9%), in part because they tend to live longer and reach advanced ages when they are most likely to need the physical care and the financial help others can provide (authors' calculations from U.S. Census Bureau,

2012). In the United States, 43% of adults over 65 will reside in assisted living facilities at some point in their lives. In Canada, a larger proportion of women (33%) than men (22%) aged 85 and older lived in institutional settings in 2011 (Statistics Canada, 2011b). Elderly men who need help with activities of daily living (ADLs) such as eating, bathing, or getting around generally receive informal care from their wives, whereas elderly women with disabilities are more likely to rely on assistance from grown children, to live with other family members, or to enter a nursing home (Silverstein, Gans, & Yang, 2006).

To explain trends in living arrangements among elderly persons, researchers have focused on a variety of constraints and preferences that shape people's living arrangement decisions (Bianchi, Hotz, McGarry, & Seltzer, 2008). The number and sex of children generally affect the likelihood that an elderly person will live with relatives. The greater the number of children, the greater the chances that there will be a son or daughter who can take care of an elderly parent. Daughters are more likely than sons to provide housing and care for an elderly parent, presumably as an extension of the traditional female caretaker role and stronger norms of filial responsibility. Geographical distance from children is also a key factor; having children who live nearby promotes co-residence when living independently is no longer feasible for the elderly person (Haxton & Harknett, 2009; Silverstein et al., 2006).

Older Americans with higher income and better health are more likely to live independently (Klinenberg, 2012). In the United States, since 1940, growth in Social Security benefits accounted for half of the increase in independent living among elderly persons (McGarry & Schoeni, 2000). By contrast, elderly Americans in financial need are more likely to live with relatives (Klinenberg, 2012).

Social norms and personal preferences also determine the choice of living arrangements for elderly persons (Seltzer, Lau, & Bianchi, 2012; Silverstein et al., 2006). Many elderly individuals are willing to pay a substantial part of their incomes to maintain their own residence, which suggests strong personal preferences for privacy and independence (Klinenberg, 2012). Social norms involving family obligations and ties may be especially important when examining racial and ethnic differences in the living arrangements of elderly persons. Immigrants and ethnic minorities are more likely than whites to live with an elderly relative not only because of their often limited economic circumstances, but also because their cultural norms and values stipulate moral obligations to care for the elderly (Cohen & Casper, 2002; Glick & Van Hook, 2002).

Despite the trend toward independent living among older Americans, many of them are not able to live alone without assistance. Many families who have older kin in frail health provide extraordinary care. One study in New York City, for example, found that 40% of those who reported caring for an elderly relative devoted 20 or more hours per week to such informal care, and 80% of caregivers had been providing care for more than a year (Navaie-Walsier et al., 2001).

Despite the growth of home-health services and adult day-care centers, most long-term care consists of care provided informally, usually by spouses or younger relatives (Stone, 2000). Adult women, in particular, are likely to have primary responsibility for home care of frail elderly persons, often including parents-in-law. Some evidence suggests that female caregivers experience greater levels of stress than do male caregivers (Yee & Schulz, 2000). Research has shown that even relatively low-cost interventions, such as support groups and telephone counseling, to assist informal caregivers can greatly reduce the harmful effects of such stress on caregivers' health (Belle & REACH II Investigators, 2006).

Living Arrangements of Young Adults

The young-adult years (ages 18–30) have been described as "demographically dense" because these years involve many interrelated life-altering transitions (Rindfuss, 1991). Between these ages, young people usually finish their formal schooling, leave home, develop careers, marry, and begin families, but these events do not always occur in this order. Delayed marriage extends the period during which young adults can experiment with alternative living arrangements before they adopt family roles. Young adults may experience any number of independent living arrangements before they marry, as they change jobs, pursue education, and move into and out of intimate relationships. They may also return to their parents' homes for periods of time, if money becomes tight or at the end of a relationship.

In 1890, half of American women had married by age 22, and half of American men had married by age 26. The ages of entry into marriage dipped to an all-time low during the post–World War II baby-boom years, when the median age at first marriage reached 20 years for women and 23 years for men in 1956. Age at first marriage then began to increase and reached 26 years for women and 28 years for men by 2009 (Kreider & Ellis, 2011b). In Canada, the average age at marriage increased from 25 years in 1972 to 31 years in 2008 for men and from 23 years to 29 years for women (Statistics Canada, 2008). In 1960, it was unusual for a woman to reach age 25 without marrying; only 10% of women aged 25 to 29 had never married (Casper & Bianchi, 2002). In 2011, 50% of women aged 25 to 29 in the United States and 64% of men in the same age group had never been married (U.S. Census Bureau, 2011h).

This delay in marriage has shifted the family and living arrangement behaviors in young adulthood in three important ways. First, later marriage coincides with a greater diversity and fluidity in living arrangements in young adulthood. Second, delaying marriage has accompanied an increased likelihood of entering a cohabiting union before marriage. Third, the trend to later marriage affects childbearing; it tends to delay entry into parenthood and, at the same time, increases the chances that a birth (sometimes planned but more often unintended) occurs before marriage (Bianchi & Casper, 2000).

Many demographic, social, and economic factors influence young adults' decisions about where and with whom to live (Casper & Bianchi, 2002). Family and work transitions are influenced greatly by fluctuations in the economy, as well as by changing ideas about appropriate family life and roles for men and women. Since the 1980s, the transition to adulthood has been hampered by recurring recessions, tight job markets, slow wage growth, and soaring housing costs, in addition to the confusion over roles and behavior sparked by the gender revolution. Even though young adults today may prefer to live independently, they may not be able to afford to do so (Rosenfeld, 2007). Many entry-level jobs today offer low wages, yet housing costs have soared, putting independent living out of reach for many young adults. Higher education, increasingly

necessary in today's labor market, is expensive, and living at home may be a way for families to curb higher education expenses. Even when young adults attend school away from home, they still frequently depend on their parents for financial help and may return home after graduation if they cannot find a suitable job.

The percentage of young men living in their parents' homes was 59% in 2011, about the same as in 1970, whereas the percentage increased for young women from 39% to 50% (U.S. Census Bureau, 2011i). In Canada, the proportion of young adults who resided with their parents increased dramatically from 28% in 1981 to 44% in 2006 (Statistics Canada, 2007).

Young adults who leave home to attend school, join the military, or take a job have always had, and continue to have, high rates of "returning to the nest" and have become known as "boomerang children." Those who leave home to get married have had the lowest likelihood of returning home, although returns to the nest have increased over time even in this group.

American parents often take in their children after they return from the military or school, or when they are between jobs. In the past, however, many American parents apparently were reluctant to take children in if they had left home simply to gain "independence." This is not true today. Before the 1970s, leaving home for simple independence was probably the result of friction within the family, whereas today, leaving and returning home seems to be a common part of a successful transition to adulthood (Klinenberg, 2012; Rosenfeld, 2007). In the past, a young adult may have been reluctant to move back in with parents because a return home implied failure; fewer stigmas are attached to returning home these days (Casper & Bianchi, 2002).

Changing demographic behaviors among young adults and their living arrangements have implications for family health care nursing. In contrast to the situation in Canada, in the United States, young adults often lack health insurance and, in many cases, are not financially independent, reducing the likelihood that they will receive routine checkups or seek medical care when the need arises (Casper & Haaga, 2005). The increasing numbers of people showing up in emergency rooms and urgent care settings put additional pressure on the health care providers, especially nurses. Also, the acuity level of the medical problems in these young adults is greater because they did not seek earlier treatment.

Unmarried Opposite-Sex Couples

One of the most significant household changes in the second half of the 20th century in North America was the increase in men and women living together without marrying. The increase of cohabitation outside marriage appeared to counterbalance some of the delay of marriage among young adults and the overall increase in divorce. Unmarried-couple households made up less than 1% of U.S. households in 1960 and 1970 (Casper & Cohen, 2000). This share increased just over 2% by 1980, and to nearly 9% by 2011, representing 7.6 million family groups (U.S. Census Bureau, 2011m). Unmarried-couple households also are increasingly likely to include children. In 1978, 24% of unmarried-couple households included children younger than 15; by 2011, 40% of unmarried-partner family groups included children. Although the percentage of U.S. households consisting of an unmarried couple is small, many Americans have lived with a partner outside marriage at some point. Nearly 62% of the couples who married between 1997 and 2002 had lived together before marriage, up from 49% in 1985 to 1986, and a big jump from just 8% of first marriages in the late 1960s (Bumpass & Lu, 2000; Kennedy & Bumpass, 2008).

In Canada, cohabiting couples are known as common-law couples. The 2001 Canadian Census showed that increasing proportions of families were headed by common-law couples, from 5.6% in 1981 to 13.8% in 2001. By 2011 this figure increased to 17% (Statistics Canada, 2012e). As in the United States, more Canadian children are living with common-law (cohabiting) parents. Nearly 44% of common-law couples in 2011 have children under age 24 residing with them. In 2011, about 910,700 children aged 0 to 14 (16.3% of the total) lived with common-law parents, up from 12.8% in 2001 (Statistics Canada, 2012e). In both countries, the pace of the increase in cohabitation has slowed somewhat since the rapid rise in the 1970s and 1980s.

Why has cohabitation increased so much? Researchers have offered several explanations, including increased uncertainty about the stability of marriage, the erosion of the stigma associated with cohabitation and sexual relations outside of marriage, the wider availability of reliable birth control, economic changes, and increased individualism and secularization (Bianchi et al., 2012; Cherlin, 2009). Youths reaching adulthood in the past two decades are much more likely to have witnessed their parents' divorce than any generation before them. Some have argued that cohabitation allows a couple to experience the benefits of an intimate relationship without committing to marriage. If a cohabiting relationship is not successful, one can simply move out; if a marriage is not successful, one suffers through a sometimes lengthy and difficult divorce.

Nevertheless, most adults in the United States eventually do marry. In 2011, 90% of women aged 50 to 54 had been married at least once (U.S. Census Bureau, 2011h). An estimated 88% of U.S. women born in the 1960s will eventually marry; however, considerable differences exist by race/ethnicity (Raley, 2000). For example, 88% of African American women reaching adulthood in the 1960s would eventually marry, compared with only 66% coming of age in the 2000s. The meaning and permanence of marriage may be changing, however. Marriage used to be the primary demographic event that marked the formation of new households, the beginning of sexual relations, and the birth of a child. Marriage also implied that an individual had one sexual partner, and it theoretically identified the two individuals who would parent any child born of the union. The increasing social acceptance of cohabitation outside marriage has meant that these linkages can no longer be assumed. Couples began to set up households that might include the couple's children, as well as children from previous marriages or other relationships (Casper & Bianchi, 2002). Similarly, what it meant to be single was no longer always clear, as the personal lives of unmarried couples began to resemble those of their married counterparts.

Cohabiting households can pose unique challenges for health care providers, especially in the United States. Because cohabiting relationships are not legally sanctioned in most states, partners may not have the right to make health care decisions on behalf of each other or of the other's children (Casper & Haaga, 2005). Cohabiting couples report poorer health and have lower incomes than do married couples, on average (Waite & Gallagher, 2000). Thus, although they are more likely to need health care services, they may be less likely to have the financial ability to secure them.

Same-Sex Couples

The number of same-sex couples has increased substantially in North America over the past couple of decades. A conservative estimate shows that the number of same-sex couples in the United States grew by 80% from 358,390 in 2000 to 646,464 in 2010 (Lofquist, Lugaila, O'Connell, & Feliz, 2012). In Canada, the number of same-sex couples increased by 42.4% from 45,345 in 2006 to 64,575 in 2011, of which nearly a third were married couples (Statistics Canada, 2012e). The vast majority of same-sex couples live in common-law or cohabiting relationships. Before 2000, same-sex marriage was not legally recognized. In 2005, however, after the Netherlands and Belgium, Canada became the third country to legalize same-sex marriage. Following legalization, the number of same-sex married couples in Canada almost tripled from 7,465 in 2006 to 21,015 in 2011 (Statistics Canada, 2012e). In the United States, federal law provides each state with autonomy to grant marriage recognition and legal rights to same-sex couples. In 2004, Massachusetts became the first state to legalize same-sex marriage; since then, a number of states and jurisdictions have followed suit. Nevertheless, same-sex marriage is still not legally recognized in most states.

Although the division of labor for parenting and household chores in same-sex families tends to be more egalitarian than among opposite-sex couples, same-sex couples are not as "genderless" as has been previously suggested. This equality often changes as couples transition to parenthood, when one of the partners usually becomes more involved in child rearing, assumes more responsibility for housework, and often becomes the partner in charge of caring for the health of the children and seeking health services for them.

PARENTING

Even with the increase in divorce and cohabitation, postponement of marriage, and decline in childbearing, most North American adults have children, and most children live with two parents. In 2011, 64% of families with children were two-parent, married families and an additional 5% were two-parent, unmarried families (U.S. Census Bureau, 2011a). In Canada, in 2011, the level was comparable: 62% of Canadian families with children were married two-parent families, 14% were two-parent common-law families, and 24% were lone-parent (single-parent) families (authors' calculations from Statistics Canada, 2011c). In 2011, 26% of American families were mother-only families and only 4% were father-only families. "Lone-parent families" in Canada increased from 9% of all families (including those with no children) in 1971 to about 16% in 2011, including 13% lone mothers and 3% lone fathers. The changes in marriage, cohabitation, and nonmarital childbearing over the past few decades have had a profound effect on North American families with children and are changing our images of parenthood.

This section discusses individuals' and couples' transitions into parenthood, beginning with current trends in fertility, the increased use of assisted reproductive technologies (ARTs) to achieve parenthood, and trends and patterns in adoption. As individuals become parents, different types of family forms emerge. The section explores single motherhood, fathering, and child rearing within cohabitation and same-sex couple families. The section concludes with a discussion of the important role grandparents are playing in rearing and caring for grandchildren.

Fertility

In the United States and Canada, fertility has exhibited a trend of long-term decline for more than a century, interrupted by the baby-boom period and other small fluctuations. In recent decades, fertility rates in most developed countries have fallen below the level required to replace the population. Replacement-level fertility refers to the required number of children each woman in the population would have to bear on average to replace herself and her partner, and it is conventionally set at 2.1 children per woman for countries with low mortality rates. This threshold is set slightly above 2 in order to account for a negligible rate of childhood mortality and a small proportion of individuals who do not survive to their reproductive age (Preston, Heuveline, & Guillot, 2001).

The U.S. fertility decline has not been very drastic; thus, the United States is an atypical case among developed countries. Figure 2-1 shows the trends in fertility rates since the 1930s for the United States and Canada, respectively. As this graph shows, both countries experienced a post-WWII baby boom during the 1950s and 1960s,

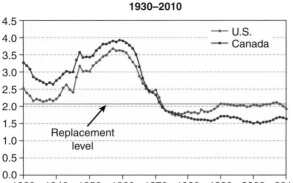

Total Fertility Rate for the U.S. and Canada: 1930–2010

FIGURE 2-1 Total fertility rate for the United States and Canada: 1930–2010. *(Data from Martin et al., 2012; Statistics Canada, 2011d.)*

after which fertility began to decline again. Since the 1980s, the United States has exhibited fertility rates close to replacement level. In 2010, the total U.S. fertility rate was 1.93 children per woman (Martin et al., 2012). In Canada, however, the fertility decline has been of greater magnitude; in 2010, the fertility rate was 1.63 (Statistics Canada, 2012a). Persistent levels of below replacement fertility have raised concerns regarding population shrinkage. Fewer births also imply a subsequent contraction of the working-age population that, coupled with increases in life expectancy, reduces the tax base that supports health care and retirement benefits for the aging population (Lee, 2003). In the United States and Canada, a significant proportion of population growth during recent decades has come from immigration.

Fertility varies by demographic characteristics. In the United States, except for Asians, immigrants tend to exhibit higher fertility rates than the native-born population. In 2010, native-born women had on average 1.8 children, whereas foreign-born women had 2.2 children (U.S. Census Bureau, 2010d). Fertility also varies by race and ethnicity. In 2010 in the United States, fertility was the highest among Hispanic women (2.3), followed by African Americans (2.0), and the lowest rate was observed among white and Asian women (1.80) (U.S. Census Bureau, 2010d). The differences are greater by educational level. Women with less than a high school education had on average 2.56 births, whereas women with a graduate or professional degree had only 1.67 births (U.S. Census Bureau, 2010d).

The causes behind the secular trends in fertility decline can be grouped into socioeconomic, ideological, and institutional factors. Among socioeconomic factors are the increase in women's opportunity costs and the rising cost of rearing children. The socioeconomic position of women has drastically changed since the 1960s. Economic changes have also made it more difficult to maintain a family on the income of a single earner. Women's education and labor force participation increased considerably during this period. In addition, changes in laws and civil rights have reduced discriminatory practices against women. All of these changes have resulted in increases in women's wages, although they have not yet reached parity with men's. As women's incomes and career opportunities have improved, women's opportunity costs of not participating in the labor market have increased, thus reducing women's fertility intentions. At the same time, higher educational expectations for children and rising living standards have substantially increased the costs of raising children (Lino, 2012).

Cultural and ideological changes, such as the growth in individualism and the desire for self-realization, have decreased the appeal of long-term commitments, including childbearing (Bianchi et al., 2012; Cherlin, 2009). The accentuation of individual autonomy and the rise of feminism have increased the desirability for more symmetrical gender roles. However, institutions dealing with family life still exhibit high levels of gender inequality. Equal opportunities for women in education and employment are often curtailed within families as women continue to pay a penalty for having children in the form of reduced career involvement and income prospects. This asymmetry accentuates the incompatibility of childbearing and labor force participation (McDonald, 2000).

In addition, in the 1960s more effective birth control methods became available, providing couples with better means to control their fertility. Moreover, favorable attitudes toward nonmarital sex and cohabitation have also weakened the link between sex, marriage, and childbearing (Casper & Bianchi, 2002). Thus, most developed countries have experienced a considerable rise in nonmarital births to single and cohabiting mothers. In 2010, 41% of all births in the United States were to unmarried women, of which 58% were to cohabiting women (Martin et al., 2012). In Canada, births to unmarried women have also increased, representing 27.3% of all births in 2007 (U.S. Census Bureau, 2012).

The birth rate for teenagers has decreased substantially in both countries, although in the United States this rate is more than twice that observed in Canada. In Canada in 2008, only 4% of all births were to women ages 15 to 19, compared with 9% in the United States in 2010. The birth rate for teenagers in Canada was 14.3 births per 1,000 women in 2008, down from 26.1 in 1981 (Milan, 2011). The U.S. teenage birth rate for women ages 15 to 19 was 34.3 births per 1,000 women in 2010, down from 52.2 in 1981 (Martin et al., 2012). The United States still exhibits one of the highest rates of teenage pregnancy in the industrialized world.

Nonetheless, women increasingly have been delaying childbearing since the 1960s; thus, the average age at first birth has risen in both countries. In 2010, the average age at first birth in the United States was 25.4 (Martin et al., 2012). In 2008 in Canada, the average age at first birth was 28.1, up from 23.5 in the mid-1960s (Milan, 2011). However, the onset of fertility varies by race/ethnicity in the United States. Whereas the average age at first birth for African American and Hispanic women was slightly above 23 years in 2010, for white women it was 26.3. Asian and Pacific Islanders exhibited the highest average age at first birth at 29.1 (Martin et al., 2012). Thus, childbearing for middle-class whites and Asians is increasingly becoming concentrated in the late twenties and early thirties.

Overall, these trends imply not only that women are having fewer children, but also that they are increasingly having children at older ages. Nurses are more likely to encounter more educated and mature mothers and pregnant women. However, as women wait longer to have their first child, complications in pregnancies and deliveries will become more common. Moreover, age-related infertility will be more likely to affect these women, increasing the rate of involuntary infertility. As delays in fertility continue, a larger pool of women approaching the end of their reproductive years will seek the services of assisted reproductive technology.

Assisted Reproductive Technologies (ARTs)

Although various definitions have been used for assisted reproductive technologies (ARTs), the current definition used by the U.S. Centers for Disease Control and Prevention (CDC) is based on the 1992 Fertility Clinic Success Rate and Certification Act. According to this definition, ARTs include all fertility treatments in which both eggs and sperm are handled. In general, ART procedures involve surgically removing eggs from a woman's ovaries, combining them with sperm in the laboratory, and returning them to the woman's body or donating them to another woman. According to this definition, treatments in which only sperm are handled are not included (i.e., intrauterine—or artificial—insemination), nor are procedures in which a woman takes medications only to stimulate egg production without the intention of having eggs retrieved (U.S. Centers for Disease Control and Prevention, 2012).

ARTs have been used in the United States since 1981 to help women become pregnant, most commonly through the transfer of fertilized human eggs into a woman's uterus (in vitro fertilization). Deciding whether to undergo this expensive and time-consuming treatment can be difficult. Worldwide, an estimated 9% of couples meet the definition of infertility, with 50% to 60% of them seeking care (Boivin, Bunting, Collins, & Nygren, 2007). In the United States, approximately 7% of married couples reported at least 12 months of unprotected intercourse without conception, while 2% of women reported having visited an infertility-related clinic within the past year (Chandra, Martinez, Mosher, Abma, & Jones, 2005). In Canada, the estimated percentage of couples experiencing infertility in 2010 ranged from 11.5% to 15.7%, depending on the definition of infertility used. Infertility treatment costs sum up to well over three billion dollars annually in the United States (Myers et al., 2008). As women wait longer to have their first child, the likelihood of age-related infertility increases. Although there is some controversy about whether the proportion of the population with self-reported infertility is increasing, stable, or decreasing, there has been a clear increase in the use of ARTs (Stephen & Chandra, 2006; Sunderam et al., 2012).

The number of in vitro fertilization (IVF) cycles performed in the United States increased from approximately 30,000 in 1996 (Myers et al., 2008) to over 147,000 in 2010, resulting in 47,090 live births (deliveries of one or more living infants) and 61,564 infants (U.S. Centers for Disease Control and Prevention, 2012). Over this time, the proportion of deliveries in the United States resulting from ARTs has increased from 0.37% in 1996 to 0.94% in

2005. In 2009, ARTs accounted for 1.4% of U.S. births (Sunderam et al., 2012). In Canada 3,428 babies were born through ARTs in 2007 (Assisted Human Reproduction Canada, 2011). ARTs often result in multiple births, such as twins, triplets, and so on, which increases health risks for children and mothers. In the United States and Canada, nearly 30% of all ART births result in multiple births. Due to high costs and increased health risks, the Assisted Human Reproduction Canada (AHRC) agency has set as a goal to reduce the rate of multiple births resulting from ARTs (AHRC, 2011).

A growing number of same-sex couples seeking to become parents are also turning to ARTs to achieve this goal: in the case of lesbians, usually through the use of a sperm donor and artificial insemination; and in the case of gay men, through the use of an egg donor and/or a surrogate. It is worth noting that male same-sex couples face greater challenges than female same-sex couples to become parents, not only because fertility centers are less likely to accept male gay patients, but also because the procedure is more expensive as it involves obtaining both an oocyte donor and a gestational surrogate, that is, a woman who will carry the zygote and take the pregnancy to term (Greenfeld, 2007).

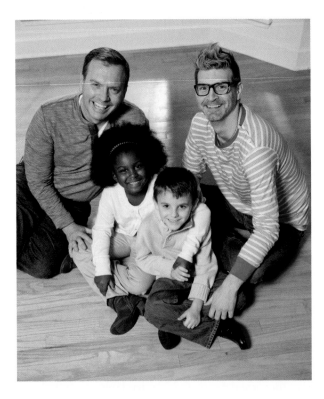

Although data on psychological outcomes of women who become pregnant after infertility treatment are quite limited, the available data suggest that women have outcomes as good as, and perhaps better than, women who get pregnant from spontaneous conception. Based on the available literature, there are no differences in parenting skills when comparing singleton pregnancies resulting from ART to spontaneous conceptions (Myers et al., 2008). In fact, mothers of infants resulting from ART appear to have better outcomes. By contrast, there is some evidence that fathers may do worse on some scales. The multiple gestations and preterm births that frequently result with ART significantly increase stress and depressive symptoms, especially for mothers of infants with chronic disabilities.

Births resulting from ART are more likely to involve multiple births, pregnancy complications, preterm delivery, and low birth weight, all of which may pose substantial risks to the health of mothers and infants. Additionally, children born as a result of ART experience relatively worse neurodevelopmental outcomes, higher rates of hospitalization, and more surgeries than other children. There is little evidence, however, that the relatively worse outcomes for ART babies are a direct result of infertility treatments; infertility treatments are more likely to be used by couples with a history of subfertility—difficulty achieving and sustaining pregnancy without medical assistance—and worse outcomes typically result for the children of these couples, irrespective of whether they have received infertility treatments (Myers et al., 2008).

In sum, family nurses will likely encounter a growing number of opposite-sex couples seeking infertility treatment, as well as same-sex couples who wish to become parents. This process is time consuming, expensive, and stressful for all of the parties involved. Unsuccessful attempts to become pregnant are likely to be met with sorrow, anger, and regret. Nurses should be aware of the delicate circumstances surrounding this type of care. They should also be aware of the heightened risk of multiple births, potential birth defects, and increased women's health risks.

Adoption

Accurate trends on adoption in the United States are difficult to obtain, but U.S. Census Bureau data indicate that the number of adopted children increased in the 1990s from about 1.6 million in 1991 to 2.1 million in 2004 and then decreased to 1.4 million in 2009 (Kreider & Ellis, 2011a). Other data show that in 2007 there were approximately 1.7 million adopted children living in the United States (Vandivere, Malm, & Radel, 2009). Box 2-2 illustrates the three primary forms of adoption in the United States: foster care adoption, private domestic adoption, and international adoption.

According to the U.S. Administration for Children and Families, the number of adoptions from foster care has ranged from 50,000 to 57,000 annually between 2002 and 2011, with some fluctuations and no clear trend (U.S. Department of Health and Human Services, 2011). In 2007, 661,000 children were adopted from foster care, representing 37% of all adopted children. Of foster care–adopted children, 23% were adopted by relatives, 40% were adopted by someone who knew them before the adoption (including relatives), and 69% were adopted by someone who was previously their foster parent (Vandivere et al., 2009). Because these children were removed from their homes due to abuse or neglect, they are more likely than other children, and even than those adopted through different means, to have special health care needs—in 2007 54% had special needs.

In 2007, about 677,000 or 38% of adopted children were adopted privately from sources other than foster care. Of these, 41% were adopted by relatives and 44% were adopted by someone who knew them before the adoption (including relatives). Almost one-third of these children have special health care needs. The majority of children adopted privately in the United States were placed with their adoptive family as newborns or when they were younger than 1 month old (62%).

International adoptions increased from about 15,700 in 1999 to about 23,000 children in 2004. Since 2004, they have been steadily decreasing to 9,300 in 2011 due to stricter laws and regulations

---

BOX 2-2

Three Primary Forms of Adoption in the United States

Foster Care Adoption

Children adopted from foster care are those who were removed from their families due to their families' inability or unwillingness to provide appropriate care and were placed under the protection of the state by the child protective services system. Public child welfare agencies oversee such adoptions, although they sometimes contract with private adoption agencies to perform some adoption functions.

Private Domestic Adoption

These children were adopted privately from within the United States and were not part of the foster care system at any time before their adoption. Such adoptions may be arranged independently or through private adoption agencies.

International Adoption

This group includes children who originated from countries other than the United States. Typically, adoptive parents work with private U.S. adoption agencies, which coordinate with adoption agencies and other entities in children's countries of origin. Changes in international adoption laws have made it more difficult to adopt children from abroad. Starting in 2008, the Hague Convention on Protection of Children and Co-operation in Respect of Intercountry Adoption has been regulating adoptions from several countries. Its purpose is to protect children and to ensure that placements made are in the best interests of children. For adoptions from countries not part of the Hague Convention, U.S. law dictates that children have to be orphans in order to immigrate into the United States. The Hague Convention seems to have contributed to the decrease in international adoptions. For example, in 2007 24% of all international adoptions of children under age 18 were from Guatemala, but in March 2008, the U.S. Department of State announced that it would not process Guatemalan adoptions until further notice, due to concerns about the country's ability to adhere to the guidelines of the Hague Convention. Additionally, in 2008, Guatemala stopped accepting any new adoption cases (U.S. Department of State, 2011).

Other countries have also implemented stricter regulations for international adoptions. For example, as of May 2007, China enacted a rigorous policy requiring adoptive parents be married couples between the ages of 30 and 50 with assets of at least $80,000 and in good health (including not being overweight). In November 2012 a bilateral adoption agreement between the United States and Russia increased safeguards for and monitoring of Russian children adopted by U.S. parents (U.S. Department of State, 2011). In addition, China and other countries, such as Russia and Korea, are attempting to promote domestic rather than international adoption (Lee, 2007; Voice of Russia World Service in English, 2007).

(U.S. Department of State, 2011). Internationally adopted children make up the smallest group, numbering about 444,000 or 25% of all adopted children. Of these adopted children, 29% have special health care needs. More than 7 in 10 adopted children in 2011 came from just five countries—China (28%), Ethiopia (19%), Russia (10%), South Korea (8%), and the Ukraine (7%). In Canada, international adoptions have also slightly decreased from an average of 2,000 adoptions per year during the 1990s and early 2000s. In 2010, 1,946 children were adopted from abroad. In the same year, nearly 6 in 10 international adoptions to Canada came from China (24%), Haiti (9%), the United States (8%), Vietnam (7%), Ethiopia (6%), and Russia (5%) (Hilborn, 2011).

Since 2008, the Hague Convention on Protection of Children and Co-operation in Respect of Intercountry Adoption has been regulating adoptions from approximately 75 countries. The stricter law adopted by the Hague Convention has probably contributed to the decline in international adoption (see Box 2-2). In the past several years, many countries have changed their adoption requirements, thus making it harder to adopt. All of these legal changes have reduced the number of international adoptions in the United States.

Social and demographic changes coupled with changing laws have altered the context of adoption. Recent developments in reproductive medicine, such as intrauterine insemination and in vitro fertilization, seem to have contributed to the decline in adoption in recent years by reducing the demand for adoption. At the same time, never-married mothers have become less likely to put their infants up for adoption—in 1973, 9% of births were placed for adoption compared to just 1% in the 1990s and 2000s, reducing the supply of infants for domestic adoptions (Jones, 2008).

According to a recent study conducted at the U.S. Department of Health and Human Services, overall, 87% of adopted children have parents who said they would "definitely" make the same decision to adopt their child, knowing everything then that they now know about their child. More than 90% of adopted children ages 5 and older have parents who perceived their child's adoption experience as "positive" or "mostly positive" (Vandivere et al., 2009).

According to this study, overall, 40% of the adopted children are in transracial adoptions; either one or both adoptive parents are of a different race, culture, or ethnicity than their child. The majority of adopted children have non-Hispanic white parents but are not themselves non-Hispanic white. Transracial adoptions are most common for children whose families adopted internationally. Overall, about half of adopted children are male (49%)—33% of internationally adopted children are male, while 57% of children adopted from foster care are male (Vandivere et al., 2009). Adopted children are less likely than biological children in the general population to live in households below the poverty line (12% compared with 18%). However, nearly half of children adopted from foster care (46%) live in households with incomes no higher than two times the poverty threshold. Over two-thirds of adopted children (69%) live with two married parents; they are just as likely to do so as children in the general population (Vandivere et al., 2009).

The majority of adoptive children engage in enrichment activities with their families, and in fact they are more likely to have some of these positive experiences than all children in the population (Vandivere et al., 2009). As youngsters, adopted children are more likely than all children to be read to every day (68% compared with 48%), to be sung to or told stories every day (73% compared with 59%), and to participate in extracurricular activities as school-age children (85% compared with 81%). A small percentage of adopted children have parents who report parental aggravation (for example, feeling the child was difficult to care for, or feeling angry with the child). Parental aggravation is more common among parents of adopted children than among all parents (11% compared with 6%).

This socioeconomic and demographic portrait of adopted children has implications for family nursing. First, although most adoptive children fare well with regard to health, educational achievement, and social and cognitive development, those who are adopted through foster care are disproportionately disadvantaged. Second, because most parents of adopted children do not share with them their genetic endowment and because the medical histories of the biological parents are often unknown, diagnosis for these children can be more challenging than for biological children. Third, the substantial proportion of transracial adoptive families requires special attention. For decades, adoptive parents who were of a different race than their child were taught to be color blind regarding their adoptive children and to raise them according to the culture of the parent. More recently, adoption social workers have encouraged adoptive parents to embrace the child's culture of origin and to help their children develop positive racial and ethnic identities. As most of these parents are white, however, they may be unaware of the nuances of the culture the child is coming from and may not have the capacity to teach their children how to deal with bias and discrimination (Shiao, Tuan, & Rienzi, 2004). Nurses should be sensitive to these differences and help guide the parents in understanding how to help their children.

Finally, unlike biological families, many adoptive families emerge out of loss for all members—for example, foster parents who are not able to have biological children; biological parents who are relinquishing their children; and adoptive children who are losing or have lost their biological parents. This unique family form requires an adjustment period for all of those involved. Separations of adoptive children from biological parents at birth deprive children of the bioregulatory channels that exist between a mother and her baby—from breathing, to respiration, to heart rate and blood pressure. Taking away a baby at birth cuts off this regulation and may cause children to cry more often, become angry or confused, or behave badly simply because they do not understand the separation (Verrier, 1993). Nurses should be aware that unusual behaviors such as these among adoptive children may not stem from illness or health-related causes.

Single Mothers

How many single mothers are there? This turns out to be a more difficult question to answer from official statistics than it would first appear. Over time, it is easiest to calculate the number of single mothers who maintain their own residence. In the United States between 1950 and 2011, the number of such single-mother families increased from 1.3 million to 8.7 million (U.S. Census Bureau, 2011c). These estimates do not include single mothers living in other persons' households but do include single mothers who are cohabiting with a male partner. The most dramatic increase was during the 1970s, when the number of single-mother families was increasing at 8% per year. The

average annual rate of increase slowed considerably during the 1980s and was near 0% after 1994 (Casper & Bianchi, 2002). By 2011, single mothers who maintained their own households accounted for 25% of all families with children, up from 6% in 1950 (U.S. Census Bureau, 2011c). Almost 1.4 million more single mothers lived in someone else's household, bringing the total number of single mothers to over 10 million (U.S. Census Bureau, 2011c). In 2011 in Canada, there were 1.2 million lone mothers and 328,000 lone fathers with children of any age living with them (Statistics Canada, 2012e).

Single mothers with children at home face a multitude of challenges. They usually are the primary breadwinners, disciplinarians, playmates, and caregivers for their children. They must manage the financial and practical aspects of a household and plan for the family's future. Many mothers cope remarkably well, and many benefit from financial support and help from relatives and from their children's fathers.

Women earn less than men, on average, and because single mothers are usually younger and less educated than other women, they are often at the lower end of the income curve. Never-married single mothers are particularly disadvantaged; they are younger, less well educated, and less often employed than are divorced single mothers and married mothers. Single mothers often must curtail their work hours to care for the health and well-being of their children.

Despite the fact that the majority of American single mothers are not poor, they are much more likely to be poor than other parents. Single-parent families are officially defined as poor if they have incomes under the poverty line, which for a single mother with two children translates into an annual income of less than $18,123 in 2011. Overall, 20% of U.S. children lived in poverty in 2009. Children in two-parent families had the lowest rate at 13.3%, followed by children living in father-only families at 19.9%. Children in mother-only families had the highest poverty rate at 38.1%. Poverty and family structure are highly correlated with race in the United States. Children in black and Hispanic single-mother families exhibit the highest poverty rate at about 45% compared with white children in two-parent families, who have the lowest rate at 8.6% (Kreider & Ellis, 2011a).

The family income of children who reside with a never-married single mother is less than one-fourth that of children in two-parent families (Bianchi & Casper, 2000). Almost three of every five children who live with a never-married mother are poor. Mothers who never married are much less likely to get child support from the father than are mothers who are divorced or separated. Whereas 43% of divorced mothers with custody of children younger than 21 received some child support from the children's father, fewer than 25% of never-married mothers reported receiving regular support from their child's father (U.S. Census Bureau, 2010c).

Children who live with a divorced mother tend to be much better off financially than are children of never-married mothers. Divorced mothers are substantially better educated and more often employed than are mothers who are separated or who never married. Even so, the average incomes of families headed by divorced mothers is less than half that of two-parent families.

In 2010, three million Canadians lived in low income and about 546,000 or 8.1% of children younger than 18 lived in low-income families (Statistics Canada, 2012c). Canadian lone-parent families with children younger than 18 are much more likely to have low incomes, and thus, more likely to be poor (First Call: BC Child and Youth Advocacy Coalition, 2011). Among children living in female lone-parent families, 187,000, or 21.8%, were low income, whereas the incidence of low income was 5.7% among children living in two-parent families (Statistics Canada, 2012c).

In the United States, single mothers with children in poverty are particularly affected by major welfare reform legislation, such as the Personal Responsibility and Work Opportunity Reconciliation Act (PRWORA) (Box 2-3). President Clinton claimed in his 1993 State of the Union Address that the 1996 law would "end welfare as we know it," and the changes embodied in PRWORA—time limits on welfare eligibility and mandatory job-training requirements, for example—seemed far-reaching (Hays, 2003). Some argued that this legislation would end crucial support for poor mothers and their children; several high-level government officials resigned because of the law. Others heralded PRWORA as the first step toward helping poor women gain control of their lives and making fathers take responsibility for their children. Many states had already begun to experiment with similar reforms. The success of this program is open to dispute because it has been and continues to be such a political issue.

Why have mother-child families increased in number and as a percentage of North American families? Explanations tend to focus on one of two trends. First is women's increased financial independence. More women entered the labor force and women's incomes increased relative to those of men, and welfare benefits for single mothers expanded during the 1960s and 1970s. Women today are less dependent on a man's income to support themselves and their children, and many can afford to live independently rather than stay in an unsatisfactory relationship. Second, the job market for men has tightened, especially for less-educated men. As the North American economy experienced a restructuring in the 1970s and 1980s, the demand for professionals, managers, and other white-collar workers expanded, whereas wages for men in lower-skilled jobs declined in real terms (Casper & Bianchi, 2002). Over the past two decades, this pattern has continued due to technological advances and outsourcing displacing manufacturing and other lower-skilled jobs (Bianchi et al., 2012). Men still earn more than women, on average, but the earnings gap narrowed steadily between the 1970s and 2000 as women's earnings increased and men's earnings remained flat or declined. In the past decade, the gender-earnings gap has been relatively constant because both men's and women's average earnings have stagnated. In 2011 in the United States, full-time, year-round female workers earned 77 cents for every dollar earned by full-time, year-round male workers (DeNavas-Walt, Proctor, & Smith, 2012).

In the early years of the 20th century, higher mortality rates made it more common for children to live with only one parent (Uhlenberg, 1996). As declining death rates reduced the number of widowed single parents, a counterbalancing increase in single-parent families occurred because of divorce. For example, at the time of the 1960 Census, almost one-third of American single mothers living with children younger than 18 were widows (Bianchi, 1995). As divorce rates increased precipitously in the 1960s and 1970s, most single-parent families were created through divorce or separation. Thus, at the end of the 1970s, only 11% of American single mothers were widowed and two-thirds were divorced or separated. In 1978, about one-fifth of single American mothers had never married but had a child and were raising that child on their own (Bianchi & Casper, 2000). By 2011, 46.5% of single mothers had never married (U.S. Census Bureau, 2011k).

BOX 2-3
Welfare Reform in the United States

Federal and state programs in the United States to aid low-income families have been transformed during the past two decades. The 1996 PRWORA was the legislative milestone at the federal level.

- PRWORA replaced the Aid to Families With Dependent Children program, an entitlement for poor families, with a program of block grants to the states called Temporary Assistance to Needy Families (TANF).
- It requires states to impose work requirements on at least 80% of TANF recipients.
- It forbids payments to single mothers younger than 18 unless they live with an adult or in an adult-supervised situation.
- It set limits of 60 months on TANF for any individual recipient (and 22 states have used their option to impose shorter lifetime limits).
- It gives states more latitude to let TANF recipients earn money or get child support payments without reduction of benefits and to use block grants for child care.

Welfare-reform proponents often supported efforts to "make work pay," as well as to discourage long-term dependence on welfare. The Earned Income Tax Credit, for example, was expanded several times during the 1980s and 1990s and now provides twice as much money to low-income families, whether single- or two-parent families. Funding for child care was also expanded during the decade, though child care remains a problem for low-income working families in most places.

PRWORA accelerated a decline in welfare caseloads throughout the country. Because of a concern that former welfare recipients entering the workforce would lose insurance coverage through Medicaid for their children, the 1997 Balanced Budget Act set up the new State Child Health Insurance Program (SCHIP), providing federal money to states in proportion to their low-income population and recent success in reducing the proportion of uninsured children.

Lack of health insurance remains an important concern for children in the United States, however. The Census Bureau estimated that in 2011 about 1 of every 10 children in the United States was not covered by any health insurance (and one in five adults between ages 18 and 64 were uninsured) (DeNavas-Walt et al., 2012).

In 1996, Congress also made the following statements: (1) Marriage is the foundation of a successful society. (2) Marriage is an essential institution of a successful society which promotes the interests of children. To support healthy marriage, in conjunction with TANF, the Deficit Reduction Act of 2005 was implemented providing $150 million per year of funding to support healthy marriage and responsible fatherhood promotion. The goal of the Healthy Marriage Initiative (HMI) is to help couples, "who have chosen marriage for themselves, gain greater access to marriage education services, on a voluntary basis, where they can acquire the skills and knowledge necessary to form and sustain a healthy marriage" (U.S. Department of Health and Human Services, 2012).

Key requirements of the law specify that HMI funds may be used for competitive research and demonstration projects to test promising approaches to encourage healthy marriages and promote involved, committed, and responsible fatherhood by public and private entities and also for providing technical assistance to states and tribes:

- Applicants for funds must commit to consult with experts in domestic violence; applications must describe how programs will address issues of domestic violence and ensure that participation is voluntary.
- Healthy marriage promotion awards must be used for eight specified activities, including marriage education, marriage skills training, public advertising campaigns, high school education on the value of marriage, and marriage mentoring programs.

Not more than $50 million each year may be used for activities promoting fatherhood, such as counseling, mentoring, marriage education, enhancing relationship skills, parenting, and activities to foster economic stability (U.S. Department of Health and Human Services, 2012).

The remarkable increase in the number of single-mother households with women who have never married was driven by a dramatic shift to childbearing outside marriage. The number of births to unmarried women grew from less than 90,000 per year in 1940 to nearly 1.6 million per year in 2010 (Martin et al., 2012). Less than 4% of all births in 1940 were to unmarried mothers compared with 41% in 2010. The rate of nonmarital births—the number of births per 1,000 unmarried women—increased from 7.1 in 1940 to 47.6 in 2010. The nonmarital birth rate peaked in 1994 at 46.2, leveled out in the latter 1990s, and has increased slightly since the mid-2000s (Bianchi & Casper, 2000; Martin et al., 2012). Births to unmarried women have increased in Canada as well, from 12.8% in 1980 to 27.3% of all births in 2007 (U.S. Census Bureau, 2012).

The proportion of births that occur outside marriage is even higher in some European countries than in the United States and Canada. But unmarried parents in European countries and Canada are more likely to be living together with their biological children than are unmarried parents in the United States (Heuveline, Timberlake, & Furstenberg, 2003). In the United States, the tremendous variation in rates of unmarried childbearing among population groups suggests that there may be a constellation of factors that determine whether women have children when they are not married. In 2010, the percentage of births to unmarried mothers was the highest for blacks at 73%, followed by Native Americans (66%), Hispanics (53%), and white non-Hispanics (29%). Asian and Pacific Islanders reported the lowest percentage at 17% (Martin et al., 2012, Tables 13 and 14). Overall, 25% of all family groups with children under 18 are maintained by single mothers. The percentage of mother-only family groups is much higher for African American families (52%) than for Hispanic (28%), white non-Hispanic (19%), and Asian (12%) families (U.S. Census Bureau, 2011m).

Single-mother families present challenges for family health care nurses providing care to this vulnerable group. Single mothers today are younger and less educated than they were a few decades ago. This presents problems because these mothers have less experience with the health care system and are likely to have more difficulty reading directions, filling out forms, communicating effectively with doctors and nurses, and understanding their care instructions. In the U.S., these mothers are also more likely to be poor and uninsured, making it less likely they will seek care and more likely they will not be able to pay for it. Consequently, when the need arises, these women are more likely to resort to emergency rooms for noncritical illnesses and injuries. Time is also in short supply for single mothers. With the advent of welfare reform in the United States, more of them are working, which conceivably reduces the time they used in the past to care for themselves and their children (see Box 2-3). Moreover, although many of these mothers can rely on their families for help, they are apt to have tenuous ties with their children's fathers.

Fathering

A new view of fatherhood emerged out of the feminist movement of the late 1960s and early 1970s. The new ideal father was a co-parent who was responsible for and involved in all aspects of his children's care. The ideal has been widely accepted throughout North American society; people today, as opposed to those in earlier times, believe that fathers should be highly involved in caregiving (Hernandez & Brandon, 2002). In the U.S. and Canada, although mothers still spend nearly twice as much time caring for children than fathers do, fathers are spending more time with their children and are doing more housework than in earlier decades. In 1998, married fathers in the United States reported spending an average of 4 hours per day with their children, compared with 2.7 hours in 1965 (Bianchi, 2000). In 2010, in Canada, fathers spent on average 24.4 hours per week (3.5 hours per day) taking care of children (Statistics Canada, 2012f). These estimates vary by employment status of both parents and by the children's age. Fathers spend more time caring for children when mothers are employed and when children are young.

At the same time, other trends increasingly remove fathers from their children's lives. When the mother and father are not married, for example, ties between fathers and their children often falter. Fathers' involvement with children differs by marital status and living arrangements. Among fathers residing with their children, biological married fathers spend more time with their children, followed by fathers in cohabiting relationships. Stepfathers exhibit the lowest level of involvement among all resident fathers. Nonresidential fathers exhibit the lowest involvement in child rearing. They also provide less financial support to their children (Hofferth, Pleck, Stueve, Bianchi, & Sayer, 2002). Family demographer Frank Furstenberg (1998) used the label "good dads, bad dads" to describe the parallel trends of increased commitment to children and child rearing on the part of some fathers at the same time that there seems to be less connection to and responsibility for children on the part of other fathers.

Fathers' involvement is associated with improved child well-being, including better cognitive development, fewer behavioral problems, and better emotional health. However, fathers' involvement and child support significantly decrease when parents separate, especially if the father or mother forms a new family or if the custodial mother poses obstacles for a father's contact with his children (Carlson & McLanahan, 2010). As a result, union disruption not only hurts children's cognitive and emotional well-being, but also reduces children's contact with fathers, decreasing the parental and financial resources available to children (Amato & Dorius, 2010). Nonetheless, when fathers re-partner and acquire stepchildren, they usually assume new responsibilities and provide for their stepchildren, a fact that is often overlooked when assessing fathers' involvement (Hernandez & Brandon, 2002).

How many years do men spend as parents? Demographer Rosalind King (1999) estimated the number of years that American men and women will spend as parents of biological children or stepchildren younger than 18 if the parenting patterns of the late 1980s and early 1990s continue throughout their lives; her estimations have not been refuted to date. Almost two-thirds of the adult years will be "child-free" years in which the individual does not have biological children younger than 18 or responsibility for anyone else's children. Men will spend, on average, about 20% of their adulthood living with and raising their biological children, whereas women will spend more than 30% of their adult lives, on average, raising biological children. Whereas women, regardless of race, spend nearly all of their parenting years rearing their biological children, men are more likely to live with stepchildren or a combination of their own children and stepchildren. Among men in the United States, white men will spend about twice as much time living with their biological children as African American men.

One of the new aspects of the American family in the last 50 years has been an increase in the number of single fathers. Between 1950 and 2011, the number of households with children that were maintained by an unmarried father increased from 229,000 to 2.2 million (U.S. Census Bureau, 2011c). During the 1980s and 1990s, the percentage of single-father households nearly tripled for white and Hispanic families and doubled for African American families (Casper & Bianchi, 2002). Recent demographic trends in fathering have changed the context of family health care nursing. The growth in single fatherhood and joint custody, together with the increased tendency for fathers to perform household chores, means that family health care nurses are more likely today than in decades past to be interacting with the fathers of children.

Unmarried Parents Living Together

In the United States, changes in marriage and cohabitation tend to blur the distinction between one-parent and two-parent families. The increasing acceptance of cohabitation as a substitute for marriage, for example, may reduce the chance that a premarital pregnancy will lead to marriage before the birth (Casper & Bianchi, 2002). Greater shares of children today are born to a mother who is not currently married than in previous decades. Some of those children are born to cohabitating parents and begin life in a household that includes both their biological parents. Data from the 2006–2010 National Survey of Family Growth show that 58% of recent nonmarital births were to cohabitating women (Martin et al., 2012). Cohabitation increased for unmarried mothers in all race and ethnic groups, but especially among whites. Cohabitating couples account for up to 13% of all single-parent family groups. In 2011, 13% of white single parents were actually cohabitating compared with 9% of black, 13% of Asian, and 19% of Hispanic single parents (U.S. Census Bureau, 2011d). In 2011 in Canada, 17% of all families consisted of common-law couples, and among families with children under age 14, 14% were common-law families (Statistics Canada, 2012e).

Same-Sex Couple Families

An increasing number of same-sex couples are now raising children. In the United States, nearly 17% of same-sex couples had children in 2010 (author's own calculations based on Lofquist et al., 2012). In Canada, 9.4% of same-sex couples were raising children in 2011 (Statistics Canada, 2012e). Same-sex couples, especially gay male couples, face considerable obstacles and need to overcome negative public attitudes to become parents (Biblarz & Savci, 2010). Female couples are more likely than male couples to be parents (Statistics Canada, 2012e). Many same-sex couples bring children into their households from previous heterosexual relationships; others become parents through the use of assisted reproductive technology and surrogacy, yet an increasing number of them become parents through adoption as same-sex couples obtain legal adoption rights (Biblarz & Savci, 2010; Greenfeld, 2007).

Although some people have raised concerns about the parenting styles of same-sex parents and the potential negative effect for children's outcomes and well-being, recent research has found that, for the most part, the parental skills of same-sex couples are comparable to if not better than those of heterosexual couples (Biblarz & Savci, 2010). This finding is partly explained by the fact that although many same-sex couples are very eager to become parents, they face several obstacles that require them to invest more time, money, and effort to achieve this goal. Their higher initial investments make them more likely to devote a great deal of time to their children when they finally become parents (Biblarz & Savci, 2010).

Research on children's outcomes has focused on different dimensions of well-being, including psychological well-being, emotional development, social behavior, and school performance. Overall, these studies have found that children of same-sex parents fare relatively as well, if not better, compared with children raised by heterosexual couples. The gender of the child is an important moderating factor. Sons of same-sex couples are more likely to experience disapproval from their peers and face greater homophobic teasing than girls; boys may be at greater risk of experiencing emotional distress. This effect seems to depend on the level of social tolerance in their surrounding environments (Biblarz & Savci, 2010).

Nurses and health workers should be aware that same-sex couples often face particular challenges to safeguarding their well-being and that of their children. Although children raised by same-sex couples generally exhibit similar outcomes and levels of well-being, these children may be more sensitive to judgmental attitudes of individuals with whom they interact, including health workers.

Stepfamilies

Stepfamilies are formed when parents bring together children from a previous union. By contrast, remarriages or cohabiting unions in which neither partner brings children into the marriage are conceptualized and measured similarly to first marriages. The U.S. Census Bureau uses the term *blended families* to denote families with children that are formed when remarriages occur or when children living in a household share only one or no biological parents. The presence of a stepparent, stepsibling, or half-sibling designates a family as blended; these families can include adoptive children who are not the biological child of either parent if there are other children present who are not related to the adoptive child. In 2009, 13.3% of households with children under 18 were blended-family households, numbering 5.3 million (Kreider & Ellis, 2011a). Almost 16% of U.S. children

(11.7 million) lived in blended families in 2009. Blended families were the least common among Asian children (7%) and the most common among black and Hispanic children (17% each). Although the number of children living in blended families has increased by almost 2 million since 1991, the percentage increase has been negligible (from 15% to 16%) (Furukawa, 1994; Kreider & Ellis, 2011a). In 2011, the Census of Population in Canada identified stepfamilies for the first time. Nearly 13% of couple families with children were stepfamilies, and almost 10% of children aged 14 and under were living in stepfamilies in 2011 (Statistics Canada, 2012g).

Parental and financial responsibilities for biological parents are upheld by law, customs, roles, and rules that provide a cultural map of sorts for parents to follow in raising their children. Because no such map is available for stepfamilies, stepparents' roles, rules, and responsibilities must be defined, negotiated, and renegotiated by stepparents. Through these negotiations, many different types of stepfamilies are formed, resulting in a variety of configurations and different patterns of everyday living. The ambiguity surrounding roles in stepfamilies and the lack of a shared family history and kinship system provide opportunities to build new traditions and family rituals; however, they also open the door for greater conflict. Consider the following scenarios.

When asked by researchers, members of families who are all related by either blood or partnership (marriage or cohabitation) can very easily tell you and agree upon who is in their family. By contrast, members within stepfamilies often do not share a common definition of who is included in their family. Common omissions include stepchildren, biological children not living in the household, biological parents not living in the household, and stepparents (Furstenberg & Cherlin, 1991). Even biological siblings can have different ideas regarding who they consider to be family members depending on the degree of closeness they feel toward stepparents, biological parents, biological siblings, half-siblings, and stepsiblings, especially if the biological siblings are living in different households; a girl living with her biological mother and stepfather may consider her brother living with his biological father and a stepmother as a separate family.

Negotiations must occur with ex-spouses or ex-partners, as well as with former in-laws. Researchers have found that the ex-spouse relationship can play an important role in the well-being of stepfamilies (Golish, 2003) and may affect the relationship between the new stepparents, especially in the beginning of the relationship. Couples' relationships in stepfamilies and remarriages are informed and shaped by experiences in previous unions, leading to increased expectations in the remarriage. Remarried women expect and have more say in decision making than women in first marriages. In stepfamilies, the division of labor in the household is more egalitarian between spouses, as are economic roles and responsibilities (Allen, Baucom, Burnett, Epstein, & Rankin-Esquer, 2001).

Step-relationships in particular are often weak or ambivalent, and stress arises around various issues such as perceptions of playing favorites, or jealousy among biological children, of former spouses, and of stepchildren toward stepparents. These tensions arise because in some families stepparents are not viewed by stepchildren as real parents (Furstenberg & Cherlin, 1991). The level of conflict also depends on the age of children, increasing as children approach adolescence. Unlike in biological families where the role of parent emerges with the birth of the child (ascribed), stepparent roles must be earned (achieved). As a result, discipline in stepfamilies is often a problem. Additionally, it is more difficult to be a stepparent than a biological parent because new family cultures are being developed.

Like children growing up in single-parent families, children with stepparents have lower levels of well-being than children growing up with biological parents (Coleman, Ganong, & Fine, 2000). Thus, it is not simply the presence of two parents, but the presence of two biological parents that seems to promote children's healthy development. Despite these challenges, positive changes can occur when stepfamilies are formed. For example, a stepfather's income can compensate for the negative economic slide that tends to occur for divorced mothers, and a stepparent can alleviate the demands of single parenting (Smock, Manning, & Gupta, 1999).

Because stepfamilies comprise a significant proportion of families with children, nurses are likely to deal with parents whose roles and responsibilities are not well defined and with children who have behavioral problems, especially among recently formed blended families. Obtaining legal authorization for medical procedures can be challenging when legal obligations are unclear. Family nurses should take care to identify which parent(s) have legal responsibility for medical decision making. Health care workers should be aware that they may also need to notify nonresidential parents when their children require medical attention as these parents may share the legal right to make medical decisions.

Grandparents

One moderating factor in children's well-being in single-parent families can be the presence of grandparents in the home. Although the image of single-parent families is usually that of a mother living on her own and trying to meet the needs of her young child or children, many single mothers live with their parents. For example, in the United States in 2011, about 12% of children of single mothers lived in the homes of their grandparents compared with 8% of children of single fathers (U.S. Census Bureau, 2011g). An additional 5.2% of children of single mothers had a grandparent living with them compared with 4.7% of children of single fathers. This is a snapshot at one point in time, however. A much higher percentage of single mothers (36%) live in their parents' home *at some point* before their children are grown. African American single mothers with children at home are more likely than are others to live with a parent at some time.

Several studies have shown that the presence of grandparents has beneficial effects on children's outcomes and can buffer some of the disadvantages of living in a single-parent family (DeLeire & Kalil, 2002). This beneficial effect, however, seems to be more pronounced among whites than among African Americans, probably because white grandparents in the United States have more education and resources than black grandparents (Dunifon & Kowaleski-Jones, 2007). The involvement of grandparents in the lives of their children has even become an issue for court cases, as there have been several rulings in recent years on grandparents' visitation rights. The 2000 U.S. Census included a new set of questions on grandparents' support of grandchildren. Children whose parents cannot take care of them for one reason or another often live with their grandparents. In 1970, 2.2 million, or 3.2% of all American children, lived in their grandparents' households.

By 2011, this number increased to nearly 5 million, or 6.6% of all American children (U.S. Census Bureau, 2011f). Since the Great Recession in 2008 the number of children living with grandparents increased by 14%, from 4.3 million in 2008 to nearly 5 million in 2011. In 2011 in Canada, 4.8% of children aged 0 to 14 resided with at least one grandparent, up from 3.3% in 2001 (Statistics Canada, 2012e). In addition, in 2010 in the United States, grandparents were the regular child care providers for 15% of gradeschoolers and 23% of preschoolers (U.S. Census Bureau, 2010a, 2010b).

The prevalence of grandparent families is a result of demographic factors, socioeconomic conditions, and cultural norms. Increases in life expectancy have expanded the supply of potential kin support across generations, resulting in more multigenerational households. At the same time, changes in work and family life have increased parents' need for child care, which, coupled with pressing economic circumstances, has made multigenerational households a strategic symbiotic arrangement, especially among single-mother, low-income, and immigrant families (Glick & Van Hook, 2002). Grandparents often provide financial, emotional, child care, and residential support and, in turn, receive emotional and physical support (Bengtson, Giarrusso, Mabry, & Silverstein, 2002). Nonetheless, after practical and economic factors are taken into account, racial and ethnic differences in the prevalence of grandparent households remain. Strong kinship ties and family norms also seem to explain the prevalence of grandparent households, especially among African American, Native American, Hispanic, and immigrant families (Florian & Casper, 2011; Haxton & Harknett, 2009). Thus, norms stressing familial obligations may also be an important factor explaining differences in the formation of grandparent families.

Emerging research reveals that grandparents play an important role in multigenerational households, which is at odds with the traditional image of grandparents as family members who themselves require financial and personal support. Although early studies assumed that financial support flowed from adult children to their parents, more recent research suggests that the more common pattern is for parents to give financial support to their adult children (Bengtson, 2001; Bianchi et al., 2008). In

multigenerational households, it is more common for adult children and grandchildren to move into a house that grandparents own or rent. In 2007 in the United States, 64% of multigenerational households were headed by grandparents (Florian & Casper, 2011). Nearly 37% of all the grandparent-maintained families were skipped generation, that is, grandparents living with their grandchildren without the children's parents (authors' calculations based on data from U.S. Census Bureau, 2011f). Nearly 3.1% or 413,490 of all households in Canada contained a grandparent in 2011. Of these households, 53% also contained both parents, 32% contained a lone parent (mostly the mother), and 12% were skipped-generation households comprised of children residing with their grandparents without a parent (Statistics Canada, 2012e).

Grandparents who own or rent homes that include grandchildren and adult children are younger, healthier, and more likely to be in the labor force than are grandparents who live in a residence owned or rented by their adult children. Grandparents who maintain multigenerational households are also better educated (more likely to have at least a high-school education) than are grandparents who live in their children's homes (Casper & Bianchi, 2002). Nevertheless, supporting grandchildren can drain grandparents' resources. A recent study indicated that grandfathers who are primary caretakers of grandchildren are at higher risk of experiencing poverty if they are in a skipped-generation household, are ethnic minorities, or are not married (Keene, Prokos, & Held, 2012).

The structure of grandparent households differs by nativity. Although co-residential grandparent families are more common among immigrant families, immigrant grandparent families are less likely to be maintained by grandparents and less likely to be skipped generation. Thus, while the flow of support in native-born multigenerational families more often runs from older to younger generations, in immigrant grandparent families support more often flows from adult children to their older parents (Florian & Casper, 2011).

Parents who support both dependent children and dependent parents have been referred to as the "sandwich" generation, because they provide economic and emotional support for both the older and younger generations. Although grandparents in parent-maintained households tend to be older, in poorer health, and not as likely to be employed, many are in good health and are, in fact, working (Bryson & Casper, 1999). These findings suggest that, at the very least, the burden of maintaining a co-residential "sandwich family" household may be somewhat overstated in the popular press. Many of the grandparents who are living in the houses of their adult children are capable of contributing to the family income and helping with the supervision of children.

Many grandparents step in to assist their children in times of crisis. Some provide financial assistance or child care, whereas others are the primary caregivers for their grandchildren. Although grandmothers comprise the majority of grandparent caregivers, a sizable number of grandfather caregivers exist who are likely to experience more challenges than grandmothers as primary caregivers (Keene et al., 2012).

The recent increase in the numbers of grandparents raising their grandchildren is particularly salient to health care providers because both grandparents and grandchildren in this situation often suffer significant health problems (Casper & Bianchi, 2002). Researchers have documented high rates of asthma, weakened immune systems, poor eating and sleeping patterns, physical disabilities, and hyperactivity among grandchildren being raised by their grandparents (Kelley, Whitley, & Campos, 2011; Minkler & Odierna, 2001). Grandparents raising grandchildren tend to be in poorer health than their counterparts. They have higher levels of stress, higher rates of anxiety and depression, poorer self-rated health, and more multiple chronic health problems, especially if the grandchildren exhibit behavioral problems (Leder, Grinstead, & Torres, 2007). Other studies suggest, however, that these negative outcomes may not necessarily be a result of caring for grandchildren; instead, they may reflect grandparents' preexisting health conditions and economic circumstances before they began to raise their grandchildren (Hughes, Waite, LaPierre, & Luo, 2007). It is important to keep in mind that, although many of the grandparents who live in their adult children's homes are in good health, some of these grandparents require significant care. Nurses should also be aware that there are also adult children who provide care for their parents who are not living with them. Adults who provide care for both generations are likely to face both time and money concerns.

SUMMARY

Families change in response to economic conditions, cultural change, and shifting demographics, such as the aging of the population and immigration. North America has gone through a particularly tumultuous period in the last few decades, resulting in rapid changes in family structure, functions, and processes. Families have grown more diversified.

- More single-mother families, single-father families, same-sex parent families, and families with both parents in the labor force exist today than in the past. This translates into less time for parents to take care of the health needs of family members.
- Single mothers may find it particularly challenging to meet the health care needs of their families because they tend to have the least time and money to do so.
- More fathers are taking responsibility for being primary caretakers of their children and will be more likely than in the past to be the parent with whom nurses will interact.
- Changes in childbearing behaviors have also altered family life.
- Persistent levels of below replacement fertility in Canada have raised concerns about the future contraction of the population, which would reduce the tax base to support children and the growing number of senior citizens.
- As more couples delay childbearing, they are more likely to seek assistance to conceive from health care providers.
- The growing number of same-sex couples who aspire to become parents has further increased the demand for assisted reproductive technology.
- Nurses should be aware that this is a stressful time in families' lives, as more adults and children live in nontraditional family forms.
- Nurses also should be aware that the roles of parents and responsibility for children in these households may be ambiguous.
- Many North American families adopt children. These children are likely to face a period of adjustment and are also more likely than other children to have special health care needs.
- More grandparents are raising their grandchildren, and these grandchildren may suffer

from more health problems compared with other children.

- Many families maintained by grandparents are in poverty, and many of the grandparents in these families suffer from poor health themselves. Nurses will increasingly be likely to provide care to grandparent families, and they should be aware of the unique health and financial challenges these families face.

- As mortality rates at older ages continue to improve, and as baby boomers move into their retirement years, the proportions of the population of elderly persons will continue to increase. This demographic shift will increase the need for nurses who specialize in caring for elderly persons.

- More adults will have children and parents for whom they must care, increasing the need for care in both directions, that of the younger and the older.

- Working with health care needs of both generations will be a challenge for health care professionals, especially nurses who are on the front line in most health care systems.

- Today, more North Americans come from other countries than in the past.

- Health care providers will be serving a more ethnically and culturally diverse population.

- Many of these individuals speak a language other than English.

- Economics and family relationships remain intertwined. Family issues growing in importance include balancing paid work with child rearing, income inequality between men and women, fathers' parenting roles, the expected increase in the number of frail elderly persons, and intergenerational relationship changes due to the increase in life expectancy.

- The Great Recession has put economic strain on many families, increasing the likelihood of stress-related illness and decreasing the ability to afford appropriate care.

Families have been amazingly adaptive and resilient in the past; one would expect them to be so in the future.

REFERENCES

Allen, E. S., Baucom, D. H., Burnett, C. K., Epstein, N., & Rankin-Esquer, L. A. (2001). Decision-making power, autonomy, and communication in remarried spouses compared with first-married spouses. *Family Relations, 50,* 326–334.

Amato, P. R., & Dorius, C. (2010). Fathers, children, and divorce. In M. E. Lamb (Ed.), *The role of the father in child development* (5th ed., pp. 177–200). Hoboken, NJ: John Wiley & Sons.

Assisted Human Reproduction Canada (AHRC). (2011). Making a difference. AHRC annual report 2010–2011. Retrieved from http://www.ahrc-pac.gc.ca/v2/pubs/ar-ra-2010-2011-eng.php

Belle, S. H., & REACH II Investigators. (2006). Enhancing the quality of life of dementia caregivers from different ethnic or racial groups. *Annals of Internal Medicine, 145*(10), 727–738.

Bengtson, V. (2001). The Burgess Award lecture: Beyond the nuclear family: The increasing importance of multigenerational bonds. *Journal of Marriage and Family, 63*(1), 1–16.

Bengtson, V. L., Giarrusso, R., Mabry, J. B., & Silverstein, M. (2002). Solidarity, conflict, and ambivalence: Complementary or competing perspectives on intergenerational relationships. *Journal of Marriage and Family, 64,* 568–576.

Bianchi, S. M. (1995). The changing demographic and socioeconomic characteristics of single-parent families. *Marriage and Family Review, 20,* 71–97.

Bianchi, S. M. (2000). Maternal employment and time with children: Dramatic change or surprising continuity? *Demography, 37*(4), 401–414.

Bianchi, S. M., & Casper, L. M. (2000). American families. Population Bulletin, 55(4), 1–44. Retrieved from http://www.prb.org/source/acfac41.pdf

Bianchi, S. M., Hotz, V. J., McGarry, K., & Seltzer, J. A. (2008). Intergenerational ties: Alternative theories, empirical findings and trends, and remaining challenges. In A. Booth, N. Crouter, S. Bianchi, & J. Seltzer (Eds.), *Intergenerational caregiving* (pp. 3–43). Washington, DC: Urban Institute Press.

Bianchi, S. M., Raley, S. B., & Casper, L. M. (2012). Changing American families in the 21st century. In P. Noller & G. C. Karantzas (Eds.), *The Wiley-Blackwell handbook of couples and family relationships* (pp. 36–47). New York, NY: Wiley-Blackwell.

Biblarz, T. J., & Savci, E. (2010). Lesbian, gay, bisexual, and transgender families. *Journal of Marriage and Family, 72*(3), 480–497.

Boivin, J., Bunting, L., Collins, J. A., & Nygren, K. G. (2007). International estimates of infertility prevalence and treatment seeking: Potential need and demand for infertility medical care. *Human Reproduction, 22*(6),1506–1512.

Bryson, K., & Casper, L. M. (1999). *Coresident grandparents and grandchildren* (Current Population Reports, P23–198). Washington, DC: U.S. Census Bureau.

Bumpass, L. L., & Lu, H. (2000). Trends in cohabitation and implications for children's family contexts in the United States. *Population Studies, 54*(1), 29–41.

Carlson, M. J., & McLanahan, S. S. (2010). Fathers in fragile families. In M. E. Lamb (Ed.), *The role of the father in child development* (5th ed., pp. 241–269). Hoboken, NJ: John Wiley & Sons.

Casper, L. M., & Bianchi, S. M. (2002*). Continuity and change in the American family.* Thousand Oaks, CA: Sage.

Casper, L. M., & Cohen, P. (2000). How does POSSLQ measure up? Historical estimates of cohabitation. *Demography, 37*(2), 237–245.

Casper, L. M., & Haaga, J. G. (2005). Family and health demographics. In S. M. H. Hanson, V. Gedaly-Duff, & J. R. Kaakinen (Eds.), *Family health care nursing: Theory, practice and research* (3rd ed., pp. 39–68). Philadelphia, PA: F. A. Davis.

Chandra, A., Martinez, G. M., Mosher, W. D., Abma, J. C., & Jones, J. (2005). Fertility, family planning, and reproductive health of U.S. women: Data from the 2002 National Survey of Family Growth. *Vital & Health Statistics, Series 23*(25), 1–160.

Cherlin, A. J. (2009). *The marriage-go-round: The state of marriage and the family in America today.* New York, NY: Vintage Books.

Citizenship and Immigration Canada. (2011). Canada—Permanent residents by category, 2007–2011. Retrieved from http://www.cic.gc.ca/english/resources/statistics/facts2011-summary/01.asp

Citizenship and Immigration Canada. (2012). Health care—Refugees. Retrieved from http://www.cic.gc.ca/english/refugees/outside/arriving-healthcare.asp

Cohen, P. N., & Casper, L. M. (2002). In whose home? Multigenerational families in the United States, 1998–2000. *Sociological Perspectives, 45*(1), 1–20.

Coleman, M., Ganong, L., & Fine, M. (2000). Reinvestigating remarriage: Another decade of progress. *Journal of Marriage and the Family, 62*(4), 1288–1307.

DeLeire, T., & Kalil, A. (2002). Good things come in threes: Single-parent multigenerational family structure and adolescent adjustment. *Demography, 39,* 393–413.

DeNavas-Walt, C., Proctor, B. D., & Smith, J.C. (2012). Income, poverty, and health insurance coverage in the United States: 2011. Current population reports. Retrieved from http://www.census.gov/prod/2012pubs/p60-243.pdf

Dunifon, R., & Kowaleski-Jones, L. (2007). The influence of grandparents in single-mother families. *Journal of Marriage and Family, 69*(2), 465–481.

Farley, R. (1996). *The new American reality: Who we are, how we got here, where we are going.* New York, NY: Russell Sage Foundation.

First Call: BC Child and Youth Advocacy Coalition. (2011). 2011 BC child poverty report card. Retrieved from http://intraspec.ca/BC_ReporCard2011.pdf

Florian, S. M., & Casper, L. M. (2011, October). Structural differences in native-born and immigrant intergenerational families in the U.S. Paper presented at the annual meetings of the American Sociological Association, Las Vegas, NV.

Furstenberg, F., Jr. (1998). Good dads–bad dads: Two faces of fatherhood. In A. J. Cherlin (Ed.), *The changing American family and public policy* (pp. 193–218). Washington, DC: Urban Institute.

Furstenberg, F. F., & Cherlin, A. J. (1991). *Divided families: What happens to children when parents part.* Cambridge, MA: Harvard University Press.

Furukawa, S. (1994). *The diverse living arrangements of children: Summer 1991* (Current Population Reports, Series P70, No, 38). Washington, DC: U.S. Census Bureau.

Glick, J. E., & Van Hook, J. (2002). Parents' coresidence with adult children: Can immigration explain racial and ethnic variation? *Journal of Marriage and Family, 64,* 240–253.

Golish, T. (2003). Stepfamily communication strengths: Understanding the ties that bind. *Human Communication Research, 29*(1), 41–80.

Greenfeld, D. A. (2007). Gay male couples and assisted reproduction: Should we assist? *Fertility and Sterility, 88*(1), 18–20.

Grieco, E. M., Acosta, Y. D., De la Cruz, G. P., Gambino, C., Gryn, T., Larsen, L. J., ... Walters, N. P. (2012). The foreign-born population in the United States: 2010. U.S. Census Bureau. American Community Survey Reports. Retrieved from http://www.census.gov/prod/2012pubs/acs-19.pdf

Haxton, C. L., & Harknett, K. (2009). Racial and gender differences in kin support: A mixed-methods study of African American and Hispanic couples. *Journal of Marriage and Family, 30*(8), 1019–1040.

Hays, S. (2003). *Flat broke with children: Women in the age of welfare reform.* New York, NY: Oxford University Press.

Hernandez, D. J., & Brandon, P. D. (2002). Who are the fathers of today? In C. S. Tamis-LeMonda & N. Cabrera (Eds.), *Handbook of father involvement. Multidisciplinary perspectives* (pp. 33–62). Mahwah, NJ: Lawrence Erlbaum Associates.

Heuveline, P., Timberlake, J. M., & Furstenberg, F. F., Jr. (2003). Shifting child rearing to single mothers: Results from 17 Western nations. *Population and Development Review, 29*(1), 47–71.

Hilborn, R. (2011). Canadians go abroad to adopt 1,946 children in 2010. Retrieved from http://www.familyhelper.net/news/111027stats.html

Hoefer, M., Rytina, N., & Baker, B. C. (2011). Estimates of the unauthorized immigrant population residing in the United States: January 2010. Retrieved from http://www.dhs.gov/xlibrary/assets/statistics/publications/ois_ill_pe_2010.pdf

Hofferth, S. L., Pleck, J., Stueve, J. L., Bianchi, S., & Sayer, L. (2002). The demography of fathers: What fathers do. In C. S. Tamis-LeMonda & N. Cabrera (Eds.), *Handbook of father involvement. Multidisciplinary perspectives* (pp. 63–90). Mahwah, NJ: Lawrence Erlbaum Associates.

Hughes, M. E., Waite, L. J., LaPierre, T. A., & Luo, Y. (2007). All in the family: The impact of caring for grandchildren on grandparents' health. *Journal of Gerontology, 62B*(2), S108–S119.

Jones, J. (2008). Adoption experiences of women and men and demand for children to adopt by women 18–44 years of age in the United States, 2002. *Vital and Health Statistics, 23*(27), 1–36.

Keene, J. R., Prokos, A. H., & Held, B. (2012). Grandfather caregivers: Race and ethnic differences in poverty. *Sociological Inquiry, 82*(1), 49–77.

Kelley, S. J., Whitley, D. M., & Campos, P. E. (2011). Behavior problems in children raised by grandmothers: The role of caregiver distress, family resources, and the home environment. *Children and Youth Services Review, 33*(11), 2138–2145.

Kennedy, S., & Bumpass, L. (2008). Cohabitation and children's living arrangements: New estimates from the United States. *Demographic Research, 19*(47), 1663–1692.

King, R. B. (1999). Time spent in parenthood status among adults in the United States. *Demography, 36*(3), 377–385.

Klinenberg, E. (2012). *Going solo. The extraordinary rise and surprising appeal of living alone.* New York, NY: Penguin Press.

Kreider, R. M., & Ellis, R. (2011a). Living arrangements of children: 2009. Household economic studies. Retrieved from http://www.census.gov/prod/2011pubs/p70-126.pdf

Kreider, R. M., & Ellis, R. (2011b). Number, timing, and duration of marriage and divorces: 2009. Household economic studies. Retrieved from http://www.census.gov/prod/2011pubs/p70-125.pdf

Leder, S., Grinstead, L. N., & Torres, E. (2007). Grandparents raising grandchildren: Stressors, social support, and health outcomes. *Journal of Family Nursing, 13*(3), 333–352.

Lee, B. J. (2007). Adoption in Korea: Current status and future prospects. *International Journal of Social Welfare, 16,* 75–83.

Lee, R. (2003). The demographic transition: Three centuries of fundamental change. *Journal of Economic Perspectives, 17*(4), 167–190.

Levy, F. (1998). *The new dollars and dreams.* New York, NY: Russell Sage Foundation.

Lino, M. (2012). *Expenditures on children by families, 2011.* U.S. Department of Agriculture, Center for Nutrition Policy and Promotion, Miscellaneous Publication No. 1528-2011.

Lofquist, D., Lugaila, T., O'Connell, M., & Feliz, S. (2012). *Households and families: 2010*. 2010 Census briefs No. C2010BR-14, U.S. Census Bureau, Department of Commerce Economics and Statistics Administration. Retrieved from http://www.census.gov/prod/cen2010/briefs/c2010br-14.pdf

Martin, J. A., Hamilton, B. E., Ventura, S. J., Osterman, M. J. K., Wilson, E. C., & Mathews, T. J. (2012). Births: Final data for 2010. *National Vital Statistics Reports, 61*(1), 1–100. Retrieved from http://www.cdc.gov/nchs/data/nvsr/nvsr61/nvsr61_01.pdf

McDonald, P. (2000). Gender equity, social institutions and the future of fertility. *Journal of Population Research, 17*(1), 1–16.

McGarry, K., & Schoeni, R. F. (2000). Social security, economic growth, and the rise in elderly widows' independence in the twentieth century. *Demography, 37*(2), 221–236.

McLanahan, S., & Casper, L. (1995). Growing diversity and inequality in the American family. In R. Farley (Ed.), *State of the union: America in the 1990s* (pp. 1–46). New York, NY: Russell Sage Foundation.

Milan, A. (2011). Fertility: Overview, 2008. Component of Statistics Canada Catalogue no. 91-209-X, Report on the Demographic Situation in Canada. Retrieved from http://www.statcan.gc.ca/pub/91-209-x/2011001/article/11513-eng.htm

Minkler, M., & Odierna, D. (2001). California's grandparents raising children: What the aging network needs to know as it implements the national family caregiver support program. Center for the Advanced Study of Aging Services, University of California, Berkeley. Retrieved from http://cssr-pw01.berkeley.edu.libproxy.usc.edu/pdfs/CAgrandparents_entire.pdf

Myers, E. R., McCrory, D. C., Mills, A. A., Price, T. M., Swamy, G. K., Tantibhedhyangkul, J., ..., Matchar, D. B. (2008). *Effectiveness of assisted reproductive technology*. Rockville, MD: Agency for Healthcare Research and Quality.

National Center for Health Statistics. (2008). *Health, United States 2008, with chartbook on trends in the health of Americans*. Hyattsville, MD: Public Health Service.

Navaie-Walsier, M., Feldman, P. H., Gould, D. A., Levine, C., Kuerbis, A. N., & Donelan, K. (2001). The experiences and challenges of informal caregivers: Common themes and differences among whites, blacks, and Hispanics. *Gerontologist, 41*(6), 733–741.

Popenoe, D. (1993). American family decline, 1960–1990: A review and appraisal. *Journal of Marriage and the Family, 55*(3), 527–555.

Preston, S. H., Heuveline, P., & Guillot M. (2001). *Demography: Measuring and modeling population processes*. Oxford, England: Blackwell Publishers.

Raley, R. K. (2000). Recent trends and differentials in marriage and cohabitation. In L. Waite (Ed.), *Ties that bind: Perspectives on marriage and cohabitation* (pp. 19–39). New York, NY: Aldine de Gruyter.

Reinhardt, U. E. (2003). Does the aging of the population really drive the demand for health care? *Health Affairs, 22*(6), 27–39.

Rindfuss, R. R. (1991). The young adult years: Diversity, structural change, and fertility. *Demography, 28*(4), 493–512.

Rosenfeld, M. J. (2007). *The age of independence: Interracial unions, same-sex unions, and the changing American family*. Cambridge, MA: Harvard University Press.

Ruggles, S. (1994). The transformation of American family structure. *American Historical Review, 99*(1), 103–127.

Ruggles, S. (1996). Living arrangements of the elderly in America: 1880–1990. In T. Harevan (Ed.), *Aging and generational relations: Historical and cross-cultural perspectives* (pp. 254–263). New York, NY: Aldine de Gruyter.

Saenz, R. (2004). *Latinos and the changing face of America*. Washington, DC: Population Reference Bureau.

Schoen, R., & Canudas-Romo, V. (2006). Timing effects on divorce: 20th century experience in the United States. *Journal of Marriage and Family, 68*, 749–758.

Seltzer, J. A., Lau C. Q., & Bianchi, S. M. (2012). Doubling up when times are tough: A study of obligations to share a home in response to economic hardship. *Social Science Research, 41*, 1307–1319.

Service Canada. (2012). Changes to Old Age Security. Retrieved from http://www.servicecanada.gc.ca/eng/isp/oas/changes/index.shtml

Shiao, J. L., Tuan, M., & Rienzi, E. (2004). Shifting the spotlight: Exploring race and culture in Korean-White adoptive families. *Race and Society, 7*(1), 1–16.

Shin, H. B., & Kominski, R. A. (2010). Language use in the United States: 2007. American Community Survey Reports, ACS-12. Retrieved from www.census.gov/prod/2010pubs/acs-12.pdf

Silverstein, M., Gans, D., & Yang, F. (2006). Intergenerational support to aging parents: The role of norms and needs. *Journal of Family Issues, 27*(8), 1068–1084.

Singer, A. (2004). The rise of new immigrant gateways. Retrieved from http://www.brookings.edu/~/media/research/files/reports/2004/2/demographics%20singer/20040301_gateways.pdf

Smock, P. J., Manning, W. D., & Gupta, S. (1999). The effect of marriage and divorce on women's economic well-being. *American Sociological Review, 64*(6), 794–812.

Stacey, J. (1993). Good riddance to "The Family": A response to David Popenoe. *Journal of Marriage and the Family, 55*(3), 545–547.

Statistics Canada. (2007). Indicators of well-being in Canada: Family life—Young adults living with their parent(s). Retrieved from http://www4.hrsdc.gc.ca/.3ndic.1t.4r@-eng.jsp?iid=77

Statistics Canada. (2008). Indicators of well-being in Canada: Family life—Marriage. Retrieved from http://www4.hrsdc.gc.ca/.3ndic.1t.4r@-eng.jsp?iid=78

Statistics Canada. (2010). Women in Canada: Paid work 1976 to 2009. Retrieved from http://www.statcan.gc.ca/daily-quotidien/101209/dq101209a-eng.htm

Statistics Canada. (2011a). The Canadian population in 2011: Age and sex. Retrieved from http://www12.statcan.gc.ca/census-recensement/2011/as-sa/98-311-x/98-311-x2011001-eng.cfm

Statistics Canada. (2011b). Living arrangements of seniors. 2011 census in brief No. 4. Retrieved from http://www12.statcan.gc.ca/census-recensement/2011/as-sa/98-312-x/98-312-x2011003_4-eng.cfm

Statistics Canada. (2011c). Private households by household type, 2011 counts, for Canada, provinces and territories. Retrieved from http://www12.statcan.gc.ca/census-recensement/2011/dp-pd/hlt-fst/fam/Pages/highlight.cfm?TabID=1&Lang=E&Asc=1&PRCode=01&OrderBy=999&View=1&tableID=302&queryID=1

Statistics Canada. (2011d). Total fertility rate, 1926 to 2008 and completed fertility rate, 1911 to 1979. Retrieved from http://www.statcan.gc.ca/pub/91-209-x/2011001/article/11513/figures/desc/desc05-eng.htm

Statistics Canada. (2012a). Births and total fertility rate, by province and territory: 2006–2010. Retrieved from http://

www.statcan.gc.ca/tables-tableaux/sum-som/l01/cst01/hlth85b-eng.htm

Statistics Canada. (2012b). Divorce cases in civil court, 2010/2011. Retrieved from http://www.statcan.gc.ca/pub/85-002-x/2012001/article/11634-eng.htm

Statistics Canada. (2012c). Income in Canada 2010. Retrieved from http://www.statcan.gc.ca/pub/75-202-x/75-202-x2010000-eng.htm

Statistics Canada. (2012d). Population by sex and age group, 2012. Retrieved from http://www.statcan.gc.ca/tables-tableaux/sum-som/l01/cst01/demo10a-eng.htm

Statistics Canada. (2012e). Portrait of families and living arrangements in Canada. Retrieved from http://www12.statcan.gc.ca/census-recensement/2011/as-sa/98-312-x/98-312-x2011001-eng.cfm

Statistics Canada. (2012f). Time spent on unpaid care of a child in the household, by working arrangement and age of youngest child, Canada, 2010 (Table 6). Retrieved from http://www.statcan.gc.ca/pub/89-503-x/2010001/article/11546/tbl/tbl006-eng.htm

Statistics Canada. (2012g). 2011 census of population: Families, households, marital status, structural type of dwelling, collectives. Retrieved from http://www.statcan.gc.ca/daily-quotidien/120919/dq120919a-eng.htm

Statistics Canada. (2012h). 2011 census of population: Linguistic characteristics of Canadians. Retrieved from http://www.statcan.gc.ca/daily-quotidien/121024/dq121024a-eng.htm

Stephen, E. H., & Chandra, A. (2006). Declining estimates of infertility in the United States: 1982–2002. *Fertility and Sterility*, *86*(3), 516–523.

Stone, R. I. (2000). *Long-term care for the elderly with disabilities: Current policy, emerging trends, and implications for the twenty-first century*. New York, NY: Milbank Memorial Fund.

Sunderam, S., Kissin, D. M, Flowers, L., Anderson, J. E., Folger, S. G., Jamieson, D. J., & Barfield, W. D. (2012). Assisted reproductive technology surveillance—United States, 2009. *Surveillance Summaries*, *61*(SS7), 1–23. Retrieved from http://www.cdc.gov/mmwr/preview/mmwrhtml/ss6107a1.htm

Treas, J., & Torrecilha, R. (1995). The older population. In R. Farley (Ed.), *State of the union: America in the 1990s* (pp. 47–92). New York, NY: Russell Sage Foundation.

Uhlenberg, P. (1996). Mortality decline in the twentieth century and supply of kin over the life course. *Gerontologist*, *36*, 681–685.

U.S. Census Bureau. (2008). Estimated median age at first marriage, by sex: 1890 to the present (Table MS-2). Retrieved from http://www.census.gov/population/www/socdemo/hh-fam.html

U.S. Census Bureau. (2010a). Child care arrangements of grade-schoolers 5 to 14 years old living with mother, by employment status of mother and selected characteristics: Spring 2010 (Table 3A). Retrieved from http://www.census.gov/hhes/childcare/data/sipp/2010/tables.html

U.S. Census Bureau. (2010b). Child care arrangements of preschoolers under 5 years old living with mother, by employment status of mother and selected characteristics: Spring 2010 (Table 1A). Retrieved from http://www.census.gov/hhes/childcare/data/sipp/2010/tables.html

U.S. Census Bureau. (2010c). Child support payments agreed to or awarded custodial parents by selected characteristics and sex: 2009 (Table 4). Retrieved from http://www.census.gov/hhes/www/childsupport/cs09.html

U.S. Census Bureau. (2010d). Completed fertility for women 40 to 44 years old by single race in combination with other races and selected characteristics: June 2010 (Detailed Table 7). Retrieved from http://www.census.gov/hhes/fertility/data/cps/2010.html

U.S. Census Bureau. (2010e). Women who had a child in the last year per 1,000 women, by race, Hispanic origin, nativity status, and selected characteristics: June 2010. Detailed fertility tables (Table 4). Retrieved from http://www.census.gov/hhes/fertility/data/cps/2010.html

U.S. Census Bureau. (2011a). All parent/child situations, by type, race, and Hispanic origin of householder or reference person: 1970 to present (Table FM-2). Retrieved from http://www.census.gov/hhes/families/data/families.html

U.S. Census Bureau. (2011b). America's families and living arrangements: 2011. Family status and household relationship of people 15 years and over, by marital status, age, and sex: 2011 (Table A2). Retrieved from http://www.census.gov/population/www/socdemo/hh-fam/cps2011.html

U.S. Census Bureau. (2011c). Families, by presence of own children under 18: 1950 to present (Table FM-1). Retrieved from http://www.census.gov/hhes/families/data/families.html

U.S. Census Bureau. (2011d). Family groups: 2011 (Table FG10). Retrieved from http://www.census.gov/hhes/families/data/cps2011.html

U.S. Census Bureau. (2011e). Family status and household relationship of people 15 years and over, by marital status, age, and sex: 2011 (Table A2). Retrieved form http://www.census.gov/hhes/families/data/cps2011.html

U.S. Census Bureau. (2011f). Grandchildren under age 18 living in the home of their grandparents: 1970 to present (Table CH-7). Retrieved from http://www.census.gov/hhes/families/data/children.html

U.S. Census Bureau. (2011g). Living arrangements of children under 18 years/1 and marital status of parents, by age, sex, race, and Hispanic origin/2 and selected characteristics of the child for all children: 2011 (Table C3). Retrieved from http://www.census.gov/hhes/families/data/cps2011.html

U.S. Census Bureau. (2011h). Marital status of people 15 years and over, by age, sex, personal earnings, race, and Hispanic origin/1, 2011 (Table A1). Retrieved from http://www.census.gov/hhes/families/data/cps2011.html

U.S. Census Bureau. (2011i). More young adults are living in their parents' home. Census Bureau Reports, Newsroom. Retrieved from http://www.census.gov/newsroom/releases/archives/families_households/cb11-183.html

U.S. Census Bureau. (2011j). One-parent unmarried family groups with own children/1 under 18, by labor force status of the reference person: 2011 (Table FG5). Retrieved from http://www.census.gov/hhes/families/data/cps2011.html

U.S. Census Bureau. (2011k). One-parent unmarried family groups with own children/1 under 18, by marital status of the reference person: 2011 (Table FG6 One). Retrieved from http://www.census.gov/population/www/socdemo/hh-fam/cps2011.html

U.S. Census Bureau. (2011l). Population 65 years and over in the United States: 2011. American Community Survey. Retrieved from http://factfinder2.census.gov/faces/tableservices/jsf/pages/productview.xhtml?pid=ACS_11_1YR_S0103&prodType=table

U.S. Census Bureau. (2011m). Unmarried partners of the opposite sex, by presence of children: 1960 to present (Table UC-1).

Retrieved from www.census.gov/population/socdemo/hh-fam/uc1.xls

U.S. Census Bureau. (2012). Statistical abstract of the United States 2012 (Table 1335). Washington, DC: U.S. Government Printing Office.

U.S. Centers for Disease Control and Prevention (CDC). (2010). Immigrant and refugee health. Retrieved from http://www.cdc.gov.libproxy.usc.edu/immigrantrefugeehealth/about-refugees.html

U.S. Centers for Disease Control and Prevention (CDC). (2012). What is assisted reproductive technology? Retrieved from http://www.cdc.gov/art/

U.S. Department of Health and Human Services. (2009). Summary of immigrant eligibility restrictions under current law. Retrieved from http://aspe.hhs.gov/hsp/immigration/restrictions-sum.shtml

U.S. Department of Health and Human Services. (2011). *Trends in foster care and adoption—FY 2002–FY 2011*. Washington, DC: Administration for Children and Families, Administration Children's Bureau. Retrieved from www.acf.hhs.gov/programs/cb

U.S. Department of Health and Human Services. (2012). *Healthy marriage initiative*. Washington, DC: Administration for Children and Families Archives. Retrieved from http://archive.acf.hhs.gov/healthymarriage/

U.S. Department of Homeland Security. (2012). *Annual flow report. U.s. legal permanent residents: 2011*. Washington, DC: Office of Immigration Statistics.

U.S. Department of State. (2011). *Intercountry adoption*. Washington, DC: Office of Children's Issues, United States. Retrieved from http://adoption.state.gov/about_us/statistics.php

Vandivere, S., Malm, K., & Radel, L. (2009). *Adoption USA: A chartbook based on the 2007 National Survey of Adoptive Parents*. Washington, DC: U.S. Department of Health and Human Services, Office of the Assistant Secretary for Planning and Evaluation.

Verrier, N. N. (1993). *The primal wound: Understanding the adopted child* (reprinted 2011). Baltimore, MD: Gateway Press.

Voice of Russia World Service in English (RUVR). (2007). Russian families' change of heart on adoption. Retrieved from http://www.ruvr.ru/main.php?lng=eng&q=18909&cid=59&p=16.11.2007

Waite, L. J., & Gallagher, M. (2000). *The case for marriage: Why married people are happier, healthier and better off financially*. Garden City, NY: Doubleday.

World Health Organization. (2011). Life tables for WHO member states 2009. Retrieved from http://apps.who.int/ghodata/?vid=720

Yee, J. L., & Schulz, R. (2000). Gender differences in psychiatric morbidity among family caregivers: A review and analysis. *Gerontologist, 40*(2), 147–164.

Suggested Readings

Baker, M. (Ed.). (2009). *Families: Changing trends in Canada* (6th ed.). Toronto, Canada: McGraw-Hill Ryerson.

Bianchi, S. M., & Casper, L. M. (2005). Explanations of family change: A family demographic perspective. In V. L. Bengtson, A. C. Acock, K. R. Allen, P. Dilworth-Anderson, & D. M. Klein (Eds.), *Sourcebook of family theory and research* (pp. 93–117). Thousand Oaks, CA: Sage.

Brown, S. L. (2004). Family structure and child well-being: The significance of parental cohabitation. *Journal of Marriage and Family, 66*(2), 351–367.

Brown, S. L. (2010). Marriage and child well-being: Research and policy perspectives. *Journal of Marriage and Family, 72*(5), 1059–1077.

Burton, P., & Phipps, S. (2011). Families, time, and well-being in Canada. *Canadian Public Policy, 37*(3), 395–423.

The decade in review. (2000). *Journal of Marriage and Family, 62*(4), 873–1307.

The decade in review. (2010). *Journal of Marriage and Family, 72*(3), 401–803.

Edin, K., & Kefalas, M. (2005). *Promises I can keep: Why poor women put motherhood before marriage*. Berkeley, CA: University of California Press.

Ellwood, D. T., & Jencks, C. (2004). The uneven spread of single-parent families: What do we know? Where do we look for answers? In K. M. Neckerman (Ed.), *Social inequality* (pp. 3–77). New York, NY: Russell Sage Foundation.

Farley, R., & Haaga, J. (Eds.). (2004). *The American people*. New York, NY: Russell Sage Foundation.

Federal Interagency Forum on Aging-Related Statistics. (2012). *Older Americans 2012: Key national indicators of well-being*. Washington, DC: U.S. Government Printing Office.

Federal Interagency Forum on Child and Family Statistics. (2012). *America's children: Key national indicators of well-being, 2012*. Washington, DC: U.S. Government Printing Office.

Jacobs, J., & Gerson, K. (2004). *The time divide: Work, family, and gender inequality*. Cambridge, MA: Harvard University Press.

Kennedy, S., & Bumpass, L. (2008). Cohabitation and children's living arrangements: New estimates from the United States. *Demographic Research, 19*(47), 1663–1692.

McLanahan, S. (2004). Diverging destinies: How children are faring under the second demographic transition. *Demography, 41*(4), 607–627.

McLanahan, S. (2009). Fragile families and the reproduction of poverty. *Annals of the American Academy of Political and Social Science, 621*, 111–131.

National Center for Health Statistics. (2001). *Healthy people 2000 final review*. Hyattsville, MD: Public Health Service.

Nock, S. L. (1998). *Marriage in men's lives*. New York, NY: Oxford University Press.

Pettit, B., & Hook, J. (2009). *Gendered tradeoffs: Family, social policy, and economic inequality in twenty-one countries*. New York, NY: Russell Sage.

Stewart, S. D. (2006). *Brave new stepfamilies: Diverse paths. Toward stepfamily living*. Thousand Oaks, CA: Sage Publications.

Waite, L. J., Bachrach, C. A., Hinden, M., Thomson, E., & Thornton, A. T. (2000). *The ties that bind: Perspectives on marriage and cohabitation*. New York, NY: Aldine de Gruyter.

Contacts

- *Child Trends: www.childtrends.org*
- *Designing New Models for Explaining Family Change and Variation: www.soc.duke.edu/~efc/*
- *Federal Interagency Forum on Aging-Related Statistics: www.agingstats.gov*
- *Federal Interagency Forum on Child and Family Statistics: www.childstats.gov*
- *Fragile Families and Child Wellbeing Study: www.fragilefamilies.princeton.edu/*
- *Kaiser Commission on Medicaid and the Uninsured: www.kff.org*
- *Kids Count: The Annie E. Casey Foundation: www.aecf.org/kidscount*

- *National Center for Health Statistics, U.S. Department of Health and Human Services, Centers for Disease Control and Prevention: www.cdc.gov/nchs*
- *National Institute on Aging, National Institutes of Health: www.nia.nih.gov*
- *National Center for Marriage and Family Research: ncfmr.bgsu.edu/*
- *National Institute of Child Health and Human Development, National Institutes of Health: www.nichd.nih.gov*
- *The National Longitudinal Study of Adolescent Health: www.cpc.unc.edu/projects/addhealth*

- *Population Reference Bureau: www.prb.org*
- *Statistics Canada/Statistique Canada: www.statcan.gc.ca*
- *U.S. Census Bureau: www.census.gov*
- *Welfare, Children, & Families: A Three City Study: web.jhu.edu/threecitystudy/index.html*

chapter 3

Theoretical Foundations for the Nursing of Families

Joanna Rowe Kaakinen, PhD, RN

Shirley May Harmon Hanson, PhD, PMHNP/ARNP, FAAN, CFLE, LMFT

Critical Concepts

- Theories inform the practice of nursing. Practice informs theory and research. Theory, practice, and research are interactive, and all three are critical to the profession of nursing and family care.

- The major purpose of theory in family nursing is to provide knowledge and understanding that improves the quality of nursing care of families.

- By understanding theories and models, nurses are prepared to think more creatively and critically about how health events affect family clients. Theories and models provide different ways of comprehending issues that may be affecting families, and offer choices for action.

- The theoretical/conceptual frameworks and models that provide the foundations for nursing of families have evolved from three major traditions and disciplines: family social science, family therapy, and nursing.

- No single theory, model, or conceptual framework adequately describes the complex relationships of health events on family structure, function, and process.

- Nurses who use an integrated theoretical approach build on the strengths of families in creative ways. Nurses who use a singular theoretical approach to working with families limit the possibilities for families they serve. By integrating several theories, nurses acquire different ways to conceptualize problems, thus enhancing thinking about interventions.

By understanding theories and models, nurses are prepared to think creatively and critically about how health events affect the family client. The reciprocal or interactive relationship between theory, practice, and research is that each aspect informs the other, thereby expanding knowledge and nursing interventions to support families. Theories and models extend thinking to higher levels of understanding problems and circumstances that may be affecting families and, thereby, offer more choice and options for nursing interventions.

Currently, no single theory, model, or conceptual framework adequately describes the complex relationships of family structure, function, and process. Nor does one theoretical perspective give nurses a sufficiently broad base of knowledge and understanding to guide assessment and interventions with families. No one theoretical perspective is better, more comprehensive, or more correct than another (Doane & Varcoe, 2005; Kaakinen & Hanson, 2010). The goal for nurses is to have a deep understanding of the stresses that families experience when their family clients have a health event and to support and implement family interventions based on theoretical perspectives that best match the needs identified by the family.

Many theoretical approaches exist to understanding families. The purpose of this chapter is to demonstrate how families who have members experiencing a health event are conceptualized differently depending on the theoretical perspective. In this chapter, nurses seek different data depending on which theory is being used, both to understand the family experience and to determine the interventions offered to the family to help bring them back to a state of stability.

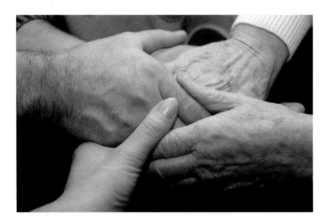

This chapter begins with a brief review of the components of a theory and how the components contribute to the nursing of families. It then presents five theoretical approaches for working with families, ranging from a broader to a more specific perspective:

- Family Systems Theory
- Developmental and Family Life Cycle Theory
- Bioecological Theory
- Chronic Illness Framework
- Family Assessment and Intervention Model

The chapter utilizes a case study of a family with a member who is experiencing progressive multiple sclerosis (MS) to demonstrate these five different theoretical approaches to nursing care.

RELATIONSHIP BETWEEN THEORY, PRACTICE, AND RESEARCH

In nursing, the relationship of theory to practice constitutes a dynamic feedback loop rather than a static linear progression. Theory, practice, and research are mutually interdependent. Theory grows out of observations made in practice and is tested by research; then tested theory informs practice, and practice, in turn, facilitates the further refinement and development of theory. Figure 3-1 depicts the dynamic relationship between theory, practice, and research.

Theories do not emerge all at once; they build slowly over time as data are gathered through practice, observation, and analysis of evidence. Relating together the various concepts that emerge from observation and evidence occurs through a purposeful, thoughtful reasoning process. *Inductive reasoning* is a process that moves from specific pieces of information toward a general idea; it is thinking about how the parts create the whole. *Deductive reasoning* goes in the opposite direction from inductive reasoning. Deductive reasoning is where the general ideas of a given theory generate more specific questions about what filters back into the cycle; it helps refine understanding of the theory and how to apply the theory to practice (Smith & Hamon, 2012; White & Klein, 2008).

Theories are designed to make sense of the world, to show how one thing is related to another and how together they make a meaningful pattern that can predict the consequences of certain clusters of characteristics or events. Theories are abstract, general ideas that are subject to rules of

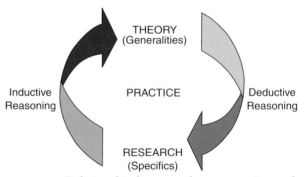

FIGURE 3-1 Relationship between theory, practice, and research. *(Adapted from Smith, S. R., Hamon, R. R., Ingoldsby, B. B., & Miller, J. E. [2008]. Exploring family theories [2nd ed.]. New York, NY: Oxford University Press.)*

organization. Theories provide a general framework for understanding data in an organized way, as well as showing us how to intervene. We live in a time when tremendous amounts of information are readily available and quickly accessible in multiple forms. Therefore, theories provide ways to transform this huge volume of information into knowledge and to integrate/organize the information to help us make better sense of our world (White, 2005). Ideally, nursing theories represent logical and intelligible patterns that make sense of the observations nurses make in practice and enable nurses to predict what is likely to happen to clients (Polit & Beck, 2011). Theories can be used as a level of evidence on which to base nursing practice (Fawcett & Desanto-Madeya, 2012). The major function of theory in family nursing is to provide knowledge and understanding that improves nursing services to families.

Most important, theories explain what is happening; they provide answers to "how" and "why" questions, help to interpret and make sense of phenomena, and predict or point to what could happen in the future. All scientific theories use the same components: *concepts*, *relationships*, and *propositions*. We will discuss hypotheses and conceptual models as well.

Concepts, the building blocks of theory, are words that create mental images or abstract representations of phenomena of study. Concepts, or the major ideas expressed by a theory, may exist on a continuum from empirical (concrete) to abstract (Powers & Knapp, 2010). The more concrete the concept, the easier it is to figure out when it applies or does not apply (White & Klein, 2008). For example, one concept in Family Systems Theory is that families have boundaries. A highly abstract aspect of this concept is that the boundary reflects the energy between the environment and the system. A more concrete aspect of this concept is that families open or close their boundaries in times of stress.

Propositions are statements about the relationship between two or more concepts (Powers & Knapp, 2010). A proposition might be a statement such as the following: Families as a whole influence the health of individual family members. The word *influence* links the two concepts of "families as a whole" and "health of individual family members." Propositions denote a relationship between the subject and the object. Propositions may lead to

hypotheses. Theories are generally made up of several propositions that emphasize the relationships among the concepts in that specific theory.

A *hypothesis* is a way of stating an expected relationship between concepts or an expected proposition (Powers & Knapp, 2010). The concepts and propositions in the hypothesis are derived from and driven by the original theory. For example, using the concepts of family and health, one could hypothesize that there is an interactive relationship between how a family is coping and the eventual health outcome of family members. In other words, the family's ability to cope with stress affects the health of individual family members and, in turn, the health of this individual family member influences the family's ability to cope. This hypothesis may be tested by a research study that measures family coping strategies and family members' health over time and that uses statistical procedures to look at the relationships between the two concepts.

A *conceptual model* is a set of general propositions that integrate concepts into meaningful configurations or patterns (Fawcett & Desanto-Madeya, 2012). Conceptual models in nursing are based on the observations, insights, and deductions that combine ideas from several fields of inquiry. Conceptual models provide a frame of reference and a coherent way of thinking about nursing phenomena. A conceptual model is more abstract and more comprehensive than a theory. Like a conceptual model, a conceptual framework is a way of integrating concepts into a meaningful pattern, but conceptual frameworks are often less definitive than models. They provide useful conceptual approaches or ways in which to look at a problem or situation, rather than a definite set of propositions.

In this chapter, the terms *conceptual model or framework* and *theory or theoretical framework* are often used interchangeably. In part, that is because no single theoretical base exists for the nursing of families. Rather, nurses typically draw from many theoretical conceptual foundations using a more pluralistic and eclectic approach. The interchangeable use of these various terms reflects the fact that there is considerable overlap among ideas in the various theoretical perspectives and conceptual models/frameworks and that many "streams of influence" are important for family nurses to incorporate into practice. As might be expected, a substantial amount of cross-fertilization among disciplines has occurred, such as between social science and nursing, and concepts originating in one theory or discipline have been translated into similar concepts for use in another discipline. Currently, no one theoretical perspective gives nurses a sufficiently broad base of knowledge and understanding to guide assessment and interventions with families.

THEORETICAL AND CONCEPTUAL FOUNDATIONS FOR THE NURSING OF FAMILIES

Nursing is a scientific discipline; thus, nurses are concerned about the relationships between ideas and data. Nurse scholars explain empirical observations by creating theories, which can be used as evidence in evidence-based practice (Fawcett & Garity, 2008). Nurse researchers investigate and test the models and relationships. Nurses in practice use theories, models, and conceptual frameworks to help clients achieve the best outcomes (Kaakinen & Hanson, 2010). In nursing, evidence, in the form of theory, is used to explain and guide practice. The theoretical foundations, theories, and conceptual models that explain and guide the practice of nursing families have evolved from three major traditions and disciplines: family social science theories, family therapy theories, and nursing models and theories. Figure 3-2 shows the theoretical frameworks that influence the nursing of families.

Family Social Science Theories

Of the three sources of theory, *family social science theories* are the best developed and informative

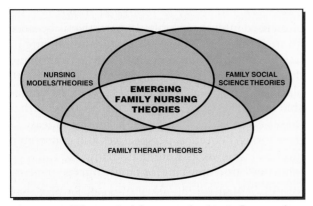

FIGURE 3-2 Theoretical frameworks that influence the nursing of families.

about family phenomena; examples of such theories include the following: family function, the environment-family interchange, interactions and dynamics within the family, changes in the family over time, and the family's reaction to health and illness. Table 3-1 summarizes the basic family social science theories and provides some classic references where these theories originate. It is somewhat challenging to use the purist form of family social science theories as a basis for nursing assessment and intervention because of their abstract nature. Despite this challenge, in recent years, nursing and family scholars have made strides in extrapolating and morphing these theories for use in clinical work (Fine & Fincham, 2012; Kaakinen & Hanson, 2010).

Family Therapy Theories

Family therapy theories are newer than and not as well developed as family social science theories. Table 3-2 lists these theories and the names of some foundational scholars who first developed them. These theories emanate from a practice discipline of family therapy, rather than from an academic discipline of family social science. Family therapy theories were developed to work with troubled families and, therefore, focus primarily on family pathology. Nevertheless, these conceptual models describe family dynamics and patterns that are found, to some extent, in all families. Because these models are concerned with what can be done to facilitate change in "dysfunctional" families, they are both descriptive and prescriptive. That is, they not only describe and explain observations made in practice but also suggest treatment or intervention strategies.

Nursing Conceptual Frameworks

Finally, of the three types of theories, *nursing conceptual frameworks* are the least developed "theories" in relation to the nursing of families. Table 3-3 lists several of the theories and theorists from within the nursing profession. During the 1960s and 1970s, nurses placed great emphasis on the development of nursing models. Other than the Neuman Systems Model (Neuman & Fawcett, 2010) and the Behavioral Systems Model for Nursing (Johnson, 1980), both of which were based on family social science theories, the majority of the classic nursing

Table 3-1	Family Social Science Theories Used in Family Nursing Practice
Family Social Science Theory	**Summary**
Structural Functional Theory Artinian (1994) Friedman, Bowden, & Jones (2003) Nye & Berardo (1981)	The focus is on families as an institution and how they function to maintain family and social network.
Symbolic Interaction Theory Hill & Hansen (1960) Nye (1976) Rose (1962) Turner (1970)	The focus is on the interactions within families and the symbolic communication.
Developmental Theory and Family Life Cycle Theory Carter & McGoldrick (2005) Duvall (1977) Duvall & Miller (1985)	The focus is on the life cycle of families and representing normative stages of family development.
Family Systems Theory von Bertalanffy (1950, 1968)	The focus is on the circular interactions among members of family systems, which result in functional or dysfunctional outcomes.
Family Stress Theory Hill (1949, 1965) McCubbin & McCubbin (1993) McCubbin & Patterson (1983)	The focus is on the analysis of how families experience and cope with stressful life events.
Change Theory Maturana (1978) Maturana & Varela (1992) Watzlawick, Weakland, & Fisch (1974) Wright & Leahey (2013) Wright & Watson (1988)	The focus is on how families remain stable or change when there is change within the family structure or from outside influences.
Transition Theory White (2005) White & Klein (2008)	The focus is on understanding and predicting the transitions families experience over time by combining Role Theory, Family Development Theory, and Life Course Theory.

theorists from the 1970s focused on individual patients and not on families as a unit of care/analysis. The nursing models, in large part, represent a deductive approach to the development of nursing science (general to specific). Although they embody an important part of our nursing heritage, these nursing conceptual frameworks and their deductive approach are viewed more critically today. As the science of nursing has evolved, more inductive approaches to nursing theory development (specific to the general) are now being advocated.

Table 3-4 shows the differences between family social science theories, family therapy theories, and nursing models/theories as they inform the practice of nursing with families. The following case study is used to demonstrate how the five different theoretical approaches may inform a nurse's work with one particular family.

Table 3-2	Family Therapy Theories Used in Family Nursing Practice

Family Therapy Theories	Summary
Structural Family Therapy Theory Minuchin (1974) Minuchin & Fishman (1981) Minuchin, Rosman, & Baker (1978) Nichols (2004)	This systems-oriented approach views the family as an open sociocultural system that is continually faced with demands for change, both from within and from outside the family. The focus is on the whole family system, its subsystems, boundaries, and coalitions, as well as family transactional patterns and covert rules.
International Family Therapy Theory Jackson (1965) Satir (1982) Watzlawick, Beavin, & Jackson (1967)	This approach views the family as a system of interactive or interlocking behaviors or communication processing. Emphasis is on the here and now rather than on the past. Key interventions focus on establishing clear, congruent communication and clarifying and changing family rules.
Family Systems Therapy Theory Freeman (1992) Kerr & Bowen (1988) Toman (1961)	This approach focuses on promoting differentiation of self from family and promoting differentiation of intellect from emotion. Family members are encouraged to examine their processes to gain insight and understanding into their past and present. This therapy requires a long-term commitment.

Table 3-3	Nursing Theories and Models Used in Family Nursing Practice

Nursing Theories and Models	Summary
Nightingale Nightingale (1859)	Family is described as having both positive and negative influences on the outcome of family members. The family is seen as a supportive institution throughout the life span for its individual family members.
Rogers's Science of Unitary Human Beings Casey (1996) Rogers (1970, 1986, 1990)	The family is viewed as a constant open system energy field that is ever-changing in its interactions with the environment.
Roy's Adaptation Model Roy (1976) Roy & Roberts (1981)	The family is seen as an adaptive system that has inputs, internal control, and feedback processes and output. The strength of this model is understanding how families adapt to health issues.
Johnson's Behavioral Systems Model for Nursing Johnson (1980)	The family is viewed as a behavioral system composed of a set of organized interactive interdependent and integrated subsystems that adjust and adapt with internal and external forces to maintain stability.
King's Goal Attainment Theory King (1981, 1983, 1987)	The family is seen as the vehicle for transmitting values and norms of behavior across the life span, which includes the role of a sick family member. Family is responsible for addressing the health care function of the family. Family is seen as both an interpersonal and a social system. The key component is the interaction between the nurse and the family as client.

Table 3-3	Nursing Theories and Models Used in Family Nursing Practice—cont'd

Nursing Theories and Models	Summary
Neuman's Systems Model Neuman (1983, 1995)	The family is viewed as a system. The family's primary goal is to maintain its stability by preserving the integrity of its structure by opening and closing its boundaries. It is a fluid model that depicts the family in motion and not a static view of family from one perspective.
Orem's Self-Care Deficit Theory Gray (1996) Orem (1983a, 1983b, 1985)	The family is seen as the basic conditioning unit in which the individual learns culture, roles, and responsibilities. Specifically, family members learn how to act when one is ill. The family's self-care behavior evolves through interpersonal relationships, communication, and culture that is unique to each family.
Parse's Human Becoming Theory Parse (1992, 1998)	The concept of family and who makes up the family is viewed as continually becoming and evolving. The role of the nurse is to use therapeutic communication to invite family members to uncover their meaning of the experience, to learn what the meaning of the experience is for each other, and to discuss the meaning of the experience for the family as a whole.
Friedemann's Framework of Systemic Organization Friedemann (1995)	The family is described as a social system that has the expressed goal of transmitting culture to its members. The elements central to this theory are family stability, family growth, family control, and family spirituality.
Denham's Family Health Model Denham (2003)	Family health is viewed as a process over time of family member interactions and health-related behaviors. Family health is described in relation to contextual, functional, and structural domains. Dynamic family health routines are behavioral patterns that reflect self-care, safety and prevention, mental health behaviors, family care, illness care, and family caregiving.

Table 3-4	Family Social Science Theories, Family Therapy Theories, and Nursing Models/Theories		
Criteria	Family Social Science Theories	Family Therapy Theories	Nursing Models/Theories
Purpose of theory	Descriptive and explanatory (academic models); to explain family functioning and dynamics.	Descriptive and prescriptive (practice models); to explain family dysfunction and guide therapeutic actions.	Descriptive and prescriptive (practice models); to guide nursing assessment and intervention efforts.
Discipline focus	Interdisciplinary (although primarily sociological).	Marriage and family therapy; family mental health; new approaches focus on family strengths.	Nursing focus.
Target population	Primarily "normal" families (normality-oriented).	Primarily "troubled" families (pathology-oriented).	Primarily families with health and illness problems.

Source: Kaakinen, J. R., & Hanson, S. M. H. (2010). Theoretical foundations for nursing of families. In J. R. Kaakinen, V. Gedaly-Duff, D. P. Coehlo, & S. M. H. Hanson (Eds.), *Family health care nursing: Theory, practice and research* (4th ed.). Philadelphia, PA: F. A. Davis, with permission.

Family Case Study: Jones Family

Setting: Inpatient acute care hospital

Nursing Goal: Work with the family to assist them in preparation for discharge that is planned to occur in the next 2 days.

Family Members:

The Jones family is a nuclear family. The Jones family genogram and ecomap are illustrated in Figures 3-3 and 3-4.

- Robert: 48 years old; father, software engineer, full-time employed.
- Linda: 43 years old; mother, stay-at-home homemaker, has progressive multiple sclerosis, which recently has worsened significantly.
- Amy: 19 years old; oldest child, daughter, freshman at university in town 180 miles away.
- Katie: 13 years old: middle child, daughter, sixth grade, usually a good student.
- Travis: 4 years old: youngest child, son, just started attending an all-day preschool because of his mother's illness.

Jones Family Story:

Linda was diagnosed with multiple sclerosis (MS) at age 30 when Katie was 3 months old. After she was diagnosed with MS, Linda had a well-controlled, slow progression of her illness. Travis was a surprise pregnancy for Linda at

age 39, but he is described as "a blessing." Linda and Robert are devout Baptists, but they did discuss abortion in light of the fact that Linda's illness could progress significantly after the birth of Travis. Their faith and personal beliefs did not support abortion. They made the decision to continue with Linda's pregnancy, knowing the risk that it might exacerbate and speed up her MS. Linda had an uncomplicated pregnancy with Travis. She felt well until 3 months postpartum with Travis when she noted a significant relapse of her MS.

Over the last 4 years, Linda has experienced development of progressive relapsing MS, which is a progressive disease from onset with clear, acute relapses without full recovery after each relapse. The periods between her relapses are characterized by continuing progression of the disease. She now has secondary progressive multiple sclerosis because of her increased weakness. Robert and Linda are having sexual issues with decreased libido and painful intercourse for Linda. Both are experiencing stress in their marital roles and relationship.

Currently, Linda has had a serious relapse of her MS. She is hospitalized for secondary pneumonia from aspiration. She has weakness in all limbs, left foot drag, and increasing ataxia. Linda will be discharged with a wheelchair (this aid is new as she has used a cane up until this admission). She has weakness of her neck muscles and cannot hold her head steady for long periods. She has difficulty swallowing, which probably caused her

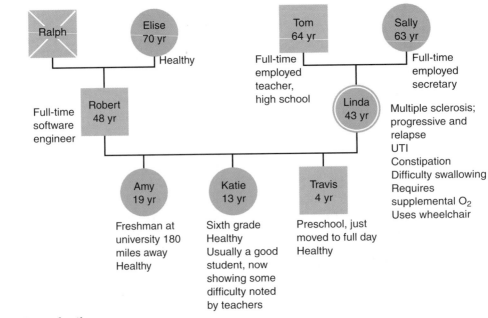

FIGURE 3-3 Jones family genogram.

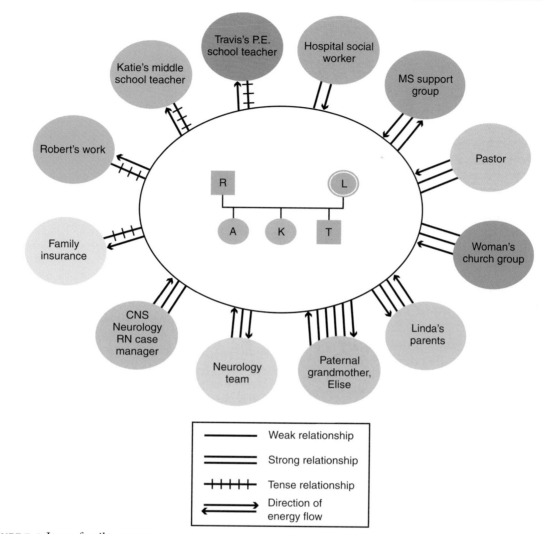

FIGURE 3-4 Jones family ecomap.

aspiration. She has numbness and tingling of her legs and feet. She has severe pain with flexion of her neck. Her vision is blurred. She experiences vertigo at times and has periodic tinnitus. Constipation is a constant problem, together with urinary retention that causes periodic urinary tract infections.

Health Insurance:

Robert receives health insurance through his work that covers the whole family. Hospitalizations are covered 80/20, so they have to pay 20% of their bills out of pocket. Although Robert is employed full-time, this cost adds heavily to the financial burden of the family. Robert has shared with the nurses that he does not know whether he should take his last week of vacation when his wife comes home, or whether he should save it for a time when her condition

worsens. Robert works for a company that offers family leave, but without pay.

Family Members:

Robert reports being continuously tired from caring for his wife and children, as well as working full-time. He asked the doctor for medication to help him sleep and decrease his anxiety. He said he is afraid that he may not hear Linda in the night when she needs help. He is open to his mother moving in to help care for Linda and the children. He began counseling sessions with the pastor in their church.

Amy is a freshman at a university that is 180 miles away in a different town. Her mother is proud of Amy going to college on a full scholarship. Amy does well in her coursework but travels home weekends to help the

(continued)

family and her mother. Amy is considering giving up her scholarship to transfer home to attend the local community college. She has not told her parents about this idea yet.

Katie is in the sixth grade. She is typically a good student, but her latest report card showed that she dropped a letter grade in most of her classes. Katie is quiet. She stopped having friends over to her home about 6 months ago when her mother began to have more ataxia and slurring of speech. Linda used to be very involved in Katie's school but is no longer involved because of her illness. Katie has been involved in Girl Scouts and the youth group at church.

Travis just started going to preschool 2 months ago for full days because of his mother's illness. This transition to preschool has been difficult for Travis because he had been home full-time with Linda until her disease worsened. He is healthy and developmentally on target for his age.

Linda's parents live in the same town. Her parents, Tom and Sally, both work full-time and are not able to help. Robert's widowed mother, Elise, lives by herself in her own home about 30 minutes out of town and has offered to move into the Jones' home to help care for Linda and the family.

Discharge Plans: Linda will be discharged home in 2 days.

THEORETICAL PERSPECTIVES AND APPLICATION TO FAMILIES

The case of the Jones family is used throughout the rest of this chapter to demonstrate how assessments, interventions, and options for care vary based on the particular theoretical perspective chosen by nurses caring for this family.

Family Systems Theory

Family Systems Theory has been the most influential of all the family social science frameworks (Kaakinen & Hanson, 2010; Wright & Leahey, 2013). Much of the understanding of how a family is a system derives from physics and biology perspectives that organisms are complex, organized, and interactive systems (Bowen, 1978; von Bertalanffy, 1950, 1968). Nursing theorists who have expanded the concept of systems theory include Hanson (2001), Johnson (1980), Neuman (1995), Neuman and Fawcett (2010), Parker and Smith (2010), Walker (2005), and Wilkerson and Loveland-Cherry (2005).

The Family Systems Theory is an approach that allows nurses to understand and assess families as an organized whole and/or as individuals within family units who form an interactive and interdependent system (Kaakinen & Hanson, 2010). Family Systems Theory is constructed of concepts and propositions that provide a framework for thinking about the family as a system. Typically, in family nursing, we look at three-generational family systems (Goldenberg & Goldenberg, 2012).

One of the major assumptions of Family Systems Theory is that family system features are designed to maintain stability, although these features may be adaptive or maladaptive. At the same time, families change constantly in response to stresses and strains from both the internal and external environments. Family systems increase in complexity over time and increase their ability to adapt and to change (Smith & Hamon, 2012; White & Klein, 2008). The family systems theoretical perspective encourages nurses to see individual clients as participating members of a larger family system. Figure 3-5 depicts a mobile showing how family systems work. Any change in one member of the family affects all members of the family. As it applies to the Jones family, nurses who are using this perspective would assess the impact of Linda's illness on the entire family, as well as the effects of family functioning on Linda. The goal of nurses is to help maintain or restore the stability of the family, to help family members achieve the highest level of functioning that they can. Therefore, emphasis should be on the whole, rather than on any given individual. Some of the concepts of systems theory that help nurses working with families are explained in the following sections.

Concept 1: All Parts of the System Are Interconnected

What influences one part of the system influences all parts of the system. When an individual in a family experiences a health event, all members are affected because they are connected. The effect on each family member varies in intensity and

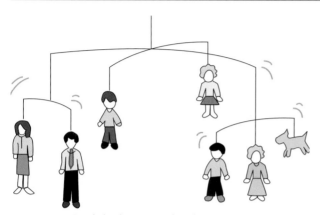

FIGURE 3-5 Mobile depicting family system.

quality. In the Jones case study, all members of the Jones family are touched when Linda's health condition changes, requiring her to be hospitalized. Linda takes on the role of a sick person and must give up some of her typical at-home mother roles; she is physically ill in the hospital. She feels guilty about not being at home for her family. Robert is affected because he has to assume the care of Katie and Travis. These tasks require getting them ready for school, transporting them to school and other events, and making lunches. Katie gives up some after-school activities to help Travis when he gets home from preschool. Travis misses the food his mother prepared for him, his afternoon alone time with his mother when they read a story, and being tucked into bed at night with songs and a back rub. Amy, who is a freshman in college, finds it difficult to concentrate while reading and studying for her college classes. The formal and informal roles of all these family members are affected by Linda's hospitalization. What affects Linda affects all the members of the Jones family in multiple ways.

Concept 2: The Whole Is More Than the Sum of Its Parts

The family as a whole is composed of more than the individual lives of family members. It goes beyond parents and children as separate entities. Families are not just relationships between the parent-child but are all relationships seen together. As we look at the Jones family, it is a nuclear family—mother, father, and three children. They are a family system that is experiencing the stress of a chronically ill mother who is deteriorating over time; each of them is individually affected, but so is the family as a

whole affected by this unexpected (nonnormative) family health event. The individuals in this family may, at times, wonder what will happen to them as a family (whole) when Linda dies.

One way of visualizing the family as a whole is to think of how the Jones family has built the concept of the "Jones Family Easter." Even though Linda always decorates the house and bakes several special dishes for the family for this holiday, this year she has been too ill to decorate or cook for Easter. The family as a whole feels stressed by the loss of routine and ritual as it represents a change in their family tradition and beliefs. Thus, the family loss is larger than individual loss of this tradition.

Concept 3: All Systems Have Some Form of Boundaries or Borders Between the System and Its Environment

Families control the in-flow of information and people coming into its family system to protect individual family members or the family as a whole. Boundaries are physical or abstract imaginary lines that families use as barriers or filters to control the impact of stressors on the family system (Smith & Hamon, 2012; White & Klein, 2008). Family boundaries include levels of permeability in that they can be closed, flexible, or too open to information, people, or other forms of resources. Some families have closed boundaries as exemplified by statements such as, "We as a family pull together and don't need help from others," or "We take care of our own." For example, if the Jones family were to have a *closed boundary*, they would not want to meet with the social worker or, if they did, they would reject the idea of a home-health aide and respite care.

Some families have *flexible boundaries*, which they control and selectively open or close to gain balance or adapt to the situation. For example, the Jones family welcomes a visit from the pastor but turns down visits from some of the women in Linda's Bible study group. Some families have *too open boundaries* in which they are not discriminating about who knows their family situation or the number of people from whom they seek help. Open boundaries can invite chaos and unbalance if the family is not selective in the quantity or quality of resources. If the Jones family were to have truly *open boundaries*, it may reach out to the larger community for resources and have different church members come stay with the children every evening. The permeability of boundaries resides on a continuum and varies from family to family.

Concept 4: Systems Can Be Further Organized Into Subsystems

In addition to conceptualizing the family as a whole, nurses can think about the subsystems of the family, which may include husband to wife, mother to child, father to child, child to child, grandparents to parents, grandparents to grandchildren, and so forth. These subsystems take into account the three dimensions of families discussed in Chapter 1: structure, function (including roles), and processes (interconnection and dynamics). By understanding these three dimensions, family nurses can streamline interventions to achieve specific family outcomes. For example, the Jones family has the following subsystems: parents, siblings, parent-child, a daughter subsystem, an in-law subsystem, and a grandparent subsystem. The nurse may work to decrease family stress by focusing on the marital spouse subsystem to help Linda and Robert continue couple time, or the nurse may focus on the sibling subsystem of Katie and Travis and their after-school activities.

Application of Family Systems Theory to the Jones Family

The focus of the nurses' practice from this perspective is family as the client. Nurses work to help families maintain and regain stability. Assessment questions of family members are focused on the family as a whole. While planning for Linda's discharge that is scheduled in the next couple of days, a nurse would ask questions such as the following to explore with Linda or with Linda and Robert:

- Who are members of your family? (See Concept 1.)
- How do you see your family being involved in your care once you go home? (See Concept 1.)
- Who in your family will experience the most difficulty coping with the changes, especially now that you will be using a wheelchair? (See Concept 1.)
- How are the members of your family meeting their personal needs at this time? (See Concept 1.)
- The last time your condition worsened, what helped your family the most? (See Concept 2.)

- The last time your condition worsened, what was the least help to your family? (See Concept 2.)
- Who outside of your immediate family do you see as being a potential person to help your family during the next week when you go home? (See Concept 3.)
- How do you feel your family would react to having a home-health aide come to help you twice a week? (See Concept 3.)
- Are there some friends, church members, or neighbors who might be able to help with some of the everyday management issues, such as carpooling to school, or providing some after-school care for Travis so Katie could go to her after-school activities? (See Concepts 3 and 4.)
- What are your thoughts about how the children will react to having Grandma Elise here to help the family? (See Concept 4.)

Interventions by family nurses must address individuals, subsystems within the family, and the whole family all at the same time. One strategy would be to assess family process and functioning and then offer intervention strategies to assist the family in its everyday functioning. Nurses could ask the following types of questions about functioning:

- Linda and Robert, from what you have told me, it appears that your oldest daughter, Amy, has been able to help take on some of the parental jobs in the family by being the errand runner, chauffeur, and grocery shopper. Now that Amy is off to college, which of your family roles will need to be covered by someone else for a while when you and Linda first come home: cooking, laundry, chauffeur, cleaning the house?
- Because you both shared with me that your family likes to go bowling on family night out, how do you envision how Linda being in a wheelchair might affect family night out?
- Robert and Linda, have the two of you discussed legal durable power of attorney for health care so Robert can make health care decisions when the time comes that Linda may not be able to do this for herself? Linda, who would you prefer to make health care decisions for you, should you not be able to do so? Let's discuss what those health care decisions might involve.

■ Tell me about your personal/sexual relationship that you, Linda, are experiencing now that you are more disabled.

The goal of using a family systems perspective is to help the family reach stability by building on their strengths as a family, using knowledge of the family as a social system, and understanding how the family is an interconnected whole that is adapting to the changes brought about by the health event of a given family member.

Strengths and Weaknesses of Family Systems Theory

The strengths of the general systems framework are that this theory covers a large array of phenomena and views the family and its subsystems within the context of its suprasystems (the larger community in which it is embedded). Moreover, it is an interactional and holistic theory that looks at processes within the family, rather than at the content and relationships between the members. The family is viewed as a whole, not as merely a sum of its parts. Another strength of this approach is that it is an excellent data-gathering method and assessment strategy, such as using a family genogram to gather a snapshot of the family as a whole or other family system assessment instruments discussed in Chapter 4.

Systems theory also has its limitations (Smith & Hamon, 2012). Because this theoretical orientation is so global and abstract, it may not be specific enough for beginners to define family nursing interventions. It is important for family nurses to be able to understand conceptually how important the family as a whole is to the practice of family nursing. As health care systems continue to emphasize the autonomy of the individual, it takes time and practice to develop ways to deeply understand how a family, as a whole, is greater than the members of the family.

Developmental and Family Life Cycle Theory

Developmental Theory provides a framework for nurses to understand normal family changes and experiences over the members' lifetimes; the theory assesses and evaluates both individuals and families as a whole. Developmental stages for individuals have been detailed by psychologists and sociologists, such as Erikson, Piaget, and Bandura.

Families are seen as a system in that what happens at one level has powerful ramifications at other levels of the system. Families are seen as the basic social unit of society and as the optimal level of intervention.

The family developmental theories are specifically geared to understanding families and not individuals (Smith & Hamon, 2013; White & Klein, 2008). Families, like individuals, are in constant movement and change throughout time—the family life cycle. Family developmental theorists who inform the nursing of families include Duvall (1977); Duvall and Miller (1985); and McGoldrick, Carter, and Garcia-Preto (2010). The original work of Duvall (1977), and later Duvall and Miller (1985), examined how families were affected or changed cognitively, socially, emotionally, spiritually, and physically when all members experienced developmental changes. The relationships among family members are affected by changes in individuals, and changes in the family as a whole affected the individuals within the family. These theorists recognized that families are stressed at common and predictable stages of change and transition and need to undergo adjustment to regain family stability. This early theoretical work was primarily based on the experiences of white Anglo middle-class nuclear families, with a married couple, children, and extended family.

McGoldrick et al. (2010) expanded on the original Developmental and Family Life Cycle Theory because they recognized the dramatically changing landscape of family structure, functions, and processes that was making it increasingly difficult to determine normal predictable patterns of change in families. They replaced the concept of "nuclear family" with "immediate family," which takes into consideration all family structures, such as stepfamilies, gay families, and divorced families. Instead of addressing the legal aspects of being a married couple, they viewed the concept of couple relationships and commitment as a focal point for family bonds.

Concept 1: Families Develop and Change Over Time

According to Family Developmental Theory, family interactions among family members change over time in relation to structure, function (roles), and processes. The stresses created by these changes in family systems are somewhat predictable for different stages of family development.

The first way to view family development is to look at predictable stresses and changes as they relate to the age of the family members and the social norms the individuals experience throughout their development. The classic traditional work of Duvall (1977) and Duvall and Miller (1985) identified overall family tasks that need to be accomplished for each stage of family development, as related to the developmental trajectory of the individual family members. It starts with couples getting married and ends with one member of the couple dying. Refer to Table 3-5 for a detailed list of the traditional family life cycle stages and developmental tasks. McGoldrick et al. (2010) expanded the traditional developmental and family life cycle theory to address changes in the family that undergoes a divorce. Table 3-6 outlines the emotional process of a family undergoing a divorce and describes the developmental tasks the family deals with at different stages.

According to this theory, families have a predictable natural history. The first stage involves the simple husband-wife pairing, and the family group becomes more complex over time with the addition of new members. When the younger generation leaves home to take jobs or marry, the original family group becomes less complex again.

The second way to view family development is to assess the predictable stresses and changes in families based on the stage of family development and how long the family is in that stage. For example, suppose each of the following couples have made a choice to be childless: a newly married couple, a couple who have been married for 3 years, and a couple who have been married for

Table 3-5	Traditional Family Life Cycle Stages and Developmental Tasks
Stages of Family Life Cycle	**Family Developmental Tasks**
Married couple	Establishing relationship as a married couple.
	Blending of individual needs, developing conflict-and-resolution approaches, communication patterns, and intimacy patterns.
Childbearing families with infants	Adjusting to pregnancy and then infant.
	Adjusting to new roles, mother and father.
	Maintaining couple bond and intimacy.
Families with preschool children	Understanding normal growth and development.
	If more than one child in family, adjusting to different temperaments and styles of children.
	Coping with energy depletion.
	Maintaining couple bond and intimacy.
Families with school-age children	Working out authority and socialization roles with school.
	Supporting child in outside interests and needs.
	Determining disciplinary actions and family rules and roles.
Families with adolescents	Allowing adolescents to establish their own identities but still be part of family.
	Thinking about the future, education, jobs, working.
	Increasing roles of adolescents in family, cooking, repairs, and power base.
Families with young adults: launching	After member moves out, reallocating roles, space, power, and communication.
	Maintaining supportive home base.
	Maintaining parental couple intimacy and relationship.
Middle-aged parents	Refocusing on marriage relationship.
	Ensuring security after retirement.
	Maintaining kinship ties.
Aging families	Adjusting to retirement, grandparent roles, death of spouse, and living alone.

Table 3-6 Family Life Cycle for Divorcing Families

Phase	Emotional Process of Transition: Prerequisite Attitude	Developmental Issues
Divorce		
The decision to divorce	Acceptance of inability to resolve marital tensions sufficiently to continue relationship.	Acceptance of one's own part in the failure of the marriage.
Planning the breakup of the system	Supporting viable arrangements for all parts of the system.	a. Working cooperatively on problems of custody, visitation, and finances.
		b. Dealing with extended family about the divorce.
Separation	a. Willingness to continue cooperative co-parental relationship and joint financial support of children.	a. Mourning loss of intact family.
	b. Work on resolution of attachment to spouse.	b. Restructuring marital and parent-child relationships and finances; adaptation to living apart.
		c. Realignment of relationships with extended family; staying connected with spouse's extended family.
The divorce	More work on emotional divorce: overcoming hurt, anger, guilt, among other emotions.	a. Mourning loss of intact family.
		b. Retrieval of hopes, dreams, expectations from the marriage.
		c. Staying connected with extended families.
Postdivorce Family		
Single parent (custodial household or primary residence)	Willingness to maintain financial responsibilities, continue parental contact with ex-spouse, and support contact of children with ex-spouse and his or her family.	a. Making flexible visitation arrangements with ex-spouse and family.
		b. Rebuilding own financial resources.
		c. Rebuilding own social network.
Single parent (noncustodial)	Willingness to maintain financial responsibilities and parental contact with ex-spouse, and to support custodial parent's relationship with children.	a. Finding ways to continue effective parenting.
		b. Maintaining financial responsibilities to ex-spouse and children.
		c. Rebuilding own social network.

Source: Adapted from Carter, B., & McGoldrick, M. (2005). The divorce cycle: A major variation in the American family life cycle. In B. Carter & M. McGoldrick (Eds.), *The expanded family life cycle: Individual, family, and social perspectives* (3rd ed.). New York, NY: Allyn & Bacon.

15 years (White & Klein, 2008). The stresses each couple experiences from this decision would be different.

Concept 2: Families Experience Transitions From One Stage to Another

Disequilibrium occurs in the family during the transitional periods from one stage of development to the next stage. When transitions occur, families experience changes in kinship structures, family roles, social roles, and interaction. Family stress is considered to be greatest at the transition points as families adapt to achieve stability, redefine their concept of family in light of the changes, and realign relationships as a result of the changes (McGoldrick et al., 2010). For example, marriage changes the status of all family members, creates new relationships for family members, and joins two different complex family systems.

Family developmental theorists explore whether families make these transitions "on time" or "off time" according to cultural and social expectations

(Smith & Hamon, 2012; White & Klein, 2008). For example, it is "off time" for a couple in their forties to have their first child. It is still considered "on time" in North America to have a couple be married before the birth of a child, but that norm may be changing given the increased numbers of babies born to couples who are not married but cohabitate.

Even though some family developmental needs and tasks must be performed at each stage of the family life cycle, developmental tasks are general goals, rather than specific jobs that must be completed at that time. Achievement of family developmental tasks enables individuals within families to realize their own individual tasks. According to family developmental theory, every family is unique in its composition and in the complexity of its expectations of members at different ages and in different roles. Families, like individuals, are influenced by their history and traditions and by the social context in which they live. Furthermore, families change and develop in different ways because their internal/external demands and situations differ. Families may also arrive at similar developmental levels using different processes. Despite their differences, however, families have enough in common to make it possible to chart family development over the life span in a way that applies to most, if not all families (Friedman, Bowden, & Jones, 2003). Families experience stress when they transition from one stage to the next. The predictable changes that are based on these family developmental steps are called *normative* changes. When changes occur in families out of sequence, "off time," or are caused by a different family event, such as illness, they are called *nonnormative*.

In contrast with the Duvall (1977) and later Duvall and Miller's (1985) traditional developmental approach, Carter and McGoldrick (1989) and McGoldrick et al. (2010) built on this work by approaching family development from the perspective of family life cycle stages. They explored what happens within families when family members enter or exit their family group; they focus on specific family experiences, such as disruption in family relationships, roles, processes, and family structure. Examples of a family member leaving would be divorce, illness, a miscarriage, or death of a family member. Examples of family members entering would include birth, adoption, marriage, or other formal union.

Today, the Developmental and Family Life Cycle Theory remains useful as long as it is viewed generally for use with families, despite all the current variations of families. McGoldrick et al. (2010) recently expanded the Family Life Cycle to incorporate the changing family patterns and broaden the view of both development and the family.

Application of Developmental and Family Life Cycle Theory to the Jones Family

In conducting family assessments using the developmental model, nurses begin by determining the family structure and where this family falls in the family life cycle stages. Using the developmental tasks outlined in the developmental model, the nurse has a ready guide to anticipate stresses the family may be experiencing or to assess the developmental tasks that are not being accomplished. Family assessment would also entail determining whether the family is experiencing a "normative" or "nonnormative" event in the family life cycle.

According to Duvall and Miller (1985), the Jones family is in the *Families With Young Adults: Launching Phase* because Amy left home and is now a freshman at a college. She is living away from home for the first time. Regardless of the fact that the Jones family is experiencing a nonnormative event (unexpected, developmental stressor) because Linda, the mother, is now in the hospital, the family is also experiencing the normative or expected challenges for a family when the oldest child leaves home. This is a good example of where major individual and whole family events coincide and present challenges for families. Questions to explore with the family might include the following:

1. How has the family addressed the reallocation of family household physical space since Amy left for school? (For example, the allocation of bedrooms or the arrangement of space within the bedroom if Katie and Amy shared the bedroom).
2. How has Amy developed as an indirect caregiver (such as calling home to chat with dad and see how he is doing, talking with the siblings and teasing or supporting their efforts, or sharing with parents her school life to reduce their worry about her adjustment)?
3. How have family roles changed since Amy left for school? What roles did Amy perform

for the family that someone else needs to pick up now? For example, who will perform such roles as chauffeur, grocery shopper, errand runner, and babysitter now that Linda is not able and Amy is gone?

4. How has the power structure of the family shifted now that Katie is more responsible for the care of Travis?

5. How has the parents' couple time changed since Amy went off to college?

With the developmental approach, nursing interventions may include helping the family to understand individual and family developmental tasks. Interventions could also include helping the family understand the normalcy of disequilibrium during these transitional periods. Another intervention is to help the family mitigate these transitions by capitalizing on family rituals. Family rituals serve to decrease the anxiety of changes in that they help link the family to other family members and to the larger community (Imber-Black, 2005).

Family nurses must recognize that every family must accomplish both individual and family developmental tasks for every stage of the Developmental and Family Life Cycle. Events at one stage of the cycle have powerful effects at other stages. Helping families adjust and adapt to these transitions is an important role for family nurses. It is important for nurses to keep in mind the needs and requirements of both the family as a whole and the individuals who make up the family.

Strengths and Weaknesses of the Developmental and Family Life Cycle

A major strength of the developmental approach is that it provides a systematic framework for predicting what a family may be experiencing at any stage in the family life cycle. Family nurses can assess a family's stage of development, the extent to which the family has achieved the tasks associated with that stage of family development, and problems that may or may not exist. It is a superb theoretical approach for assisting nurses who are working with families on health promotion. Family strengths and available resources are easier to identify because they are based on assisting families to achieve developmental milestones.

A primary criticism of family development theory is that it best describes the trajectory of intact, two-parent, heterosexual nuclear families. The original eight-stage model was based on a nuclear family, assumed an intact marriage throughout the life cycle of the family, and was organized around the oldest child's developmental needs. It did not take into account divorce, death of a spouse, remarriage, unmarried parents, childless couples, or cohabitating or gay and lesbian couples. It normalized one type of family and invalidated others (Smith & Hamon, 2012). Today's families vary widely in their makeup and in their roles. The traditional view of families moving in a linear direction from getting married, tracking children from preschool to launching, middle-aged parents, and aging families is no longer so clear-cut and applicable. Carter and McGoldrick (1989, 2005), Carter (2005), and McGoldrick et al. (2010) expanded the family developmental model to include stresses in the remarried family. As family structures continue to change in response to the culture and ecologic system, trajectories of families likely will not fit within the traditional developmental framework (White & Klein, 2008).

Bioecological Systems Theory

Urie Bronfenbrenner was one of the world's leading scholars in the field of developmental psychology (Bronfenbrenner, 1972a, 1972b, 1979, 1981, 1986, 1997; Bronfenbrenner & Morris, 1998). He contributed greatly to the ecological theory of human development, which concentrated on the interaction and interdependence of humans—as biological and social entities—with the environment. Originally this idea was called the Human Ecology Theory, then it was changed to Ecological Systems Theory, and it finally evolved into the *Bioecological Systems Theory* (Bronfenbrenner & Lerner, 2004). The Bioecological System is the combination of children's biological disposition and environmental forces coming together to shape the development of human beings. This theory combines both Developmental Theory and Systems Theory to understand individual and family growth.

Before Bronfenbrenner, child psychologists studied children, sociologists examined families, anthropologists analyzed society, economists scrutinized the economic framework, and political scientists focused on political structures. Through Bronfenbrenner's groundbreaking work in "human ecology," environments from the family to larger economic/political structures have come to be viewed as part of the life course from childhood through adulthood. This "bioecological" approach to human development crosses over barriers among the social sciences and builds bridges among the disciplines, allowing for better understanding to emerge about key elements in the larger social structure that are vital for optimal human development (both individual and family) (Boemmel & Briscoe, 2001).

The human ecology framework brings together other diverse influences. From evolutionary theory and genetics comes the view that humans develop as individual biological organisms with capacities limited by genetic endowment (*ontogenetic development*) that lead to hereditary familial characteristics. From population genetics comes the perspective that populations change by means of natural selection. For the individual, this means that individuals/families demonstrate their fitness by adapting to ever-changing environments. From ecological theories come the notion that human and family development is "contextualized" and "interactional" (White & Klein, 2008, p. 247). All of this leads to the never-ending debate related to the dual nature of humans as constructions of both biology and culture, hence the argument nature versus nurture. Although this debate has never been resolved, scientists have moved beyond debate to the realization that the development of most human traits depends on a nature/nurture interaction rather than on one versus the other (White & Klein, 2008). Thus, Bronfenbrenner moved his own theory and ideas from the concept and terminology of ecology (environment) to bioecology (both genetics and society) as a way of embracing two developmental origins for this theory. His Bioecological Systems Theory emphasizes the interaction of both the biological/genetics (ontologic/nature) and the social context (society) characteristics of development (Smith & Hamon, 2012; White & Klein, 2008).

The human bioecological perspective consists of a framework of four locational/spatial contexts and one time-related context (Bengtson, Acock, Allen, Dilworth-Anderson, & Klein, 2005). A primary feature of this theory is the premise that individual and family development is contextual over time. According to Bronfenbrenner, individual development is affected by five types or levels of environmental systems (Figure 3-6) (Emory University, 2008). Family Bioecological Theory describes the interactions and influences on the family from systems at different levels of engagement.

Microsystems are the settings in which individuals/families experience and create day-to-day reality. They are the places people inhabit, the people with whom they live, and the things they do together. In this level, people fulfill their roles in families, with peers, in schools, and in neighborhoods where they are in the most direct interaction with agents around them.

Mesosystems are the relationships among major microsystems in which persons or families actively participate, such as families and schools, families and religion, and families to peers. For example, how does the interaction between families and school affect families? Can the relationship between families and their religious/spiritual communities be used to help families?

Exosystems are external environments that influence individuals and families indirectly. The person may not be an active participant within these systems, but the system has an effect on the persons/families. For example, a parent's job experience affects family life, which, in turn, affects the children (parent's job's travel requirements, job stress, salary). Furthermore, governmental funding to other microsystems environments—schools, libraries, parks, health care, and day care—affect the experiences of children and families.

Macrosystems are the broad cultural attitudes, ideologies, or belief systems that influence institutional environments within a particular culture/subculture in which individuals/families live. Examples include the Judeo-Christian ethic, democracy, ethnicity, and societal values. Mesosystems and exosystems are set within macrosystems, and together they are the "blueprints" for the ecology of human and family development.

Chronosystems refer to time-related contexts where changes occur over time and have an effect on the other four levels/systems of development mentioned earlier. Chronosystems include the patterning of environmental events and transitions over the life course of individuals/families. These effects are created by time or critical periods in development and are influenced by sociohistorical conditions, such as parental divorce, unexpected death of a parent, or a war. Individuals/families have no control over the evolution of such external systems over time.

Within each one of these levels are roles, norms, and rules that shape the environment.

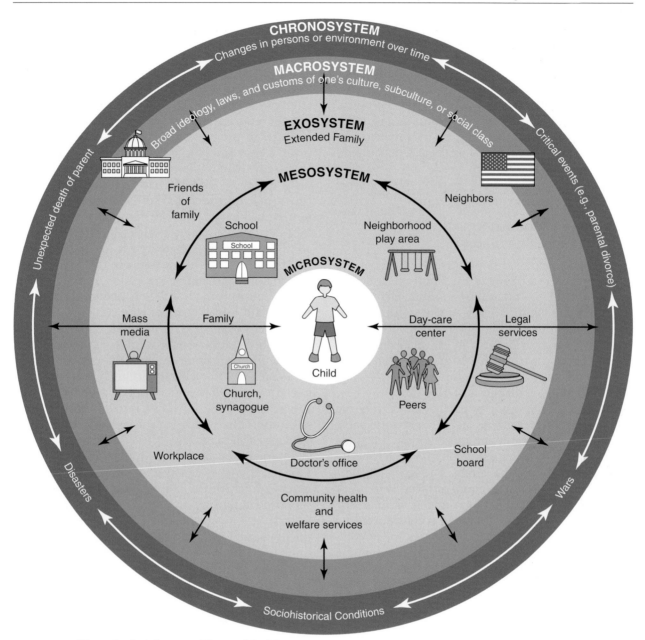

FIGURE 3-6 Bioecological Systems Theory Model.

Bronfenbrenner's model of human/family development acknowledges that people develop not in isolation, but rather in relation to their larger environment: families, home, schools, communities, and society. All of these interactive, ever-changing, and multilevel environments over time are key to understanding human/family development.

Bronfenbrenner uses the term *bidirectional* to describe the influential interactions that take place between children and their relationships with parents, teachers, and society. All relationships among humans/families and their environment are bidirectional or interactional. The environment influences us as individuals or families, but, in turn, individuals/families influence what happens in their own environments. This kind of interaction is also basic to family systems theory.

In the bioecological framework, what happens outside family units is as important as what happens inside individual members and family units.

Developing families are on center stage as an active force shaping their social experiences for themselves. The ecological perspective views children/families and their environments as mutually shaping systems, each changing and adapting over time (again, a systems perspective). The bioecological approach addresses both opportunities and risks. Opportunities mean that the environment offers families material, emotional, and social encouragement compatible with their needs and capacities. Risks to family development are composed of direct threats or the absence of opportunities.

Application of the Bioecological Systems Theory to the Jones Family

Assessment consists of looking at all levels of the system when interviewing the family in a health care setting. Assessment of the *microsystem* reveals that the Jones family consists of five members: two parents and three children. They live in a two-story home with four bedrooms in an older suburban section of the town. Mother Linda had been a full-time homemaker before experiencing health problems related to her diagnosis of MS. The *mesosystem* assessment for the family consists of identifying the schools the children attend, neighborhood/friends, extended family, and religious affiliation. The oldest daughter is a college student who travels home on weekends to help the family. The second daughter is in a local middle school and can walk back and forth to her school. The youngest child, a boy, attends an all-day preschool and is transported by his parents or other parents from the preschool. The family has attended a Protestant church in the neighborhood. The family lives in a house in an older established neighborhood, and has made friends through the schools, church, and neighborhood contacts. Part of the extended family (grandparents) live nearby, and all of the family members get together for the holidays; neither parent has siblings who live nearby. The *exosystem* assessment shows that father Robert works 40 hours a week for an industrial plant at the edge of town, and he drives back and forth daily. The father has some job stress, because he is in a middle-management position. His salary is average for middle-class families in the United States. State and county funding to the area schools, libraries, and recreational facilities are always a struggle in this community. The town has physicians/clinics of all specialties and has one community hospital. An assessment of the

macrosystem shows that this community is largely white, with only 10% of residents from ethnic backgrounds. Most people in the community embrace a Christian ethic.

The value system includes a family focus and a strong work ethic. Many of the people prefer the Democratic Party. In terms of the time-related contexts of the *chronosystem*, a few things are notable. These time-related events put more stress on the family than usual nonnormative events. Linda's disease process with MS has exacerbated in recent times, placing additional strain on the family system. Robert's own dad died in the past year, leaving him extra responsibility for his widowed mother in addition to his responsibility for his own children and now ill wife. The economy in the country and region is going through a recession, leading people to feel some fear about their economic futures. Robert had hoped that his wife could go to work part-time when their youngest child went to school, but that no longer seems to be a possibility. The family assessment would include how the family at each of the earlier-mentioned levels is influenced by the changes brought about by Linda's progressing debilitative disease and recent hospitalization. The family is experiencing disturbance at many of these levels.

Interventions include the following possibilities. In general, nurses can also look for additional systems with which the family could interact to help support family functioning during this family illness event. Nurses could make home visits to assess the living arrangements of the family and to determine how the home could be changed to accommodate a wheelchair/walker. The nurses should talk with the parents about their relationship to the schools, church, and extended family support systems. The parents might be advised to inform the school(s), church, workplace, and grandparents of what is happening to their family. The nurses could make suggestions relative to Travis's current behavior with having to go to all-day preschool. The nurses also could explore with the family the larger external environment, including community resources (e.g., Multiple Sclerosis Society, visiting nurse service, or counseling services). The nurses should contact the medical doctor(s) and discharge planning nurse at the hospital to obtain information to interpret the diagnosis, prognosis, and treatment of MS to the family. The nurses might talk to the family about how their faith can be of help during these tough times and what their primary concerns are as a family. The nurses should get in touch with the social workers at the hospital to co-ordinate care and social well-being strategies for the posthospitalization period, as well as in the future. Strategies may involve application to social security for the disabled. A family care planning meeting should be set up to involve as many care-takers and stakeholders as possible.

Evaluation of the interventions would consist of follow-up with the family through periodic home visits and telephone contact. The nurses would be interested in how the family is adapting to its situation, how the father is dealing with the extra responsibility, how the children are coping, and the physical and mental health of the mother. Because MS is a chronic progressive relapsing dis-order, a plan would be put into place for periodic evaluations that might involve changing the plan of care.

Strengths and Weaknesses of the Bioecological Systems Theory

The strength of the bioecological perspective is that it represents a comprehensive and holistic view of human/family development—a bio/psycho/socio/cultural/spiritual approach to the understanding of how humans and families develop and adapt to the larger society. It includes both the *nature* (biological) and *nurture* (environmental contexts) aspects of growth and development for both individuals and families. It directs our attention to factors that occur within, as well as to the layered influences of factors that occur outside individuals and families. The bioecological perspective provides a valuable complement to other theories that may offer greater insight into how each aspect of the holistic approach affects individuals and families over time.

The strength of this theory is also part of the weakness of this approach. The different systems show nurses what to think about that may affect the family, but the direction of how the family adapts is not specifically delineated in this theory. In other words, the bio/psycho/socio/cultural/spiritual as-pects of human/family growth and development are not detailed enough to define how individuals/families can accomplish or adapt to these contextual changes over time. Aspects of the theory require further delineation and testing, that is, the influence of biological and cognitive processes and how they interact with the environment.

Chronic Illness Framework

The Chronic Illness Framework was proposed by Rolland (1987, 1994) to help foster understanding of how chronic illness affects the family. Chronic illness is a complex concept that has vast implica-tions for the individual and the family. Rolland's conceptual framework has evolved over time and helps nurses think about multiple factors of the ill-ness and how these influence family functioning. This framework, sometimes called the Family Sys-tems and Chronic Illness Framework (Rolland, 1987), has three major elements:

- Illness types
- Time phases of the illness
- Family functioning

The illness types include the following aspects of chronic illness: onset of the illness, the course of the disease, the outcome of the illness, and the degree of incapacitation of the family member. The aspect of time addresses how issues facing families and individuals vary depending on the timing in the course of the illness, such as initial diagnosis, long chronic illness day-to-day adjust-ment phase, or terminal phase. All of these factors influence the third major concept of family func-tioning. Family functioning includes the demands of managing the illness and the family strengths and vulnerabilities. All of these aspects of the Chronic Illness Framework are detailed in the fol-lowing section. Figure 3-7 depicts the different factors that influence how the family experiences the chronic illness of a family member. The over-arching factor for families living with chronic ill-ness is the degree of uncertainty about how the illness will present and affect the family. According to the Chronic Illness Framework, it is possible to have at a minimum 24 different configurations of the factors that influence chronic illness and family systems (Rolland, 1987).

Illness Types

Onset of Illness: Gradual or Acute

When chronic illness has an acute onset (e.g., a spinal cord injury, a traumatic brain injury, or an amputation), the family reacts by rapid mobi-lization of crisis mode strategies to manage the situation. These strategies include short-term role flexibility, accessing previously used problem-solving approaches in other crises, and the ability

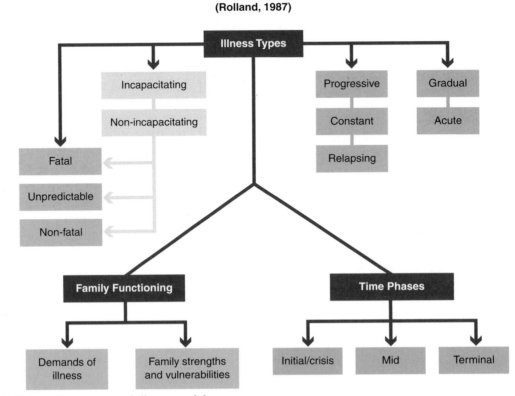

FIGURE 3-7 Family systems and illness model.

to use outside resources. As the acute phase of a chronic condition morphs into a chronic illness—or if a chronic illness has a gradual onset, such as multiple sclerosis, Parkinson's disease, or renal failure—the family adaptation occurs over a prolonged period of time.

Course of Illness: Progressive, Constant, or Relapsing/Episodic

The issues families manage are affected by the course of the illness. Chronic disease, however, is seldom a pure typology and over time it often changes from one course to another. When individual family members have a progressive chronic illness, the disability occurs in a stepwise fashion. It requires families to make gradual changes in their roles to adapt to the losses and needs of the family member as the illness progresses in severity. The families must address perpetual symptoms, which requires continual adaptation mixed with minimal periods of relief. Thus, families usually experience exhaustion from the demands of the illness. As the disease progresses, new family roles

develop and family caregiving tasks evolve over time. Examples of a progressive chronic illness are amyotrophic lateral sclerosis (ALS), Huntington's disease, and Parkinson's disease.

Chronic illness is considered constant when, after the initial chaos and stress caused by the acute illness/injury, it evolves into a semipermanent change in condition that is stable and somewhat predictable. The potential for family stress and exhaustion are present, but to a lesser degree than in a progressive chronic illness. Examples of a constant chronic illness are spinal cord injuries, cerebrovascular stroke, and myocardial infarction.

With a relapsing/episodic chronic illness, families alternate between stable low symptomology periods and periods of exacerbation with flare-up. Families are strained by both the frequency of the transition between stable and unstable crisis modes of functioning and the ongoing uncertainty of when the remission and exacerbation will occur. The uncertainty and unpredictability of relapsing is very taxing on families. Examples of relapsing/episodic chronic illness are multiple sclerosis, bipolar disorder, schizophrenia, and lupus.

Outcome: Trajectory of Illness

The trajectory of the illness and the possible outcome affect family functioning. Stress is constant and adaptation strained when the chronic illness has a fatal outcome that results in a shortened life span, such as metastatic cancers, ALS, Huntington's disease, or cystic fibrosis. Other chronic illnesses do not shorten the individual's life span, so they do not generate the same amount of family adjustment as other outcomes. Types of chronic illness that do not shorten a person's life span are arthritis, chronic fatigue syndrome, and gluten intolerance. Some chronic illnesses both shorten the life span of the individual and have the potential for sudden death. Examples of these types of chronic illness include congestive heart failure and autonomic dysreflexia with a high spinal cord injury. These types of chronic illness present with a different set of family stressors and adaption needs than either of the two other possible outcomes or trajectories.

Outcome: Incapacitation

The extent and kind of incapacitation of the illness places different stressors on the family and the individual living with chronic illness. Incapacitation can present in a variety of ways, such as cognitive (Alzheimer's disease, Parkinson's disease), energy production or expenditure (congestive heart failure, chronic obstructive pulmonary disease), impaired mobility (stroke, multiple sclerosis, cerebral palsy), disfigurement (amputation, scars), or social stigma (mental health disorders or HIV).

Time Phases

The stress responses and needs of the family change depending on the time phase of the illness. The needs of the family when a chronic illness is newly diagnosed are different than when a person adjusts and lives with the illness over time. The needs change again when ill family members enter the terminal phase of their chronic illness. Specific family stressors or needs for each time phase are outlined below.

Initial/Crisis Time Phase

When family members are first diagnosed with a chronic illness they must (1) establish a positive working relationship with health care providers, (2) gather information about the diagnosis, and (3) accept the diagnosis (Danielson, Hamel-Bissell, & Winstead-Fry, 1993). All diagnoses have the potential to create stress. The diagnostic process creates stress and uncertainty in families. Families vary in their ability to seek resources or information and to understand the ramifications of the diagnosis. For some families, the diagnosis is unexpected and can put the family in a crisis mode. For other families, the diagnosis is confirmation of their observations and concerns and so may result in relief. Families may or may not accept the diagnosis. Some families may deny the diagnosis, and others will question the diagnosis and seek other opinions. Once a medical diagnosis is given to families, the diagnosis becomes public knowledge, which means that everyone who knows the diagnosis has a reaction and response. Families may choose to keep the information within their family unit or be discriminating about whom they tell. Nurses have a central role in providing information to families with new diagnoses and helping them navigate the health care system. Family education is critical to the health outcomes, specifically integrating the medical treatment plan into family life and family roles.

Mid–Time Phase

The mid–time phase is considered the "long haul" of chronic illness (Rolland, 1987, 2005a). Rolland (2005a) outlined the salient issues in this phase: (1) pacing and avoiding burnout, (2) minimizing relationship skew between the patient and other family members, (3) sustaining autonomy for all members of the family, (4) preserving or redesigning individual and family development goals within the constraints of the illness, and (5) sustaining intimacy in the face of threatened loss. According to Danielson, Hamel-Bissell, and Winstead-Fry (1993), this time phase also includes the following challenges: (1) accept the treatment plan, (2) reorganize family roles, and (3) maintain a positive relationship with health care providers. Once families accept the diagnosis, they move into what Danielson et al. (1993) called "illness career," which is a way that families adapt and adjust to the illness on a day-by-day basis. The major challenge of the family is to redefine what is a normal balanced family life while also facing uncertainty about the future (Rolland, 2005a, 2005b). During this phase, families are constantly adjusting to the situation caused by the illness. Families vary in their ability to adjust to the illness situation—the more problems adjusting, the more stress families will experience. Family role stress, role strain, and role overload can occur when the family lives with illness over a long period.

Family tasks in this phase are to redefine normal, adjust to social stigma or altered relationships caused by the disability or illness, continue to maintain positive relationships with the health care team, and successfully grieve the loss caused by the disability or chronic condition. The family must adjust continually to the remission and exacerbations of the illness. One of the major tasks is to balance the needs of the family and the needs of ill family members (Danielson et al., 1993).

Families must adapt to the demands of the chronic condition; thus, a whole body of information has evolved around family coping and family adaptation with medical regimens. How do families promote the recovery of ill members while preserving their energy to nurture other family members and perform other family functions? An example of an appropriate intervention would be to help families find respite care for family caregivers so that caregivers do not "burn out." The family relationship with the health care provider(s) is a critical component of this phase. Families expect that they will be active members of the treatment team.

Terminal Time Phase

The nursing tasks in the terminal time phase consist of working with the family through the dying of the family member, through the grieving process, to integrating the loss into the family and family life. Nurses can work with families to change focus from managing the illness to comfort care strategies and working on the concept of "letting go" (Rolland, 2005a). During this time, an important nursing role is to help families with the cascade of decisions that occur in the terminal phase. Each family member will respond differently to the loss, and the family will be forever changed by the loss. The loss requires the family to adjust and adapt to the finality and to develop or generate a different sense of identity of family without the person (see Chapter 10).

Family Functioning

Families, as a whole, experience health events. When family members become ill, it triggers a stress response in the family to adapt to the needs of the individual and the family member. As presented earlier in the chapter, the *demands of the illness* can take multiple forms, depending on the illness type and the time phases of the illness. As each family is unique in its *strengths and vulnerabilities*, the ways in which families adapt to the challenge of chronic illness are vast and too numerous to list, which reinforces the opening statements of this chapter that nurses who bring knowledge of a variety of models, theories, and conceptual frameworks to their practice tailor their practice to the family needs by building on the strength of families in creative ways.

Application of the Chronic Illness Framework to the Jones Family

The Jones family is living with, adjusting to, and stressed and influenced by Linda's chronic illness of multiple sclerosis (MS). The course of MS is a gradual *onset* of symptoms. Linda was diagnosed after the birth of her second child, Katie; therefore, the Jones family has been living with her chronic illness for 13 years. The *course of illness* for Linda is typical of many individuals with MS. For the first 10 years, or in the Jones' case 13 years, of the disease, the most common type of MS is relapsing MS (RMS), which is characterized by exacerbation (relapses and attacks) followed by partial recovery periods (remission) and no disease progression between exacerbations. For most people with MS, after this initial course of disease, the presentation changes to progressive. At this point in time, Linda's illness has morphed to secondary progressive MS (SPMS), which is characterized by a steadily worsening disease course with or without occasional exacerbations, minor partial recoveries, or plateaus until death. Approximately 50% of people with RMS will convert to SPMS within 10 years (Lewis, Dirksen, Heitkemper, Bucher, & Camera, 2011). The Jones family remains in the *mid–time phase* of the illness trajectory, but the change in the course of Linda's illness brings with it increased *incapacitation* and an *unpredictable outcome*.

The Jones family is constantly adjusting and adapting to the course of Linda's illness and increasing incapacitation. The family is exhausted with managing this change; solutions that have worked for this family in the past are not working now. The family roles need to be supported, redefined, or renegotiated. Each of the members is experiencing role stress and strain. Linda is having to "let go" of more of her mothering role and actions. Her self-concept regarding her illness has been changed. Robert is having role overload with all the changes in his life. The intimacy needs of the couple are stressed by these changes. Amy is thinking of staying home and not going to college in another town. Katie is now a struggling student. Travis is a full-day student in a preschool. Grandmother, Elise, will no longer be living independently as she moves into the Jones family home to assume new roles as caretaker to the children and Linda. All the role changes, and seeing Linda get worse or more incapacitated, creates uncertainty about the future for each member and the family as a whole. Each family member experiences uncertainty differently based on age, family roles, role expectations, and the developmental needs of each person.

Family functioning is of central concern for the family nurse as he helps Linda and the family learn to adapt to new treatment and regimen management issues and establish a new normal day-to-day long-haul balance. One aspect of family functioning the nurse can help with revolves around family roles. The nurse can assist by exploring options for care and potential future decisions the family may face as Linda's health continues to decline and the time phase changes to terminal.

Strengths and Weaknesses of the Chronic Illness Framework

The strength of this descriptive framework is that it outlines how multiple factors of a chronic illness can be grouped in a variety of ways that affect family functioning. Rolland's (1987, 1994) conceptual framework depicts the complexity of chronic illness and the diversity of potential family responses to chronic illness. It may appear at first glance that families have similar circumstances given the same chronic illness, but on closer assessment it becomes clear that families' experiences of the different components of this framework result in different family stressors and strengths.

The weakness of this model is the same as the strengths in that the complexity of chronic illness is not predictive. Because this framework depicts how the individual's illness progresses from more of a medical model, it is easy for nurses to focus only on that part of the framework and not think about the overarching aspect of the family as a whole.

Family Assessment and Intervention Model

The *Family Assessment and Intervention Model*, originally developed by Berkey and Hanson (1991), is based on Neuman's Health Care Systems Model (Hanson, 2001; Hanson & Mischke, 1996; Kaakinen & Hanson, 2010). Neuman's model and theoretical constructs are based on systems theory and were extended and modified to focus on the family rather than on the individual (Neuman & Fawcett, 2010). Figure 3-8 depicts the Family Assessment and Intervention Model.

According to the Family Assessment and Intervention Model, families are viewed as a dynamic, open system interacting with their environment. One of the roles for families is to help buffer their members, or protect the family as a whole, from perceived threats to the family system. The core of the family system comprises basic family structure, function, processes, and energy/strength resources. This basic family structure must be protected at all costs, or the family ceases to exist. The family develops normal lines of defense as an adapting mechanism and abstract flexible protective lines of defense when the system is threatened by significant stressors. Family systems are vulnerable to tensions produced when stressors in the form of problems or concerns penetrate the family's lines of defenses. Families also have lines of resistance to help prevent penetration into the basic family core. The lines of defense and resistance depicted in the model (see Fig. 3-8) demonstrate how unexpected/unwanted health status changes can affect the basic family unit or core.

Families are subject to imbalance from normal homeostasis when stressors (e.g., physical or mental health problems) penetrate families' flexible and normal lines of defense. Furthermore, the stressors can challenge the families' lines of resistance, which have been put in place to maintain stability and to prevent penetration of the basic family defense system. In other words, health events cause families to react to stressors created by changes in the health status of a family member. Families vary in their response to the stressors and in their ability to cope, depending on how deeply the stressors penetrate the basic family unit and how capable or experienced the family is in adapting to maintain its stability.

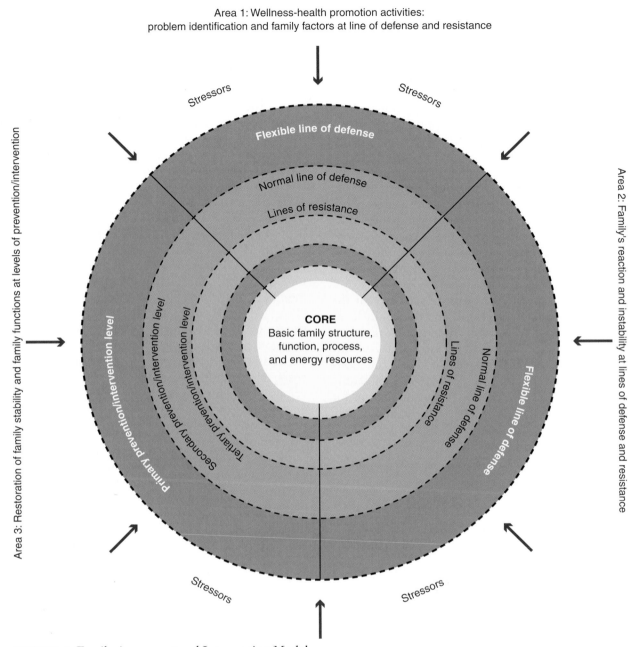

FIGURE 3-8 Family Assessment and Intervention Model.

Reconstitution or adaptation is the work the family undertakes to preserve or restore family stability after stressors penetrate the family lines of defense and resistance. This process alters the whole of the family. The model addresses three areas: (1) wellness–health promotion activities—problem identification and family factors at lines of defense and resistance, (2) family reaction and instability at lines of defense and resistance, and (3) restoration of family stability and family functioning at levels of prevention and intervention. The Family Assessment and Intervention Model focuses specifically on what causes family stress and how families react to this stress. One critical concept is to build on the family's strengths by helping the family identify its problem-solving strategies. The basic assumptions of this family-focused model are listed in Box 3-1.

BOX 3-1

Basic Assumptions for Family Assessment and Intervention Model

- Although each family has a unique family system, all families have a common basic structure that is a composite of common, known factors or innate characteristics within a normal given range of response.
- Family wellness is on a continuum of available energy to support the family system in its optimal state.
- The family, in both a state of wellness or illness, is a dynamic composite of interrelationships of variables (physiological, psychological, sociocultural, developmental, and spiritual).
- A myriad of environmental stressors can affect the family. Each stressor differs in its potential for disturbing the family's stability level or normal line of defense. The specific family interrelationships (physiological, psychological, sociocultural, developmental, and spiritual) affect the degree to which a family is protected by its flexible lines of defense against possible reactions to the stressors.
- Families evolve a normal range of response to the environment, which is called a *normal line of defense*. The normal line of defense is flexible or accordion-like as it moves to protect the family.

- When the flexible line of defense is no longer capable of protecting the family or family system against the environmental stressor, the stressor is said to break through the normal line of defense.
- Families have an internal resistance factor called the *line of resistance* that functions to stabilize and return the family to its usual wellness state (normal line of defense), or possibly to a higher level of stability after an environmental stressor reaction.
- Primary prevention is general knowledge that is applied in family assessment and intervention for identification and mitigation of risk factors associated with environmental stressors to prevent possible reaction.
- Secondary prevention is symptomatology after reaction to stressors, appropriate ranking of intervention priorities, and treatment to reduce their noxious effects.
- Tertiary prevention is the adjusting processes that take place as reconstitution begins and maintenance factors move the client back in the circular manner toward primary prevention.
- The family is in a dynamic, constant energy exchange with the environment.

Adapted from Berkey, K. M., & Hanson, S. M. (1991). *Pocket guide to family assessment and intervention.* St. Louis, MO: Mosby–Year Book.

Family Systems Stressor-Strength Inventory

Berkey and Hanson (1991) developed an assessment, intervention, and measurement tool, the Family Systems Stressor-Strength Inventory (FS³I), to help guide nurses working with families who are undergoing stressful health events and to build on the strengths of the family. The FS³I is divided into three sections: (1) family systems stressor—general, (2) family stressors—specific, and (3) family system strengths. The tool helps nurses assess family stability by gathering information on family stressors and strengths. The assessment of general, overall stressors is followed by an assessment of specific issues or problems, such as birth of first child, automobile accident, or family divorce. The tool helps to identify family strengths to help determine potential or actual problem-solving abilities of the family system. Examples of family strengths could include supportive extended family, health insurance, and availability of family counseling.

The FS³I is intended for use with multiple family members. Individual members of the family can complete the FS³I, or the entire family can sit together and complete the assessment. The nurse meets with family members and interviews them to clarify their perceived general stressors, specific stressors, and family strengths as identified by the family members.

After the interview, the nurse completes the quantitative summary and enters each respondent's score on the graph. Recording individual scores on the graph allows for a comparison of the family responses and visually shows the variability among family members' perceptions of general and specific health stressors. The nurse synthesizes the interview information gleaned from all the family participants on the qualitative summary. Together, the nurse and family develop a family care plan with intervention strategies tailored to the individual family needs and built on the strengths of the family.

A major benefit of using the FS³I for family assessment and intervention planning is that both quantitative and qualitative data are used to determine the level of prevention and intervention needed: primary, secondary, or tertiary (Pender, Murdaugh, & Parsons, 2006). Primary prevention focuses on moving the individual and family toward a state of improved health or toward health-promotion activities. *Primary interventions* include providing families with information about their strengths, supporting their coping and functioning capabilities, and encouraging movement toward health through family education. *Secondary interventions* attain system stability after stressors or problems have invaded the family core. Secondary interventions include helping the family to handle its problems, helping family members to find and use appropriate treatment, and intervening in crises. *Tertiary prevention* is designed to maintain system stability through intervention strategies that are initiated after treatment has been completed. Coordination of care after discharge from the hospital and postdischarge rehabilitation services are examples of tertiary prevention.

The Family Assessment and Intervention Model focuses on the family as client. The Family Systems Stressor-Strength Inventory (FS³I) was developed to provide a concrete, focused assessment and intervention instrument that helps families identify current family stressors and strengths and that assists nurses and families in planning interventions to meet family needs. The model and inventory represent a nursing model made for nursing care of families. An updated blank copy of the instrument, with instructions for administration and a scoring guide, can be found in Appendix A. A summary of a completed instrument applied to the case study follows.

Application of the Family Assessment and Intervention Model With the Jones Family

The FS³I was used to assess stressors (problems) and strengths (resources) that the Jones family had to cope with their situation. Robert and Linda were interviewed together by the nurse, but each person completed a separate FS³I. Scores were tallied using the scoring guide for the FS³I. Amy was away attending college, and Katie and Travis were too young to complete the assessment instrument.

The general stressors were viewed similarly by both Robert and Linda, and these stressors were assessed as more serious by the nurse than by the couple. Robert, Linda, and the nurse concurred that the general stress level was high. The specific stressors were perceived slightly differently by Robert and Linda. The following figures summarize information gained from the Jones family: Figure 3-9, which applies the FS³I to the Jones

Family; Figure 3-10, which presents an FS³I quantitative summary of family system stressors, general and specific, for the Jones family; Figure 3-11, which lists FS³I family and clinician perception scores of the Jones family; Figure 3-12, which is an FS³I qualitative summary, family and clinician, of the Jones family; and Figure 3-13, which provides an FS³I family care plan for the Jones family.

The qualitative summary, family and clinician form in Figure 3-12, serves as the groundwork for the family care plan. This form synthesizes information pertaining to general stressors, specific stressors, family strengths, and the overall functioning and physical and mental health of the family members. The nurse completed this form using her assessment skills with information obtained from the verbal exchange and the FS³I.

The family members and the nurse perceived that the chronic and debilitating diagnosis of MS was the major general stressor. Linda's specific stressors included her growing inability to function as a wife and mother; her physical problems, such as increasing physical weakness, swallowing challenges, pain, vision impairment, vertigo/tinnitus, constipation, urinary infections; and her mental health issues, such as guilt, anxiety, and depression. Specific stressors for Robert included his worry about Linda's health; loss of his life's partner in taking care of the family, household maintenance, and raising children; fear of the unknown future and health outcomes; loss of sexual expression with his wife; and financial worries. The strengths of the family were seen as communication between the couple, religious faith, the social support network of extended family, and the availability of good health providers. The overall family functioning was considered to be as good as could be expected under the circumstances. Where the mother's physical health was compromised, the father's physical health was good. Both Linda and Robert expressed mental health concerns. Overall, the nurse perceived that this family had the strengths it needed to deal with both the general and specific stressors. After completing a genogram (Fig. 3-3) and ecomap (Fig. 3-4) of this family unit, the nurse concluded that the family was being supported by community/family resources. These social support systems are important factors in coping with stress, and the nurse concluded that this family could use assistance in utilizing these resources.

INSTRUCTIONS FOR ADMINISTRATION

The Family Systems Stressor-Strength Inventory (FS³I) is an assessment and measurement instrument intended for use with families (see Chapter 14). It focuses on identifying stressful situations occurring in families and the strengths families use to maintain healthy family functioning. Each family member is asked to complete the instrument on an individual form before an interview with the clinician. Questions can be read to members unable to read.

After completion of the instrument, the clinician evaluates the family on each of the stressful situations (general and specific) and the strengths they possess. This evaluation is recorded on the family member form.

The clinician records the individual family member's score and the clinician perception score on the Quantitative Summary. A different color code is used for each family member. The clinician also completes the Qualitative Summary, synthesizing the information gleaned from all participants. Clinicians can use the Family Care Plan to prioritize diagnoses, set goals, develop prevention and intervention activities, and evaluate outcomes.

Family Name _Jones_   **Date** _April 18, 2009_

Family Member(s) Completing Assessment _Robert and Linda_

Ethnic Background(s) _"American all mixed up"_

Religious Background(s) _Protestant_

Referral Source _Neurologist For Linda_

Interviewer _Meredith Rowe, RN_

Family Members	Relationship in Family	Age	Marital Status	Education (highest degree)	Occupation
1. _Robert_	_Father_	_48 yr_	_Married_	_MS_	_Software engineer_
2. _Linda_	_Mother_	_43 yr_	_Married_	_____	_Home maker_
3. _Amy_	_Daughter_	_19 yr_	_Single_	_____	_____
4. _Katie_	_Daughter_	_13 yr_	_Single_	_____	_____
5. _Travis_	_Son_	_4 yr_	_Single_	_____	_____
6._____	_____	_____	_____	_____	_____

Family's current reasons for seeking assistance:

Linda MS is progressing family feels stressed.

FIGURE 3-9 Family System Stressor-Strength Inventory: Jones family. *(Source: Hanson, S. M. H. [2001]. Family health care nursing: Theory, practice, and research [2nd ed.]. Philadelphia, PA: F. A. Davis, with permission.)*

The family care plan for the Jones family was developed by the nurse in concert with the family members who completed the FS³I (see Fig. 3-13). The family care plan addresses the diagnosis of general and specific family systems stressors and family systems strengths that support the family care plan and the goals of the family and the clinician(s): interventions/prevention activities—primary/secondary/tertiary, and outcome/evaluation/replanning proposed for this family. The goal of this family care plan was to achieve a restoration of optimum health that could provide homeostasis and stability for this family, as well as more positive health outcomes than the family could reach at the beginning of their health challenges. The outcome/evaluation/replanning

QUANTITATIVE SUMMARY OF FAMILY SYSTEMS STRESSORS: GENERAL AND SPECIFIC FAMILY AND CLINICIAN PERCEPTION SCORES

DIRECTIONS: Graph the scores from each family member inventory by placing an "X" at the appropriate location. (Use first name initial for each different entry and different color code for each family member.)

	FAMILY SYSTEMS STRESSORS (GENERAL)			FAMILY SYSTEMS STRESSORS (SPECIFIC)	
SCORES FOR WELLNESS AND STABILITY	FAMILY MEMBER PERCEPTION SCORE	CLINICIAN PERCEPTION SCORE	SCORES FOR WELLNESS AND STABILITY	FAMILY MEMBER PERCEPTION SCORE	CLINICIAN PERCEPTION SCORE
5.0			5.0		
4.8			4.8	X√1	
4.6			4.6		
		X			X
4.4			4.4		
	X√1			X√2	
4.2			4.2		
4.0	X√2		4.0		
3.8			3.8		
3.6			3.6		
3.4			3.4		
3.2			3.2		
3.0			3.0		
2.8			2.8		
2.6			2.6		
2.4			2.4		
2.2			2.2		
2.0			2.0		
1.8			1.8		
1.6			1.6		
1.4			1.4		
1.2			1.2		
1.0			1.0		

*PRIMARY Prevention/Intervention Mode: Flexible Line   1.0-2.3   √1 = Robert
*SECONDARY Prevention/Intervention Mode: Normal Line   2.4-3.6
*TERTIARY Prevention/Intervention Mode: Resistance Lines   3.7-5.0   √2 = Linda
*Breakdowns of numerical scores for stressor penetration are suggested values.

FIGURE 3-10 Quantitative summary of family systems stressors, general and specific: Jones family.

FAMILY SYSTEMS STRENGTHS FAMILY AND CLINICIAN PERCEPTION SCORES

DIRECTIONS: Graph the scores from the inventory by placing an "X" at the appropriate location and connect with a line. (Use first name initial for each different entry and different color code for each family member.)

SUM OF STRENGTHS AVAILABLE FOR PREVENTION/ INTERVENTION MODE	FAMILY SYSTEMS STRENGTHS	
	FAMILY MEMBER PERCEPTION SCORE	CLINICIAN PERCEPTION SCORE
5.0		
4.8		
4.6		
4.4		X
4.2		
4.0	√2	
3.8		
3.6		
3.4	√1	
3.2		
3.0		
2.8		
2.6		
2.4		
2.2		
2.0		
1.8		
1.6		
1.4		
1.2		
1.0		

*PRIMARY Prevention/Intervention Mode: Flexible Line   1.0-2.3   √1 = Robert
*SECONDARY Prevention/Intervention Mode: Normal Line   2.4-3.6
*TERTIARY Prevention/Intervention Mode: Resistance Lines   3.7-5.0   √2 = Linda
*Breakdowns of numerical scores for stressor penetration are suggested values.

FIGURE 3-11 Family and clinician perception scores: Jones family.

QUALITATIVE SUMMARY FAMILY AND CLINICIAN REMARKS
PART I: FAMILY SYSTEMS STRESSORS (GENERAL)

Summarize general stressors and remarks of family and clinician. Prioritize stressors according to importance to family members.

The major general stressor of the family is the DX of MS and the impact of the progressive disabling illness on the entire family.

PART II: FAMILY SYSTEMS STRESSORS (SPECIFIC)

A. Summarize specific stressors and remarks of family and clinician.

    Linda's specific stressors: growing disability to function as wife/mother, physical signs of impairment and guilt, anxiety, and depression. Robert's specific stressors: loss of fully functional wife, fear of unknown; loss of sexual expression and finances.

B. Summarize differences (if discrepancies exist) between how family members and clinicians view effects of stressful situation on family.

    Each family member has some different stressors, but share in common the fears, anxiety, helplessness, sadness over their losses due to Linda's condition. Nurse views general and specific stressors higher than family rates them.

C. Summarize overall family functioning.

    Functioning as best as can be expected. Physical health in question. Mental health standing up so far. Family addressing issues one by one.

D. Summarize overall significant physical health status for family members.

    Mother's physical health compromised. Father's physical health is okay.

E. Summarize overall significant mental health status for family members.

    Mother is frustrated and anxious. Expressed guilt, which makes her depressed. Father is also frustrated and worried about Linda, the children, and finances.

PART III: FAMILY SYSTEMS STRENGTHS

Summarize family systems strengths and family and clinician remarks that facilitate family health and stability.

    Couple communication, religious faith, social support of extended family and believe they have competent caring health care providers.

FIGURE 3-12 Qualitative summary, family and clinician: Jones family.

Diagnosis: General and Specific Family System Stressors	Family Systems Strengths Supporting Family Care Plan	Goals for Family and Clinician	Prevention/Intervention Mode		Outcomes Evaluation and Replanning
			Primary, Secondary, or Tertiary	Prevention/ Intervention Activities	
Dx of MS weakness of swallowing, pain, vision impairment, vertigo/tinnitus, constipation, urinary infections, guilt/anxiety, depression, sexual dysfunction, over-load for caregiver father.	Couple communication, religious faith, social support of extended family, good medical care.	Restoration of stability and homeostasis at each level of progressive chronic illness.	Support of family changes, connect family with MS family support group, locate part-time family helper for home, coordinate with other medical groups involved, set up rehabilitation, and physical therapy.	Couple receives counseling, pain and symptom management; involve social worker to look at community agencies to offer assistance.	Evaluation to be done once plan implemented.

FIGURE 3-13 Family care plan: Jones family.

section of the family care plan remains blank for now because it is dependent on feedback from the interventions proposed for the family, as well as the physical and mental health status of the entire family.

Strengths and Weaknesses

The strength of the FS³I approach is that both quantitative and qualitative data are used to determine the level of prevention and intervention needed: primary, secondary, or tertiary. The instrument is brief, is easy to administer, and yields data to compare one family member with another member and one family with another family. The weakness of this model and instrument is that they focus only on family strengths and stressors rather than all the dimensions of the family as a unit. This model and instrument hold much promise for nursing assessment of families, but more work needs to be done on this approach. See Box 3-2 for a comparison of the approaches.

SUMMARY

By understanding theories and models, nurses are better prepared to think creatively and critically about how health events affect the family. This chapter introduced nurses to the concept of theory-guided, evidence-based family nursing practice. It presented the relationship between theory,

practice, and research, and explained crucial aspects of theory. The chapter then explored five theories and models for the nursing care of families and applied the theories to the case study in the chapter:

- Family Systems Theory
- Developmental and Family Life Cycle Theory
- Bioecological Theory
- Chronic Illness Framework
- Family Assessment and Intervention Model

The chapter revealed how nurses can practice family nursing differently with the Jones family according to the different theoretical perspectives.

The following points highlight critical concepts that are addressed in this chapter:

- No single theory, model, or conceptual framework adequately describes the complex relationships of family.
- No one theoretical perspective gives nurses a sufficiently broad base of knowledge and understanding to guide assessment and interventions with all families.
- No one theoretical perspective is better, more comprehensive, or more correct than another.
- Nurses who draw from multiple theories are more effective in tailoring their nursing practice and family interventions. Using multiple theories substantially increases the

BOX 3-2

Comparison of Theories as They Apply to the Jones Family

Family Systems Theory

Conceptual

Family is viewed as a whole. What happens to the family as a whole affects each individual family member, and what happens to individuals affects the totality of the family unit. Focus is on the circular interactions among members of the family system, resulting in functional or dysfunctional outcomes.

Assessment

The family may be assessed together or individually. Assessment questions relate to the *interaction* between the individual and the family, and the *interaction* between the family and the community in which the family lives.

Intervention Examples

- Complete a family genogram to understand patterns and relationships over several generations over time.
- Complete family ecomap to see how individuals/family relate to the community around them.
- Collect data about the family as a whole and about individual family members.
- Conduct care-planning sessions that include family members.

Strengths

Focus is on family as a whole or its subsystems, or both. It is a generally understood and accepted theory in society.

Weaknesses

Theory is broad and general. It does not give definitive prescriptions for interventions.

Application to Jones Family

All members of the Jones family are affected by the mother's progressive chronic health condition and changes. Family structure, functions, and processes of the family are influenced, changing family roles and dynamics. Everyone in the family has his or her own concerns and needs attention from health care professionals.

Family Developmental and Life Cycle Theory

Conceptual

Family is viewed as a whole over time. All families go through similar developmental processes starting with the birth of the first child to death of the parents. Focus is on the life cycle of families and represents normative stages of family development.

Assessment

The family may be assessed together or individually. Assessment questions relate to the normative predictable events that occur in family life over time. It also includes nonnormative, unexpected events.

Intervention Examples

- Conduct family interview to determine where family is in terms of cognitive, social, emotional, spiritual, and physical development.
- A family genogram and ecomap should be completed.
- Determine the normative and nonnormative events that have occurred to the family as a whole or to individuals within the family.
- Analyze how an individual's growth and developmental milestones may affect the family developmental trajectory.

Strengths

Focus is on the family as a whole. The theory provides a framework for predicting what a family will experience at any given stage in the family life cycle so that nurses can offer anticipatory guidance.

Weaknesses

The traditional linear family life cycle is no longer the norm. Modern families vary widely in their structure and roles. Divorce, remarriage, gay parents, and never-married parents have changed the traditional trajectory of growth and developmental milestones. The theory does not focus on how the family adapts to the transitions from one stage to the other; rather, it simply predicts what transitions will occur.

Application to Jones Family

The Jones family is in the stages of "families with adolescents" and "launching young adults." The nonnormative health condition of the mother is changing the predictable normative course of development for the individuals and for the family as a whole. These health events will change the cognitive, social, emotional, spiritual, and physical development as the family shifts to integrate new roles into their lives as family members.

Bioecological Systems Theory

Conceptual

Bioecological systems theory combines children's biological disposition and environmental forces that come together to shape the development of human beings. This theory has a basis in both developmental theory and systems theory to understand individual and family growth. It combines the influence of both genetics and environment from the individual and family with the larger economic/political structure over time. The basic premise is that individual and family development are contextual over time. The different levels of the theory that apply to the family at any one point in time vary depending on what is happening at that time. Therefore, the interaction of the systems vary over time as the situation changes.

BOX 3-2

Basic Assumptions for Family Assessment and Intervention Model—cont'd

Assessment

Assess all levels of the larger ecological system when interviewing the family. Determine the microsystem, mesosystem, exosystem, macrosystem, and chronosystem of the individual and of the family as a whole.

Intervention Examples

- Conduct a family interview to determine the family's status in relationship to four locational/spatial contexts and one time-related context.
- A family genogram and ecomap should be completed.
- Determine how individuals are doing in relationship to their entire environment, which includes immediate family, extended family, home, school, and community.
- Analyze the family in its smaller and larger contextual aspects.

Strengths

Focus is on a holistic approach to human/family development. A bio/psycho/socio/cultural/spiritual approach to understanding how individuals and families develop and change/adapt over time in their society is a more complete approach.

Weaknesses

This holistic approach is not specific enough to define contextual changes over time. Nor can the larger context in which individuals/families are embedded be predicted or controlled.

Application to Jones Family

- Microsystem: The Jones family consists of school-age children living at home. The parental roles have been traditional until recent health events.
- Mesosystem: Family has much interaction with schools, church, and extended family.
- Exosystem: Family influenced by father's work at the factory and other institutions in the community.
- Macrosystem: Family consistent with community culture, attitudes, and beliefs. Their community is largely Caucasian, middle class, and Christian.
- Chronosystem: At this time in the illness story of the Jones family with the mother's illness changing, the family situation changes and moves between stability and crisis.

Chronic Illness Framework

Conceptual

This is a conceptual framework and not a theory. Therefore, each aspect of the framework represents several fields of inquiry relative to chronic illness. The framework has been built and data have been organized to provide a coherent way of thinking about families when a member

has a chronic illness. The areas of inquiry that inform this model are onset of the chronic illness, course of illness, outcome or trajectory of the chronic illness, outcome relative to degree of incapacitation from the illness, time phase of the illness, and family functioning.

Assessment

In this framework, it is important first to analyze the various aspects of the specific type of chronic illness. Each aspect presents a different type of stress or challenge for the family based on the particular chronic illness. The last aspect of the framework, family function, requires the family nurse to explore how the specific chronic illness affects this specific family based on the demands of the illness and the family strengths and vulnerabilities.

Intervention Examples

- Complete a family genogram and ecomap.
- Implement a plan of care to help facilitate family adaptation and coping strategies.
- Work with families by building on the family strengths to adjust family roles to help the family with managing the stressors identified in this specific chronic illness for this specific family.

Strengths

The Chronic Illness Framework is designed to support family-centered nursing care. Focus is on family strengths and vulnerabilities through identified predictable stressors experienced by families who are in that aspect of the chronic illness. Anticipatory guidance can be provided as the chronic illness may progress through typical trajectories or times phases.

Weaknesses

The model is not specific enough to identify precise ways families adapt; rather, it is more of a guideline to typical stressors and coping tasks that may happen when a family member develops a chronic illness.

Application to Jones Family

The Jones family is struggling to adapt during the rocky chronic illness phase. As the mother's illness has changed from being episodic to progressive in nature, the family is stressed with adapting to the mother losing ambulation and needing more physical support than in the past. The family is in a constant state of stress as it adjusts to the new patterns, regimens, and roles. The family is grieving as Linda becomes more disabled.

Family Assessment and Intervention Model

Conceptual

Families are viewed as dynamic, open systems in interaction with their environment. A major role of family is to

Continued

BOX 3-2

Basic Assumptions for Family Assessment and Intervention Model–cont'd

help protect itself from events such as illness that may threaten the family's inner core. The inner core of the family consists of family structure, function, process, and energy/strength resources and must be protected or the family ceases to exist. Adaptation is the work the family undertakes to preserve/restore family stability. This model evolved out of nursing and builds on general systems theory, stress theory, and change theory.

Assessment

Family may be assessed together, but all individuals are asked to complete the measurement instrument. The Family Systems Stressor-Strength Inventory (FS³I) is administered to determine general family stressors, specific family stressors, and family system strengths. The stressors that affect the balance of the family strengths are analyzed to assist the family to achieve stability.

Intervention Examples

- The FS³I is completed by all adult individuals in the family. Scores are derived from the measurement scales and then analyzed. Health care providers meet with families to review results and provide different intervention strategies based on the specific stressors, how the family is coping, and what strengths are brought to the situation.
- A family genogram and ecomap should be completed.

Strengths

The model and instrument provide a structured approach to family assessment and intervention based on both quantitative and qualitative data. These data help determine the primary, secondary, and tertiary levels of prevention and intervention. The focus on family strengths is unique to this model and approach.

Weaknesses

This model is used specifically when families enter the health care system. It is applicable when health problems have come up that cause stressors. Although the model per se is applicable to all families in terms of life stressors and strengths, the administration of the FS³I is specific to only these two aspects of the health events.

Application to Jones Family

The adults in this family were interviewed together, with each person completing the FS³I. General stressors and specific stressors were rated similarly by each member of the couple. The nurse also rated her perceptions of the family stressors and strengths. Overall family physical and mental functioning were also rated. The nurse concluded that this family had the strengths it needed to deal with both the general and specific stressors.

---

likelihood that the family will be able to achieve stability and health as a family unit.
- Theories that inform the nursing of families should be the "gold standard" of nursing practice (Segaric & Hall, 2005); hence, family nursing is a theory-guided, evidence-based nursing practice.

This chapter presents ways of providing excellent family health care nursing that is theory driven and evidence based. By using different lenses to view family care problems, different solutions and options for care and interventions become available. Clearly, no one theoretical perspective gives all nurses in all settings a sufficiently broad base of knowledge on which to assess and intervene with the complex health events experienced by families. What is crucial is that nurses use multiple theoretical perspectives to guide their practice with the nursing care of families.

REFERENCES

Artinian, N. T. (1994). Selecting model to guide family assessment. *Dimensions of Critical Care Nursing, 14*(1), 4–16.

Bengtson, V. L., Acock, A. C., Allen, K. R., Dilworth-Anderson, P., & Klein, D. M. (Eds.). (2005). *Sourcebook of family theory and research.* Thousand Oaks, CA: Sage.

Berkey, K. M., & Hanson, S. M. H. (1991). *Pocket guide to family assessment and intervention.* St. Louis, MO: Mosby.

Boemmel, J., & Briscoe, J. (2001). Web Quest Project theory fact sheet of Urie Bronfenbrenner. Retrieved from http://blog.lib.umn.edu/cpstudy/cpstudy/Bronfenbrenner%20article%205.9.2001.pdf

Bowen, M. (1978). *Family therapy in clinical practice.* New York, NY: Jason Aronson.

Bronfenbrenner, U. (1972a). *Influences on human development.* Hinsdale, IL: Dryden Press.

Bronfenbrenner, U. (1972b). *Two worlds of childhood.* New York, NY: Simon & Schuster.

Bronfenbrenner, U. (1979). *The ecology of human development.* Cambridge, MA: Harvard University Press.

Bronfenbrenner, U. (1981). *On making human beings human.* Thousand Oaks, CA: Sage.

Bronfenbrenner, U. (1986). Ecology of the family as a context for human development: Research perspectives. *Developmental Psychology, 22,* 723–742.

Bronfenbrenner, U. (1997). Ecology of the family as a context for human development: Research perspectives. In J. L. Paul et al. (Eds.), *Foundations of special education* (pp. 49–83). Pacific Grove, CA: Brooks/Cole.

Bronfenbrenner, U., & Lerner, R. M. (Eds.). (2004). *Making human beings human: Bioecological perspectives on human development.* Thousand Oaks, CA: Sage.

Bronfenbrenner, U., & Morris, P.A. (1998). The ecology of developmental processes. In W. Damon (Series Ed.) & R. M. Lerner (Vol. Ed.), *Handbook of child psychology: Vol. 1. Theoretical models of human development* (pp. 993–1028). New York, NY: John Wiley & Sons.

Carter, B. (2005). Becoming parents: The family with young children. In B. Carter & M. McGoldrick (Eds.), *The expanded family life cycle: Individual, family and social perspectives* (3rd ed., pp. 249–273). New York, NY: Allyn & Bacon.

Carter, B., & McGoldrick, M. (1989). *The changing family life cycle: A framework for family therapy.* New York, NY: Gardner Press.

Carter, B., & McGoldrick, M. (2005). The divorce cycle: A major variation in the American family life cycle. In B. Carter & M. McGoldrick (Eds.), *The expanded family life cycle: Individual, family, and social perspectives* (3rd ed., pp. 373–380). New York, NY: Allyn & Bacon.

Casey, B. (1996). The family as a system. In C. Bomar (Ed.), *Nurses and family health promotion: Concepts, assessment, and interventions* (2nd ed., pp. 49–59). Philadelphia, PA: Saunders.

Danielson, C. B., Hamel-Bissell, B., & Winstead-Fry, P. (1993). *Families, health and illness: Perspectives on coping and intervention.* St. Louis, MO: Mosby.

Denham, S. (2003). *Family health: A framework for nursing.* Philadelphia, PA: F. A. Davis.

Doane, G. H., & Varcoe, C. (2005). *Family nursing as relational inquiry: Developing health-promoting practice.* Philadelphia, PA: Lippincott Williams & Wilkins.

Duvall, E. M. (1977). *Marriage and family development* (5th ed.). Philadelphia, PA: Lippincott.

Duvall, E. M., & Miller, B. (1985). *Marriage and family development* (6th ed.). Philadelphia, PA: J. B. Lippincott.

Emory University. (2008). Urie Bronfenbrenner. Retrieved from www.des.emory.edu/mfp/302/302bron.PDF

Fawcett, J., & Desanto-Madeya, S. (2012). *Contemporary nursing knowledge: Analysis and evaluation of nursing models and theories* (3rd ed.). Philadelphia, PA: F. A. Davis.

Fawcett, J., & Garity, J. (2008). *Evaluating research for evidenced-based nursing practice.* Philadelphia, PA: F. A. Davis.

Fine, M. A., & Fincham, F. D. (Eds.). (2012). *Handbook of family theories: A content-based approach.* New York, NY: Routledge Academic Press.

Freeman, D. S. (1992). *Multigenerational family therapy.* New York, NY: Haworth Press.

Friedemann, M. L. (1995). *The framework of systemic organization: A conceptual approach to families and nursing.* Thousand Oaks, CA: Sage.

Friedman, M. M., Bowden, V. R., & Jones, E. G. (2003). *Family nursing: Research, theory and practice* (5th ed., pp. 103–150). Upper Saddle River, NJ: Prentice Hall.

Goldenberg, H., & Goldenberg, I. (2012). *Family therapy: An overview* (8th ed.). Belmont, CA: Wadsworth.

Gray, V. (1996). Family self-care. In C. Bomar (Ed.), *Nurses and family health promotion: Concepts, assessment, and interventions* (2nd ed., pp. 83–93). Philadelphia, PA: Saunders.

Hanson, S. M. H. (2001). *Family health care nursing: Theory, practice and research* (2nd ed.). Philadelphia, PA: F. A. Davis.

Hanson, S. M. H., & Mischke, K. M. (1996). Family health assessment and intervention. In P. J. Bomar (Ed.), *Nurses and family health promotion: Concepts, assessment and intervention* (2nd ed., pp. 165–202). Philadelphia, PA: W. B. Saunders.

Hill, R. (1949). *Families under stress.* New York, NY: Harper & Brothers.

Hill, R. (1965). *Challenges and resources for family development: Family mobility in our dynamic society.* Ames, IA: Iowa State University.

Hill, R., & Hansen, D. (1960). The identification of conceptual frameworks utilized in family study. *Marriage and Family Living, 22*(4), 299–311.

Imber-Black, E. (2005). Creating meaningful rituals for new life cycle transitions. In B. Carter & M. McGoldrick (Eds.), *The expanded family life cycle: Individual, family and social perspectives* (3rd ed., pp. 202–214). New York, NY: Allyn & Bacon, Pearson Education.

Jackson, D. D. (1965). Family rules: Marital quid quo. *Archives of General Psychiatry, 12,* 589–594.

Johnson, D. (1980). The behavioral system model for nursing. In J. P. Riehl & C. Roy (Eds.), *Conceptual models for nursing practice* (2nd ed., pp. 207–216). New York, NY: Appleton-Century-Crofts.

Kaakinen, J. R., & Hanson, S. M. H. (2010). Theoretical foundations for nursing of families. In J. R. Kaakinen, V. Gedaly-Duff, D. P. Coehlo, & S. M. H. Hanson (Eds.), *Family health care nursing: Theory, practice and research* (4th ed., pp. 63–102). Philadelphia, PA: F. A. Davis.

Kerr, M., & Bowen, M. (1988). *Family evaluation: An approach based on Bowen's theory.* New York, NY: Norton.

King, I. (1981). *Family therapy: A comparison of approaches.* Bowie, MD: Brady.

King, I. (1983). King's theory of nursing. In I. W. Clements & J. B. Roberts (Eds.), *Family health: A theoretical approach to nursing* (pp. 177–187). New York, NY: John Wiley & Sons.

King, I. (1987, May). *King's theory* [Cassette recording]. Recording presented at the Nursing Theories Conference, Pittsburgh, PA.

Lewis, S. L., Dirksen, S. R., Heitkemper, M. M., Bucher, L., & Camera, I. M. (2011). *Medical-surgical nursing* (Vols. I and II). St. Louis, MO: Elsevier.

Maturana, H. (1978). Biology of language: The epistemology of reality. In G. Millar & E. Lenneberg (Eds.), *Psychology and biology of language and thought* (pp. 27–63). New York, NY: Academic Press.

Maturana, H. R., & Varela, F. J. (1992). *The tree of knowledge: The biological roots of human understanding.* Boston, MA: Shambhala (Random House).

McCubbin, H. I., & Patterson, J. M. (1983). The family stress process: The double ABCX model of adjustment and adaptation. In H. I. McCubbin, M. B. Sussman, & J. M. Patterson (Eds.), *Social stress and the family: Advances in developments in family stress theory and research* (pp. 7–27). New York, NY: Haworth.

McCubbin, M. A., & McCubbin, H. I. (1993). Family coping with illness: The Resiliency Model of Family Stress, Adjustment, and Adaptation. In C. Danielson, B. Hamel-Bissell, & P. Winstead-Fry (Eds.), *Families, health and illness: Perspectives on coping and intervention* (pp. 21–64). St. Louis, MO: Mosby.

McGoldrick, M., Carter, B., & Garcia-Preto, N. (Eds.). (2010). *The expanded family life cycle: Individual, family and social perspectives* (4th ed.). New York, NY: Allyn & Bacon.

Minuchin, S. (1974). *Families and family therapy.* Cambridge, MA: Harvard University Press.

Minuchin, S., & Fishman, H. G. (1981). *Family therapy techniques.* Cambridge, MA: Harvard University Press.

Minuchin, S., Rosman, B. L., & Baker, L. (1978). *Psychosomatic families: Anorexia nervosa in context.* Cambridge, MA: Harvard University Press.

Neuman, B. (1983). Family intervention using the Betty Neuman health care systems model. In I. W. Clements & F. B. Roberts (Eds.), *Family health: A theoretical approach to nursing care* (pp. 239–254). New York, NY: John Wiley.

Neuman, B. (1995). *The Neuman systems model* (3rd ed.). Stanford, CT: Appleton & Lange.

Neuman, B., & Fawcett, J. (2010). *The Neuman systems model* (5th ed.). Upper Saddle River, NJ: Prentice Hall.

Nichols, M. P. (2004). *Family therapy: Concepts and methods* (6th ed.). Boston, MA: Pearson/Allyn & Bacon.

Nightingale, F. (1859). *Notes on nursing: What it is, and what it is not.* London: Harrison. (Reprinted 1980, Edinburgh, NY: Churchill Livingtone.)

Nye, F. I. (1976). *Role structure and analysis of the family* (Vol. 24). Beverly Hills, CA: Sage.

Nye, F. I., & Berardo, F. (Eds.). (1981). *Emerging conceptual frameworks in family analysis.* New York, NY: Praeger.

Orem, D. (1983a). The family coping with a medical illness: Analysis and application of Orem's theory. In I. Clements & F. Roberts (Eds.), *Family health: A theoretical approach to nursing care* (pp. 385–386). New York, NY: John Wiley.

Orem, D. (1983b). The family experiencing emotional crisis: Analysis and application of Orem's self-care deficit theory. In I. Clements & F. Roberts (Eds.), *Family health: A theoretical approach to nursing care* (pp. 205–217). New York, NY: John Wiley.

Orem, D. (1985). *Nursing: Concepts of practice* (3rd ed.). New York, NY: McGraw-Hill.

Parker, M., & Smith, M. (2010). *Nursing theories and nursing practice* (3rd ed.). Philadelphia, PA: F. A. Davis.

Parse, R. R. (1992). Human becoming: Parse's theory of nursing. *Nursing Science Quarterly, 5,* 35–42.

Parse, R. R. (1998). *The human becoming school of thought: A perspective for nurses and other health professionals.* Thousand Oaks, CA: Sage.

Pender, N. J., Murdaugh, C. L., & Parsons, M. A. (2006). *Health promotion in nursing practice* (5th ed.). Upper Saddle River, NJ: Prentice Hall.

Polit, D., & Beck, C. (2011). *Nursing research: Generating and assessing evidence for nursing practice* (9th ed.). Philadelphia, PA: Lippincott Williams & Wilkins.

Powers, B., & Knapp, T. (2010). *A dictionary of nursing theory and research* (4th ed.). New York, NY: Springer.

Rogers, M. (1970). *Introduction to the theoretical basis of nursing.* Philadelphia, PA: F. A. Davis.

Rogers, M. (1986). Science of unitary human beings. In V. Malinski (Ed.), *Explorations on Martha Rogers' science of unitary human beings* (pp. 3–8). Norwalk, CT: Appleton-Century-Crofts.

Rogers, M. (1990). Nursing: Science of unitary, irreducible, human being: Update, 1990. In E. Barret (Ed.), *Visions of Rogers' science-based nursing* (pp. 5–11). New York, NY: National League for Nursing.

Rolland, J. S. (1987). Chronic illness and the life cycle: A conceptual framework. *Family Process, 26*(2), 203–221.

Rolland, J. S. (1994). *Families, illness and disability: An integrated treatment model.* New York, NY: Basic Books.

Rolland, J. S. (2005a). Cancer and the family: An integrative model. *Cancer Supplement, 104*(11), 2584–2595.

Rolland, J. S. (2005b). Chronic illness and the family life cycle. In B. Carter & M. McGoldrick (Eds.), *The expanded family life cycle: Individual, family and social perspectives* (3rd ed., pp. 492–511). New York, NY: Allyn & Bacon, Pearson Education.

Rose, A. M. (1962). *Human behavior and social processes.* Boston, MA: Houghton Mifflin.

Roy, C. (1976). *Introduction to nursing: An adaptation model.* Englewood Cliffs, NJ: Prentice-Hall.

Roy, C., & Roberts, S. (1981). *Theory construction in nursing: An adaptation model.* Englewood Cliffs, NJ: Prentice-Hall.

Satir, V. (1982). The therapist and family therapy: Process model. In A. M. Horne & M. M. Ohlsen (Eds.), *Family counseling and therapy* (pp. 12–42). Itasca, IL: F. E. Peacock.

Segaric, C., & Hall, W. (2005). The family theory-practice gap: A matter of clarity? *Nursing Inquiry, 12*(3), 210–218.

Smith, S. R., & Hamon, R. R. (2012). *Exploring family theories* (3rd ed.). New York, NY: Oxford University Press.

Toman, W. (1961). *Family constellation: Its effects on personality and science behavior.* New York, NY: Springer.

Turner, R. H. (1970). *Family interaction.* New York, NY: John Wiley & Sons.

von Bertalanffy, L. (1950). The theory of open systems in physics and biology. *Science, 111,* 23–29.

von Bertalanffy, L. (1968). *General systems theory: Foundations, development, and applications.* New York, NY: George Braziller.

Walker, P. H. (2005). Neuman's systems model. In J. J. Fitzpatrick & A. L. Whall (Eds.), *Conceptual models of nursing: Analysis and application* (4th ed., pp. 194–224). Upper Saddle River, NJ: Pearson Prentice Hall.

Watzlawick, P., Beavin, J., & Jackson, D. (1967). *Pragmatics of human communication.* New York, NY: W. W. Norton.

Watzlawick, P., Weakland, J., & Fisch, R. (1974). *Change: Principles of problem formulation and problem resolution.* New York, NY: W. W. Norton.

White, J. M. (2005). *Advancing family theories.* Thousand Oaks, CA: Sage.

White, J. M., & Klein, D. M. (2008). *Family theories* (3rd ed.). Los Angeles, CA: Sage.

Wilkerson, S., & Loveland-Cherry, C. (2005). Johnson's behavioral systems model. In J. J. Fitzpatrick & A. L. Whall (Eds.), *Conceptual models of nursing: Analysis and application* (4th ed., pp. 83–103). Upper Saddle River, NJ: Pearson Prentice Hall.

Wright, L., & Leahey, M. (2013). *Nurses and families: A guide to family assessment and intervention* (6th ed.). Philadelphia, PA: F. A. Davis.

Wright, L. M., & Watson, W. L. (1988). Systemic family therapy and family development. In C. J. Falicox (Ed.), *Family transitions: Continuity and change over the life cycle* (pp. 407–430). New York, NY: Guilford Press.

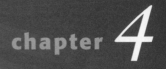
Family Nursing Assessment and Intervention

Joanna Rowe Kaakinen, PhD, RN

Aaron Tabacco, BSN, RN, Doctoral Candidate

Critical Concepts

- Families are complex social systems with which nurses interact in many ways and in many different contexts; the use of a logical systematic family nursing assessment approach is important.

- In the context of family nursing, the creative nurse thinker must be aware of possibilities, be able to recognize the new and the unusual, be able to decipher unique and complex situations, and be inventive in designing an approach to family care.

- Nurses determine through which theoretical and practice lens(es) to analyze the family event.

- Knowledge about family structures, functions, and processes inform nurses in their efforts to optimize and provide individualized nursing care, tailored to the uniqueness of every family system.

- Nurses begin family assessment from the moment of contact or referral.

- Family stories are narratives that nurses construct in framing, contextualizing, educating, communicating, and providing interpretations of their family clients' needs as they exercise clinical judgment in their work.

- Interacting with families as clients requires knowledge of family assessment and intervention models, as well as skilled communication techniques so that the interaction will be effective and efficient for all parties.

- The family genogram and ecomap are both assessment data-gathering instruments. The therapeutic interaction that occurs with the family while diagramming a genogram or ecomap is itself a powerful intervention.

- Families' beliefs about health and illness, about nurses and other health care providers, and about themselves are essential for nurses to explore in order to craft effective approaches to family interventions and promote health literacy.

- Families determine the level of nurses' involvement in their health and illness journeys, and nurses seek to tailor their work and approach accordingly.

- Nurses and families who work together and build on family strengths are in the best position to determine and prioritize specific family needs; develop realistic outcomes; and design, evaluate, and modify a plan of action that has a high probability of being implemented by the family.

- The final step in working with families should always be for nurses to engage in critical, creative, and concurrent reflection about the family, their work with the family, and professional self-reflection of their practice.

Families are complex social systems. Therefore, the use of logical, systematic approaches to assess and intervene with family clients is essential for several reasons: (1) to ensure that the needs of the family are met, (2) to uncover any gaps in the family plan of action, and (3) to offer multiple supports and resources to the family. Nurses use a variety of assessment models to collect information about families. In concert with the family, this information is used to develop the interventions families use to manage their current health event. Some assessment and intervention instruments are based on theoretical models, and some are developed using a psychometric approach to instrument development. Built on the traditional nursing process as visualized by Doenges, Moorhouse, and Murr (2013) (Fig. 4-1) and combined with the Outcome Present State Testing Model (Pesut & Herman, 1999), this chapter presents a dynamic systematic critical reasoning method to conducting a family assessment and tailoring interventions to meet family needs (Fig. 4-2) and applies it to a case study. The chapter explores assessment strategies, including how to select assessment instruments, determine the need for interpreters, assess for health literacy, diagram family genograms, and develop family ecomaps. Intervention strategies follow assessment strategies to assist nurses and families in shared decision making. The chapter concludes with a brief introduction to three family assessment and intervention models that were developed by nurses.

FAMILY NURSING ASSESSMENT

Central to the delivery of safe and effective family nursing care is the nurse's ability to make accurate assessments, identify health problems, and tailor plans of care. Each step of working with families, whether applied to individuals within the family or the family as a whole, requires a thoughtful, deliberate reasoning process. Nurses decide what data to collect and how, when, and where those data are collected. Nurses determine the relevance of each new piece of information and how it fits into the emerging family story. Before moving forward, nurses decide whether they have obtained sufficient information on problem and strength identification, or whether gaps exist that require additional data gathering.

Nurses must always be aware that "common" interpretations of data may not be the "correct" interpretation in any given situation, and that commonly expected signs and symptoms may not appear in every case or in the same data pattern presentation. The ability of nurses to be open to the unexpected and to be alert to unusual or different responses is critical to determining the primary

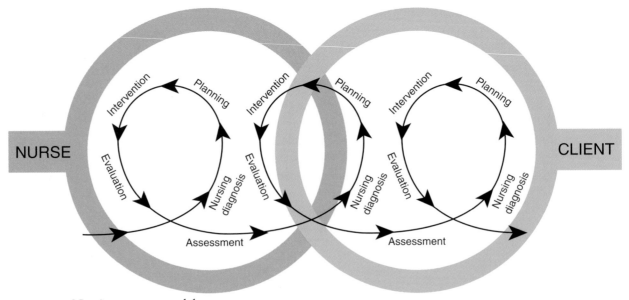

FIGURE 4-1 Nursing process model.

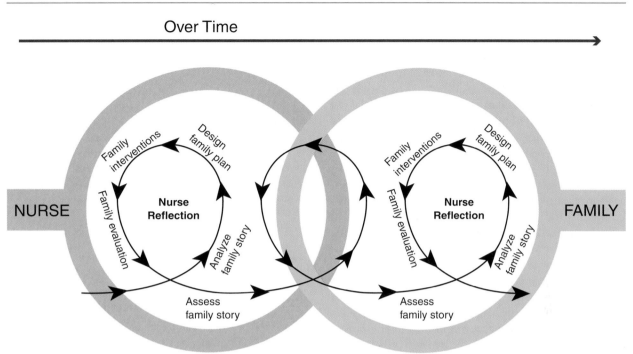

FIGURE 4-2 Family nursing assessment model.

needs confronting the family. Nurses should be able to perceive that which is not obvious and to understand how this family story is similar to or different from other family stories.

The family nursing assessment includes the following steps:

- Assessment of the family story: The nurse gathers data from a variety of sources to see the whole picture of the family experience.
- Analysis of family story: The nurse clusters the data into meaningful patterns to see how the family is managing the health event. The family needs are prioritized using a Family Reasoning Web.
- Design of a family plan of care: Together, the nurse and family determine the best plan of care for the family to manage the situation.
- Family intervention: Together, the nurse and family implement the plan of care incorporating the most family-focused, cost-effective, and efficient interventions that assist the family to achieve the best possible outcomes.
- Family evaluation: Together, the nurse and family determine whether the outcomes are being reached, are being partially reached, or need to be redesigned. Is the care plan

working well, does a new care plan need to be put into place, or does the nurse/family relationship need to end?

- Nurse reflection: Nurses engage in critical, creative, and concurrent reflection about themselves and their own family experiences, the family client, and their work with the family.

Engaging Families in Care

Background and First Contact

Nurses encounter families in diverse health care settings for many different kinds of problems and circumstances. Every family has a story about how the potential or actual health event influences its individual members, family functioning, and management of the health event. Nurses are charged with gathering, sifting, organizing, and analyzing the data to craft a clear view of the family's story. Nurses filter data gathered in the story through different views or approaches, which affects how they think about the family as a whole and each individual family member. For example, a family who is faced with a new diagnosis of a chronic illness would have different needs than a family who is faced with a member dying of an end-stage chronic illness. Nurses might use different strategies if the patient is in the acute hospital setting, is in an assisted living center, or is living at home.

The underlying theoretical approach used by the nurses working with families influences how they ask questions and collect family data. For example, if the family is worried about how their 2-year-old child will react to a new baby, such as in the Bono family case study presented later in this chapter, the nurse may elect to base the assessment and interventions on a family systems theoretical view, or the developmental family life cycle theoretical view. Refer to Chapter 3 for a detailed discussion of working with families from different theoretical perspectives.

Data collection, which is the first part of assessment, involves both subjective and objective family information that is obtained through direct observation, examination, or in consultation with other health care providers. In all cases, family assessment begins from the first moment that the family is referred to the nurse. Following are some circumstances in which a family is referred to a nurse:

- A family is referred by the hospital to a home health agency for wound care on the feet of a client with diabetes.
- A couple seeks advice for managing their busy life with three children as the mother returns home from the hospital following an unplanned cesarean section.
- A family calls the Visiting Nurse Association to request assistance in providing care to a family member with increasing dementia.
- A school nurse is asked by the school psychologist to conduct a family assessment with a family who is suspected of child neglect.
- A physician requests a family assessment with a child who has nonorganic failure to thrive.
- A family with a member with critical care needs is asked to make decisions about life-sustaining treatments in the intensive care unit.

Making Community-Based Appointments

As soon as a family is identified, the nurse begins to collect data about the family story. Sources of data that can be collected before contacting a family for a home or clinic appointment are listed in Box 4-1. Specifically, the nurse needs to know the following information:

- The reason for the referral or requested visit
- The family knowledge of the visit or referral

> **BOX 4-1**
> ### Sources of Pre-encounter Family Data
>
> - Referral source: includes data that indicated a problem for this family, as well as demographic information
> - Family: includes family members' views of the problem, surprise that the referral was made, reluctance to set up the meeting, avoidance in setting up the appointment
> - Previous records: in the health care systems or that are sent by having the client sign a release for information form, such as process logs, charts, phone logs, or school records

- Specific medical information about the family member with the health problem
- Strategies that have been used previously
- Insurance sources for the family
- Family problems identified by other health providers
- Family demographic data, when available, such as the number of people and ages of family members or basic cultural background information
- The need for an interpreter

Before contacting the family to arrange for the initial appointment, the nurse decides whether the most appropriate place to conduct the appointment is in the family's home or the clinic/office. The type of agency where the nurse works may dictate this decision. Advantages and disadvantages of a home setting and a clinic setting are listed in Table 4-1.

Contacting the family for the appointment provides valuable information about the family. It is imperative that the nurse be confident and organized when making the initial contact. Information that is important for the nurse to note is whether the family acts surprised that the referral was made, shows reluctance in setting up a meeting, or expresses openness about working together. The family also gathers important information about the nurse during the initial interaction. For example, family members will notice whether the nurse takes time to talk with them, uses a lot of words they do not understand, or appears organized and open to working with the family. To facilitate the best possible outcomes in engaging families for the first time to learn about their health and illness story, effective nurses consider the family and its needs as central to starting a successful collaboration.

Table 4-1	**Advantages and Disadvantages of Home Visits Versus Clinic Visits**
Home Visit	**Clinic Visit**
Advantages • Opportunity to see the everyday family environment. • Observe typical family interactions because the family members are likely to feel more relaxed in their physical space. • More family members may be able to attend the meeting. • Emphasizes that the problem is the responsibility of the whole family and not one family member.	• Conducting the family appointment in the office or clinic allows for easier access to consultants. • The family situation may be so strained that a more formal, less personal setting will facilitate discussions of emotionally charged issues.
Disadvantages • Home may be the only sanctuary or safe place for the family or its members to be away from the scrutiny of others. Therefore, conducting the meeting in the home would invade or violate this sanctuary and bring the clinical perspective into this safe world. • The nurse must be highly skilled in communication, specifically setting limits and guiding the interaction, or the visit may have a more social tone and not be efficient or productive.	• May reinforce a possible culture gap between the family and the nurse.

This relationship of trust begins from the moment of first contact with families. As a guide, Box 4-2 outlines steps to follow when making an appointment with a family.

Family Assessments in Acute Care Settings

Nurses in acute care settings encounter families of their individual patients on a daily basis. The degree to which nurses feel comfortable and to which they demonstrate clinical competence engaging families varies widely. Because cost (which is constrained) determines length of stay, and because of the increasing population of people with chronic illnesses who experience poor symptom management, nurses in acute care settings often feel there is little time to engage families effectively. Lack of time, in fact, has been identified by nurses as the primary barrier to engaging families, though there are many other barriers as well, including nurse bias, safety concerns, and negative nurse attitudes about working with families (Duran, Oman, Abel, Koziel, & Szymanski, 2007; Gurses & Carayon, 2007; Svavarsdottir, 2008). It is critical that nurses gain skill and comfort with families in acute care settings as families are the primary caregivers following the discharge of their family members. Families need the help of nurses in order to learn how to provide effective postdischarge care tasks; engage in shared decision making with health care providers; understand the current health status of their ill family member; balance admission and postdischarge family life demands; assist families during critical events such as resuscitation; and solve ethical dilemmas that arise in the care of their loved one. With this extensive list of needs, it is essential that nurses in acute care settings intentionally and effectively engage families.

Nurses in acute care settings encounter a number of challenges, including caring for several acutely ill persons simultaneously, managing the informational needs of interdisciplinary providers, and coping with a host of distractions that often keep nurses away from the bedside. Therefore,

---

BOX 4-2
Setting Up Family Appointments

■ Introduce yourself.
■ State the purpose of the requested meeting, including who referred the family to the agency.
■ Do not apologize for the meeting.
■ Be factual about the need for the meeting but do not provide details.
■ Offer several possible times for the meeting, including late afternoon or evening.
■ Let the family select the most convenient time that allows the majority of family members to attend.
■ Offer services of an interpreter, if required.
■ Confirm date, time, place, and directions.

nurses seeking to engage families, complete family assessments, and implement family interventions must be highly efficient and creative. A number of specific strategies and tools must be used to accomplish a meaningful and effective experience. For an in-depth discussion of acute care family nursing needs, refer to Chapter 14.

Using Interpreters With Families

It is critical for the nurse to determine whether an interpreter is needed during the family meeting, because the number of families who do not speak English is increasing. For 55.4 million Americans, English is not the primary language spoken in the home, and 13.6 million of these people speak English poorly or not at all (U.S. Census Bureau, 2010). Language barriers have been found to complicate many aspects of patient care, including comprehension and adherence to plans of care. Furthermore, language barriers have been found to contribute to adverse health outcomes, compromised quality of care, avoidable expenses, dissatisfied families, and increased potential for medical mistakes (Flores, Abreu, Barone, Bachur, & Lin, 2012; Schenker, Wang, Selig, Ng, & Fernandez, 2007). Thus, it is essential that nurses who are not bilingual use interpreters when working with non–English-speaking families.

The types of interpreters that nurses solicit to help work with families have the potential to influence the quality of the information exchanged and the family's ability to follow the suggested plan of action. One of the most common types of interpreters used are bilingual family members or friends, called *ad hoc family interpreters*. The problems with using family members as interpreters are that they have been found to buffer information, alter the meaning of the content, or make the decision for the person for whom they are interpreting (Flores et al., 2012; Ledger, 2002). The ad hoc family member interpreter also has been found to lack important language skills, especially when it comes to medical interpretation (Flores et al., 2012; Khwaja et al., 2006; Ledger, 2002). If the ad hoc family member interpreter is a child, the information that is being discussed may be frightening or the topic may be too personal and sensitive (Ledger, 2002). Using ad hoc family interpreters also raises confidentially issues (Gray, Hilder, & Donaldson, 2011). Therefore, it is not ideal for nurses to use a family member for interpretation, especially if another choice is available.

If a qualified medical interpreter cannot come to the meeting in the family home, the nurse should plan to use a speaker phone so that the professional interpreter can be involved in the conversation with the family. One of the problems with using an interpreter on the phone is that interpreters do not have the advantage of seeing the family members in person and cannot observe nonverbal communication (Bethell, Simpson, & Read, 2006; Gray et al., 2011; Herndon & Joyce, 2004). Also, the nurse should be aware that using a telephone interpreter introduces another outside person into the family setting, which may be perceived as impersonal by the family (Bethell et al., 2006).

Family-Centered Meetings and Care Conferences

Family-centered care (FCC) principles should be applied in all interactions between nurses and families or other health care providers. According to the Institute for Patient and Family Centered Care (IPFCC) (2013), the core principles of FCC are respect and dignity, information sharing, participation, and collaboration. The goal of FCC is to increase the mutual benefit of health care provision for all parties, with a focus on improving the satisfaction and outcomes of health care for families (IPFCC, 2013). By utilizing these principles in all aspects of the family nursing approach from assessment through intervention and evaluation, nurses can facilitate exchanges of shared expertise, which lead to better holistic health outcomes.

During the initial interaction with families, it is critical for nurses to introduce themselves to the family, meet all the family members present, learn about the family members not present, clearly state the purpose for working with the family, outline what will happen during this session, and indicate the length of time the meeting will last. Taking these actions demonstrates respect for family members and their unique story. To continue with this precedent, the nurse needs to develop a systematic plan for the first and all following family meetings. This focus on respect, dignity, and collaboration in initial meetings helps to establish relationships that are therapeutic; effective, satisfying partnerships between nurses and families are critical as they work together toward health-related goals.

Nurses who use a therapeutic approach to family meetings have found that their focus on family-centered care increased, and that their communication skills with families became more fluid with experience (Harrison, 2010; Martinez, D'Artois, & Rennick, 2007). When nurses use therapeutic communication skills with families, the families report feeling a stronger rapport with the nurse, an increased frequency of communication between families and the nurse occurs, and families perceive these nurses to be more competent (Harrison, 2010; Martinez et al., 2007).

Conducting family meetings not only requires skilled communication strategies but also requires knowledge of family assessment and intervention models. Nurses use a variety of data collection and assessment instruments to help gather information in a systematic and efficient manner. Therefore, it is important that the instruments be carefully selected so they are family friendly and render information pertinent to the purpose of working with the family.

FAMILY NURSING ASSESSMENT MODELS AND INSTRUMENTS

Nurses practice family nursing using a variety of tools. The following three family assessment models have been developed by family nurses. The Family Assessment and Intervention Model and the FS^{3}I were developed by Berkey-Mischke and Hanson (1991). Friedman developed the Friedman Family Assessment Model (Friedman et al., 2003). The Calgary Family Assessment Model (CFAM) and Calgary Family Intervention Model (CFIM) were developed by Wright and Leahey (2013). These three approaches vary in purpose, unit of analysis, and level of data collected. Table 4-2 has a detailed comparison of the essential components of these three family assessment models.

Table 4-2 Comparison of Family Assessment Models Developed by Family Nurses			
Name of model	Family Assessment and Intervention Model and the Family System Stressor-Strength Inventory (FS^{3}I)	Friedman Family Assessment Model	Calgary Family Assessment and Intervention Model
Citation	Berkey-Mischke & Hanson (1991) Hanson (2001)	Friedman, Bowden, & Jones (2003)	Wright & Leahey (2013)
Purpose	Concrete, focused measurement instrument that helps families identify current family stressors and builds interventions based on family strengths	Concrete, global family assessment interview guide that looks primarily at families in the larger community in which they are embedded	Conceptual model and multidimensional approach to families that looks at the fit among family functioning, affective, and behavioral aspects
Theoretical underpinnings	Systems: Family systems Neuman systems Model: Stress-coping theory	Developmental Structural-functional Family stress-coping Environmental	Systems: Cybernetics Communication Change Theory
Level of data collected	Quantitative: Ordinal and interval Qualitative: Nominal	Qualitative: Nominal	Qualitative: Nominal
Settings in which primarily used	Inpatient Outpatient Community	Outpatient Community	Outpatient Community
Units of analysis	Family as context Family as client Family as system Family as component of society	Family as client Family as component of society	Family as system

(continued)

Table 4-2	Comparison of Family Assessment Models Developed by Family Nurses—cont'd		
Strengths	Short Easy to administer Yields data to compare one family member with another family member Assess and measure focused presenting problem	Comprehensive list of areas to assess family	Conceptually sound
Weaknesses	Narrow variable	Large quantities of data that may not relate to the problem No quantitative data	Not concrete enough to be useful as a guideline unless the provider has studied this model and approach in detail

Family Assessment and Intervention Model

The Family Assessment and Intervention Model, originally developed by Berkey-Mischke and Hanson (1991), is presented in greater detail in Chapter 3, but is worth exploring in this context as well. The Family Assessment Intervention Model is based on Neuman's health care systems model (Kaakinen & Hanson, 2005).

According to the Family Assessment and Intervention Model, families are subject to tensions when stressed. The family's reaction depends on how deeply the stressor penetrates the family unit and how capable the family is of adapting to maintain its stability. The lines of resistance protect the family's basic structure, which includes the family's functions and energy resources. The family core contains the patterns of family interactions and strengths. The basic family structure must be protected at all costs or the family ceases to exist. Reconstitution or adaptation is the work the family undertakes to preserve or restore family stability. This model addresses three areas: (1) health promotion, wellness activities, problem identification, and family factors at lines of defense and resistance; (2) family reaction and instability at lines of defense and resistance; and (3) restoration of family stability and family functioning at levels of prevention and intervention.

The FS^{3}I is the assessment and intervention tool that accompanies the Family Assessment and Intervention Model. The FS^{3}I is divided into three sections: (1) family systems stressors—general; (2) family stressors—specific; and (3) family system strengths. An updated copy of the instrument, with instructions for administration and a scoring guide, can be found in Appendix A.

Nurses can assess family stability by gathering information on family stressors and strengths. The nurse and family work together to assess the family's general, overall stressors, and then specific family problems. Identified family strengths give an indication of the potential and actual problem-solving abilities of the family system. A plus to the FS^{3}I approach is that both quantitative and qualitative data are used to determine the level of prevention and intervention needed. The family is actively involved in the discussions and decisions. Moreover, this assessment and intervention approach focuses on family stressors and strengths, and provides a theoretical structure for family nursing.

Friedman Family Assessment Model

The Friedman Family Assessment Model (Friedman et al., 2003) is based on the structural-functional framework and developmental and systems theory. This assessment model takes a macroscopic approach to family assessment by viewing families as subsystems of the wider society, which includes institutions devoted to religion, education, and health. Family is considered an open social system and this model focuses on family's structure, functions (activities and purposes), and relationships with other social systems. The Friedman model is commonly used when the family-in-community is the setting for care (e.g., in community and public health nursing). This approach enables family nurses to assess the family system as a whole, as a subunit of the society, and as an interactional system. Box 4-3 delineates the general assumptions of this model (Friedman et al., 2003, p. 100).

BOX 4-3
Underlying Assumptions of Friedman's Family Assessment Model

- A family is a social system with functional requirements.
- A family is a small group possessing certain generic features common to all small groups.
- The family as a social system accomplishes functions that serve the individual and society.
- Individuals act in accordance with a set of internalized norms and values that are learned primarily through socialization.

Source: Friedman, M. M., Bowden, V. R., & Jones, E. G. (2003). *Family nursing: Research, theory & practice* (5th ed.). Upper Saddle River, NJ: Prentice Hall/Pearson Education.

Structure refers to how a family is organized and how the parts relate to each other and to the whole. The four basic structural dimensions are role systems, value systems, communication networks, and power structure. These dimensions are interrelated and interactive, and they may differ in single-parent and two-parent families. For example, a single mother may be the head of the family, but she may not necessarily take on the authoritarian role that a traditional man might in a two-parent family. In turn, the value systems, communication networks, and power structures may be quite different in the single-parent and two-parent families as a result of these structural differences.

Function refers to how families go about meeting the needs of individuals and meeting the purposes of the broader society. In other words, family functions are what a family does. The functions of the family historically are discussed in Chapter 1, but the following specific family functions are considered in this approach:

- Pass on culture, religion, ethnicity.
- Socialize young people for the next generation (e.g., to be good citizens, to be able to cope in society through education).
- Exist for sexual satisfaction and reproduction.
- Provide economic security.
- Serve as a protective mechanism for family members against outside forces.
- Provide closer human contact and relations.

The Friedman Family Assessment Model form consists of six broad categories of interview questions: (1) identification data, (2) developmental stage and history of the family, (3) environmental data, (4) family structure (i.e., role structure, family values, communication patterns, power structure), (5) family functions (i.e., affective functions, socialization functions, health care functions), and (6) family stress and coping. Each category has several subcategories (Friedman et al., 2003).

Friedman's assessment was developed to provide guidelines for family nurses who are interviewing a family. The guidelines categorize family information according to structure and function. Friedman's Family Assessment Form exists in both a long form and a short form. The long form is quite extensive (13 pages), and it may not be possible to collect all of the data in one visit. Moreover, all the categories of information listed in the guidelines may not be pertinent for every family. Like other approaches, this model has its strengths and weaknesses. One problem with this approach is that it can generate large quantities of data with no clear direction as to how to use all of the information in diagnosis, planning, and intervention. The strength of this approach is that it addresses a comprehensive list of areas to assess the family, and that a short assessment form has been developed to highlight critical areas of family functioning. The short form, which is included in Appendix B, outlines the types of questions the nurse can ask.

Calgary Family Assessment Model

The CFAM by Wright and Leahey (2013) blends nursing and family therapy concepts that are grounded in systems theory, cybernetics, communication theory, change theory, and a biology of recognition. The following concepts from general systems theory and family systems theory make up the theoretical framework for this model (Wright & Leahy, 2013, pp. 21–44):

- A family system is part of a larger suprasystem and is also composed of many subsystems.
- The family as a whole is greater than the sum of its parts.
- A change in one family member affects all family members.
- The family is able to create a balance between change and stability.
- Family members' behaviors are best understood from a perspective of circular rather than linear causality.

Cybernetics is the science of communication and control theory; therefore, it differs from systems theory. Systems theory helps change the focus of one's conceptual lens from parts to wholes. By contrast, cybernetics changes the focus from substance to form. Wright and Leahey (2013) pull two useful concepts from cybernetics theory:

■ Families possess self-regulating ability.
■ Feedback processes can simultaneously occur at several system levels with families.

Communication theory in this model is based on the work of Watzlawick and colleagues (Watzlawick, Weakland, & Fisch, 1967, 1974). Communication represents the way that individuals interact with one another. Concepts derived from communication theory used in the CFAM are as follows (Wright & Leahey, 2013):

■ All nonverbal communication is meaningful.
■ All communication has two major channels for transmission: digital (verbal) and analogical (nonverbal).
■ A dyadic relationship has varying degrees of symmetry (similarity) and complementarity (divergence, contrast, or complementary characteristics).
■ All communication has two levels: content and relationship.

Helping families to change is at the very core of family nursing interventions. Families need a balance between change and stability. Change is required to make things better, and stability is required to maintain some semblance of order. A number of concepts from change theory are important to this family nursing approach (Wright & Leahey, 2013):

■ Change is dependent on the perception of the problem.
■ Change is determined by structure.
■ Change is dependent on context.
■ Change is dependent on co-evolving goals for treatment.
■ Understanding alone does not lead to change.
■ Change does not necessarily occur equally in all family members.
■ Facilitating change is the nurse's responsibility.
■ Change occurs by means of a "fit" or meshing between the therapeutic offerings (interventions of the nurse) and the bio-psycho-social-spiritual structures of family members.

■ Change can be the result of a myriad of causes.

Figure 4-3 shows the branching diagram of the CFAM (Wright & Leahey, 2013, p. 48). The assessment questions that accompany the model are organized into three major categories: (1) structural, (2) developmental, and (3) functional. Nurses examine a family's structural components to answer these questions: Who is in the family? What is the connection between family members? What is the family's context? Structure includes family composition, sex, sexual orientation, rank order, subsystems, and the boundaries of the family system. Aside from interview and observation, strategies recommended to assess structure include the genogram and the ecomap.

The second major assessment category in the Calgary approach is family development, which includes assessment of family stages, tasks, and attachments. For example, nurses may ask, "Where is the family in the family life cycle?" Understanding the stage of the family enables nurses to assess and intervene in a more purposeful, specific, and meaningful way. There are no actual instruments for assessing development, but nurses can use developmental tasks as guidelines.

The third area for assessment in the CFAM is family functioning. Family functioning reflects how individuals actually behave in relation to one another, or the "here-and-now aspect of a family's life" (Wright & Leahey, 2013, p. 116). Aspects of family functioning include activities of daily life, such as eating, sleeping, meal preparation, and health care, as well as emotional communication, verbal and nonverbal communication, communication patterns (the way communication and responses are passed back and forth between members), problem solving, roles, influence and power, beliefs, and alliances and coalitions. Wright and Leahey indicate that nurses may assess in all three areas for a macroview of the family, or they can use any part of the approach for a microassessment. Wright and Leahey (2013) developed a companion model to the CFAM, the CFIM. This intervention model provides concrete strategies by which nurses can promote, improve, and sustain effective family functioning in the cognitive, affective, and behavioral domains. The strength of the Calgary Assessment and Intervention Model is that it is a conceptually sound model that incorporates

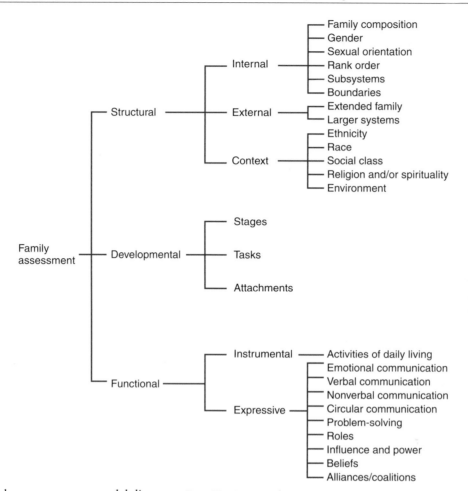

FIGURE 4-3 Calgary assessment model diagram. *(From Wright L. M., & Leahey, M. [2009]. Nurses and families: A guide to family assessment and intervention [5th ed.]. Philadelphia, PA: F. A. Davis, with permission.)*

multiple theoretical aspects into working with families. The strength of this approach is also its weakness in that unless you are intimately knowledgeable with the model and the interventions, it is difficult to implement in acute care settings.

Family Assessment Instruments

Because there are approximately 1,000 family-focused instruments that have been developed and used in assessing family-related variables (Touliatos, Perlmutter, & Straus, 2001), the selection of the appropriate instrument can be complex. Sometimes, a simple questionnaire or instrument can be completed in just a few minutes. One such example is the Patient/Parent Information and Involvement Assessment Tool (PINT), which is an instrument

that Sobo (2004) designed to assess the family's perspective on shared decision making. Other times, more comprehensive family assessment instruments are necessary, such as the Family Systems Stressor-Strength Inventory (FS³I) (Berkey-Mischke & Hanson, 1991; Hanson, 2001; Kaakinen, Hanson, & Denham, 2010). The FS³I is an instrument designed by nurses to provide quantitative and qualitative data pertinent to family stressors, family strengths, and intervention strategies (see Appendix A). To select the most appropriate assessment instrument, be sure the instrument has the following characteristics:

- Written in uncomplicated language at a fifth-grade level
- Only 10 to 15 minutes in length
- Relatively easy to score

- Offers valid data on which to base decisions
- Sensitive to sex, race, social class, and ethnic background

Regardless of which assessment/measurement instrument is used, families should always be informed of how the information gathered through the instruments will be used by the health care providers.

Two other family data-gathering instruments that should be used in working with families are the family genogram and the family ecomap. Both are short, easy instruments and processes that supply essential family data and engage the family in therapeutic conversation.

Family Genogram and Family Ecomap

Genograms and ecomaps provide care providers with visual diagrams of the current family story and situation (Harrison & Neufeld, 2009; Kaakinen, 2010). The information gathered from both the genogram and ecomap help guide the family plan of action and the selection of intervention strategies (Ray & Street, 2005). One of the major benefits of working with families with these two instruments is that family members can feel and visualize the amount of energy they are expending to manage the situation, which in itself is therapeutic for the family (Harrison & Neufeld, 2009; Holtslander, 2005; Rempel, Neufeld, & Kushner, 2007).

The use of genograms and ecomaps among nurses and other disciplines is growing and these useful tools are being applied in a number of practice and research contexts. Genograms, used historically in the context of genetic prediction and counseling, have been applied alongside ecomaps as primary assessment and decision-making tools in acute centers (Leahey & Svavarsdottir, 2009; Svavarsdottir, 2008). Examples of how other providers have applied the use of these tools include enhancing health promotion (Cascado-Kehoe & Kehoe, 2008); increasing provider cultural competence and spiritual assessment of families (Hodge & Limb, 2010); and assessment of child social support systems (Baumgartner, Burnett, DiCarlo, & Buchanan, 2012). It is clear that generating and annotating visual data in these diagrammatic forms will be increasingly useful to nurses caring for families in many settings and contexts.

Family Genogram

The *family genogram* is a format for drawing a family tree that records information about family members and their relationships over at least three generations (McGoldrick, Gerson, & Petry, 2008).

This diagram offers a rich source of information for planning intervention strategies because it displays the family visually and graphically in a way that provides a quick overview of family complexities. Family genograms help both nurses and families to see and think systematically about families and the impact of the health event on family structure, function, and processes.

The three-generational family genogram had its origin in Family Systems Theory (Bowen, 1985; Bowen & Kerr, 1988). According to family systems, people are organized into family systems by generation, age, sex, or other similar features. How a person fits into his or her family structure influences its functioning, relational patterns, and what type of family he or she will carry forward into the next generation. Bowen incorporated Toman's (1976) ideas about the importance of sex and birth order in shaping sibling relationships and characteristics. Furthermore, families repeat themselves over generations in a phenomenon called the *transmission of family patterns* (Bowen, 1985). What happens in one generation repeats itself in the next generation; thus, many of the same strengths and problems get played out from generation to generation. These include psychosocial and physical and mental health issues.

Nurses establish therapeutic relationships with families through the process of asking questions while collecting family data. Families become more engaged in their current situation during this interaction as their family story unfolds. Both the nurse and the family can see the "big picture" historically on the vertical axis of the genogram and horizontally across the family (McGoldrick et al., 2008). This approach can help families see connectedness, and help identify potential and missing support people.

The diagramming of family genograms must adhere to specific rules and symbols to ensure that all parties involved have the same understanding and interpretations. It is important not to confuse family genograms with a family genetic pedigree. A family pedigree is specific to genetic assessments (see Chapter 7), whereas a genogram has broader uses for family health care practitioners. Olsen, Dudley-Brown, and McMullen (2004) have suggested, however, that given the advancement of genomics in driving health care, nursing should consider blending pedigrees with genograms and ecomaps as a way to offer a more comprehensive holistic nursing care perspective. Creative blended models built upon these ideas are emerging in practice with innovative applications such as the use of color coding for enhancing multimodal understanding of children and families (Driessnack, 2009).

Figure 4-4 provides a basic genogram from which a nurse can start diagramming family members over the first, second, and third generations (McGoldrick, Gerson, & Schellenberger, 1999). Figure 4-5 depicts the genogram symbols used to describe basic family membership and structure, family interaction patterns, and other family information of particular importance, such as health status, substance abuse, obesity, smoking, and mental health comorbidities (McGoldrick et al., 2008). The health history of all family members (e.g., morbidity, mortality, and onset of illness) is important information for family nurses and can be the focus of analysis of the family genogram. An example of a family genogram developed from one interview is contained in the Bono family case study below.

The structure of the interview for gathering the genogram information is based on the reasons why the nurse is working with the family. For example, if the context of creating a genogram is that of obtaining a health history aimed at uncovering family patterns of illness, the nurse may wish to explore more fully the health history of each generational family member. If, on the other hand, the context of the nursing care is determining the nature of social relationships and roles among family members to craft an acute care plan of discharge, the nurse may wish to focus the interview more closely on determining who is directly in the home and how

their relationships function to aid in the recovery of the ill family member. A suggested format for conducting a concise, focused family genogram interview is outlined in Box 4-4. Most families are cooperative and interested in completing their genogram, which becomes a part of their ongoing health care record. The genogram does not have to be completed at one sitting. As the same or a different nurse continues to work with a family, data can be added to the genogram over time in a continuing process. Families should be given a copy of their own genogram.

Family Ecomap

A *family ecomap* provides information about systems outside of the immediate nuclear family that are sources of social support or that are stressors to the family (Olsen et al., 2004). The ecomap is a visual representation of the family unit in relation to the larger community in which it is embedded (Kaakinen, 2010). It is a visual representation of the relationship between an individual family and the world around it (McGoldrick et al., 2008). The ecomap is thus an overview of the family in its current context, picturing the important connections among the nuclear family, the extended family, and the community around it.

The blank ecomap form consists of a large circle with smaller circles around it (Fig. 4-6). A simplified version of the family is placed in the center of the larger circle to complete the ecomap. This circle marks the boundary between the family and its extended external environment. The smaller outer circles represent significant people, agencies, or

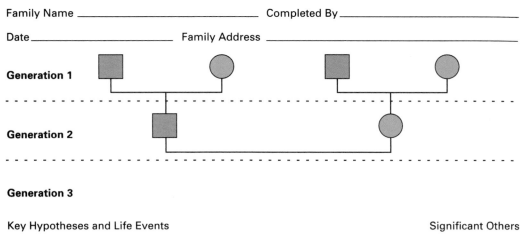

FIGURE 4-4 Basic genogram format.

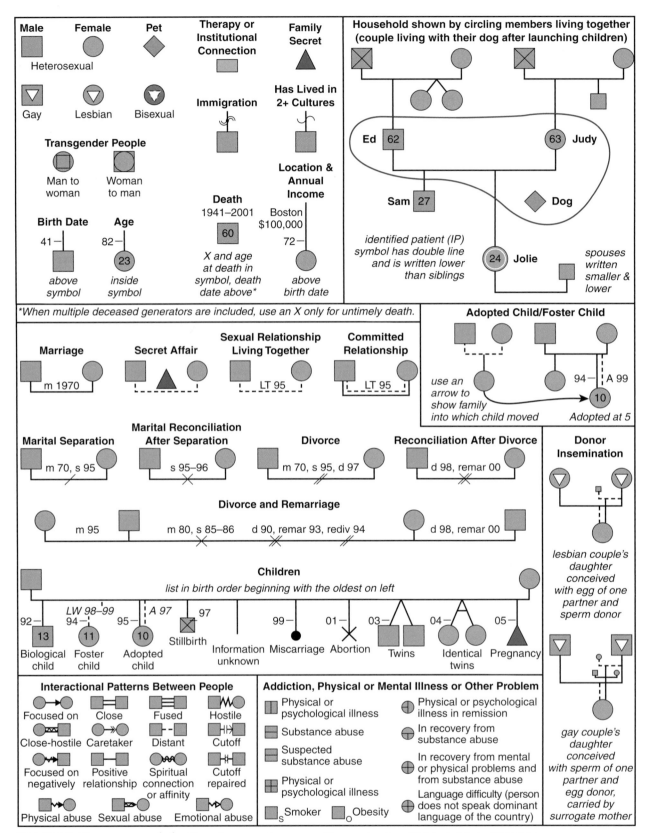

FIGURE 4-5 Genogram symbols. *(From Genograms: Assessment and Intervention, Second Edition by Monica McGoldrick, Randy Gerson, and Sylvia Shellenberger. Copyright © 1999 by Monica McGoldrick and Sylvia Shellenberger. Copyright © 1985 by Monica McGoldrick and Randy Gerson. Used by permission of W. W. Norton & Company, Inc.)*

BOX 4-4
Family Genogram Interview Data Collection

1. Identify who is in the immediate family.
2. Identify the person who has the health problem.
3. Identify all the people who live with the immediate family.
4. Determine how all the people are related.
5. Gather the following information on each family member.
   - Age
   - Sex
   - Correct spelling of name
   - Health problems
   - Occupation
   - Dates of relationships: marriage, separation, divorce, living together, living together/committed
   - Dates and age of death
6. Seek the same information for all family members across each generation for consistency and to reveal patterns of health and illness.
7. Add any information relative to the situation, such as geographical location and interaction patterns.

institutions with which the family interacts. Lines are drawn between the circles and the family members to depict the nature and quality of the relationships, and to show what kinds of energy and resources are moving in and out of the immediate family. Straight lines show strong or close relationships; the more pronounced the line or greater the number of lines, the stronger the relationship is. Straight lines with slashes denote stressful relationships, and broken lines show tenuous or distant relationships. Arrows reveal the direction of the flow of energy and resources between individuals, and between the family and the environment. Ecomaps not only portray the present situation but also can be used to set goals, for example, to increase connections and exchanges with individuals and agencies in the community. See the Bono family case study later in this chapter for an example of a completed ecomap.

The value of using a genogram and ecomap in family nursing practice is expansive. By creating a visual picture of the system in which the family

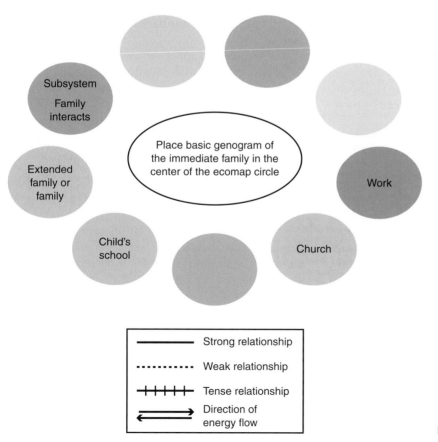

FIGURE 4-6 Blank ecomap.

exists, families are more able to envision alternative solutions and possible social support networks (Ray & Street, 2005; Yanicki, 2005). In addition, the process of this data collection itself helps to expose a clearer picture of the supportive or unsupportive family relationships that are going on in a family system (Neufeld, Harrison, Hughes, & Stewart, 2007). This information will enhance understanding of the family's social network with their caregivers (Ray & Street, 2005).

Family Health Literacy

Health literacy is the ability to use health information to make informed decisions through the comprehension of reading material, documents, and numbers. Functional health literacy incorporates all of these elements, but it also implies that the client (family) has the ability to act on health care decisions. Concepts of health literacy include the comprehension of medical words, the ability to follow medical instructions, and the understanding of the consequences when instructions are not followed (Speros, 2005). Nurses who understand the concept of health literacy will actively seek to collect ongoing assessment data about the learning needs of family members in their meetings, interviews, or conferences. This data about the family members' abilities and preferences for learning will help guide the nurse to provide education, materials, and other supports, such as videos or Web sites, that are accessible to the family.

Through interactions with the family and when completing the genogram and ecomap, nurses have the opportunity to determine whether there is an issue of health literacy for any member of the family. Health literacy is an important measure for health care practitioners because lower health literacy is strongly associated with poor health outcomes (Berkman, Sheridan, Donahue, Halpern, & Crotty, 2011; Sentell & Halpin, 2006; Speros, 2005). Health literacy plays a primary role in people's ability to gain knowledge, make decisions, and take actions that result in positive health outcomes (Berkman et al., 2011; DeWalt, Boone, & Pignone, 2007; Speros, 2005), especially when managing a chronic illness (Gazmararian, Williams, Peel, & Baker, 2003). Assessment is particularly important when low literacy or low language proficiency exists, because such individuals are more likely to attempt to hide their inability to read or understand

because of shame or embarrassment (Bass, 2005; Dreger & Tremback, 2002; Osborn et al., 2007).

When nurses design written material for the family, the following common elements make it easier to understand from a health literacy perspective (Bass, 2005; Peters, Dieckmann, Dixon, Hibbard, & Mertz, 2007):

- All written information should be in at least 14-point font using high-contrast Arial or sans serif print with plenty of blank space on glossy paper.
- Uppercase and lowercase letters should be used.
- Information is most easily seen when using black ink on white paper. Use short sentences with bullets or lists no longer than seven items (Peters et al., 2007).

Written information presented at the third-grade reading level will reach the largest audience, but it may be necessary to write at the fifth-grade level to retain the meaning of the content (Mayer & Rushton, 2002; Peters et al., 2007). Using multiple forms of communication, including visual aids, will help families retain the information (Bass, 2005; Dreger & Tremback, 2002; Osborn et al., 2007).

Nurses need to approach assessment of the family health literacy with sensitivity and understanding. It is a crucial element to take into consideration during the analysis of the family story and in the development of the family action plan.

ANALYSIS OF THE FAMILY STORY

One of the challenges of data collection is organizing the individual pieces of information so that the "big picture" or whole family story can be understood and analyzed. To understand the family picture, the nurse must consolidate the data that were collected into meaningful patterns or categories so as to visualize the relationships between and among the patterns of how the family is managing the situation. Diagramming the family and the relationships between the data groups assists identifying the most pressing issues or problems for the family. If the family and nurse focus on solving these major family problems, the outcome will have a ripple effect by positively influencing the other areas of family functioning.

The Family Reasoning Web (Fig. 4-7) is an organizational tool to help analyze the family story, by clustering individual pieces of data into meaningful family categories. The components of the Family Reasoning Web have been pulled from various theoretical concepts, such as Family Structure and Function Theory, Family Developmental Theory, Family Stress Theory, and family health promotion models. This systematic approach to collecting and analyzing information helps structure the information collection process to ensure inclusion of important pieces of information. The categories of the Family Reasoning Web are as follows:

1. Family routines of daily living (i.e., sleeping, meals, child care, exercise)
2. Family communication
3. Family supports and resources
4. Family roles
5. Family beliefs
6. Family developmental stage
7. Family health knowledge
8. Family environment
9. Family stress management
10. Family culture
11. Family spirituality

Once the data have been placed into the categories of the Family Reasoning Web template, the nurse assigns a family nursing diagnosis to each category. "A nursing diagnosis is defined as a clinical judgment about individuals, families, or community responses to actual or potential health problems/life processes. Nursing diagnoses link information to care planning. Nursing diagnoses provide the basis for selecting nursing interventions to help achieve outcomes for which nurses are accountable" (Doenges et al., 2013, p. 11). The case study below presents more information on nursing diagnoses.

The North American Nurses Diagnosis Association (NANDA) (2007) is the most global nursing classification system. NANDA nursing diagnoses that are specific to families are listed in Box 4-5. If the pattern of family data in the specific category in the Family Reasoning Web does not match one of the NANDA nursing diagnoses, nurses are encouraged to create a family nursing diagnosis that captures the family problem. Nursing diagnosis manuals are extremely important resources for nurses because family nursing diagnoses are readily linked with both the Nursing Intervention Classification (NIC) (Bulechek, Butcher, Dochterman, & Wagner, 2013) and Nursing Outcomes Classification (NOC) (Moorhead, Johnson, Maas,

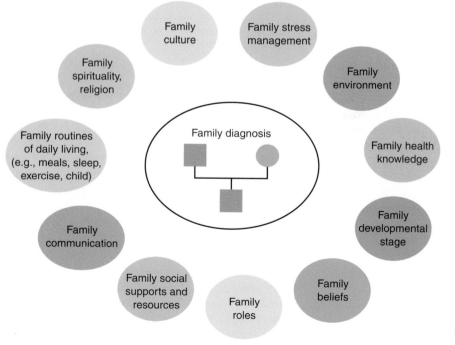

FIGURE 4-7 Family Reasoning Web template.

BOX 4-5

NANDA Nursing Diagnoses Relevant to Family Nursing

- Risk for impaired parent/infant/child attachment
- Caregiver role strain
- Risk for caregiver role strain
- Parental role conflict
- Compromised family coping
- Disabled family coping
- Readiness for enhanced family coping
- Dysfunctional family processes: alcoholism
- Readiness for enhanced family processes
- Interrupted family processes
- Readiness for enhanced parenting
- Impaired parenting
- Risk for impaired parenting
- Relocation stress syndrome
- Ineffective role performance
- Ineffective family therapeutic regimen management

Source: Doenges, M. E., Moorhouse, M. F., & Murr, A. C. (2013). *Nursing diagnosis manual: Planning, individualizing, and documenting client care* (3rd ed.). Philadelphia, PA: F. A. Davis, with permission.

Table 4-3	Selected Family-Centered Diagnoses From *Diagnostic and Statistical Manual of Mental Disorders, Fifth Edition*
V61.9	Relational problem related to a mental disorder or general medical condition
V61.20	Parent-child relational problem
V61.10	Partner relational problem
V61.8	Sibling relational problem
V71.02	Child or adolescent antisocial behavior
V62.82	Bereavement
V62.3	Academic problem
V62.4	Acculturation problem
V62.89	Phase-of-life problem

Source: American Psychiatric Association. (2013). *Diagnostic and statistical manual of mental disorders (DSM-5)* (5th ed.). Washington, DC: Author.

Table 4-4	Selected Family-Centered Diagnoses From ICD-9-CM
313.3	Relationship problems
313.8	Emotional disturbances of childhood or adolescence
V61.0	Family disruption
V25.09	Family planning advice
V61.9	Family problem
94.41	Group therapy
94.42	Family therapy

Source: American Medical Association. (2013). *International classification of diseases: Clinical modifications (IDC-9-CM)*. Dover, DE: Author.

& Swanson, 2012) data sets. These resources provide many new ideas for family interventions and suggest focused family outcomes that can be explored with families.

Other diagnostic classification systems that can be used to identify problems include the Omaha System–Community Health Classification System (Martin, 2004), the *Diagnostic and Statistical Manual of Mental Disorders, Fifth Edition* (DSM-5; American Psychiatric Association, 2013), and the *International Classification of Diseases: Clinical Modifications, Ninth Edition* (ICD-9-CM; American Medical Association, 2012). See Tables 4-3 and 4-4, respectively, for examples of selected family diagnoses from the DSM and ICD-9-CM sources.

A rapidly growing system of diagnostic language relevant to nursing in North America is that of the World Health Organization ICD companions, the International Classification of Functioning (ICF) and its related child and youth version (ICF-CY) (World Health Organization, 2013). This broad schema of classification focuses on making diagnostic statements of health impact in four domains: body structure, body function, activity and participation, and environment (World Health Organization, 2013). Family nursing practice greatly involves the focus on the domains of activity and participation and the environmental context of family life. Given that nurses' primary focus with individuals and families is the functional aspect of health in daily life, this system of categorizing and coding functional outcomes of health is compelling. The ICF and ICF-CY approaches are being used with expanded focus in Europe and Canada particularly (Florin, Björvell, Ehnfors, & Ehrenberg, 2012; Raggi, Leonardi, Cabello, & Bickenbach, 2010).

After the categories have been assigned and a family nursing diagnosis determined, the next step in analyzing the family story is for the nurse and family to work together to determine the relationships between the categories. Arrows are drawn between the family categories showing the direction of influence if the data in one category influence the data in another category. The important family problems or issues surface by systematically working through all of the relationships because they are the ones that have the most arrows indicating the strongest relationships to all other areas of family functioning. The step reveals the primary family problems.

Another dimension of the family story that is of importance to nurses is the dimension of beliefs. Family and family member beliefs about health, illness, health care providers, and even their own roles and processes are of great importance for nurses to assess in planning to provide optimal care. The Beliefs and Illness Model by Wright and Bell (2009) suggests that nurses should assess families' beliefs in a number of areas, specifically, family structure, roles, communication, and decision-making authority; beliefs about health and illness (how they are defined, why they occur, how they are managed); and beliefs about health care providers (their intentions, motivations, and knowledge and the meaning of their presence and actions to the families and their health or illness experience). Individuals and families often behave based upon their beliefs and thus any attempt for nurses to engage families in health promotion, health literacy, or health intervention in any setting requires an exploration of these key areas. After verifying all of these findings with the family, the next step is to work with the family to understand their preferences for decision making and design a family plan of care accordingly.

Shared Decision Making

Family nurses should explore how involved the family would like to be in the decision-making processes. Universal needs of families include consistency, clarity, comprehensive information, and involvement in shared decision making with the health care provider (Salmond, 2008; Schattner, Bronstein, & Jellin, 2006; Whitmer, Hughes, Hurst, & Young, 2005). Nurses, consciously and otherwise, affect the family stress level by controlling how much (and how quickly) they involve the family in the care of their family members (Corlett & Twycross, 2006). Nurses control how much information they share with families, how much they involve the family in the daily routine, visiting

hours, and even discussions with/among family members. Families have expressed fears of alienating health care providers (Taylor, 2006), thus compromising their loved ones' care. All of this may interfere with nurses being able to be effective family advocates (Leske, 2002).

Health care providers underestimate the extent that families want to be involved in the care of and decision making about loved ones (Bruera, Sweeny, Calder, Palmer, & Benisch-Tolly, 2001; Pierce & Hicks, 2001). Although most families prefer a shared decision-making approach (de Haes, 2006; Schattner et al., 2006; Whitmer et al., 2005), families vary relative to the amount of information they want and their role in the decision-making process (Sobo, 2004). The amount of information families seek or need changes over the course of the health event, the stage of the illness, and the likelihood of a cure (Butow, Maclean, Dunn, Tattersall, & Boyer, 1997).

An option grid is one strategy for implementation of shared decision making (Elwyn et al., 2012). An option grid is developed by the family nurse keeping health literacy principles at the fifth-grade level. Elwyn et al. specifically developed the grid format as a decision-making paper worksheet addressing common therapeutic approaches to specific health conditions where patients and families could view the benefits or drawbacks associated with different possible treatment decisions. On the worksheet, the most relevant, frequently asked questions about a specific condition make up the rows of the grid, and the specific options available for the decision make up the columns. Patients are given the paper grid and talked through the options available to them with their provider. For example, see Box 4-6, an option grid that a nurse could design to help parents determine respite placement for their 12-year-old daughter who is medically fragile with severe cerebral palsy. This specific tool shows promise for nurses working with families because not only does it represent the principles of family-centered care in practice, but also because families often have difficulties understanding their options and the potential benefits or consequences associated with their choices.

Another approach to shared decision making is to use the Patient/Parent Involvement Information Assessment Tool (PINT) developed by Sobo (2004). The PINT is a self-administered survey that can be kept in the medical record to facilitate and target information for communication between the health care team and the family. In the

BOX 4-6
Example of Option Grid

The following is an example of an option grid for helping a family to decide about 1-week respite placement for their 12-year-old medically fragile child:

Option 1: Home	Option 2: Grandmother's home	Option 3: Nursing home
Child knows own home and is around familiar surroundings.	Child has been to grandmother's home only a couple of times because it is in a different city.	New setting for child.
Home is adapted to the child's needs and wheelchair.	Home is not adapted to the physical care needs of child, such as wheelchair and bathing.	Setting can accommodate the child's special needs and wheelchair.
Caregiver would be the skills trainer who knows the child.	Caregiver is grandmother, who the child knows well and has spent considerable time with.	No personal relationship with caregivers in this setting. Grandmother could visit during day.
Parents are comfortable with the child being with the skills worker during the day, but do not have experience with this person at night.	Parents are comfortable with the child being with grandmother. Grandmother has helped take care of child for short times before, such as a weekend.	Parents do not have a relationship with the caregivers in this setting.
Cost: $250 a day for 7 days for a total of $1,750. This would come out of the parents' pocket because insurance does not cover this care.	Cost: nothing.	Cost: Covered by insurance.

challenge to collaborate in the care and meet the needs of individuals and family members, nurses may ask the following two sample questions from the PINT tool (Sobo, 2004, p. 258):

1. When possible, what level of information would you prefer to receive?
   - The simplest information possible
   - More than the simplest, but want to keep it on everyday terms
   - In-depth information that you can help me understand
   - As much in-depth and detailed information as can be provided

2. When possible, what decision-making role do you want to assume?
   - Leave all decisions to the health care team
   - Have the care team make the decisions about care with serious consideration of our views
   - Share in the making of the decisions with the health care team
   - Make all the decisions about care with serious consideration of the health care team advice

Supporting the hypothesis that not all families and family members want full involvement in making

health care decisions, Makoul and Clayman (2006) have outlined the following nine options for shared decision making (p. 307):

- Doctor alone
- Doctor led and patient acknowledgment sought or offered
- Doctor led and patient agreement sought or offered
- Doctor led and patient views/option sought or offered
- Shared equally
- Patient led and doctor views/opinions sought or offered
- Patient led and doctor agreement sought or offered
- Patient led and doctor acknowledgment sought or offered
- Patient alone

One of the problems with the implementation of shared decision making is that every health care provider has a different definition and understanding of the components of this concept, as well as personal biases and beliefs about how individuals and families may or may not wish to participate (Elwyn et al., 2012; Makoul & Clayman, 2006). Shared decision making is not just informing the family of the decisions and keeping the lines of communication open, nor is it the health care providers determining what decisions the family can make. Shared decision making requires that health care providers tailor their communication, accommodate their talk to the level of the family, and present information in a way that allows the family to make informed choices. Shared decision making includes the following steps as outlined by Makoul and Clayman (2006, pp. 305–306):

- The family and health care provider must define and agree on the health problem that is confronting the family member.
- The health care provider presents and discusses options of care in a way that invites family questions.
- The family and health care provider discuss pros and cons of options, including cost benefits, convenience, and financial costs.
- The family and health care provider discuss values and preferences, including ideas, concerns, and outcome expectations.
- The family and health care provider discuss ability and confidence to follow through with steps or regimen for each option.
- Both the health care provider and family should check and clarify for understanding the discussion and information shared.
- Both the health care provider and family should reach a decision or defer decisions until an agreed-on, specified time.
- The health care provider should follow up to track the outcome of the decision.

FAMILY NURSING INTERVENTION

The family plan of action (or care) is designed by the nurse and the family to focus on the concerns that were identified in the Family Reasoning Web as the most pressing or causing the family the most stress. The plan should account for the family preferences for decision making and should meet their health literacy needs. The more specific the family plan of action and the interventions, the more positive the outcomes. The role of the nurse is to offer guidance to the family, provide information, and assist in the planning interventions. Working with families from an outcome perspective helps to clarify what information and resources are necessary to address the family need.

The following four points will help the family break the plan into action steps:

1. We need the following type of help.
2. We need the following information.
3. We need the following supplies or resources.
4. We need to involve or tell the following people about our family action plan.

For the purposes of clarity and evaluation, this plan should be a written document. The action steps or interventions should be clear and concise. The plan should outline specifically who needs to do what by when and also articulate the timeframe in which the nurse will follow up. The last step of any family action plan should entail evaluation that involves the nurse and family reflecting and sharing ideas about what worked well, what needs to continue to be addressed by the family, and avenues for seeking help in the future.

Working with families to improve health and adapt to illness is the primary goal of family health care nursing. Nevertheless, there has been little direct evidence of the potential outcomes and effects associated with family nursing intervention because nurses are not often leading such research and/or tend to focus more on descriptive rather than interventional research (Chesla, 2010). What has been distilled from the bodies of literature on family health care intervention, however, is that family intervention does seem to produce better effects than usual, individual-focused medical care; greater effects have been shown in improving child health than adult health in some chronic conditions; and family-focused intervention examples found in childhood obesity efforts reveal the most compelling effects (Chesla, 2010).

Chesla (2010) also articulated that the means of interventions varied and ranged from simple home visits to coach families to much more complex educational and skill-developing strategies. Nurses were involved in relationship-based interventions to improve family communication, problem solving, and skill building as they related to illness or health management. The more tools nurses tended to use to assist families (multimodal) as part of their care plans, the better the outcomes seemed to be, particularly in managing complex health conditions that required numerous lifestyle changes. Family members were sometimes noted to be beneficiaries of interventions, experiencing unique and improved outcomes that were separate from the health of the patient (Chesla, 2010). The field requires additional intervention strategies and resulting evidence of outcomes, though more frequent examples are beginning to emerge in practice (Svavarsdottir & Jonsdottir, 2011).

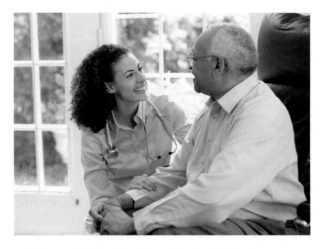

Nurses help families in the following ways: (1) providing direct care, (2) removing barriers to needed services, and (3) improving the capacity of the family to act on its own behalf and assume responsibility. Family nursing interventions can be directed toward improving the health outcomes of the member with the illness or condition, the family members' health-related outcomes of caregiving, or a combination of both. One of the important aspects of working with the family is the nurse-family relationship, which is an intervention in and of itself as families can experience a sense of strength, comfort, and confidence that can be therapeutic and useful (Friedman, Bowden, & Jones, 2003).

The nurse is responsible for helping the family implement the plan of care. The nurse can assume the role of teacher, role model, coach, counselor, advocate, coordinator, consultant, and evaluator in helping the family to implement the plan of the care they jointly created. The types of interventions are limitless because they are designed with the family to meet its needs in the context of its family story. Three examples below illustrate different family nursing interventions in various contexts.

Brief Therapeutic Conversations in Acute Care

Brief family conversations or interviews can be considered a family intervention. These brief interviews could include nurses making introductions to family members, collecting focused data to complete simple genograms and ecomaps, and opening pathways of knowing about families' self-defined needs and priorities (Wright & Leahey, 2013). Svavarsdottir, Tryggvadottir, and Sigurdardottir (2012) conducted a study measuring families' perceptions of nurse support and their own reports of family functioning. The study compared families who received brief family intervention interviews with nurses and those who did not. Predictably, families who received the nursing intervention interview reported feeling more supported than those who did not. Surprisingly, this finding was true for families with a child with an acute health crisis but was not true for those coping with chronic conditions. Expressive family functioning did not seem to change in the latter situation. Families of acutely ill children may experience significant benefits, however, when nurses take small amounts of time to enact simple family health care strategies (Svavarsdottir et al., 2012).

Home Visits and Telephone Support

Nursing visits to family homes are part of the early historical tradition of nursing and are appropriate to use today in family nursing. Northouse et al. (2007) utilized a clinical trial design to provide three in-home support visits along with two follow-up telephone calls to partnered couples where men were living through prostate cancer treatment. In the study, both patients and partners who received the in-home visits and phone calls reported that their communication and relationship with one another improved. Nurses offered these families coaching in communication, facilitated discussions that identified the beliefs and needs of both partners, and helped the families make decisions about care tasks and life balance. The partners seemed to benefit by demonstrating improved quality of life, increased self-efficacy, and less overall caregiving negativity than partners who did not receive the intervention. Additionally, some spouses continued to report these effects for up to 8 months following the intervention, suggesting that the act of providing access to nurses in the home and via telephone helped spouses long after the contact ended (Northouse et al., 2007).

Self-Care Talk for Family Caregivers

Nurses caring for families can intervene to promote health by helping families to identify potential health risks that stress the health of the family, such as when a 45-year-old father and husband with metabolic syndrome refused to comply with diet and exercise interventions. Parker, Teel, Leenerts, and Macan (2011) proposed a unique family nursing intervention for developing self-care motivation and implementation in family caregivers of people with high-acuity health needs; it is widely known that intensive periods of caregiving can result in worsening health of caregivers. In this intervention, family nurses made a series of six extended telephone calls that helped the family caregivers identify the barriers they faced in taking care of themselves and then used a theory-based framework to remove those barriers and implement self-care strategies to improve their own health. Clinical trial research is needed to demonstrate the efficacy and effectiveness of this intervention, but early evidence from similar approaches indicates that the ideas have promise for improving caregiver health. Moreover, the relational nature of the intervention, supplied entirely by telephone, is creative and has implications for nurses serving families in a variety of settings, including those in rural locations.

FAMILY NURSING EVALUATION

In making clinical judgments, nurses engage in critical thinking to determine whether and to what extent they have met an outcome. The means of measuring desired changes in outcomes varies with the specific problem upon which the action plan is focused. For example, if the family has identified that a primary focus problem is disrupted sleep routines for their young child with attention-deficit/hyperactivity disorder, the nurse may propose that the family create a simple chart to measure their new routine of sleep hygiene practices on a daily basis. The family determines that at present, the child is not able to fall asleep with ease on any given night and they set a goal to have the child falling asleep with ease 3 nights a week initially. Using the simple daily charting concept, the nurse and family can easily look to the collected data at a specified time to determine if the goal has been met. The team makes the decision about whether to proceed as originally planned, to modify the family action plan, or to revisit the family story in total. As indicated previously, the critical reasoning approach of thinking about families

and their needs is not linear. In practice, a constant flow occurs between the components of the family assessment and intervention strategy with plans being continually evaluated and modified through reflection.

There can be many reasons underlying a lack of success in meeting desired outcomes when working with families, some of which may be related to family factors, others to nurse factors, and even others to additional environmental factors. Apathy and indecision are examples of potential family barriers. Family apathy may occur because of value differences between the nurse and the family. The family may be overcome with a sense of hopelessness, may view the problems or bureaucracy as too overwhelming, or may have a fear of failure. Nurses also should consider whether they themselves imposed barriers. Examples of nurse barriers to achieving desired family outcomes could include discrepant values or beliefs from the family, resulting in a lack of follow-through on the part of the nurse; not listening to family concerns about the problems of importance, leading to two separate, rather than one unified, outcome goal; or even lack of time and resources needed for the nurse to address the family needs in a timely fashion. Examples of additional environmental factors that act as barriers to desired outcomes can be things such as a change in the prescription formulary that limits access to the effective drug of choice on a family's insurance plan, lack of access to an appropriate specialty care provider because of rural geography, or the loss of a job by the primary wage earner in the family. A more detailed list of possible barriers to family outcomes can be found in Box 4-7.

BOX 4-7
Barriers to Family Outcomes

- Family apathy
- Family indecision about the outcome or actions
- Nurse-imposed ideas
- Negative labeling
- Overlooking family strengths
- Neglecting cultural or gender implications
- Family perception of hopelessness
- Fear of failure
- Limited access to resources and support
- Limited finances
- Fear and distrust of health care system

Aside from evaluating outcomes, another important part of the family evaluation is the decision when to end the relationship with the family. Sometimes care with a family ends suddenly. In this case, it is important for nurses to determine the forces that brought about the closure. The family may seek to end the relationship prematurely, which may require a renegotiating process. The insurance or agency requirements may place a financial constraint on the amount of time nurses can work with a family. Other times, the family-nurse relationship comes to an end more naturally, as when the nurse and family together determine that the family has achieved the intended outcomes. Whatever the reason for the end of the nurse-family relationship, it is crucial that closure be achieved between the parties.

Building closure into the family action plan will benefit the family by providing for a smooth transition process. Strategies often used in this transition include decreasing contact with the nurse, extending invitations to the family for follow-up, and making referrals when appropriate. If possible, this process should include a summary evaluation meeting where the nurse and family put formal closure to their relationship. Following up with a therapeutic letter can encourage families to continue positive adaptation. The therapeutic letter should include recognition of the family achievement, a summary of the actions, commendations to each family member, and an insightful question for the family to think about in the future that may provide the family a future direction (Wright & Bell, 2009). An example of a therapeutic family letter is found in Box 4-8.

BOX 4-8
Example of Therapeutic Family Letter

Dear W, H, and T,

First, I want to thank all of you for allowing me the opportunity to get acquainted with your family. I appreciated your openness and willingness to talk with me.

During our time together, we discussed several issues that were important to your family. One of these issues was the ongoing possibility of H losing his job because of the seasonal nature of his work. We explored the effects of potential job loss on a personal and family level.

H, you expressed some concern about your ability to provide adequately for your family. You indicated a personal constraining belief that a lack of steady employment meant that you were letting your family down and not providing for them. We discussed the idea that a paying job is only one part of the entire family support system that you provide. We explored some examples of noneconomic means of support, such as specific tasks related to farm chores, household management, and child care. If your job situation changes again, I hope you will find some of these suggestions helpful.

W, I was so impressed with your ability to juggle your caregiving job with home, farm, kids, and spouse. I can't think of many women who could handle all of that with such strength and grace. With all that you do, it's not surprising that there isn't much time left over for your own personal endeavors. We discussed your constraining belief that you had to be responsible for everything. You envisioned the possibility of letting go of certain tasks and suggesting ways to share other tasks more equitably

among family members. If you and your family choose to implement some task-sharing ideas, I sincerely hope this will work for all of you.

T, you have mapped out a path to higher education and a future career. You have every reason to expect success. We briefly touched upon what "success" might mean for you and whether success depends on the university attended. I hope you will consider my thoughts in this regard. Whatever the outcome, you have the love and support of your parents.

Finally, I would like to commend all of you for your deep devotion to each other and for putting family first. You value family time, and you strive to communicate in a way that sustains your close relationship with each other.

I would like to invite W and H to consider a suggestion regarding making time for just the two of you. "Couple time" is easy to overlook when you are focused on creating a loving, stable home for E and helping to launch T into higher education. Please remember that you two are the solid foundation of your family; the stronger your relationship is, the stronger your whole family can be.

As a result of our time spent together, I came away with the feeling that your family is exceptionally strong, deeply committed to one another, and fully capable of adapting to any of life's challenges. Thank you again for your time.

Best wishes to you and your family,
Nursing student signature here

NURSE AND FAMILY REFLECTION

The final step in critically thinking about family nursing is for nurses and families to engage in vital, creative, and concurrent reflection about their work together. There are two purposes of engaging in individual and collaborative reflection: to facilitate evaluation of progress toward the desired family outcomes and to increase expertise of the nurse.

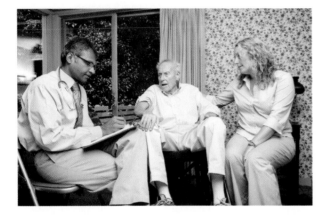

The first purpose is for the nurse to reflect on the success of the family outcome in collaboration with the family as part of outcome evaluation. Reflection entails thinking about your thought process relative to this family client. Nurses can link ideas and consequences together in logical sequences by using an "if (describe a situation) ... then (explain the outcome)" exercise, which can help the

family member articulate concerns. A comparative analysis approach of the family problem can be used to analyze the strengths and weaknesses of competing alternatives. The nurse may decide to reframe the family problem or priority need by attributing a different meaning to the content or context of the family situation based on testing, judgment, or changes in the context or content of the family story (Pesut & Herman, 1999). While this process of reflecting with the family results in new co-created evaluation and knowledge related to the collaborative work, the nurse can also engage in this comparative reflective reasoning individually in preparation for and follow-up to the discussions with the family.

The second purpose of reflection is for nurses to build on their expertise by reflecting on client stories and their practice with each family. In essence, nurses create a library of family stories so that each time they come upon a similar family story, they can pull ideas from previous experiences. This aspect of reflection assists nurses with pattern recognition.

Yet another, more individual purpose of reflection is to engage in self-reflection and self-evaluation. By using this critical thinking strategy, nurses learn from mistakes and cement patterns of action that assist them to advance in their nursing practice from novice to expert family nurse.

A family case study follows that demonstrates critical reasoning about a family, assessment to identify concerns, and interventions to meet family needs.

Family Case Study: Bono Family

In preparation for her appointment with the Bono family in the mother-baby clinic, Vicki reviews the chart notes written by the nurse midwife about the family. Vicki sees that the Bono family is coming in for a 1-week well-baby checkup of newborn infant Hannah and a follow-up for Libby, the mother, after her cesarean section (C-section) delivery 7 days ago. The note from the receptionist indicates that Libby expressed some concerns with her effectiveness in breastfeeding Hannah. The appointment book notes that the whole Bono family is coming for this visit. Vicki notes that the Bonos are a nuclear family that consists of a married couple with two biological children. Figure 4-8 shows the Bono family genogram.

Knowing that this is a nuclear family coming in for a well-baby checkup, Vicki decides to use a Developmental Family Life Cycle theoretical approach to this family with a

new member. (See Chapter 3 for details about this theoretical model.) Based on this approach, Vicki has many questions in her mind as she prepares for her appointment with the Bono family. The questions Vicki has about each family member and the whole family are presented in bulleted lists after a brief description of each family member.

Libby Bono is a 35-year-old mother recovering from a cesarean section delivery 7 days ago. She does not have any existing health problems. Libby's roles in the family are primary child-rearer, events planner, disciplinarian, and health expert. Libby is a hairdresser and is independently contracted with a hair salon. She has planned to take off 3 months for maternity leave.

- How might Libby's recovery from the cesarean section be affecting her roles in the family, especially with an active 2-year-old and a newborn?

(continued)

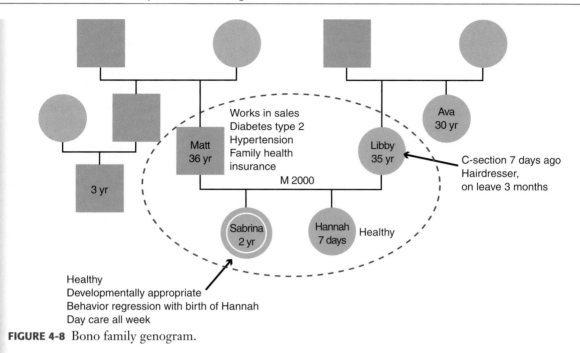

Works in sales
Diabetes type 2
Hypertension
Family health
insurance

Matt
36 yr

M 2000

Libby
35 yr

Ava
30 yr

C-section 7 days ago
Hairdresser,
on leave 3 months

3 yr

Sabrina
2 yr

Hannah
7 days

Healthy

Healthy
Developmentally appropriate
Behavior regression with birth of Hannah
Day care all week

FIGURE 4-8 Bono family genogram.

- What are Libby's thoughts or plans for returning to work after her maternity leave?
- How is Libby adjusting to her expanded mother role? Assess Libby for postpartum depression.

Matt Bono, 36 years old, works for Frito Lay Company in sales and distribution. His primary roles in the family are decision maker, maintenance person, pioneer, and information provider. He reports feeling little attachment to his occupation and welcomes this new birth as a change in routine and an opportunity to consider a change in his place of employment. His current medical problems include type 2 diabetes and mild hypertension; both are well managed and controlled by oral diabetic and antihypertensive medications. Currently, he is following the Weight Watchers diet to reduce his weight and to control the symptomatology experienced from his health conditions.

- How is Matt adjusting to the expanded role of father of two daughters?
- What are Matt's plans for employment, specifically about financial support for the family if he leaves his job? How would this affect health insurance for the family?

Sabrina Bono is a healthy 2-year-old girl who is developmentally appropriate. Psychologically, Sabrina is in the autonomy versus shame-and-doubt developmental stage. Her parents report that she often attempts to try new things on her own, and they frequently praise her efforts to

promote independence. Her interest in potty training is developing, but still intermittent. Her immunizations are current. She normally goes to a day-care center that is close to her mother's work.

- How is Sabrina adjusting to the new baby?
- Is Sabrina showing any regression in her skills and abilities?
- Are each of the parents finding time to spend with Sabrina alone?
- How are the parents talking with Sabrina about her role as big sister?

Hannah Bono, 7 days old, was delivered after 42 weeks' gestation and was proved to be adequate for gestational age (AGA; 10th–90th percentile), 53.75 cm and 3,966 g, with American Pediatric Gross Assessment Record (APGAR) scores of 8 at 1 minute and 9 at 5 minutes.

- Is Hannah developing on target for her age and gestational age at birth?
- How often is Hannah eating, and is she gaining weight?
- How is Hannah nursing?

The Bono family is a nuclear family with the addition of second child.

- What are the major concerns for the family at this time?
- Who in the family is having the most difficult adjustment to the changes brought about by the addition of a new family member?

- How is the family adjusting to these changes?
- Who or what are the support systems for this new family?

Bono Family Story:

During the appointment, Vicki confirms that family life for the Bono family has changed. Hannah was found to be healthy and developmentally appropriate. Libby is healing well from the C-section, but reported occasional discomfort when she "overdoes it." Libby's concerns about breastfeeding were easily relieved as Vicki validated her breastfeeding technique. An assessment for postpartum depression revealed that Libby is not demonstrating any signs of depression at this time. Throughout the examination of Hannah, the parents demonstrated overwhelming signs of bonding, such as talking with the infant and bragging about her beauty and temperament. During the appointment, Vicki noted that Sabrina was throwing toys and attempting to crawl onto her mother's lap while Libby was nursing Hannah. Sabrina would say "baby back" when she was upset. When Matt attempted to coddle or praise the baby, Sabrina became extremely angry with her father. They were not ignoring Sabrina but were not focused on her during the appointment. The parents' nonverbal actions showed frustration with Sabrina's behaviors. When asked, they reported that Sabrina has been very temperamental and inconsolable at day care. They reported that she had begun to show progress with toilet training before Hannah's birth but had now lost all interest.

Analysis of Bono Family Story:

To help everyone see the larger family picture, Vicki uses the Family Reasoning Web (see Fig. 4-7). Based on the responses from using the Family Reasoning Web, she uncovered the following family information for analysis:

- Family routines of daily living: Matt and Libby are both tired from Hannah's every-3-hour breastfeeding schedule. They share some of the responsibility for comforting Hannah and seeing to her needs. Meals have been challenging as Matt has had to assume this responsibility because Libby has not recovered from her C-section. At this time, they do not have extended family support. Sabrina is still going to day care but is evidencing difficulty there.
- Family communication: Communication has been identified as a strength of the couple. They have a shared decision-making style. They appear nurturing with their children. Sabrina is emotionally up and down. She is clingy with her dad and ignores her mother except when she is breastfeeding Hannah. Sabrina was throwing toys when upset or frustrated. She periodically pointed to Hannah and said, "Take back."

- Family supports and resources: This family is fully covered under Matt's health insurance through his work. They have some family they can call on to help them. Ava, Libby's sister, volunteered to come for a visit and stay for 2 weeks. Matt's brother, his wife, and their 3-year-old child live in the same city. They have informally talked about sharing some child care. Both parents need to work to sustain their family lifestyle. Libby does not have benefits in her contracted hairdresser job. When she is off work, she does not make money. She does not have paid maternity leave. The couple planned for Libby to take 3 months off from work. The needs identified are for some immediate family support with everyday living and some financial concern at the end of the 3 months, given that the family had not planned for a longer period of reduced income than this.
- Family roles: All of the family members are experiencing role ambiguity with their new roles. Matt and Libby are now parents of two daughters. Sabrina is a big sister, and Hannah is the new infant. Matt expressed some role overload because he is assuming many of the typical daily household chores of meals, laundry, food shopping, and primary care provider for Sabrina.
- Family beliefs: They strongly state that "family comes first." This was a planned pregnancy. They see themselves as loving parents. They express some confusion about disciplining Sabrina given her recent behaviors.
- Family developmental stage: This is a nuclear family in the family-with-toddler stage. They also have a new infant; therefore, they are in two developmental stages at the same time.
- Family health knowledge: The family expressed that it needed more help in knowing how to help Sabrina. The parents do not know how to work with Sabrina to help her adjust to being a big sister. They are confused with Sabrina's behavior of aggression, mood swings, clinging, and pointing at the baby and saying "take back." They feel that she has lost some of her skills. Health literacy does not appear to be an issue.
- Family environment: At this time, they have enough room in their home for a family of four. They live in a safe neighborhood, but they do not know their neighbors well.
- Family stress management: They express feeling stressed about Sabrina's behaviors. They are both tired. Sabrina is stressed, as evidenced by her behaviors and changes in behavior. They are dealing with the current situation on their own but are open to asking for help from family for the immediate assistance with daily living routines. They are open to learning more about how to help Sabrina.

(continued)

- Family culture: They are white with an Italian Catholic background. They are of working lower-middle-class socioeconomic status.
- Family spiritually: They were both raised Catholic but are not practicing their religion. They do not belong to a church. They describe themselves as spiritual.

The parents identified that both of them and Sabrina are having difficulty adjusting to the expansion of their family and the shift in their family roles. They state that they are most concerned with Sabrina's adjustment to the new baby. They state that they just do not know the best way to help her. They shared that they thought that since this was the "second time around" they believed they could be even better parents. They have been frustrated thinking about how to cope with what to do with two young children. The nursing diagnosis *Readiness for Enhanced Parenting* is related to the new role of parents of two children and is evidenced by the parents' subjective statements about parenting, Sabrina's reactions to the new baby, and parents asking for information and help on sibling rivalry.

Bono Family Intervention:

Together, the nurse, along with Matt and Libby, review the family genogram (see Fig. 4-8), which helps the couple visualize the family. The parents decide that Ava is the best person to come to help at this time. They say they will talk later with Matt's brother and family about sharing some childcare. They complete a family ecomap (Fig. 4-9) to help assess what is creating stress and determine what could help alleviate family stress.

Vicki provides Matt and Libby with several educational packets about toddlers and new infants. She directs them to several online Web sites after she confirms that they have computer skills. They discuss ideas on how both parents can make personal time to spend with each daughter. They brainstorm ways to help Sabrina interact with Hannah but to keep Hannah safe from aggressive toddler behavior

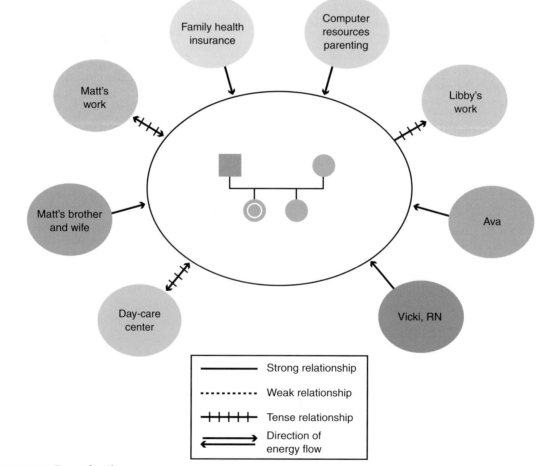

FIGURE 4-9 Bono family ecomap.

to a new sibling. They plan to talk with the day-care providers so they can be effective with their help for Sabrina. They will call Ava as soon as they get home to plan for her visit. Vicki makes a follow-up appointment with the Bono family for their next well-baby visit and to see how they are progressing with both children.

Bono Family Evaluation:

Vicki plans a follow-up phone call to check in with Libby and Matt. At the next visit, Vicki will revisit the family action plan with Libby and Matt to see whether their priority family concerns remain the same, or have decreased/increased or disappeared. Vicki plans to observe Sabrina's behaviors to see how she is coping and whether she is adapting in more positive ways. She will talk with the parents to assess their anxiety level. She will observe the parents and their interactions with both children.

Nurse Reflection:

Vicki reflects about her work with the Bono family. She determines that her therapeutic communication skills were excellent. She showed empathy and validated the family's concern for the added stresses that a newborn child creates for a family. The 7-day-old well-baby visit in the clinic setting presented an ideal time to observe and address parenting techniques and ease parental concerns. Learning how to shift focus from the more medical concern of the well-baby to family dynamics was the most challenging aspect, yet also the most rewarding. The interventions were appropriate and truly empowered their overall ability to cope and function as a family.

SUMMARY

- Conducting a family assessment includes the following components: assessment strategies, including how to select assessment instruments, determining the need for interpreters, assessing for family health literacy, and diagramming family genograms and ecomaps.
- Family nurses must work in partnership with families as they build from a strengths model and not a deficit model.
- Using the family assessment approach outlined in this chapter, nurses and families together identify the family priorities.
- The Family Reasoning Web is a systematic method used to ensure that families are viewed in a holistic manner, which also helps to keep the interventions oriented to family strengths.
- Family interventions need to be tailored to each individual family, with consideration of the family's structure, function, and processes.
- By subscribing to and selecting a theory-based approach to assessment, and formulating mutually derived intervention strategies, families are more likely to be committed and follow through with family plans and interventions.
- Family nurses serve as the catalyst for assessment, intervention, and evaluation that are specific to family identified needs.

REFERENCES

American Medical Association. (2012). *International classification of diseases: Clinical modifications* (ICD-9-CM). Dover, DE: Author.

American Psychiatric Association. (2013). *Diagnostic and statistical manual of mental disorders, fifth edition* (DSM-5). Washington, DC: Author.

Bass, L. (2005). Health literacy: Implications for teaching the adult patient. *Journal of Infusion Nursing, 28*(1), 15–22.

Baumgartner, J., Burnett, L., diCarol, C., & Buchanan, T. (2012). An inquiry of children's social support networks using eco-maps. *Child & Youth Care Forum, 41*, 357–369.

Berkey-Mischke, K. M., & Hanson, S. M. H. (1991). *Pocket guide to family assessment and intervention*. St. Louis, MO: Mosby–Year Book.

Berkman, N. D., Sheridan, S. L., Donahue, K. E., Halpern, D. J., & Crotty, K. (2011). Low health literacy and health outcomes: An updated systematic review. *Annals of Internal Medicine, 155*(2), 97–107.

Bethell, C., Simpson, L., & Read, D. (2006). Quality and safety of hospital care for children from Spanish-speaking families with limited English proficiency. *Journal for Healthcare Quality, 28*(3), W3.

Bowen, M. (1985). *Family therapy in clinical practice*. Norvale, NJ: Jason Aronson.

Bowen, M., & Kerr, M. (1988). *Family evaluation: An approach based on Bowen's Theory*. New York, NY: W. W. Norton.

Bruera, E., Sweeney, C., Calder, C., Palmer, L., & Benisch-Tolley, S. (2001). Patient preferences versus physician perceptions of treatment decisions in cancer care. *Journal of Clinical Oncology, 19*(11), 2883–2885.

Bulechek, G., Butcher, H., Dochterman, J., & Wagner, C. (2013). *Nursing interventions classification* (6th ed.). St. Louis, MO: Mosby.

Butow, P. N., Maclean, M., Dunn, S. M., Tattersall, M., & Boyer, M. J. (1997). The dynamics of change: Cancer patients' preferences of information, involvement and support. *Annals of Oncology, 8*(9), 857–863.

Cascade-Kehoe, M., & Kehoe, M. (2008). Using genograms creatively to promote healthy lifestyles. *Journal of Creativity in Mental Health, 3*(4), 19–29.

Chesla, C. A. (2010). Do family interventions improve health? *Journal of Family Nursing, 16*(4), 355–377.

Corlett, K., & Twycross, A. (2006). Negotiation of parental roles within family-centered care: A review of the research. *Journal of Clinical Nursing, 15*(10), 1308–1316.

de Haes, H. (2006). Dilemmas in patient centeredness and shared decision making: A case for vulnerability. *Patient Education and Counseling, 62*(3), 291–298.

DeWalt, D. A., Boone, R. S., & Pignone, M. P. (2007). Literacy and its relationship with self-efficacy, trust and participation in medical decision making. *American Journal of Health Behavior, 31*(Suppl 3), S27–S35.

Doenges, M. E., Moorhouse, M. F., & Murr, A. C. (2013). *Nursing diagnosis manual: Planning, individualizing, and documenting client care* (3rd ed.). Philadelphia, PA: F. A. Davis.

Dreger, V., & Tremback, T. (2002). Optimize patient health by treating literacy and language barriers. *Association of Operating Room Nurses Journal, 75*(2), 280–293.

Driessnack, M. (2009). Using the colored eco-genetic relationship map with children. *Nursing Research, 58*(5), 304–311.

Duran, C., Oman, K., Abel, J., Koziel, V., & Szymanski, D. (2007). Attitudes toward and beliefs about family presence: A survey of health care providers, patients' families and patients. *American Journal of Critical Care, 16*(3), 270–282.

Elwyn, G., Lloyd, A., Joseph-Williams, N., Cording, E., Thomson, R., Durand, M. A., & Edwards, A. (2012). Option grids: Shared decision making made easier. *Patient Education and Counselling, 90*, 207–212.

Flores, G., Abreu, M., Barone, C. P., Bachur, R., & Lin, H. (2012). Errors of medical interpretation and their potential clinical consequences: A comparison of professional versus ad hoc versus no interpreters. *Annals of Emergency Medicine, 60*(5), 545–553.

Florin, J., Björvell, C., Ehnfors, M., & Ehrenberg, A. (2012). Comparison of the ability of VIPS and ICF to express nursing content in the health record. In 2012 11th International Congress on Nursing Informatics, June 23–27, Montreal, Canada, Proceedings (p. 529).

Friedman, M. M., Bowden, V. R., & Jones, E. G. (2003). *Family nursing: Research, theory and practice* (5th ed.). Upper Saddle River, NJ: Prentice Hall/Pearson Education.

Gazmararian, J. A., Williams, M. V., Peel, J., & Baker, D. W. (2003). Health literacy and knowledge of chronic disease. *Patient Education and Counseling, 52*(3), 267–275.

Gray, B., Hilder, J., & Donaldson, H. (2011). Why do we not use trained interpreters for all patients with limited English proficiency? Is there a place for using family members? *Australian Journal of Primary Health, 17*(3), 240–249.

Gurses, A., & Carayon, P. (2007). Performance obstacles of intensive care nurses. *Nursing Research, 56*(3), 185–194.

Hanson, S. M. H. (2001). Family nursing assessment and intervention. In *Family health care nursing: Theory, practice and research* (2nd ed., pp. 170–195). Philadelphia, PA: F. A. Davis.

Harrison, M., & Neufeld, A. (2009). *Nursing and family caregiving: Social support and nonsupport.* New York, NY: Springer.

Harrison, T. M. (2010). Family centered pediatric nursing care: State of the science. *Journal of Pediatric Nursing, 25*(5), 335.

Herndon, E., & Joyce, L. (2004). Getting the most from language interpreters. American Academy of Family Physicians. Retrieved from http://www.aafp.org/fpm/2004/0600/p37.html

Hodge, D., & Limb, G. (2010). A Native American perspective on spiritual assessment: the strengths and limitations of a complementary set of assessment tools. *Heatlh & Social Work, 35*, 121–131.

Holtslander, L. (2005). Clinical application of the 15-minute family interview: Addressing the needs of postpartum families. *Journal of Family Nursing, 11*(1), 217–228.

Institute for Patient and Family Centered Care (IPFCC). (2013). FAQs. Retrieved from http://www.ipfcc.org/faq.html

Kaakinen, J. R. (2010). Family nursing process: Family nursing assessment models. In J. R. Kaakinen, V. Gedaly-Duff, D. Coehlo, & S. M. H. Hanson (Eds.), *Family health care nursing: Theory, practice and research* (4th ed., pp. 103–131). Philadelphia, PA: F. A. Davis.

Kaakinen, J.R., & Hanson, SM.H. (2005). Family nursing assessment and intervention. In S.M.H. Hanson, V. Gedaly-Duff, & J.R. Kaakinen (Eds.). *Family health care nursing: Theory, practice & research* (3rd ed.). Philadelphia, PA: F.A. Davis

Kaakinen, J. R., Hanson, S. M. H., & Denham, S. A. (2010). Family health care nursing: An introduction. In J. R. Kaakinen, V. Gedaly-Duff, D. Coehlo, & S. M. H. Hanson (Eds.), *Family health care nursing: Theory, practice and research* (4th ed., pp. 3–33). Philadelphia, PA: F. A. Davis.

Khwaja, N., Sharma, S., Wong, J., Murray, D., Ghosh, J., Murphy, M. O., & Walker, M. G. (2006). Interpreter services in an inner city teaching hospital: A 6-year experience. *Annals of the Royal College of Surgeons of England, 88*(7), 659–662.

Leahey M., & Svavarsdottir, E. K. (2009). Implementing family nursing: How do we translate knowledge into clinical practice? *Journal of Family Nursing, 15*(4), 445–460.

Ledger, S. D. (2002). Reflections on communicating with non-English-speaking patients. *British Journal of Nursing, 11*(11), 773–780.

Leske, J. S. (2002). Interventions to decrease family anxiety. *Critical Care Nurse, 22*(6), 61–65.

Makoul, G., & Clayman, M. L. (2006). An integrative model of shared decision making in medical encounters. *Patient Education and Counseling, 60*(3), 301–312.

Martin, K. S. (2004). *The Omaha System: A key to practice, documentation and information management* (2nd ed.). St. Louis, MO: Elsevier Health Sciences.

Martinez, A., D'Artois, D., & Rennick, J. E. (2007). Does the 15 minute (or less) family interview influence family nursing practice? *Journal of Family Nursing, 13*(2), 157–178.

Mayer, B. B., & Rushton, N. (2002). Writing easy-to-read teaching aids. *Nursing, 32*(3), 48–49.

McGoldrick, M., Gerson, R., & Petry, S. S. (2008). *Genograms: Assessment and intervention* (3rd ed.). New York, NY: W. W. Norton.

McGoldrick, M., Gerson, R., & Schellenberger, S. (1999). *Genograms in family assessment* (2nd ed.). New York, NY: W.W. Norton.

Moorhead, S., Johnson, M., & Maas, M. (Eds.). (2004). *Nursing outcomes classification* (3rd ed.). St. Louis, MO: Mosby.

Moorhead, S., Johnson, M., Maas, M., & Swanson, E. (2012). *Nursing outcomes classification* (5th ed.), St Louis, MO: Mosby.

Neufeld, A., Harrison, M. J., Hughes, K., & Stewart, M. (2007). Nonsupportive interaction in the experience of women family caregivers. *Health and Social Care in the Community, 15*(1), 530–541.

North American Nursing Diagnosis Association. (2007). *Nursing diagnosis: Definitions and classifications, 2007–2008.* Philadelphia, PA: Nursecom, Inc.

Northouse, L. L., Mood, D. W., Schafenacker, A., Montie, J. E., Sandler, H. M., Forman, J. D., & Kershaw, T. (2007). Randomized clinical trial of a family intervention for prostate cancer patients and their spouses. *Cancer, 110*(12), 2809–2818.

Olsen, S., Dudley-Brown, S., & McMullen, P. (2004). Case for blending pedigrees, genograms and ecomaps: Nursing's contribution to the big picture. *Nursing and Health Sciences, 6*(4), 295–308.

Osborn, C. Y., Weiss, B. D., Davis, T. C., Skripkauskas, S., Rodrigue, C., Bass, P. F., & Wolf, M. S. (2007). Measuring adult literacy in health care: Performance of the newest vital sign. *American Journal of Health Behavior, 31*(Suppl 1), S36–S46.

Parker, C., Teel, C., Leenerts, M. H., & Macan, A. (2011). A theory-based self-care talk intervention for family caregiver-nurse partnerships. *Journal of Gerontological Nursing, 37*(1), 30.

Pesut, D. J., & Herman, J. (1999). *Clinical reasoning: The art and science of critical and creative thinking.* Boston, MA: Delmar.

Peters, E., Dieckmann, N., Dixon, A., Hibbard, J., & Mertz, C. K. (2007). Less is more in presenting quality information to consumers. *Medical Care Research and Review, 64*(2), 169–190.

Pierce, P. E., & Hicks, J. D. (2001). Patient decision making behavior. *Nursing Research, 50*(5), 267–274.

Raggi, A., Leonardi, M., Cabello, M., & Bickenbach, J. E. (2010). Application of ICF in clinical settings across Europe. *Disability & Rehabilitation, 32*(S1), S17–S22.

Ray, R. A., & Street, A. F. (2005). Ecomapping: An innovative research tool for nurses. *Journal of Advanced Nursing, 50*(5), 545–552.

Rempel, G. R., Neufeld, A., & Kushner, K. E. (2007). Interactive use of genograms and ecomaps in family caregiving research. *Journal of Family Nursing, 13*(4), 403–419.

Salmond, S, (2008). Who is family? Family and decision making. In S. B. Lewenson & M. Truglio-Londrigan (Eds.), *Decision-making in nursing: Thoughtful approaches for practice* (pp. 89–104). Sudbury, MA: Jones & Bartlett.

Schattner, A., Bronstein, A., & Jellin, N. (2006). Information and shared decision-making are top patients' priorities. *BMC Health Services Research, 6*, 21.

Schenker, Y., Wang, F., Selig, S. J., Ng, R., & Fernandez, A. (2007). The impact of language barriers on documentation of informed consent at a hospital with on-site interpreter services. *Journal of General Internal Medicine, 22*(2), 294–299.

Sentell, T. L., & Halpin, H. A. (2006). Importance of adult literacy in understanding health disparities. *Journal of General Internal Medicine, 21*(8), 862–866.

Sobo, E. J. (2004). Pediatric nurses may misjudge parent communication preferences. *Journal of Nursing Care Quality, 19*(3), 253–262.

Speros, C. (2005). Health literacy: Concept analysis. *Journal of Advanced Nursing, 50*(6), 633–640.

Svavarsdottir, E. (2008). Excellence in nursing: A model for implementing family systems nursing in nursing practice at an institutional level in Iceland. *Journal of Family Nursing, 14*(4), 456–468.

Svavarsdottir, E.K. (2008). Excellence in nursing: A model for implementing family systems nursing in nursing practice at an institutional level in Iceland. *Journal of Family Nursing, 14*(4), 456–468.

Svavarsdottir, E., & Jonsdottir, H. (2011). *Family nursing in action.* Reykjavik, Iceland: University of Iceland Press.

Svavarsdottir, E. K., Tryggvadottir, G. B., & Sigurdardottir, A. O. (2012). Knowledge translation in family nursing: Does a short-term therapeutic conversation intervention benefit families of children and adolescents in a hospital setting? Findings from the Landspitali University Hospital family nursing implementation project. *Journal of Family Nursing, 18*(3), 303–327.

Taylor, B. (2006). Giving children and parents a voice: The parents' perspective. *Paediatric Nursing, 18*(9), 20–23.

Toman, W. (1976). *Family constellation: Its effect on personality and social behavior* (3rd ed.). New York, NY: Springer.

Touliatos, J., Perlmutter, B., & Straus, M. (2001). *Handbook of family measurement techniques.* Newbury Park, CA: Sage.

U.S. Census Bureau (2010). Language use in the United States: 2007. Author. Retrieved March 15, 2013, from http://www.census.gov/prod/2010pubs/acs-12.pdf

Watzlawick, P., Weakland, J. H., & Fisch, R. (1967). *Pragmatics of human communication.* New York, NY: W. W. Norton.

Watzlawick, P., Weakland, J. H., & Fisch, R. (1974). *Change: Principles of problem formulation and problem resolution.* New York, NY: W. W. Norton.

Whitmer, M., Hughes, B., Hurst, S. M., & Young, T. B. (2005). Innovative solutions: Family conference progress note. *Dimensions of Critical Care Nursing, 24*(2), 83–88.

World Health Organization. (2013). *International classification of functioning disability and health (ICF).* Author. Geneva, Switzerland.

Wright, L. M. & Bell, J. (2009). *Beliefs and illness: A model for healing.* Calgary, Canada: 4th Floor Press, Inc.

Wright, L. M., & Leahey, M. (2013). *Nurses and families: A guide to family assessment and intervention* (6th ed.). Philadelphia, PA: F. A. Davis.

Yanicki, S. (2005). Social support and family assets: The perceptions of low-income lone-mother families about support from home visitation. *Canadian Journal of Public Health, 96*(1), 46–49.

chapter 5

Family Social Policy and Health Disparities

Isolde Daiski, RN, BScN, EdD

Casey R. Shillam, PhD, RN-BC

Lynne M. Casper, PhD

Sandra M. Florian, MA, PhD Candidate

Critical Concepts

- Health disparities arise from complex, deeply rooted social issues, and are directly related to the social and political structure of a society.
- Many factors contribute to (determine) health status, including educational level, socioeconomic status, and physical surroundings.
- It is critical for nurses to recognize the link between the determinants of health and health disparities.
- The social and political structures of a society influence how health care is delivered to and restricted from those in need. An upstream approach of health promotion and disease prevention is more effective than a downstream approach of reactive treatment of disease.
- For those who are sick, access to quality, affordable health care should be considered a basic human right from a societal perspective. All aspects of health care should be designed to minimize disparities.
- The policy decisions made by a society or government about families and how they are legally defined, what constitutes a legal relationship, and how health care is delivered have a profound effect on families and their health. Defining families from a legal perspective may contribute to health disparities by restricting access to social and health care services. Ethical issues can arise if we restrict care to families by how they are defined legally.
- In the past, the profession of nursing had a well-defined role in advocating for vulnerable populations. Recently, nursing involvement in the development of health policy from either professional organization or individual perspectives has declined, resulting in increased health disparities for families.
- Nursing professionals can benefit from theoretical and practical education about social policy issues, resulting in resounding effects on the health of a family.
- Nurses can participate in advocacy related to family policies at all levels of health care systems in the context of society.
- Illness of one member affects all members of the family, and in turn, family health affects all of society. Therefore, nurses have to consider the whole family unit within the context of the changed health situation and larger social system.

This chapter exposes the nurse to social issues, behavioral risks, and disparities that affect the health of families. Threaded throughout the chapter is the role of the nurse providing care within a framework of family nursing. Specifically, this chapter presents the key components that contribute to health disparities between families in the health care system. It explores health disparities in the context of health determinants, social policy, and the nurse's role with respect to social policy. This chapter also discusses the unique factors that affect health policy and family health in both Canada and the United States. At the completion of this chapter, the nurse will have developed a broad understanding of social policy and how it can contribute to or mitigate health disparities. Armed with this knowledge, nurses can assist families to adopt health promotion and disease prevention strategies and can advocate for families in their organizations, communities, and nations for policies that minimize disparities and maximize access to resources.

DEFINING SOCIAL POLICY AND HEALTH DISPARITIES

It is critical first to create a common understanding of and foundation for the concepts underlying the substance of the chapter, such as health determinants, health disparities, and family social policy. This section also provides a brief overview of where both the United States and Canada stand in terms of health care coverage for all citizens.

Determinants of Health

The determinants of health are defined as factors that directly influence the health of individuals, families, and communities (World Health Organization [WHO], 2012a). WHO (2012a) defines *social determinants of health* as "the conditions in which people are born, grow, live, work and age, including the health system. These circumstances are shaped by the distribution of money, power and resources at global, national and local levels" (paragraph 1). More specifically, determinants include a person's demographic characteristics, such as gender, race, and ethnicity, which cannot be changed, but to which societal responses can be altered. They also include characteristics that can be changed. These changeable characteristics are considered behavioral

or social. Behavioral determinants include activities such as eating habits, smoking, substance use, physical activity, and coping skills. Social determinants include physical, social, and economic environments, which further break down into income, housing, education, employment, access to health care, public safety, transportation, and availability of community-based resources (Hunter, Neiger, & West, 2011; Mikkonen & Raphael, 2010; U.S. Department of Health and Human Services [USDHHS], 2010). Along with demographic and behavioral ones, these social determinants have a strong, indelible influence on the health of families and will continue to contribute to health disparities within family systems. An uneven distribution of the social determinants of health is often reported as the root problem of health disparities. Without the necessary financial resources for a healthy lifestyle, for example, it is difficult or even impossible to overcome such disparities.

Health Disparities

Health disparities are defined in the United States and Canada as follows: (a) health differences for particular populations that are (b) closely linked to social or economic disadvantage and (c) result in distinct differences in the presence of disease, health outcomes, or access to care (Public Health Agency of Canada, 2012; USDHHS, 2010). Health and health status are complex concepts, and no universal agreement has been reached on the definitions. WHO defines *health* as a "state of complete physical, mental, and social well-being and not merely the absence of disease or infirmity" (WHO, 2012b). This basic definition has not been changed since it was published in 1948. Later, the WHO (1986) added the following: "Health is seen as a resource for living, a positive concept" that affects the extent an individual is able to change and cope with the environmental factors. These definitions, combined, will be used for the purposes of this chapter.

Family Social Policy

An exploration of health determinants and health disparities logically begins with a discussion of social policy and its impact on families. But what constitutes social policy? Policy can be understood broadly as a course of action. Social policies are those policies that include social concepts, such as health, education, housing, and employment affecting people's everyday lives. Multiple social issues affect the health of families; in effect, they both create and mitigate health disparities. Nevertheless, social policies are developed for the purpose of *mitigating* health disparities and promoting equity and social justice. *Social justice* has been defined as "full participation in society and the balancing of benefits and burdens by all citizens, resulting in equitable living and a just ordering of society" (Buettner-Schmidt & Lobo, 2012, p. 948). Some examples of social policies adopted in the United States that have had resounding effects on the health of families include the State Child Health Insurance Program (SCHIP), Medicare Part D, and the Welfare-to-Work program. These programs, enacted during the 2000s, were intended to improve access to health care, manage costs, reduce taxpayer burden, and thereby ultimately address health disparities. Interestingly, however, the very policies created to mitigate health disparities often result in the most vulnerable of these populations experiencing even further challenges. For example, Medicare Part D was enacted in 2006 to increase prescription coverage for older adults. Although mean annual out-of-pocket medication expenditures have decreased by 30% to 50%, older adults with persistent pain experience additional disparities (Millett, Everett, Matheson, Bindman, & Mainous, 2010). Multiple factors contribute to these disparities: pain medications are often more expensive than many other medications, Medicare part D reimburses a lower percentage of pain medications than other medications, and Medicare does not cover complementary or alternative therapies often used for pain management such as massage therapy, acupuncture, or transcutaneous electrical nerve stimulation. Currently, tremendous social policy changes are underway in the United States with respect to health care access, changes that will bear heavily on the health of the population.

Briefing on the Current State of Health Care Policy

The United States is in the midst of a transition to a more affordable and accessible health care system. The Affordable Care Act (ACA), passed in March 2010 (USDHHS, 2011b), seeks to enhance access to health insurance. Despite much legislative and legal wrangling, the ACA was upheld by the U.S. Supreme Court in 2012 and implementation efforts began in 2013 (USDHHS, 2011b). The immediate benefit of the law will be to decrease disparities in access to health care insurance (and hence in health) by, for example, providing expanded coverage to young adults, addressing inconsistencies in Medicare drug benefits, and disallowing coverage denial for many pre-existing health conditions. Additionally, beginning in 2013, the approximately 40 million uninsured U.S. citizens will be able to access health coverage through the Health Insurance Marketplace. The Marketplace, a set of government-regulated and standardized health care plans, will allow those without insurance to submit one application to choose from multiple private-sector policies. The selection is based on their individual eligibility, but there is no possibility of being denied coverage or being charged a higher premium due to pre-existing treatments or conditions (USDHHS, 2011b).

Despite the progress sure to be wrought by these recent changes to the health care system, the United States will continue to face health disparity issues for many years to come. The long-standing lack of a universally available health care system has resulted in the development of social systems that will continue to influence determinants of health (Mikkonen & Raphael, 2010; Raphael, Curry-Stevens, & Bryant, 2008). In fact, on an annual basis, it is estimated that nearly 50 million residents of the United States have no health insurance (Kaiser Family Foundation, 2011). More than three-quarters of those uninsured are from working families whose employers do not offer such coverage. Young adults are further disproportionately affected, as their low incomes make it more difficult to afford coverage if it is not provided by the employer (Kaiser Family Foundation, 2011). Women and children are also disproportionately affected because they are more likely to be living below the poverty level. Without a payment system for health coverage, many people delay seeking health care services, which increases the likelihood that illness or need for services will be at a crisis level when they enter the system and require intensive downstream care. When this delay occurs, costs for health care increase.

The Centers for Medicare and Medicaid Services is a governmental agency in the United States with responsibility for Medicare, Medicaid, SCHIP, the Health Insurance Portability and Accountability Act (HIPAA), and the Clinical Laboratories Improvement Amendment. Medicare is a health insurance program for people older than 65 years, certain disabled individuals younger than 65 years, and those with end-stage renal disease. Medicare covers nearly 50 million persons on an annual basis (Kaiser Family Foundation, 2012). Medicaid is a federal–state partnership health insurance program for eligible low-income groups and is managed by individual states. SCHIP was enacted in 1997 to address the lack of health insurance coverage of children who did not qualify for Medicaid. In 2009, President Obama signed the Children's Health Insurance Program Reauthorization Act (CHIPRA) into law, providing new financial resources and options to expand and improve health coverage for children through both Medicaid and SCHIP (USDHHS, 2011c). This restructuring of the program has been successful in delivering coverage to more than 40 million children compared to only roughly 10 million in the earlier part of the century (USDHHS, 2011c). Enrollment growth is attributed both to the restructuring of the program and the economic downturn that began in early 2008.

Also worth noting is the Prenatal Care Assistance Program (PCAP), which targets pregnant women who meet certain income requirements and are eligible for part of the Medicaid system. The PCAP program includes prenatal care; delivery services; postpartum care up to 2 months after the birth of the baby; referral to the Women, Infants, and Children Program (WIC); and infant care for 1 year.

Because in the United States the majority of government health care programs are managed and delivered by individual states with only partial support by the federal program, the burden to state budgets is enormous. Some unique programs have been implemented to help individual states bridge this gap in costs of health care coverage. The state of Massachusetts now mandates that residents have some form of health insurance, similar to the common requirement that anyone with a car have collision insurance. Residents who do not have coverage are at risk for fines and tax penalties. A Massachusetts state-subsidized plan, Commonwealth Care, was established to offer affordable health care to residents. Still, the potential exists of posing an additional burden on the poor, especially if they are fined for not enrolling in something they can ill afford.

Canada

By way of contrast, Canada has boasted universal, federally funded health care access for physicians' services, hospital care, and diagnostics since 1966 (Medical Care Act, Canada, 1966). Canada's Medical Care Act (1966) has had a major influence on social policy affecting health care. It ensures that on a national level, hospital care, doctor's visits, and diagnostic services are accessible to everyone, without charge. Many people also have additional extended benefit plans through their employers, for medication coverage, dental care, and other therapies. Persons who are on social assistance programs, such as welfare or disability pensions, as well as those receiving old-age pensions, have additional publicly funded coverage for essential medications and basic dental care. These additional benefits do not, however, extend to those working for low wages with no additional benefits, who often cannot afford their medications (Pilkington et al., 2010). Although some provincially funded coverage is available for this group, obtaining it is very difficult; it is only meant for dire situations of need, and disqualifies most of those working for low wages. As a result, many prescriptions remain unfilled as choices have to be made between paying the rent, feeding the family, and buying medications (Pilkington et al., 2010). Although universal health care exists, it does not cover all aspects of health.

So the system is not perfect. There is a gap in the health care delivery for those who lack private insurance. Provinces and municipalities provide long-term care for persons in need, but there are never enough facilities. At various times, some cash-strapped provinces have attempted to implement user fees for doctor and emergency department visits. Due to immense public pressure, the federal government so far has stepped in to prevent this from happening. One policy, severely curtailing federal health care funding for refugees, was implemented in 2012 by the federal government, leaving this vulnerable and often traumatized group unprotected (Canadian Association of Community Health Centres [CACHC], 2012; Service Canada, 2012). This move was seen as a major injustice by the public—physicians' and nurses' associations, as well as hospitals and community health centers, have voiced a strong unified opposition to this policy. In the meantime, much of needed care for this group is provided free by volunteer health providers, while individual hospitals and provinces are absorbing the costs for emergency treatments within their general budgets. Care is provided first and questions are asked later (CACHC, 2012).

MODELS

There are several models that pertain to health determinants and implementation of social policy that are worth mentioning briefly here. The Social Determinants of Health Model (Dahlgren & Whitehead, 1991; Institute of Medicine [IOM], 2002, p. 404) conceptualizes an approach to assessment and planning care using a foundation of family nursing theory. This model, depicted in Figure 5-1, can assist the nurse in understanding how—aside from the behaviors of individuals—physical, social, environmental, and psychological components influence and affect the state of family health. In this model the general social, economic, cultural, and environmental conditions are the context and give rise to the next layer, which consists of the social determinants of health, the specific social and physical factors representing healthy or unhealthy living conditions. In turn, these factors influence social and community networks, which then influence the lifestyles possible within this context. The center of the model finds the individual/family with their age and gender, enabled/restricted by the contextual layers. Nurses must

take into consideration the family within context to provide holistic care. Changing any of the determinants depicted can bring about changes in family health, as they impinge upon the primary underlying conditions of health and illness (Canadian Nurse Association, 2012). Using this model provides an overview of how all factors interrelate and what possibilities for health promotion may emerge at the institutional and community/societal levels.

The Care Model (Fig. 5-2), pertaining specifically to health care delivery, can be used to guide nurses' care for families/communities in the context of implementing social policy. Initially developed by the Robert Wood Johnson Foundation to deliver quality care to those with chronic illness, the Care Model has since been adapted to assist health care teams change the wider health care delivery systems with a goal of eliminating health disparities (Dahlgren & Whitehead, 1991). Components of the Care Model include the health care organization, community resources and policies, decision support, delivery system support, clinical information systems, and self-management support. Further, the Care Model has the potential to frame the work necessary to address complex self-management problems with a social-policy approach, which includes forming community partnerships to support self-management. Acknowledging the importance of family and community is essential in order to implement a successful program, as humans are relational social beings depending on each other. A proactive health care team employing the Care Model, for example, might initiate an intervention policy of a community garden and kitchen within a poor neighborhood, where many clients have

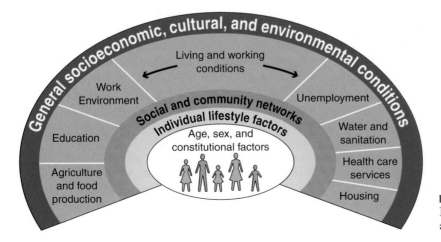

FIGURE 5-1 Social Determinants of Health Model suggested by Dahlgren and Whitehead (1991).

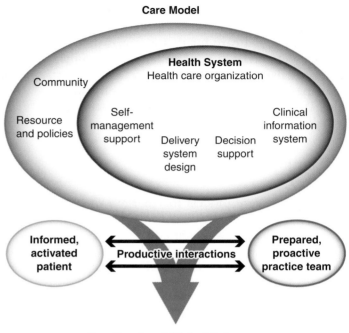

Care Model

FIGURE 5-2 The Care Model. (From Texas Association of Community Health Centers. (2008). *The care model*. Retrieved April 29, 2009, from http://www.tachc. org/HDC/Overview/Care Model.asp, with permission.)

type 2 diabetes and lack the resources to buy healthy foods. Clients referred to this program can share growing food and cooking meals together. This innovative policy adds new resources, while enhancing client skills and self-management support. At the same time, the program also strengthens community ties and cohesion.

Similarly, Canadian scholars Doane and Varcoe (2005) describe a socio-environmental approach to nursing care focused on relationships within families, communities, and health care systems. Health is seen by these authors as a socio-relational experience that is shaped by contextual factors. As in the models discussed earlier, nurses need to take into consideration not only the clients and their families but also all of their physical and social surroundings. Working closely with families and communities and building on the concept of health as a resource for living, the socio-environmental approach recognizes that health is deeply rooted in human nature and environmental structures (WHO, 1986). Knowing their needs and situations, empowered communities therefore are able to promote health with the capacity "to define, analyse and act on concerns in one's life and living conditions" (Doane & Varcoe, 2005, p. 29). This approach, like the Care Model, functions under the premise that a comprehensive social-health-policy approach must be utilized for

optimal delivery of health care, as change is most effectively brought about at the level of physical and social environments.

SOCIAL DETERMINANTS AND RESULTING HEALTH DISPARITIES

Health disparities are such an overwhelming problem in the United States that Congress charged the Institute of Medicine (IOM) to investigate and develop a report on the subject. The landmark IOM report, *Unequal Treatment: Confronting Racial and Ethnic Disparities in Health Care* (2003), detailed long-standing and deeply rooted inequalities in health care directly related to race and ethnicity. Despite the IOM providing a comprehensive review of the contributing factors to health disparities and recommendations to promote health equity, a 2012 evaluation on the progress toward reducing health disparities reveals continued health disparities (IOM, 2012). For instance, African Americans continue to experience higher rates of death from heart disease and cancer than white Americans, and children who live in urban areas are more likely to have asthma than children living in less population dense areas (IOM, 2012). These health disparities continue to correlate with certain environments and lack of adequate resources in multiple areas, such as limited access to health care, exposure to environmental toxins in impoverished environments, personal behaviors related to substance abuse, inadequate nutrition, lack of physical exercise, and lack of treatment for mental illnesses (IOM, 2012). This section will discuss key social determinants of health, their direct outcomes and effects, and the associated health disparities.

Poverty

Social determinants of health are interrelated and mutually reinforcing. Poverty is likely the most fundamental social determinant contributing to health disparities. It influences the other social determinants, such as housing, food and job security, education, and lifestyle choices, and is related to racism and chronic illness. So, it is impossible to discuss one without delving into the others. For instance, poor-quality housing or overcrowding—a result of poverty—affects health by contributing to stress and safety issues, while mildew and dampness might trigger asthma or other respiratory conditions. Unemployment/employment insecurity, which can result in poverty, limits the choice of affordable housing, and living in a low-resource community further adds to unhealthy lifestyle choices. For example, areas where affordable housing is located tend to lack public transportation and grocery stores, and they have less access to fresh fruits and vegetables, which makes shopping for, and eating, healthy foods difficult. Often, the only choice is to buy unhealthy processed foods from the local variety stores, and frequently at high prices (Hilmers, Hilmers, & Dave, 2012).

Poverty creates serious issues when it comes to housing and can result in homelessness for many families who live below the poverty level. Homeless children are three times more likely to have been born to a single mother than their nonhomeless counterparts (National Center on Family Homelessness, 2008). Education is a strong predictor of eventual stability, success, and health, yet education is not (or cannot be) emphasized within homeless communities (National Alliance to End Homelessness, 2006). In the end, homeless children are less healthy—they are more likely to have developmental delays, to have learning disabilities, and to repeat a grade in school (National Center on Family Homelessness, 2008).

In the United States today, as well as in Canada, concern exists over a widening income gap leaving many families and individuals below the poverty level. Interestingly, although the annual median household income for 2011 experienced a continued decline by 1.5% to $50,054, the national poverty rate only declined 0.1%, indicating that the top-income-earning Americans continue to increase in wealth and the middle- and lower-middle-class Americans are experiencing significant declines in income (Luhby, 2012). This widening income inequality between the wealthy and the middle class poses a serious threat of more Americans heading toward poverty. Today, more than 4.9 million Americans, including 1.2 million children, live in poverty in the United States. As explored further below in the sections on race and gender, African American families and those with female heads of households disproportionately account for those living at or below the poverty level. African Americans earn 61% ($31,969) of what non-Hispanic white individuals earn ($52,423). Women continue to earn approximately 77% of what men earn overall (DeNavas-Walt, Proctor, & Smith, 2007).

Canada fares only slightly better, as there is a widening income disparity too. Whereas the top 10% of incomes represent more than a quarter of total incomes, the bottom 10% only represents 1/40th of total incomes. The 80% in between earn the remaining 75% (Canadian Centre for Policy Alternatives [CCPA], 2013). The Canadian Index of Wellbeing [CIW] (2012, p. 2), reported that Canada, since 2008, is experiencing an economic backslide. From 1994 to 2010, even though Canada's Gross Domestic Product (GDP) grew by an impressive 28.9%, improvements in Canadians' wellbeing grew by a significantly smaller 5.7%. The key message is that despite years of steady economic growth in Canada, this prosperity has not been fairly distributed among the Canadian population (CIW, 2012), as income disparities continue to rise. CIW further pointed out that income inequality, measured as the difference between the richest 20% and the poorest 20% of Canadian families, is particularly problematic, as this gap has grown by over 40% since 1994.

In the United States, availability of employment-based health coverage has declined from 64.4% in 1997 to 56.5% in 2010 (U.S. Census Bureau, 2010). This decline has left many more workers and their dependents without health coverage. The cost of health coverage is well beyond the means of those living in or close to the poverty level. Meanwhile, the public debate on an appropriate level of support for families who lack basic housing, food, health services, or social stability continues. Another important factor that affects poor families is a lack of affordable day care. To relieve stress on the families and to escape poverty, families need reliable and quality day care allowing both parents to work.

Multiple other factors worsen the influence of poverty on health outcomes (Woolf, Johnson, Phillips, & Philipsen, 2007), factors such as access to resources, health literacy, gender, ethnicity, and education. All of these factors are considered major contributors to poor health, particularly cardiovascular disease (Shikatani et al., 2012), type 2 diabetes (Chaufan, Constantino, & Davis, 2011; Pilkington et al., 2011), and mental illness (Mental Health Strategy of Canada, 2012; Mental Health Commission of Canada, nd). It is important that nurses and other health professionals support policies that help to eradicate poverty and the resulting health disparities (Kirkpatrick & Tarasuk, 2009).

Gender

Gender is a social determinant everywhere, with women and sexual minorities experiencing disparities in access to resources and well-paying jobs (Mikkonen & Raphael, 2010). Women earn less than men when performing the same job, approximately 77% of men's wages (Devas-Walt, Proctor & Smith, 2007), yet they are more likely than men to be heads of single parent households. In fact, gender is one of the factors that further exacerbates poverty and, in turn, contributes to even greater health disparities. Gender affects health care in other ways as well. For example, women with cardiovascular disease are more likely to receive a misdiagnosis, as their symptoms do not follow the typical presentation men demonstrate, and most tests for cardiovascular disease were developed based on male physiology (Schiff, Kim, Abrams, Cosby, & Lambert, 2005). Women are also less likely to receive referrals for surgical procedures, pain management, and other health conditions even when displaying comparable symptoms as male controls.

Race and Ethnicity

Racial and ethnic minorities, or those of First Nation status, tend to have lower incomes and lower-quality jobs (Mikkonen & Raphael, 2010), factors that contribute directly to health disparities. Recent Canadian data show that the health of non-European immigrants of color deteriorates over time whereas the health of European immigrants is actually superior to that of Canadian-born residents. Hispanic/Latino men are three times as likely to contract HIV as white men, and Latino populations are disproportionately affected by HIV, accounting for nearly 20% of new infections in the United States (Centers for Disease Control and Prevention [CDC], 2013a). Other examples of disparities based on race and ethnicity are as follows: African American, American Indian, and Puerto Rican infants have higher death rates than white infants; African Americans, Hispanics, American Indians, and Alaska Natives are twice as likely to have diabetes than non-Hispanic whites; and Hispanic and African American older adults are less likely than non-Hispanic whites to receive influenza and pneumococcal vaccines (CDC, 2013a; Rodriguez, Chen, & Rodriguez, 2010).

Additionally, members of these groups may experience overt or subtle differences in treatment in the health care system, due to discrimination against minority populations. Self-reported racial/ethnic discrimination encountered by health care providers is significantly associated with lower quality of care indicators, such as development of foot disorders and regulation of HbA1c (Peek, Wagner, Tang, Baker, & Chin, 2011). Other recent studies indicate that although minorities are more likely to require health care, they are less likely to receive health services. Further, even when access is equal, minorities are far less likely to receive surgical or other therapies. Nurses have the moral obligation to advocate for clients who are faced with discrimination in the system and ensure that they receive the same care and treatment as everyone else.

Presence of Chronic Illness

The presence of chronic illness is a determinant that leads to health disparities beyond the mere presence of the chronic illness. It often results in poor quality of life and increased financial strain, especially for those who have no or limited access to health care and resources. In severe cases chronic illness also leads to inability to work and therefore forces those who are ill to rely on the social safety net, which has been increasingly cut back over the last 20 years (Mikkonen & Raphael, 2010). Despite improvements in treatment and management strategies for chronic illness improving both quantity and quality of life, social determinants continue to place disadvantaged populations at risk of poor outcomes from chronic illness. Likewise, the presence of chronic illness itself is a determinant that leads to health disparities for and between families. If one family member is ill the whole family is affected and often has to pick up the financial and care burden. This is true for the United States but also in Canada where medications and home care, for example, are not covered by universal health care. Unless a patient has private insurance benefits, these costly treatments place a burden on families. The following section explores several common chronic illnesses and the ways that they contribute to health disparities.

Type 2 Diabetes

Type 2 diabetes is on the rise and is four times more likely in low-income communities than in their higher-income counterparts. Lower-income communities often also coincide with high proportions of immigrant population and people on social assistance (Mikkonen & Raphael, 2010). Health promotion efforts involving diet and exercise to ward off obesity have a significant influence on disease rates; however, they require sufficient resources (Webster, Sullivan-Taylor & Turner, 2011). Due to lack of resources, preventive measures, such as keeping a healthy weight, are much less likely in lower-income groups (Chaufan et al., 2011; Dinca-Panaitescu et al., 2012; Pilkington et al., 2011; Raphael, 2008; Raphael, Daiski, Pilkington, Bryant, Dinca-Panaitescu & Dinca-Panaitescu, 2011). Aboriginal peoples, for example, only developed diabetes when they started to eat Western foods, instead of their traditional diets. Before the 1940s, this disease was virtually unknown in that group (Health Canada, 2011).

Dinca-Panaitescu et al. (2012), however, present research showing that even with obesity levels the same, diabetes rates were four times higher among those persons who lived in lower-income

neighborhoods, confirming that the reasons for this disparity are complex and multilayered. These layers include lack of needed resources for a healthy lifestyle, such as healthy diets; lack of exercise; inability to pay for prescription drugs; lower incomes; unhealthy environments; racial and/or ethnic discrimination; and stress. Researchers have found evidence that worry and chronic stress, which leads to high cortisol levels, plays a role in chronic disease (Brunner & Marmot, 2006). Chronic stress disproportionately affects most minority ethnic groups who are often subject to discrimination and the constant worries attached to low incomes. When people have to cope with the added expenses of the illness, it increases stress further, creating a cycle and exacerbating chronic illness. As stated earlier, the social determinants that create health disparities are multilayered, complex and mutually reinforcing.

Asthma and Other Lung Diseases

According to the American Lung Association (2008), approximately 34.1 million Americans report a diagnosis of asthma, and the incidence of asthma is increasing, with similar reports from Canada (Public Health Agency of Canada, 2012). Direct health costs for treating asthma are estimated to be $10 billion annually. Asthma is the leading chronic illness among children and is the third leading cause of hospitalization for children younger than 15 (American Lung Association, 2008). It is associated with poor-quality physical environments, such as increased air pollution and substandard housing. Major asthma attack triggers include secondhand tobacco smoke, dust, pollution, cockroaches, pets, and mold. Less common triggers include exercise, extremes of weather, food, and hyperventilation (National Center for Environmental Health, 2013).

In adults we find chronic obstructive pulmonary disease (COPD) and lung cancer to be serious chronic diseases that shorten life and decrease its quality. Lung diseases, like all other diseases, are associated with social determinants such as poverty, as well as with considerable health care costs.

HIV/AIDS

More than 1 million people live with HIV/AIDS today in the United States. AIDS is now seen as a chronic, treatable disease in America and other developed countries (AIDS in America, n.d.). With the introduction of antiretroviral drugs in the 1990s, HIV has been treated as a chronic illness, and more people are living longer with the infection. Unfortunately, the treatability has contributed to an "unsafe sex problem" leading to complacency, and the infection rate, instead of declining, has remained stable since 2006 (AIDS in America, n.d.).

Mental Illness

Mental illness is widespread and very debilitating, particularly due to the stigma attached. It often leads to homelessness and family breakup, two other significant health determinants. It is estimated that one in five persons in North America will have a mental illness at some point in their lives and it can strike at any age, including childhood. Those with mental illness who are poor are more likely to end up homeless and destitute (Canadian Mental Health Association [CMHA], 2009).

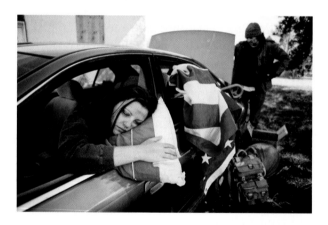

In North America it is estimated that 4 persons out of 10 will develop cancer in their lifetime. In recent years, with improved detection and treatments, many cancers are now cured or, like AIDS, can become chronic diseases that people live with for some time. Similarly, cardiovascular disease is becoming a chronic health condition (Hemingway, 2007; Shikatani et al., 2012), with those affected needing support to manage their disease. As persons with chronic illnesses live and work within their communities, they need to learn how to self-manage their conditions (Health Council of Canada, 2012). Nurses as advocators and coaches have a large role to play here, when they care for individuals and families within the context of their physical and social environments. One of the roles

of nurses to help clients with chronic diseases is teaching health literacy.

Health Literacy

Health literacy, first noted in the *Healthy People 2010* objectives, is defined as "the degree to which individuals have the capacity to obtain, process, and understand basic health information and services needed to make appropriate health decisions" (National Network of Libraries of Medicine, n.d.). Health literacy is one of the social determinants that contributes to health disparities; but though a relationship between health disparities and health literacy has been established, it is complex. The IOM found that approximately 9 out of 10 adults have difficulty understanding health information (IOM, 2011), and the Canadian Council on Learning (2007) found 60% of Canadians are health illiterate. Individuals with low health literacy do not understand health information, so it affects their health outcomes disproportionately because they seek fewer health screenings, they use urgent or emergency care, they experience errors in medication dosing and scheduling, they lack alternatives in treatment regimens, and they are unable to access accurate health-related information.

Nurses, as educators and advocates, must consider the health literacy of the patients and families that they serve. Explaining health-related concepts in plain language will help to ensure that patients understand the information correctly. Nurses may also assist families by filling out complicated forms when applying for social support or filing insurance claims (Street Health Report, 2007).

The Definition of Family

The definition of family, rarely challenged until recent times in the United States, has major social implications in terms of health disparities. Most directly, the definition of family can influence who is able to access health care and social support resources and who is not. The typical definition of family is "two or more people who are related by blood, marriage/partnership or adoption, that live together for a certain period of their lives" (Statistics Canada, 2011). In Canada "the traditional family, a married couple with 2.5 children, has been reconfigured to include cohabiting couples (with or without children), lone parent families, blended or step-families, same-sex couples, couples who remain childless by choice, and intergenerational families" (Statistics Canada, 2011). The definition is evolving as families evolve, but perhaps not as quickly as necessary.

Members of a "family" can be given access to or denied health insurance, housing, and access to social and health programs. In the United States, the Administration for Children and Families, overseen by the USDHHS, "is responsible for federal programs that promote the economic and social well-being of families, children, individuals, and communities in the U.S." (USDHHS, 2013a). Such programs include, for example, Temporary Assistance to Needy Families (TANF), the Healthy Marriage Initiative, and Head Start (USDHHS, 2008). But because of how families are legally defined, many individuals who consider themselves part of a family unit would be ineligible for these programs. In fact, a limited legal definition of family can have devastating results. Take, for example, one instance in Black Jack City, Missouri, where a family composed of two parents and three children was denied an occupancy permit simply because the parents were not legally married and the male parent was not the biological father of the oldest child residing in the household (Coleman, 2006).

Canada is somewhat more liberal in this regard. The provinces, with exception of the Province of Quebec, legally recognize the common-law family, meaning two people cohabiting without being officially married (Statistics Canada, 2011). In 1967, former Prime Minister Pierre Elliott Trudeau, then Justice Minister, declared: "The state has no business in the bedrooms of the nation" (cited by Overall, 2004, p. 1). Today, same-sex marriage is legally recognized in that "a couple may be of the opposite or same sex" (Statistics Canada, 2011). Canada's recognition of both same-sex and common-law families results in major implications for access to spousal benefits and pensions, child custody, and other traditionally family-oriented rites of inheritance. Previously, only traditionally married couples of the opposite sex were recognized as beneficiaries, leaving many nontraditional spouses destitute after their life partners died or divorced them. Legal definitions of family in the United States will continue to be blurred as families continue to evolve through adoption, same-sex marriage, cohabitation, and blended families.

Education

Education is another key social determinant of health. Schools in affluent areas have better resources for the most part. In poor areas, poor quality education and high drop-out rates contribute further to poverty, preventing access to high-quality jobs and incomes. School districts vary greatly, as does the quality of education they provide. They may be as small as a single grade school or as large as the multimillion-pupil New York City system. In the United States, the historical expectation is that a locally elected or appointed school board will determine the way in which the community's children will be educated. Federal funds, often for special education or programs for impoverished students, account for only about 7% of school expenditures (Ramirez, 2002). The reporting about schools without texts, without modern science laboratories or computers, and cutting back on "frills" such as music, art, and gym has stimulated an active search for ways to make equitable funding available. Given the high positive correlation between health status and level of education, this determinant of health and associated policies should be an area of concern to every nurse. Education makes it possible to obtain a better job and higher income and is the best way out of poverty.

Health Resources

Despite the presence of the universal health insurance program in Canada, some major inequities remain. For example, in rural areas, access to health care is often very limited. This is of particular concern in Canada's far north, inhabited mainly by First Nations people. Communities there are served mostly by nurses. Although the nurses have the opportunity to provide primary health care, resources are limited. For major health problems requiring surgical or other complex interventions, or even to give birth, patients are routinely flown out to larger centers, resulting in family separation and lack of community support for the patient. Using technology such as telemedicine provides hope for improvements of health care in these underserviced communities.

RISKS AND BEHAVIORS THAT CONTRIBUTE TO DISPARITIES

This section focuses on the behavioral health determinants that contribute to health disparities. In popular discussions, and sometimes among professionals, health-related behaviors are treated as resulting solely from conscious choice by individuals, who are to blame if their risky behavior leads to poor health outcomes. Many health activists, by contrast, seek to place blame on commercial interests that profit from these behaviors or on government policies that protect them. Research on the causes of risky behaviors is much less developed than is research on the consequences of such behaviors. But even so, it is clear that these risky behaviors are the result of multiple causes and can be influenced by health policy in multiple ways (Berkman & Mullen, 1997; Singer & Ryff, 2001). This section explores obesity, alcohol use, smoking, and other risk factors specifically pertinent to adolescents.

Obesity

In North America, one of the most disturbing trends in health over the past decade has been the increase in the proportion of the population that is overweight or obese. Obesity is defined as body mass index (BMI) at or above the 95th percentile of the sex-specific BMI, according to the CDC's BMI-for-age growth charts (CDC, 2010). BMI is calculated as weight in kilograms divided by the square of height in meters. Obese people are more likely than are those of normal weight to suffer from heart disease, stroke, diabetes, gallstones, sleep apnea, and some types of cancer (USDHHS, 2009). Hypertension, musculoskeletal problems, and arthritis tend to be more severe in obese people. Obesity increased little in the U.S. population between the early 1960s and 1980. Since 1980, however, obesity has increased dramatically in the United States. Fifteen percent of American adults were obese in the mid-to-late 1970s. The prevalence of obesity doubled in the two subsequent decades to 31% by 2000, and by 2009–2010, nearly 36% of adults were obese (CDC, 2012). Women (36.2%) are more likely than men (32.6%) to be obese (Shields, Carroll, & Ogden, 2011).

Obesity rates are lower in Canada than in the United States, but Canadian rates have also increased rapidly in recent years. Approximately 24% of Canadian adults were obese in 2007–2009 (Shields et al., 2011). In contrast to the United States, in Canada men were more likely to be obese than women; trends in the incidence of obesity are now similar for both: in 2007–2009 24.3% of men and 23.9% of women were obese in Canada (Shields et al., 2011).

In 2009–2010, over one-third of adults age 65 and older in the United States were obese (CDC, 2012). Since 1999, the incidence of obesity among older adults has increased, especially among men. With projections for the number of older adults to more than double from 44.2 to 88.5 million by 2050, obesity in this group will contribute significantly to health care costs (Fakhouri, Ogden, Carroll, Kit, & Flegal, 2012).

The percentage of children and teenagers who are obese has been increasing dramatically since the 1980s. In the mid-1980s in the United States, only 5% of children were obese, yet by the early 2000s, obesity increased to 18% among children and adolescents (Federal Interagency Forum on Child and Family Statistics, 2012). A recent report in August 2013 by the CDC (2013b) reveals for the first time in decades that there is a slight improvement in obesity rates in the United States among preschool children who live in low poverty. From 2008 through 2011, data were collected in 43 states and territories for preschool children who participate in the Women, Infants, and Children (WIC) federally funded program. There was a slight drop in the obesity rates in 19 of these states, with the largest drop of 1% in Florida, Georgia, Missouri, New Jersey, and South Dakota. One factor that could contribute to this new trend is changes in the WIC program, which include eliminating juice from food packets, less food with saturated fats, and easier access to fruits and vegetables. Along with these changes, the breastfeeding rates in the United States continue to increase. Whereas this is an excellent trend, childhood obesity remains of deep concerns as one in eight children are obese, with one in five African American children and one in six Hispanic children still obese. Boys and girls have been historically about equal in their likelihood to be overweight, but in 2007–2008, a higher percentage of boys (21.2%) were obese than girls (17.3%). Mexican American and African American teenagers are more likely to be overweight than are non-Hispanic white teenagers.

By 2007–2008, the percentage of overweight Mexican American teenagers was 24.2%, compared with 22.4% for African Americans and 17.4% for whites (Federal Interagency Forum on Child and Family Statistics, 2012).

By comparison, in 2011, 24% of 12- to 17-year-old Canadian boys were obese and about 17% of girls (Human Resources and Social Development Canada, 2013). Over the past quarter century, the percentage of Canadian adolescents ages 12 to 17 who are overweight has more than doubled, and the percentage of those who are obese has tripled. North American children who eat fruits and vegetables frequently are less likely to be overweight. By contrast, those who watch TV, play video games, or spend time on the computer are more likely to be overweight (USDHHS, 2010).

U.S. medical expenditures related to obesity are estimated to be as high as $147 billion dollars annually (Finkelstein, Trogdon, Cohen & Dietz, 2009). The most common recommendations for the treatment of overweight and obesity include participating in physical exercise and following dietary guidelines for healthy eating. Although healthy diets and exercise are part of the solution to the obesity epidemic, nurses must consider constraining social and policy factors determining health, including lack of access to healthy foods, unsafe neighborhoods with limited facilities for physical exercise, and cultural beliefs and attitudes about weight and health. Overall, we know that losing weight reduces and sometimes corrects type 2 diabetes. Obesity plays a major role in cardiovascular diseases and puts unnecessary stress on joints, which causes them to become deteriorated with painful arthritic symptoms. In general this condition leads to debilitating health problems and may also lead to self-esteem issues, particularly in younger people.

Tobacco

Smoking and substance abuse are critical behavioral health determinants that lead to multiple health disparities among families in the United States and Canada. Although smoking is still prevalent, it has declined steadily among adults in the United States. In 1965, more than half of adult men smoked, as did a third of adult women. Smoking has declined more rapidly for men than for women, and the gap between sexes has narrowed. By 2011, approximately 21.5% of adult men and 17.3% of adult women were current smokers. Prevalence of cigarette smoking is highest among American Indians/Alaska Natives (31.4%), followed by whites (21.0%), African Americans (20.6%), Hispanics (12.5%), and Asians (excluding Native Hawaiians and other Pacific Islanders) (9.2%) (USDHHS, 2011a). In Canada, the proportion of daily smokers decreased from 24% to 15.1% between 1995 and 2011. In 2011, another 5% of Canadians reported being occasional smokers. As in the United States, more men (22.3%) were smokers than women (17.5%) (Human Resources and Social Development Canada, 2013).

Smoking is a significant behavioral health determinant. It harms most body organs, reduces circulation, and causes several diseases, including coronary heart disease, chronic obstructive lung diseases, lung cancer, leukemia, and other types of cancer. Smoking also has adverse reproductive effects and is associated with infertility problems, low birth weight, and stillbirth. Smokers are at higher risk than nonsmokers of developing many other diseases and chronic health conditions (USDHHS, 2011a). The myriad of health implications from smoking are of critical importance for nurses to consider when planning care for families with members who smoke. The impact of the behavior on the entire family should be included in all health teaching, with realistic goals set by the nurse and family in collaboration with one another.

Alcohol

Use of alcohol is a risk factor and determinant for a wide range of poor physical and mental health outcomes. Alcohol use is legal for adults, though impaired driving (DUI) and, to a lesser extent, public drunkenness are banned. Alcohol use is illegal for minors, though widely tolerated in both the United States and Canada. In 2011, 62.6% of American adult men (age 21 or older) and 50.9% of American adult women reported that they currently drank alcohol. Almost one-third of men and 16% of women reported "binge drinking" (defined as the consumption of five or more drinks on one occasion for men, and four or more drinks for women) during the preceding month. In the United States, non-Hispanic whites were more likely than other race groups to be current drinkers, whereas Native Americans were more likely than other race groups to be binge drinkers (USDHHS, 2011b). In Canada in 2011, 18.7% of those who consumed alcohol engaged in chronic drinking, defined as 10 or more drinks per week for women and 15 or more for men; and 13.1% engaged in acute drinking, defined as three or more drinks during a single occasion for women, and four or more drinks for men (Health Canada, 2012).

The prevalence of illegal drug use, the particular drugs used, and the methods in which they are taken vary considerably over time, among racial and ethnic groups, across social and economic classes, and among regions of the country or even neighborhoods. In 2011, 21.4% of Americans ages 18 to 25 reported that they were current users of illicit drugs; this rate lessened to 6.3% among adults age 26 or older (USDHHS, 2012). In 2011, illicit drug use of one of five substances was reported to have decreased from 11.3% in 2004 to 4.8% in 2011 among the Canadian population age 15 or older (Health Canada, 2012). Alcohol consumption can result in malnutrition, liver disease, and both short- and long-term cognitive impairment (Antai-Otong, 2006).

Alcohol and substance abuse have serious consequences for individual health. Individuals who engage in excessive drinking are more likely to suffer from high blood pressure and to develop chronic diseases such as liver cirrhosis, pancreatitis, and different types of cancers. Excessive drinking also affects psychological health. Substance abuse also causes unintentional injuries produced by car accidents, drowning, falls, and other types of incidents.

Adolescence

Once children survive the first year of life, the risk of death decreases dramatically (Federal Interagency Forum on Child and Family Statistics, 2012). The risk of death increases again in the teen years as youths, especially male and minority youths, are subject to heightened risk of fatal motor vehicle accidents and homicides. In the United States, African American teenage men are more often victims of homicide than teens in other racial and ethnic groups (Federal Interagency Forum on Child and Family Statistics, 2012). For young Americans ages 15 to 24, the most common causes of death in 2009 were unintentional injuries and homicide, accounting for more than three-fourth of deaths to young people. Additionally, the risk of dying for

those between 15 and 24 years of age was more than twice as high for boys as for girls. Asian or Pacific Islander teenage girls have the lowest mortality rates, and African American teenage boys have the highest. Automobile accidents account for more deaths among American Indians or Alaskan Natives, followed by white male and female adolescents, than among other minority adolescents (Federal Interagency Forum on Child and Family Statistics, 2012). These distressing statistics can be attributed to the fact that adolescents experiment more with risky behaviors that result in health consequences.

Still, in the United States, from 1991 to 2011, adolescent smoking and alcohol consumption significantly declined (Federal Interagency Forum on Child and Family Statistics, 2012). And though the use of illicit drugs increased substantially in the mid-1990s, these rates likewise decreased during the 2000s. Despite some historical fluctuations in the rate of smoking over the last several decades, by 2011 only 10% of high-school seniors reported regular cigarette use (Federal Interagency Forum on Child and Family Statistics, 2012). The risky behaviors of smoking, alcohol use, and drug use are all much more likely among white than among minority youths (Casper & Bianchi, 2002). African Americans were the least likely to report engaging in most of these behaviors. The rates of alcohol use for Canadian adolescents remained relatively stable during the 1990s, but decreased in the 2000s. During 2007–2008, the rates of alcohol use hovered between 46% and 62% for both boys and girls ages 12 to 18, depending on the province (Drug & Alcohol Use Statistics, 2012). Similar to the United States, 12th-graders in Canada also exhibit the highest rates of alcohol and drug use among adolescents (Canadian Centre on Substance Abuse, 2011). Fewer Canadian adolescents smoke today than was the case a decade ago. In 2011, slightly more than 9% of adolescents ages 15 to 19 smoked daily or occasionally compared with nearly 30% in 1994 (Human Resources and Social Development Canada, 2013).

Researchers evaluating large data sets of representative samples of young people over time, such as the National Study of Adolescent Health, are beginning to untangle the effects of peer influences, family factors, school climate, and neighborhood contexts on youth risk-taking behavior (Duncan, Harris, & Boisjoly, 2001; National Center for

Health Statistics, 2012). As this section reflects, multiple, complex, and challenging factors contribute to the nurse's ability to evaluate risks and behaviors that lead to health disparities. Families comprised of members demonstrating one or more of these risks or behaviors may present challenges to the nurse developing a comprehensive plan of care that meets all needs of all family members. Nevertheless, it is critically important that each family member be assessed and evaluated when creating a family plan of care.

SOCIAL POLICY

As discussed earlier, the U.S. Public Health Service has set a target goal to eliminate health disparities among the poor, minority groups, and genders. The U.S. Department of Health and Human Services Bureau of Primary Health Care has developed the Health Disparities Collaborative as a mechanism to change the delivery of care to populations at risk and meet this goal (Gillis, 2004). The greatest impact will be achieved through an upstream approach of primary prevention and health promotion (Falk-Rafael & Betker, 2012; Smith Battle, 2012). This section presents some current social policy aimed at mitigating health disparities and then explores several key areas in need of additional social policy to minimize disparities.

Educational Policy

Education is a crucial social determinant of health and illness disparities. Educated individuals are more likely to follow health practice advice that substantially reduces adult and children health risk factors. Better-educated individuals are also more likely to look for medical care when they get sick, and thus they receive more health care (Cutler, Deaton, & Lleras-Muney 2006). As a consequence, a gradient in health disparities exists by educational level. This section explores some of the educational policies in place to minimize disparities and promote health.

Every child in the United States and Canada has a right to an education, up through the completion of high school. This social policy is one of the few guarantees given to residents of the United States. The majority of American and Canadian children attend a school that is in the same community in which they reside with their family. When a school is community based, it can also serve as a community center, providing after-school programs for working parents and evening educational programs to community members. Schools can support and improve the lives of children and their families by serving community needs. The school system also functions as a social gatekeeper and may be held accountable for enforcing many public health laws and regulations, such as the requirement for vaccination before children enter the system.

Nurses, social workers, and psychologists in U.S. and Canadian schools are now well established as integral providers of services for children and families. Psychological testing and services, speech and language therapy, occupational therapy, and physical therapy are a legal right for all children assessed as having special health care or learning needs and are administered under such legislation at Section 504 of the Americans with Disabilities Act. In Canada, the provincial Ministry of Education is responsible for administering the public funds of children's education (Canadian Encyclopedia, 2012).

Nevertheless, educational equity is not always easy to achieve, and educational inequity leads ultimately to health disparities. For example, the No Child Left Behind (NCLB) law was enacted in 2001 and was a reauthorization of the Elementary and Secondary Education Act originally adopted in 1965. This educational plan has four pillars: accountability, flexibility, proven methods, and parental ability to transfer their children out of low-performing schools after 2 years. On paper, the NCLB does not appear to hinder the educational process, but there are many concerns about this law. The title of the law is intentionally inclusive and brings to mind equity in education, but when put into practice, equity was elusive among disabled students and students from ethnic and racial minorities (Thompson & Barnes, 2007, p. 12). The process of grading schools and requiring continuous improvement in test scores as a condition of economic support may prove impossible to manage. Some schools starting with high scores may not be able to make substantial increases, and other schools starting with very low scores may make meaningful improvement without meeting the stated standards. In Canada too, recent cutbacks to education have resulted in curtailing some programs considered "frills," such as sports and music.

They have met with public outcries from parents, often reversing the decision to cut back.

School Nursing

The National Association of School Nurses (NASN) in the United States holds the position that each school nurse plays an active role in assisting children to optimize health, wellness, and development as a foundation to achieve educational success (NASN, 2003). This organization supports the need for a nurse in every school and acknowledges the role of the nurse that extends to family nursing, often the only health care resource in a community. As a resource, the school nurse should function as a case manager with knowledge of available insurance programs, health care providers, and community-based health-related services.

Traditionally, the school nurse has been responsible for managing emergency situations, providing mandatory screenings and immunization surveillance, dispensing prescribed medications, and serving as a resource for health-related information (American Academy of Pediatrics [AAP], 2001). The role of the school nurse, as part of a comprehensive school-based health care team, has expanded into many communities as a source of health care for the uninsured. Many large cities employ registered nurses and advanced practice nurses who provide primary care services in school-based clinics, not only because children lack a source of care but because school-based care is accessible and comfortable for young people.

The AAP (2001) describes the role of the school nurse as one who provides care to children, including acute, chronic, episodic, and emergency care. The nurse is also responsible for the provision of health education and health counseling, and serves as the advocate for all students, including those with disabilities. The school nurse should work in collaboration with community-based doctors, organizations, and insurers to ensure that each child has access to health care (AAP, 2001). This recommendation is an exceptional expectation, especially when many schools function without a full-time nurse. Far too many schools have no nurse, only a part-time nurse, or a nurse whose only role is to ensure that children with special health care needs receive their medications, catheter care, or other prescribed services.

In Canada, where all permanent residents have universal health coverage, most individuals and families have a family physician and therefore better access to health care. School nursing falls under the purview of public health nurses who visit schools as part of their roles determined by various provincial government mandates. These nurses have an opportunity to connect with children and families and mediate their needs and available resources and practice health promotion. They play an important role in primary health care with an emphasis on upstream approaches of health promotion and disease prevention (Butterfield, 2002; Falk-Rafael & Betker, 2012; Smith Battle, 2012). Recently, with a push from governments to focus more strongly on the "three Rs" (reading, writing, and arithmetic) and increasing standardization and testing, time allotted for public health nurses to service the individual schools is being cut. School health today falls under a consensus statement of many public agencies, rather than nursing alone (Canadian Consensus Statement on Comprehensive School Health, 2007). In Ontario, for example, if specific nursing services are required today, the trend is to provide services by nurses attached to a Community Care Access Centre (CCAC), an agency that delivers nursing care in the community in general. These nurses are only looking after specific children with specific health care needs, which range from physical problems to learning disabilities. Therefore, the coordinated health promotion aspect of school nursing is disappearing in Canada too.

The variability in the presence or expectations of school nurses is a source of concern in the United States. In some districts (and by law in some states), every school has full-time nurses with both knowledge and time to work with children and parents to support or improve physical or mental health. According to the NASN, schools that provide "adequate nursing coverage" have lower dropout rates, higher test scores, and fewer absences, which translate into better health outcomes for children and families. The U.S. government recommends one nurse for every 750 students as outlined in the *Healthy People 2020* objectives, with adjustment depending on community and student needs (USDHHS, 2010). To date, only 45% of public schools have a school nurse all day every day, and an additional 30% have a nurse part-time in one or multiple schools (NASN, 2010).

School nurses are in a unique position to provide many health-related services to school-age children and their families. Unfortunately, in many communities in both the United States and Canada, social policy and funding shortfalls are constricting these resources. If given the appropriate resources and backing, school nurses are well positioned to promote and facilitate family health and creatively bring needed services to schools such as can be seen in the establishment of school-based community health centers.

Housing and Poverty Reduction Policies

The Canadian Centre for Policy Alternatives (CCPA, 2012) points to the lack of national policies on housing and poverty reduction, creating an urgent need for developing policies to mitigate income disparities, by (a) increasing minimum wages to a "living wage," meaning a wage large enough to live comfortably with a healthy lifestyle; (b) increasing social support payments to allow for the necessities of life; and (c) a fairer system of taxation in which higher incomes are taxed progressively more. The public good should come before the individual good in this vision based in principles of social justice and dignity (CCPA, 2012). Nurses should advocate for policies ensuring quality housing, including subsidized housing for low-income families. Since Canada has no national housing policy, creating one seems to be of utmost priority.

Policy Related to Chronic Illness

As discussed earlier in the chapter, chronic illness is both a social determinant of health for families and a creator of health disparities between families. A number of chronic health-related policies have been created that have the potential to reduce disparities in this area. This section explores several of these policies.

Asthma Policy

The objective of policy makers now is to create "asthma-friendly communities." These communities would offer better access to and quality of treatment for all populations, but especially those in poorer communities; increased awareness of asthma and its risks; and environmentally safe schools and homes (Lara et al., 2002). New York City, for example, began an Asthma Initiative in 1999 that includes an Asthma Institute, a comprehensive program called Managing Asthma in Schools and Daycare, a Community Integrated Pest Management

program, and an Asthma Care Coordinator program that provides follow-up care and support to children hospitalized for asthma. The Asthma Institute provides free education to health care providers, community educators, and homeless shelter workers on asthma signs and symptoms, asthma self-management, and other clinical topics related to asthma. This initiative helped reduce hospitalizations for asthma by 9% in 2005 (New York City Department of Health and Mental Hygiene, 2008). No-smoking policies, legislation on emission controls for industries and car exhausts, and cleaner electricity generation initiatives also make a difference in terms of asthma health.

HIV/AIDS Policy

As discussed earlier, with the introduction of antiretroviral drugs in the 1990s, HIV has been treated as a chronic illness, and people are living longer with the infection. Therefore, an increased need for nurses exists to offer prevention education and promote testing for all men and women. Moreover, nurses should join the campaign to continue to encourage the safer-sex practices that helped to reduce the rates of infection in the earlier days of the illness. As stated earlier, with the successful introduction of the antiretroviral drugs, safer-sex practices have been relaxed and rates of infection are no longer decreasing. The CDC currently recommends routine screening and testing for all adults, adolescents, and pregnant women (CDC, 2006). It is believed that when a person infected with HIV is aware of his or her sero-status, he or she can live a healthy and long life by adopting healthy behaviors and using antiretroviral drugs. Knowing HIV status also helps to reduce transmission by practicing safer sex. Prevention education, screening, and counseling are priorities for the family nurse. Policies that prevent the spread of AIDS would also include sex education in schools and for the public at large.

Mental Illness Policy

As a first step, Canada is about to introduce its first national mental health strategy (Mental Health Strategy of Canada, 2012). The Housing First program for individuals with mental illnesses who are homeless, which gets them into supportive housing without demanding that they first be treated, seems to have made a big difference to this vulnerable population, reducing the numbers of unhoused and sick individuals living on the street and in shelters (Mental Health Strategy of Canada, 2012).

Aging Population Policy

Many chronic and debilitating illnesses in the elderly are preventable or can be delayed. Early adoption of a healthy lifestyle and prevention of obesity decreases the prevalence of illnesses such as diabetes, cardiovascular disease, pulmonary disease, and physical disabilities. Hence, it is important to create policies that promote health in an upstream approach before illness sets in, making healthy lifestyles affordable for all. This calls for policies to mitigate the root causes, such as poverty, unhealthy living conditions, food insecurity, lack of access to early interventions when ill, and all other relevant social determinants of health. For nurses it means, once again, advocating for their clients and helping them attain the necessary resources within the complicated systems of health care and social support.

Health Promotion Policies

Health promotion generates health improvements through multiple approaches of research, public education, changes in the physical and social environment, regulation of disease- and injury-promoting activities or behaviors, and improved access to high-quality health care through policies that mitigate disparities and promote equity. For effective outcomes, these policies must consider the social determinants of health as the foundational concepts influencing health (Marmot, 1993; Mikkonen & Raphael, 2010). In 1990, at the urging of the Surgeon General of the United States, the U.S. federal government published a national agenda for health promotion, titled *Healthy People 2000*, which identified 319 objectives for health promotion and set measurable goals for achieving them. Many of the objectives for the decade dealt with health behaviors such as physical activity and exercise; tobacco, alcohol, and drug use; violent and abusive behaviors; safer sexual practices; and behaviors designed to prevent or mitigate injuries. These objectives were set as national goals to be realized through a combination of public sector, private sector, community, and individual efforts (see National Center for Health Statistics [2011] for a complete list of objectives and an assessment of progress toward their achievement). The outcomes to date appear to be mixed, with considerable

success in some areas, including increases in moderate physical activity; moderate improvements in some others, including decreases in "binge drinking" and increases in safer sexual practices; and little progress in some other behavioral objectives, including marijuana use and tobacco use during pregnancy (National Center for Health Statistics, 2011). A new set of objectives and measurable goals were established in *Healthy People 2010* and revised again in *Healthy People 2020*. The relevant *Healthy People* goals provide a standardized approach to assess changes in behaviors that determine health outcomes. Numerous tables in the statistical yearbooks published by the National Center for Health Statistics form a "scorecard" for this national health promotion effort.

Ensuring access to health and illness care services is one way to improve the health of individuals and families. Using upstream approaches, children should receive necessary immunizations and should be evaluated on a regular basis for normal growth and development. Likewise, it is important that adults be adequately immunized and screened for hypertension, diabetes, and cancer at appropriate ages and intervals. The absence of a comprehensive commitment to access or assurance of universal health insurance coverage for all, until now, has made achieving the desired level of interaction with health professionals extremely difficult in the United States (Bernstein, Gould, & Mishel, 2007). Community health centers (CHCs), offering a wide range of services, could hold possibilities for more coordinated care in the United States, as well as in Canada.

Although much emphasis has been on the roles parents have in ensuring that their children receive needed services, many adults also have responsibilities for the health care of aging parents. Adults with both children and aging parents dependent for support struggle with access to health care and management of illnesses, and therefore experience a particularly difficult burden in today's world. They are referred to as the sandwich generation and are in danger of caregiver burnout (Drew, 2012). Adequate supports for families are needed so they do not have to shoulder the burden of care alone. Suggestions for promising approaches are health coaches, particularly registered nurses (RNs), who develop a trusting relationship with their clients and act as advisors and resources for the clients. The RN–Health Coach was recently introduced in the United States with good results and is currently piloted in Canada as well (Change Foundation, 2013).

Areas in Need of Additional Social Policy to Avoid Growing Disparities

There are a number of areas in particular need of additional social policy to help stem growing disparities.

Elder Care

The Administration on Aging (USDHHS, 2012) predicts that by 2020, 19.2% of the 15.2 million persons older than 65 living alone will need help with daily living. The provision of care to the elderly is growing both as a family responsibility and as a profession. More women are caregivers than men. Policies such as the Family and Medical Leave Act are written as gender neutral, but women experience a general expectation that they will be the caregivers regardless of the burden that places on them. Lay caregivers are unpaid, which benefits social programs, especially Medicare and Medicaid. Home care in Canada is also poorly funded and benefits enormously from free labor by family members. Women who provide lay home health care experience much greater levels of stress than their other family members, as well as more alienation from those outside of the home (Armstrong, 1996). Respite care and increased home health nursing and other supports are needed here to ease the burden (Bookman, Harrington, Pass, & Reisner, 2007; Change Foundation, 2013). Recently, some parts of Canada introduced compassionate care benefits, which apply when the death of a family member is expected within the next 6 months. A family caregiver can be granted up to 6 weeks leave from work, during which time she receives Employment Insurance benefits (Employment Insurance Compassionate Care Benefits, 2013). Day care for elders and increasing funding for community-based care in the home would make it easier for older people to stay out of costly institutional care and increase their quality of life. This type of care needs to include house calls by doctors, nurses, physical therapists, and other health care professionals if clients are unable to go to appointments. It also needs to focus on home safety (Change Foundation, 2013). It could go a long way toward reducing health disparities

imposed by chronic illness by providing access to optimal care for vulnerable older persons.

Women's Reproduction

Women's reproduction is another area where social policy could help stem health disparities. In 2006, for example, the state of South Dakota banned access to abortion services. This ban was seen as a direct challenge to federal precedent set in *Roe v. Wade*. In South Dakota, it is now a felony for a health care provider to perform an abortion unless there is proof that the mother's life is at risk. At the time of the ban, only one provider of abortion services, Planned Parenthood, operated in the state. The clinic was reliant on physicians who would fly in from other states because no local physician was willing to provide abortions to women. As a result of this law, women do not have access to abortions unless they have the resources to leave the state for care. In Canada, in the small province of Prince Edward Island, many doctors have refused to perform abortions, which forces women to seek them outside of the province, even though it is a legalized procedure there.

On a similar note, some pharmacists across both countries have refused to fill prescriptions for contraceptives, including emergency contraception, stating that doing so is in direct conflict with their moral and personal beliefs (Stein, 2005). Women, who are often unaware of these reproductive health issues until they are directly affected, are outraged when pharmacists' beliefs override their right to services. Women have a legal right to access prescription medications. The question is, whose rights prevail? In Canada, religious-based health care institutions, as well as individuals, can also refuse abortions and birth control counseling, although women have the right to these services under the Canadian Charter of Rights and Freedoms. Those who are refusing to provide the services are legally required to refer the women to another practitioner who is willing to perform the service. In underserviced areas, this might mean traveling long distances, which not all women can afford.

In the United States, according to the Guttmacher Institute (2005), 47 states have a policy that allows health care providers, including nurses and pharmacists, to refuse to participate in the delivery of reproductive health services, which could leave many women with no choice regarding their reproductive health. Once again, gender, socioeconomic position, and geography seem to be determinants of health that disproportionately disadvantage women by denying them access to care. Both countries are in need of social policy to help mitigate these disparities.

LGBT Health Disparities

Arguably one of the most significant areas of current relevance to family health in North America relates to families with nonheterosexual or gender-conforming identities. Lesbian, gay, bisexual, and transgendered (LGBT) families characterize a growing number of households in the United States (U.S. Census Bureau, 2011). Some estimates from these data suggest that there has been as much as a 51.8% increase in the number of formal same-sex households from the previous decade, though the prevalence in the overall population is still quite small at approximately 1% of U.S. households. The majority of these households, approximately 81%, do house children (U.S. Census Bureau, 2011). This prevalence is significant because with the definition of family currently in flux, these couples and parents face a number of challenges with insurance access, financial benefits and death planning, decision-making abilities, and other key social policy related family health challenges. In Canada, where same-sex marriages are legalized, same-sex marriages have all the rights, duties, and privileges that come with being a married couple. Nevertheless, the stigma associated with homosexuality remains in varying degrees, so the issues cited below in both countries are similar.

According to data presented by the *Healthy People 2020* initiative, LGBT individuals face a number of specific health disparities, such as stigma and discrimination-related mental health disorders, and increased rates of suicide and substance abuse (USDHHS, 2013b). As a result of systemic and policy-related stigma and barriers, these individuals experience significant differences in health-seeking and health-promoting behaviors: they are far more likely to delay accessing health care; they are less likely to receive preventive screens such as mammograms; and they experience greater alcohol and tobacco use, as well as physical violence, than their heterosexual counterparts (Krehely, 2009). Families with LGBT youth are particularly vulnerable and experience significant family life challenges related to stigma and acceptance. As such, LGBT adolescents experience much higher rates of homelessness, prostitution, and substance use, and they are at increased risk of infectious diseases such as HIV, hepatitis, and a host of sexually transmitted infections (Ryan, Huebner, Diaz, & Sanchez, 2009). Both the United States and Canada need additional social policies to decrease these disparities.

To combat these individual and family health problems, San Francisco State University completed a significant family-based intervention project to assist families to develop skills and attributes of acceptance, particularly among families with high degrees of religiosity (Ryan, Russell, Huebner, Diaz, & Sanchez, 2010). Their Family Acceptance Project provides an entire evidence-based family intervention plan and resources available to the general public, along with links to peer-reviewed research aimed to assist families, that can be accessed at http://familyproject.sfsu. edu. Efforts such as these, aimed at assisting families at the individual and community level, in combination with systems of health research, provide an important link between social policy development and LGBT individual and family health issues.

THE NURSE'S ROLE IN ADVOCACY FOR SOCIAL POLICY

This section will look at the role of the nurse historically and today in advocating for social policies to promote the health of clients and families, particularly those who are disadvantaged. As holistic care providers, nurses are in an excellent position to inform the public, including politicians, about what policies are needed and why, and to negotiate for, and help clients and families obtain, the best possible resources.

Historical Involvement in Social Policy

Historically, nurses have worked closely with vulnerable populations and developed unique solutions to challenging health care problems. Many of these interventions took place in the community setting and focused on the family, not just the individual. The profession of nursing historically has been involved in social issues and has worked tirelessly to advocate and provide a voice to many vulnerable populations, starting with the Grey nuns in the 18th century in Canada. The Grey nuns were Catholic, religious sisters who established themselves in the city of Montreal. Their mission was to care for the poor and destitute (Hardill, 2006). In England, in the mid-19th century, Florence Nightingale began to reform the Poor Houses of London and stressed the importance of the environment in health care (Hardill, 2006; Monteiro, 1985). The Henry Street Settlement (HSS) in New York City, founded by Lillian Wald, likewise demonstrated nursing's role as an advocate for vulnerable populations. Founded in the late 19th century, the mission of the HSS was to provide "health teaching and hygiene to immigrant women" (Henry Street Settlement, 2004). Today, the HSS continues to function as a community center for families in New York through its midwifery and nurse practitioner program. Mary Breckinridge established the Frontier Nursing Service (FNS) in Hyden, Kentucky, in 1925. The FNS introduced community-based midwifery care to the women of Appalachia, a vulnerable population with distinct health care needs. These nurses were serving the needs of women and vulnerable minority populations who, at the time, had no human rights, such as voting or owning property.

In the early 20th century, as nursing care moved into the hospital setting, the role of the nurse changed. Nurses lost their autonomous practice as healers and became subordinated to physicians (Ashley & Wolf, 1997). Care became increasingly centered on the medical model and focused on curing the sick individual as opposed to caring for the human response to illness in the context of the physical and social environments. Assessing the influence of the determinants of health and evaluating their effects on the overall health of the individual and family lost much of its importance, as care delivery became focused on the individual's medical diagnosis.

Nursing Today

Today most front-line nurses in the United States and Canada function primarily in the acute care setting, a practice that breeds an inadequate perspective on the role of the social determinants of health and an associated limitation in advocacy. This limited involvement, however, will be forced to change with the looming transformation of health care through the Affordable Care Act in the United States and talk on both sides of the border to move care from institutions into the community.

In 2011, the IOM released a report outlining key recommendations for preparing the nursing workforce to meet the needs of the population: *The Future of Nursing: Leading Change, Advancing Health*. This landmark report describes the need to harness the power of nurses to realize the objectives set forth in the Affordable Care Act by transforming the health care system from one that focuses on the provision of acute care services to one that delivers health care where and when it is needed, ensuring access to high-quality preventive care in the community. The IOM committee explains that nurses will need to be full partners in redesigning efforts, to be accountable for their own contributions to delivering high-quality care, and to work collaboratively with leaders from other health professions by taking responsibility for identifying problems, devising and implementing solutions to those problems, and tracking improvements over time to ensure the health of the population (IOM, 2011).

Numbering over 3 million in the United States and just over 250,000 in Canada, RNs comprise the largest segment of the U.S. and Canadian health care workforce and must be active leaders in improving the access to and quality of health care. Advancing health care will require a cultural shift in the expectations of the nursing profession regarding education, practice, and advocacy for vulnerable populations. In Canada, Pilkington, et al. (2011) found that, even in community-based health care centers, many nurses failed to take into account the clients' social and housing conditions, as these concepts were not included in the standard nursing assessment forms. The allotted time spent with clients was mostly focused on traditional health teaching about lifestyle changes, despite the fact that these same nurses indicated that assessment of access to necessary resources was a critically important component for success in meeting clients' needs promoting their health (Ministry of Community and Social Services, 2012).

Although nurses today may have difficulty making the link between clinical practice and social policy, nursing leaders are pressing for greater involvement in such efforts. On a professional level, many nursing organizations advocate for vulnerable populations and attempt to solve health disparity issues. In fact, in 1992 the American Nurses Association moved the national office to

Washington, DC, to increase visibility of the profession of nursing among U.S. legislators (Milstead, 1999). Similarly, the Canadian Nurses Association (CNA) and provincial professional associations, such as the Registered Nurses Association of Ontario (RNAO) (2012), play an increasingly stronger advisory role, advocating with the federal and provincial governments regarding health policies.

Most nurses currently may not possess the knowledge and skills to interact with policy makers, an activity that must be learned if the needs of the population are to be met. Although few studies exist to describe this complex topic, undergraduate students report limited knowledge of how to engage in a dialogue with legislators or how the role of the nurse relates to such activity (Schofield, 2007). Hewison (2007) acknowledges the lack of policy involvement among nurses and concludes that this may be related to the complexity of the policy process. In Canada too there is very little focus on policy in nursing education. This lack of preparation in policy development is due in part to the traditional focus of curriculum to be foremost on the competencies necessary to obtain licensure. Another reason contributing to this omission in nursing education is the biomedical institutional focus associated with nursing, even in community settings. Advocacy work is mostly not recognized as part of the nursing job description or scope of responsibility (Pilkington et al., 2011).

Brewah (2009) recommends integrating advocacy into nursing curricula and staff education. Primomo (2007) studied the influence of an educational intervention on political awareness in a group of graduate nursing students and found that perceived competence among the students increased after the intervention. Hewison (2007) describes an organized method for policy analysis to be used by nurse managers. This method involves a process by which a summary of the policy is developed, including its origin and status, a history and link to other policy initiatives, and, finally, themes and elements of nursing practice affected by the policy. Once the analysis is concluded, the nurse can take a position on whether this policy will meet the needs of the constituency. Nurses with strong policy analysis skills are critical to improving health for all citizens and to closing the health disparities gap.

Professional nurses with an interest in learning more about their role in the policy arena can find resources through professional associations or can enroll in a health care policy course. One example is the Washington Health Policy Institute conducted by George Mason University in Arlington, Virginia. Nurses and other health care professionals spend 1 week learning about health and social policy, strategies to advocate for at-risk populations, and how to influence policy makers. Similarly, in Canada, the CNA and provincial associations such as the RNAO also offer information, workshops, and training for nurses to gain skill in health care policy development. Social policies are a major contributing factor to the mitigation of health disparities. Nurses have the ability to influence policy on many levels, but not all policies are focused on interactions with governments.

Nursing Policy, Research, and Education

Many important policies are at the institutional level, where nurses work; nursing practice, research, and education should reflect this orientation.

Nurses Influencing Social Policy

The implications of becoming involved in the influence of social policy as a context for nursing care of families are limitless, especially in community and institutional settings. Nurse involvement in policy development can constitute a wide range of activities, from a micro level, where nurses can inform institutional policies in the workplace, to a macro level, where nurses may petition government representatives regarding development of needed or modification of harmful policies.

Nurses can influence policy in small ways. Beginning by using open-ended questions that do not assume marital status, gender of partner, relationships with children, and sources of financial support will yield a much more complete assessment. Discharge planning for return to the community should begin with an open exploration of potential support and resources, without assuming that any are automatically available. Here are some ways in which nurses can get involved in influencing policy from micro to macro levels:

■ Join committees in your institution to change relevant policies (e.g., include questions regarding available resources in assessment forms; make sure needed resources are

available before discharge; ensure follow-up after discharge/referrals)
- Join professional association and advocate for needed social policies
- Write to or phone elected representatives regarding needed policies or changes to those that are harmful
- Join community advocacy groups, such as those requesting affordable day care
- Join boards of directors for agencies, such as social housing, CHCs

Nursing Research

Nursing research has already developed useful tools and frameworks for providing nursing care across cultural barriers and under difficult circumstances. The recent development of community-based participatory research models (Minkler & Wallerstein, 2008) provides a methodology for studies more respectful of the potentially diverse views of family in a community. This approach requires the nurse researcher to establish a relationship with the community in which the study is to occur *before* the development of the research question. Sharing all stages of the research process with the members of the community, nurse scientists using this collaborative approach to examining health disparities can directly affect community improvement based on the results of the study. Adopting this level of respect for reshaping nursing studies of "family" helps nurses gain a more complete understanding of health care for all types of families. This approach is particularly important as trends in care move away from acute care institutions toward community-based care delivery provided by CHCs and home care delivery in both the United States and Canada. Nurses will be particularly well positioned to participate in policy changes and program development in collaboration with an interdisciplinary team, including their clients and families, providing comprehensive health care where and when the community needs it (Hankivsky & Christoffersen, 2008).

Nursing Education

As discussed earlier, there is currently very little inclusion of policy development and advocacy work in nursing curricula. Opportunities for learning experiences in settings that have established services for vulnerable populations provide the nursing student with clinical situations in which to practice assumption-free assessment skills and learn about diverse life situations and needs. Homeless shelters, services for gay and lesbian adolescents, shelters for victims of intimate partner abuse, outreach centers for sex workers, and street syringe and needle exchange programs all reach a disproportionate share of individuals whose family experiences are not the idealized norm (Hunt, 2007). Working in coalition with clients and other health care providers, nurses can ensure the maximum beneficial influence of such policies on the needs of families, communities, and society (Bergan & While, 2012; Brewah, 2009).

The inclusion of health policy in nursing education has the potential to increase the sensitivity of nurses to social and health policy issues. Policy involvement is about empowering others through leadership, not exerting power over others (Brewah, 2009). Nurses must understand that it is not sufficient to provide care in isolation from the forces that increase risk for disease or limit access to medical services. Electives in history, economics, and political science inform nurses' understanding of policy. The IOM recommends that nurses engage in lifelong learning, thereby speaking to the need for nurses to engage in professional practice that strives to stay current on the state of the science in health care and the influences of public policy on the delivery of that health care (IOM, 2011). Nurses, at all levels, must be able to understand current affairs, join nursing and other advocacy organizations, and participate in local, state/provincial, or national political processes. Nurses should be educated to take on responsibility of advocating for equity and social justice to help develop family-friendly policies.

SUMMARY

This chapter has focused on health disparities and how they can be mitigated by social policies. As nursing care shifts from institutions into the community, nurses wanting to deliver the most effective care need to return to historical role models in nursing. They need to become knowledgeable about the influence of the political social structures that are facilitating or hindering health promotion and particularly affect those families who are vulnerable. Promoting health and mitigating disparities, nurses have to be aware of and keep in mind the following:

- Health disparities arise from complex, deeply rooted social issues.

- Health disparities are directly related to the social and political structure of a society, which gives rise to the determinants of health.
- The social determinants of health include poverty, housing, education, employment and food security, accessibility to health care, presence of chronic illness, gender, and being of an ethnic, racial, or sexual minority.
- All these social determinants of health intersect and mutually reinforce each other.
- The social determinants are the root causes of illness and health, as they affect lifestyle possibilities and limitations and access to health care resources.
- The policy decisions made by a society or government about families and what constitutes a legal relationship, and how health care is delivered, have a profound effect on families and their health.
- In the past, the profession of nursing had a well-defined role in advocating for vulnerable populations. In the last century, nursing involvement in the development of health policy has declined, due to a focus on medical diagnosis rather than whole individuals and families in their environmental and social contexts.
- Nurses today need again to get involved in policy development at institutional and societal levels to promote health and well-being for families.
- Nursing professionals can benefit from theoretical and practical education about social policy issues that are broad and complex, but result in resounding effects on the health of a family.
- Family nursing practice has the potential to improve the health of all families, regardless of definition and composition, by closely collaborating with clients and interdisciplinary health care teams.
- Nursing education needs to include teaching policy development and advocacy.
- Nursing research should include collaborative, community-based participatory research with families for best meeting their needs, as they are the experts of their own lives.

REFERENCES

AIDS in America. (n.d.). Retrieved from http://www.ask.com/web?q=hiv+and+aids+in+america&askid=126009d6-f7bc-49a7-9e45-90338b9ea324 us_gsb&kv=sdb&gc=0&dqi=AIDS%2520in%2520America&qsrc=999&o=4800&l=dir

American Academy of Pediatrics. (2001). The role of the school nurse in providing school health services. Retrieved from http://www.nasn.org/Portals/0/statements/aapstatement.pdf

American Lung Association. (2008). What is asthma? Retrieved from http://www.lungusa.org/site/apps/s/content.asp?c=dvI.UK9O0E&b=40611738&ct=534727

Antai-Otong, D. (2006). Women and alcoholism: Gender-related medical complications: Treatment considerations. *Journal of Addictions Nursing, 17*(1), 33–45.

Armstrong, P. (1996). Resurrecting the family: Interring the state. *Comparative Family Studies, 27*(2), 221–248.

Ashley, J., & Wolf, K. (Eds.). (1997). *Selected readings.* New York, NY: National League for Nursing.

Bergen, A., & While, A. (2012). "Implementation deficit" and "street-level bureaucracy": Policy, practice and change in the development of community nursing issues. *Health & Social Care in the Community, 13*(1), 1–10.

Berkman, L. F., & Mullen, J. M. (1997). How health behaviors and social environment contribute to health differences between black and white older Americans. In L. G. Martin & B. J. Soldo (Eds.), *Racial and ethnic differences in the health of older Americans* (pp. 163–182). Washington, DC: National Academy Press.

Bernstein, J., Gould, E., & Mishel, L. (2007). Poverty, income and health insurance needs 2006. Retrieved from http://www.epi.org/content.cfm/webfeatures_ecoindicators_income20070828

Bookman, A., Harrington, M., Pass, L., & Reisner, E. (2007). *Family caregiver handbook: Finding elder care resources in Massachusetts.* Cambridge, MA: Massachusetts Institute of Technology.

Brewah, H. (2009). Policy formulation and implementation. *Primary Health Care, 19*(2), 35–38.

Brunner, E., & Marmot, M. (2006). Social organization, stress and health. In M. Marmot & R. G. Wilkinson (Eds.), *Social determinants of health* (2nd ed.) Oxford: Oxford University Press.

Buettner-Schmidt, K., & Lobo, M. L. (2012). Social justice: A concept analysis. *Journal of Advanced Nursing, 68*(4), 948–958. doi:10.1111/j.1365-2648.2011.05856.x

Butterfield, P. G. (2002). Upstream reflections on environmental health: An abbreviated history and framework for action. *Advances in Nursing Science, 25*(1), 32–39.

Canadian Association of Community Health Centres. (2012). Retrieved from http://www.cachc.ca

Canadian Centre for Policy Alternatives. (2012). Retrieved from http://www.policyalternatives.ca

Canadian Centre for Policy Alternatives. (2013). Retrieved from http://www.policyalternatives.ca/newsroom/updates/income-inequality-numbers

Canadian Centre on Substance Abuse. (2011). Cross-Canada report on student alcohol and drug use. Retrieved from http://www.ccsa.ca/Eng/Priorities/Research/StudentDrugUse/Pages/default.aspx

Canadian Consensus Statement on Comprehensive School Health. (2007). Schools and communities working in partnership to create and foster health-promoting schools. Retrieved from http://www.safehealthyschools.org/CSH_Consensus_Statement2007.pdf

Canadian Council on Learning. (2007). Health literacy in Canada: A healthy understanding. Report. Retrieved from http://www.ccl-cca.ca/CCL/Reports/HealthLiteracy/index.html

Canadian Encyclopedia. (2012). Education policy. Retrieved from http://www.thecanadianencyclopedia.com/articles/education-policy

Canadian Index of Wellbeing. (2012). Measuring what matters. Retrieved from https://uwaterloo.ca/canadian-index-wellbeing/sites/ca.canadian-index-wellbeing/files/uploads/files/CIW2012-HowAreCanadiansReallyDoing-23Oct2012_0.pdf

Canadian Mental Health Association. (2009). Homelessness. Retrieved from http://www.cmha.ca/public-policy/subject/homelessness

Canadian Nurses Association. (2012). Advocacy inside the maze. Retrieved from http://www.cna-aiic.ca

Casper, L. M., & Bianchi, S. M. (2002). *Continuity and change in the American family.* Thousand Oaks, CA: Sage.

Centers for Disease Control and Prevention (CDC). (2006). Revised recommendations for HIV testing of adults, adolescents, and pregnant women in health-care settings. *MMWR, 55*(RR14), 1–17. Retrieved from http://www.cdc.gov/mmwr/preview/mmwrhtml/rr5514a1.htm

Centers for Disease Control and Prevention (CDC). (2010). Overweight and obesity: Defining overweight and obesity. Retrieved from http://www.cdc.gov/obesity/adult/defining.html

Centers for Disease Control and Prevention (CDC). (2012). NCHS Data Brief: Prevalence of obesity in the United States. No. 82, January 2012. Retrieved from http://www.cdc.gov/obesity/adult/defining.html

Centers for Disease Control and Prevention (CDC). (2013a). Hispanic or Latino populations. Retrieved from http://www.cdc.gov/minorityhealth/populations/REMP/hispanic.html

Centers for Disease Control and Prevention (CDC). (2013b, August). Progress on childhood obesity. Retrieved from http://www.cdc.gov/vitalsigns/childhoodobesity

Change Foundation. (2013). Summary and reflections safety at home: A pan-Canadian home care safety study. Retrieved from www.changefoundation.com

Chaufan, C., Constantino, S., & Davis, M. (2011): "It's a full time job being poor": Understanding barriers to diabetes prevention in immigrant communities in the USA. Critical Public Health. doi:10.1080/09581596.2011.630383. Retrieved from http://dx.doi.org/10.1080/09581596.2011.630383

Coleman, T. (2006). Eye on unmarried America. Column one. Retrieved from http://www.unmarriedamerica.org/column-one/-2-27-06-definition-of-family.html

Cutler, D., Deaton, A., & Lleras-Muney, A. (2006). The determinants of mortality, *Journal of Economic Perspectives, 20*(3), 97-120.

Dahlgren, G., & Whitehead, M. (1991). Policies and strategies to promote social equity in health. Stockholm: Institute of Future Studies.

DeNavas-Walt, C., Proctor, B., & Smith, J. (2007). U.S. Census Bureau: Income, poverty and health insurance coverage 2006. Retrieved from http://www.census.gov/prod/2007pubs/p60-233.pdf

Dinca-Panaitescu, M., Dinca-Panaitescu, S., Raphael, D., Bryant, T., Pilkington, B., & Daiski, I. (2012). The dynamics of the relationship between diabetes incidence and low income: Longitudinal results from Canada's national population health survey. *Maturitas, 72,* 229–235.

Doane, G. J., & Varcoe, C. (2005). *Family nursing as relational inquiry: Developing health promoting practice.* Baltimore, MD: Lippincott Williams & Wilkins.

Drew, S. (2012). Avoiding care giver burnout. Retrieved from http://www.everydayhealth.com/cancer-center/avoiding-caregiver-burnout.aspx

Drug and Alcohol Use Statistics. (2012). Health Canada. Retrieved from http://www.hc-sc.gc.ca/hc-ps/drugs-drogues/stat/index-eng.php

Duncan, G. J., Harris, K. M., & Boisjoly, J. (2001). Sibling, peer, neighbor and schoolmate: Correlations as indicators of the importance of context for adolescent development. *Demography, 38*(3), 437–447.

Employment Insurance Compassionate Care Benefits. (2013). Retrieved from http://www.servicecanada.gc.ca/eng/ei/types/compassionate_care.shtml

Fakhouri, T. H. I., Ogden, C. L., Carroll, M. D., Kit, B. K., & Flegal, K. M. (2012). Prevalence of obesity among older adults in the United States, 2007–2010. U.S. Department of Health and Human Services: National Center for Health Statistics, Brief No. 106. Retrieved from http://www.cdc.gov/nchs/data/databriefs/db106

Falk-Rafael, A., & Betker, C. (2012). Witnessing social injustice downstream and advocating for health equity upstream: "The trombone slide" of nursing. *Advances in Nursing Science, 35*(2), 98–112.

Federal Interagency Forum on Child and Family Statistics. (2012). America's children in brief: Key National indicators of well-being, 2012. Detailed tables. Retrieved from http://www.childstats.gov/americaschildren/tables.asp

Finkelstein, E., Trogdon, J., Cohen, J., & Dietz, W. (2009). Annual medical spending attributable to obesity: Payer-and-service-specific estimates. *Health Affairs, 28,* 822–831.

Gillis, L. (2004). The health disparities collaborative. In J. O'Connell (Ed.), *The healthcare of homeless persons: A manual of communicable diseases and common problems in shelters and on the streets.* Boston, MA: Guthrie Nixon Smith Printers.

Guttmacher Institute. (2005). Striking a balance between a provider's right to refuse and a patient's right to receive care. Retrieved from http://www.guttmacher.org/media/presskits/2005/08/04/index.html

Hankivsky, O., & Christoffersen, A. (2008, September). Intersectionality and the determinants of health: A Canadian perspective. *Critical Public Health, 18*(3), 271–283. doi:10.1080/09581590802294296

Hardill, K. (2006). From the Grey Nuns to the streets: A critical history of outreach nursing in Canada. *Public Health Nursing, 24*(1), 94–97.

Health Canada. (2011). Communities in action: Aboriginal diabetes initiative. Retrieved from http://celarc.ca.ezproxy.library.yorku.ca/cppc/233/233707.pdf

Health Canada. (2012). Canadian Alcohol and Drug Use Monitoring Survey. Summary of results. Retrieved from http://www.hc-sc.gc.ca/hc-ps/drugs-drogues/stat/index-eng.php

Hemingway, A. (2007). Determinants of coronary heart disease risk for women on a low income: Literature review. *Journal of Advanced Nursing, 60*(4), 359–367. doi:10.1111/j.1365-2648. 2007.04418.x

Henry Street Settlement. (2004). About our founder, Lillian Wald. Retrieved from http://www.henrystreet.org/site/ PageServer?pagename=abt_lwald

Hewison, A. (2007). Policy analysis: A framework for nurse managers. *Journal of Nursing Management, 15*(7), 693–699.

Hilmers, A., Hilmers, D. C., & Dave, J. (2012). Neighborhood disparities in access to healthy foods and their effects on environmental justice. *American Journal of Public Health, 102*(9), 1644–1654.

Human Resources and Social Development Canada. (2013). Indicators of well-being in Canada: Health. Retrieved from http://www4.hrsdc.gc.ca/d.4m.1.3n@-eng.jsp?did=1

Hunt, R. (2007). Service learning: An eye-opening experience that provokes emotions and challenges stereotypes. *Journal of Nursing Education, 46*(6), 277–281.

Hunter, B. D., Neiger, B., & West, J. (2011). The importance of addressing social determinants of health at the local level: The case for social capital. *Health & Social Care in the Community, 19*(5), 522–530. doi:http://dx.doi.org/10.1111/j.1365-2524. 2011.00999.x

Institute of Medicine (IOM). (2003). *Unequal treatment: Confronting racial and ethnic disparities in health care.* Washington, DC: National Academies Press.

Institute of Medicine (IOM). (2011). *The future of nursing: Leading change, advancing health.* Washington, DC: National Academies Press.

Institute of Medicine (IOM). (2012). *How far have we come in reducing health disparities? Progress since 2000: Workshop summary.* Washington, DC: National Academies Press.

Kaiser Family Foundation. (2011). *The uninsured: Key facts about Americans without health insurance.* Washington, DC: Author. Retrieved from http://www.kff.org/uninsured/ upload/7451-07.pdf

Kaiser Family Foundation. (2012). State health facts. Retrieved from http://www.statehealthfacts.org/profileind.jsp?ind= 290&cat=6&rgn=1

Kirkpatrick, S. I., & Tarasuk, V. (2009). Food insecurity and participation in community food programs among low-income Toronto families. *Canadian Journal of Public Health, 100*(2), 135–139.

Krehely, J. (2009). How to close the LGBT health disparities gap. Center for American Progress. Retrieved April 13, 2013, from http://www.americanprogress.org/wp-content/ uploads/issues/2009/12/pdf/lgbt_health_disparities.pdf

Lara, M., Nicholas, W., Morton, S., Vaiana, M. E., Emont, S., Branch, M. . . . Weiss, K (2002). Improving childhood asthma outcomes in the United States: A blueprint for policy action. Washington, DC: RAND.

Luhby, T. (2012). Median income falls, but so does poverty. CNN Money Report. Retrieved from http://money.cnn. com/2012/09/12/news/economy/median-income-poverty/ index.html

Marmot, M. (1993). *Explaining socioeconomic differences in sickness absence: The Whitehall II study.* Toronto, ON: Canadian Institute for Advanced Research.

Medical Care Act Canada. (1966). History commons. Retrieved from http://www.historycommons.org/entity.jsp?entity= medical_care_act__canada__1966__1

Mental Health Strategy of Canada. (2012). Retrieved from http://strategy.mentalhealthcommission.ca/pdf/strategy- summary-en.pdf

Mikkonen, J., & Raphael, D. (2010). *Social determinants of health: The Canadian facts.* Toronto, ON: York University School of Health Policy and Management. Retrieved from http://www. thecanadianfacts.org

Millett, C., Everett, C. J., Matheson, E. M., Bindman, A. B., & Mainous, A. G. (2010). Impact of Medicare Part D on seniors' out-of-pocket expenditures on medications. *Archives of Internal Medicine, 170*(15), 1325–1330.

Milstead, J. (1999). *Health policy and politics: A nurse's guide.* Gaithersburg, MD: Aspen.

Minkler, M., & Wallerstein, N. (2008). *Community-based participatory research for health: From process to outcome.* San Francisco, CA: Jossey-Bass.

Monteiro, L. A. (1985). Then and now: Florence Nightingale on public health nursing. *American Journal of Public Health, 75,* 181–186.

National Alliance to End Homelessness, (2006). *Housing first.* Retrieved from: http://www.endhomelessness.org/library/ entry/what-is-housing-first

National Association of School Nurses. (2003). Access to a school nurse. Retrieved from http://www.nasn.org/Portals/0/ statements/resolutionaccess.pdf

National Association of School Nurses. (2010). Caseload assignments. Retrieved from http://www.nasn.org/portals/ 0/binder_papers_reports.pdf

National Center for Environmental Health. (2013). CDC's national asthma control. Retrieved from http://www.cdc. gov/asthma/default.htm

National Center for Health Statistics. (2011). *Healthy people 2010 final review.* Hyattsville, MD: Public Health Service.

National Center for Health Statistics. (2012). Data resource center for child and adolescent health. Retrieved from http:// www.childhealthdata.org/home

National Center on Family Homelessness. (2008). America's homeless children. Retrieved from http://www.familyhome- lessness.org/pdf/fact_children.pdf

National Network of Libraries of Medicine. (n.d.). Health literacy. Retrieved May 9, 2008, from http://nnlm.gov/ outreach/consumer/hlthlit.html

New York City Department of Health and Mental Hygiene. (2008). Asthma initiative. Retrieved from http://www. nyc.gov/html/doh/html/asthma/asthma.shtml

Overall, C. (2004, June 28). The state's role in marriage (part 2). *Kingston Whig Standard.* Retrieved from https://christiangays. com/marriage/overall2.shtml

Peek, M. E., Wagner, J., Tang, H., Baker, D. C., & Chin, M. H. (2011). Self-reported racial discrimination in health care and diabetes outcomes. *Medical Care, 49*(7), 618–625. doi:10.1097/ MLR.0b013e318215d925

Picketty, T., & Saez, E. (2004). Income inequality in the United States, 1913–2002. Retrieved from http://elsa.berkeley.edu/ ~saezOUP04US.pdf

Pilkington, F. B., Daiski, I., Bryant, T., Dinca-Panaitescu, M., Dinca-Panaitescu, S., & Raphael, D. (2010). The experience of living with diabetes for low-income Canadians. *Canadian Journal of Diabetes, 34*(2), 119–126.

Pilkington, F. B., Daiski, I., Lines, E., Bryant, T., Raphael, D., Dinca-Panaitescu, M., & Dinca-Panaitescu, S. (2011). Type 2 diabetes in vulnerable populations: Community healthcare providers' perspectives on health service needs and policy implications. *Canadian Journal of Diabetes, 35*(5), 503–511.

Primomo, J. (2007). Changes in political astuteness after a health systems and policy course. *Nurse Educator, 32*(6), 260–264.

Public Health Agency of Canada. (2012). Reducing health disparities—Roles of the health sector: Recommended policy directions and activities. Retrieved from www.publichealth.gc.ca

Ramirez, A. (2002). The shifting sands of school finance. *Educational Leadership, 60*(4), 54–58.

Raphael, D. (2008). Social determinants of health: An overview of key issues and themes. In D. Raphael (Ed.), *Social determinants of health* (2nd ed., pp. 2–19). Toronto, ON: Canadian Scholars' Press.

Raphael, D., Curry-Stevens, A., & Bryant, T. (2008). Barriers to addressing the social determinants of health: Insights from the Canadian experience. *Health Policy, 88,* 222–235. Retrieved from http://dx.doi.org/10.1016/j.healthpol.2008.03.015

Raphael, D., Daiski, I., Pilkington, F. B., Bryant, T., Dinca-Panaitescu, M., & Dinca-Panaitescu, S. (2011). Toxic combination of poor social policies and programmes, unfair economic arrangements, and bad politics: The experiences of poor Canadians with type 2 diabetes. Critical Public Health. Retrieved from http://www.tandfonline.com/doi/abs/10.1080/09581596.2011.607797

Registered Nurses Association of Ontario. (2012). Topic: Advocacy. Retrieved from http://rnao.ca/category/topics/advocacy

Rodriguez, H. P., Chen, J., & Rodriguez, M. A. (2010). A national study of problematic care experiences among Latinos with diabetes. *Journal of Healthcare for the Poor and Underserved, 21*(4), 1152–1168.

Ryan, C., Huebner, D., Diaz, R. M., & Sanchez, J. (2009). Family rejection as a predictor of negative health outcomes in white and Latino lesbian, gay, and bisexual young adults. *Pediatrics, 123*(1), 346–352.

Ryan, C., Russell, S. T., Huebner, D., Diaz, R., & Sanchez, J. (2010). Family acceptance in adolescence and the health of LGBT young adults. *Journal of Child and Adolescent Psychiatric Nursing, 23*(4), 205–213.

Schiff, G. D., Kim, S., Abrams, R., Cosby, K., Lambert, B., & Elstein, A. . . . McNutt, R. (2005). Diagnosing diagnosis errors: Lessons from a multi-institutional collaborative project. In K. Henriksen, J.B. Battles, E.S. Marks & D. I. Lewin (Eds.) *Advances in patientssafety: From research to implementation* (Volume 2). Rockville, MD: Agency for Healthcare Research and Quality.

Schofield, T. (2007). Health inequity and its social determinants: A sociological commentary. *Health Sociology Review, 16*(2), 105–114.

Service Canada. (2012). Interim federal health program. Retrieved on October 10, 2012, from http://www.servicecanada.gc.ca/eng/goc/interim_health.shtml

Shields M, Carroll MD, Ogden CL. (2011) Adult obesity prevalence in Canada and the United States. NCHS data brief, no 56. Hyattsville, MD: National Center for Health Statistics.

Shikatani, E. A., Trifonova, A., Mandel, E. R., Liu, S. T. K., Roudier, E., Krylova, A., . . . Haas, T.(2012). Inhibition of proliferation, migration and proteolysis contribute to corticosterone-mediated inhibition of angiogenesis. *PLoS ONE, 7*(10), e46625. Public Library of Science. doi:10.1371/journal.pone.0046625

Singer, B., & Ryff, C. D. (2001). New horizons in health: An integrative approach. No. 277. Washington DC, National Academies Press.

Smith Battle, L. (2012). Moving policies upstream to mitigate the social determinants of early childbearing. *Public Health Nursing, 29*(5), 444–454.

Statistics Canada. (2011). Concept: Census family. Retrieved from www.statcan.gc.ca

Stein, R. (2005). Pharmacists' rights at front of new debate. *Washington Post.* Retrieved from http://www.washingtonpost.com/wp-dyn/articles/A5490-2005March27.html

Street Health Report. (2007). Toronto. Retrieved from www.streethealth.ca/Downloads/SHReport2007.pdf

Thompson, T. G., & Barnes, R. E. (2007). Beyond no child left behind. Aspen Institute. Retrieved from www.aspeninstitute.org/site/c.hul.WJeMRKpH/b.938015

U.S. Census Bureau. (2010). Employment-based health insurance. Retrieved August 9, 2013, from http://www.census.gov/prod/2013pubs/p70-134.pdf

U.S. Census Bureau. (2011). Same-sex households. Retrieved April 11, 2013, from http://www.census.gov/prod/2011pubs/acsbr10-03.pdf

U.S. Department of Health and Human Services. (2008). National survey of family growth. Centers for Disease Control and Prevention. Retrieved from http://www.cdc.gov/nchs/nsfg.htm

U.S. Department of Health and Human Services. (2010). *Healthy people 2020: Social determinants of health.* Washington, DC. Retrieved from http://www.healthypeople.gov/2020/topicsobjectives2020/overview.aspx?topicid=39#one

U.S. Department of Health and Human Services. (2011a). Adult cigarette smoking in the United States: Current estimate. Retrieved from http://www.cdc.gov.libproxy.usc.edu/tobacco/data_statistics/fact_sheets/adult_data/cig_smoking

U.S. Department of Health and Human Services. (2011b). HealthCare.gov. Washington, DC. Retrieved from http://www.healthcare.gov/index.html

U.S. Department of Health and Human Services. (2011c). 2011 annual CHIPRA report. Washington, DC. Retrieved from http://www.insurekidsnow.gov/chipraannualreport.pdf

U.S. Department of Health and Human Services. (2012). Results from the 2011 National Survey on Drug Use and Health: Summary of national findings. Retrieved from http://www.samhsa.gov/data/NSDUH/2k11Results/NSDUHresults2011.htm#2.3

U.S. Department of Health and Human Services. (2013a). Administration for children and families: What we do. Retrieved from http://www.acf.hhs.gov/about

U.S. Department of Health and Human Services. (2013b). Lesbian, gay, bisexual, and transgender health. *Healthy People 2020.* Retrieved April 11, 2013, from http://www.healthypeople.gov/2020/topicsobjectives2020/overview.aspx?topicId=25

Woolf, S. H., Johnson, R. E., Phillips, R. L., Jr., & Philipsen, M. (2007). Giving everyone the health of the educated: An examination of whether social change would change more lives than medical advances. *American Journal of Public Health, 97*(4), 679–683.

World Health Organization. (1986). The Ottawa charter for health promotion: Retrieved from http://www.who.int/healthpromotion/conferences/previous/ottawa/en/index.html

World Health Organization. (2012a). The determinants of health. Retrieved October 10, 2012, from http://www.who.int/hia/evidence/doh/en/index.html

World Health Organization. (2012b). A human rights–based approach to health. Retrieved September 29, 2012, from http://www.who.int/hhr/news/hrba_info_sheet.pdf

Families Across the Health Continuum

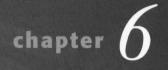

Relational Nursing and Family Nursing in Canada

Colleen Varcoe, PhD, RN

Gweneth Hartrick Doane, PhD, RN

Critical Concepts

- Relational inquiry rests in a socio-environmental understanding of health and health promotion (World Health Organization, 1986). A socio-environmental understanding of health incorporates sociological and environmental aspects, as well as medical and lifestyle choices. Thus, a person's/family's capacity to define, analyze, and act on concerns in one's life and living conditions joins treatment and prevention as an essential goal of family nursing practice.

- Families, health, and family nursing are understood to be shaped by the historical, geographical, economic, political, and social diversity of the particular person's/family's context. By purposefully working with this diversity when providing care, nurses are prepared to take into account the contextual nature of people's/families' health and illness experiences, and how their lives are shaped by their intrapersonal, interpersonal, and contextual circumstances to provide more appropriate care.

- "Context" is not something outside or separate from people; rather, contextual elements (e.g., socioeconomic circumstances, family and cultural histories) are literally embodied in people and within their actions and responses to particular situations.

- Similar to other Western countries, Canada is prosperous, but has a significant and growing gap between rich and poor, along with a biomedical- and corporate-oriented health care system. These influences shape Canadians' health, experiences of family, and experiences of health care and nursing care. By understanding how these economic and political influences shape family experiences and nursing situations, nurses can promote health more effectively.

- Dominant expectations and discourses about families in Canada are similar to other Western countries. These expectations and discourses shape Canadians' health, their experiences of family, and their experiences of health care and nursing care. By examining how families and nurses themselves draw on these expectations and discourses, nurses can improve their responsiveness to families.

- Multiculturalism is part of Canada's national identity and is enshrined in Canadian state policy. Multiculturalism is understood in Canada to promote equality and tolerance for diversity, especially as it relates to linguistic, ethnic, and religious diversity. Tensions exist between this understanding and the lived experiences of families, however, particularly those who are racialized, do not have French or English as their first language, and are from nondominant religions. *Racialization* refers to the social process by which people are labeled according to particular physical

(continued)

characteristics or arbitrary ethnic or racial categories, and then dealt with in accordance with beliefs related to those labels (Henry, Tator, & Mattis, 2009). Nurses who understand these tensions and how they shape families and experiences are better prepared to provide responsive nursing care.

■ As a colonial country, Canada has an evolving history of oppressive and genocidal practices against Canada's indigenous people, and an evolving history of varied immigration practices. Understanding how migration and colonization affect both indigenous and newcomer families, and the health and lives of people within those families, is fundamental to providing effective family nursing care.

■ Competent, safe, and ethical family nursing involves taking the intrapersonal, interpersonal, and contextual aspects of families' lives into account. Nurses also need to consider how their own contexts shape their understandings and responses to particular families and situations. Together, these actions enable nurses to tailor their understanding and care to the specific circumstances of families' lives and mitigate the possibility of making erroneous assumptions about the families they serve.

■ Without a careful consideration of context and its influence on families' health and illness experiences, nurses typically draw uncritically on stereotypes in ways that limit possibilities for families they serve. By inquiring into the context of families' and nurses' own lives, nurses are able to provide responsive, ethical, and appropriate care.

Relational inquiry, the process of understanding and assessing the importance of relationships in order to support optimal health, is a valuable approach to family nursing. This approach rests in a socio-environmental understanding of health and health promotion (World Health Organization, 1986). This understanding of health incorporates sociological and environmental aspects, as well as medical and lifestyle (behavioral) ones. From this perspective, health is considered to be "a resource for living . . . a positive concept . . . the extent to which an individual or group is able to realize aspirations, to satisfy needs, and to change or cope with the environment" (World Health Organization, 1986, p. 1). Subsequently, promoting health and the capacity of people/families to define, analyze, and act on their concerns is the central goal of family nursing practice.

Relational inquiry family nursing practice is oriented toward enhancing the capacity and power of people/families to live a meaningful life (meaningful from their own perspective). Although this may involve treating and preventing disease or modifying lifestyle factors, the primary focus is to enhance peoples' well-being, as well as their capacity and resources for meaningful life experiences. Thus, relational inquiry focuses very specifically on how *health is a socio-relational experience* that is strongly shaped by contextual factors.

Understanding and working directly with context provides a key resource and strategy for responsive, health-promoting family nursing practice. Having an appreciation for the range of diverse experiences and how the dynamics of geography, history, politics, and economics shape those experiences allows nurses to provide more effective care to particular families, better understand the stresses and challenges families face, and better support families to draw on their own capacities. Developing such an appreciation requires that nurses consider how the varied circumstances of their own lives shape their understanding.

Grounded in a relational inquiry approach, this chapter focuses on the significance of context in family nursing practice. Specifically, we highlight the interface of socio-political, historical, geographical, and economic elements in shaping the health and illness experiences of families in Canada and the implications for family nursing practice. This chapter begins by discussing why consideration of context is integral to family nursing. The chapter then covers some of the key characteristics of Canadian society, and how those characteristics shape health, families, health care, and family nursing. Finally, informed by a relational inquiry approach to family nursing, the chapter turns to the ways nurses might practice more responsively and effectively based on this understanding.

CONTEXT IS INTEGRAL TO FAMILY NURSING

Whereas "context" is often conceptualized as a sort of container of people, something that surrounds people but is somewhat distinct and separate from people, this chapter encourages readers to think of context as something that is integral to the lives of people, as something that shapes not only people's external circumstances and opportunities but their physiology at the cellular level. In other words, context is embodied. For example, if a person is born into a middle-class, English-speaking, Euro-Canadian family, the very way that person speaks—accent, intonation, vocabulary—is shaped by that context. The way that person's body grows is influenced by the nutritional value of the food and quality of water available, the level of stress in the family, the quality of housing the family has, the opportunities for rest and physical activity. Similarly, the person's sense of self and expectations for her life are shaped by the circumstances into which the person is born. The individual's success in education will depend not only on what educational opportunities are available, but on how the person comes to that education—for example, how well fed or hungry, well rested or tired, or confident and content he is—and the economic resources available that shape which school the person attends. It will also be affected by how education is valued within the person's family or community. Thus, a person's/family's multiple contexts cannot be "left" or understood as being outside or separate from one's self or necessarily under one's control. Rather, people/families embody their circumstances, and their circumstances embody them. Although they have some influence over their circumstances, such influence generally is more limited than we would like to imagine. Moreover, the contextual elements, and the experiences to which those elements give rise, live on in people. That is, past contexts go forward within people, shaping how they experience present and future situations.

People are both influenced *by* their context and live *within* contexts. Throughout nursing careers, nurses provide care in specific contexts, and families will live in their own diverse contexts. Consciously considering the interface of these differing contexts and how they are shaping families' health and illness experiences is vital to providing responsive, health-promoting care. Also foundational to this process is the need to inquire into how "context" is shaping your own life and practice as a nurse. This enables you to choose more intentionally how to draw on those influences to enhance your responsiveness to families. For example, many nurses practice in health care settings, surrounded by well-educated and financially stable professionals. This context contrasts with many clients, who may lack education and live in low-income and unstable housing due to financial instability. When a nurse recognizes this difference, care includes sensitivity to the disparity between these two contexts.

CANADA IN CONTEXT

Canada is diverse in multiple ways. This section considers five key areas of diversity that are significant to families and family nursing: geographical, economic, ethnocultural, linguistic, and religious diversity. These contextual elements overlap and intersect, shaping health, experiences of family, and experiences of health care and nursing.

Geographical Diversity

Canada's varied geography, encompassing differing terrains and climates, and ranging from dense urban settings to sparsely populated remote rural areas, shapes Canadian life. Across the prairies, the various coastal regions, the remote areas of the north, and the different mountain ranges are varied resources and climatic conditions that shape the lives of Canadians in differing ways. The population of Canada is concentrated primarily in urban centers in the south. In 2011, Statistics Canada reported that less than 20% of Canadians (about 6.5 million people) were living in rural areas (areas located outside urban centers and that have a population of 10,000 or more people). A continuing trend exists toward urbanization as more people move from less to more urban settings. In 2011, more than 27 million Canadians (81%) lived in urban areas, a reversal from over a century ago. The three largest urban areas in Canada—Toronto, Vancouver, and Montréal—made up just over one-third (35%) of Canada's entire population in 2011 (Human Resources and Social Development Canada, 2012).

Geographical differences influence other aspects of life. For example, incomes in rural settings are lower than in urban settings (Canadian Population Health Initiative, 2006), and health indicators are generally poorer in rural settings. In 2001, a lower proportion of Canadians living in small towns, rural regions, and northern regions rated their health as "excellent" compared with the national average and had a greater prevalence of being overweight and smoking (Mitura & Bollman, 2003; Williams & Kulig, 2012). People living in northern regions had greater unmet health care needs compared with the national average, whereas people in major urban regions had lower unmet health care needs. Life expectancy is lower and mortality rates are greater, particularly from diabetes, injuries, suicide, and respiratory disease, in rural settings compared with urban settings (Canadian Population Health Initiative, 2006; Williams & Kulig, 2012).

Geographical diversity shapes health through multiple pathways, including different access to food, housing, and other health resources; the kinds of employment available; environmental conditions and hazards; and social patterns. The health disparities across geographical areas continue to be a challenge to the quality of nursing care. Rural areas of Canada, in particular, lack sufficient numbers of nurses to meet the complex needs of rural and poor clients (Williams & Kulig, 2012). Family nursing is challenged by the distance between clients, the difficulty clients have in reaching health care centers, and the lack of resources needed to provide quality care. Nurses are often faced with having to provide care in a shortened amount of time with fewer resources. Yet, if nurses recognize these challenges, they can work on a micro level to incorporate relational inquiry into even the briefest contact, asking family members how they support healthy living patterns, and at a macro level by being advocates for improved rural health.

Economic Diversity

Although Canada is a wealthy, developed nation, a large and steadily widening income gap exists between rich and poor (Conference Board of Canada, 2012; Statistics Canada, 2006), with many Canadians living in poverty. Statistics Canada estimated that in 2009, nearly 3.2 million Canadians, or 9.6% of the population, lived in low-income families (Statistics Canada, 2011b). About 634,000 children age 17 or under, or 9.5%, lived in low-income families in 2009. About 196,000 of these children, or 31%, lived in a lone-parent family headed by a woman. Roughly 22% of children living with a single mother were in low-income households in 2009. Among 29 of the "richest countries" in the world, Canada's child poverty rate is about midway between those with the lowest child poverty rates (less than 5% in the Netherlands) and those with the highest, with over 15% in Greece, the United States, Lithuania, Latvia, and Romania (UNICEF Office of Research, 2013).

The economic prosperity of Canada is disproportionately distributed, and the inequities between those who are wealthy and those who are poor, and between those who are healthy and those who are not, continue to grow (Coburn, 2010). For example, a study analyzing the Canadian Community Health Survey found that, compared with white people, minorities were more likely to earn less than $30,000 Canadian per year (Quan et al., 2006). A study of Aboriginal people in urban settings found that approximately 30% of Aboriginal households are headed by a lone parent compared with 13.4% for non-Aboriginal households in the same communities (Canada Mortgage and Housing Corporation, 2006). More than 50% of urban Aboriginal children in the Prairie and Territories Regions live in single-parent households versus 17% to 19% for non-Aboriginal children. Of those Aboriginal single-headed households, 43% lived in poverty compared with 28% of non-Aboriginal single-headed households (Collin & Jensen, 2009). This information is critical because income is a key determinant of health, affecting multiple dimensions of well-being. People who are racialized, are new immigrants, live in rural settings, and have disabilities are more likely to be poor, and are therefore more affected by the health consequences of poverty. For example, the *2011 Child Poverty Report Card* (First Call, 2011) reports that despite an overall national "child poverty" rate of about 9.5%, particular groups are at greater risk for poor health outcomes, including children of recent immigrants (42%), Aboriginal children (36%), children of lone female parents (33%), and children with disabilities (27%). The reported measured poor outcomes, including health, education, and long-term employment achievement. A review of these outcomes from the Canadian Child Welfare Research Portal

(Boer, Rothwell, & Lee, 2013) indicated that those individuals in poverty, especially during the first 3 years of life, had lower developmental skills, had poorer reading skills during school age, and were more likely to be unemployed or underemployed as adults.

Ethnocultural Diversity

Canada is one of the most ethnically diverse countries in the world, and the ethnic diversity of the Canadian population is increasing (Statistics Canada, 2009). More than 200 different ethnic origins were reported in the 2006 Canadian Census (Human Resource and Development Canada, 2012). In 2006, nearly 2 million people, or 6.3% of the total population, were immigrants who had arrived during the previous 10 years. In 2006, there were 1,172,785 Aboriginal people in Canada, comprising 3.8% of the Canadian population. Of the three Aboriginal groups, First Nations people (698,025) had the largest population, followed by Métis (389,780), and Inuit people (50,480).

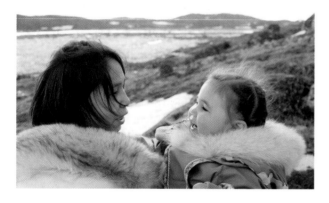

Approximately 250,000 people immigrate to Canada annually. Of the more than 13.4 million immigrants who came to Canada during the 20th century, the largest number arrived during the 1990s. The 2006 census showed that one in five (19.8% of the total population) Canadians were foreign born, the highest proportion since the 1930s (Statistics Canada, 2009). The origins of immigrants to Canada have changed in recent decades, with increasing numbers coming from non-European countries. Between 2001 and 2006, the majority of immigrants arrived from Asia (58.3%), whereas only 16.1% of immigrants came from European countries (Human Resource and Development Canada, 2012).

Although Canada has official state policy that advocates equality and promotes tolerance through multiculturalism, many argue that the rhetoric of multiculturalism masks inequities and discrimination based on ethnicity and racism (Thobani, 2007). The Ethnicity Diversity Survey (Statistics Canada, 2003a) found that 2.2 million people, or 10%, reported that they felt uncomfortable or out of place sometimes, most of the time, or all of the time because of their ethnocultural characteristics. Those people who were identified as "visible minorities" were most likely to feel out of place. Recently a large study found that many newcomer children and youth feel mistreated and isolated by both peers and teachers (Oxman-Martinez et al., 2012). Henry et al. (2009) argue that in Canada a form of racism is practiced wherein policies and rhetoric simultaneously promote equity and justice and tolerate widespread discrimination.

Racism has significant health effects (Harris et al., 2006). Discrimination based on race has been linked with health outcomes such as hypertension and other chronic diseases (Krieger, Chen, Coull, & Selby, 2005), mental health problems such as depression and suicide (Borrell, Kiefe, Williams, Diez-Roux, & Gordon-Larsen, 2006; McGill, 2008), and low birth weight (Mustillo et al., 2004). For example, Veenstra's (2009) analysis of the Canadian Community Health Survey found significant relative risks for poor health for people identifying as Aboriginal, Aboriginal/White, Black, Chinese, or South Asian that were not explained by socioeconomic status, gender, age, immigrant status, or location, suggesting that experiences with institutional and everyday racism and discrimination play an important role.

Changing immigration patterns and increasing ethnic diversity coupled with discriminatory policies and attitudes influence families' experiences and health. Migration processes are stressful, and this stress is intensified when combined with language barriers and downward economic mobility (Papademetriou, Somerville, & Sumption, 2009). These factors, combined with a gap between health care providers' lack of understanding of cultural differences and clients' lack of understanding of cultural health practices in Canada, add to the risks for poor health care. Nurses are key in minimizing these risks by continually striving to assess and understand cultural differences and assisting families in understanding Canadian health care practices. Nurses can also be advocates for families by assisting family members in protecting important cultural practices in an unfamiliar health care setting.

Linguistic Diversity

Consistent with its history as a colonial nation and destination for immigrants from around the globe, Canada is linguistically diverse. The 2011 Census recorded more than 60 Aboriginal languages, grouped into 12 distinct language families, and more than 213,000 people reported an Aboriginal mother tongue. Most Canadians speak one or both of the official languages: French and English. Yet, in 2011, about one of every five people reported having a mother tongue other than English or French (Statistics Canada, 2012). Of these, one-third reported that the only language they spoke at home was a language other than English or French, that is, a nonofficial language. Over the past few decades, language groups from Asia and the Middle East increased in number, and Chinese is now the third largest language group after English and French.

Language affects health in many ways. First, because language is connected to identity, language loss is related to the loss of cultural identity experienced in an ongoing manner by Aboriginal peoples and immigrants to Canada. When individuals and families lose their cultural identity, they are at risk of increased isolation and depression. This outcome threatens not only their desire and ability to seek health care, but also increases their risk for secondary poor mental health outcomes. Second, language barriers profoundly affect access to resources, including employment, social, and health resources. Finally, language barriers can be direct barriers when receiving health care and communicating with health care providers.

Some people who speak the dominant languages of Canada presume that everyone should learn French or English, without considering the resources it requires to do so and the barriers (such as poverty, transportation, discrimination, ability) to doing so. Very limited supports are available for language acquisition, and in the case of immigrant families, the priority for who accesses language classes is often the person who is most likely to be able to obtain employment. This pattern leads to higher health risks for those unemployed and without the ability to speak the dominant languages, including single parents, disabled adults, and children. Nurses can be advocates for these family members by assisting families with the use of interpreters, connecting families to community resources that teach languages, and using visual pictures and icons to explain health care procedures rather than just verbal instructions.

Religious Diversity

Canada is also a country of considerable religious diversity. Although Canada is predominantly Christian, with 7 of every 10 Canadians identifying themselves as either Roman Catholic or Protestant in 2003 (Statistics Canada, 2003b), this pattern is changing. Over the past decades, fewer people have identified as Protestant and more have identified with religions such as Islam, Hinduism, Sikhism, and Buddhism, and more have reported no religion, with 35% in 2010 saying they do not affiliate with any religion (Statistics Canada, 2011d). These shifts are the result of changing sources of immigrants, and the decline in major Protestant denominations since the 1930s, as their members age and fewer young people identify with these denominations. Despite this changing profile, Christianity continues to dominate many Canadian public institutions, including health care.

Religious affiliation affects health and nursing practice in multiple ways, including fostering social inclusion and community support, and, depending on the religion, serving as a basis for discrimination and negative effects on health practices, access to care, and acceptance of care. Despite Canada's professed tolerance for diversity, acts of anti-Semitism and discrimination against other non-Christian religious groups are not uncommon, including escalating discrimination against Muslims and presumed Muslims since 2001 (Mojab & El-Kassem, 2008). This discrimination is brought on in part by the dramatic increase in immigration to Canada from a variety of individuals from diverse religious backgrounds. Canada now leads the world in accepting immigrants, with 20.6% of Canadians now foreign born, with the next country accepting immigrants being Germany, at 13% of the population being foreign born. This acceptance of immigration brings religious diversity and a weakening of the majority culture, including religious affiliation. The largest share of immigrants to Canada (57%) came from Asia and the Middle East, and these immigrants are predominately Buddhist, Muslim, and Hindu in religious affiliation. At the same time, many Canadians are claiming no religious affiliation, with as many as 24% of Canadians claiming no connection to religious groups, up from 15% a decade earlier. Still, 64% of Canadians affiliate with Christian religious groups, with the largest group (39%) being Catholics (Welcome/Bienvenue, 2011).

This increase in religious diversity means that in order to offer culturally appropriate nursing care, family nurses need to be familiar with major values and beliefs of each religious group. For example, families within certain religious groups participate regularly in individual and group prayer as part of the healing process (e.g., Catholics), whereas families without a religious affiliation do not generally participate in religious prayer. Family nurses can provide appropriate care by asking about religious affiliations and how the families' religious beliefs affect their values and beliefs about healing. Nurses should also seek families' expectations of how health care professionals can incorporate religious beliefs into their treatment plan when appropriate and possible. Nurses must also be knowledgeable about not insulting religious beliefs unknowingly. For example, males in the Muslim religion generally do not tolerate being naked in front of females. It may be necessary to ask a male nurse to provide care to a male patient. Likewise, females of the Muslim religion are not allowed to be cared for by male nurses. This religious value should be respected whenever possible. If it is not possible, then for females, the husband should be present. Having a Muslim provider is ideal and should be sought when possible to provide optimal and ethical care. This holds true for all major religious groups (Chicago Healthcare Council, 1999).

HOW FAMILY IS UNDERSTOOD IN CANADA

Given this incredible geographical, economic, ethnocultural, and religious diversity, what constitutes "family" in Canada, and how family is lived and experienced, varies greatly. Despite this diversity, age-old assumptions about family continue to dominate. These ideas shape our expectations about families, such that families are "normally" nuclear and comprise a mother, father, and two children. They shape policies, such as the idea that people receiving social assistance should turn to extended family and "exhaust" family resources before accepting social assistance. And they also shape health care providers' expectations and practices, such as in the belief that families should provide care to elderly members. Exploring and critically scrutinizing these dominant ideas in light of the diverse contextual elements that shape any particular family assists nurses to understand their own and families' expectations, the differences between those expectations, and tensions that might arise among different stakeholders.

Three general assumptions/expectations about family are especially useful for nurses to explore in order to understand families in Canada and similar industrialized Western countries. First, families are generally assumed to be "nuclear," that is, to consist of two generations, including parents (generally assumed to be heterosexual) and children. Second, women generally are expected to do the majority of parenting and caregiving. Third, family is generally held to be a safe and nurturing experience. In reality, however, people's experiences vary greatly and differ from these assumptions.

Heterosexual Nuclear Family as the Norm

The idea that the heterosexual nuclear family is the norm is belied by statistics; for example, in 2006, 16.5% of families with children in Canada's metropolitan areas and 13.3% of families in rural areas and small towns were lone-parent families. The rate of lone-parent families increased by 8% by 2011, with 1,527,000 children being raised by lone parents (Statistics Canada, 2011a). Statistics Canada notes that throughout the 20th century and into the 21st century, the proportion of large households has decreased with each successive census, and there has been a steadily increasing trend toward smaller households. The 2006 census found that there were more than three times as many one-person households as households with five or more persons. Of the 12,437,500 private households, 26.8% were one-person households, whereas 8.7% were households of five or more persons. In 2006, women living in a same-sex union represented 0.6% of all women in couples in Canada (or 41,200), and the 49,500 men living in a same-sex union accounted for 0.7% of all men in couples. In 2006, 16% of women in same-sex couples had children age 24 and under present in the home, representing a smaller share than for women in opposite-sex unions (49%) but a much higher percentage than for men in same-sex couples (2.9%) (Statistics Canada, 2011a).

Although some people construe living in households with larger numbers of people as a "cultural" preference, doing so often increases financial strain. For example, the Longitudinal Survey of Immigrants to Canada (LSIC) (Statistics Canada, 2005) notes that, although the average size of a Canadian household was 2.6 persons, the average household size for LSIC immigrants was 3.4 persons, ranging from 3.1 for skilled worker immigrants to 4.0 persons for refugees. Most LSIC immigrants reported living in two- (21%), three- (24%), or four-person (22%) households, and were more likely to report living in a household of six or more people (12%) as compared with the Canadian average (3%). Aboriginal households were somewhat more crowded than the general population, with an average of 2.9 occupants and 2.6 bedrooms, compared with 2.5 and 2.8, respectively, for non-Aboriginal households.

It is important for nurses to understand the economic and social influences that shape housing for families. For example, the number of lone mothers heading families is, in part, a reflection of the prevalence of violence against women and the social expectation for women to "leave" abusive partners. The largest population-based survey focused on violence in Canada revealed that 50.7% of women reported physical assault from a former partner, and that violence is a significant factor in many separations and divorces (Varcoe et al., 2011). If society could decrease violence in the homes, the number of lone-parent families, particularly those run by women and at higher risk for poverty, would in turn decrease.

Canada continued to study other family structures in the 2011 census, including same-sex parents, common-law parents, stepfamilies, children living with grandparents, children living in foster homes, and young adults (ages 20 to 29 years) still living in a parental home. Although traditional nuclear families with opposite-sex parents remain the majority, at two-thirds of all family structures, other structures are growing. Common-law parents account for 16.3% of families, and 10% of children under 14 years of age live in stepfamilies. A growing number of children are living with their grandparent(s), with 4.8% of children under 14 years of age living with one or more grandparents, and 0.5% of those children do not have a biological parent in the home. Foster children make up another 0.5% of the children living in families, and 0.8% of children are living with same-sex parents. Finally, the age for independence is increasing, similar to other Westernized countries. Forty-two percent of young adults 20 to 29 years of age are still living or have returned to living in a parental home. This trend is more true for males than females.

These trends have important implications for nursing care. For example, family nurses can no longer expect children to have two opposite-sex parents in their home. Family nurses need to assess the current family structure and avoid assumptions or biases regarding expected norms. Each family structure has benefits and risks, and family nurses need to both assess these within individual families, and educate families about changing structures and how those changes influence child development. Nurses also need to be familiar with, and connect families to, appropriate support services to help families do the best they can for their children regardless of the family structure. For example, although grandparents raising grandchildren poses risks to the grandparents' economic stability and connection with peers, the grandchildren have an opportunity to learn more about their family's history and family tradition than those children not raised by grandparents, and grandparents receive more support from their grandchildren compared with those grandchildren not raised by their grandparents (Rosenthal & Gladstone, 2000). Although grandparents often struggle with the isolation and economic hardship, most provinces in Canada provide financial support, health care, and legal support for grandparents raising their grandchildren.

Ideals of Motherhood and Women

In Canada, prevalent ideas about mothering and women shape families' experiences, their health, and health care provider expectations. These ideas include mothers living with their husbands and being the primary caretaker for their children. Despite the diversity of family structures and roles, the "gold standard" continues to be mothering within a two-parent family (Ford-Gilboe, 2000), with the ideal being exclusive mothering, or mothering without work outside the home. Another social expectation for women is primary responsibility for family caregiving for dependent elders or those who are ill or have disabilities, especially in the wake of changes to the health care and social services systems that include deinstitutionalization of care.

These expectations are at odds with other social forces, however, including financial forces and changes to views about women's interests and capabilities. Women, including mothers, increasingly are expected and desire to work outside the home (Statistics Canada, 2012). In 2009, 72.9% of women with children under 16 living at home were part of the employed workforce; 64.4% of women with children less than age 3 were employed, more than double the figure in 1976, when only 27.6% of these women were employed. Similarly, 69.7% of women whose youngest child was from 3 to 5 years of age were working in 2009, up from 36.8% in 1976. Social policy, such as "workfare" social assistance policies, increasingly only provides financial assistance to women with dependent children if they seek employment, making many of these women feel that they are forced into waged labor, even when the work available is not adequate to cover the costs of safe child care. At the same time, policies such as cuts to minimum wage levels have deepened women's poverty even as they attempt to participate in the waged labor force (Pulkingham, Fuller, & Kershaw, 2010). Women are also seeking higher education and more professional careers. A study by Caponi and Plesca (2009), looking at trends in education, wages, and work hours, found that 50% of women were graduating from college and universities compared with only 44% of men. This trend has also contributed to women shifting away from the more traditional role of full-time caregiving to the more common role of shared responsibilities between work and career and home.

As described earlier, the "ideal" of the nuclear family is often just that, an ideal. Women are increasingly lone parents, often living below the poverty line and often on social assistance (Statistics Canada, 201a). At the same time, changing expectations of men as fathers mean that fathers are somewhat more actively engaged in child care and somewhat more likely to be the head of lone-parent families than in previous decades. In 2006, there were about four times as many female lone-parent families (1.1 million) as male lone-parent families (281,800) (Statistics Canada, 2011a). This ratio has been fairly consistent over the past several decades, but from 2001 to 2006, male lone-parent families grew more rapidly (15%) than did female lone-parent families (6.3%). At least partly because of gender economics, many children are not being raised by their mothers. For example, the 2006 Canadian census reported that over 28,000 grandchildren younger than 18 years were living with their grandparents without parents in the home, with implications for the health of older men and women. Based on federal and provincial and territorial reports from 2000, Farris-Manning and Zandstra (2004) estimated that approximately 76,000 children in Canada were under the protection of Child and Family Services across the country. These trends, juxtaposed against ideals of good mothering, have contributed to phrases such as "working mother" and "welfare mom" that convey negative judgments.

In fact, when families are judged against the ideal of "exclusive" mothering, or against the ideals of family caregiving, they are often found wanting. That is, when women do not devote themselves to mothering exclusively or take up caregiving for a parent, spouse, or other dependent person and forego labor force participation, they are often judged as providing inadequate mothering. Still, the economic and social conditions do not exist for most women to care for children and other dependents without also participating in waged work. In Canada, as in most Western countries, the "typical" mother is working outside the home and is often the lone head of a household and may also be living under or near the poverty line, while at the same time being responsible for mothering and/or caregiving of other family members.

Family as Safe and Nurturing

In Canada, as in many Western countries, family is portrayed generally as positive, supportive, and safe. But statistics belie this ideal as well. Canada is similar to other Western countries in the levels of violence perpetrated within families and levels of substance use. According to the most conservative estimates, 7% of female individuals and 6% of male individuals in current or previous spousal relationships reported having experienced some form of spousal violence during the previous 5 years (Statistics Canada, 2006). Violence against women tends to be much more severe than against men. Between 1995 and 2004, male individuals perpetrated 86% of one-time incidents, 94% of repeat (two to four) incidents, and 97% of chronic incidents (Statistics Canada, 2006). In that same time frame, the rate of spousal homicide against female individuals was three to five times greater than the rate of male spousal homicide, a ratio that remains consistent up to 2009 (Zhang, Hoddenbagh, McDonald, & Scrim, 2012). In 2009, 46,918 spousal violence incidents were brought to the attention of police, 81% involving female victims and 19% involving male victims (Zhang et al., 2012). Using population surveys, lifetime rates of physical assault by an intimate partner have been estimated at 25% to 30% in Canada and the United States (Johnson & Sacco, 1995; Jones et al., 1999). Physical assault is often accompanied by sexual violence or emotional abuse, and many women experience intimate partner violence in more than one relationship over their lifetime (Johnson, 1996).

Estimates of child abuse rely primarily on cases reported to child welfare authorities and are thus gross underestimates. Based on data from child welfare authorities, the Canadian Incidence Study (CIS) of Reported Child Abuse and Neglect estimated a rate of 21.52 investigations of child maltreatment per 1,000 children (Public Health Agency of Canada, 2001). Importantly, the greatest proportion of reported and substantiated child abuse cases involved neglect, which often overlaps with the social conditions created by poverty. Socioeconomic status has been shown consistently to be related to parenting effectiveness (Wekerle, Wall, Leung, & Trocmé, 2007). Despite the prevalence of neglect, less attention is paid to neglect in research, policy, and practice than to severe physical abuse and child sexual abuse, possibly in part because those forms of abuse are more sensational (McLean, 2001) and more visible. Child welfare authorities tend to focus on risk assessment and urgent intervention for severe cases of child physical abuse, rather than on the more frequent situations of neglect. Trocmé, MacMillan, Fallon, and De Marco (2003) argue that because the CIS found severe physical harm (severe enough to warrant

medical attention) in about 4% of substantiated cases, assessment and investigation priorities need to be revised and include consideration of long-term needs for housing, income, child care, and so on. Health care providers should focus on helping families to access longer-term and broader social support.

Although it is difficult to estimate the extent of elder abuse in Canada, it is purported to be a significant problem (Walsh & Yon, 2012). Almost 2% of older Canadians indicate that they had experienced more than one type of abuse (Canadian Centre for Justice Statistics, 2011). Elder abuse and neglect encompasses intimate partner violence that continues into older adulthood, and forms of abuse and neglect that arise as persons become more vulnerable with age. As with any form of intimate partner violence, in older adults it is gendered—that is, older women are at greater risk than men. Statistics Canada (2011c) reported that in 2009 although the overall rate of violent victimization was higher for senior men than senior women, family-related violent victimization was higher among senior women. Spouses and grown children were the most common perpetrators of family violence against senior women, and grown children were most often the perpetrators of family violence against senior men.

Substance abuse within families is another factor that may make the experience of family less than safe and nurturing. Most problematic use in Canada involves alcohol. The Canadian Addiction Survey found that, although most Canadians drink in moderation, 6.2% of past-year drinkers engaged in heavy drinking (five drinks or more in a single sitting for male individuals and four or more drinks for female individuals) at least once a week and 25.5% at least once a month (Collin, 2006). Using the Alcohol Use Disorder Identification Test, which identifies hazardous patterns of alcohol use and indications of alcohol dependency, Collin (2006) identified 17% of current drinkers as high-risk drinkers. Although most heavy and hazardous drinkers were male individuals younger than 25, this pattern suggests that harmful alcohol use is fairly common. According to the 2002 Canadian Community Health Survey, 2.6% of Canadians age 15 and older (3.8% male and 1.3% female) reported symptoms consistent with alcohol dependence at some time during the 12 months before the survey. Rehm et al. (2006)

estimate that 9% of disease and disability in Canada is caused by alcohol use. A range of problems are associated with problematic alcohol use, including violence and neglect. In 2004, 14% of Canadians reported using cannabis in the past year and 1% or less reported using other illegal drugs other than cannabis. For those who do use drugs, the effects on families can be profound. For example, one of the most common reasons stated for grandparents raising grandchildren is paternal drug abuse and addiction (Rosenthal & Gladstone, 2000). For those children raised in a family with active addiction, the risk for all types of abuse increases. Further, several studies in both Canada and the United States document long-term negative outcomes for children being raised by parents addicted to alcohol and other drugs, including mental health risks, higher rates of unemployment, and poor relationship success. For example, a study of 8,472 families in Canada by Walsh, MacMillan, and Jamieson (2003) found that children exposed to drug-addicted parents were twice as likely to be abused than those without drug addiction in their family.

Given the statistics on violence, neglect, and substance use, although many families are safe and nurturing, nurses cannot safely make this assumption. Indeed, in light of the levels of violence against women, children, and older persons, and the levels of substance use, nurses can anticipate that many families they meet are experiencing some form of violence, neglectful parenting, or problematic substance use. In Canada, it is mandatory to report child abuse, but it is not recommended to screen for child abuse. Because of the high rate of false-positive results in screening tests for child maltreatment and the potential for incorrectly labeling people as child abusers, the possible harms outweigh the benefits (MacMillan, 2000). Similarly, insufficient evidence of benefit has been reported to warrant screening for other forms of violence (Coker, 2006; MacMillan et al., 2009; Ramsey, Richardson, Carter, Davidson, & Feder, 2002) and there are no reporting requirements for other forms of abuse outside of child abuse. Nevertheless, nurses need to be aware that family is not always a safe and nurturing experience for people, and to be responsive to indications of harm. Alternatives to screening include "case finding" in which nurses have a clear understanding of the dynamics of

violence and abuse, and develop their practice based on that understanding, using such knowledge to attend to each family's presentation (Ford-Gilboe, Varcoe, Wuest, & Merritt-Gray, 2010). Case finding does not stop at identifying families at risk and in need of further evaluation and intervention, but rather begins the assessment phase to identify and explore the incidence of family violence.

CANADIAN HEALTH CARE CONTEXT

The funding and structure of the Canadian health care system influences families, health, and family nursing. Although Canada has "universal" health care and all Canadian citizens have access to what are termed *medically necessary* services, considerable inequities are present in access to health care, and these inequities are deepening as the health care system is increasingly privatized. The privatized portion of health care primarily includes funding for services and products not covered by the public services and not considered medically necessary, such as vision and dental care, cosmetic surgery, most home health services, and pharmaceuticals. The amount covered and uncovered by the public health care system varies from province to province. Currently, the health care system in Canada is approximately 70% publicly funded and 30% privately funded. This means that many important elements of health care are paid for by individuals or by private insurance. Therefore, in most provinces, medications outside of hospital, many types of treatments such as physiotherapy, and services such as home care are paid for privately in whole or in part. In contrast, the government discourages physicians from providing private care through disincentives such as requiring physicians to choose either private or public clients, charging patients the same fee whether paid by public or private insurance, and in some provinces, banning privatized medical care for any essential medical services.

Thus, despite commitment to universal access, access to health care in Canada is inequitable along many dimensions (Asada & Kephart, 2007; Barr, Pedersen, Pennock, & Rootman, 2008). Families in rural settings have access to fewer services and must pay for their own transportation, accommodation, and loss of income to access services.

Families without private insurance and those with lower incomes face more financial hardship associated with illness. Because some groups of people are more likely to have lower incomes, such as those who are elderly, those with disabilities, and women, families from such groups are more likely to face greater barriers.

Although the Canadian health care system has been dominated by hospital care, over the past several decades fiscal concerns have stimulated shifts to decrease hospital care and increase the care provided at home. From mental illness, to surgery, to maternity care, to elder care, to end-of-life care, the trend has been to deinstitutionalize care, shorten length of stay, and shift to care "in the community." Such care mostly means care by family members, primarily women (Statistics Canada, 2011a), which affects family well-being and health, and, in turn, affects patterns of family nursing (Funk et al., 2010; Williams, Forbes, Mitchell, & Corbett, 2003). Family nurses need to provide added support to all family members in teaching home health care to avoid women in the family suffering from role overload and caregiver burnout. Family nurses can also help advocate for families needing hospitalized care longer when family members are unable to care for the individual at home.

Family nursing is not funded or identified as a separate area of practice in Canada, with most nurses still practicing in hospital settings. Because government health care funding only covers what is deemed to be medically necessary, only a very small proportion of nursing care in homes and communities is funded, leaving families to pay directly. Increasingly, in some areas, the shortage of primary care physicians has made room for family nurse practitioners to provide primary care and enhance health care access. These trends shape families' experiences of health and affect their health care.

FAMILY NURSING PRACTICE: ATTENDING TO CONTEXT

To this point, this chapter has spoken to the significance of context and offered details on the specific context in which nurses operate in Canada. As the discussion earlier has highlighted, families in Canada live diverse lives that are shaped by the interface of geography, economics, culture, language, and religion. Similarly, their lives and their health and illness experiences are shaped by differing understandings and forms of "family" and by the imperfect health care system in place in Canada. This health care system, including policies and norms that dominate health care practices, has been built on limited understandings of family and health. For example, understandings of family most often reflect Eurocentric, post–World War II notions of the nuclear two-parent, heterosexual family. It is the discrepancy between the reality of families' lives and the normative expectations and understandings of family that often dominate health care settings and practices that make attending to context not only important but ethically essential in family nursing practice.

Overall, attending to context requires taking a relational inquiry stance as a family nurse. It involves listening carefully to families; inquiring into their health/illness situations; paying attention to, observing, and critically considering the ways in which contextual elements are embodied in people/families and shape their experiences; and reflecting on how current contextual aspects might be addressed to promote health. An essential feature of this inquiry process is reflexive consideration of your own contextual location, including the values, norms, and assumptions of family, health, and nursing that you act both from and within.

The following story illustrates the significance of context to families' health experiences and how attending to context enhances family nursing practice. As you read Sharon's story, stay mindful of the contextual elements that seem to be shaping the experiences of the two families she meets. Focus on how the elements discussed earlier (e.g., geography, economics, culture, language, religion, understandings of family, health care policies, and normative practices) are shaping the experience and responses of the different family members and of Sharon as a nurse. Also note how Sharon is or is not attending to those elements as she engages with the families. Ask yourself how your own context is similar to or different from Sharon's, and from the two families'. Furthermore, reflect on how those similarities and differences might affect how you would respond as a nurse.

Family Case Study: Sharon's Story

After several years of experience on a pediatric medical unit, Sharon has begun to work in a pediatric diabetic teaching clinic. She just completed her 1-week orientation, and this morning is about to do an "intake" on two families new to the clinic. It is clinic policy to have a half-hour appointment for "intake" and 15 minutes for subsequent appointments. Families usually attend the clinic for about three or four sessions, biweekly, depending on their needs. The referral information Sharon has on the two families is as follows:

- *Family 1:* Justin Henderson, 11 years old, is from Stony Life Reserve (designated land for Native Americans). Justin has been newly diagnosed with diabetes. He began an insulin regimen on Tuesday (3 days ago) that was ordered by the general practitioner in a walk-in clinic close to where he lives; Justin was referred to the clinic for diabetic teaching and counseling. This is his first visit to the clinic.
- *Family 2:* Greg Stanek, 12 years old, is from Belcarra. Greg has been newly diagnosed with diabetes. His insulin regimen was started yesterday by the family's general practitioner, who referred Greg to the clinic for diabetic teaching and counseling. This is his first visit.

Justin's appointment was scheduled for 9:00, but he does not arrive on time. At 9:15, Sharon decides to see her other new client, Greg Stanek, because he and his father arrived early. Greg seems small for his age; he is thin and looks quite pale. He is very quiet and barely looks at Sharon. Greg's father speaks with heavily accented English that Sharon recognizes as Czech, in part because she associates Belcarra with the large community of people who emigrated from the Czech Republic. Sharon does a brief physical assessment, noting that Greg is 4 feet 8 inches tall, but weighs only 41 kg (about 90 lb). Sharon attempts to take the family history as outlined on her intake form, but Greg's father wants to address the fact that he cannot bring his son to clinic. Greg's father tells Sharon that he was just laid off from his job as a carpet layer and is required by unemployment insurance policies to be searching for work. Mr. Stanek says bitterly that when he came to Canada he had been promised he could find work in his field as a mining engineer. Greg's mother works in a local meat processing plant, and she cannot take time off to bring Greg to the clinic without risking the loss of her job.

Sharon reinforces with the father how important it is for Greg to learn about his diabetes and how to manage it,

and how important supportive family is. Mr. Stanek becomes annoyed and insists that they cannot come to clinic again. As Greg's father becomes more frustrated, Sharon finds it more difficult to understand what he is saying because of his heavy accent and rapid talking. Sharon tries to engage Greg by asking him how he is feeling and how it is going at school, but Greg answers Sharon's questions by shrugging his shoulders and saying "OK." Greg's father attempts to return the conversation back to his own concerns. Eventually, Sharon says that she will "see what she can do." The half-hour clinic visit ends with little of the intake form completed, all parties feeling frustrated, and no follow-up appointment scheduled. As Sharon walks out of the room, the clinic receptionist lets her know that Justin and a woman, who turns out to be his grandmother, have been waiting to see her for their appointment.

Sharon reviews what she knows about Justin from reading his intake information. She remembers that the Stony Life Reserve is located several hours from the hospital in which her clinic is located, and that Jackson is a small town near the reserve. Sharon wonders how Justin and his grandmother got to the clinic today. As she walks in the room, Sharon apologizes for keeping them waiting and asks if they drove to the appointment. Justin's grandmother says one of her brothers drove them because the appointment was too early to be able to come by bus. She also shares that she had to borrow money to pay her brother for gas. Sharon does a brief physical assessment on Justin. Justin, like Greg, barely looks at Sharon, even when she is addressing him directly. Justin appears somewhat overweight, as does his grandmother, and on assessment Sharon notes that he is 4 feet 5 inches tall and weighs 55 kg (121 lb). With Justin and his grandmother, who introduces herself as Rose Tarlier, the intake assessment goes more smoothly for Sharon. Mrs. Tarlier tells her that she has had custody of Justin and his two younger sisters since he was 4 years old and the sisters were infants. She shares with Sharon that Justin's mother, her daughter, has had problems with alcohol for many years, is now living in Montreal, and has not seen her children for several years. Mrs. Tarlier makes it a point to tell Sharon that she herself has been "clean and sober" for more than 20 years. As Sharon continues with the intake assessment, she finds out that Justin's grandmother gives Justin his insulin and helps him check his blood sugar. Sharon listens as the grandmother describes what she has been doing, and Sharon provides positive feedback and encouragement. Although Sharon tries to bring Justin into the conversation, he does not look at her and does not answer her questions. Sharon reviews what subsequent appointments will cover, and

(continued)

thinking about the distance and gas money, asks if they need one longer appointment next week rather than the usual two short ones a week apart. She schedules the next appointment.

Taking a Relational Inquiry Stance:

Attending to context begins by taking a relational inquiry stance to understand what is meaningful and significant to a particular family, and inquiring into the family's current experience and the contextual intricacies shaping the family's life. In taking this stance with the two families in the earlier story, what becomes immediately apparent is the way that contextual forces have contributed to and are shaping each of the family's situations. For example, although Justin's family may want to live in the Aboriginal community for cultural and social reasons, it may have little choice for economic reasons. Justin's grandmother may well be one of many Aboriginal women living on low income or in poverty. At the time of the 2001 census, based on before-tax incomes, more than 36% of Aboriginal women, compared with 17% of non-Aboriginal women, were living in poverty (Townson, 2005). High rates of poverty among Aboriginal people have overwhelming effects on health, with the life expectancy of Aboriginal people being 7 years less than the overall Canadian population. Also, as Townson notes, there are almost twice as many infant deaths among Aboriginal peoples compared to the national norm. As noted, Aboriginal children are much more likely to live in poverty than other Canadian children.

The fact that Justin lives on a reserve may negatively influence his health care access and ability to adhere to recommendations. The matrix of policies related to Aboriginal people in Canada has ensured that many reserve communities have been denied access to traditional foods (fish, game, naturally growing plants) and have substandard housing, poor water supplies, and insufficient income opportunities. Justin's grandmother's attendance at residential school, both his mother's and grandmother's experiences with alcohol, and the current situation with Justin's grandmother being his primary caregiver present a clear example of the impact colonization has on family well-being. Historical colonizing policies and practices in Canada included the creation of the Indian Act; removal of entire communities onto reserves, often with insufficient resources to sustain the community; government appropriation of Aboriginal lands; forced removal of children into residential schools; outlawing of cultural and spiritual practices; and widespread discriminatory attitudes toward Aboriginal peoples. The effects of colonization continue to shape people's health, social, and economic status today (Kubik, Bourassa, &

Hampton, 2009). Colonizing practices continue as Aboriginal people are racialized by wider society and governed by race-based policies, including those related to land ownership, banking, and health care.

Although Justin and his grandmother's situation may not reflect all of these contextual challenges, this historical and current contextual backdrop shapes their situation and responses to health care providers, including their willingness and ability to attend clinic. Moreover, the challenges they face accessing the clinic (e.g., appointment times that are out of sync with bus schedules, having younger children to care for, the cost of travel) may make coming to clinic seem less than positive in terms of the effect on Justin's and the family's overall health.

Similarly, Greg's family experience has been shaped by multiple factors. Both parents are facing significant job insecurity. The family has experienced immigration laws and policies that limit employment opportunities and contribute to the "downward mobility" experienced by many well-educated immigrants. As described, children in recent immigrant families and racialized families are most likely to live in poverty because of overrepresentation of racialized groups in low-paying jobs, market failure to recognize international work experience and credentials, and racial discrimination in employment (*2011 Child Poverty Report Card,* First Call, 2011).

Canada is a country of considerable ethnic diversity, but despite national commitment to tolerance and multiculturalism, racialized groups experience considerable discrimination both in policies and institutions, and in the attitudes expressed toward them at an interpersonal level. Was this playing out during the clinic visit? Although it may not have been Sharon's intent to be discriminatory, the way in which she disregarded the contextual reality of Mr. Stanek's employment and its implications for future clinic visits and the frustration she felt toward him was a form of intolerance. Taking a stance of inquiry to attend to context would have enabled Sharon to be aware of the likelihood of discriminatory experiences and of the potential health effects.

Listening and Paying Attention to Experience and Context:

Attending to context involves listening carefully to families, and to what is meaningful and significant within the current context of their lives. For Justin and his grandmother, who live in a rural setting, and for Greg's family, where both parents need to work, it becomes apparent that geography, economics, and health are intricately intertwined. For example, although for Sharon what is most significant is getting Greg's family to attend clinic so Greg's diabetes can be monitored and addressed, for Greg's father, finding and maintaining employment is of greatest concern. Moreover, the experience of being told that he would be able to work in his profession and then finding that this was not the case may well be influencing his response and willingness to engage with yet another authority and institution that does not seem to be recognizing the importance of his employment or interested in what is most pressing for him. Although Sharon cannot address the employment concern directly within her current role (i.e., she cannot help find him a job), it is obvious that those concerns will ultimately affect Greg's experience and management of diabetes. Thus, listening to and recognizing the interrelationship of those concerns regarding how the family will be able and willing to care for Greg and his diabetes is crucial.

In fact, the well-intended clinic may be heightening health challenges for families by not considering these contextual elements. Even how clinic appointments have been structured as short, frequent sessions affects both families' ability to attend clinic and ignores the socio-environmental elements affecting families' health on a day-to-day basis. Thus, attending to family context involves also attending to the health care context. Depending on the setting of care, the nurse would have to work within that context to support more responsive care. For example, is it possible to have fewer, longer appointments? Is a longer intake visit possible—not just for Greg's family, but for others as well? Even within the prescribed time frame, the nurse should acknowledge what is of meaning and significance to the family.

Attending to context involves acknowledging Greg's father's distress about his employment and inviting him to talk about what it has been like for different family members as they have sought employment and attempted to build a life with limited resources, support, or both. As part of this process, it would be important to communicate respect and genuine interest and concern, asking what might be helpful from their perspective, how the clinic could assist them in caring for Greg's diabetes in light of the other challenges they are experiencing. On the surface, focusing on the father's concerns might not seem to be the top nursing priority (or even relevant to diabetic care), but doing so might reduce frustration for both Sharon and Greg's father, make better use of time, and allow them to attend to Greg's diabetes more effectively. If the family concerns are not addressed, Greg's care is jeopardized, because he may not come back to the clinic.

Listening and paying attention to experience and context with Justin's family brings attention to the geographical distance between the family's home and the clinic, and raises questions about other possibilities for supporting the family in diabetes care. For example, knowing the economic statistics for Aboriginal women, the cost of travel to the clinic might have an impact on the family. If the family is on a limited income, frequent travel may be impossible and may take money from other essential needs. In response, Sharon might look into resources at the local level, such as a community health representative or local community health nurse, who might be able to provide face-to-face care to the family while liaising with the clinic so that the family does not need to travel such a great distance so frequently.

Overall, attending to context sets one up to be curious, to be interested, and to inquire, rather than make judgments and assumptions based on surface characteristics and behaviors. For example, both Greg and Justin were quiet, did not make eye contact, and did not respond very much to Sharon. Rather than making assumptions about the children based on her own location and context, Sharon might intentionally reflect on the contexts in which they have been living recently. As a result, their responses might be viewed through a range of possibilities, including everything from wondering about the physiological effect of diabetes, to the immediate effect of the diagnosis of diabetes, to the experience of coming to the clinic for the first time, to the multiple contextual experiences and challenges they and their families have been living. Part of assessing the context includes the awareness of cultural differences, which affect eye contact, reaction to health professionals, reaction to genders, and behavior toward adults and elders. Attending to context can cue nurses to stay open to possibilities, gently and thoughtfully reaching out to connect with people and families as they are in the moment. Rather than focusing on behavior or lack of response as a problem or frustration, any response is viewed contextually. People and families are not measured against any norms; rather, the goal is to understand their reactions contextually and to respond in a meaningful and relevant manner using inquiry rather than judgment.

Attending to context also moves us beyond the immediate situation of particular patients to question how larger policies and structures governing our practice and agency are affecting families. That is, the contextual particularities of these families reveal limitations of the policies and structures of the clinic more generally. Clinic policies and structures might need to be changed to be more responsive to families. For example, offering home visits, evening appointments, or both for families who have both parents working and are unable to make daytime appointments might enhance the clinic's responsiveness. Similarly, seeing

(continued)

the family in context draws attention to the importance of working with the contexts within which the families live. This could include everything from intentionally establishing relationships with government departments and community agencies that are part of the family's context that might liaise with the clinic in providing services and resources, to lobbying for increased access and resources for particular groups or particular services and supplies.

In regard to these particular families, first, the nurse would want to optimize her ability to provide optimal care given the restrictions within the current system. She must prioritize her care to both acknowledge the families' circumstances and begin to support Greg and Justin within their families and those circumstances. Beyond a more flexible pattern of appointments, are there other providers who might be involved? A social worker, child and youth care worker, or other resources may be available. Ways to enhance access to health care, such as resources for transportation, may be available. The nurse would want to draw on broader social resources, such as those related to immigration and employment, resources for working parents (i.e., evening hours, weekend hours, online care, etc.), and resources for parents (i.e., counseling, support groups, other forms of diabetic care education such as local classes, online classes, books, home health services). Acknowledging Greg's father's concerns and supporting him through referrals will allow the nurse to integrate attention to the family while focusing on Greg and his diabetes. In so doing, Sharon will develop approaches and knowledge of resources for a range of other families as well.

Reflexivity:

Reflexivity, meaning intentional and critical reflection on one's own understanding and actions in context, is central to using contextual knowledge. Reflexivity draws attention to a nurse's own contextual background, including taken-for-granted assumptions, stereotypes, and knowledge one draws on when engaging with families. Examining how a nurse's own context and social location shape and structure her nursing is a first step to attending to families' contexts. For example, if Sharon had grown up in a rural setting or in poverty, it would be important for her to consider reflexively how those experiences influence her when working with families who share that context and social location. Her background might lead her to see herself as successful despite those constraints, and to overlook how the challenges she faced and privileges she enjoyed might differ from the experiences of the families with whom she is working. Or, if she had grown up in a middle-class urban setting,

she may find that she is somewhat oblivious to or does not think to consider the challenges that poverty and geography raise in accessing health care. Similarly, as a nurse working within a diverse milieu, it is important for Sharon to consider how her own family history might be shaping her attitudes toward immigrants, people whose first language is not English, racialized groups, Aboriginal people, and other groups. Perhaps she herself is an immigrant, perhaps she is a member of a racialized group, or perhaps she is a member of dominant groups—English speaking, Euro-Canadian, middle class. It is important that she ask herself how her religious affiliations (or lack thereof) shape how she thinks religion is relevant to health and to her nursing practice.

Although each aspect of Sharon's social location may shape her thinking, as Applebaum (2001) notes, one's social location "does not imply that we are inevitably locked within a particular perspective. White feminists can be anti-racist, men can be feminists, and heterosexuals can be 'straight but not narrow'" (p. 416). By reflexively scrutinizing our own social locations, we can examine our understandings and make explicit decisions about how to draw on (or not) various views and assumptions.

Examining our own contexts and social locations to see how we are limiting our views of families can be challenging. We can see more easily our own disadvantages than our privileges. For example, Sharon might have to work harder to see how her privilege as a securely employed, fluent English-speaking health care provider gives her an advantage that Greg's father does not have. If she has experienced employment disadvantages based on her gender, she might see him as a privileged man and have difficulty recognizing the challenges he faces.

Overall, reflexivity in family nursing involves developing a critical awareness of our own context and social location, scrutinizing how that context/location is shaping our view of a particular family, and intentionally looking *beyond* that location to consider the family within its own context. In Sharon's situation, this would involve her examining how the rural context, economics, language, ethnicity, and religion, and her understandings of these, shape how she is engaging with the families. She might ask how her own experiences of family are shaping her ability to see and accept the differing forms of family—for example, a family in which the parents are separated, such as Greg's, and a grandmother-led family such as Justin's. How does her own location enable or limit her ability to understand how difficult it might be for Greg's father and mother to get him to the clinic appointments given their current family situation?

Engaging in such reflexive examination also enables consideration of the wider sociopolitical elements shaping families' experiences, such as contextual factors (e.g., the stress of immigration), that may have contributed to Greg's parents separating from one another. At the same time, approaching her work in this reflexive manner highlights areas where she may need to learn more. For example, how well does Sharon understand the history of the Aboriginal people with whom she is working? How well does she understand the relationship between historical trauma and diabetes? How is diabetes cared for in Czechoslovakia versus the Aboriginal culture versus the broader Canadian culture? What are the roles of children in understanding and participating in their care across these multiple overlapping cultures?

Family Case Study: Attending to Context

Mrs. Dickson, a 40-year-old woman admitted with a diagnosis of bowel cancer, is a single mother of four children who is experiencing postoperative complications. Discharged home 3 days prior, Mrs. Dickson has been readmitted via ambulance with undiagnosed pain and extreme nausea. Her eldest daughter Sandra (age 21 years and married) and her third daughter Simone (age 17 years), who are present in the room, describe how their mother collapsed at home after screaming out in pain. Throughout Mrs. Dickson's illness, Simone, who is the eldest child at home (their middle sister lives in another city), has taken the role of primary caregiver for her mother, her 13-year-old brother, and her 86-year-old grandfather, who lives with them. As you enter the room, they are sitting beside their sedated mother. They look up with strained expressions and ask whether the doctors have figured out what is wrong with their mom.

What Intervention Strategies Might You Employ?

A relational inquiry approach to family nursing rests on the assumption that what constitutes high-quality nursing care can only be determined in the relational situation. Because the experiences of people/families vary so greatly, as do the realities within which health care occurs, there is no linearly laid out sequence or prescribed method. There are no prescriptions for assessment or action because it all depends on the situation. What constitutes contextually responsive care depends on the particularities of specific nursing situations. Because we work with particular people/families in particular situations, it is impossible to

present standardized action steps. The same action may in one case be responsive and health promoting and in another case not be. Thus, the question of how to intervene is one that needs to be asked in and tailored to each and every situation: How might I best relate to this family in a way that is meaningful and significant and promotes their health and healing capacity?

Consider how you might respond as a family nurse in the situation above. Where would you begin? What would you focus on? For example, it is evident from their facial expressions and the question they pose that the daughters are very worried about their mother. That might be an effective place to start because the question points to their immediate concern, to what is of meaning and significance to them. "Following their lead" (their worried expressions) is a form of both assessment and intervention in a relational inquiry approach. Acknowledging Sandra and Simone's worry could be a way of joining them in their experience and furthering your understanding of both the immediate family situation and the context of their lives.

As you follow their lead and inquire into their living experience and what is of meaning and significance to them, focus too on picking up contextual cues. For example, you might respond by sharing your observations in a tentative manner by stating, "You look pretty worried," or, "It's hard not knowing what is wrong with your mom," to invite them to confirm, expand, or modify your understanding. Making inclusive observations, asking open-ended questions, and being interested to "know more" invites people/families to lead the way. By working in this collaborative manner, you work with the family to make connections between experiences and context and discern the "so what" for action. This involves recognizing the patterns of capacity and of adversity that are simultaneously part of the person's/family's illness experience. It also enables you to understand how contextual elements are shaping the situation and what their immediate needs might be. For example, as you look contextually you might be concerned about the caregiving load that Simone is carrying (looking after her mother, brother, and grandfather). If you were working from a relational inquiry approach that nursing concern is not something you know, you inquire into its relevance in terms of capacity/adversity; keep in mind that what might be considered to be adversity to one person/family, may not be adversity to another. Asking "How has it been for you to be caring for your mom, brother, and grandfather while your mom is ill?" enables you to learn how contextual elements are meaningfully experienced by the person/family. By inquiring, you might find that nothing

(continued)

has changed—that since her mother works long hours Simone is used to assuming a lot of the domestic chores or that she has a lot of support from friends or relatives. Or, you may find that the added responsibility of caring for her mother while her mother is ill is more than she can handle, and she may open up and ask for more assistance in problem solving.

As you "listen to and for context" you might learn of other socio-contextual structures and processes (economics, health care policies, values, norms, traditions, history) that are shaping the family's experience. Knowing the population you serve (e.g., income levels, employment opportunities, social financial assistance) you are attuned to listen for a range of possibilities without assuming how this particular family "fits" with population norms. So, this family might be fine in terms of managing household and caregiving needs, but they might not have access to money or transportation to get to the hospital. Or, the worry for her mother may be affecting Simone's ability to do schoolwork or hold down her part-time job that contributes to the family's income. Thus, as you listen contextually you are listening and inquiring into resources—the resources they have, need, and/or can access. You also listen for what has enabled them to live in adversity—that is, what capacities they have within them and/or have accessed or enlisted. Similarly, you check your own view and your own capacities. Are your immediate nursing concerns obscuring your understanding of broader contextual issues and/or longer-term concerns? For example, given that you are located in an acute care setting, is Mrs. Dickson's physical well-being your primary concern? Are you able to extend your view to consider the longer-term health impact of this illness situation? How do you balance your need to care for Mrs. Dickson's acute health needs, while simultaneously consider her family contextual needs?

Evaluating Family Nursing Action:
Specifically, relational inquiry involves asking the person/family for *their* version of the story and purposefully opening the space for *their* decision making. Thus, evaluation of your nursing intervention involves an ongoing reflexive process where you "check in" with both families and yourself. Evaluation is centered in continually asking the following questions: How might I be as responsive as possible? How are my actions expanding (or constraining) the choice and capacity of this family? How might I support this family in ways that are meaningful to them and in ways that enable them to address their

concerns and realize their aspirations? Relational inquiry helps you to evaluate nursing effectiveness in the longer as well as the shorter term. For example, a quick discharge may result in a readmission for Mrs. Dickson if the context of the family situation is not taken into account. It also helps you to provide *family* nursing care, beyond the immediate individual patient and beyond the immediate acute health care needs.

SUMMARY

- One of the few predictable characteristics of families is diversity. By understanding and intentionally attending to diversity when providing care, family nurses in Canada are prepared to take into account the contextual nature of families' health and illness experiences, and how their lives are shaped by their circumstances.
- Contexts are literally embodied in people; both nurses and families live their contexts and circumstances.
- For family nurses in Canada to work responsively with a range of different families, it requires understanding the particular families.
- Understanding the families entails taking a stance of inquiry, listening and paying attention to the specific experiences of particular families, reflexively attending to one's own understandings, and continuously developing new knowledge and cultural awareness. This process embraces the complexity of family nursing care and provides more relational, and thereby more appropriate and successful, care for families.
- Family nurses in Canada must also be aware of the risks facing families, including changing family structures, risks for health disparities, risks for family violence, and risks for families living in poverty, especially in rural communities.
- Family nurses in Canada must optimize family care within a structure that limits out-of-hospital care and limits access to care in rural communities. Family nurses need to collaborate with other providers and resources to help families optimize their health and long-term health outcomes.

REFERENCES

Applebaum, B. (2001). Locating one's self, I-dentification and the trouble with moral agency. *Philosophy of Education Year Book*, 412–422.

Asada, Y., & Kephart, G. (2007). Equity in health services use and intensity of use in Canada. *BMC Health Services Research*, 7, 41.

Barr, S., Pedersen, G., Pennock, R., & Rootman, I. (2008). Health equity through intersectoral action: An analysis of 18 country case studies. Ottawa, Ontario, Canada: Public Health Agency of Canada and World Health Organization.

Boer, K., Rothwell, D., & Lee, C. (2013). Home. Canadian Child Welfare Research Portal. Retrieved June 21, 2013, from http://cwrp.ca

Borrell, L. N., Kiefe, C. I., Williams, D. R., Diez-Roux, A. V., & Gordon-Larsen, P. (2006). Self-reported health, perceived racial discrimination, and skin color in African Americans in the CARDIA study. *Social Science & Medicine*, 63(6), 1415–1427.

Canada Mortgage and Housing Corporation. (2006). Urban Aboriginal households: A profile of demographic, housing and economic conditions in Canada's prairie and territories region. Retrieved September 18, 2008, from http://dsp-psd. pwgsc.gc.ca/Collection/NH18-23-106-024E.pdf

Canadian Centre for Justice Statistics. (2011). *Family violence in Canada: A statistical profile 2009*. Ottawa, ON: Statistics Canada.

Canadian Population Health Initiative. (2006). *How healthy are rural Canadians? An assessment of their health status and health determinants—A component of the initiative Canada's rural communities: Understanding rural health and its determinants*. Ottawa, ON: Canadian Institute for Health Information.

Caponi, V., & Plesca, M. (2009). Post-secondary education in Canada: Can ability bias explain the earnings gap between college and university graduates? *Canadian Journal of Economics/ Revue Canadienne D'économique*, 42(3), 1100–1131. doi:10.1111/j.1540-5982.2009.01540.x

Chicago Healthcare Council. (1999). International Strategy and Policy Institute (ISPI). Retrieved June 23, 2013, from http:// www.ispi-usa.org/guidelines.htm

Coburn, D. (2010). Health and health care: A political economy perspective. In D. Raphael, T. Bryant, & M. Rioux (Eds.), *Staying alive: Critical perspectives on health, illness and health care* (pp. 65–92). Toronto, ON: Canadian Scholar's Press.

Coker, A. L. (2006). Preventing intimate partner violence: How we will rise to this challenge. *American Journal of Preventive Medicine*, 30(6), 528–529.

Collin, C. (2006). *Substance abuse and public policy in Canada: Alcohol and related harms*. Ottawa, ON: Political and Social Affairs Division, Library of Parliament, Canada.

Collin, C., & Jensen, H. (2009, September). Current publications: Social affairs and population: A statistical profile of poverty in Canada (PRB 09-17E). Retrieved June 27, 2013, from http://www.parl.gc.ca/content/lop/researchpublications/ prb0917-e.htm

Conference Board of Canada. (2012). Canadian income inequality. Retrieved January 4, 2013, from http://www.conferenceboard. ca/hcp/hot-topics/caninequality.aspx

Farris-Manning, C., & Zandstra, M. (2004). *Children in care in Canada: A summary of current issues and trends with recommendations for future research*. Ottawa, ON: Child Welfare League of Canada, Foster LIFE Inc.

First Call: BC Child and Youth Advocacy Coalition. (2011). *2011 child poverty report card*. Vancouver, BC: First Call: BC Child and Youth Advocacy Coalition.

Ford-Gilboe, M. (2000). Dispelling myths and creating opportunity: A comparison of the strengths of single-parent and two-parent families. *Advances in Nursing Science*, 23(1), 41–58.

Ford Gilboe, M., Varcoe, C., Wuest, J., & Merritt-Gray, M. (2010). Nursing practice and family violence. In J. Humphreys & J. C. Campbell (Eds.), *Family violence and nursing practice* (2nd ed., pp. 115–154). New York, NY: Springer.

Funk, L., Stajduhar, K., Toye, C., Aoun, S., Grande, G., & Todd, C. (2010). Part 2: Home-based family caregiving at the end of life: A comprehensive review of published qualitative research (1998–2008). *Palliative Medicine*, 24(6), 594–607.

Harris, R., Tobias, M., Jeffreys, M., Waldegrave, K., Karlsen, S., & Nazroo, J. (2006). Racism and health: The relationship between experience of racial discrimination and health in New Zealand. *Social Science & Medicine*, 63(6), 1428–1441.

Henry, F., Tator, C., & Mattis, W. (2009). *Racism and human-service delivery. The colour of democracy: Racism in Canadian society*. Toronto, ON: Harcourt Brace.

Human Resources and Social Development Canada. (2012). Indicators of well being in Canada: Canadians in context. Retrieved January 5, 2013, from http://www4.hrsdc.gc.ca/ d.4m.1.3n@-eng.jsp?did=6

Johnson, H. (1996). *Dangerous domains: Violence against women in Canada*. Scarborough, ON: International Thomson Publishing.

Johnson, H., & Sacco, V. (1995, July). Researching violence against women: Statistics Canada's national survey. *Canadian Journal of Criminology*, 281–304.

Jones, A. S., Gielen, A. C., Campbell, J. C., Schollenberger, J., Dienemann, J. A., Kub, J., . . . , & Wynne, E. C. (1999). Annual and lifetime prevalence of partner abuse in a sample of female HMO enrollees. *Women's Health Issues*, 9(6), 295–305.

Krieger, N., Chen, J. T., Coull, B. A., & Selby, J. V. (2005). Lifetime socioeconomic position and twins' health: An analysis of 308 pairs of United States women twins. *PLoS Medicine*, 2(7), 0645–0653.

Kubik, W., Bourassa, C., & Hampton, M. (2009). Stolen sisters, second class citizens, poor health: The legacy of colonization in Canada. *Humanity & Society*, 33, 18–34.

MacMillan, H. L. (2000). Preventive health care, 2000 update: Prevention of child maltreatment. *Canadian Medical Association Journal/Journal De L'association Medicale Canadienne*, 163(11), 1451–1458.

MacMillan, H., Wathen, C., Jamieson, E., Boyle, M., Shannon, H., Ford-Gilboe, M., . . . McMaster Violence Against Women Research Group. (2009). Screening for intimate partner violence in health care settings: A randomized trial. *Journal of the American Medical Association*, 302(5), 493–501.

McGill, J. (2008). An institutional suicide machine: Discrimination against federally sentenced Aboriginal women in Canada. *Race/Ethnicity: Multidisciplinary Global Perspectives*, 2(1), 89–119.

McLean, C. (2001). Less sensational but more dangerous. *Report/Newsmagazine (National Edition)*, 28(22), 44.

Mitura, V., & Bollman, R. D. (2003). The health of rural Canadians: A rural-urban comparison of health indicators. *Rural and Small Town Canada Analysis Bulletin*, 4(6), 1–23.

Mojab, S., & El-Kassem, N. (2008). *Cultural relativism: Theoretical, political and ideological debates. Canadian Muslim women at the crossroads: From integration to segregation?* Gananoque, ON: Canadian Council of Muslim Women.

Mustillo, S., Krieger, N., Gunderson, E. P., Sidney, S., Mc-Creath, H., & Kiefe, C. I. (2004). Self-reported experiences of racial discrimination and black-white differences in preterm and low-birthweight deliveries: The CARDIA Study. *American Journal of Public Health, 94*(12), 2125–2131.

Oxman-Martinez, J., Rummens, A. J., Moreau, J., Choi, Y. R., Beiser, M., Ogilvie, L., & Armstrong, R. (2012). Perceived ethnic discrimination and social exclusion: Newcomer immigrant children in Canada. *American Journal of Orthopsychiatry, 82*(3), 376–388. doi:10.1111/j.1939-0025.2012.01161.x

Papademetriou, D. G., Somerville, W., & Sumption, M. (2009). *The social mobility of immigrants and their children.* Washington, DC: Migration Policy Institute.

Public Health Agency of Canada. (2001). The Canadian Incidence Study of reported child abuse and neglect: Highlights. Retrieved April 15, 2008, from http://www.phac-aspc.gc.ca/cm-vee/cishl01

Pulkingham, J., Fuller, S., & Kershaw, P. (2010). Lone motherhood, welfare reform and active citizen subjectivity. *Critical Social Policy, 30*(2), 267–291.

Quan, H., Fong, A., De Coster, C., Wang, J., Musto, R., Noseworthy, T. W., & Ghali, W. A. (2006). Variation in health services utilization among ethnic populations. *CMAJ: Canadian Medical Association Journal, 174*(6), 787–791.

Ramsey, J., Richardson, J., Carter, Y. H., Davidson, L. L., & Feder, G. (2002). Should health professionals screen women for domestic violence? Systematic review. *British Medical Journal, 325*(7359), 314–318.

Rehm, J., Baliunas, D., Brochu, S., Fischer, B., Gnam, W., Patra, J., … & Taylor, B. (2006). *The costs of substance abuse in Canada 2002.* Ottawa, ON: Canadian Centre on Substance Abuse.

Rosenthal, C. J., & Gladstone, J. (2000). *Contemporary family trends: Grandparenthood in Canada.* Ontario: Vanier Institute of the Family

Statistics Canada. (2003a). *Ethnic diversity survey: Portrait of a multicultural society.* Ottawa, ON: Statistics Canada.

Statistics Canada. (2003b). Religions in Canada. Ottawa, ON: Statistics Canada.

Statistics Canada. (2005). Longitudinal Survey of Immigrants to Canada (LSIC): A portrait of early settlement experiences. Retrieved September 15, 2008, from http://www.statcan.ca/bsolc/english/bsolc?catno=89-614-X

Statistics Canada. (2006). *Family violence in Canada: A statistical profile 2006.* Ottawa, ON: Canadian Centre for Justice Statistics.

Statistics Canada. (2009). Immigration in Canada: A portrait of the foreign-born population, 2006 census: Immigration: Driver of population growth. Retrieved January 4, 2013, from http://www12.statcan.ca/census-recensement/2006/as-sa/97-557/p2-eng.cfm

Statistics Canada. (2011a). Canadian social trends. Ottawa, ON: Statistics Canada. Available at http://publications.gc.ca/collections/collection_2012/statcan/11-008-x/11-008-x2011002-eng.pdf

Statistics Canada. (2011b, June 15). Statistics Canada—The Daily. Income of Canadians. Retrieved January 4, 2013, from http://www.statcan.gc.ca/daily-quotidien/110615/dq110615b-eng.htm

Statistics Canada. (2011c). *Women in Canada: A gender-based statistical report* (6th ed.). Ottawa, ON: Statistics Canada.

Statistics Canada, (2011d). *National Household Survey,* Statistics Canada Catalogue no. 99-010-X2011032. Retrieved from http://www12.statcan.gc.ca/nhs-enm/2011

Statistics Canada. (2012). 2011 census of population: Linguistic characteristics of Canadians. The Daily, October 24. Retrieved January 4, 2013, from http://www.statcan.gc.ca/daily-quotidien/121024/dq121024a-eng.htm

Thobani, S. (2007). *Exalted subjects: Studies in the making of race and nation in Canada.* Toronto, ON: University of Toronto Press.

Townson, M. (2005). *Poverty issues for Canadian Women.* Ottawa, ON: Status of Women Canada.

Trocmé, N., MacMillan, H., Fallon, B., & De Marco, R. (2003). Nature and severity of physical harm caused by child abuse and neglect: Results from the Canadian Incidence Study. *Canadian Medical Association Journal/Journal De L'association Medicale Canadienne, 169*(9), 911–915.

UNICEF Office of Research. (2013). *Child well-being in rich countries: A comparative overview. Innocenti Report Card 11.* Florence, Italy: UNICEF Office of Research.

Varcoe, C., Hankivsky, O., Ford Gilboe, M., Wuest, J., Wilk, P., Hammerton, J., & Campbell, J. C. (2011). Attributing selected costs to intimate partner violence in a sample of women who have left abusive partners: A social determinants of health approach. *Canadian Public Policy, 37*(3), 359–380.

Veenstra, G. (2009). Racialized identity and health in Canada: Results from a nationally representative survey. *Social Science & Medicine, 69*(4), 538–542. doi:10.1016/j.socscimed.2009.06.009

Walsh, C., MacMillan, H. L., & Jamieson, E. (2003). The relationship between parental substance abuse and child maltreatment: Findings from the Ontario Health Supplement. *Child Abuse & Neglect: The International Journal, 27*(12), 1409–1425.

Walsh, C. A., & Yon, Y. (2012). Developing an empirical profile for elder abuse research in Canada. *Journal of Elder Abuse & Neglect, 24*(2), 104–119. doi:10.1080/08946566.2011.644088

Wekerle, C., Wall, A.-M., Leung, E., & Trocmé, N. (2007). Cumulative stress and substantiated maltreatment: The importance of caregiver vulnerability and adult partner violence. *Child Abuse & Neglect, 31*(4), 427–443.

Welcome/Bienvenue. (2011). Government of Canada, Statistics Canada. Retrieved June 27, 2013, from http://www.statcan.gc.ca

Williams, A., Forbes, D., Mitchell, J., & Corbett, B. (2003). The influence of income on the experience of informal caregiving: Policy implications. *Health Care for Women International, 24*(4), 280–292.

Williams, A. M., & Kulig, J. C. (2012). Health and place in rural Canada. In J. C. Kulig & A. M. Williams (Eds.), *Health in rural Canada.* Vancouver, BC: UBC Press.

World Health Organization. (1986). *Ottawa charter for health promotion.* Geneva, CH: World Health Organization.

Zhang, T., Hoddenbagh, J., McDonald, S., & Scrim, K. (2012). *An estimation of the economic impact of spousal violence in Canada, 2009.* Ottawa, ON: Department of Justice Canada.

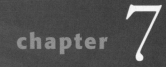

chapter 7

Genomics and Family Nursing Across the Life Span

Dale Halsey Lea, MPH, RN, CGC, FAAN

Critical Concepts

- Genomics refers to the study of all genes in the human genome and their interactions with each other and the environment.

- Genetics refers to the study of individual genes and their effect on clinical disorders.

- Biological members of a family may share the risk for disease because of genetic factors.

- Families are unique and respond to genetic discoveries differently based on personal coping styles, family values, beliefs, and patterns of communication. Even within the same family, members react differently.

- In every case, it is the nurse's role to support families to make decisions that are most appropriate for their particular circumstances, cultures, and beliefs.

- The two major nursing responsibilities when a genetic risk is identified are to help families understand that the risk is present and to help families make decisions about management and surveillance.

- Results of genetic tests are private and cannot be disclosed to other family members without the tested individual's consent.

- Nurses identify accurate information and access resources for families with concerns regarding genetic and genomic health risks.

- All nurses, regardless of their areas of practice, apply an understanding of the effects of genetic risk factors when conducting assessments, planning, and evaluating nursing interventions.

Some illnesses "run in families" and people commonly wonder if they, or their children, will develop a disease that is present in their parents or grandparents. The ability to apply an understanding of genetics in the care of families is a priority for nurses and for all health care providers. As a result of genomic research and the resultant rapidly changing body of knowledge regarding genetic influences on health and illness, more emphasis has been placed on involving all health care providers in this field. This integration of genetic knowledge, attitudes, and skills is especially important for nurses, and is reflected in the *Essential Nursing Competencies and Curricula Guidelines for Genetics and Genomics* (Consensus Panel, 2008), hereafter referred to in this chapter as "essential nursing competencies." Essential nursing competencies include both the ability to apply genetic and genomic knowledge in conducting nursing assessments and the ability to assess responses to genetic and genomic information (Consensus Panel, 2008). These competencies are also identified in documents for general practitioners in the United Kingdom (National Genetics Education and Development Centre, 2008).

It is important for family nurses to be aware of the effect of genetics on families because biological family members share genetic risk factors. In addition, families function as systems with shared health risks that affect the whole family, and family processes mediate coping and adaptation of both individual family members and the family unit as a whole (Walsh, 2003). Family members inevitably have an effect on each other's lives, and in many cases, they support each other in seeking and maintaining healthy growth and development, regardless of their biological kinship. Much of what is known about the health care needs of persons with genetic conditions has focused on the individual, with less attention directed toward the person's biological and socially defined family. All nurses, regardless of their areas of practice, apply an understanding of the effects of genetic risk factors when conducting assessments, planning, and evaluating nursing interventions.

This chapter describes nursing responsibilities for families of persons who have, or are at risk for having, genetic conditions. These responsibilities are described for families before conception, with neonates, teens in families, and families with members in the middle to elder years. The goal of the chapter is to describe the relevance of genetic information within families when there is a question about genetic aspects of health or disease for members of the family. Family nursing knowledge is incomplete without attention to the effects of genetic factors on health and functioning of individuals, as well as on family units.

GENETICS AND GENOMICS

The term *genomics* is commonly used to reflect the study of all genes in the human genome, as well as interactions among genes and with environmental and other psychosocial or cultural factors (Feetham & Thomson, 2006). The human genome consists of approximately 3.1 billion bases of DNA sequence, some of which are unique to each person (National Human Genome Research Institute,

2012). Individuals inherit genetic material from their parents and pass it on to their children. Some conditions result from a change or mutation in a DNA sequence of a gene. A *gene* is defined as the basic physical unit of inheritance (National Human Genome Research Institute, 2013). For example, Huntington's disease results from a specific change within the DNA sequence in a particular gene. This is an example of a condition traditionally referred to as a "Mendelian" or "single-gene disorder" and is one that follows an identified pattern of traditional inheritance in families, in this case, autosomal dominant inheritance. Persons who are biologically related may have inherited many of the same DNA sequences in addition to having shared common environments with other family members; this combination ultimately increases risks for having similar specific illnesses.

Researchers also identify common genetic variations known as single-nucleotide polymorphisms. These variations may not cause an actual disruption in the DNA coding but can often be used as tools that help scientists and clinicians recognize DNA variations that may be associated with disease. These conditions include common disorders, such as diabetes, that are observed to occur more frequently in families but do not follow a traditional pattern of inheritance.

A core competency for nurses is to maintain knowledge of the relationships of genetic and genomic factors to the health of individuals and their families. Cancer provides an example of the relationships between genes, environment, and health. The development of a malignant tumor is the result of a complex series of changes at the cellular level. A number of genes protect against cancer by regulating cell division (during mitosis), and mutations in those genes can occur over the course of a person's lifetime, affecting one's predisposition to cancer. A person may be at increased risk of developing cancer if an inherited mutation occurs in one of those genes or if exposed to environmental factors that influence genetic mutations. For example, tumor suppressor genes help protect against the development of breast cancer. If a woman inherits a mutation in a tumor suppressor gene (such as the *BRCA1* gene), she has lost some of her protection against breast cancer from birth, but she will not necessarily develop cancer unless other cellular changes (some of which are influenced by factors such as her reproductive history) occur during her lifetime (Bougie & Weberpals, 2011). Others in her family also may have inherited the same mutation and are similarly at risk. If she subsequently becomes a smoker, she has an additional increased risk for lung cancer because of the environmental influence of smoking on cell division in her lungs. In families where smoking is the norm, there may be a perceived "familial" condition because of the shared environmental and genetic influences on a number of members of the family. Box 7-1 lists inherited and multifactor inherited genetic conditions.

GENETIC TESTING

Genetic testing can be performed for several purposes, including prenatal diagnosis, detection of carrier status, predictive testing for familial disorders, and presymptomatic testing. See Table 7-1 for types of genetic tests. Prenatal testing is available to pregnant women during a pregnancy, such as prenatal testing for Down syndrome. Carrier testing can tell people if they have (carry) a gene alteration for a particular kind of inherited disorder called an autosomal recessive genetic disorder, such as cystic fibrosis or sickle cell anemia. Predictive testing can identify individuals who have a higher chance of getting a disease before the symptoms appear. Predictive testing is available for inherited genetic risk factors that make it more likely for someone to develop certain cancers, such as colon or breast cancer. Presymptomatic genetic testing can indicate which family members are at risk for a certain genetic condition that is already known to be present in their family. This type of testing is

performed for people who have not yet shown symptoms of a disease, such as Huntington's disease (National Human Genome Research Institute, 2011).

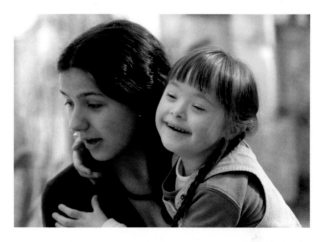

The National Comprehensive Cancer Network (2008) continually updates guidelines that specify what kind of screening is indicated for a person who has a gene mutation that increases the chances of cancer developing. For example, family members may seek testing if they are at greater risk for familial colon cancer (Madlensky, Esplen, Gallinger, McLauglin, & Goel, 2003). In some cases, clinical practice guideline criteria recommend that genetic testing be done to determine whether a person is at risk.

A new type of genetic testing, called pharmacogenetic testing, is performed to examine an individual's genes to determine how medications are absorbed, move through the body, and are metabolized by the body. The purpose of pharmacogenetic testing is so that health professionals can create tailored drug treatments that are individualized and specific to each person. For example, there is a test that is used in patients who have chronic myelogenous leukemia. The test indicates which patients will benefit from the medication Gleevec (National Human Genome Research Institute, 2011). In addition, gene changes can affect how an individual's body metabolizes some medications. For instance, patients can be tested to see if they are poor metabolizers, intermediate metabolizers, or ultrarapid metabolizers. Based on the pharmacogenetic test results, patients would be prescribed the right amount of the medication for their body. For instance, pharmacogenetic testing can help determine the best dose of the blood-thinning medication warfarin. A patient who is a

Table 7-1	Types of Genetic Tests
Diagnostic	Performed when signs and/or symptoms of a genetic condition are present. Confirms whether or not an individual has the suspected condition.
Carrier	Detects whether a person is a carrier of either an autosomal recessive or an X-linked disorder.
	A carrier of an autosomal recessive condition usually has no signs of the condition and will be at risk for having an affected child if the other parent is also a carrier. He has one normal copy of the gene in question and one mutated copy.
	A female carrier of an X-linked condition has one normal copy of the gene on the X chromosome and one mutated copy of the gene on the other X chromosome, and generally has no signs or very mild signs of the condition. Her sons have a 50% chance of having the condition, and her daughters have a 50% chance of being carriers.
Predictive or presymptomatic	Performed on healthy individuals; detects whether they inherited a mutation in a gene and, therefore, whether they will or may develop a condition in the future.
Prenatal diagnosis	Genetic test performed on the fetus. Indicates whether the fetus has inherited the gene mutation that causes a specific condition and, therefore, whether the child will develop that condition.
Pharmacogenetic testing	Analyzes a person's genes to understand how drugs may move through the body and be broken down. The purpose of pharmacogenetic testing is to help select drug treatments that are best suited for each person.
Direct-to-consumer genetic testing	Direct-to-consumer (DTC) genetic tests are marketed directly to the general public, usually via the Internet. DTC genetic testing provides access to an individual's genetic information, usually without involving a health care professional.

poor metabolizer will be prescribed a lower dose of warfarin, and a person who is an ultrarapid metabolizer will be prescribed a higher dose of warfarin (National Human Genome Research Institute, 2011).

Another new type of genetic test, called direct-to-consumer (DTC) genetic testing, is now available to the general public. DTC genetic tests are offered over the Internet. They usually involve receiving a packet in the mail for DTC genetic testing, which includes instructions and materials for individuals to scrape a few cells from the inside of their cheek and mail the sample to a particular laboratory to perform the genetic tests (National Human Genome Research Institute, 2012). Several companies offer DTC genetic testing, including the company 23andMe, which claims that its testing can "help you manage risk and make informed decisions" (23andMe, 2012).

The market for DTC genetic tests may increase individuals' awareness of genetic diseases and allow them to take a more proactive role in their health care (Genetics Home Reference, 2012). The types of DTC tests that are offered include those that evaluate parts of a person's genome for variants that may have an influence on that person's risk for developing particular diseases such as Alzheimer's disease. The DTC genetic tests offered by companies also claim they can test for particular genetic markers that may indicate a person's ancestry, personality, or physical traits, some of which may have implications for the person's health.

It is important that nurses are aware of DTC so that they can advise patients interested in DTC to meet with health care providers or genetic counselors to learn more about this type of testing and its accuracy and applicability to health care. Furthermore, nurses and other health care professionals should be aware of the reliability of DTC genetic testing. In 2010, the U.S. Government Accountability Office (GAO) conducted a study of DTC genetic testing to determine its reliability. Using fictitious names for consumers, they submitted samples to several DTC companies. The results that the donors received about disease risk predictions varied across the companies, showing that the identical DNA samples submitted yielded contradictory results. Sometimes, the DNA-based predictions conflicted with their actual medical conditions (U.S. Government Accountability Office, 2010). People who are considering a DTC genetic test should first talk about this type of testing with their health care provider or a genetic counselor. The concern is that without guidance from a health care provider or genetic counselor, the individual may make significant decisions about prevention or a particular treatment that is based on incomplete or inaccurate information (Genetics Home Reference, 2012; National Human Genome Research Institute, 2013).

Disadvantages of Predictive Genetic Tests

Nurses should understand the differences in the types of genetic tests that families may consider and the potential advantages or disadvantages of predictive genetic tests summarized in Box 7-2. Nurses who participate in discussions about genetic testing

---

BOX 7-2
Potential Advantages and Disadvantages of Predictive Genetic Tests

Potential advantages of testing include:

- Opportunity to learn whether one has an increased likelihood of developing an inherited disease; in those who prefer certainty, this can help resolve feelings of discomfort, even if the result shows the person has inherited the condition
- Relief from worry about future health risks for a specific disease if the test is negative
- Information that can be used for making reproductive decisions
- Information to inform lifestyle choices (e.g., food choices, smoking, alcohol use, contraceptive choice)
- Information to guide clinical surveillance or management of the condition
- Information for other family members about their own status
- Confirmation of a diagnosis that has been suspected (i.e., that early or nonspecific signs and symptoms are due to a specific condition)

  Potential disadvantages are that the test results may provide:

- A source of increased anxiety about the future
- Guilt at having survived when others in the family are affected, if the result is negative ("survivor's guilt")
- Concern about potential discrimination based on genetic test results
- Regret about past life decisions (such as not having children)
- Changes in family attitudes toward the person who has been tested (such as less reliance on them for support)

---

must maintain current knowledge on these tests, as well as on new technology for testing and interpretations of results.

Genetic tests have limitations that vary according to the specific test. For some tests, not all persons who want the test may qualify, which occurs when their family history does not suggest that the disease has a major genetic component, or where the genetic mutation that causes the disease has not been identified. For some tests, it is possible that a result may be difficult to interpret. For some conditions, genetic mutations have been discovered that are associated with the disease in that family. Because many genes may be associated with one condition, or a number of different mutations may be possible in a gene, it is often necessary to test an affected family member first to try to identify which gene is involved and which type of mutation is causing the disease in that family. A sample is taken from the affected person to determine whether a genetic mutation can be identified that is associated with that disease. This may not be possible if the affected person in the family has passed away or if the affected person refuses to undergo the genetic testing to help other family members.

Another limit to genetic testing is the fact that results may not be definitive. For example, a test result of an infant screened for cystic fibrosis may be in the positive range for a screening test. A positive screening test simply means, however, that a diagnostic test is required to determine whether the infant has the condition. It is important for parents to understand that, in some infants, a diagnostic test result can indicate that the infant has a genetic condition and will need further evaluation and treatment, and in other cases, subsequent tests will be normal. When an infant has further evaluation, and is found not to have the condition, the first test result is sometimes referred to as a false positive, or an out-of-range result that required further testing. Parents who understand the reason for the repeated testing tend to experience less stress than those who do not (Hewlett & Waisbren, 2006). When a family receives an abnormal newborn screening test result, it is crucial for the nurse to help the family understand that abnormal results from a screening test do not necessarily mean that the child is ill or has the disease (Hewlett & Waisbren, 2006). The waiting period between the newborn screening result and the diagnostic testing is known to be especially difficult for parents (Tluczek, Koscik, Farrell, & Rock, 2005).

FAMILY DISCLOSURE OF GENETIC INFORMATION

Communicating information about the genetic aspects of a condition to families at the time of diagnosis and over time is an important role for nurses and other health care professionals (Gallo, Angst, Knafl, Twomey, & Hadley, 2010). Having an effective partnership and communication between health care professionals and families is essential to the success of developing both collaborative and therapeutic working relationships (Levetown & American Pediatric Committeee, 2008). Nurses work with families through a cascade of decisions and information about the genetic disorder (Reid Ponte & Peterson, 2008).

Gallo et al. (2010) describe four main themes relative to how health care professionals share genetic information with parents of children with a genetic condition:

■ Sharing information with parents
■ Taking into account parental preferences
■ Understanding the condition
■ Helping the parents inform others about the genetic condition

Sharing information with parents should be initiated at the time of diagnosis and then tailored over time based on the parents' particular needs, the characteristics of the child's condition, and the environmental factors (Gallo et al., 2010). Important roles of nurses in this process include reinforcing the information to help parents understand the condition, coordinating the patient's care, educating parents on expectations, discussing potential management of the care for their child at home, and helping the parents to inform others about their child's genetic condition (Gallo et al., 2010).

Access to genetic information gained from genetic testing, as well as from family history, raises a host of questions for the family regarding confidentiality that includes the following: who to tell, what and when to tell them, and how much to share. Nurses must maintain the confidentiality of each family member's genetic testing information. It is completely up to the individual to determine whether or not to reveal information about genetic

risks, testing, disease, or management. Results of genetic tests are private, and in the United States, they cannot be disclosed to other family members without the tested person's consent (U.S. Department of Health and Human Services, 1996). In the United States, the Health Insurance Portability and Accountability Act (HIPAA) permits disclosures of health information if there is an immediate and serious threat to the person and if the disclosure could reasonably lessen or prevent the threat (U.S. Department of Health and Human Services, 1996). In most cases, however, the choice of disclosure of genetic information is an individual decision that is made in the context of the family.

Discovery of health problems in more than one family member should be accompanied by a discussion with family members regarding their understanding of risks for potentially inherited disorders. Disclosure can be a challenging task, as the person with the genetic mutation must decide who to inform, what to say, and when to talk about this finding (Gaff et al., 2007).

Family members may prefer to maintain privacy regarding their decision about predictive testing, even within the family. This decision may reflect an attempt to avoid disagreements within the family, an attempt to protect others in the family from sadness or worry, or an attempt to prevent discrimination or bias. For example, people who have predictive Huntington's disease testing may be reluctant to share this information with their primary care provider. This reluctance may be because they fear that any notation in their medical record may be accessed by an employer or insurance provider, which may lead to loss of employment or insurance. Although laws have been passed that prohibit insurance or employment discrimination based on a person's genotype, some individuals may be concerned that revealing their genotype may place them at risk for discrimination (Penziner et al., 2008).

When one person in a family has a condition that is caused by an alteration in a single gene, such as a gene associated with hereditary breast or ovarian cancer, the person with the mutation is asked to notify others in the family that they too may have this same DNA mutation. In general, the family members themselves pass on this information, but occasionally, with the consent of all concerned, direct conversations can occur between the nurse and other family members. Because families vary in their adaptability regarding health challenges, families vary in how they decide to share information (McDaniel, Rolland, Feetham, & Miller, 2006).

Both individual and family relationship factors can influence communication among family members. Nurses should, therefore, have a good understanding of their patient's personal beliefs about sharing genetic risk information with family members. Nurses work closely with the individual to explore relationships with relatives to identify potential areas of difficulty and provide support for communication of accurate genetic information (Wiseman, Dancyger, & Michie, 2010). The family communication style may affect disclosure and sharing of genetic information. For example, a family with a disengaged communication pattern may share affection for each other but actually speak relatively infrequently with each other (McDaniel et al., 2006). For families with this style of communication and lack of closeness, sharing information about one's personal medical history may be especially difficult (Stoffel et al., 2008). In contrast, families with an enmeshed style of family communication frequently talk with others in the family about personal health matters (McDaniel et al., 2006). Gender may influence the sharing of genetic information with family members. Women were noted to have more difficulty in sharing genetic information with older parents, brothers, or fathers (Patenaude et al., 2006). Men expressed difficulty disclosing genetic information to all family members (Gaff, Collins, Symes, & Halliday, 2005). Box 7-3 depicts an example of family communication of genetic information.

Parents: To Tell or Not to Tell

Parents of a child with a genetic disorder take into consideration what to tell their children about the condition based on the developmental level of the child and the child's extent of interest in knowing about the genetic condition. Thus, parents whose children had a single gene disorder described sharing genetic information with their children as an unfolding process that was not a one-time occurrence but continued throughout childhood as their cognitive stage of development progressed (Gallo, Angst, Knafl, Hadley, & Smith, 2005).

Parents, usually, believe that they are the most appropriate people to inform their children about genetic risks. Still, when no current effective treatment

---

BOX 7-3
Family Communication of Genetic Information

Brian, a 46-year-old man, is the oldest of three siblings. He is married but has no biological children. Brian was aware that his mother died of bowel cancer at the age of 38 years, and although this worried him, he hid his anxiety from both friends and relatives. He never discussed his mother's death with his wife or siblings. Brian had been experiencing abdominal pain for some months when he collapsed at work one day and was taken to his local hospital emergency department. He was found to be anemic and suffering a bowel obstruction. A tumor located near the hepatic flexure of the large colon was removed successfully. Brian was informed that his family and medical history indicated that it was likely he had inherited a mutation in an oncogene that predisposed him to bowel cancer. He was advised to share this finding with his siblings, and recommend that they seek advice and screening for themselves. Brian was reluctant to discuss the issue with his siblings but did tell his wife. Brian chose not to disclose this information to his siblings. Several months later, at the encouragement of his wife, they met with the cancer nurse to discuss the situation. The cancer nurse helped Brian decide what information to share with his siblings. They created a plan for how and when to share the information. Subsequently, both Brian's sister and brother had genetic testing. Brian's sister was found to carry the mutation. She was screened, and she worked with the nurse to devise a plan to tell her children about their possible risk when they reached 18 years of age.

---

or cure exists, parents struggle with balancing "the right" of individuals to know about their potential genetic risks with their natural instinct as parents to spare their children from undue anxiety (Tercyak et al., 2007). In some cases, individuals delay telling other adults in the family because they worry that they will accidently say something to the child or that they may be overheard by the child (Speice, McDaniel, Rowley, & Loader, 2002).

Parents of children with genetic conditions may choose not to share information because they have concerns about school issues, obtaining health care for their children, and insurability or employability of their children. Parents worry that their child could feel different from other children because of food or activity restrictions, or visible signs of the genetic condition (Gallo, Hadley, Angst, Knafl, &

Smith, 2008). Nurses have a significant role in helping parents decide what information to share with their children about their genetic condition based on their developmental level. Another role of family nurses is helping parents determine how much information to share with outside sources, such as schools, day care, or employers, about their child's genetic condition.

Concealing Information: Family Secrets

Some families are quite open, whereas others choose to keep genetic information a secret, even from other immediate family members (Peters et al., 2005). Families choose to keep genetic information a secret for a variety of reasons. Sometimes information is kept a secret out of a desire to protect other family members. Some keep a secret because they feel shame. Still other families may choose to keep information secret because the exploration of genetic inheritance may reveal other personal information. For example, consider a family with four sisters who want health advice because their father has a form of familial colon cancer. In the course of obtaining the family history, the mother confides to the nurse that her husband is not the biological parent of the oldest daughter, and that others in the family do not know this history. In this situation, the nurse recognizes that the oldest daughter does not share the same risk for this disease as her sisters, but the nurse would not be permitted to reveal that information to any family member without the mother's permission. This family secret can create conflict for the nurse, because the lack of disclosure might mean the eldest daughter is exposed to unnecessary procedures, such as a colonoscopy (which carries a risk for morbidity). The nurse would discuss the issue of risks for procedures with the mother so that the she can consider all the information in deciding to tell her daughter the family secret. The mother would have to decide if the benefits of disclosure outweigh the distress the daughter may experience by learning about her parentage.

Family Reactions to Disclosure of Genetic Information

Families are unique and respond to genetic discoveries differently. Even within the same family, family members will respond differently. Some members seek predictive testing to determine whether they have inherited the genetic condition.

Others choose not to seek testing. Some members react to genetic discoveries with grief, loss, and denial. The nurse's role is to support all family members in their reactions and ultimate choices.

Children, regardless of age, may wonder if they will have the same condition as their parent. For example, this may be the case for teens who have a parent or grandparent with Huntington's disease, an autosomal dominant condition. Guidelines do not recommend predictive testing until a teen is old enough to provide informed consent. Teens may want to protect their parents from their concerns and are reluctant to share their thoughts with their parents (Sparbel et al., 2008). Thus, nurses should offer the opportunity for them to ask questions and discuss their concerns, including offering to facilitate a family discussion. Box 7-4 depicts a family managing decisions about teenager.

Elders in the family often are keen to contribute to genetic studies to help their offspring (Skirton,

---

BOX 7-4

Working With an Adolescent About Genetic Testing

Susan is a 17-year-old young woman whose mother developed breast cancer at age 42 and had to have a double mastectomy. She is now recovering from her surgery and doing well. Susan's maternal grandmother and one of her maternal aunts died from breast cancer in their forties. Susan's mother chose to have genetic testing to learn about the possible genetic cause of her breast cancer. The test results revealed that she has a *BRCA1* gene mutation, which significantly increases a woman's lifetime risk of developing breast cancer. At her annual health care appointment Susan tells the nurse about her family history of breast cancer and that her mother has a *BRCA1* gene mutation. Susan says that she would like to know what her risk is for inheriting this gene and that she would like to have the genetic testing to find out if she carries the same *BRCA1* gene as her mother. She says that she is worried about her younger sister too. She tells the nurse that she does not want to worry her mother or family by talking with them about her concerns. The nurse informs Susan that she is free to express her concerns with her and her physician and that they can talk with her about how best to talk with her mother and express her concerns. She also lets Susan know that when she is 18 she will be old enough to provide informed consent to have genetic testing for the *BRCA1* mutation that her mother has. She recommends that when she is 18, she consider genetic counseling with a genetic specialist to learn more about her risk and the *BRCA1* genetic testing.

Frazier, Calvin, & Cohen, 2006) and serve as an information source of family history. Advances in genomics will make susceptibility testing for common diseases of middle and old age (such as coronary artery disease or cancer) more common.

Family members possess beliefs about their own risks and who in the family will develop a genetic condition. These beliefs are termed *preselection* (Tercyak, 2010). Preselection beliefs are often based on the family's previous experience. For example, if only male relatives have been affected by an autosomal dominant condition that could affect either sex, female members in the family may believe they are not at risk. Sometimes preselection beliefs are based on the fact that the person thought to have inherited the condition physically resembles the affected parent or shares a physical characteristic (such as hair color) with other affected relatives. A preselection belief may influence the person's self-image and overall functioning. For example, those who believe they will develop a condition may make different career choices, avoid long-term relationships, or decide not to have children. Box 7-5 depicts a case study that demonstrates preselection beliefs.

DECISION TO HAVE GENETIC TESTING

In some circumstances, family members may want to know the likelihood that they will develop a condition in the future, which is referred to as either *predictive* or *presymptomatic testing*. Typically the physical risk for undergoing genetic testing is minimal, but not so for the emotional risk. The test results may have a significant effect on a person emotionally, influence medical decisions, and result in discrimination. Undergoing genetic predictive testing requires nurses to work with clients so that they make this decision in a way that meets their specific needs, alert to the nonphysical risks. Nurses involved with these families should be able to identify the sources of emotional distress and offer effective strategies to help mediate distress, make informed decisions about medical interventions, and handle possible discrimination (Williams et al., 2009).

Emotional Health

Family members seek or avoid genetic testing for a variety of reasons. Some elect to know whether or not they carry a mutation so they can reduce

---

BOX 7-5
Preselection Beliefs

John is a 21-year-old young man who has recently graduated from college and is trying to decide what career he wants to pursue. John has a family history of Huntington's disease (HD) on his mother's side. His mother's brother and her father have both passed away from HD. His mother, age 45, is currently in good health. John is very worried that he will develop HD because it is in his mother's family. John makes an appointment with his health care provider so that he can talk with him about his concerns. As the nurse is taking his vital signs, John tells her about his concerns that he will develop HD. He says that he doesn't know if his mother has it and he is worried because it seems to be in the males of the family, and he looks like his uncle who died from HD. John says that he would like to go to medical school but he is scared that he will develop HD when he is young and it will greatly affect his career. He also tells the nurse that he has a girlfriend to whom he is very attached, but he is afraid to consider getting married because he does not want to put her through the experience of losing him to HD. He says that he has not even told her about his family history. The nurse tells John that she understands his concerns and encourages John to talk with his doctor about how he can learn more about his risk for HD. She tells him that he could consider having genetic counseling to talk further about his risks and available genetic testing for HD to learn more. John thanks her for her support and suggestions and says that he will surely talk with his doctor further about his concerns and options.

---

their fear of the unknown, or make life choices, such as having children. Some people decide not to have predictive testing because they believe this knowledge would increase their level of anxiety and would prompt a constant watch for developing symptoms (Soltysiak, Gardiner, & Skirton, 2008). Test results mean different things in different situations, which makes these decisions to undergo testing even more complex and multifaceted. For example, a positive test for a *BRCA1* or *BRCA2* breast cancer mutation does not mean the individual has a 100% chance of developing breast cancer, so taking precautionary measures requires weighing costs and benefits. In other situations, such as in the case of Huntington's disease, if an individual carries the autosomal dominant condition, he will develop the disease. Some choose not to be tested for fear that they would lose hope.

Even adjustment to a negative result—meaning that a person does not have the genetic pattern of the disease—can be difficult. Some people who find that they are not at risk of developing a genetic condition experience "survivor guilt," which can be described as a sense of self-blame or remorse felt by a person who, in this case, will not develop a condition that others in the family will develop.

Evidence exists that when individuals have a genetic test that indicates that they will develop a condition, other family members may rely on them less than previously, in an emotional sense. These individuals experience feelings of loss of place in the family well before developing disease symptoms (Williams & Sobel, 2006). Some experience a deep sense of grief and loss of a potential future.

Medical Decisions

Physicians and nurse practitioners are in an excellent position to work closely with clients in making medical decisions about their health based on the individual's genetic and genomic information. These health care providers have the ability to refine and personalize medical care that is based on the client's genetic makeup. For example, there is an increased probability that treatment outcomes will result in fewer adverse effects from medications, such as pain management being determined on the basis of whether a client is a known fast metabolizer or slow to metabolize certain kinds of drugs. But just because there are many tests available does not mean that the best option is for the client to have genetic testing done. Advanced practice nurses need to work closely with the individual and family in deciding to have genetic testing that would include what the test would show, how specific the results might or might not be, and explore what options are possible based on the outcome of the testing.

After conferring with the health care provider, some clients may not choose to have genetic testing at that time. Instead, these clients may elect to undergo regular checkups and screenings, such as more frequent mammograms. In contrast, when a person has genetic testing and tests positive for a specific disease, a cascade of decisions then befalls that person, including and involving preventive or prophylactic treatments, degrees of treatment, risks of treatment, and benefits of treatment. For example, a woman may decide to undergo surgery, such as sterilization, so as to not pass on to offspring a condition such as cystic fibrosis or sickle cell anemia; or someone with positive results for *BRCA1* breast cancer mutation may elect to have a bilateral mastectomy.

Discrimination

Even though there is little evidence that genetic discrimination is a current problem (Feldman, 2012), many individuals choose not to undergo genetic testing because they fear discrimination. For example, a person may have concerns that she may be bypassed for promotion if it was known she tested positive for a medical condition. The Genetic Information Nondiscrimination Act (GINA) of 2008 protects individuals from discrimination initiated by an employer or health insurance company.

Under GINA, insurers may not use genetic information to set or adjust premiums, deny coverage, or impose preexisting conditions, and they may not require any genetic testing. Unfortunately, the GINA law does not apply to employers with less than 15 employees and it does not include protection against discrimination when an individual seeks to obtain life insurance, short-term disability insurance, or long-term care insurance. GINA does not protect members of the military, veterans, federal employees, or the Indian Health Service. Each of these sectors of society is protected against discrimination by other laws and statutes.

Under GINA, an employer may not make any decisions about hiring, firing, promoting or pay or assignment based on any genetic information. The Patient Protection and Affordable Care Act of 2010 also prohibits denial of insurance coverage based on genetic information. The GINA law is significantly more stringent and specific in preventing discrimination by employers and health care insurance agencies (Feldman, 2012), however, because it defines genetic information as including medical history.

ROLES OF THE NURSE

When there exists a genetic risk, nurses, together with others on the health care team, have two major responsibilities: (1) to help families understand that the risk is present, and (2) to help family members make decisions about management or surveillance. In every case, the nurse's role is to support families to make decisions that are most appropriate for their particular circumstances, cultures, and beliefs (International Society of Nurses in Genetics, 2010). This section suggests ways that nurses should review their own beliefs and values when working with families. It covers how to conduct a risk assessment and genetic family history, the importance of working with a couple in preconception education, and the role of nurses as genetic information managers.

Personal Values: A Potential Conflict

Nurses must become aware of cultural values that differ from their own family cultural values. Cultural awareness allows nurses to tailor their practices to meet the needs of the family. Box 7-6 demonstrates how a nurse who does not understand a family's cultural values could contribute to a poor outcome.

It is a difficult emotional situation when nurses' personal values conflict with those of families. One example of this type of conflict occurs when the nurse personally does not agree with the family decisions relative to the potential risks of having a child who is genetically predisposed to having a terminal disease. It is unethical, however, for nurses to

---

BOX 7-6

Cultural Awareness

Kate is a genetic nurse working in a pediatric clinic for children with inherited metabolic conditions. She was scheduled to see a family whose son had a rare inherited metabolic disorder to discuss the parents' future reproductive options, including prenatal diagnosis. When the family entered the room, she noted with surprise that the parents and the child were accompanied by both sets of grandparents. She quickly arranged for more chairs to be brought into the room. Kate was quite disconcerted to find that the paternal grandfather repeatedly answered questions that were directed to the parents, and she continued to address the parents. Eventually, the child's father explained that, according to his culture, the oldest male relative on the father's side was responsible for making the decision that would affect the family; therefore, it was critical that the grandfather be fully involved in all discussions. While reflecting with her mentor, Kate realized that, in the future, she would ask the family at the beginning of the family conference to share any specific cultural needs she should know about in order to help meet their family needs.

---

try to influence the decisions of the family or family members because of their own personal views.

Another type of conflict occurs when opinions within the family vary. In this type of situation, the role of the nurse is to facilitate family members expressing their views. In clinical genetics, more than one family member may be involved in decision making, and nurses should respect each person's autonomy.

Conducting a Genetic Family History

All nurses should be able to conduct a risk assessment that includes obtaining a genetic family history (Consensus Panel, 2008). As described in Chapter 4, a genogram collects useful information about family structure and relationships. Nurses can use a three-generation family pedigree to provide information about a potential genetic inheritance pattern and recurrence risks. The genetic risk assessment enables nurses to identify those family members who may be at risk for disorders with a genetic component so that they can be provided appropriate lifestyle advice, screening recommendations, and possibly reproductive options. Information on standardized pedigree symbols and the construction of a genetic family pedigree is available to the public through the U.S. Surgeon General's Family History Initiative (U.S. Department of Health and Human Services, 2005), and resources are available through the National Genetics Education and Development Centre (2008).

The purpose of drawing the family tree using a genetic family pedigree is to enable medical information to be presented in context of the family structure. Obtaining a genetic family history in this systematic manner helps ensure inclusion of all critical information in the analysis (Skirton, Patch, & Williams, 2005). The process of obtaining a detailed health history and causes of family deaths is as follows:

- Start with the client
- Client's immediate family members
- Client's mother's side of the family
- Client's father's side of the family
- Relatives who have died, including their cause of death

Relatives who are not biologically related, such as those joining the family through adoption or marriage, should also be noted with the appropriate

BOX 7-7
Genetic/Genomic Nursing Assessment

A genetic nursing assessment includes the following information:

- Three-generation pedigree using standardized symbols
- Health history of each family member
- Reproductive history
- Ethnic background of family members (as described by the family)
- Documentation of variations in growth and development of family members
- Individual member and family understanding of causes of health problems that occur in more than one family member
- Identification of questions family members have about potential genetic risk factors in the family
- Identification of communication of genetic health information within the family

should be treated as personal and private information (U.S. Department of Health and Human Services, 1996, 2005).

Drawing the genetic family pedigree or family tree for at least three generations often provides important data about the potential inheritance pattern. When a condition affects both male and female members, and is present in more than one generation, a *dominant condition* is suspected (Fig. 7-1). Conditions that affect mainly male relatives, with no evidence of male-to-male transmission, increase suspicion of an *X-linked recessive condition* (Fig. 7-2). When more than one child is affected of only one set of parents, it may be evidence of an *autosomal recessive condition* (Fig. 7-3).

Nurses should not assume that a condition is genetic merely because more than one family member has it. Family members who are subject to similar environmental influences may have similar conditions without a genetic basis. One such example is a family with a strong history of lung cancer. Bob, a 62-year-old man, was affected by lung cancer. His two brothers and father all died of lung cancer. Bob expressed deep concern about having a genetic predisposition that he could pass on to his grandsons. The family history revealed that Bob's father and every male member of his family worked underground as coal miners from the age of 14 years. In addition, they all smoked at least 20 cigarettes a day from when they were teenagers. None of the women smoked, nor did they work in the mines, and none developed lung cancer. In this family, the cancer could likely be attributed to environmental rather than inherited causes.

pedigree symbol. The reason that relatives who are not biologically related are noted in a pedigree with a special symbol is to identify them as family members who are not at risk for passing on or inheriting harmful genes from the family they have joined.

Obtaining a family genetic history is a nursing skill that requires technical expertise and knowledge of what needs to be asked, as well as sensitivity to personal or distressing topics and an awareness of the ethical issues involved. Box 7-7 outlines the components of a genetic nursing assessment. Information given by patients is considered part of their personal health record and

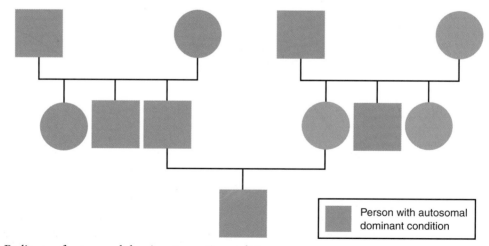

FIGURE 7-1 Pedigree of autosomal dominant genetic condition.

Person with autosomal dominant condition

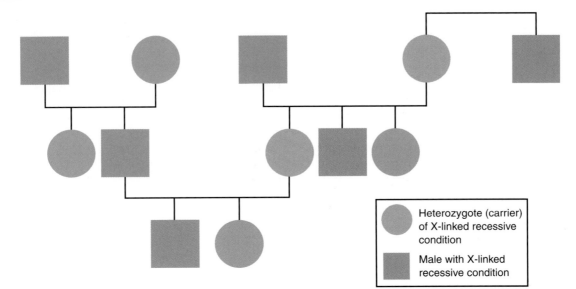

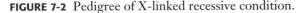

FIGURE 7-2 Pedigree of X-linked recessive condition.

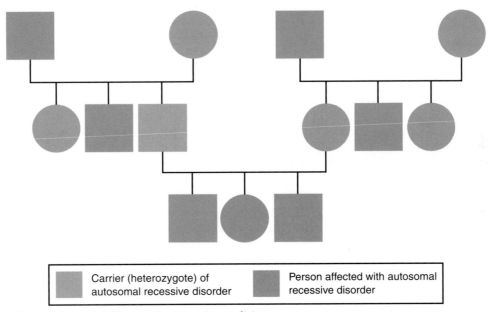

FIGURE 7-3 Pedigree of autosomal recessive genetic condition.

Preconception Assessment and Education

Preconception counseling is an intervention that includes providing information and support to individuals before a pregnancy to promote health and reduce risks (Walfisch & Koren, 2011). It is ideal when a family has the opportunity to discuss difficult genetic decisions before a pregnancy. During a pregnancy, the emotional ties to the existing fetus may complicate the decision-making process for the parents. Preconception counseling enables a couple to explore options without time pressures.

One aspect of preconception education is conducting a health risk profile that includes family history, prescription drug use, ethnic background, occupational and household exposures, diet, specific genetic disorders, and habits such as smoking, alcohol, or street drug use. When nurses identify information that may present a health risk in future offspring, they should explore whether the woman or family wants a more extensive evaluation from a genetic specialist. Box 7-8 provides an example of preconception education for a couple concerned about genetic risks for offspring.

In addition to identifying inherited conditions, preconception counseling includes education regarding other risk factors that could change the outcome of a pregnancy. During preconception counseling, family nurses explain the importance, for instance, of taking an adequate amount of folic acid, one of the B vitamins, which is known to decrease the number of babies born with neural tube defects (NTDs) (Centers for Disease Control and Prevention, 2006). Box 7-9 provides more information about NTDs.

Risk Assessment in Adult-Onset Diseases

Genetic history taking is important in the adult population to assess for risk factors that are pertinent to common diseases, such as cancer and coronary heart disease. The risk assessment is based on the genetic family pedigree, but additional genetic

---

BOX 7-9
Folic Acid Recommendations to Prevent Neural Tube Defects

In 1992, the U.S. Public Health Service recommended that all women capable of becoming pregnant take 0.4 mg/400 g folic acid daily, which is the amount of folic acid in most multivitamins. Although a daily intake of folic acid does not completely rule out the possibility that an infant will have neural tube defects (NTDs), studies have reported an 11% to 20% reduction in cases of anencephaly and a 21% to 34% reduction in cases of spina bifida since this recommendation was issued (Mosley et al., 2009).

---

or biochemical testing may be used to clarify the potential risk to each individual. To ensure privacy, health care providers must obtain consent from all living relatives before accessing their medical records and confirming relevant medical history. Family members who are seeking information are advised of their risks and options for clinical screening and follow-up. One example is the assessment of risk for cancer when there is a strong history of cancer in the family (Gammon, Kohlmann, & Burt, 2007). Individuals who find through counseling and testing that they have an increased risk for cancer may experience psychological difficulties (Kenen, Ardern-Jones, & Eeles, 2006). Nurses must explore feelings of grief and anxiety about the future, as well as beliefs about the inheritance pattern. Providing explanations enables families to understand the information and helps them learn possible options to reduce the risk for cancer in their family members.

BOX 7-8
Preconception Education

Jay and Sara are college students who are planning to be married. Both are of Ashkenazi Jewish ancestry. Although both have heard about Tay-Sachs disease, and the availability of carrier testing, neither has had the carrier test. When Sara visited the student health office, she talked with the nurse about her fears that she may not be able to have healthy babies. She knew that Tay-Sachs disease, a degenerative neurological condition, is more common in Ashkenazi Jewish families, and that no treatment will alter the course of the disease. Sara was interested in learning more about the carrier test. The nurse offered to refer Sara to a genetics specialist, who would help the couple explore the following childbearing options:

- Decide to have or not have biological children
- Have a pregnancy with no form of genetic testing
- Have a preimplantation genetic diagnosis
- Have a pregnancy and have a prenatal genetic diagnosis with an option to terminate an affected fetus
- Have a pregnancy using a donor gamete from a non-carrier donor
- Adopt a child

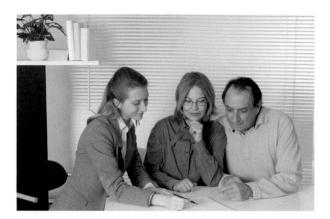

Increasingly, women with a family history of breast or ovarian cancer, or both, are seeking to reduce their risks for these conditions. This is especially true for women whose own mothers died at a relatively young age from breast or ovarian cancers (van Oostrom et al., 2006). All women have a risk for breast cancer (a lifetime risk of about 1 in 11 in the U.S. population) and may be offered mammography screening according to the standards of care or regional health policy (National Institute for Clinical Excellence, 2006). For women with a genetic family history that is consistent with familial breast and ovarian cancer, genetic and familial cancer specialists should discuss earlier and more frequent screening.

With appropriate treatment, some health problems with a major genetic component may improve or at least remain stable. But many genetic conditions lead to increasing loss of health and function throughout the person's life span. These genetic conditions require more and more complex care from both health care providers and the family. In the chronic phase of a genetic condition, individuals and the family not only come to terms with the permanent changes that come with the onset of illness symptoms (Biesecker & Erby, 2008; Truitt, Biesecker, Capone, Bailey, & Erby, 2012), but also must adapt their family routines and roles, and locate needed resources to meet changing health care needs.

Providing Information and Resources

An essential nursing competence includes the need for nurses to be able to identify resources that are useful, informative, and reliable for patients and families. Knowledge of genetics is rapidly changing, and Web-based resources may provide the most current information. Families value the recommendations of health professionals on suitable resources of information (Skirton & Barr, 2008). It is the role of nurses to ensure that recommended Web sites include relevant and evidence-based information. Patients and families have a need for psychosocial and medical information about genetics; therefore, any information that is prepared for distribution should include material on both types of needs (Lewis, Mehta, Kent, Skirton, & Coviello, 2007).

Evaluation of Genomic and Genetic Nursing Interventions

Genomics and genetics are relatively new fields in nursing, but some work has assessed the value of genetic services, including nursing input, for patients and their families. Researchers conducted a study to define nursing outcomes relative to genetics in both the United States and the United Kingdom (Williams et al., 2001). The views of nurses indicated that enhancing patient knowledge of the disease and the genetic risks associated with the disease were important aspects of care. Nurses also believed that offering families psychosocial support was an integral part of their practice. In Skirton's study (2001), patients reported that they gained peace of mind from the care they received, and that increasing their knowledge about the condition, being treated as an individual, and having a warm relationship with the health professionals caring for them were important to the overall outcome of the consultation. Nurses should aim not only to be knowledgeable about genomics but also provide individualized care, and address the needs and specific agendas of each family. Box 7-10 provides

---

BOX 7-10
Evaluation of Nursing Intervention

Fiona is a 5-year-old child who is attending kindergarten. Her teacher is concerned that she does not appear to be progressing as well as expected, and asks the school nurse, Cindy, to check her hearing. Cindy arranges for Fiona's parents to bring her for a hearing test. She asks Fiona's mother about her medical history; the mother says she has always been a well child and has not had any ear infections but has developed some "funny patches" on her skin. They have not caused a problem, but the mother has wondered what they are and if they could turn cancerous. Cindy checks these and notes that they seem to be café-au-lait patches—small, pale brown pigmented areas of the skin. She reassures the parents that the café-au-lait patches are not harmful but could indicate an underlying cause for Fiona's slight learning problems. She draws a genetic family pedigree or family tree (Fig. 7-4) and notes that Fiona's

(continued)

BOX 7-10
Evaluation of Nursing Intervention—cont'd

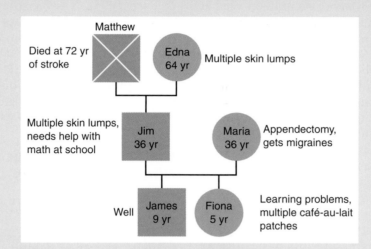

Matthew

Died at 72 yr
of stroke

Edna
64 yr — Multiple skin lumps

Multiple skin lumps,
needs help with
math at school — Jim
36 yr

Maria
36 yr — Appendectomy,
gets migraines

Well — James
9 yr

Fiona
5 yr — Learning problems,
multiple café-au-lait
patches

FIGURE 7-4 Genetic pedigree: Fiona's family tree.

father and his mother (Fiona's paternal grandmother) had unusual skin lumps, but no other medical problems.

When the pediatrician sees the family, she measures Fiona's head circumference and examines her skin. She confirms that the skin marks are café-au-lait patches and that Fiona has eight of them. Fiona's head circumference is larger than average, on the 97th percentile for her age. A diagnosis of neurofibromatosis type 1 is made. The pediatrician explains that this is a genetic condition, but that it could have arisen for the first time in Fiona or may have been inherited from one of her parents. Neither parent is aware of the condition in the family. The pediatrician examines both parents and finds that Fiona's father has a large head circumference and has several raised lumps on the skin, called *neurofibromas.* He tells the pediatrician he needed extra help with math at school, but he finished college and works teaching French. He has never been

concerned about the lumps because his own mother had dozens of them, and apart from having one removed because her shoe was rubbing against it, they did not cause her a problem.

The pediatrician is aware that children with this condition may have learning problems. She recommends that Fiona be evaluated to identify whether Fiona would benefit from extra help at school. As high blood pressure and malignancies can occur as a result of the condition, she also makes arrangements for Fiona and her father to have an annual checkup. Fiona's brother, James (9 years old), is also examined but has no signs of the condition and does not require any further assessment.

When Cindy is informed of the diagnosis, she helps the family to identify reliable sources of information on the Web and provides Fiona's parents with information about neurofibromatosis organizations.

an example of a nurse's evaluation of interventions with a family whose child has a genetic condition.

Although it is not possible for health professionals to have current knowledge about every condition, nurses exhibit competence in this area by having an awareness of their limitations, being open to discussion, finding appropriate resources, and referring to specialists when required. It is essential that nurses working in all types of settings be prepared with an adequate knowledge base to explain the basis and implications of genetics and genomics.

SUMMARY

- Families share both social and biological ties. Identifying biological risk factors is an essential component of professional nursing practice, and a nursing assessment is incomplete without identifying biological factors that may place individuals or their offspring at risk for genetic conditions.
- Nurses providing care to families across all health care settings and throughout the life

span must maintain current knowledge of genomic aspects of health and risks for illness to assist families in obtaining information and further evaluation if needed.

■ Nurses work with families on assessment, identification of issues influencing family members' health, facilitating appropriate referrals, and evaluating the effect of these activities on the family's health and well-being.

■ Family values, beliefs, and patterns of communication are integral components of how families cope with and respond to family members with medical conditions that have a genetic component.

REFERENCES

Biesecker, B. B., & Erby L. (2008). Adaptation to living with a genetic condition or risk: A mini-review. *Clinical Genetics, 74*(5), 401–407.

Bougie, O., & Weberpals, J. I. (2011). Clinical considerations of *BRCA1*- and *BRCA2*-mutation carriers: A review. *International Journal of Surgical Oncology, Vol 2011*(2011), Article ID 374012.

Centers for Disease Control and Prevention. (2006). Recommendations to improve preconception health and health care: United States. *Morbidity and Mortality Weekly Report, 55* (RR-6), 1–23.

Consensus Panel. (2008). *Essential nursing competencies and curricula guidelines for genetics and genomics.* Retrieved from http://www.genome.gov/Pages/Careers/HealthProfessionalEducation/geneticscompetency.pdf

Feetham, S. L., & Thomson, E. J. (2006). Keeping the individual and family in focus. In S. M. Miller, S. H. McDaniel, J. S. Rolland, & S. L. Feetham (Eds.), *Individuals, families, and the new era of genetics* (pp. 3–33). New York, NY: W. W. Norton.

Feldman, E. A. (2012). Health policy: The Genetic Information Nondiscrimination Act (GINA): Public policy and medical practice in the age of personalized medicine. *Journal of General Internal Medicine, 27*(6), 743–746.

Gaff, C. L., Clarke, A. J., Atkinson, P., Sivell, S., Elwyn, G., Iredale, R., . . ., & Edwards, A. (2007). Process and outcome in communication of genetic information within families: A systematic review. *European Journal of Human Genetics, 15*, 999–1011.

Gaff, C. L., Collins, V., Symes, T., & Halliday, J. (2005). Facilitating family communication about predictive genetic testing: Probands' perceptions. *Journal of Genetic Counseling, 14*(2), 133–139.

Gallo, A. M., Angst, D., Knafl, K. A., Hadley, E., & Smith, C. (2005). Parents sharing information with their children about genetic conditions. *Journal of Pediatric Health Care, 19*(5), 267–275.

Gallo, A. M., Angst, D. B., Knafl, K. A., Twomey, J. G., & Hadley, E. (2010). Health care professionals' views of sharing information with families who have a child with a genetic condition. *Journal of Genetic Counseling, 19*(3), 296–304.

Gallo, A. M., Hadley, E. K., Angst, D. B., Knafl, K. A., & Smith, C. A. M. (2008). Parents' concerns about issues related to their children's genetic conditions. *Journal of the Society for Pediatric Nursing, 13*(1), 4–14.

Gammon, A., Kohlmann, W., & Burt, R. (2007). Can we identify the high-risk patients to be screened? A genetic approach. *Digestion, 76*(1), 7–19.

Genetics Home Reference. (2012). Your guide to understanding genetic conditions. What is direct-to-consumer genetic testing? Retrieved from http://www.ghr.nlm.nih.gov/handbook/testing/directtoconsumer

Hewlett, J., & Waisbren, S. E. (2006). A review of the psychosocial effects of false-positive results on parents and current communication practices in newborn screening. *Journal of Inherited and Metabolic Diseases, 29*, 677–682.

International Society of Nurses in Genetics. (2010). Position statement: Access to genomic healthcare: The role of the nurse. Retrieved from http://www.isong.org/ISONG_PS_access_genomic_healthcare.php

Kenen, R., Ardern-Jones, A., & Eeles, R. (2006). "Social separation" among women under 40 years of age diagnosed with breast cancer and carrying a *BRCA1* or *BRCA2* mutation. *Journal of Genetic Counseling, 15*(3), 149–162.

Levetown & American Pediatric Committee on Bioethics. (2008). Communicating with children and families: From everyday interactions to skill in conveying distressing information. *Pediatrics, 121*(5), e1441–e1160.

Lewis, C., Mehta, P., Kent, A., Skirton, H., & Coviello, D. (2007). An assessment of written patient information relating to genetic testing from across Europe. *European Journal of Human Genetics, 15*, 1012–1022.

Madlensky, L., Esplen, M. J., Gallinger, S., McLauglin, J. R., & Goel, V. (2003). Relatives of colorectal cancer patients: Factors associated with screening behavior. *American Journal of Preventive Medicine, 25*(3), 187–194.

McDaniel, S., Rolland, J., Feetham, S., & Miller, S. (2006). "It runs in the family": Family systems concepts and genetically linked disorders. In S. M. Miller, S. H. McDaniel, J. S. Rolland, & S. L. Feetham (Eds.), *Individuals, families, and the new era of genetics* (pp. 118–138). New York, NY: W. W. Norton.

Mosley, B. S., Cleves, M. A., Siega-Riz, A. M., Shaw, G. M., Canfield, M. A., Waller, D. K., . . ., & Hobbs, C. A. (2009). Neural tube defects and maternal folate intake among pregnancies conceived after folic acid fortification in the United States. *American Journal of Epidemiology, 169*(1), 9–17.

National Comprehensive Cancer Network. (2008). NCCN clinical practice guidelines in oncology. Retrieved from http://www.nccn.org

National Genetics Education and Development Centre. (2008). A competence framework for general practitioners with a special interest in genetics. Retrieved from http://www.geneticseducation.nhs.uk

National Human Genome Research Institute. (2011). Frequently asked questions about genetic testing. Retrieved from http://www.genome.gov/19516567

National Human Genome Research Institute. (2012). Genetics 101 for health professionals. Retrieved from http://www.genome.gov/27527637

National Human Genome Research Institute. (2013). Gene. Retrieved from the Talking Glossary of Genetic Terms at http://www.genome.gov/Glossary/index.cfm?id=70

National Institute for Clinical Excellence. (2006). CG41 familial breast cancer—full guideline (the new recommendations and the evidence they are based on). Retrieved from http://www.nice.org.uk/nicemedia/pdf/CG41fullguidance.pdf

Patenaude, A. F., Dorval, M., DiGianni, L. S., Schineider, K. A., Chiteenden, A., & Garber, J. E. (2006). Sharing *BRCA1/2* test results with first-degree relatives: Factors predicting who women tell. *Journal of Clinical Oncology, 24*(4), 700–706.

Penziner, E., Williams, J. K., Erwin, C., Wallis, A., Bombard, Y., Beglinger, L., . . ., & Paulson, J. S. (2008). Perceptions of genetic discrimination among persons who have undergone predictive testing for Huntington disease. *American Journal of Medical Genetics Part B, 147B,* 320–325.

Peters, K., Apse, K., Blackford, A., McHugh, B., Michalic, D., & Biesecker, B. (2005). Living with Marfan syndrome: Coping with stigma. *Clinical Genetics, 68*(1), 6–14.

Reid Ponte, P., & Peterson, K. (2008). A patient- and family-centered care model paves the way for a culture of quality and safety. *Critical Care Nursing Clinics of North America, 20*(4), 451–464.

Skirton, H. (2001). The client's perspective of genetic counseling—A grounded theory study. *Journal of Genetic Counseling, 10*(4), 311–329.

Skirton, H., & Barr, O. (2008). Antenatal screening: Informed choice and parental consent. Retrieved from http://www.learningdisabilities.org.uk/content/assets/pdf/publications/ANSPAC_Briefing_paper_FINAL_Approved_(2).pdf?view=Standard

Skirton, H., Frazier, L. Q., Calvin, A. O., & Cohen, M. Z. (2006). A legacy for the children: Attitudes of older adults in the United Kingdom to genetic testing. *Journal of Clinical Nursing, 15,* 565–573.

Skirton, H., Patch, C., & Williams, J. (2005). *Applied genetics in healthcare: A handbook for specialist practitioners.* New York, NY: Taylor & Francis.

Soltysiak, B., Gardiner, P., & Skirton, H. (2008). Exploring supportive care for individuals affected by Huntington disease and their family caregivers in a community setting. *Journal of Clinical Nursing, 17*(7B), 226–234.

Sparbel, K. J. H., Driessack, M., Williams, J. K., Schutte, D. L., Tripp-Reimer, T., & McGonigal-Kenney, M. (2008). Experiences of teens living in the shadow of Huntington disease. *Journal of Genetic Counseling, 17*(4), 327–335.

Speice, J., McDaniel, S. H., Rowley, P. T., & Loader, S. (2002). Family issues in a psychoeducation group for women with a *BRCA* mutation. *Clinical Genetics, 62*(2), 121–127.

Stoffel, E. M., Ford, B., Mercado, R. C., Punglia, D., Kohlmann, W., Conrad, P., . . ., & Syngal, S. (2008). Sharing genetic test results in Lynch syndrome: Communication with close and distant relatives. *Clinical Gastroenterology & Hepatology, 6*(3), 333–338.

Tercyak, K. P. (2010). *Handbook of genomics and the family: Psychosocial context for children and adolescents.* Family myths about inheritance. Springer. Retrieved from http://books.google.com/books?id=v8mPfjFpd5QC&pg=PA175&lpg=PA175&dq=family's+pre-selection++beliefs+about+which+members+will+inherit+a+genetic+disorder&source

Tercyak, K. P., Peshkin, B. N., Demarco, T., Patenaude, A. F., Schneider, K. A., Garber, J. E., . . ., & Schwartz, M. D. (2007). Information needs of mothers regarding communicating *BRCA1/2* cancer genetic test results to their children. *Genetic Testing, 11*(3), 249–255.

Tluczek, A., Koscik, R. L., Farrell, P. M., & Rock, M. J. (2005). Psychosocial risk associated with newborn screening for cystic fibrosis: Parents' experience while awaiting the sweat-test appointment. *Pediatrics, 115*(6), 1692–1704.

Truitt, M., Biesecker, M., Capone, G., Bailey, T., & Erby, L. (2012). The role of hope in adaption to uncertainty: The experience of caregivers of children with Down syndrome. *Patient Education and Counseling, 87*(2), 233–238.

23andMe, Inc. (2012). Personal Genome Service. Retrieved from https://www.23andme.com/welcome

U.S. Department of Health and Human Services. (1996). Office for Civil Rights—HIPAA. Medical privacy: National standards to protect the privacy of personal health information. Retrieved from http://www.hhs.gov/ocr/privacy/index.html

U.S. Department of Health and Human Services. (2005). Surgeon General's family history initiative. Retrieved from http://www.hhs.gov/familyhistory

U.S. Government Accountability Office. (2010). *Direct to consumer genetic tests: Misleading test results are further complicated by deceptive marketing and other questionable practices.* Retrieved from http://www.gao.gov/assets/130/125079.pdf

van Oostrom, I., Meijers-Heijboer, H., Duivenvooden, H. J., Brocker-Vriends, A. H., van Asperen, C. J., Sijmons, R. H., . . ., & Tibben, A. (2006). Experience of parental cancer in childhood is a risk factor for psychological distress during genetic cancer susceptibility testing. *Annals of Oncology, 17*(7), 1090–1095.

Walfisch, A., & Koren, G. (2011). Preconception counseling: Rational, practice and challenges. *Minerva Ginecologica, 63*(5), 411–419.

Walsh, F. (2003). *Normal family processes* (3rd ed.). New York, NY: Guilford.

Williams, J. K., Skirton, H., Paulsen, J. S., Tripp-Reimer, T., Jarmon, L., McGonigal Kenney, M., . . ., & Honeyford, J. (2009). The emotional experience of family carers in Huntington disease. *Journal of Advanced Nursing, 65*(4), 789–798.

Williams, J. K., Skirton, H., Reed, D., Johnson, M., Maas, M., & Daack-Hirsch, S. (2001). Genetic counseling outcomes validation by genetics nurses in the UK and US. *Journal of Nursing Scholarship, 33*(4), 369–374.

Williams, J. K., & Sobel, S. (2006). Neurodegenerative genetic conditions: The example of Huntington disease. In S. M. Miller, S. H. McDaniel, J. S. Rolland, & S. L. Feetham (Eds.), *Individuals, families, and the new era of genetics* (pp. 231–247). New York, NY: W. W. Norton.

Wiseman, M., Dancyger, C., & Michie, S. (2010). Communicating genetic risk information within families: A review. *Familial Cancer, 9,* 691–703.

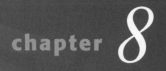

chapter 8

Family Health Promotion

Yeoun Soo Kim-Godwin, PhD, MPH, RN

Perri J. Bomar, PhD, RN

Critical Concepts

- Family health promotion refers to activities that families engage in to strengthen the family unit and increase family unity and quality of family life.

- Health promotion is learned within families, and patterns of health behaviors are formed and passed on to the next generation.

- A major task of the family is to teach health maintenance and health promotion.

- The role of the family nurse is to help families attain, maintain, and regain the highest level of family health possible.

- Family health promotion is the by-product of family interactions with factors outside the home and internal family processes: microsystem, mesosystem, exosystem, and macrosystem.

- Positive, reinforcing interaction between family members leads to a healthier family lifestyle.

- Different cultures define and value health, health promotion, and disease prevention differently. Clients may not understand or respond to the family nurses' suggestions for health promotion because the suggestions conflict with their health beliefs and values.

- Family health promotion should become a regular part of taking a family history and a routine aspect of nursing care.

- A primary goal of nursing care for families is empowering family members to work together to attain and maintain family health; therefore, family health promotion should focus on strengths, competencies, and resources.

Fostering the health of the family as a unit and encouraging families to value and incorporate health promotion into their lifestyles are essential components of family nursing practice. *Family health promotion* refers to the activities that families engage in to strengthen the family as a unit. Family health promotion is defined as achieving maximum family well-being throughout the family life course and includes the biological, emotional, physical, and spiritual realms for family members and the family unit (Fiese & Everhart,

2011; Kim-Godwin & Bomar, 2010). Health promotion is learned within families, and patterns of health behaviors are formed and passed on to the next generation. Families are primarily responsible for providing health and illness care, being a role model, teaching self-care and wellness behaviors, providing for care of members across their life course and during varied family transitions, and supporting each other during health-promoting activities and acute and chronic illnesses. A major task of families is to make efforts toward health maintenance and health promotion, regardless of age. For families, maintaining health and well-being is a collective effort whereby routines are established, relationships are formed that foster health in others, and quality of life is promoted when better health is experienced by multiple members of the household (Fiese & Everhart, 2011).

One of the major functions of the family is to provide health care for its members, including how to promote healthful lifestyles among the family members and the way the family functions together as a whole.

The purpose of this chapter is to introduce the concepts of family health and family health promotion. The chapter presents models to represent these concepts, including the Model of Family Health, Family Health Model, McMaster Model of Family Functioning, Developmental Model of Health and Nursing, Family Health Promotion Model, and Model of the Health-Promoting Family. The chapter also examines internal and external factors through a lens of the bioecological systems theory that influence family health promotion, family nursing intervention strategies for health promotion, and two family case studies demonstrating how different theoretical approaches can be used for assessing and intervening in the family for health promotion.

WHAT IS FAMILY HEALTH?

Definitions of *family health* have evolved from anthropological, biopsychosocial, developmental, family science, cultural, and nursing paradigms. The concept of family health is often used interchangeably with the terms *family functioning, healthy families, resilient families,* and *balanced families* (Alderfer, 2011; Kaakinen & Birenbaum, 2012; Walsh, 2006, 2011a). Family scientists define healthy families as resilient (Black & Lobo, 2008), and as possessing a balance of cohesion and adaptability that is facilitated by good communication (Smith, Freeman, & Zabriskie, 2009). According to Black and Lobo (2008), family resilience factors include a positive outlook, spirituality, family member accord, flexibility, communication, financial management, time together, mutual recreational interests, routines and rituals, and social support (p. 38).

Family therapy definitions of family health often emphasize optimal family functioning and freedom from psychopathology (Goldenberg & Goldenberg, 2007; McGoldrick, Gerson, & Petry, 2008). Furthermore, within the developmental framework, healthy families complete developmental tasks at appropriate times (Carter & McGoldrick, 2005; Duval & Miller, 1985; McGoldrick, Carter, & Garcia-Preto, 2011).

Other definitions of family health focus on the totality, or *gestalt*, of the family's existence, and include the internal and external environment of the family. The health of a family is best described in interactional traits for optimal growth, functioning, and well-being of the family as a whole (Black & Lobo, 2008). A holistic definition of family health encompasses all aspects of family life, including interaction and health care function. A healthy family has a sense of well-being. Different aspects of family functioning that nurses can assess or help promote to encourage overall family health care functions include family nutrition, recreation, communication, sleep and rest patterns, problem solving, sexuality, use of time and space, coping with stress, hygiene and safety, spirituality, illness care, health promotion and protection, and emotional health of family members (Alderfer, 2011; Novilla, 2011).

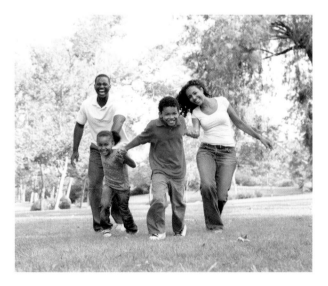

For the purposes of this chapter, *family health* is a holistic, dynamic, and complex state. Family health is more than the absence of disease in an individual family member or the absence of dysfunction in family dynamics. Rather, it is the complex process of negotiating and solving day-to-day family life events and crises, and providing for a quality life for its members (Novilla, 2011). Table 8-1 lists the characteristics of healthy families, illustrating how families can promote health.

COMMON THEORETICAL PERSPECTIVES

Many models and theories are applicable to family health and family health promotion. This section introduces a variety of models or views of family health and family health promotion followed by selected models:

- Family Health Model
- McMaster Model of Family Functioning
- Developmental Model of Health and Nursing
- Family Health Promotion Model
- Model of the Health-Promoting Family

Models of Family Health

Building on Smith's (1983) models of health and illness, Loveland-Cherry and Bomar (2004) suggest

Table 8-1　**Characteristics of Healthy Family**	
Unity **Commitment**	**Time Together**
Has a sense of trust traditions.	Shares family rituals and traditions.
Teaches respect for others.	Enjoys each other's company.
Exhibits a sense of shared responsibility.	Shares leisure time together.
Affirms and supports all of its members.	Shares simple and quality time.
Flexibility **Ability to Deal With Stress**	**Spiritual Well-Being**
Displays adaptability.	Encourages hope.
Sees crises as a challenge and opportunity.	Shares faith and religious core.
Shows openness to change.	Teaches compassion for others.
Grows together in crisis.	Teaches ethical values.
Seeks help with problems.	Respects the privacy of one another.
Opens its boundaries to admit and seek help.	
Communication **Positive Communication**	**Appreciation and Affection**
Communicates well and listens to all members.	Cares for each other.
Fosters family table time and conversation.	Exhibits a sense of humor.
Shares feelings.	Maintains friendship.
Displays nonblaming attitudes.	Respects individuality.
Is able to compromise and disagree.	Has a spirit of playfulness/humor.
Agrees to disagree.	Interacts with each other has a balance in the interactions.

Source: Modified from Kaakinen, J. R., Gedaly-Duff, V., Coehlo, D. P., & Hanson, S. M. H. (Eds.). (2010). *Family health care nursing: Theory, practice and research* (4th ed.). Philadelphia, PA: F. A. Davis; Olson, D. H. L., & Defrain, J. (2003). *Marriage and the family: Diversity and strengths* (4th ed.). New York: McGraw-Hill; and Psychological Studies Institute. (2004, September 15). New study identifies specific behaviors linked to family health. Physician Law Weekly. Retrieved from http://www.newsrx.com/newsletters/Mental-Health-Law-Weekly/2004-08-18/091320043331272MHL.html

that there are four views toward or philosophies of family health:

1. *Family Health—Clinical Model.* The family unit is viewed from this perspective. The family is healthy if its members are free of physical, mental, and family dysfunction.
2. *Family Health—Role-Performance Model.* This view of family health is based on the idea that family health is the ability of family members to perform their routine roles and achieve developmental tasks.
3. *Family Health—Adaptive Model.* In this view, families are healthy if they have the ability to change and grow and possess the capacity to rebound quickly after a crisis.
4. *Family Health—Eudaimonistic Model.* Professionals who use this view as their philosophy of practice focus on a holistic approach to family care to maximize the family's well-being and self-actualization in order to support the entire family and individual members in reaching their maximum health potential.

Table 8-2 reveals how the four models of family health define "family health." Rather than being separate, Smith (1983) suggests that the four views can be viewed as a continuum with the person (or family), going back and forth depending on the circumstances and life events. According to Loveland-Cherry and Bomar (2004), these family health models (views) are useful in three ways: (1) they provide frameworks for understanding the level of health that families are experiencing; (2) they help design interventions to assist families in maintaining or regaining good health, or in coping with illness; and (3) the specific model of family health can facilitate organization of the family nursing literature and to categorize family research.

Family Health Model

Based on family health studies with Appalachian families (Denham 1999a, 1999b, 1999c), and a broad base of literature and existing research about family health, Denham (2003a) has proposed the Family Health Model. Family health is viewed as a process over time of family members' interactions and health-related behaviors. Denham (2011) defines family health as a complex phenomenon comprised of diverse members, systems, interactions, relationships, and processes that hold the potential to maximize well-being, the household production of health, and contextual resources (p. 900). The model emphasizes the biophysical, holistic, and environmental factors that influence health.

In her Family Health Model, Denham (2003a, 2003b) suggests that family health routines offer the means of connecting with health promotion. Family routines are behavior patterns related to events, occasions, or situations that are repeated with regularity and consistency. Family routines have been identified as key structural aspects of family health that can be assessed by nurses, provide a focus for family interventions, and have potential for measuring health outcomes (2003a). Routines supply information about behaviors and

Table 8-2	**Models of Family Health**
Model	**Definition of Family Health**
Clinical model	Lack of evidence of physical, mental, social disease or deterioration, or dysfunction of the family system.
Role-performance model	Ability of the family system to conduct family functions effectively and to achieve family developmental tasks.
Adaptive model	Family patterns of interaction with the environment characterized by flexible, effective adaptation or ability to change and grow.
Eudaimonistic model	The most comprehensive view of health, a holistic view. It includes the ongoing provision of resources, guidance, and support for realization of the family's maximum well-being, self-actualization, and potential throughout the family life span.

Source: Modified from Bomar, P. J. (2004). Introduction to family health nursing and promoting family health. In P. J. Bomar (Ed.), *Promoting health in families: Applying family research and theory to nursing practice* (3rd ed., pp. 3–37). Philadelphia, PA: WB Saunders.

their predictability, member interactions, family identity, and specific ways families live. Denham (2003a) makes the following propositions about family health routines (p. 191):

- Families that tend toward moderation in family health routines are healthier than families who are highly ritualized and those who lack rituals.
- Families with clearer ideas about their goals are more likely to accommodate health needs effectively through their family routines than families who are less certain about their goals.
- Families and individuals are more likely to accommodate changes related to health concerns when family routines are supported over time by embedded contextual systems than families whose routines are not supported.
- Families with routines that support individual health care needs are more likely to achieve positive care outcomes in an individual with health concerns than families who do not have routines that support the needs of family members with health concerns.
- Children who are taught routines in the home and are supported by the embedded context are more likely to practice health routines in the home than those not supported by the embedded context. *Embedded context* is defined as "the ecological environments and nested relationships that affect the family health over the life course" (p. 277).

Denham lists the diverse types of routines, including individual routine, family routine, family health routine, family ritual, family tradition, and family celebration (Denham, 2003a, 2011). Health routines are described as interactions affected by biophysical, developmental, interactional, psychosocial, spiritual, and contextual realms, with implications for the health and well-being of members and family as a whole. Kushner (2007) has said that health routines are the means by which family members deal with everyday health needs in the household context, the way that they teach children health behaviors, and the way they support stress management. In the Family Health Model, Denham (2003a) identifies six categories of family health routines. See Table 8-3.

McMaster Model of Family Functioning

The health of a family is best described as the interactional traits of optimal growth, functioning, and well-being of the family as a whole (Black & Lobo, 2008). The McMaster Model of Family Functioning (MMFF) identifies the elements of the family group and the patterns of transactions among family members that have been found to distinguish between healthy and unhealthy families. The model specifies six domains of functioning proposed to have the greatest impact on the ability of the family to meet basic needs (needs such as food, money, transportation, and shelter), developmental needs of family members and the family unit, and emerging needs ("crises that arise for the family such as job loss, illness, etc.") (Alderfer, 2011, p. 82):

- Problem solving
- Communication
- Roles
- Affective responsiveness
- Affective involvement
- Behavioral control

The McMaster Clinical Rating Scale (MCRS) and Family Assessment Device (FAD) have been developed to assess family health across the six dimensions described by the MMFF. The MCRS is used by clinicians well trained in the McMaster Model, and the FAD is a self-report measure that can be completed by families and scored on each of the MMFF dimensions (Alderfer, 2011). Whereas the MCRS can be rated by observers during a semistructured family interview, the FAD was designed to be completed by family members and their scores averaged. The FAD is widely used and has been translated into approximately 20 different languages (Alderfer, 2011).

Models for Family Health Promotion

A great need exists to encourage health promotion of the whole family unit because health behaviors, values, and patterns are learned within a family context. Family health promotion activities are crucial both during wellness and during illness of a family member. Family health promotion increases family unity and quality of life. According to Pender, Murdaugh, and Parsons (2011), family health promotion involves a family's lifelong efforts to nurture its members, to maintain family cohesion, and

Table 8-3	Types of Family Health Routines	
Family Health Routine	**Aspects of the Routine**	**Description of the Routines**
Self-care routines	Dietary Hygiene Sleep-rest Physical activity and exercise Gender and sexuality	These routines involve patterned behaviors related to usual activities of daily living experienced across the life course.
Safety and prevention	Health protection Disease prevention Smoking Abuse and violence Alcohol and substance abuse	These routines pertain to health protection, disease prevention, avoidance and participation in high-risk behaviors, and effort to prevent unintended injury across the life course.
Mental health behaviors	Self-esteem Personal integrity Work and play Stress levels	These routines have to do with the ways individuals and families attend to self-efficacy, cope with daily stresses, and individuate.
Family care	Family fun (e.g., relaxation, activities, hobbies, vacations) Celebrations, traditions, special events Spiritual and religious practices Pets Sense of humor	These routines include daily activities, traditional behaviors, and special celebrations that give meaning to daily life, and provide shared enjoyment, pleasure, and happiness for multiple members.
Illness care	Decision making related to medical consultation Use of health care services Follow-up with prescribed medical regimens	These routines are the various ways members make decisions related to health care needs; choose when, where, and how to seek supportive health services; and determine ways to respond to medical directives and health information.
Member caregiving	Health teaching (i.e., health, prevention, illness, disease) Member roles and responsibilities Providing illness care Support of member actions	These routines pertain to the ways family members act as interactive caregivers across the life course as they socialize children and adolescents about a wide variety of health-related ideals, participate in specific health and illness care needs, and support members' individual routine patterns.

Source: Denham, S. A. (2003). *Family health: A framework for nursing.* Philadelphia, PA: F. A. Davis, with permission.

to reach a family's greatest potential in all aspects of health.

Family Health Promotion Model

Most models of health promotion focus on the individual. Adapting Pender's (1996) health promotion model, Loveland-Cherry and Bomar (2004) present a family health promotion model. In this model, the likelihood of a family engaging in health-promoting behaviors is influenced by the following general, health-related, and behavior-specific factors:

1. *General influences*
   - Family systems patterns, such as values, communication, interactions, and power
   - Demographic characteristics, such as family size, structure, income, and culture
   - Biological characteristics

2. *Health-related influences*
- Family health socialization patterns
- Family definition of "health"
- Perceived family health status

3. *Behavior-specific influences*
- Perceived barriers to health-promoting behavior
- Perceived benefits to health-promoting behavior
- Prior related behavior
- Family norms regarding health-promoting behavior
- Intersystem support for behavior
- Situational influences
- Internal and environmental family cues

How a family defines family health promotion will influence the likelihood of them planning family unit activities that promote family well-being and cohesion. Family behavioral influences such as perceived barriers or benefits of health-promoting activities of the entire family affect how committed a family will be to continuing or initiating activities that promote health. For example, to encourage a health-promoting family lifestyle, each family member must value and believe there is a benefit to eating together, sharing in activities to maintain the home, or balancing family power. Figure 8-1 depicts the Family Health Promotion Model.

Developmental Model of Health and Nursing

The Developmental Model of Health and Nursing (DMHN) constructed by Canadian scholar F. Moyra Allen in the mid-1970s and 1980s (Allen & Warner, 2002) has a goal of increasing the capacity of families and individuals in health promotion in everyday life situations. The DMHN supports the concept of empowering partnerships, as the model emphasizes health as a process and the capacities all families have, including their potential for growth and change (Black & Ford-Gilboe, 2004). In this interaction model, the nurse's role changes at each phase of the health promotion process, thereby empowering clients toward improving their health status. Examples of nursing functions include the following:

- Focuser, stimulator, and resource producer who involves clients in such tasks as clarifying concerns and goals and thinking about their learning style

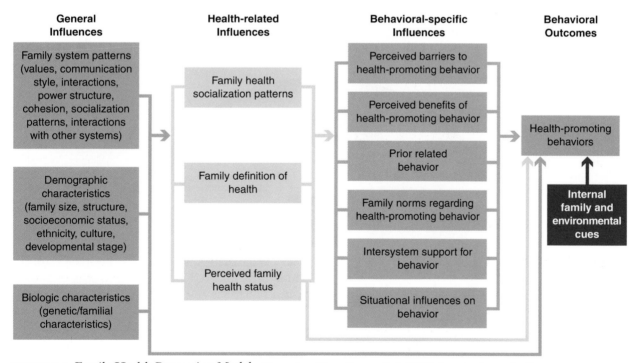

FIGURE 8-1 Family Health Promotion Model. (Reproduced from Bomar, P. J. [2004]. Introduction to family health nursing and promoting family health. In P. J. Bomar [Ed.], *Promoting health in families: Applying family research and theory to nursing practice* [3rd ed., pp. 3–37]. Philadelphia: WB Saunders, by permission.)

- Integrator and awareness raiser who assists clients with analyzing the situation, identifying additional resources, and seeking potential solutions
- Role model, instructor, coach, guide, and encourager as clients make decisions on alternatives and try new behaviors
- Role "reinforcer" and reviewer as clients review and evaluate outcomes (Allen & Warner, 2002, p. 122)

Ford-Gilboe (2002) summarizes six studies that tested the propositions of Allen's DMHN. The studies tested four concepts: health potential, health work, competence in health behavior, and health status. Results indicate significant relationships between health potential and health work. *Health work* is defined "as a process of active involvement though which families develop or learn ways of coping with health situations and using strengths and resources to achieve goals for individual and family development" (pp. 145–146). *Health potential* is defined as "a reservoir of internal and external capacities (i.e., strengths, motivation, resources) that can be drawn on to support health work" (p. 146). In essence, health work reflects what families do in response to health situations rather than who they are or what they have access to (i.e., aspects of health potential). The level of family health potential, health work, and health competence all were found

to be significant predictors of family functioning. Monteith and Ford-Gilboe (2002) also report that health work predicted 24% of the mother's health-promoting lifestyle practices. Similarly, moderate correlations also showed health work and the mother's health-promoting lifestyle practices among 41 adolescent mothers, and the mother's resilience and health work explained 30.2% of the mother's health-promoting lifestyle practices (Black & Ford-Gilboe, 2004).

Model of the Health-Promoting Family

The primary concern of Christensen's (2004) Model of the Health-Promoting Family is the "health practices of the family." The model addresses how families can play a part in promoting both the health of children and their capacities as health-promoting actors. The model draws on contemporary social science approaches to health, family, and children, suggesting a new emphasis on the family's ecocultural pathway, family practices, and the child as a health-promoting factor.

As shown in Figure 8-2, this model is analytically divided into two parts to distinguish factors external to the family and factors internal to it. The external factors are further divided into societal and community-level factors. The societal factors provide the material base for the family and will, therefore, to a large degree shape the resources

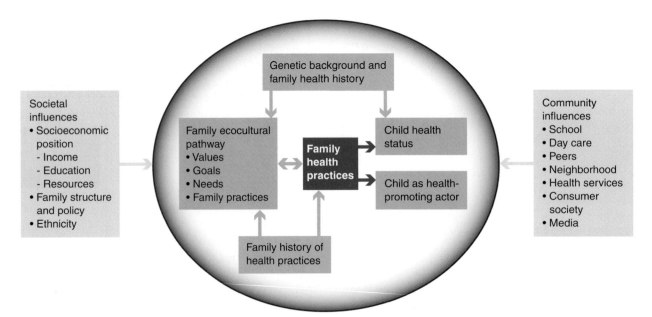

FIGURE 8-2 Model of the Health-Promoting Family. (Reproduced from Christensen, P. [2004]. The health-promoting family: A conceptual framework for future research. *Social Science & Medicine, 59,* 377–387, by permission.)

available to the family. These include, for example, income and wealth, education and knowledge, family structure and housing, ethnicity, social networks, and time. The community level is the configuration of social spheres that contribute to child health. These include the consumer society, local community, schools, health services, mass media, peer groups, and day-care institutions.

The components of the model central to the conception of the family and the processes that may be thought of as going on "inside" it are indicated with a semipermeable boundary—the circle. These are linked to and influenced by the processes and factors "outside" of the family. The internal level has the "family ecocultural pathway" and "family health practices" as the main elements. By interacting with each other, these elements lead to collective patterns of health action, practice, and forms of knowledge. An important feature of the model is that it will allow differences between families to be revealed by identifying the conditions for a family to act in an optimal way for health. It also highlights the obstacles for families in promoting the health and well-being of children, and the barriers to enabling the child's development as a health-promoting actor during her growth.

Family health practices fall into the center of the circle (internal factors), and include all those activities of everyday life that shape and influence the health of family members. These consist of the traditional health practices around food and healthy eating, physical activity, alcohol and smoking, and care and connection, as well as other key factors that can be shown to affect young people's health and well-being.

Although family health promotion has received considerable emphasis in nursing in the past decade, reports on the effectiveness of family-focused health promotion continue to be scanty. Therefore, continued research is required using family health promotion models to evaluate the effectiveness of interventions to promote family health.

ECOSYSTEM INFLUENCES: BIOECOLOGICAL SYSTEMS THEORY

The ecological approach, first proposed by Bronfenbrenner (1977), is useful to understand the multidimensional aspect of family health promotion. (See Chapter 3 for a conceptual understanding and explanation of this model.) Family health promotion is one of the by-products of family interactions with factors and systems outside the home and internal family processes. This approach attends to the interactions among the system levels:

- Microsystem
- Mesosystem
- Exosystem
- Macrosystem

The microsystem pertains to individual factors, such as biology, personal experience, and general demographics (e.g., age, gender, and education). The mesosystem refers to the interactions between the individuals and their close relationships with partners, peers, and families. The exosystem refers to the community contexts for the family, such as schools, places of work, and neighborhoods. Macrosystems are considered the broad cultural attitudes, ideologies, and belief systems that have influence on the family health choices (Lucea, Glass, & Laughon, 2011). This section explores how the ecosystem influences the quality of family life and family health.

Exosystem and Macrosystem Influences on Family Health

Both the exosystem and the macrosystem influence family decisions, actions, and interactions that contribute to the health of family members. Some specific external influences include the national economy, family and health policy, societal and cultural norms, media, and environmental hazards such as noise, air, soil, crowding, and chemicals. We explore some specific exosystem and macrosystem influences below.

Economic Resources

The national economy directly affects the family's ability to promote health. As a general matter, during economic downturns, health promotion initiatives tend to take a back seat to other, more pressing needs. More pointedly, the availability of jobs and, in turn, discretionary funds, directly affects the quality of a family's lifestyle. Clear disparities exist between health promotion in middle-class families and in low-income families (Edburg, 2013). See Chapter 5 for more on family social policy and health disparities.

Socioeconomic class is a determinant of health promotion. When a family has economic health, it has the resources needed for family health promotion. Adequate family income contributes to emotional well-being and supplies resources for adequate family space, recreation, and leisure. Low-income families, by contrast, are less likely to engage in health-promoting and preventive activities than middle- and upper-class families. The cost of buying recreational and exercise equipment, for example, is often beyond the means of low-income families. The activities of low-income families (and government policy aimed at them) are often directed toward meeting basic needs—providing for food, shelter, and safety, and curing acute illness—rather than preventing illness or promoting health. Low-income families often have disproportionately high utilization of emergency department (ED) and hospital services, and low utilization of preventive visits (Holland et al., 2012).

Governmental Health and Family Policies

Health and family policies at all governmental levels affect the quality of individual and family health. Many of the objectives in *Healthy People 2020* are couched in terms of the individual; many of these objectives, however, can be attained only by providing access to health care and require changing family health lifestyles (Holland et al., 2012; Wang, Orleans, & Gortmaker, 2012). For example, local communities provide water and monitor its quality, maintain sanitation, develop and maintain parks for recreation, and provide health services to low-income and elderly families. Such local services enhance the health of individuals and, thus, enhance family health. At the state level, services include assistance with medical care through Medicaid, the maintenance of state recreational areas and parks, health promotion and prevention programs, and economic assistance for low-income families and children (Anderson, Ward, & Hatton, 2008).

Federal-level policies and fiscal support are needed to improve the quality of family health. Because of the number of different government agencies involved in health care and family issues, a need exists for collaboration among these policy-making bodies. Box 8-1 summarizes the brief historical perspectives of family health promotion.

Environment

Awareness of the quality of the family living environment is crucial because the family and its members are exposed to public, occupational, and residential hazards. Environmental health is one of the areas of emphasis of the *Healthy People 2020* objectives. Box 8-2 lists the major objectives specific to families. Many environmental hazards are not monitored consistently by families or organizations. Therefore, it is imperative to increase the capacity of families to recognize environmental hazards and to teach strategies to prevent, remove, or cope with environmental hazards such as pollution of air, water, food, and soil from numerous chemicals, occupational hazards, and violence (Cowan, 2008). For instance, to prevent exposure to lead and pesticides, families could be taught to wash fruits and vegetables before eating. Workers should be taught to monitor chemicals and infectious materials that might be transmitted to them and their families on work clothing or skin. In addition, paint in older homes and outside play areas should be inspected for lead contamination. Families with young children and workers who work around metals and chemicals need to be especially cautious of lead poisoning, and should consult Web sites such as the Centers for Disease Control and Prevention (CDC) for additional information.

Media

Another influence on family health is the visual and print media. Media influence on children has steadily increased as new and more sophisticated types of media have been developed and made available to the public. Recent evidence raises concerns about the media influence on aggression, sexual behavior, substance use, disordered eating, and academic difficulties. Consistent evidence has been reported that violent imagery in television, film and video, and computer games has substantial short-term effects on arousal, thoughts, and emotions, increasing the likelihood of aggressive or fearful behavior in younger children (Strasburger, Jordan, & Donnerstein, 2010).

Long-term mental health risk for early childhood violent media exposure was reported by Fitzpatrick, Barnett, and Pagani (2012). They examined whether preschool child exposure to what

BOX 8-1
Historical Perspectives of Family Health Promotion

Although the majority of health care professionals continue to focus their activities on prevention and treatment of illness in individuals and dysfunctional families, key social forces, including the wellness and self-care movement started in 1979, continue to stimulate the nursing profession to focus on health promotion for families. The 1980 White House Conference on Families pointed out the need to improve family functioning and encourage healthy family lifestyles. The conference brought to light the importance of disease prevention and health promotion for improving the quality of family life in the United States. Three documents from the U.S. DHHS—*Healthy People: The Surgeon General's Report on Health Promotion and Disease Prevention* (1979); *Promoting Health/Preventing Disease: Objectives for the Nation* (1980); and *Healthy People 2000: National Health Promotion and Disease Prevention Objectives* (1990)—provided overall goals for the nation regarding health promotion for individuals and families.

Although there were many improvements in the health status of the nation as a whole, *Healthy People 2010* (USDHHS, 2000) builds on the lessons learned from the three previous initiatives. The goals for 2010 through 2020 are to eliminate health disparities and to increase the quality and years of life. Major objectives for the millennium include promoting healthy behaviors, promoting healthy and safe communities, improving systems for personal and public health, and preventing and reducing diseases and disorders.

Since the first report by the surgeon general in 1979 and the continued national interest in health promotion in the 1990s, health professionals, family scientists, sociologists, psychologists, religious leaders, and social workers have made considerable strides in understanding and intervening to improve the quality of family health. Another example of this continuing national interest in health promotion is the increasing use of parish nurses, who provide health care and health promotion to individuals and families in faith communities (Solari-Twadell, McDermott, & Matheus, 1999).

BOX 8-2
Healthy People 2020 Environmental Objectives Specific to Families

Objective Short Title

WATER QUALITY

EH-4: Increase access to safe drinking water
EH-5: Reduce waterborne disease outbreaks
EH-6: Increase water conservation
EH-7: Reduce surface water health risks

TOXICS AND WASTE

EH-8: Reduce blood lead levels in children
EH-9: Reduce risks posed by hazardous sites
EH-10: Reduce pesticide exposures
EH-11: Reduce toxic pollutants in the environment

HEALTHY HOMES AND HEALTHY COMMUNITIES

EH-13: Reduce indoor allergens
EH-14/15: Increase homes tested for radon

EH-16: Implement school policies to protect against environmental hazards
EH-17/18: Increase lead-based paint testing
EH-19: Reduce the number of occupied substandard housing

OTHER ENVIRONMENTAL OBJECTIVES SPECIFIC TO CHILDREN

24-2a: Reduce asthma-related hospitalizations of children younger than 5
TU-11: Reduce the proportion of nonsmokers exposed to secondhand smoke
TU-14: Increase the proportion of smoke-free homes

Source: U.S. Department of Health and Human Services. (2012). *Healthy People 2020.* Washington, DC. Retrieved from http://healthypeople.gov/2020/topicsobjectives2020/objectiveslist.aspx?topicId=12

parents generally characterize as violent television programming predicts a range of second-grade mental health outcomes, and reported that child exposure to televised violence was associated with teacher-reported antisocial symptoms, emotional distress, inattention, and lower global academic achievement in second grade. Violent viewing also was associated with less child-reported academic self-concept and intrinsic motivation in second grade (Fitzpatrick et al., 2012).

Many advertisements advocate drinking alcohol, using tobacco products, and consuming foods that are high in sugar, salt, and fat. Increasingly, tobacco, alcohol, and illicit drugs have been glamorized in the media. Tobacco manufacturers spend $6 billion per year and alcohol manufacturers $2 billion per year in advertising that appeals to children ("Influence on Children Media," 2008). Movies and television programs often show the lead character or likeable characters using and enjoying tobacco and alcohol products.

At the same time, the readily available and rapidly increasing media outlets put more emphasis on health in a positive way (Lee, 2008). Relatively recent tobacco advertising regulations, for instance, take a small step in the right direction toward promoting healthier families. The regulations prohibit tobacco advertisements near schools, on T-shirts, and in magazines for teens. Many states require that cigarettes not be in the reach of minors in retail stores (CDC, 2012). In fact, one of the *Healthy People 2020* objectives is to reduce the proportion of adolescents and young adults in grades 6 through 12 who are exposed to tobacco advertising and promotion (U.S. Department of Health and Human Services [USDHHS], 2012).

The American Academy of Pediatrics (AAP) (2010) has offered comprehensive recommendations to address the issue of media influence on children. Included in these recommendations are suggestions for parents, practitioners, schools, entertainment industry, advertising industry, researchers, and government to protect children and adolescents from harmful media effects and to maximize the powerfully prosocial aspects of modern media. In addition, the AAP urges media producers to be more responsible in their portrayal of violence. It advocates for more useful and effective media ratings. Specifically, it recommends proactive parental involvement in children's media experiences. By monitoring what children hear and see, discussing issues that emerge, and sharing media time with their children, parents can moderate the negative influences and increase the positive effects of media in the lives of their children (AAP, 2010).

Science and Technology

Advances in science and technology have increased the life span of Americans, decreased the length of hospital stays, and contributed to our understanding of how to prevent, reduce, and treat disease. The development of more effective medications and advanced medical equipment technology has greatly increased the feasibility of home health care for chronically ill family members of all ages. Families are often the caregivers for ill members, and they provide the majority of care to older adults. Many valuable sources of information on health promotion for families and individuals are now available. The Internet and the use of the worldwide Web is one forum that has come of age in the areas of family life education and nutrition education (Silk et al., 2008; Välimäki, Nenonen, Koivunen, & Suhonen, 2007).

Other technological advances are changing how we provide health care. The use of remote patient monitoring, often referred to as telehealth, has been widely adopted by health care providers, particularly home care agencies (Suter, Suter, & Johnston, 2011). Most agencies have invested in telehealth to facilitate the early identification of disease exacerbation, particularly for patients with chronic diseases such as heart failure and diabetes. For example, telehealth permits families to transmit heart rates via telemedicine to health care providers and for specialists to consult with family physicians, making it easier for individuals to access health care and for practitioners to provide it (Gregoski et al., 2012). Suter et al. (2011) proposed that the use of telehealth by home care agencies and other health care providers be expanded to empower patients and promote disease self-management with resultant improved health care outcomes. Telehealth has the potential to improve health care access, quality, and efficiency.

Microsystem and Mesosystem Influences on Family Health

Internal ecosystem influences on family health include family type and developmental stage, family lifestyle patterns, family processes, personalities of family members, power structure, family role models, coping strategies and processes, resilience, and culture. All of these factors are interrelated. For example, a family's lifestyle cycle stage influences a family's structural pattern, and family structures affect the family interaction process and relationships (McGoldrick et al., 2011). Therefore, nurses working with families in the area of health promotion must be sensitive to these various factors to recommend successful family health promotion interventions.

Family Structure

Families in this millennium are quite different structurally from the families of the 1970s. Family structures are more diverse; there are more dual-career/dual-earner families, blended families, same-sex couples, and single-parent families (Kaakinen & Birenbaum, 2012). Recently, increasing numbers of grandparents raising grandchildren have been reported (Leder, Grinstead, & Torres, 2007). Families in both the middle and lower classes are in such economic strain that they both struggle with health promotion. The number of vulnerable families has also increased, including low-income traditional families, low-income migrant families, homeless families, and low-income older adults. Included in the vulnerable population are low-income, single-parent families and single-parent teen families. Vulnerable families are coping with a pileup of stressors and may be unable to focus on activities to enhance health (Walsh, 2011a). As stated earlier, low-income families may focus less on health promotion and more on basic needs of obtaining shelter, adequate food, and health care.

Health promotion for these different families presents various challenges. For example, a single, working parent may lack parent-child time, experience role stress, and have poor lifestyle patterns and poor life satisfaction (Walsh, 2011a). Data from the 2002, 2006, and 2010 Scottish Health Behavior in School-aged Children (HBSC) surveys indicate that in single-mother homes, having a working mother was also positively associated with irregular breakfast consumption (Levin, Kirby, & Currie, 2012). Similarly, the findings of the Canadian Community Health Survey indicated that there is an association between household structure and smoking among adolescents in Canada. The odds of youth smoking in the single-parent household was 1.78 times greater than the odds of youth smoking in two-parent households (Razaz-Rahmati, Nourian, & Okoli, 2011). Family structure is associated with a range of adolescent risk behaviors, including smoking, drinking, cannabis use, having sex, and fighting (Levin et al., 2012). Those adolescents living in a family with both parents present fared better than those who lived with single parents.

Family Processes

Family processes are continual actions, or a series of changes, that take place in the family experience. Essential processes of a healthy family include functional communication and family interaction (Smith et al., 2009). Through both verbal and nonverbal communication, parents teach behavior, share feelings and values, and make decisions about family health practices. It is through communication that families adapt to transitions and develop cohesiveness (Smith et al., 2009). Positive, reinforcing interaction between family members leads to a healthier family lifestyle. For example, when family members encourage, express affection, and show appreciation to each other, the family tends to be more functional (healthier).

Family Culture

Cultures define and value health, health promotion, and disease prevention differently (Meyer, Toborg, Denham, & Mande, 2008; Spector, 2013). One of the most evident features of families today is the growing cultural diversity (Walsh, 2011b). A mounting trend is toward a global society with ever-increasing diversity among the populations; therefore, an expanded worldview is necessary for health care students and providers (Purnell, 2013). Clients may not understand or respond to a family nurse's suggestions for health promotion because the suggestions conflict with their own health beliefs and values. Hence, it is crucial to assess and understand the family culture and health beliefs before suggesting changes in health behavior (Spector, 2013). An important component of family assessment is the consideration of cultural health practices. These practices influence all aspects of the nursing process, and understanding them helps the nurse evaluate client behavior and plan more effective interventions that are consistent with client health beliefs.

Keep in mind with regard to family culture that cultural tension or an acculturation gap may emerge between immigrant children and their parents relative to beliefs about healthful behavior (Birman & Poff, 2011). Children become involved in the new culture relatively quickly, particularly if they attend school, but their parents may never acquire sufficient comfort with the new language and culture to become socially integrated into their new country. In addition, immigrant children may have few opportunities to participate in and learn about their heritage culture (Birman & Poff, 2011). Therefore, nurses need to be aware that parents and children may misunderstand one another because of cultural differences in expectations for parent and child behaviors and family relationships. In addition, immigrant parents may have strict and controlling parenting styles in their heritage culture that are considered warm and attentive to the child, but that in the host culture are considered authoritarian (Farver, Xu, Bhadha, Narang, & Lieber, 2007). At the same time, children may embrace the opportunity to engage in unsupervised activities and behaviors that may be normative in the host society (such as sexual activity, drinking alcohol, eating fast foods, or recreational drug use) but unacceptable in their heritage culture and to their parents (Birman & Poff, 2011). The children taking on unhealthful behaviors of the new culture interferes with the health promotion function of the parents, so there is a tension between society and the family socialization function.

Family Lifestyle Patterns

Lifestyle patterns affect family health. In North America, hundreds of thousands of unnecessary deaths occur each year that can be directly attributed to unhealthy lifestyles. These deaths can be traced back to heart disease, hypertension, cancer, cirrhosis of the liver, diabetes, suicide, mental health, and homicide. For example, parental smoking is associated with a significantly higher risk of their adolescent children smoking (Gillman et al., 2009).

Likewise, positive lifestyle patterns affect families in positive ways. For instance, when family members engage often in leisure activities, recreation, and exercise, they are able to cope with day-to-day problems better (Smith et al., 2009). Time together promotes family closeness. Healthy lifestyle practices such as good eating habits, good sleep patterns, proper hygiene, and positive approaches to stress management are passed from one generation to another (McGoldrick et al., 2008). In addition, when one family member initiates a health behavior change, other family members often make a change too. For example, when an individual family member changes eating patterns, perhaps by going on a diet, other family members often change their eating patterns as well.

Family Nutrition

Family nutrition is a crucial aspect of 21st century family health promotion and health protection. A major issue today for American families is the tendency toward overweight and lack of exercise among family members of all ages. Major factors that influence nutritional health are societal trends (technology, media, fast food, status), the family system (rituals, mealtime, environment, culture, values, communication, finances, marital status), and individual characteristics (self-concept, age, activity levels) (Epstein, Roemmich, &, Robinson, 2008; Levin et al., 2012; Musick & Meier, 2012; Smith et al., 2008; Spector, 2013).

"Overnutrition" in American families is often the issue rather than malnutrition (Levin et al., 2012). A result of societal and family changes is that obesity in children and adolescents is a key 21st-century issue (USDHHS, 2011). Effective parenting, health teaching about nutrition, physical activity, and consideration of the family context are reported to be essential to reducing childhood obesity (Kitzmann, 2008). For example, lowering TV-viewing time by 1 hour per day could reduce approximately 100 kcal/day through reducing eating while watching, exposure to food and beverage advertising, and sedentary behavior. Increasing physical activity and reducing sedentary behaviors are clearly important strategies to restore youth energy balance (Epstein et al., 2008; Sonneville & Gortmaker, 2008).

The nurses' role in family nutrition is to assess the quality of nutrition for individuals and the family system, provide anticipatory guidance, teach about nutrition, and support changes in the individual and family nutritional lifestyle. For example, one of the primary issues for people is large portion size. To promote weight loss and control, the family cook and members could be taught the appropriate portion size according to age and nutritional guidelines. The nurse can become familiar with the most current guidelines in the *Dietary Guidelines for Americans 2010* published by the USDHHS (2011).

Religion and Spirituality

Religion and spirituality are factors that influence the quality of family life. Many fundamental family beliefs are founded in religion and spirituality. Spirituality and religious beliefs appear to serve as powerful protectors embraced by resilient families (Black & Lobo, 2008).

Although often used interchangeably, the terms *religion* and *spirituality* are different (Koenig, 2012). Religion tends to relate to the expression of beliefs and includes a relationship with God or some supernatural power. Spirituality provides transcendence, meaning, and compassion for others. Pivotal life events such as births, marriage, life-threatening illness, tragedy, and death are situations that may spark a family's interest in spirituality (Burkhart, 2011).

Religion aids in family coping responses and is reported to provide support for selected caregivers (Burkhart, 2011). Membership in a church is often an avenue to gain supportive networks for family members (Carson & Koenig, 2011; Koenig, 2012; Walsh, 2011a). The social support of religion and the clergy can be particularly helpful during family transitions. Many faith communities sponsor support groups that are a valuable resource for single parents, stepfamilies, single adults, the bereaved, widows and widowers, the unemployed, and parents of young children.

Spirituality may or may not be religion based, but whatever the spiritual orientation, families associated with a shared internal value system that provides meaning tend to feel a connection with the family, community, and universe (Walsh, 2011a). Family spirituality provides the basis for harmony, communication, and wholeness among family members (Black & Lobo, 2008). A shared belief system of hope and triumph enables families to make sense of crisis or change. When confronted with problems, many families foster an optimistic attitude with spirituality, seeking purpose in faith. Spirituality has also been found to be an essential factor of resilience, as it provides families with the ability to unite, understand, and overcome stressful situations (Black & Lobo, 2008). Religiosity is reported to have a strong positive relationship to parent-adolescent attachment, family functioning, and adolescent psychological adjustment in the United States and Ireland (Goeke-Morey et al., 2013; Kim-Spoon, Longo, & McCullough, 2012).

The positive effect of spirituality is pervasive in health care for the lives of many families; therefore, a need exists to integrate spiritual assessment and interventions in total family care (Black & Lobo, 2008). Four nursing diagnoses related to family spiritual health are (1) spiritual distress, (2) readiness for enhanced spiritual well-being, (3) risk for spiritual distress, and (4) impaired religiosity, both risk for and actual (NANDA International, 2012). Spiritual distress is a disruption in the harmony of life and pervades the entire person's or family's universe. To provide holistic care, nurses should assess a family's spiritual health in a nonjudgmental manner by supporting the family's spiritual beliefs, assisting families to meet their spiritual needs, providing spiritual resources for family transitions and lifestyle changes, and assisting families to find meaning in their circumstances (Carson & Koenig, 2011). Last, to foster a family's spiritual well-being, the nurse should listen, be encouraging and empathetic, show vulnerability, and demonstrate commitment.

FAMILY NURSING INTERVENTIONS FOR FAMILY HEALTH PROMOTION

Family health promotion has been defined as the process by which families work to improve or maintain the physical, social, emotional, and spiritual well-being of the family unit and its members (Loveland-Cherry, 2011). Family nurses have a crucial role in facilitating health promotion and wellness within the family context across the life span. Enhancing the well-being of the family unit is essential during periods of wellness, as well as during illness, recovery, and stress. A primary goal of nursing care for families is empowering family members to work together to attain and maintain family health; therefore, family health promotion should focus on strengths, competencies, and resources (Gottlieb, 2013; Wright & Leahey, 2013). Family nursing that focuses on health promotion should be logical, systematic, and include the client(s). The outcomes of health promotion of the family include family unity, flexibility, communication, and quality of care (Loveland-Cherry, 2011).

A myriad of strategies and interventions facilitate family health promotion, such as empowerment, promotion of family integrity, maintenance of family process, exercise promotion, environmental management, mutual goal setting, parent education, offering information, drawing forth family support, and anticipatory guidance (Loveland-Cherry, 2011; Wright & Leahey, 2013). The interventions have focused on building resources in families and promoting changes in families. A number of the interventions center on fostering the development of parents' self-efficacy in effective parenting and accessing resources to meet family health needs

(Loveland-Cherry, 2011). The following strategies will be discussed for promoting family health: family self-care contract, family empowerment and family strengths-based nursing care, anticipatory guidance and offering information, use of rituals/routines and family time, and family meal and healthy eating.

Family Self-Care Contract: Involvement of All Family Members

The family and nurse must collaborate and set mutual goals by establishing a nursing contract. The nursing contract is a working agreement that is continuously renegotiable and may or may not be written depending on the situation (Anderson et al., 2008). The premise of contracting is that it is under the family's control, it increases the family's ability to make healthy choices, and this process facilitates family empowerment by collaborating with a health professional (Anderson et al., 2008).

Once the nurse and family have identified family strengths and areas for growth and change, the family should prioritize its goals. The commitment of all family members directed toward achieving a goal is crucial to the family's success. Nurses can assist a family to develop a self-care contract to improve health behaviors, independently or with a nurse. Table 8-4 provides components and sample items of a family self-care contract. The contracts are more effective when the components are negotiated and signed by all family members (Kim-Godwin & Bomar, 2010).

Family provides resources for health behaviors and health care. These resources include monetary support, information, emotional support, skills to navigate systems, and direction on desirable or healthy behaviors (Loveland-Cherry, 2011). Families are responsible for the health care of their members. These responsibilities include required immunizations and health checks; providing adequate shelter, clothing, and food; and seeking health care when warranted (Loveland-Cherry, 2011). Socialization of family members is another major function in families and is accomplished in a variety of ways. Parents are important role models for children.

| Table 8-4 | Components of a Family Self-Care Contract |

Component of the Contracting Process (Mutually Agreed on By Family Members and Health Professional or By Family Alone)	Example of Item in a Family Contract
Family assessment of wellness and identification of area for improvement	Our family feels a sense of always being hurried with no time to relax, and we are irritable with each other.
Set the goal, environmental planning, and reinforcement	We want to have more relaxing time together as a family and to enjoy our time together.
Develop a plan	Have a family meeting to evaluate barriers and create a plan. The outcome might be to reduce sports activities for children. Specify a family fun night/afternoon.
Assign responsibilities	Plan an evening game night with no television or phone calls allowed.
	All members agree on the game or recreation activity. No one else but the family should participate. Evaluate the budget for games. The family nurse will assist the family to create the plan. Family members will agree to take part in the family fun time.
Determination of time frame	We plan to do this for 2 months, one night a week on Sunday evening from 4:00 p.m. to 7:00 p.m.
Evaluate the outcomes	After each week, we will spend 5 minutes talking about what was good and what could be improved. How are we relating to each other the remainder of the week?
Modify, renegotiate, or terminate	We will evaluate the family fun time after 2 months and mutually agree on changes.

Source: Kim-Godwin, Y. S., & Bomar, P. (2010). Family health promotion. In J. R. Kaakinen, V. Gedaly-Duff, D. P. Coehlo, & S. M. H. Hanson (Eds.), *Family health care nursing* (4th ed.). Philadelphia, PA: F. A. Davis, with permission.

Family members provide both negative and positive role models. For example, smoking, use of drugs and alcohol, poor nutrition, and inactivity are often intergenerational patterns. Stress management, exercise, and communication are also learned from parents, siblings, and extended family members such as grandparents (McGoldrick et al., 2008). One interesting finding of note to nurses is that fathers' involvement is especially important for vulnerable families. Marsiglio (2009) reported that fathers' lack of exercise, poor eating, excessive drinking, and smoking predicts the same behaviors among adolescents. Shapiro, Krysik, and Pennar (2011) analyzed mother-reported data in families eligible for the Healthy Families Arizona prevention program ($N = 197$) and found that families with greater father involvement had better prenatal care, higher incomes, less maternal involvement in Child Protective Services, less physical domestic violence, and greater maternal mental health reflected through less loneliness. Therefore, nurses need to make an effort to include fathers when developing plans for family health promotion and to assist fathers to develop positive role models for their children. By teaching healthy lifestyle in the community, faith-based centers, homes, and the workplace, nurses promote positive role modeling.

Family Empowerment and Family Strengths-Based Nursing Care

A primary goal of nursing care for families is empowering family members to work together to attain and maintain family health; therefore, family health promotion should focus on strengths, competencies, and resources (Gottlieb, 2013; Wright & Leahey, 2013). The nurse collaborates with the family and provides information, encouragement, and strategies to help the family make lifestyle changes. This process is termed *empowerment*. The underlying assumption of empowerment is one of partnership between the professional and the client as opposed to one in which the professional is dominant. Families are assumed to be either competent or capable of becoming competent (Anderson et al., 2008).

The primary emphasis in family empowerment is involvement of the family in goal setting, planning, and acting, not on having the nurse do this for the family. A key role of family nurses in family health promotion is to empower family members to value their "oneness," to appreciate family togetherness, and to plan activities to foster their unity (Gottlieb, 2013).

One way of empowering a family is the use of commendation because it enables families to view the family problems differently and move toward solutions that are more effective. Wright and Leahey (2013) recommend that nurses routinely commend family and individual strengths, competencies, and resources observed during the family interview. According to Wright and Leahey (2013), commendations to families regarding their strengths are "powerful, effective and enduring therapeutic interventions" (p. 150). While this intervention is important for all families, it is especially important for vulnerable families. Often, a family has unique strengths that are temporarily overshadowed by the health needs, so these strengths lie outside of the family's awareness (Walsh, 2011a). By commending a family's competence and strengths, and offering it a new opinion of itself, a context for change is created that allows families to discover their own solutions to problems (Gottlieb, 2013; Wright & Leahey, 2013).

The strengths-based approach has been used in health promotion, to enhance wellness and well-being. Working with strengths enables a person to get the most out of living in order to cope, recover, heal, and discover a new purpose and meaning in living. Strengths-based nursing care does not ignore or negate problems; neither does it turn a blind eye to weaknesses or deficits. Instead, it uses strengths to balance or overcome them (Gottlieb, 2013, p. 24). Working with the person's and family's strengths allows patients to maximize and support their responses in order to deal with everyday events and difficult life challenges (including illness, injury, disability, and trauma) and to meet their goals (Gottlieb, 2013). Strengths can be biological, intrapersonal and interpersonal, and social. Biological strengths are related to the biochemical, genetic, hormonal, and physical qualities within each individual or family. Intrapersonal and interpersonal strengths reside in the person and define one's personhood and are considered a part of a person's or a family's inner resources. Social strengths, commonly known as resources or assets, reside in the person's environment and are available to individuals or the family (Gottlieb, 2013).

Anticipatory Guidance and Offering Information

During their life course, families inevitably experience crises and either normative or nonnormative stress. The family's resilience, unity, and resources influence how they cope with crisis and stress. The goal of the family nurse is to facilitate family adaptation by empowering the family to promote resilience, reduce the pileup of stressors, make use of resources, and negotiate necessary changes to enhance the family's ability to rebound from stressful events or crises. The nurse can teach families to anticipate life changes, make the necessary adjustments in family routines, evaluate roles and relationships, and cognitively reframe events.

Nurses should offer information based on family abilities and should encourage family members to seek resources independently (Wright & Leahey, 2013). Families usually desire information about developmental issues and health promotion. For example, helping parents to understand and help their children is an important intervention for families (Wright & Leahey, 2013). Nurses can teach families about physiological, emotional, and cognitive characteristics, as well as identify developmental tasks or goals of children and adolescents that can be affected or altered during times of illness (Wright & Leahey, 2013, p. 152).

Nurses working with well families can teach family awareness, encourage family enrichment, and provide information on community agencies and Web sites that are resources for strengthening and enriching families. The family could be encouraged to agree on a goal to attend or find out more about resources or programs. By offering opportunities for family members to express feelings about family experiences, the nurse enables the family to draw forth its own strengths and resources to support one another (Wright & Leahey, 2013). Drawing forth family support is especially important in primary health care settings (Wright & Leahey, 2013).

Use of Rituals/Routines and Family Time

Denham (2011) emphasizes the use of family rituals and routines for health promotion. The findings of previous research have indicated that predictable routines and meaningful rituals are related to healthier outcomes and that establishing routines is vital to managing demands in households with many extended family members (Hall, 2007).

Family nurses know that routines are observable and repeated behavior patterns that have great consistency and regularity. Family routines are collective events that occur on a daily, weekly, or annual basis. They typically include a set time and place, assignment of roles, and an element of planning ahead. Nurses can work with families to establish or help them maintain daily routines that are created around mealtimes, taking medications, and sleep (Fiese & Everhart, 2011). Families are able to plan ahead and provide a sense of stability to daily routines, yielding lower levels of stress and better family life. Family routines can be disrupted for expected developmental transitions (such as having a new baby in the house or moving to a new geographical location) and unexpected family situations (such as a diagnosis of a chronic health condition or strained economic resources). Therefore, family nurses can help prospective parents discuss family routines so they can be established when the new family member arrives. The key preservative function of routines appears to be not only maintaining a sense of order in daily life, but also staying connected as a group (Fiese & Everhart, 2011). Routines provide family members the opportunity to communicate about events important to them. For example, at family holiday gatherings, memories about past gatherings are shared, communicating a shared heritage and sense of belonging to a larger group. Over time, these communication patterns expressed during family gatherings come to cement relationships shown to be associated with healthy family functioning (Fiese & Everhart, 2011).

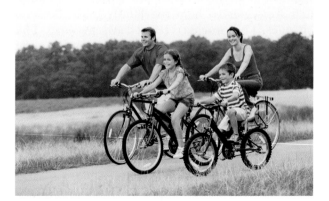

Family ritual is a repetitive pattern of prescribed formal behavior pertaining to some specific event, occasion, or situation, which tends to be repeated over and over again (Imber-Black, 2011). Family rituals often surround secular (such as birthday) and ceremonial occasions linked to religion (such as baby baptism), faith or some form of canonical principles that distinguish ordinary from extraordinary and celebrate value ideals (Denham, 2011). Rituals are best introduced when there is an excessive level of confusion, as they provide clarity in a family system (Imber-Black, 2011).

Family routines/rituals may be perceived as being a fairly reliable index of family collaboration, accommodation, and synergy (Denham, 2011). To use rituals and routines as therapeutic interventions, nurses must identify ways to use intentionality to assist family members as they create, amend, and adjust routines so that they are relevant to families' unique health and illness needs. Nurses need to be educated to observe or consider the impact of family rituals and routines on management of chronic illness. For example, diabetes is a disease greatly influenced by adherence to a prescribed medical regimen that usually includes a dietary plan, exercise, compliance in medicine usage, blood glucose monitoring, physician visits, and other care modalities. When adherence to a medical regimen is a concern, family members must identify the critical care aspects, key member duties for essential activities, and necessary actions to be included in family routines (Denham, 2011).

Family Meal and Healthy Eating

Factors in the family environment that promote healthful eating include the healthfulness of foods available in the home and consumed at meals, the frequency of family meals, and parental modeling of and support for children's healthful eating (Fruh et al., 2012; Haerens et al., 2008; Hammons & Fiese, 2011). Employed mothers are noted to purchase prepared foods more frequently, including fast food and carry-out meals, consume more food away from home, and commonly report missing out on family meals (Devine et al., 2009).

Bauer, Hearst, Escoto, Berge, and Neumark-Sztainer (2012) analyzed the data from Project F-EAT, a population-based study of a sociodemographically diverse sample of 3,709 parents of adolescents living in a metropolitan area in the Midwestern United States. They reported that full-time employed mothers reported fewer family meals, less frequent encouragement of their adolescents' healthful eating, lower fruit and vegetable intake, and less time spent on food preparation when compared to part-time and not employed mothers. Full-time employed fathers reported significantly fewer hours of food preparation. In addition, higher work-life stress between both parents was associated with less healthful family food environment characteristics, including less frequent family meals and more frequent sugar-sweetened beverage and fast food consumption by parents.

Research on family mealtime reveals that frequency of family meals is a protective factor that may curtail high-risk behaviors among youth (Fruh et al., 2012). For example, frequency of eating a family meal was associated with a reduced likelihood of all risk behaviors (e.g., smoking, drinking, cannabis use, bullying) among girls and all but fighting and having sex among boys (Levin et al., 2012). Fruh et al. (2012) listed the following outcomes from families eating together:

- Teenagers who eat meals with their families frequently are less likely to be depressed or use drugs than those who do not eat with their families as often. They are also less likely to be violent, to have sex, and to experience emotional stress. Adolescents who eat meals with their families are likely to be more highly motivated in school and have better peer relationships.
- Regular shared mealtimes can increase children's sense of belonging and stability, and the entire family's feeling of group connection. Many adolescents in a large national study reported that they want to be with their parents for most evening meals.
- Teenagers who share meals with their families on a regular basis tend to eat healthier foods than those who do not. They consume fewer high-fat, high-sugar prepared and packaged foods, and more fruits and vegetables and other foods high in important nutrients and fiber.

In addition, family mealtimes facilitate improving family communication, fostering family tradition, and teaching life skills to children. Encouraging shared meals when possible is a way nurses can enhance family bonding as this gives families an opportunity to be together and communicate with each other.

FAMILY CASE STUDIES

The following family case studies are used in the next sections of the chapter to demonstrate how different theoretical approaches can be used for assessing and intervening in the family for health promotion.

Family Case Study: Budd Family

Setting: Prenatal clinic (regular prenatal checkup).

Family Nursing Goals: Work with the family members to assist them in successful family transition and balance.

Family Members:
- James: father; 32 years old; full-time but temporarily employed without benefits, expects to be promoted to a permanent position soon with benefits (married Eleanor 3 years ago).
- Eleanor: mother; 33 years old; full-time employed, a school teacher at an elementary school with benefits, considering being a "stay-at-home" mother after giving birth (6 months pregnant); first marriage, married James after giving birth to Dustin.
- Hanna: oldest child; 8 years old; daughter (from James's first marriage), third grade, usually a good student.
- Dustin: son; 3.5 years old; all-day preschool (private day-care facility), developmentally on target.
- The couple is expecting a baby girl in 3 months.

Family Story:
James (32 years old) and Eleanor (33 years old) have one daughter, Hanna (8 years old), and one son, Dustin (3.5 years old). James is a full-time worker in a sales business (see the Budd family genogram in Figure 8-3). Currently, he is a full-time employee but under temporary status; he is expected to have a permanent position soon (date is not sure) that provides benefits and covers health insurance. Eleanor has a full-time position as an elementary-school teacher. She wants to be a stay-at-home mother but is afraid of losing health insurance and family income if she quits now, so she wants to wait until James gets a permanent full-time position with benefits.

The couple married 3 years ago; they recently moved from an apartment to a house because the family needs additional space for the new baby. Although the house is spacious, it is old and needs some renovation.

This is the first marriage for Eleanor and second marriage for James (James divorced 5 years ago). Eleanor stated that the family has been successfully going through the remarriage cycle, and Hanna and Eleanor have a pretty good relationship. Hanna is usually withdrawn after visiting her biological mother (summer and winter school vacations, and several holidays—generally five times a year), who is also remarried and gave Hanna a new stepbrother (age 2) from her current marriage. Hanna is attending an after-school program at the same school where Eleanor works and returns home with Eleanor. On the way home, Eleanor picks up Dustin from the day care, which he attends from 7:30 a.m. to 4:30 p.m. during the weekdays. Hanna attends a piano lesson on Tuesdays and ballet class on Thursdays.

Because of the family's busy schedule, they often eat at fast-food restaurants during the evenings (at least twice a week), and meals at home are usually rushed and often eaten in front of the television. Although the family tries to eat meals together, it cannot do so because James's job requires frequent traveling, so the family often ends up eating meals without James.

When James is at home, he does outdoor chores, whereas Eleanor usually does indoor chores. The children usually watch television and play video games when the couple is working at home. The couple tries to do family activities each Sunday, and all family members attend a local Presbyterian church. But James is generally not home one Sunday each month because of the travel requirements for his job. With the exception of family vacations, holidays, and Sundays, the Budds rarely spend time together enjoying each other's company.

James and Eleanor seldom agree on parenting practices; whereas Eleanor is firm and detailed, James is laid-back. James has some guilty feelings toward Hanna, thus making him very lenient toward her. Hanna usually goes to her dad to escape her regular duties and whenever Eleanor asks her to complete assigned tasks. James usually accepts Hanna's request because of his guilty feelings, and this makes Eleanor uncomfortable and frustrated.

Eleanor was seen by a nurse in the OB/GYN clinic for her regular prenatal checkups. She is going through a normal pregnancy, but she recently has experienced serious fatigue. Her additional concern is that she has a difficult time putting Dustin to bed each night. Dustin used to go to bed easily when they lived in the apartment, where he shared a room with Hanna. After moving to the new house 3 months ago, where he has his own room, he has not been the same. Eleanor notices that he is more energetic at night and wants to stay with her before going to bed. In addition, Dustin has started visiting the parents at night and staying with them during the night, when he should be sleeping in his own bed. He has recently complained about his tummy being upset, and Eleanor is not sure whether he is sick or is just faking to get attention. Dustin is excited to have a baby sister, but he also shows some jealousy. For example, Dustin acted like an infant baby when his parents decorated the baby's room and bed with pink colors.

Although James helps Hanna at night, putting Dustin to bed is Eleanor's job, and she is overwhelmed with his behavior. Eleanor says that James is a good husband, but she feels that he considers parenting to be a mother's role, which sometimes leaves her feeling overwhelmed and angry. Eleanor perceives that all family members are healthy and states that they are just a busy family. Her additional concern is the family finances after she quits her job. The nurse sees only Eleanor during this time, and requests that James and the children come for the next visit. (See the Budd family ecomap in Figure 8-4.)

Assessment:

As explained in Chapter 3, models that nurses use to assess family health differ. The following illustrates how different assessments and options for interventions vary based on the theoretical perspectives of the family.

Family Systems Theory:

The focus of the nurse's practice from this perspective is family as client; therefore, assessments of family members are focused on the family as a whole. In the case study, all members of the Budd family are affected when the mother gives birth. Eleanor currently feels that her husband considers parenting as a mother's role. If James continues to be passive in his parenting role, it would cause a difficult family transition when the baby is born. In addition, the arrival of the new baby could make going to bed even more difficult for Dustin at night, if not resolved.

Developmental and Family Life Cycle Theory:

The family is a blended family and is in the stage of the "families with young children" (infancy to school age) because their oldest daughter, Hanna, is an elementary-school child. The family is experiencing an additional normative developmental stressor of adding a new family member. The tasks required for this family include adjusting to the addition of a new family member, defining and sharing childrearing, financial and household tasks, and realigning relationships with extended family, parents, and grandparents. In addition, although Dustin is

(continued)

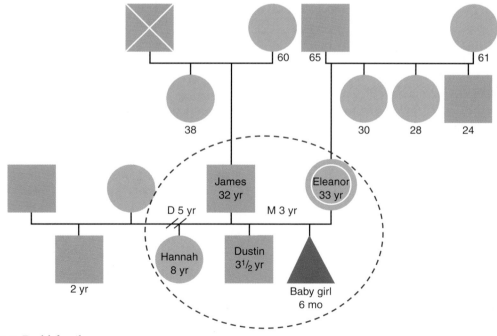

FIGURE 8-3 Budd family genogram.

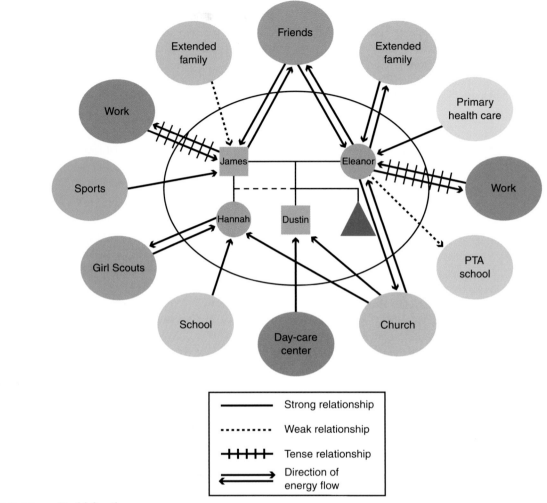

Strong relationship

---------- Weak relationship

++++++ Tense relationship

⟹ Direction of
⟸ energy flow

FIGURE 8-4 Budd family ecomap.

developmentally on target, the family is experiencing a challenge to make Dustin go to bed each night, and may face a challenge with potential sibling rivalry.

Bioecological Theory:

In the bioecological model, nurses need to assess the microsystem (i.e., family composition and home environment), mesosystem (i.e., external environment), exosystem (i.e., job and income), and macrosystem (i.e., community). The Budd family consists of two parents, two children, and a baby on the way. The couple has a white European heritage. The family lives in an old one-story house with four bedrooms in an older suburban section of town. During further interviews, the nurse found that the Budds' house was built before 1950 and is still under renovation.

The extended family (grandparents and siblings of Eleanor's side) live nearby, and Eleanor has a close relationship with them. The extended family gets together for most holidays; James and Hanna seem to have a tenuous relationship with Eleanor's family. The town is largely composed of white ethnicity with 30% African American. None of the parents or siblings of James lives nearby. James's dad passed away 10 years ago in a car accident; his mother remarried 7 years ago and lives 500 miles away. The Budds and James's mother usually meet once a year and talk once or twice a month via telephone. James has an older sister who lives out of the country because of her husband's military service.

Family Assessment and Intervention Model:

Using the Family Systems Stressor-Strength Inventory (FS³I) of the Family Assessment and Intervention Model, the major family stressors include (1) Dustin's bedtime problem, (2) Eleanor's upcoming birth, (3) insufficient couple time and family playtime, (4) insufficient "me time" (specifically Eleanor), (5) inadequate time with the children and watching television too much (children), (6) overscheduled family calendar, and (7) parenting conflict and lack of shared responsibility. Some job stress exists because James is still in a temporary position and his work requires traveling.

Family strengths include (1) shared religious core, (2) family values and encouragement of individual values, (3) affirmation and support of one another, (4) successful family transition into a new blended family, (5) trust between members, (6) support from extended family (specifically Eleanor), (7) adequate income (current-dual career family), and (8) ability to seek help.

Interventions:

Through assessment, nurses identify family strengths that foster health promotion and stressors that impede health promotion (Pender et al., 2011). Integration of the family perspective into assessment and planning facilitates more effective plans for health promotion (Wright & Leahey, 2013). Although the family has developmentally been successfully going through the remarriage cycle, it is expecting an additional life transition of adding a new family member. For this successful transition, the couple needs to define and share childrearing and household tasks. In order to resolve the current parenting and role conflicts, the couple needs to evaluate the current roles and could experiment with being responsible for the children alternately. After the birth of the baby, the couple may face a challenge with potential sibling rivalry. Spending time together as a family would promote family closeness for this blended family. When family members engage often in leisure activities, recreation, and exercise, they are able to cope with day-to-day problems better (Smith et al., 2009). The nurse should address the hurried family lifestyle and frequent unhealthful fast food eating habit.

Family Self-Care Contract:
- Involve all family members (including children) in establishing a family self-care contract.
- Assist the family members to share their perceived family health issues.
- Assist the family to prioritize the goals.
- Discuss the health promotion strategies.

Family Empowerment and Family Strengths-Based Nursing Care:
- Commend the family strengths and base interventions on the family strengths.
- Enhance and mobilize the family strengths for problem solving.

- Offer information/resources to help resolve parenting conflicts.
- Offer opportunities for the family members to express feelings about their family experiences.

Anticipatory Guidance and Offering Information:
- Help the family to anticipate/prepare for life changes after the birth of the baby girl.
- Encourage the family to make the necessary adjustments (e.g., role sharing).
- Offer information about resources for health promotion (e.g., smoking cessation, regular exercise).

Use of Rituals/Routines and Family Time:
- Assist the family to plan for family time, couple time, and individual family member alone time.
- Explore common family leisure activities, recreation, or exercise.
- Discuss ways to reduce the hurried family lifestyle by utilizing resources from extended family, church, or community.
- Assist the parents to establish bedtime routine.
- Discuss family mealtime and ways to improve healthy eating (e.g., reduction of fast food consumption, avoiding meals in front of TV).

Case Study: Matthews Family

Setting: School health nurse's office (high school).

Family Nursing Goals: Work with the family to assist it for successful family transition and balance.

Family Members:
- Andrew: father; 52 years old; part-time lecturer at a local university (married Susan 18 years ago), first marriage.
- Susan: mother; 50 years old; full-time employed at a government office, second marriage with no children from the previous marriage.
- Sophie: oldest child; 17 years old; daughter, 11th grade.
- Angela: middle child; 14 years old; daughter, 9th grade.
- Joseph: son; 11 years old; son, 6th grade.

Family Story:
Andrew (52 years old) and Susan (50 years old) have two teenage daughters, Sophie (17 years old) and Angela (14 years old) and one son, Joseph (11 years old). They have been married for 18 years.

(continued)

Andrew is a part-time college professor. Susan has a full-time position as a director at a government office. When Andrew lost his full-time job 17 years ago, the couple moved in with Andrew's mother (Lucy, age 86) and lived with her for more than 5 years until Susan's income was sufficient to cover a mortgage and family expenses. Since moving out of Lucy's house, the couple and children visit and have dinner with her every weekend, which has become the family routine. Children are expected to spend the night with their grandmother after the dinner; however, recently Sophie has refused to spend the night at grandmother's house. Andrew's sisters and their families live in the same state and visit Lucy at least once a month. Lucy has chronic health conditions, which cause unexpected emergency department (ED) visits (several times a year). After divorcing her ex-husband, Susan started to study in a graduate school in a different state, where she met Andrew. Because Susan's family lives far away, she barely sees them and sometimes feels isolation and loneliness.

Andrew has been a part-time employee at local colleges most of his life. While Andrew has spent most of his time working on computers at home (online teaching), Susan has worked at a local government agency. Since Andrew has produced minimum income, Susan provides for most of the family expenses.

The house has five rooms: master bedroom, Andrew's office (he stays at home most of the time), and three rooms for the children. The girls used to share the same room until the family added an additional room last year so the children could have their own room. Since moving to a new room upstairs, Sophie brings her friends home frequently and a couple of close friends spend the night with her on weekends and during the summer break. The parents caught Sophie and her friend leaving the house secretly to meet a group of boys after midnight; Sophie was grounded for a month as a result. Last month, Susan found Sophie and her friend on the street (instead of going to school) while she was driving to work. Sophie's boyfriend lives nearby, and they meet frequently at the park or each other's home. Susan suspects that Sophie might have a sexual relationship with her boyfriend.

This is the first marriage for Andrew and second marriage for Susan. Susan was a survivor of domestic violence from the first marriage (which lasted less than 1 year). Because Andrew has strong family-centered values, they eat dinner as a family and once or twice a week with Andrew's mother (Lucy). Sophie has started skipping the family dinners frequently, stating that she is not hungry. She also has been experiencing several fainting episodes

due to irregular eating habits. She frequently skips breakfast and lunch. The couple noticed that Sophie is eating fast food in her room or eating food after midnight by herself. Sophie's eating pattern is getting irregular, and Angela has begun to imitate her older sister's pattern and is refusing to participate in family dinners. Both girls are generally skipping breakfast, although Susan has made various attempts to get them to eat breakfast.

All children are in good health and have pleasant dispositions. The children are generally happy, but loud at home and frequently fight and yell at each other. The girls argue over clothes and cleaning and are frequently cranky and difficult for the couple to deal with. Andrew and Susan sometimes argue because of different parenting styles: whereas Susan wants to raise the children in a Christian way, Andrew opposes Susan's parenting belief. Sophie is becoming rebellious and fights with Andrew frequently. She is losing interest in her schoolwork.

Earlier in their married life, Susan mainly was responsible for household chores. Sophie expressed resentment against her father regarding his minimal house chore contribution. Over the years, as a result of numerous heated arguments, Andrew agreed to share a significant portion of household responsibilities, including outdoor chores. Still, Susan spends weekends doing grocery shopping, laundry, housecleaning, and attending to the children. During the weekdays, the couple takes the children to various lessons (piano, violin, cello, art, karate, and soccer), which sometimes causes schedule conflicts and builds marital tension.

Andrew and Susan have mutual friends, but seldom participate in social gatherings as a couple. Susan usually takes the children to church events, and Andrew takes Joseph to soccer practices or sports events. Susan feels social support and comfort by attending church and church-related activities; but Andrew considers it as his wife's overcommitment to religion. The family is affiliated with a Methodist church, which they used to attend every Sunday; Andrew stopped going to church 6 months ago. Sophie sometimes refuses to go to church as a family. Because of Susan's full-time job and frequent family gatherings with in-laws, and Lucy's frequent ED or hospital admissions, Susan has limited time to socialize with her own friends. Over the years, Susan has experienced chronic fatigue and stress from caring for the children and handling family responsibilities. She also experiences insomnia and hot flashes due to menopause. Over the last 3 years, she has gained 30 pounds and is trying to lose weight without success. (See the Matthews family genogram in Figure 8-5 and family ecomap in Figure 8-6.)

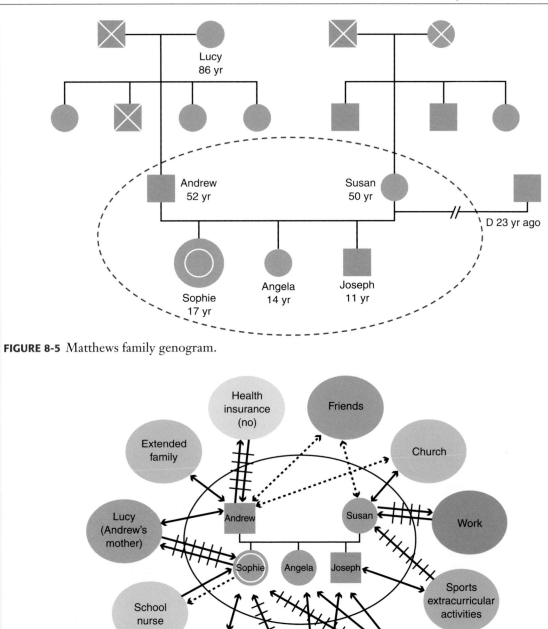

FIGURE 8-5 Matthews family genogram.

FIGURE 8-6 Matthews family ecomap.

Assessment:

Assessments of family members should be focused on the family as a whole. If Susan and/or Sophie's health status is declining and/or if Lucy's health deteriorates, the remaining members of family will experience difficulty adjusting to the changes. Andrew and Susan experience difficult family transitions raising two teenagers who show rebellious attitudes and an unhealthy lifestyle.

Developmental and Family Life Cycle Theory:

The family is a nuclear family and is in the stage of the "families with adolescents" because their oldest daughter, Sophie, is in high school. The tasks required for this family include allowing adolescents to establish their own identities but still be part of the family; thinking about the future, education, jobs, and working; and increasing roles of adolescents in family, cooking, repairs, and power bases.

Family Systems Theory:

Although the Matthews family looks healthy, there is an indication of moving to family vulnerability. When family members exhibit symptoms of an illness, other family members become aware that an individual has become ill. The Matthews family does not engage in activities to improve and maintain the health of individual members and promote family functioning. Andrew and Susan exercise infrequently. Although Susan takes the children to pediatric and dental (including orthodontic) clinics for regular checkups and maintenance, Susan skips her annual checkup. Andrew is a heavy drinker and smoker. Since Andrew does not have health insurance, he only visits a clinic when he feels sick. He does not have a plan to purchase private health insurance due to financial reasons. Sophie has recently experienced fainting episodes. Susan suspects that Sophie is becoming sexually active, but Sophie denies it and refuses to receive the human papillomavirus (HPV) vaccine. Angela and Joseph usually stay home watching TV or using the computer instead of engaging in physical activities. Due to the overscheduled family calendar and work demands, they eat fast food frequently or use frozen meals. In addition, the family does not have regularly scheduled family meetings to problem-solve for family risk reduction. Susan's increasing fatigue, Lucy's frequent ED visits, and Sophie's unhealthy lifestyle could lead to the increased vulnerability.

Bioecological Theory:

The Matthews family consists of two parents and three children. Although the family does not live with Lucy, Lucy's influence is significant. Andrew has African American

heritage with some European and Native American ancestors. Susan is biracial (50% Asian and 50% African American). The family lives in a one-story house with five bedrooms in a middle-class neighborhood. A community park is nearby the family residence, and the children hang out there with other children occasionally. The town is largely composed of white ethnicity with a small proportion of African Americans and Asian Americans.

Andrew's sisters and their families live in the same state, and the family has a close relationship with them. The extended family gets together at least once a month. The Matthews family visits Lucy every week. Susan's parents passed away and she has an older sister who lives out of the country. Susan and her sister communicate with each other via e-mail or phone, talking as needed once or twice a month. Susan has two brothers whom she usually sees once every other year.

Family Assessment and Intervention Model:

Using the Family Systems Stressor-Strength Inventory (FS³I) of the Family Assessment and Intervention Model, the family strengths include (1) family values and encouragement of individual values, (2) parents' value of children's education, (3) trust among family members, (4) support from extended family and church, (5) adequate income, (6) shared religious core, and (7) ability to seek help.

The major family stressors include (1) children's poor/irregular eating habits (including skipping meals), (2) dissolved dinnertime routine, (3) insufficient couple time and family playtime, (4) insufficient "me time" (specifically Susan), (5) inadequate time with the children and spending too much time on television and computer, (6) overscheduled family calendar, (7) Lucy's frequent ED or hospital admissions, and (8) lack of parenting skills and parental conflict. Some job stress exists because Andrew is still in a temporary part-time position.

Family Nursing Interventions:

Healthy families have both together family time and individual family member alone time (Denham, 2011; Imber-Black, 2011; Loveland-Cherry, 2011). The family experiences difficult family transitions in raising two teenagers who show rebellious attitudes and an unhealthy lifestyle.

The family needs to plan "family time." Having family activities or leisure time would bring a sense of togetherness. Considering the benefits of family mealtimes for families with teenagers, the family needs to make a concerted effort to establish family mealtime routines, and each member should make that family mealtime a priority and let no other activity interfere with it.

Families with teenagers may require help in meeting both the needs of the family as a whole and members' individual needs. To find a balance, each family member should have time alone to develop a sense of self and to focus on growth. Andrew and Susan need improved couple time by modifying the overscheduled family calendar. In addition, the family needs increased sharing of household responsibilities. There is a need to redefine and negotiate the current family roles. Many of Susan's current roles could be shared by other family members.

The parents do not seem to be good role models for the children relative to physical exercise and healthy eating style. Nurses need to address healthy lifestyle practices such as good eating habits, good sleep patterns, proper hygiene, and other positive health practices, as these are passed from one generation to another. If the couple initiates a health behavior change, the children would likely make a change too. For example, if Susan changes her eating patterns, perhaps by eating healthy meals, the children would change their eating patterns. The father's involvement is especially important for this family as a role model for the son, who will be a teenager soon.

Family Self-Care Contract:

- Involve all family members (including children) in establishing a family self-care contract.
- Assist the family members to share their perceived family heath issues.
- Encourage the family to discuss health promotion strategies.

Family Empowerment and Family Strengths-Based Nursing Care:

- List the family strengths and relate them to the characteristics of a healthy family.
- Use family strengths to balance and overcome existing problems.
- Offer opportunities for the family members to express feelings about their family experiences.
- Evaluate the current family roles and assist the family in establishing family role sharing.

Anticipatory Guidance and Offering Information:

- Offer resources to resolve the current health issues (i.e., management of menopause symptoms and eating disorders).
- Offer information for health promotion (e.g., exercise and healthy eating for the whole family; healthy eating and safer-sex education for the girls).
- Offer resources for successful parenting for teenagers and conflict resolution.

- Assist individual members in health promotion.
- *Susan:* stress management skills (e.g., exercise, Yoga, time for self).
- *Andrew:* weight loss strategies (i.e., exercise, healthy eating, and alcohol and smoking cessation).
- *Children:* time management (related to watching television and using the computer) and physical activities.

Use of Rituals/Routines and Family Time:

- Encourage the family to schedule weekly family time and/or family meeting.
- Help the family to explore family activities by consulting local newspapers, family magazines, and community agencies for activities that might interest the entire family, and afterward encourage them to continue these activities.
- Assist the parents in the family to arrange for couple time and individual time.
- Discuss ways to decrease the children's after-school activities.

Family Meals and Healthy Eating:

- Assist the family to establish family meal routines.
- Discuss ways to improve healthy eating (e.g., reduction of fast food consumption).
- Experiment with premade breakfast meals (e.g., protein bars, fruit).

SUMMARY

This chapter provides an overview of family health promotion by defining family health and health promotion, introducing family health promotion models, and describing internal and external systems that influence family health promotion. The two case studies presented in this chapter illustrate family health promotion assessment and family nursing intervention strategies. The following outlines the major learning points emphasized in this chapter on family health promotion:

- Fostering the health of the family as a unit and encouraging families to value and incorporate health promotion into their lifestyle are essential components of family nursing practice.
- Health promotion is learned within families, and patterns of health behaviors are formed and passed on to the next generation.
- A major task of the family is to teach health maintenance and health promotion.

- The role of the family nurse is to help families attain, maintain, and regain the highest level of family health possible.
- Family health is a holistic, dynamic, and complex state. It is more than the absence of disease in an individual family member or the absence of dysfunction in family dynamics. Instead, it is the complex process of negotiating day-to-day family life events and crises, and providing for quality of life for its members.
- Family health promotion refers to activities that families engage in to strengthen the family unit and increase family unity and quality of family life.
- External ecosystem influences on family health include such things as the national economy, family and health policy, societal and cultural norms, media, and environmental hazards, such as noise, air, soil, crowding, and chemicals.
- Internal ecosystem influences include family type and developmental stage, family lifestyle patterns, family processes, personalities of family members, power structure, family role models, coping strategies and processes, resilience, and culture.
- Health and family policies at all governmental levels affect the quality of individual and family health.
- Health promotion advertisements have generally targeted the more health-conscious middle class, rather than the vulnerable and underserved who are often the targets for alcohol and tobacco advertising campaigns.
- Families who are flexible and able to adjust to change are more likely to be involved in health-promoting activities.
- Vulnerable families are coping with a pileup of stressors and may be unable to focus on activities to enhance family health.
- Low-income families may focus less on health promotion and more on basic needs, such as obtaining shelter, adequate food, and health care.
- Middle-class families are skimping on health promotion, such as dental care, as they face current economic struggles.
- Through verbal and nonverbal communication, parents teach behavior, share feelings and values, and make decisions about family health practices.

- Different cultures define and value health, health promotion, and disease prevention differently. Clients may not understand or respond to the family nurses' suggestions for health promotion because the suggestions conflict with their traditional health beliefs and values.
- A primary goal of nursing care for families is empowering family members to work together to attain and maintain family health by focusing on family strengths, competencies, and resources.
- Health behaviors must be relevant and compatible with the family structure and lifestyle to be effective and useful to the family.
- The goal of the family nurse is to facilitate family adaptation by empowering the family to promote resilience, reduce the pileup of stressors, make use of resources, and negotiate necessary change to enhance the family's ability to rebound from stressful events or crises.
- Family health promotion should become a regular part of taking a family history and a routine aspect of nursing care.

REFERENCES

Alderfer, M. A. (2011). Assessing family health. In M. Craft-Rosenberg & S. Pehler (Eds.), *Encyclopedia of family* (pp. 78–85). Los Angeles, CA: Sage.

Allen, F. M., & Warner, M. (2002). A developmental model of health and nursing. *Journal of Family Nursing, 8*(2), 96–135.

American Academy of Pediatrics. (2010). Policy statement: Media education. *Pediatrics, 126*(5), 1012–1017.

Anderson, D. G., Ward, H., & Hatton, D. (2008). Family health risks. In M. Stanhope & J. Lancaster (Eds.), *Public health nursing: Population-centered health care in the community* (7th ed., pp. 578–601). St. Louis, MO: Mosby.

Bauer, K. W., Hearst, M. O., Escoto, K., Berge, J. M., & Neumark-Sztainer, D. (2012). Parental employment and work-family stress: Associations with family food environments. *Social Science & Medicine, 75*(3), 496–504.

Birman, D., & Poff, M. (2011). Intergenerational differences in acculturation. *Encyclopedia on Early Childhood Development.* Retrieved from http://www.child-encyclopedia.com/documents/Birman-PoffANGxp1.pdf

Black, C., & Ford-Gilboe, M. (2004). Adolescent mothers: Resilience, family health work and health-promoting practices. *Journal of Advanced Nursing, 48*(4), 351–360.

Black, K., & Lobo, M. (2008). A conceptual review of family resilience factors. *Journal of Family Nursing, 14*(1), 33–55.

Bomar, P. J. (Ed.). (2004). *Promoting health in families: Applying family research and theory to nursing practice* (3rd ed.). Philadelphia, PA: W. B. Saunders.

Bronfenbrenner, U. (1977). Toward an experimental ecology of human development. *American Psychologist, 32,* 513–531.

Burkhart, L. (2011). Religious/spiritual influences on health in the family. In M. Craft-Rosenberg & S. Pehler (Eds.), *Encyclopedia of family* (pp. 878–882). Los Angeles, CA: Sage.

Carson, V. B., & Koenig, H. G. (2011). *Parish nursing* (rev. ed.). Philadelphia, PA: Templeton Foundation Press.

Carter, B., & McGoldrick, M. (2005). *The expanded family life cycle: Individual, family and social perspectives* (3rd ed.). New York, NY: Allyn & Bacon, Pearson Education.

Centers for Disease Control and Prevention. (2012). Smoking and tobacco use: Legislation. Retrieved from http://www.cdc.gov/tobacco/data_statistics/by_topic/policy/legislation/index.htm

Christensen, P. (2004). The health promoting family: A conceptual framework for future research. *Social Science & Medicine, 59,* 377–387.

Cowan, M. K. (2008). Child and adolescent health. In M. Stanhope & J. Lancaster (Eds.), *Public health nursing: Population-centered health care in the community* (7th ed., pp. 602–630). St. Louis, MO: Mosby.

Denham, S. A. (1999a). The definition and practice of family health. *Journal of Family Nursing, 5*(2), 133–159.

Denham, S. A. (1999b). Family health: During and after death of a family member. *Journal of Family Nursing, 5*(2), 160–183.

Denham, S. A. (1999c). Family health in an economically disadvantaged population. *Journal of Family Nursing, 5*(2), 184–213.

Denham, S. A. (2003a). *Family health: A framework for nursing.* Philadelphia, PA: F. A. Davis.

Denham, S. A. (2003b). Relationships between family rituals, family routines, and health. *Journal of Family Nursing, 9*(3), 305–330.

Denham, S. A. (2011). Rituals, routines, and their influence on health in families. In M. Craft-Rosenberg & S. Pehler (Eds.), *Encyclopedia of family* (pp. 908–911). Los Angeles, CA: Sage.

Devine, C. M., Farrell, T. J., Blake, C. E., Jastran, M., Wethington, E., & Bisogni, C. A. (2009). Work conditions and the food choice coping strategies of employed parents. *Journal of Nutrition Education and Behavior, 41,* e365–e370.

Duval, E. M., & Miller, B. C. (1985). *Marriage and family development* (6th ed.). New York, NY: Harper & Row.

Edberg, M. (2013). *Essentials of health, culture, and diversity: Understanding people, reducing disparities.* Burlington, MA: Jones & Bartlett Learning.

Epstein, L. H., Roemmich, J. N., & Robinson J. L. (2008). A randomized trial of the effects of reducing television viewing and computer use on body mass index in young children. *Archives of Pediatrics & Adolescent Medicine, 162*(3), 239–245.

Farver, J. M., Xu, Y., Bhadha, B. R., Narang, S., & Lieber, E. (2007). Ethnic identity, acculturation, parenting beliefs, and adolescent adjustment. *Merrill-Palmer Quarterly, 53,* 184–215.

Fiese, B. H., & Everhart, R. S. (2011). Family health maintenance. In M. Craft-Rosenberg & S. Pehler (Eds.), *Encyclopedia of family* (pp. 468–472). Los Angeles, CA: Sage.

Fitzpatrick, C., Barnett, T., & Pagani, L. S. (2012). Early exposure to media violence and later child adjustment. *Journal of Developmental & Behavioral Pediatrics, 33*(4), 291–297.

Ford-Gilboe, M. (2002). Developing knowledge about family health promotion by testing the developmental model of health and nursing. *Journal of Family Nursing, 8*(2), 140–156.

Fruh, S. M., Mulekar, M. S., Hall, H., Fulkerson, J., King, A, Jezek, K., & Roussel, L. (2012). Benefits of family meals with adolescents: Nurse practitioners' perspective. *Journal for Nurse Practitioners, 8*(4), 280–287.

Gillman, S., Rende, R., Boergers, J., Abrams, D., Buka, S., Clark, M., . . . Niaura, R. (2009). Parental smoking in adolescent smoking initiation: An intergenerational perspective on tobacco control. *Pediatrics, 123*(2), e274–e281.

Goeke-Morey, M. C., Cairns, E., Merrilees, C. E., Schermerhorn, A. C., Shirlow, P., & Cummings E. M. (2013). Maternal religiosity, family resources and stressors, and parent-child attachment security in Northern Ireland. *Social Development, 22*(1), 19–37.

Goldenberg, H., & Goldenberg, I. (2007). *Family therapy: An overview* (7th ed.). Belmont, CA: Wadsworth.

Gottlieb, L. N. (2013). *Strengths-based nursing care: Health and healing for person and family.* New York, NY: Springer.

Gregoski, M. J., Mueller, M., Vertegel, A., Shaporev, A., Jackson, B. B., Frenzel, R. M., . . . Treiber, F. A. (2012). Development and validation of a smartphone heart rate acquisition application for health promotion and wellness telehealth applications. *International Journal of Telemedicine and Applications.* Article ID 696324. doi:10.1155/2012/696324

Hall, W. (2007). Imposing order: A process to manage day-to day activities in two-earner families with preschool children. *Journal of Family Nursing, 13*(1), 56–82.

Haerens, L., Craeynest, M., Deforche, B., Maes, L., Cardon, G., & De Bourdeaudhuij, I. (2008). The contribution of psychosocial and home environmental factors in explaining eating behaviours in adolescents. *European Journal of Clinical Nutrition, 62,* e51–e59.

Hammons, A. J., & Fiese, B. H. (2011). Is frequency of shared family meals related to the nutritional health of children and adolescents? *Pediatrics, 127,* e1565–e1574.

Holland, M. L., Yoo, B.-K., Kitzman, H., Chaudron, L., Szilagyi, P. G., & Temkin-Greener, H. (2012). Mother-child interactions and the associations with child healthcare utilization in low-income urban families. *Maternal and Child Health Journal, 16*(1), 83–91.

Imber-Black, E. (2011). Creating meaningful rituals for new life cycle transitions. In M. McGoldrick, B. Carter, & B. Garcia-Preto (Eds.), *The expanded family life cycle: Individual, family and social perspectives* (4th ed.). New York, NY: Allyn & Bacon, Pearson Education.

Influence on children media. (2008). History of media for children, general considerations, studies of media influence, domains of influence, recommendations. Retrieved from http://education.stateuniversity.com/pages/2212/Media-Influence-on-Children.html

Kaakinen, J. R., & Birenbaum, L. K. (2012). Family development and family nursing assessment. In M. Stanhope & J. Lancaster (Eds.), *Public health nursing: Population-centered health care in the community* (8th ed., pp. 601–623). St. Louis, MO: Mosby.

Kim-Godwin, Y. S., & Bomar, P. (2010). Family health promotion. In J. R. Kaakinen, V. Gedaly-Duff, D. P. Cohelo, & S. M. H. Hanson (Eds.), *Family health care nursing: Theory, practice and research* (4th ed., pp. 207–234). Philadelphia, PA: F. A. Davis.

Kim-Spoon, J., Longo, G. S., & McCullough, M. E. (2012). Parent-adolescent relationship quality as a moderator for the influences of parents' religiousness on adolescents' religiousness and adjustment. *Journal of Youth and Adolescence.* Advanced online publication. doi:10.107/s10964-012-9796-1

Kitzmann, K. I. (2008). Beyond parenting practices: Family context and treatment of pediatric obesity. *Family Relations, 57,* 13–23.

Koenig, H. G. (2012). *Spirituality and health research: Methods, measurements, statistics, and resources.* West Conshohocken, PA: Templeton Press.

Kushner, K. E. (2007). Meaning and action in employed mother's health work. *Journal of Family Nursing, 13*(1), 33–55.

Leder, S., Grinstead, L., & Torres, E. (2007). Grandparents raising grandchildren. *Journal of Family Nursing, 13*(3), 333–352.

Lee, C. (2008). Does the Internet displace health professionals? *Journal of Health Communication, 13,* 450–464.

Levin, K. A., Kirby, J., & Currie, C. (2012). Adolescent risk behaviours and mealtime routines: Does family meal frequency alter the association between family structure and risk behavior? *Health Education Research, 27*(1), 24–35.

Loveland-Cherry, C. J. (2011). Roles of families in health promotion. In M. Craft-Rosenberg & S. Pehler (Eds.), *Encyclopedia of family* (pp. 913–916). Los Angeles, CA: Sage.

Loveland-Cherry, C. J., & Bomar, P. J. (2004). Family health promotion and health protection. In P. J. Bomar (Ed.), *Promoting health in families: Applying research and theory to nursing practice* (3rd ed., pp. 61–89). Philadelphia, PA: WB Saunders.

Lucea, M. B., Glass, N., & Laughon, K. (2011). Theories of aggression and family violence. In J. Humphreys & J. C. Campbell (Eds.), *Family violence and nursing practice* (2nd ed., pp. 1–27). New York, NY: Springer.

Marsiglio, W. (2009). Healthy dads, healthy kids. *Contexts, 8*(4), 22–27.

McGoldrick, M., Carter, B., & Garcia-Preto, N. G. (2011). *The expanded family life cycle: Individual, family and social perspectives* (4th ed.). New York: Allyn & Bacon, Pearson Education.

McGoldrick, M., Gerson, R., & Petry, S. (2008). *Genograms: Assessment and interventions* (3rd ed.). New York: W. W. Norton.

Meyer, M. G., Toborg, M. A., Denham, S. A., & Mande, M. J. (2008). Cultural perspectives concerning adolescent use of tobacco and alcohol in the Appalachian mountain region. *Journal of Rural Health, 24*(1), 67–74.

Monteith, B., & Ford-Gilboe, M. (2002). The relationships among mother's resilience, family health work, and mother's health promoting lifestyle practices in families with preschool children. *Journal of Family Nursing, 8*(4), 383–407.

Musick, K., & Meier, A. (2012). Assessing causality and persistence in associations between family dinners and adolescent well-being. *Journal of Marriage and Family, 74*(3), 476–493.

NANDA International. (2012). *Nursing diagnosis: Definitions and Classifications, 2012–2014.* Indianapolis, IN: Wiley-Blackwell.

Novilla, M. L. B. (2011). Family health perspectives. In M. Craft-Rosenberg & S. Pehler (Eds.), *Encyclopedia of family* (pp. 472–481). Los Angeles, CA: Sage.

Olson, D. H. L., & DeFrain, J. (2003). *Marriage and the family: Diversity and strengths* (4th ed.). New York, NY: McGraw-Hill.

Pender, N. J. (1996). *Health promotion in nursing practice* (3rd ed.). Norwalk, CT: Appleton & Lange.

Pender, N. J., Murdaugh, C. L., & Parsons, M. A. (2011). *Health promotion in nursing practice* (6th ed.). Upper Saddle River, NJ: Prentice Hall.

Psychological Studies Institute. (2004, September 15). New study identifies specific behaviors linked to family health. Physician Law Weekly. Retrieved from http://www.newsrx.com/newsletters/Mental-Health-Law-Weekly/2004-08-18/091320043331272MHL.html

Purnell, L. D. (2013). *Transcultural health care: A culturally competent approach* (4th ed.). Philadelphia, PA: F. A. Davis.

Razaz-Rahmati, N., Nourian, S. R., & Okoli, C. T. (2011). Does household structure affect adolescent smoking? *Public Health Nursing, 29*(3), 191–197.

Shapiro, A. F., Krysik, J., & Pennar, A. L. (2011). Who are the fathers in Healthy Families Arizona? An examination of father data in at-risk families. *American Journal of Orthopsychiatry, 81*(3), 327–336.

Silk, K. J., Sherry, J., Winn, B., Keesecker, N., Horodynski, M. A., & Sayir, A. (2008). Increasing nutrition literacy: Testing the effectiveness of print, Web site, and game modalities. *Journal of Nutrition Educational Behaviors, 40*(1), 3–10.

Smith, J. (1983). *The idea of health: Implications for the nursing profession.* New York, NY: Teachers College Press.

Smith, K. M., Freeman, P. A., & Zabriskie, R. B. (2009). An examination of family communication within the core and balance model of family leisure functioning. *Family Relations, 58,* 79–90.

Solari-Twadell, P. A., McDermott, M., & Matheus, R. (1999). Educational preparation. In P. A. Solari-Twadell & M. McDermott (Eds.). *Parish nursing: Promoting whole-person health within faith communities.* Thousand Oaks, CA: Sage.

Sonneville, K. R., & Gortmaker, S. L. (2008). Total energy intake, adolescent discretionary behaviors and the energy gap. *International Journal of Obesity, 32*(S6), S19–S27.

Spector, R. E. (2013). *Cultural diversity in health and illness* (8th ed.). Upper Saddle River, NJ: Pearson Education, Inc.

Strasburger, V., Jordan, A. B., & Donnerstein, E. (2010). Health effects of media on children and adolescents. *Pediatrics, 125*(4), 756–767.

Suter, P., Suter, W. N., & Johnston, D. (2011). Theory-based telehealth and patient empowerment. *Population Health Management, 14*(2), 87–92.

U.S. Department of Health and Human Services. (1979). *Healthy people: The Surgeon General's report on health promotion and disease prevention* (U.S. Public Health Service, Publication No. PHS 79–55071). U.S. Department of Health, Education, and Welfare. Washington, DC: U.S. Government Printing Office.

U.S. Department of Health and Human Services. (1980). *Promoting health/preventing disease: Objectives for the nation.* Washington, DC: U.S. Government Printing Office.

U.S. Department of Health and Human Services. (1990). *Healthy people 2000: National health promotion and disease prevention objectives* (Department of Health and Human Services, Publication No. PHS 91–50213). Washington, DC: U.S. Government Printing Office.

U.S. Department of Health and Human Services. (2000). *Healthy people 2010* (vol. 1). Washington, DC: U.S. Government

Printing Office. Retrieved March 26, 2008, from http://www.health.gov/healthypeople/Document/tableofcontents.htm

U.S. Department of Health and Human Services. (2011). Dietary guidelines for Americans 2010. Retrieved from http://www.health.gov/dietaryguidelines/2010.asp

U.S. Department of Health and Human Services. (2012). Healthy people 2020. Washington, DC. Retrieved from http://healthypeople.gov/2020/topicsobjectives2020/objectiveslist.aspx?topicId=12

Välimäki, M., Nenonen, H., Koivunen, M., & Suhonen, R. (2007). Patients' perceptions of Internet usage and their opportunity to obtain health information. *Medical Informatics and the Internet in Medicine, 32*(4), 305–314.

Walsh, F. (2006). *Strengthening family resilience* (2nd ed.). New York: Guilford Press.

Walsh, F. (2011a). *Resilience and mental health: Challenges across the lifespan.* New York, NY: Cambridge University Press.

Walsh, F. (2011b). *Normal family process: Growing diversity and complexity* (4th ed.) New York: Guilford Press.

Wang, Y. C., Orleans, C. T., & Gortmaker, S. L. (2012). Reaching the healthy people goals for reducing childhood obesity: Closing the energy gap. *American Journal of Preventive Medicine, 42*(5), 437–444.

Wright, L., & Leahey, M. (2013). *Nurses and families: A guide to family assessment and intervention* (6th ed.). Philadelphia, PA: F. A. Davis.

CHAPTER WEB SITES

Government Web Sites

- *The Affordable Health Act: Key feature of the law.* http://www.healthcare.gov/law/features/index.html

- *A more secure future.* http://www.whitehouse.gov/healthreform/healthcare-overview#healthcare-menu. Retrieved December 8, 2012.

- *Dietary Guidelines for Americans—U.S. Department of Agriculture:* www.cnpp.usda.gov/DietaryGuidelines.htm

- *Dietary Guidelines for Americans 2010—Healthy People:* http://health.gov/dietaryguidelines/2010.asp

- *Dietary Guidelines for Americans 2015—Healthy People:* http://health.gov/dietaryguidelines/2015.asp

- *Low-cost insurance for children and teens—Healthy Families—California:* www.healthyfamilies.ca.gov

- *Services for Families—Administration for Children and Families:* http://www.acf.dhhs.gov/acf_services.html

- *Providing health information to prevent harmful exposures and diseases related to toxic substances—Agency for Toxic Substance and Disease Registry:* www.atsdr.cdc.gov

- *Preventing or controlling those diseases or deaths that result from interactions between people and their environment—National Center for Environmental Health:* www.cdc.gov/nceh

- *Understanding how the environment influences the development and progression of human disease—National Institute of Environmental Health:* www.niehs.nih.gov

Institution Web Sites

- *American Academy of Pediatrics: SafetyNet Resources* http://safetynet.aap.org

- *International Institute for Health Promotion:* www.american.edu/academic.depts/cas/health/iihp

- *International Union for Health Promotion and Education:* http://www.iowapublichealth.org/xr/ASPX/RecordId.10305/rx/IphiRecordDetails.htm

- *Institute of Medicine, Board on Health Promotion and Disease Prevention:* www.iom.edu/IOM/IOMHome.nsf/Pages/Health_Promotion_and_Disease_Prevention

- *Research and Training Center on Family Support and Children's Mental Health:* www.rtc.pdx.edu

- *Berkeley Center for Working Families:* http://wfnetwork.bc.edu/berkeley/outreach.html

- *Family Support America:* www.familysupportamerica.org

- *National Council on Family Relations:* www.ncfr.com

- *National Center for Families:* www.nationalcenter.com

Other Resources

- *Health Promotion in Ontario, across Canada, and in other parts of the world—Health Promotion Bookmarks/Hot Links:* www.web.net/~stirling

- *Effective family programs for prevention of delinquency—Strengthening America's Families—Office of Juvenile Justice and Delinquency Prevention:* www.strengtheningfamilies.org

- *National Clearinghouse on Families & Youth—NCFY:* www.ncfy.com

- *Families First: Making Families Last:* www.familiesfirst.org

- *Managing Your Dual Career Family:* www.dr-jane.com/chapters/Jane133.htm

- *The National Partnership for Women and Families:* www.nationalpartnership.org

- *Parents Without Partners:* www.parentswithoutpartners.org

- *Helping to support and educate stepfamilies—Stepfamily Network Inc.:* www.stepfamily.net

- *Parenting and Family:* home.about.com/parenting

- *Campaign for Tobacco-Free Kids:* www.tobaccofreekids.org

- *Family mealtime—West Virginia University Extension Service:* http://www.wvu.edu/~exten/infores/pubs/fypubs/wlg129.pdf

chapter 9

Families Living With Chronic Illness

Joanna Rowe Kaakinen, PhD, RN

Sharon A. Denham, DSN, RN

Critical Concepts

- Chronic illness is a global phenomenon with the potential to worsen the overall health of the nation's people and limit the individual's capacity to live well.

- Social determinants of health and family health routines can increase the risks for a chronic condition.

- Healthy lifestyle behaviors and early detection or screening may prevent some forms of chronic disease.

- Chronic illness presents differing challenges to individuals and their family members during the life span.

- Chronic illnesses that occur at birth or early childhood are most likely to be genetic and require special attention during developmental changes and across the life span.

- Nurses must use evidence-based knowledge to empower families with the information, skills, and abilities to manage chronic diseases over the life course and prevent complications and comorbidities.

- Family-focused care is important for prevention and management of chronic illness when it occurs; this involves intentional nursing action that meets both the individual and family needs.

- Knowledge about disease self-management and adherence to a therapeutic medical regimen is essential for individuals and their family members if they are going to prevent additional complications.

- Nurses use various actions (e.g., teach, coach, demonstrate, counsel) to assist individuals and their family members to cope with the stress of uncertainty, powerlessness, and anticipatory and ambiguous losses that accompany chronic illnesses.

The term *chronos* is the root word for "chronic" and refers to time. Chronic illness describes a health condition that lasts longer than 6 months, is not easily resolved, and is rarely cured by a surgical procedure or short-term medical therapy (Miller, 2000). When diagnosed with a chronic condition, it becomes necessary for the individual and his or her family to learn to manage the disease or disorder while living a quality life. Chronic illness not only affects the quality of life of the individual, but significantly affects all members of the family.

As individuals struggle to live with chronic conditions, family members are challenged to balance the needs of the ill family member with their own needs and the needs of the family as a whole. Individuals with a chronic condition often battle to stay healthy, live active lives, retain a high quality of life, and prevent complications. This battle primarily is waged within the confines of the family. When an individual is diagnosed with a chronic illness, whatever it might be, family members must incorporate unexpected changes into their roles and daily processes, manage disabilities imposed, and identify ways to do it with the resources they have available and within a context of uncertainty. Managing uncertainty is a significant concern for individuals and families living with chronic illness (Hummel, 2013a).

Chronic illnesses often require complex care, and many people have more than a single condition. People with chronic illnesses can experience complications or comorbidities that make situations even more difficult. For example, a person diagnosed with type 2 diabetes may also have hypertension, hyperlipidemia, and neuropathy. A person with Parkinson's disease may also have a serious sleep disorder, constipation, chronic pain, and Lewy body dementia. Often, with a chronic illness, individuals require care from multiple physicians, specialists, and a panoply of prescription drugs. Care would benefit from coordination across disciplines. The complex needs can create havoc for families with limited resources as they attempt to manage many thorny situations faced daily. The holistic approach of nurses is crucial to the individual and family adaptation and management of living with chronic illness across the life span.

Many chronic diseases are altered and sometimes worsen over the life course. Chronic illnesses affect the lives of infants, children, adolescents, young adults, older adults, elderly, and the old-old. These diseases affect the physical, emotional, intellectual, social, vocational, and spiritual functioning of the person with the condition and family members. Wide variations exist in the ways different chronic illness conditions affect physical and mental health, employment, social life, and longevity.

Differences in the ways families accommodate a chronic condition also exist and are influenced not only by the level of disability and associated symptoms, but also by individual and family factors. Families differ in their perceptions about disability, in their backgrounds, and in their access to needed resources, for example. Care responses differ depending on whether the symptoms are constant (cerebral palsy),

episodic (migraine headaches), relapsing (sickle cell anemia), worsening or progressive (Parkinson's disease or certain types of cancer), or degenerative (Alzheimer's disease or Rhett syndrome). Details of the unique individual situation vary further with the age of the individual, previous family experiences, level of disease complexity, individual's motivation or ease in managing the illness, unique family member relationships, and distinct personalities and values. Regardless of the type of chronic illness experienced, however, one thing remains the same: various family members are likely to be involved at several levels. Because family members are the most enduring care providers, they might be viewed as the biggest resource for individual care over time. Family members generally offer the constancy and continuity of care needed for the most optimal health outcome. Most health professionals come and go in the lives of persons with chronic conditions, offering medical management, education, and counseling for brief times. But it is generally family members that provide the needed ongoing and persistent care across time.

The purpose and focus of this chapter is to describe ways for nurses to think about the impact of chronic illness on families and to consider strategies for helping families manage chronic illness. The first part of this chapter briefly outlines the global statistics of chronic illness, the economic burden of chronic diseases, and three theoretical perspectives for working with families living with chronic illness. The majority of the chapter describes how families and individuals are challenged to live a quality life in the presence of chronic illness and how nurses can assist these families. Two case studies are presented in this chapter: one a family who has an adolescent with diabetes and one a family helping an elderly parent and grandparent manage living with Parkinson's disease. Although every family and illness experience is completely individual, many of the trials that these two families endure are universal to other families living with different chronic illnesses.

CHRONIC ILLNESS: A GLOBAL CONCERN

Chronic illness is a global issue and is the leading cause of mortality and disability in the world, representing 63% of all deaths (World Health Organization [WHO], 2013a). Disease rates from these conditions are accelerating globally, advancing across every region and pervading all socioeconomic classes (WHO, 2013b). "Four of the most prominent chronic diseases—cardiovascular diseases (CVD), cancer, chronic obstructive pulmonary diseases and type 2 diabetes—are linked by common and preventable biological risk factors, notably high blood pressure, high blood cholesterol and overweight, and by related major behavioral risk factors: unhealthy diet, physical inactivity and tobacco use" (WHO, 2013b).

Out of the 36 million people who died from chronic disease in 2008, 9 million were under the age of 60 years and 90% of those premature deaths occurred in low- and middle-income countries (WHO, 2013a). Cardiovascular disease is the number one cause of death globally, with 30% of all global deaths being attributed to cardiovascular disease (WHO, 2013c). Cardiovascular disease morbidity and mortality could be reduced by addressing risk factors such as tobacco use, unhealthy diet, obesity, physical inactivity, high blood pressure, diabetes, and raised lipids (WHO, 2013c).

Approximately 13% of global deaths are from cancer, with the top kinds of cancer deaths being lung, stomach, liver, colon, and breast cancer (WHO, 2013d). According to the WHO, tobacco use is the most important risk factor for cancer as it is estimated that it causes 22% of global cancer deaths and 71% of the global lung cancer deaths (2013d). In addition, tobacco use is the primary cause of chronic obstructive disease, such as emphysema and asthma, worldwide.

In 2012, approximately 347 million people globally had diabetes and it is projected to be the seventh leading cause of global deaths by 2030 (WHO, 2013e). Worldwide, obesity has doubled since 1980 (WHO, 2013f). We are at the cusp of a chronic disease epidemic that if not attended to now will result in an even more serious crisis situation in the near future.

Surveillance of Chronic Illness

How do we know how many people have chronic illness and whether the problem is getting better or worse? In public health, one approach is the availability of surveillance data that are systematically collected over time. This information is used to analyze a problem and help identify trends of change over time. In the United States and Canada,

the Behavioral Risk Factor Surveillance System (BRFSS) is a survey used to collect national information regularly. This is a state-based or province-based system of health surveys conducted through phone surveys. The survey tracks health risk factors and uses the findings to improve the health of the nation's people. For example, in 2011 in the United States, 57.1% of the population had at least one alcoholic drink within the last 30 days and 18.3% of those in the nation were binge drinkers (BRFSS, 2011). The Centers for Disease Control and Prevention ([CDC]; 2011) defines *binge drinking* as a pattern of drinking that brings a person's blood alcohol concentration (BAC) to 0.08 grams percent or above. This typically happens when men consume five or more drinks, or when women consume four or more drinks, in about 2 hours. These baseline data have not previously been tracked, but can be looked at in future years. Over the next few years, surveys will collect additional data about alcohol use and the problem of binge drinking. Therefore, it will be possible to compare and analyze alcohol abuse and bring drinking as a risk factor on chronic illness trends and concerns.

Some other survey examples follow. Another survey instrument used to collect information about chronic illness risks is the National Health and Nutrition Examination Survey (NHANES, 2011) in the United States and the Food and Nutrition Surveillance in Canada. These national surveys are used to learn about the prevalence and distribution of chronic diseases and risk factors. The National Cardiovascular Data Registry is a database used to capture information about particular individuals. The National Program of Cancer Registries in the United States and the Canadian Cancer Registry are both surveillance organizations that focus on collecting, monitoring, and interpreting trends in cancer risks among a variety of populations. Large cohort studies, such as the Framingham Heart Study (2012), provide retrospective information about groups of people that share similar experiences. The Canadian Tobacco Use Monitoring Survey (CTUMS) (2010) describes the smoking trends in Canada from 1999 to 2010. Other data regarding chronic diseases are identified through individual records, from insurance companies, and with reviews of death certificates.

Internationally, surveys have revealed that the burden of chronic disease in adults and children is increasing in low- and middle-income countries, and despite increasing awareness and commitment to address chronic illness, global actions to implement cost-effective interventions are inadequate (Alwan et al., 2010). The cause of the increase of chronic diseases in these countries is not easy to pinpoint. Most of the research on chronic illness factors has been conducted in developed countries.

Economic Burden of Chronic Illness

Chronic diseases are not only common, they are costly. In 2011, the Harvard School of Public Health released a report called *The Global Economic Burden of Non-communicable Diseases*. This report noted that more than 60% of deaths (mostly cardiovascular diseases, diabetes, cancer, and chronic respiratory diseases) occur from noncommunicable causes (Bloom et al., 2011). This report indicated that the number of worldwide cases of all sites of cancer in 2010 was 13,313,111, and predictions are that by 2030 the number of cases will likely be close to 21,503,563. In 2010, cancer medical costs were $153,697 million, with nonmedical costs at $67,072 million, and income losses at $68,969 million. It is likely that these costs will double in the next 15 years.

In 2010, diabetes cost the global economy about $500 billion in U.S. dollars with projections expected to be about $745 billion in 2030. The national economic burden of Parkinson's disease exceeded $14.4 billion in 2010 (approximately $22,800 per patient) (Kowal, Dall, Chakrabarti, Storm, & Jain, 2013). Indirect costs of Parkinson's disease (e.g., reduced employment) were conservatively estimated at $6.3 billion (or close to $10,000 per person with Parkinson's disease) (Kowal et al., 2013). When chronic illness is considered, it is useful to recognize that besides the associated dollar costs of various chronic diseases, there is also a loss in productivity and wages due to absenteeism.

In Canada, chronic diseases cost an estimated $90 billion a year in lost productivity and health care costs (Mirolla, 2004). Also in Canada, the economic burden of the three major lung diseases—cancer, asthma, and chronic obstructive pulmonary disease—was $12 billion in 2010 (Theriault, Hermus, Goldfarb, Stonebridge, & Bounajm, 2012). Given the growing number of elderly in Canada, this economic cost for chronic lung disease is expected to double by 2030. In Canada, the number of people smoking has declined; still, 37,000 people die every year related to tobacco smoke, which is one person every 12 minutes (Health Canada, 2009). As in Canada, the number of people smoking in the United States is declining; yet each year in the United States, about 443,000 people die of a smoking-related illness, and smokers die 14 years earlier than nonsmokers (Centers for Disease Control and Prevention [CDC], 2011). Indirect costs, including loss of productivity when an ill person cannot work and the loss of productivity in the workplace when family leave is taken, was estimated to be $8.6 billion. There are approximately 2 million informal family caregivers with an economic burden contribution estimated at $25 billion (Hollander, Lui, & Chappell, 2009; Keefe, 2011).

Economic costs for chronic illnesses such as diabetes are continuing to increase. In Canada, the economic cost of diabetes was approximately $12.2 billion in 2010, which accounts for about 3.5% of public health care spending in Canada (Canadian Diabetes Association, 2009). According to a study commissioned by the American Diabetes Association (2008), in 2002 diabetes was reported to cost Americans $174 billion annually. In 2007 this cost was estimated to have increased by 32% for a total cost of $218 billion (Dall et al., 2010). A disproportionate percentage of these costs result from treatment and hospitalization of persons with diabetes-related complications. The study findings suggest that one of every five health care dollars is spent caring for someone diagnosed with diabetes. Financial costs for this disease are even greater when the family pays for additional health care needs, such as over-the-counter medication and medical supplies, additional visits to optometrists or dentists, health complications that occur before the diabetes is diagnosed, lost productivity at work for the individual and family members, and costs for informal caregiving. Because of continued emphasis on treatment of disease and related complications, rather than prevention, the cost of diabetes continues to climb. In fact, only a small amount of the money spent on diabetes is on research, education, or prevention (Dall et al., 2010).

A study conducted to quantify the costs of chronic disease, the potential effects on employers, the government, and the United States economy found that the seven most common chronic diseases—cancer (broken into several types), diabetes, hypertension, stroke, heart disease, pulmonary conditions, and mental disorders—affect

133 million Americans (DeVol, 2008). These diseases have large-ticket economic costs of $1.3 trillion annually, along with potential for lost work and productivity. Findings from the DeVol (2008) study also have the following indications:

- At the current rate, a 42% increase in cases of the seven chronic diseases is predicted by 2023, with $4.2 trillion in treatment costs and lost economic output.
- Modest improvements in preventing and treating diseases could avoid 40 million cases of chronic disease by 2023, with the economic effect of chronic illness decreased by 27% or $1.1 trillion annually from the current cost.
- Decreased obesity rates, a large risk factor linked with chronic illness, could result in productivity gains of $254 billion and avoid $60 billion in annual treatment expenditures.

Many with chronic illnesses fear they will be unable to afford needed medical care, a fear not unfounded as medical costs for those with chronic illness tend to be higher. Families with a child or an adult member with a chronic condition often face economic challenges. For example, in diabetes management, although medical insurance may cover the costs of medications and supplies such as syringes and glucose testing strips, other health-promoting activities might require out-of-pocket expenses. A person with diabetes needs to eat a balanced diet, which requires the purchase of foods high in nutritional value, food that might be more expensive than less healthy foods.

Lay caregivers, although posing far less of an economic burden on the health care system, come with their own set of costs. Still, the cost of funding caregiver services and support is small compared with the value of their contributions (Feinberg, Reinhard, Houser, & Choula, 2011). Policy recommendations that can make these economically friendlier unpaid caregivers' services (Gibson & Houser, 2007) less burdensome to families include the following:

- Implementing "family-friendly" workplace policies (e.g., flextime, telecommuting).
- Preserving and expanding the protections of the Family and Medical Leave Act of 1993 and updated in 2008 (U.S. Department of Labor, 2013).

- Expanding funding for the National Family Caregiver Program, which was established in 2000 to provide funding to states and territories based on the number of people over 70 years of age. It supports families and informal caregivers to keep loved ones at home as long as possible (U.S. Department of Health and Human Services [USDHHS], 2012).
- Providing adequate funding for the Lifespan Respite Care Act (2006). This program coordinated systems of accessible, community-based respite care services for family caregivers of children and adults of all ages with special needs (Administration for Community Living, 2013).
- Providing a tax credit for caregiving.
- Permitting payment of family caregivers through consumer-directed models in publicly funded programs (e.g., Medicaid home, community-based services waivers).
- Assessing family caregivers' own needs through publicly funded home and community-based service programs and referral to supportive services.

Costs Associated With Children With Special Health Care Needs

In addition to the health care provided in clinical settings, children with chronic special health care needs (SHCN) often require illness management and health maintenance in the home. The increased time and care demands of SHCN can make it difficult for family caregivers to be employed fully; emotional stress and financial burdens can result. A child might need special therapy such as physical, speech, or occupational. Certain illnesses require constant out-of-pocket health care (such as autism, cystic fibrosis, or mental health needs) that can range from $2,669 to $69,906 per year, compared to $676 to $3,181 for families with non-SHCN children (Lindley & Mark, 2010). In addition, these families may have to pay more for everyday living expenses, such as water, heating, or special clothes or equipment, that are not included in their health plan. Parents of SHCN may lose pay as they need to take days off from work to care for their child (Lindley & Mark, 2010).

Parents working in low-income jobs often do not receive adequate health insurance benefits. Some families earn too much money to qualify for public subsidies but not enough money to cover the health care expenses of raising a child with SHCN. Compared with children in higher-income (and also lowest-income) households, children living in such "near-poor" families are more likely to have gaps in insurance coverage and more likely to be uninsured (Looman, O'Conner-Von, Ferski, & Hildenbrand, 2009). Eleven percent of uninsured children did not receive needed family support services related to chronic illness care, compared with 7.7% of children with public insurance and 2.7% of privately insured children (USDHHS, Health Resources and Services Administration, Maternal and Child Health Bureau, 2008). Families who lack health insurance are more likely to report that, although health and family support services are needed, they were not received. In addition, families can be greatly challenged as they try to balance chronic illness costs against other member and household needs. Keep in mind that costs for the individual and his or her family can also be measured in loss of quality of life.

THEORETICAL PERSPECTIVES: WAYS TO UNDERSTAND CHRONIC ILLNESS

Theory provides a common language and foundation to understand abstract concepts and their connections. This chapter explains three models that can be used by family nurses to explore the impact of chronic illness on families: Rolland's Chronic Illness Framework, the Family Management Style Framework (Knafl & Deatrick, 1990, 2003), and the Family Health Model (FHM; Denham, 2003). These models provide unique perspectives on assessment, goal planning, nursing actions, and outcome evaluation using a family-focused point of view.

Rolland's Chronic Illness Framework

Chronic illnesses can be categorized by their traits, as outlined in Rolland's (1987) Chronic Illness Framework (see Chapter 3). This framework outlines how the following aspects come together in families and explains how families with similar illness stories adapt differently:

- Onset of the illness (acute or gradual)
- Level of disability resulting from the conditions (capacitating or incapacitating)

- Outcome of the illness (fatal, unpredictable, nonfatal)
- Stability of the disease (progressive, constant vs. relapsing symptoms)
- Time phase of the chronic illness (diagnosis, mid-illness, or terminal phase).

In Rolland's framework, the above elements of chronic illness affect family functioning, strengths, and vulnerabilities. For example, although some chronic conditions involve primary disabilities, such as those occurring from birth anomalies, other conditions, such as strokes, myocardial infarctions, secondary blindness, or kidney failure, are acquired disabilities resulting from lifestyle patterns or delayed or ineffective treatment of other conditions. The reaction and adaptation of the individual and family to a chronic condition differs according to whether the disability is considered on-time and expected versus off-time and unexpected. Likewise, although some people with chronic conditions have lives fraught with pain, depression, and mental or physical difficulties, others experience satisfying lives with only minimal difficulties.

Family Management Style Framework

The Family Management Style Framework (FMSF) was designed to help nurses understand how families who have a child with a chronic condition integrate management of the chronic illness for the child into the everyday living needs and routines of the family as a whole. The original work on the development of the FMSF was conducted by Deatrick and Knafl in 1990. This original work has been refined over the last 23 years to be one of the most significant longitudinal studies of a family assessment instrument. The assessment instrument helps nurses understand the needs of families who have children with specific chronic conditions, such as brain tumors (Deatrick et al., 2006), children undergoing palliative care at home (Bousso, Miski, Mendes-Castilla, & Rossato, 2012), and adolescents who have spina bifida (Wollenhaupt, Rodgers, & Swain, 2011). In addition to investigating families with children, Beeber and Zimmerman (2012) used the FMSF to increase understanding of challenges for families who have an older adult with dementia.

Understanding the family's responses to a chronic condition provides ways for family nurses to offer effective interventions to meet both the needs of the individual and family. In this framework, there are five family management styles: *thriving, accommodating, enduring, struggling,* and *floundering.* The management style a family adopts is based on how the family members define the situation, manage the situation and perceive the consequences of the situation. In the FMSF, the parents each define what the child's chronic condition means for them individually and their family. Included in this definition is how the parents view the child. Does the parent view the child as a child who has a health issue that can be managed, or does the parent focus on the condition before the child and see the management of the health condition as tragic and difficult to manage? Influencing the definition are the parents' personal beliefs about the cause, the seriousness, the predictability, and the course of the condition. Another component in defining the illness is how disparate or similar the two parents' perceptions are on how they view their child, the condition, parenting philosophy, and overall approach to management. Table 9-1 briefly outlines the five family management styles.

Table 9-1	Family Management Style Framework			
View of the Child **Thriving**	**Accommodating**	**Enduring**	**Struggling**	**Floundering**
Parents view child from the lens of normalcy. They see the child as just as capable as other children. Their child has a chronic health condition that is incorporated into everyday life of the child and the family as a whole.	Parents usually see their child from the lens of normalcy and being capable of living everyday life.	Parents fluctuate in their view of the child between that of normalcy and tragic. Sometimes see them as capable and other times focus on vulnerabilities.	Parents are inconsistent in how they view the child relative to normalcy capabilities and vulnerabilities.	Parents have primarily a negative view of their child and see the situation as tragic. They see the child as not capable and as vulnerable.
Parents view life as normal and incorporate the management of the health condition into everyday life of the child and family.	Parents tend to view life as normal and caring for the child with a chronic condition as part of life.	Parents vary on how they view life between normal or focused on the management of the health condition.	Parents are variable in how they view everyday life, but primarily see it from a negative lens and the management overtakes their everyday life as a family.	Parents view the situation as a burden and have a sense of hatefulness about having to manage their child's chronic health condition.
Parents mutually agree in their viewpoints and definition of the child and their management approach.	Parents usually share the same viewpoints, definition, and management choices.	Parents usually share the same viewpoints, definition, and management choices.	Parents do not share the same viewpoints and definition and do not agree on management approaches, which creates much conflict between the parents.	Parents differ significantly on how they view the child, how they define the situation, and the management plan.
Management Behaviors **Thriving**	**Accommodating**	**Enduring**	**Struggling**	**Floundering**
Parents are confident in their management abilities and incorporate management regimen into the life of the family. They are proactive in their problem-solving approach.	Mothers are confident in their abilities to manage the chronic condition. Fathers are not as confident as the mothers in their abilities to manage the illness. They are usually proactive in problem solving, but sometimes are reactive.	Parents are confident in their abilities but have the viewpoint of the management regimen as burdensome. They are usually proactive in problem solving, but sometimes are reactive.	Parental conflict is the overriding theme. Mothers see the management as burdensome. Fathers express more confidence in their ability to manage the chronic condition. Both parents do not anticipate problems that are routine; therefore they are reactive to problems.	Parents view the management regimen as burdensome. They feel inadequate and overwhelmed. They are reactive to problems and often are overwhelmed or put into crisis mode when a problem occurs.

(continued)

Table 9-1	**Family Management Style Framework—cont'd**			
Perceived Consequences				
Thriving	**Accommodating**	**Enduring**	**Struggling**	**Floundering**
Parents view the child in the foreground and see the stress and hassles of the chronic health condition in the background. Parents have a positive outlook and create a new sense of "normal" for the family as a whole.	Parents usually place the child in the foreground and the stress and strains of the chronic condition in the background. In general, the parents have a positive outlook for the family as a whole.	Parents fluctuate in how they perceive the outcome and stress/strains of the chronic condition on the child and the family.	Mothers typically have a negative view of the situation and future outlook for the child. Fathers tend to be more positive in their view of the future for the child.	Parents have a negative outlook and view of the future. They worry that their future as parents will be less happy and limited.

Managing the child's condition is another piece to establishing a family's management style. To manage illness, parents combine their philosophy of parenting with their beliefs about their ability to parent a child with a chronic condition. One management approach may be that of being confident in their ability to parent and manage a chronic health condition. A second management approach may be when the parent views the child and situation as burdensome. A third approach is when parents feel they are inadequate in their abilities to parent a child with a chronic condition.

Another element of management concentrates on how the parent balances the ability to manage the chronic health condition with other aspects of family life. Parental management behaviors linked with chronic illness are often aligned with their ability to establish consistent and effective treatment routines. Parents may not be well prepared to handle the caregiving responsibilities shortly after receiving a chronic illness diagnosis; they might require some coaching (Sullivan-Bolyai, Knafl, Sadler, & Gilliss, 2004). Stable routines that allow for balance or equilibrium in daily life are essential for optimal disease management over time and through life course changes. For example, if the chronic illness requires dietary changes, family members must learn ways to balance personal food preferences and prior eating patterns with the medical needs of the ill member. Although specific management or routine activities may vary, a predictable and consistent routine seems essential.

Finally, the ways parents focus attention on and perceive consequences of a chronic illness is an important consideration in determining the family's management style. Chronic illness can be viewed as a central feature of the family, an organizing focus, or a life aspect balanced with other responsibilities.

The FMSF not only identifies cognitive and behavioral family aspects, but also points to factors that may be predictive of family strengths or problems (Knafl & Deatrick, 1990, 2003; Knafl, Deatrick, & Havill, 2012). Nurses using this model are urged to consider the unique needs of individuals within the family, those of family members or member dyads, and the family as a whole. Family nurses should use this model as a guideline that outlines ways to think about how a family is responding to having a child with a chronic illness. Nurses can use this model to help think of interventions that may help a family in the management of the situation and adaptation to living with a chronic condition. Nurses need to understand member dynamics and family processes as they assess care needs, provide education, and offer counseling.

Family Health Model

Connections between chronic illness and families are tied to ideas suggested within the Family Health Model (FHM) (Denham, 2003). This ecological model provides a lens to consider the multiple traits, interactive processes, and life experiences that influence the health and illness of interacting and developing persons. Families and individual members have infinite ways to define themselves, as they interact and exchange information with larger societal systems and institutions. The family household is the hub of action where members depart and return as individual members are nurtured and socialized. The FHM identifies member connections to each other and those beyond the household boundaries that have relevance to chronic illness. The FHM uses three domains—contextual, functional, structural—in which nurses perform assessments, plan care, provide nursing actions, and evaluate outcomes. This model encourages nurses to consider ecological factors relevant to the family members and their household. Things such as the neighborhood, community resources, community demographics, political milieu, and social environment are factors that also influence families' responses to chronic illness and disease management, and affect outcomes.

Operational definitions suggest ways to describe the complex relationships among the biophysical and holistic aspects of a chronic illness and how these aspects affect family, health, and family health. In the FHM, health is defined as an adaptive state experienced by family members as they seek to optimize their well-being and wrestle with liabilities found within self, family, households, and the various environments where they interact throughout the life course (Denham, 2003). This definition guides nursing practice roles useful for family care when a member has a chronic illness. Even when one has a chronic illness, health can still be possible and well-being can be maximized. Family health suggests that member transactions occur through system and subsystem interactions, relationships, and processes that have the potential to maximize processes of becoming, enhance well-being, and capitalize on the household production of health. Families strive to achieve a state where members are content with themselves and one another. That is, family health includes the complex interactions of individuals, family subsystems, family, and the various contexts experienced over the life course. The household becomes the pivotal point for coping with health and family health needs.

Context

Family health is depicted with contextual, functional, and structural dimensions (Fig. 9-1). The

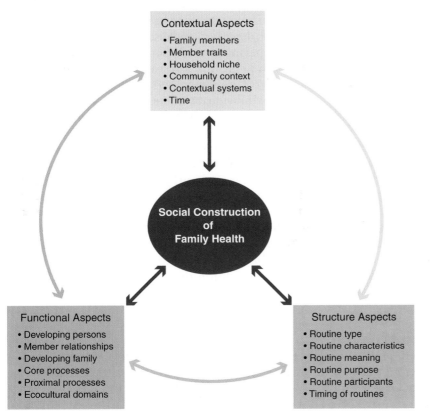

FIGURE 9-1 Contextual, functional, and structural aspects of family care.

contextual domain includes all of the environments where family members interact or have potential to be acted on, but also includes the characteristics or traits of the family (e.g., socioeconomic, educational attainment, extended kin relationships). The contextual domain is affected by the internal household environment (e.g., membership traits and qualities, culture, traditions, values) and external household environment (e.g., neighborhood, community, safety, larger society, historical period, political context). An ecological model helps nurses understand that nested life aspects can challenge or strengthen one's abilities to discern causes and outcomes. Over time, it is difficult to decipher the many powerful influencers; things overlap, intersect, and potentiate or negate important health factors.

The *family household* is a key family environment or context. The household refers to the physical structure(s), immediate neighborhood surroundings, material and nonmaterial goods, and tangible and intangible family resources of the members that live together. As people age, they often reflect back on many households where they lived and the various influences impressed upon self from those settings. The family context pervades all life aspects and affects personal interactions, values, attitudes, access to medical resources, and availability of support systems, and has influence on individual and family health routines. For example, a family living in poverty or lacking adequate health care insurance is unlikely to have the same access to medical care as a more affluent family. A rural family with a long tradition of cultural values about health or illness might minimize physical symptoms and be slower to seek medical care than an urban family with great confidence in science and the abilities of health care practitioners.

Function

The *functional domain* refers to the individual and cooperative processes family members use as they interact with and engage one another over the life course. This domain includes individual factors (e.g., values, perceptions, personality, coping, spirituality, motivation, roles), family process factors (e.g., cohesiveness, resilience, individuation, boundaries), and member or family processes (e.g., communication, coordination, caregiving, control). These dynamic factors mediate the actions of individuals, family subsystems, and families as a whole as they seek to attain, sustain, maintain, and regain health. The core family functions of caregiving, celebration, change, communication, connectedness, and coordination alter as health and illness are faced; these are areas nurses can assess, plan nursing actions, and collaborate with family members to improve chronic illness outcomes (Denham, 2003). The experiences linked with chronic illness can test and burden the functional capacities of the family and its members. In some families, individual and group strengths can be rallied to address pressing concerns, whereas other families might have member conflict that threatens the capacities of effective disease management.

Structure

The contextual and functional domains are the situational and behavioral antecedents that family members use to construct family habits or patterns linked with health and illness outcomes. The third aspect of the FHM is referred to as the *structural domain;* it is composed of six categories of family health routines: self-care, safety and precautions, mental health behaviors, family care, illness care, and member caretaking. Each routine category is comprised of complex multimember habitual actions that form interactive patterns that describe the lived health and illness experiences of family households (Denham, 2003). *Family health routines* are relatively stable but still dynamic actions or habitual patterns that can be recalled, described, and discussed from individual and family perspectives. What might initially appear as random or chaotic patterns to an outsider may represent to family members regularity, purpose, and value of individual routines.

Although routines have unique qualities and involve all household members, some aspects of them change and evolve over time. This evolution can be a voluntary and intentional act or it can be a consequence of other things occurring in the family's life. Family members tend to maintain the integrity of routines as long as they are viewed as meaningful. New life situations can cause some adaptations to occur, however. Health routines tend toward steadfastness, but the diagnosis of a chronic condition that demands medical management and the availability of new or different support or resources (i.e., contextual factors) can challenge prior valued routines. During a chronic condition, if the family uses effective modes of communication, has abilities to share roles, and is comprised of resilient personalities, it might be more capable of handling the changes than those lacking these qualities. Family members might be able to cooperate and deconstruct ineffective routines and reconstruct new ones better than a disorganized family or one where member conflict rules. Health and illness routines are ways family members can support or thwart the management of a chronic illness. Family-focused nurses who partner with individuals and families can collaborate with them to plan care, strategize ways to implement changes, and evaluate outcomes. The creation and stability of healthy family routines and lifestyles can be strengthened through cooperative efforts. Family health routines are dependent on the human and material resources needed for the individual and family to make needed changes. Functional perspectives give insight into ways families optimize health potentials and use resources to balance diverse and conflicting needs.

Well-being

Family-focused nurses strive to assist individuals and families make the most of available resources to achieve health and well-being. *Well-being*, in the Family Health Care Model (Denham, 2003), is defined as a health state with actualized opportunities, minimized liabilities, and maximized resources. Well-being includes many dimensions, including biophysical, psychological, emotional, social,

spiritual, and vocational. Well-being is achieved through accomplishment of family goals such as risk reduction, prevention, health maintenance, and self-actualization. Nurses aim to provide holistic care that enhances well-being and to partner with families to empower them when chronic illness is the concern. Nurses who provide family-focused care aid individuals and families to achieve their health goals. They also empower members to devise plans and identify ways to implement strategies, and evaluate whether goals are met. Nursing encounters become a means to target the household production of health, or holistically address related or potentially related health attributes or threats.

In chronic illness, family-focused care assists multiple family members to adapt, accommodate, and use household resources to achieve well-being for the entire family. Based on the FHM, family-focused nurses can use what are identified as core processes to consider family aspects relevant to chronic disease management and identify ways to empower individuals and families to meet care goals (Table 9-2). The FHM suggests a variety of ways to understand what happens when a member has a chronic illness from contextual, functional, and structural perspectives (Denham, 2003). Table 9-3 identifies a number of

Table 9-2	Core Family Processes and Chronic Illness		
Core Processes	**Definition**	**Areas of Concern**	
Caregiving	Concern generated from close intimate family relationships and member affections that result in watchful attention, thoughtfulness, and actions linked to members' developmental, health, and illness needs	Health maintenance Disease prevention Risk reduction Health promotion	Illness care Rehabilitation Acute episodic needs Chronic concerns
Cathexis	Emotional bonds between individuals and family that result in members' emotional and psychic energy investments into needs of the loved one	Attachment Commitment Affiliation Loss	Grief and mourning Normative processes Complicated processes
Celebration	Tangible forms of shared meanings that occur through family celebrations, family traditions, and leisure time that might be used to commemorate special times, days, and events; these times are often used to distinguish usual daily routines from special ones; they often occur across the life course and have special roles, responsibilities, and expectations	Culture Family fun Traditions Rituals	Religion Hobbies Shared activities
Change	A dynamic nonlinear process that demands an altered form, direction, and/or outcome of an expected identity, role, activity, or desired future	Control Meet expressed needs Meanings of change Contextual influences	Compare and contrast Similarities/differences Diversity

(continued)

Table 9-2	**Core Family Processes and Chronic Illness—cont'd**		
Core Processes	**Definition**	**Areas of Concern**	
Communication	The primary ways children are socialized and family members interact over the life course about health beliefs, values, attitudes, and behaviors, and incorporate or apply health information and knowledge to illness and health concerns	Language Symbolic interactions Information access Coaching Cheerleading	Knowledge and skills Emotional needs Affective care Spiritual needs
Connectedness	The ways systems beyond the family household are linked with multiple family members through family, educational, cultural, spiritual, political, social, professional, legal, economic, or commercial interests	Partner relationships Kin networks Household labor Cooperation Member roles	Family rules Boundaries Tolerance for ambiguity Marginalization
Coordination	Cooperative sharing of resources, skills, abilities, and information within the family household, among members of extended kin networks, and larger contextual environments to optimize individual's health potentials, enhance the household production of health, maintain family integrity or wellness, and achieve family goals	Family tasks Problem solving Decision making Valuing Coping Resilience	Respect Reconciliation Forgiveness Cohesiveness System integrity Stress management

Source: Modified from Denham, S. A. (2003). *Family health: A framework for nursing.* Philadelphia, PA: F. A. Davis, with permission.

Table 9-3	**Assessment Using the Family Health Model**
Categories to Assess	**Specific Areas Within Each Category**
Contextual	• Developmental stage • Family traits • Availability of health insurance • Access to care • Demographics (age, education, sex, employment) • Social support • Culture and ethnicity • Political, historical, and environmental factors
Functional	• Stressors • Coping skills • Family roles • Member responsibilities • Communication patterns
Structural	• Illness characteristics • Family organization or chaos • Routines established • Ability and willingness to alter routines

areas a family nurse might assess using this conceptual model.

PREVENTION OF CHRONIC ILLNESS THROUGH HEALTH PROMOTION

Many chronic conditions are preventable. Others, though not preventable, may be able to be delayed, thus ensuring more quality life years. Prevention is an important factor to consider when understanding chronic illnesses. For example, the CDC (2008b, p. 2) has identified several ways preventive financial investments can make important differences:

- For each dollar spent on water fluoridation, $38 is saved in dental restorative treatment costs.
- For each dollar spent on the Safer Choice Program (a school-based HIV, other sexually transmitted diseases, and pregnancy prevention program), about $2.65 is saved on medical and social costs.
- Every dollar spent on preconception care programs for women with diabetes can reduce health costs by up to $5.19, and prevent costly complications for mothers and babies.
- Implementing the Arthritis Self-Help Course among 10,000 individuals with arthritis will yield a net savings of more than $2.5 million while simultaneously reducing pain by 18% among participants.

In looking at gaps of current data collection systems, the Institute of Medicine (2011) suggests that individual and collective data are needed that helps understand the continuum of prevention, disease progression, treatment options, and their outcomes. A troubling aspect of all surveillance efforts is that we have little to no information about family roles, inputs, or outcomes in the prevention or management of chronic illness.

Nonetheless, chronic illness is often linked to behavioral and environmental risk factors that could be effectively addressed through prevention programs. For example, the increasing rates of obesity, leading to several chronic complications, could be prevented with changes in dietary and exercise behaviors and changes in our environment that encourage exercise. An optimistic scenario including weight reduction, healthy eating, a more active lifestyle, continued decrease in tobacco use, improved early detection, fewer invasive treatments, and quicker adoption of proved therapies could cut chronic illness treatment costs by $217 billion per year by 2023 (DeVol & Bedroussian, 2007). These changes could reduce the climbing chronic illness rates and reduce related complications through preventive care.

The Institute of Medicine (2012) suggests taking a "health in all policies" approach to federal regulations, legislation, and policies that improve opportunity for health and physical function for those living with chronic illness. This report also recommends that community-based services available for persons with chronic disease align with health care services and insurance reform legislation. If such an approach were to be taken, legislators and those involved in policy writing would be more conscious about health risks and the ultimate costs resulting from legislative decisions. To curb the chronic illness epidemic, it is critical to initiate innovative approaches in the ways these diseases are prevented and managed now.

HELPING FAMILIES LIVE WITH CHRONIC ILLNESS

Family-focused nurses understand that when individuals have a chronic illness, whether they are young or old, family is always involved in the care. Family members influence decision making, engage in family planning, and play roles that positively and negatively influence disease management.

Some people manage their chronic illness without much difficulty or help from others, whereas others require a great amount of assistance and significant family involvement. Many need little medical care, but others require extensive medical services that may include care from special health practitioners, regular treatments or testing, multiple medicines, or intense therapies. Life can be completely disrupted when confronting long-term or chronic illnesses that affect physical abilities, appearance, and independence. Diminished endurance capacities; continual discomfort in physical, emotional, and social realms; and financial problems are just a few of the challenges families face. New medical procedures, diagnostic tests, screening, and pharmaceuticals have improved health and the ability to live with chronic conditions and extended life span so families are living longer with chronic illness.

The Institute of Medicine (IOM) (2012) considered what it takes to live well with chronic illness and determined that it requires more than medical care and pharmaceutical treatments. The IOM suggests that there are a variety of health determinants that affect the life course (i.e., biology, genes, behavior, coping responses, physical environment, sociocultural context, peers, and family). Some of these aspects are linked with learned behaviors, family households, and the communities where families live. One might classify persons as healthy, at risk, chronically ill, functionally limited, disabled, or nearing the end of life. These health outcomes are influenced by a number of factors; some are intrinsic or controlled by the individual, and some are beyond the individual and live in the larger society (e.g., environmental risks, public policy, population surveillance, media, public health, community organizations, health care, social values). This section focuses on how to work with families to support the person with the illness to participate in his or her own self-management, and ways to help families adapt to living with a chronic illness and working with the family care provider.

Helping to Support Self-Management

Self-management is a crucial aspect to quality living and successful management of a chronic illness. Self-management includes self-efficacy, self-monitoring of illness, and symptom management that is conducted by self or as the person directs others to do for him or her (Richard & Shea, 2011). Self-management is both a process and an outcome of family nursing care. The "Self-Management Support for Canadians With Chronic Health Conditions" report (Health Council of Canada, 2012) outlines the following four recommendations to help the Canadian health care system support people living with chronic illness in a more systematic way (p. 7). These recommendations should be applied to those living with chronic illness regardless of country:

- Create an integrated, system-wide approach to self-management support.
- Enable primary health care providers to deliver self-management support as a routine part of care.

- Broaden and deepen efforts to reach more Canadians who need self-management supports.
- Engage patients and informal caregivers as a key part of any systematic approach.

Family nurses work with the individual and family to support self-management of the illness. For example, adolescents/young adults who engage in self-management at the time they transition from pediatrics to adult medical care are known to have improved health outcomes (American Academy of Pediatrics, 2011; van Staa, van der Stege, Jedeloo, Moll, & Hilberink, 2011).

Diabetes is a clear illustration. Diabetes self-management, much like self-management for any chronic illness, entails adhering to a prescribed medical regimen and making lifestyle behavior changes. Most of these actions largely occur outside nurses' and other health professionals' observation. Self-management calls for integration of prescribed treatments into the daily experience. Self-management requires highly motivated individuals to follow medically prescribed treatments and protocols that may not be understood fully. This means that the individuals must have some confidence that their doctors and other practitioners know what they are doing and trust that following these directions will improve one's quality of life.

The last several decades have produced a large body of research findings that suggest that self-efficacy is an important factor linked with a willingness to participate in specific behavior (Richard & Shea, 2011). Persons with higher self-efficacy are more likely to engage in more challenging tasks, set higher goals, and achieve them (Bandura, 1977). Individuals with the disease and their family members will have different levels of self-efficacy and may differ in their level of readiness for change. Nurses who understand self-efficacy and readiness to change can use these concepts as they collaborate with families to set goals and plan strategies for meeting them. Nurses assess families on their perceptions and abilities to make the changes and then assist them as they agree on what changes they can make together. Nurses can explore family members' desires and confidence in their ability to alter lifestyle habits that might support their family member with a chronic illness to adhere to lifestyle changes, such as diet. A nurse-led family conference might be a way for the nurse to share more information about why changes are needed, benefits that might be realized, and risks if no changes are made. Some agreement might arise on trying a few things differently each week and moving toward the goals by using small steps each week. Nurses should not be simply telling the family what needs to be done, but asking them what they need, identifying their concerns, and helping them identify what they believe will be a plan they are willing to achieve together.

Too often, persons with chronic conditions see numerous clinicians who order treatments without consulting how they might affect the whole family. Individuals and families benefit from coordinated care; this means providing treatments and medical visits in ways that integrate services and relevant communication among those providing care. Goals of coordinated care include improving health outcomes, identifying risks or problems early, avoiding crises, and ensuring cost-effectiveness of service delivery. Poorly coordinated care has risks for preventable health complications, conflicts between professionals, increased stress for the individuals and their families, unnecessary hospitalizations, added expenses, and even death. Persons who experience even a single chronic condition can receive conflicting information, numerous diagnoses, or multiple medications by different professionals. Nurses are in positions where they can facilitate care management and help individuals and family members sort out the conflicting information or directions in developing a family-focused management plan. By helping the family to develop a management plan, the nurse empowers the family and the person with the chronic illness to participate in and control self-care, with the goal of improving health outcomes for all members of the family.

Family Adaptation

Living with chronic illness is described by Arestedt, Persson, and Benzein (2013) as an ongoing process of adaptation, co-creating ways for the family members, both individually and as a family, to achieve a sense of well-being. By using this in-depth phenomenological hermeneutic analysis, family nurses can work with families to help them adjust to everyday living by developing a new rhythm of adaptation.

■ Co-creating a context for living with illness: When families are confronted with the reality of living with a family member having a chronic illness, they spend time learning how to develop different ways of accomplishing the tasks of the family and meet the needs of the family members. They accomplish this through discussion of the situation. After this initial adjustment and the establishment of how to maintain daily functioning, families report that the illness and situation is not always on their minds.

■ Communicating the illness within and outside the family: Families learn to balance discussion about the illness, the situation, and the future with chronic illness with other life events for the individual family members and the family as a whole.

■ Co-creating alternative ways for everyday life: Families learn to operate at a slower pace than before chronic illness. Families note that they are more focused on the present as there is an ever-present awareness of an uncertain future.

■ Altering relationships: The members of the family develop or adapt their relationships to include chronic illness as they have to get to know each other in a different way. In some situations, family members are interacting more often than before the onset of the chronic illness. In other situations, families report being stronger and pulling together more when the illness has exacerbations.

■ Changing roles and tasks: All roles in the family require adjustment when living in the midst of chronic illness. The family struggles to reestablish a balance in getting the needs of the family accomplished.

With many chronic illnesses, the family is continually shifting between illness being the primary focus of the family and wellness being the primary view of the family. For example, when there is an exacerbation of the illness that requires the family member to be hospitalized, the family is reminded the illness is present and needs attention. At other times, the family is focused on the wellness of everyone by, for instance, having family dinner together once a week. Co-creation of ways the family adapts and flows with this movement allows for some overlapping of these two family situations (Paterson, 2002). Nurses working with families living with chronic illness who understand this process of evolving family adaptation empower families to move from a viewpoint of "victim" of circumstances to a viewpoint of "creator" of circumstances (Arestedt et al., 2013; Paterson, 2002).

One person's chronic condition has great potential to influence the lives of many others. Those living with a family member with a chronic disability can become fatigued by the constant vigilance required to perform normal everyday activities of daily living and the stress of uncertainty (Hummel, 2013a). This fatigue is influenced by the volume of help required, the emotional strain that accompanies the daily hassles, and the relationship strain of constantly giving to another. One aspect of family nursing that is crucial to helping these families is assisting the family members to adjust to new roles, such as caregiver and care receiver. Nurses can help families explore who does what role in the family and how to use resources to help the family function well by using outside resources to fill some of the family roles. See Chapter 4 for more detail about how to work with families about role negotiation.

Family Caregiving

Family caregiver is a crucial role in providing support for those living with chronic illness. Several chapters in this book touch on family caregivers caring for family members with chronic illness. For example, Chapter 16 addresses family caregiving for families living with mental health concerns. Chapter 15 focuses on working with families who have an aging family member, and Chapter 10 offers suggestions about working with families when a member is experiencing palliative care or end-of-life care. Glasdam, Timm, and Vittrup (2012) reviewed 32 studies of professional interventions on family caregivers. The researchers found that few studies target the caregivers of family members with cancer, cardiovascular disease, or stroke. They conclude that health care providers lack knowledge about the effects of interventions on caregivers. There is a need for clear descriptions of the intensified interventions used with caregivers and the outcomes achieved in order to identify the benefits of nursing actions for caregivers. It is clear, however, that soon after the diagnosis of a chronic illness of a family member, caregivers must become proficient in many areas, including managing the illness, coordinating resources, maintaining the family unit, and caring for self. Nurses assisting

families can incorporate the following educational and counseling needs into a treatment plan, making clear who is responsible for what in the family:

- Monitoring conditions and behaviors
- Interpreting normal and expected behaviors from different and serious ones
- Providing hands-on care
- Making decisions
- Developing care routines
- Problem solving
- Teaching self-care management

This chapter will focus on two populations in terms of caregiving: one is young children providing care to the adult family member living with a chronic illness and the second is families who have a child with a chronic illness.

Child Caregiving for an Adult

One population that is growing around the world is that of young children providing care for a chronically ill adult. In the United States, there are approximately 1.3 to 1.4 million child caregivers who are between the ages of 8 and 18 (Hunt, Levine, & Naiditch). The following list provides an estimated number of children providing care for adult family members in countries or commonwealths of the United Kingdom (Caregivers Trust, 2012):

- England: Nearly 5 million people are caregivers, and of these, 145,000 are children.
- Scotland: There are 657,000 caregivers in Scotland, and of these, 16,701 are children.
- Wales: There are 340,745 people who are caregivers, and of these, 11,000 are children.
- Northern Ireland: There are 185,066 people who are caregivers, and of these, 2,300 are children.

In Australia, it is estimated that there are 300,000 young caregivers, 150,000 of them under the age of 18 years (Australian Bureau of Statistics, 2009). A 2010 Canadian high school study of 483 ethnically diverse students in grades 8 through 12 found that 12% of youth between the ages of 12 and 17, with a mean age of 14 years, self-identify as "Young Carers" (Marshall & Stainton, 2010). In response to a rising number of young caregivers, Canada created an action task force to investigate the invisible population of the young caregiver population and its needs (Bednar et al., 2013). In a similar study in the United States, Bridgeland, DiIulio, and

Morison (2006) found that a third of high school dropouts (32%) said they had to get a job and make money; 26% said they dropped out because they became a parent; and 22% said they had to care for a family member. Many of these young people reported doing reasonably well in school and had a strong belief that they could have graduated if they had stayed in school. Childhood caregiver statistics in the United States identified by Hunt et al. (2005) are listed below:

- Three in ten child caregivers are ages 8 to 11 (31%), and 38% are ages 12 to 15. The remaining 31% are ages 16 to 18.
- Child caregivers are almost evenly balanced by gender (male 49%, female 51%).
- Caregivers tend to live in households with lower incomes than non-caregivers, and they are less likely than non-caregivers to have two-parent households (76% vs. 85%).

There are both negatives and positives to being a young family caregiver. The positive effects are that they report feeling appreciated for their help and that they like helping their family member (Hunt et al., 2005). Negative outcomes from assuming the family caregiver role at a young age are reported in the literature, however. Young caregivers between 8 and 11 years old are more likely than non-caregivers to feel at least some of the time that no one loves them (Hunt et al., 2005). A 2012 study found significant effects on caregiving teens' mental health, specifically, significantly higher risk for anxiety and depression (Cohen, Greene, Toyinbo, & Siskowski, 2012). Nurses should be aware that there are several young caregiver support groups that are offered online and there are camps offered for these children where they can have some carefree time away from family responsibility. Family nurses should inquire about the involvement of children and teens in caring for family members with chronic illness.

The population of young caregivers remains an invisible population and the exact numbers are unknown. Some reasons this caregiver population is growing include the following:

- Decreasing family size
- Geographical dispersion of families
- High divorce rates
- Increasing number of single parents
- Multiple marriages and reconstituted families
- In African countries, it may be related to number of adult deaths due to AIDS

These students and young caregivers live a stressful life that has many more responsibilities when compared to age peers. In addition, the young caregivers are found to have significantly more anxiety and depression and less satisfaction when compared to non-caring age-related peers (Cohen et al., 2012). Caregiving has a negative influence on the emotional well-being of youth with dual student-caregiver roles (Cohen et al., 2012).

The UK countries have several major national laws that provide for a wide range of services and programs that include financial allocations to assess vulnerable children, provide community- and home-based services for care recipients, families, and youths, and have several support programs and resources for youth caregivers. The United States has no national policies or programs to support this vulnerable population. The American Association of Caregiving Youth (2013) was established by Connie Siskowski, a nurse. This is the only program in the United States that addresses any concerns about this vulnerable population. She designed an after-school program to help these young caregivers meet others living in similar situations, learn how to provide care for their family member safely, and learn how to seek help or resources (American Association of Caregiving Youth, 2013). This nurse also designed a week-long onsite summer camp for these young caregivers to attend so they could experience a normal childhood event and get away from the stress of everyday caregiving.

As this population of vulnerable caregivers continues to grow, one role of the family nurse is to be alert and recognize when a young child is providing care for an adult in the family. When this situation is present, the nurse should work to find supports for this caregiver and remember that the caregiver is also a child or adolescent who has normal developmental needs in addition to this caregiving family role.

Families Caring for Children Living With a Chronic Illness

According to the *National Survey of Children with Special Health Care Needs 2009–2010* (Data Resource Center for Child and Adolescent Health, 2012), 11.2 million children from 0 to 17 years of age have special health care needs, which translates to one in five American households. Children with special health care needs (SHCN) have a wide range of conditions and risk factors that underlie many shared health conditions. The top six health issues for children with SHCN, in order of prevalence, are as follows: 48.6% have allergies, 35.3% have asthma, 30.2% have attention-deficit disorder/attention-deficit hyperactivity disorder, 17.6% have developmental delays, 17.1% have anxiety, and 13.3% have behavioral problems (Data Resource Center for Child and Adolescent Health, 2012). Most of these top issues are mental health in nature, which differs from the top chronic illnesses encumbering adults noted earlier in the chapter.

Children with SHCN are like typical children in many ways: they are actively growing and developing, enjoy playing and being with peers, and thrive in cohesive family environments. Children with chronic conditions, however, have limitations that affect daily lives and contribute to challenges unique from peers without chronic conditions. Over half of the children with special health care needs report that they experience four or more functional disabilities that are related to everyday living, such as respiratory problems, eating problems, vision issues, difficulty using their hands, and communication issues.

Health care costs that exceed $250 out-of-pocket are often perceived by the family as burdensome, and even lower amounts affect families with lower socioeconomic status (Lindley & Mark, 2010). Twenty percent of families of children with SHCN report that they spend 2 to 7 hours a week providing health care for the child at home and 14% spend more than 11 hours a week. Caring for the child at home is associated with a significant increase in the odds of having a family member reducing or quitting employment outside the home because of the child's health care needs (Looman et al., 2009).

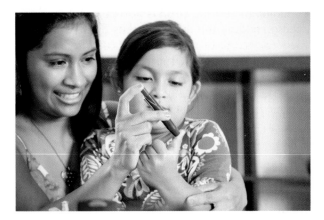

Families with children with SHCN have many needs, caregiving and otherwise. Studies have shown that mothers of chronically ill children often have greater levels of distress than fathers, a concern thought to be related to the greater care demands placed on the mothers (Spilkin & Ballantyne, 2007). It is also not unusual for parents to differ in their perceptions about the impact of the chronically ill child on the family as a whole and on the marital relationship. Although mothers may find that caregiving demands influence their role performance, fathers may perceive the impact most in their expression of feelings and emotions (Rodrigues & Patterson, 2007). A study of 173 parent dyads of children with chronic conditions found that mothers' marital satisfaction was influenced more than fathers' by perceptions about the effects of their child's condition on the family (Berge, Patterson, & Rueter, 2006). Parents' perceptions of the negative effects of the child's chronic condition were measured in terms of family social strain, role strain, and emotional strain. If parents differed in perceptions about the effects of the illness on the family or marital relationship, an increase in stress and frustration resulted. Nurses can assist couples to identify differences in perception between parents, and facilitate discussions about the effects on roles and the benefits of sharing caregiving tasks (Berge et al., 2006; Spilkin & Ballantyne, 2007).

Family-focused care involves active participation between families, nurses, and other health care professionals. Family-focused care supports partnering or collaborative relationships that value and recognize the importance of family traditions, family beliefs, and family management styles. When considering the general population of children with SHCN, approximately 35% of them received care that lacked one or more of the essential components of family-centered care (USDHHS, Health Resources and Services Administration, Maternal and Child Health Bureau, 2008), which are outlined in Table 9-4.

In general, families raising children with chronic illnesses face the joys and challenges that most typical families face, and are as unique and varied as families of typically developing children (Drummond, Looman, & Phillips, 2012). These families want their children to be happy, have a high quality of life, grow, and develop into caring adults who can live independently and contribute to society. These families

Table 9-4	Percentage of Children With Chronic Conditions Without Family-Centered Care

Family-Centered Care Component	Percentage
Health care provider does not usually spend enough time with the child	21.3
Health care provider does not usually provide enough information for the family	16.9
Health care provider does not usually make parent feel like a partner in the child's care	12.4
Health care provider is usually insensitive to the family's values and customs	11.1
Health care provider does not usually listen carefully to family's concern	11.2
Child does not have an interpreter when needed*	43.7

*This applies only to children who needed interpreter services (*N* = 36,018).

face additional stressors, and many researchers acknowledge that the children and parents in these families who care for their children at home are at increased risk for stress-related health conditions and psychosocial problems (Barlow & Ellard, 2006; Berge et al., 2006; McClellan & Cohen, 2007; Meltzer & Mindell, 2006; Mussatto, 2006). Box 9-1 provides a list of stressors likely to be experienced by families caring for a chronically ill child. Despite the risks for problems, however, most children with chronic conditions and their families, including siblings, demonstrate incredible resilience and capacity for finding positives amidst the challenges.

One approach to helping these families is to help them understand the concept of normalization.

BOX 9-1
Potential Stressors When Raising a Child With Chronic Health Conditions

- Care regimen in meeting daily caregiving demands
- Grief, loss of anticipated child events or activities
- Financial and employment strains
- Uncertainty about future
- Access to specialty services
- Reallocation of family assets (e.g., emotional, time, financial)
- Recurrent crises and crisis management
- Foregone leisure time and social interactions
- Social isolation because of stigmatizing policies and practices
- Challenges in transporting disabled children (e.g., when architectural and other barriers restrict their inclusion)
- Physiological stress of caregiving

Normalization is a lens through which families of children with chronic conditions focus on normal aspects of their lives and deemphasize those parts of life made more difficult by chronic conditions (Bowden & Greenberg, 2010; Protudjer, Kozyrskyi, Becker, & Marchessault, 2009; Rehm & Bradley, 2005). The following five attributes of normalization for families of children with chronic conditions offer foundational knowledge for nurses working with such families (Deatrick, Knafl, & Murphy-Moore, 1999):

- Acknowledge the chronic condition and its potential to threaten their lifestyle.
- View all the management of the chronic illness as just normal daily activities in the family.
- Engage in parenting behaviors and routines that are consistent with a normalcy lens.
- Develop treatment regimens that are consistent with normalcy.
- Interact with others based on a view of the child and family as normal.

Although normalization is a useful conceptual and coping strategy for many families of children with chronic conditions, in families whose children have both complex physical and developmental disabilities, normalization as a goal may be neither possible nor helpful (Rehm & Bradley, 2005). When developmental delays compound the effects of a child's physical chronic conditions, a family's ability to organize and manage its daily life is affected significantly. In this case, parents often recognize normal and positive life aspects, acknowledge the profound challenges faced by their family, and accept a "new normal" (Rehm & Bradley, 2005). This capacity to normalize adversity and to define challenging experiences as manageable and surmountable fosters family resilience.

Families with members with chronic conditions, especially those whose conditions are complicated and require care from multiple specialists, often spend a great deal of time interfacing with multiple specialists and systems. For example, a family who has a child with Down syndrome may require regular visits for cardiac, ophthalmological, developmental, and immunological evaluations, physical and occupational therapy, and orthopedic assessments. In addition, parents typically spend a significant amount of time and energy advocating for their child within the school system, attending individualized educational program (IEP) meetings, meeting with academic support professionals, and coping with worries about what is occurring when the child is out of sight (National Association for Down Syndrome, 2012).

In addition, children with chronic conditions still need well-child care similar to those without such an illness. Further, these children are susceptible to other infectious diseases or risks for injuries. It is important for children with chronic conditions to receive regular health maintenance visits with a primary care provider for anticipatory guidance, routine illness, and injury prevention discussions. Parents of children with chronic conditions expect to discuss illness concerns during the well-child care visit. Some providers may expect that care for chronic disease management will decrease opportunities for wellness discussion, but a study of primary care provision for children with SHCN demonstrated the opposite (Van Cleave, Heisler, Devries, Joiner, & Davis, 2007). For parents of children with SHCN and other parents, as more illness topics were discussed, more prevention topics were also discussed.

Researchers who have interviewed parents of children with chronic conditions report some consistent expectations that parents have for their encounters with professionals. Especially important is parents' need for information and mutual trust (Nuutila & Salantera, 2006). Parents want information to be communicated clearly, honestly, respectfully, and with empathy. To be able to give advice and guidance applicable to the lives of a family, health professionals need to know about the family's everyday living and life conditions, and must recognize parents' abilities and skills in caring for their child (Nuutila & Salantera, 2006). Whether the chronically ill person is a child or an adult, family members require useful information that can be applied directly to real family needs. A trusting environment must exist, with easy information exchange, communication directed toward meeting individual and family needs, and respect.

Families want information that will help them provide adequate care for their member with chronic illness and that will help them to anticipate future needs. A decade ago, Ray (2003) noted that excellent informational resources are available, but are not used by families because professionals assume that someone else has provided the family with the information. Parents' and others' needs for information and support change over time as they move through phases of the illness and the family life cycle (Nuutila & Salantera, 2006). At the time of diagnosis, parents want clear and consistent information, and possibly a more directive approach from the provider. For example, when a child with Down syndrome is born, the parents may want to know the immediate implications for the child's health and how that will affect their ability to care for the child at home. As the child grows older and the family gains experience in the care of the child, parents may want a less directive approach from the provider and more of a mutual exchange of information in a collaborative partnership (Nuutila & Salantera, 2006). The nurse who encounters this family at a 3-year well-child examination, for example, should acknowledge the parents' intimate understanding of the child, her reactions to the environment, and her unique needs during the clinical encounter. At this point, the most helpful advice from the nurse is likely anticipatory guidance and planning for entry into the school system. Nurses must recognize that individual and family needs will greatly differ for this child as she becomes 16, 28, or 46 years of age.

Adolescents With Chronic Illness Transition to Adult Services

Transition of care issues have been discussed in the health care industry for decades, but little attention has been allotted to studying and resolving transition problems. Transitions occur in health care in a variety of ways: when a patient moves from one health care provider to a different provider, when a person is sent home from the hospital, when a person who lives in a nursing home needs to be hospitalized, or when a person must switch from private pay to being on Medicaid. Basically a transition is any time there is a major change in the health care management. Transition of care issues for adolescents, who are required to switch from pediatric health care providers to the adult providers of care, is a global health care problem (Kralik, Visentin, & van Loon, 2011; Lugasi, Achille, & Stevenson, 2011; Sonneveld, Strating, van Staa, & Neiboer, 2013; Steinbeck, Brodie, & Towns, 2007, 2008; Wong et al., 2010). Family nurses are in a prime position to address transition issues because they work closely with families and children who have chronic illness (Jalkut & Allen, 2009). As survival rates have improved with many children who live with a chronic illness, this aspect of family nursing requires even more focus. The transition is not just about the medical care from a pediatric physician to an adult specialist. The transition also needs to include psychosocial, educational, and vocational needs of the young adult. It also needs to consider the parents who have, up until that point, orchestrated the management of the illness, communicated with the health care team, made appointments, and interfaced with school. The transition period causes anxiety for the whole family involving leaving long-term health care provider relationships, developmental psychosocial stressors of adolescences, uncertainty about health insurance coverage and issues of the Health Insurance Portability and Accountability Act (HIPAA) relative to parental knowledge, and involvement in the care process and communication (Peter, Fork, Ginsburg, & Schwarz, 2009).

What compounds the difficulty of this transition period for the family and the individual members is the fact that the adult health providers who are assuming care of the young adults with chronic illness often lack understanding of normal adolescent growth and development (Bowen, Henske, & Potter, 2010). This lack of understanding on the part of adult health care providers was recognized as a problem by the American Academy of Pediatrics (2011).

Osterkamp, Costanzo, Ehrhardt, and Gormley (2013) developed an online educational program for nurses about the transition of care for adolescent patients with chronic illness. The modules in the program are HIPAA, family-centered care and its core concepts relative to transition of care of the adolescent patient, and healthy versus chronically ill adolescent development (including information about decrease in compliance with medical regimens and feelings of isolation by being different than other teens). Of the 1,898 nurses who completed the education modules, the post-test assessment score averages were 95%. Box 9-2 lists the Principles of Successful Transition to Adult-Oriented Health Services that have been

---

BOX 9-2
Principles of Successful Transition to Adult-Oriented Health Services

1. Health care services for adolescents and young people need to be developmentally appropriate and inclusive of the young person's family where appropriate.
2. Young people with chronic illnesses and conditions share the same health issues as their healthier peers. Health services therefore need to be holistic and address a range of concerns, such as growth and development, mental health, sexuality, nutrition, exercise, and health-risking behaviors, such as drug and alcohol use.
3. Health care services require flexibility to be able to deal with young people with a range of ages, conditions, and social circumstances. The actual process of transition needs to be tailored to each individual adolescent or young person.
4. Transition is generally optimized when there is a specific health care provider who takes responsibility for helping the adolescent or young person and his or her family through the process.
5. Active case management and follow-up helps optimize a smooth transfer to adult health services, as well as promote retention within adult services.
6. Engagement with a general practitioner can address holistic health care needs and help reduce the risk of failure of transfer to adult services.
7. Close communication between pediatric and adult services will help bridge cultural and structural difference of the two health systems, resulting in smoother transition of young people to adult services.
8. An ultimate goal of transition to adult health care services is to facilitate the development of successful self-management in young people with chronic conditions.

Source: Rosen, D., Blum, R., Britto, M., Sawyer, S., & Siegel, D. (2003). Transition to adult health care for adolescents and young adults with chronic conditions. Position paper of the Society for Adolescent Medicine. *Journal of Adolescent Health, 33*, 309–311.

endorsed by the Society for Adolescent Medicine in 2003.

Nurses who work with families and their teenager with chronic illness should establish a process of "getting ready" for the transfer long before—at least a year or so in advance—the situation occurs (van Staa et al., 2011) and work with the family to design a well-thought-out purposeful plan of transition. One difficult part of this care process is working with the family and the health care team to determine when is the best time for the transition to occur. To base this transition decision solely on chronological age is not sufficient (van Staa et al., 2011). Typically, the transition occurs sometime between years 18 and 21 (American Academy of Pediatrics, 2011). The abilities of the young adult to demonstrate responsibility and to participate as much as possible in self-care management (self-efficacy) are better predictors than age of readiness to transfer (American Academy of Pediatrics, 2011; van Staa et al., 2011). Other factors nurses need to consider and address beside self-efficacy and age in this transition plan are the adolescent's attitude toward transition and the complexity of the illness and treatment plan. The transfer plan should also entail:

- Introducing the concept of transition early in the care relationship with the family. Stress that the transfer is a normative process that reflects achievement of an additional developmental task (Lugasi et al., 2011). Assure the family that transition is not a form of abandonment.
- Holding family meetings to discuss expectations regarding the move to adult care. Explore what they think will be the same or different. Discuss the timing of the transfer. Use these meetings to uncover concerns and needs of the family and each family member about the transition process (Lugasi et al., 2011).
- Assessing the adolescent's ability to provide self-care (Lugasi et al., 2011).
- Designing educational programs to meet the needs of the adolescent/young adult about the illness, how to self-monitor, how to self-manage illness and situations, and how to ask for help when needed. This should include helping the young adult to learn how to develop communication skills.
- Holding discussions about the adult health care environment, insurance coverage, and

health policy changes that will affect the care once the adolescent becomes 18 years of age and is considered a legal adult. This discussion should include differences between pediatric and adult health models of care.
- Having discussions about how the parents may need to move from acting as the primary decision makers to a more supportive and collaborative model of decision making with the young adult.
- Providing the family with a list of adult health providers they may want to consider in their selection process.
- Introducing independent visits with the pediatric health care provider without the parents present.
- Arranging for an introductory visit with the adult provider so that the first interaction is not about an exacerbation of the chronic illness, but one that is about health maintenance. If possible, plan for a joint visit of the family, the pediatric health care team, and the adult health care team.
- Identifying a transition coordinator or someone in the adult health care team who can serve in this role for the family and young adult (Lugasi et al., 2011).

Siblings of Children With Chronic Illness

Younger siblings often strive to model the behaviors of older siblings, including illness behaviors. Focus groups held with parents, siblings, and health care providers resulted in a comprehensive list of psychosocial concerns specific to the experience of school-age siblings of children with chronic illness (Strohm, 2001). These conversations identified seven significant feelings of siblings of children with chronic health care conditions (Strohm, 2001, p. 49):

- Feelings of guilt about having caused the illness or being spared the condition
- Pressure to be the "good" child and protect parents from further distress
- Feelings of resentment when their sibling with special needs receives more attention
- Feelings of loss and isolation
- Shame related to embarrassment about their sibling's appearance or behavior
- Guilt about their own abilities and success

■ Frustration with increased responsibilities and caregiving demands

Other studies reveal more positive sibling outcomes, pointing out that siblings develop improved empathy, flexibility, pride in learning about and caring for a chronic illness, and understanding of differential treatment from parents based on ability and health. Siblings are noted to be more caring, mature, supportive, responsible, and independent than their peer counterparts who do not have siblings with chronic conditions (Barlow & Ellard, 2006). Siblings are reported to have high levels of empathy, compassion, patience, and sensitivity (Bellin & Kovacs, 2006). Siblings demonstrate learning about the disease and in being supportive of their ill brother or sister, and sometimes assume parental roles (Wennick & Hallstrom, 2007). Children who learn about their chronically ill sibling's illness and its mechanisms tend to feel more confident and competent in their ability to support their sibling (Lobato & Kao, 2005; Wennick & Hallstrom, 2007).

Families face the challenge of balancing the needs of the child with a chronic condition with those of the surrounding family, including siblings. It has long been demonstrated that parents of siblings of children with disabilities often lack the ability to give needed time and attention to siblings because of the demands of caring for the child with a disability; this sometimes results in siblings resenting the child with disabilities (Rabiee, Sloper, & Beresford, 2005). Some parents rely on siblings to entertain or assist in the care of the child with disabilities, an action that puts additional stress on the other children.

Systems of Care for Children With Chronic Conditions

Often, bureaucracy and conditions in the health, education, and social services systems are sources of frustration for caregiving families. For example, many services are provided based on diagnosis or categorical determination of eligibility. Therefore, children need to fit certain categories to be eligible for services in acute care, community care, social services, or the school system. Because clinics and subspecialists are in place to serve certain populations, children with uncommon diagnoses or multiple complex chronic conditions are at a disadvantage, and families must seek scarce resources and are forced to coordinate care from multiple specialists in multiple disciplines (Ray, 2003).

When a family member has a chronic illness, the family enters into a complex network of relationships with health care providers and other professionals in the care system. Families often feel as if they are thrown into these relationships (Dickinson, Smythe, & Spence, 2006). Nurses who provide family-focused care consider implications of dynamic care systems, refer the family to appropriate care centers, and evaluate the forms of care provided. Understanding the vulnerability of families in health care provider relationships helps nurses frame their family interactions in ways that create more horizontal than hierarchical relationships. Families are truly the "experts" when it comes to the day-to-day needs of their family members with chronic conditions, and they want professionals to recognize and respect this expertise. Families want professionals and community members to be informed about their family member's diagnosis and the family implications. One parent described her frustration with staff poorly trained on sickle cell disease when she stated, "I knew we were in trouble when the nurse looked at me and said, 'so . . . how long has your daughter had sickle cell disease?' She did not even know that it was an inherited disease" (Mitchell et al., 2007). Through their multiple health care system encounters, caregivers of family members with chronic health conditions tend to develop skills that aid them in the navigation of complex systems as they advocate for their family member's needs (Mack, Co, Goldmann, Weeks, & Cleary, 2007). It is frustrating for caregivers when they encounter health care professionals who are insufficiently informed, who lack knowledge about their family member's condition, or who negate or discount their expertise in providing care (Nuutila & Salantera, 2006).

Social Support

Social support can be categorized into four types of supportive behaviors: emotional, instrumental, informational, and appraisal (House, 1981). The family's capacity to mobilize social support to manage crisis periods and chronic stressors related to a family member's health condition contributes to the well-being of all family members (Bellin & Kovacs,

2006). Table 9-5 provides examples of the four types of social support for families who have a member with a chronic health condition.

Community contexts, such as the neighborhood, school, or church, support the family's development of positive values and foster strengths (Bellin & Kovacs, 2006). Social capital is a concept that can be useful in understanding the community context of health for those with chronic illness and their families. Like social support, social capital is about resources that come from relationships with other people and institutions. Social capital includes features of social life, such as norms, networks, and trust, that enable people to act together toward shared objectives (Putnam, 1996). Looman (2006) defines social capital in terms of investments in relationships that facilitate the exchange of resources. For families who have a chronically ill family member, social capital is especially relevant.

When an individual has a chronic illness, the members of the family (particularly caregivers) are required to engage with numerous professionals and institutions in the process of managing the condition and exchanging resources. The family benefits when a mutual investment exists in their relationships with nurses, physicians, teachers, other families, and neighbors. For example, a mother might invest in her relationship with her child's teachers by providing them with information about her child's health condition, or by helping the teacher understand the child's unique learning style. The teacher, in return, might invest in a relationship with the child's family by scheduling additional parent-teacher conference sessions or by learning more about the child's specific health condition. The benefit of this investment in the family-school relationship, where the common goal is the success of the student, is an exchange of resources. The benefit of this investment may also reach other students and families if this pattern of communication becomes a norm in the school, and if the general level of trust among parents and teachers increases.

Table 9-5   Helpful Support for Families With a Chronically Ill Member

Type of Support	Definition	Activities	Example From Case Studies
Emotional support	Provision of love, caring, sympathy, and other positive feelings	Listening Offering commendations Being present	The nurse working with the Yates family commends them by saying, "I am impressed by the commitment that your family has made to making life as 'normal' as possible for Chloe and her siblings."
Instrumental support	Tangible items, such as financial assistance, goods, or services	Assisting with household chores (e.g., laundry) Providing respite care Providing transportation Assisting with physical care	Devon's parents offer to take Chloe's siblings for a weekend, providing respite for the family and giving the siblings an opportunity to share time with their grandparents.
Informational support	Helpful advice, information, and suggestions	Sharing resources (e.g., books, Web sites, provider names) Educating family members on the health needs of the ill family member Informational support groups	Sarah's brother David, who also has type 2 diabetes, recommends a Web site that provides healthy recipes for individuals with diabetes.
Appraisal support	Feedback given to individuals to assist them in self-evaluation or in appraising a situation	Reviewing daily logs Sharing written feedback from providers (e.g., laboratory results)	The nutritionist provides appraisal support to Sarah during her regular appointments, offering feedback on how Sarah is doing with her lifestyle and dietary changes.

In this way, social capital facilitates the family's ability to acquire emotional, instrumental, informational, and appraisal support in many contexts.

FAMILY NURSING INTERVENTION DURING CHRONIC ILLNESS

The role of the family nurse is to assist multiple family members to interact in ways that optimize abilities and strengths. Although chronic illness care requires consideration of individual outcomes, it must be addressed within the family environment, with consideration of long-term caregiver needs and family outcomes. Across the life course, families use management styles, functional processes, and family health routines to address actual problems, minimize risks, and maximize potentials. Nurses who assess for these styles, processes, and routines, and who then tailor their interventions accordingly to empower and collaborate with families, will be most effective in meeting chronic care needs. Nurses assist families by discussing things such as family strengths, couple time, balancing illness and family needs, developmental milestones, sibling needs, economic restraints, and caregiver well-being (Kieckhefer, Trahms, Churchill, Kratz, Uding, & Villareale, 2013). Moreover, family-focused nursing care should address prevention or reduction of additional health risks, maintenance of optimal wellness levels for all family members, development of therapeutic care management routines, goal-setting that enhances individual and family well-being and integrity, and accommodating unplanned changes. The FHM (Denham, 2003) suggests that families have *core processes* (i.e., caregiving, cathexis, celebration, change, communication, connectedness, coordination) or ways families interact with one another. Nurses can use these ideas as guides to working effectively with families who have a member with a chronic illness (see Table 9-3).

In chronic disease management, family-focused care needs that equip these individuals and their families with knowledge and tools to be effective self-managers have long been lacking (Wagner et al., 2001). Use of an empowerment model and integrative processes to respond to unique needs has been most successful (Hummel, 2013b; Tang, Funnell, & Anderson, 2006). An empowerment model involves the following types of care:

- Patient-centered care
- Problem-based care
- Strengths-based care
- Evidence-based care
- Culturally relevant care

Moreover, empowerment acknowledges that the person is central to chronic care self-management. As nurses seek to empower families for chronic illness management, they should encourage flexibility, coordinate actions of multiple caregivers, use evidence-based guidelines, help families identify community resources, and provide education that builds confidence and skills in multiple family members. A need exists for more evidence about empowerment interventions (Henshaw, 2006; Hummel, 2013b).

Family nurses will be well served by keeping in mind that families typically vary in four systematic ways in their abilities to incorporate medical regimens into their daily routines: remediation, redefinition, realignment, and reeducation (Fiese & Everhart, 2006). Remediation refers to a need to make slight alterations in daily routines to fit illness care into preexisting routines. Redefinition refers to a strategy whereby the emotional connections made during routine gatherings need to be redefined. Realignment occurs when individuals within the family disagree about the importance of different medical routines, and routines need to be realigned in the service of the child's health. The fourth form, reeducation, arises when the family has little history or experience with routines and family life is substantially disorganized (Fiese & Everhart, 2006).

Research about family health suggests that structural behaviors or family health routines are visible activities that family members can readily recall and discuss from multiple perspectives (Denham, 1997, 1999a, 1999b, 1999c). Although family members may report similarities in routines, unique variations are common. The nested family context is a powerful, persuasive, and motivating determinant that influences ways health information is shared within a family and then incorporated into daily routines. Routines have unique characteristics, they vary in rigidity and timing, and members have different expectations across families due to response to member beliefs, values, and perceived needs. Information that fits with perceived family needs is probably the most likely to be incorporated into daily actions. Thus, nursing assessment of chronic care management extends beyond the disease and should also include ways members interact and the life patterns already established.

Family health routines include a number of categorically different foci. Self-care routines involve habits linked with usual activities of daily living such as hygiene. Safety and prevention routines are primarily concerned with health protection, disease prevention, prevention of unintended injury, and avoidance. A nurse assessing this routine area might also be interested in discerning less healthy habits and considering the impact of high-risk behaviors, such as smoking, alcohol, and misuse of other substances, on a chronic condition. Mental health routines are related to self-esteem, personal integrity, work and play, shared positive experiences, stress, self-efficacy, individuation, and family identity. Family-care routines are related to valued traditions, rituals, celebrations, vacations, and other events tied to making meaning and sharing enjoyable times. Illness-care routines are related to decisions about disease, illness, and chronic health care needs, and often determine when, where, and how members seek health care services and incorporate medical directives and health information into self-care routines. Family caregiving routines pertain to reciprocal member interactions believed to assist with health and illness care needs and support during times of crisis, loss, and death.

Families use routines to arrange ordinary life and cope with health or illness events (Fiese & Wamboldt, 2000). These routines are embedded in the cultural and ecological context of families, and highlight ways to focus on family processes and individual and family dynamics (Fiese et al., 2002). Nurses aiming to provide education and counseling to individuals with a chronic illness need to understand the unique family routines of multiple household members and the ways chronic care management is going to alter patterns that are revered, cherished, and comfortable. Nurses who collaborate with families during assessment, goal setting, and outcome evaluation increase the likelihood of providing effective nursing actions that get results that are sustainable over time.

CASE STUDIES: FAMILIES LIVING WITH CHRONIC ILLNESS

It is important to recognize that all chronic diseases are not the same. When diagnosis differs, individual and family needs can differ as well. Other factors also enter into the picture. For example, the age, gender, education, culture, and race of the individual diagnosed, as well as availability of family members, can be critical factors in ways diseases are managed in family situations. This section explores the ways the Yates and Current families address chronic illness management. The Yates family has a daughter who has been diagnosed with type 1 diabetes and the family has been living with this situation for a while. The second family, the Currents, provides an example of working with a family who has an adult member living with Parkinson's disease. Although these two chronic diseases share some similar characteristics for the families living with chronic illness, some unique qualities also emerge. The ways and timing of diagnosis can differ. Treatments can be different. Living with the disease over several decades could mean that new treatments become available. Families living with these two conditions often face different challenges as a result of individual motivation and knowledge, family member characteristics, family developmental stage, and demographics. Family-focused nurses recognize that multiple factors enter into understanding why individuals successfully manage their disease and reasons why they are at risk for complications.

Case Study: Yates Family

Chloe Yates, age 13, was recently admitted to the pediatric intensive care unit with ketoacidosis, a complication of type 1 diabetes. She passed out at school after vomiting and complaining of fatigue and was transported to the hospital via ambulance. On her hospital admission, her serum glucose level was 350 mg/dL. Her glycosylated hemoglobin (Hba1c) was 11%, indicating poor metabolic control over the past 3 months. Chloe has been in the hospital for 2 days and is getting ready to be discharged home today.

Chloe's parents, Devon and Bonita Yates, were surprised when they found out how poorly Chloe's metabolic control had been before her admission. See Figure 9-2 for a detailed Yates family genogram. They believed that their family had open communication and that they knew what was happening with their children. Chloe told her parents that her glucose levels were "fine." Chloe is an honor-roll student at school, active in basketball and soccer, and well liked by her peers. Devon, an African American man, is college educated and works for a thriving law firm. Bonita, a college-educated woman with Hispanic roots, is employed as a business manager in a large firm.

The Yates family recently experienced several stressors besides this new hospitalization. Bonita's father, Henry, passed away 2 months ago after a long bout with Alzheimer's disease, and the family recently moved into a new and larger home in a racially diverse urban neighborhood. The children are enrolled in a private school, so the move did not affect their school relationships. Chloe and her younger siblings, Leslie and Trevor, appear to have adjusted to the new living location and seem content with their new neighborhood friends. Chloe has continued to receive primary care services in the clinic where the long-term pediatric nurse practitioner has come to know the family quite well.

Chloe was diagnosed with diabetes 2 years ago and was 11 years old at the time. When diagnosed, she spent several days in the hospital. Bonita accompanied her to a

series of diabetes education classes, and they shared what they learned with the rest of the family. Chloe easily assumed responsibility for monitoring her glucose levels and administering her insulin when she was diagnosed. At first, the family struggled to make needed changes to their family health routines based on Chloe's medical needs—changes in Chloe's dietary needs, daily regulation of her insulin, bouts with hypoglycemia, and frequent monitoring of blood glucose levels that required significant management. The family has tried to adopt dietary patterns that support Chloe's needs. Bonita learned some new things about counting carbohydrates, avoiding processed foods with high fructose, and preparing foods in nutritious ways. For example, Bonita avoids buying chips and now shops for more nutritious snack items that will not elevate Chloe's blood glucose level. The family incorporated the management of her diabetes into the family routines, and it seems less foreign to them now. Leslie and Trevor were unhappy with the dietary changes at first, but they have made a positive adjustment over time. The family makes a point of eating at least one meal together daily, which allows each family member to talk about their day. The family recently started "highlight/lowlight" time at dinner, during which each family member shares one high point and one low point about his or her day. Chloe's highlights focused on

(continued)

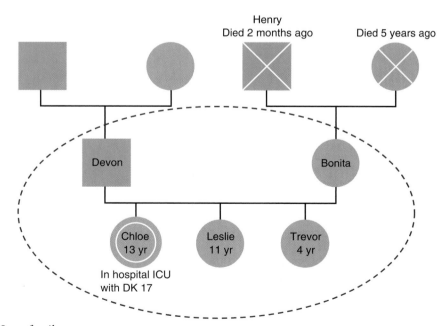

FIGURE 9-2 Yates family genogram.

her new friend at school, Brian. Her lowlights have focused on the "hassle" of checking her glucose and having to eat differently than her friends, something she is finding embarrassing.

Leslie and Trevor are staying with Devon's parents while Bonita and Devon prepare to take Chloe home from the hospital today. Leslie and Trevor have been asking about Chloe for several days, as they are worried about her "sugar." Leslie, age 11, has been especially concerned about Chloe. She and Chloe have been arguing lately and Leslie feels it might be her fault that Chloe became ill. Trevor, age 4, has been asking if he can use Chloe's "finger pokers" and saying, "I have diabetes too!" Devon and Bonita share with the nurse their beliefs that he wants some of the special attention that his sister is getting at the hospital. These parents are worried about being "spread too thin" as they try to fulfill their employment responsibilities, attend for each child's unique needs, and provide Chloe with the medical care she needs to manage the diabetes.

Chloe's parents are meeting with the nurse today as they prepare for Chloe's discharge home. When the nurse asks whether they thought Chloe fully understood how to manage her diabetes, Devon said, "She not only understands, she could teach it! We just can't figure out why she had such a setback recently." This family is experiencing a transitional stress that is typical of adolescent behavior and also typical of adolescents living with a chronic illness.

Family Nurse's Reflection on the Yates Family Using Evidence-Based Practice:

In poor-functioning families of children with type 1 diabetes, metabolic control is also likely to be poor, and this seems to be particularly true for youths older than 12 years (Fiese & Everhart, 2006). In studies of families managing childhood diabetes, reports of a parent and child working together as a team around daily management tasks were associated with better adherence (Fiese & Everhart, 2006). Mothers in families with children who have type 1 diabetes reported having less time to engage in activities with their children compared with mothers who do not have a child with diabetes (McClellan & Cohen, 2007). Parents of children with type 1 diabetes are more likely to describe their families as less achievement oriented than families without children who have diabetes (McClellan & Cohen, 2007).

Although nurses should be aware of the potential for family conflict around diabetes management, they should not assume that poor medical adherence is a product of the conflict observed, because conflict and poor medical adherence are developmentally normal processes in families

with adolescents (Dashiff, Bartolucci, Wallander, & Abdullatif, 2005). It is important to keep in mind that conflict occurs in all families, regardless of the age of individual family members. What is vital is the way conflict is handled and resolved. Nurses can assist families by suggesting effective communication techniques and developmentally appropriate strategies to address problems and areas of conflict linked with healthy functioning and development. Studies of psychosocial well-being in families of children with chronic conditions too often focus on psychopathology and lack of adjustment, with less attention given to well-functioning and positive growth after childhood illness (Barlow & Ellard, 2006). More recent research on sibling relationships measures the positive attributes that occur in families with a child with a disability, instead of only pathologizing this experience (Barlow & Ellard, 2006; Bellin & Kovacs, 2006; Lobato & Kao, 2005; Wennick & Hallstrom, 2007).

Little is known about the best ways to educate caregivers about ways to manage this disease in the family household and little to no consideration is given to individuals' social background (Glasdam et al., 2012). Findings from a recent study that considered family support and adherence to medical regimen identified that persons with diabetes felt sabotaged by family members when members knew what was needed to manage the disease, but were unmotivated to provide support needed to make changes or offered temptations to indulge in contradictory activities (Mayberry & Osborn, 2012). These researchers concluded that there is a need for nursing actions that enhance family members' motivation and assist them to choose behavioral skills that empower their family member diagnosed with diabetes.

In families with adult members who have diabetes, family health routines are instrumental in self-management (Collier, 2007; Denham, Manoogian, & Schuster, 2007). A diabetes diagnosis affects previously constructed health routines; these old behaviors often need to be deconstructed and new ones formed in accord with unique family needs (Denham & Manoogian, unpublished). In diabetes self-management, differences in family members (e.g., gender, age, motivation, relationship) have implications for member support or threats to dietary and other care routines (Schuster, 2005).

As a nurse working with persons with various types of diabetes, it is important to note that a one-size-fits-all solution is not appropriate. Nursing assessments must consider the various ways conditions might affect individual members and the family as a whole. Chronic diseases may have similar diagnostic factors involved and symptoms might be similar, but the human and family response of different households can be extremely different. Therefore, developing plans of care, nursing actions, and ideas about family empowerment must be based on the unique circumstances experienced by each family.

The Yates family case study illustrates the multiple factors that face families who have a child with a chronic illness. The Yates family has three children, ages 13, 11, and 4. Chloe, the oldest child, has had diabetes for 2 years and has done well with parental guidance and self-management until recently. As a young teen, Chloe is moving into a new developmental stage. Chloe's disease management is threatened by things outside the family household, such as peer pressure and larger periods outside of the home environment with friends that involve food choices.

In the Yates family case study, Leslie's and Trevor's reactions are typical for siblings of children with chronic conditions. Leslie, for example, feels responsible for Chloe's hospitalization, and has expressed possible guilt linked with recent arguments. Trevor's desire to have diabetes like his sister may represent his recognition that Chloe's diabetes is the source of much attention from their parents, attention that may be drawn away from him.

Chloe's parents have rearranged their lives to incorporate the management of her diabetes, but they also face the continued needs of their other children. These parents need to recognize the ways Leslie's and Trevor's developmental needs influence their actions and consider possible ways the psychosocial development of children at different ages will be attended to in the future (Bellin & Kovacs, 2006). The experience may catalyze these siblings' abilities to tap into inner resources and develop empathy, compassion, patience, and sensitivity. Leslie and Trevor will benefit from age-appropriate, accurate information about Chloe's diabetes and from knowing that their responses are normal.

The Yates family demonstrates several examples of a cohesive family unit. For example, the family members value time together at meals and encourage shared feelings. Several studies have shown that high family cohesion is associated with adherence in children and teens with treatments for type 1 diabetes (Cohen, Lumley, Naar-King, Partridge, & Cakan, 2004; Leonard, Jang, Savik, & Plumbo, 2005). Cohesiveness allows for shared understanding, respect for differences of opinions, and an emotional investment in keeping the family together (Fiese & Everhart, 2006). The Family Management Style Framework could be useful for nurses in considering the Yates family (Knafl & Deatrick, 1990, 2003; Knafl et al., 2012). Chloe's parents attempt to focus on the normal aspects of Chloe's early adolescence, and they see her as normal in many ways. For this reason, the Yates family might be viewed as

accommodating. They have, up to this point, felt confident about Chloe's ability to manage her diabetes independently, but perhaps Chloe's transition into adolescence will require the family to reassess their assumptions. The Yates family has the resources and cohesiveness to negotiate the developmental changes that occur along the way.

Chloe's parents were surprised to learn that her metabolic control is poor, as she had previously managed responsibilities linked with diabetes self-management with ease and skill. An early adolescent who has successfully managed diabetes may find it difficult to continue to manage the condition while simultaneously negotiating a move to social independence. Chloe's desire to fit in with her peers may be at odds with her need to check her blood glucose levels before meals, especially at school, and with her dietary limitations. Chloe's communication with her parents is particularly important at this transitional time. Parents are challenged to provide the adolescent with a level of autonomy that is developmentally appropriate while simultaneously monitoring abilities to adhere to complex medical regimens. Studies have shown that the more teens (particularly girls) perceive their mothers as controlling, the greater the negative effect on adherence (Fiese & Everhart, 2006).

It is possible that providers and parents may overestimate adolescents' desire for autonomy and confidentiality, especially when illness-related (Britto et al., 2007). Adolescents, who tend to be more peer oriented, may wish to reduce the power differential between themselves and their health care providers. They might prefer that providers use direct communication styles. Adolescents with chronic illnesses may actually have fewer expectations for confidentiality and greater needs for parental involvement in care than healthy peers (Britto et al., 2007). Thus, nurses should not assume that all teens are seeking independence and autonomy just because they have reached the adolescent stage. In fact, nurses should consider the uniqueness of individual and family situations before giving advice and avoid passing judgment.

The family nurse should work with Chloe's parents' mobilized resources to help them meet the needs of all their family members. See the Yates family ecomap in Figure 9-3. The grandparents provided care for their two younger children while the parents prepared to take Chloe home from the hospital. In addition, the nurse could facilitate a parents and Chloe meeting with the school nurse and teachers. By helping families to assess their resources and determine what they still need the whole family will enjoy improved health outcomes.

(continued)

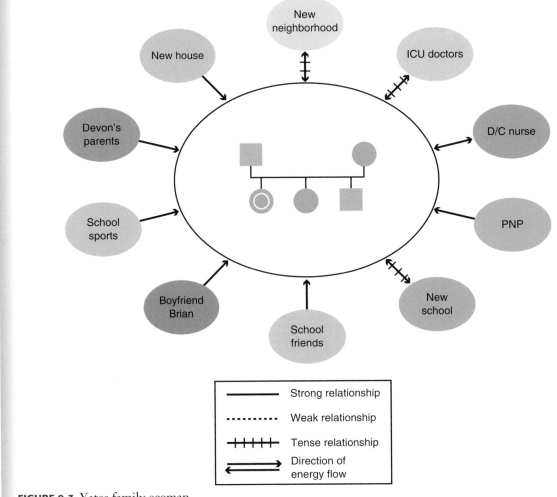

FIGURE 9-3 Yates family ecomap.

Current Family Case Study

Ben Current is a 68-year-old widow, diagnosed with Parkinson's disease at the age of 58. He owns and farms his 500-acre family ranch in eastern Oregon on which he raises cattle and hay. This case study is presented through the lens of Rolland's Chronic Illness Framework.

Illness Onset:

Parkinson's disease (PD) is a slowly progressive neurodegenerative brain disorder with motor symptoms of slowness, rigidity, and tremor. There are also a host of nonmotor symptoms that include autonomic, neuropsychiatric (e.g., dementia and depression), and sleep complaints. The cause of PD is not known and treatment is aimed at minimizing disability and maintaining optimal quality of life. At this most recent visit to the Movement Disorder Clinic, Ben

presents with a number of motor and nonmotor concerns. In addition, he has low adherence to treatment recommendations and his family is expressing strain from the growing burden of care.

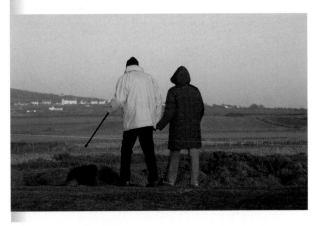

Course of Illness:

When individual family members have a progressive chronic illness, such as Ben with PD, the increasing disability requires families to make continual changes in their roles as they adapt to the losses and needs of the family member. Ben's family is at the Movement Disorder Clinic today to seek help with Ben's increasing symptoms. Several family members express feeling of stress and are exhausted with the routine and ongoing demands of his progressive symptoms.

There are two assessment tools used to evaluate the progressive aspects of PD. The first is the Hoehn and Yahr scale. This instrument identifies five stages based on motor symptoms: Stage 1 is unilateral motor involvement; Stage 2 is bilateral movement involvement; Stage 3 is mild to moderate disease with impaired balance; Stage 4 is severe disease with marked disability; and Stage 5 is confinement to bed or a wheelchair. It is important for family nurses to know that any reference to staging of PD is a quick look at the condition at that point in time during that visit and is not meant to suggest a timeframe of progression. It is also worth noting that it only evaluates motor symptoms and it is important to realize that nonmotor symptoms, such as depression, can cause as much (or more) disability as the motor symptoms. The second instrument, the Unified Parkinson's Disease Rating Scale (UPDRS), is a detailed instrument that assists family nurses to assess the daily needs of the ill family member and the family caregiver in six areas of function: functional status, level of activities of daily living, motor function, mood, cognition, and treatment-related manifestations.

Outcome—Trajectory of Illness and Incapacitation:

Typically, people with PD can live 20 years or more from the time of diagnosis. Death is usually secondary to symptoms of immobility. It is the 14th leading cause of death in the United States. There is currently no cure for PD. The stages of the illness, as discussed above, are progressive in nature. Ben has been in Stage 3 of the disease and symptoms suggest he is progressing to Stage 4. The focus of this visit is to minimize disability through symptom management and to help the family find resources in its local community to support Ben and minimize caregiver strain. If these interventions improve his compliance with medication, the family may maintain Ben in his current Stage 3.

Time Phase: Brief Review of Ben's Initial Diagnosis:

At initial diagnosis, Ben, 58 years old, was, in his words, "just not doing well." He was worried about a tremor in his left hand, but at that point it did not interfere much with his daily work or activities. Sarah, his wife, had taken over writing the paychecks for their three ranch hands and all of the bills because Ben's handwriting had started to deteriorate. He noticed that he was slowing down, but attributed his increasing stiffness of legs and arms to "getting old" and his demanding physical lifestyle. What brought him in to see his health care provider was dizziness and falls. Sarah was worried that he would get dizzy while operating the farm machines. When he came home with a cut lip, swollen ankle, and scraped-up shoulder, Sarah demanded he see the family nurse practitioner (FNP), who is located 50 miles from his ranch. The FNP suspected Ben had PD, but sent him to the Movement Disorder Clinic and specialists in Portland, Oregon, which is 330 miles from where Ben lives. Since then, Ben has been managed primarily by his FNP with consultation and supportive assistance from the specialists, who see Ben every 6 months. Due to weather and other family events, however, Ben and his family have not been to the clinic for a year.

Mid–Time Phase and Family Functioning:

Ben and his family have been living and adapting to his progressive PD for 10 years. See Figure 9-4, which shows the Current family genogram. Early on, the adaptation was relatively smooth as Ben responded well to medication intervention and his wife Sarah was the major support person. The family experienced a major change in the family involvement and management of Ben's illness when Sarah died 2 years ago from a heart attack at age 66. Since that time, 27-year-old Logan, Ben's grandson, has been living at the ranch and helping to provide support and care for Ben.

Julie, the NP specialist in the Movement Disorder Clinic, consulted the detailed family genogram in the chart. She noted that the family genogram had not been updated since Sarah's death; therefore, she updated it. At this visit, the family members who are present include Ben, his daughter Kathleen, his daughter Carole, and his grandson Logan, who is the primary caregiver. Logan expresses feeling overwhelmed with his caregiver role and work-time conflict. He feels like Ben needs more assistance. As both Kathleen and Carole are worried about Ben's safety while Logan is working on the ranch during the day, they report alternating days they come to spend with Ben. In order to facilitate uncovering the family stressors as well as the current medical condition of Ben, Julie decided to write issues in a table format that may then easily be used as a decision-making grid for the family. Julie completes her physical assessment of Ben's motor abilities, which are incorporated into the table. Ben fills

(continued)

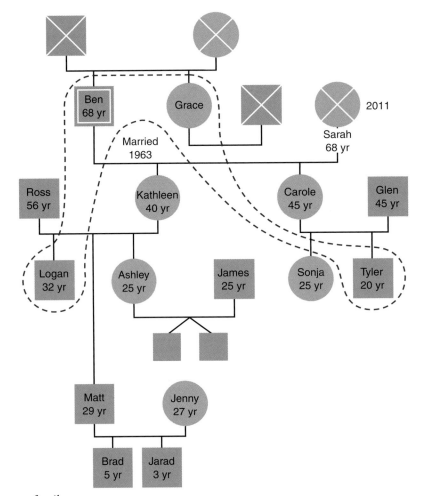

FIGURE 9-4 Current family genogram.

out a geriatric depression assessment instrument. Logan completes a caregiver strain assessment instrument.

Salient family issues in this phase for the Current family as it struggles to find a balanced family life and normalcy in functioning include the following:

1. Pacing and avoiding burnout: Logan is overwhelmed with being the primary caregiver for Ben. When Ben was more independent and the PD medications worked well at relieving Ben's motor problems, Logan primarily had to focus on cooking and being sure that Ben took his medications. With advancing executive function (short-term) memory issues, the increased number of falls, and concerns about his grandfather's safety, Logan feels that he cannot manage his own

work on the ranch and taking care of Ben. In the last month, Kathleen and Carole have been alternating days at the ranch to provide care for Ben during the day while Logan is working.

2. Reorganization of family roles: Logan, Kathleen, and Carole are all experiencing role overload as they all spend considerable time as the caregiver. Logan has expressed that he cannot continue to provide care for Ben in the home in the same way that he has in the past. The whole Current family is committed to keeping Ben at home as long as possible. Ben is clear that he does not want to leave the ranch. Tyler, 20-year-old grandson and Logan's cousin, stated that he would move into the ranch to help as he works

there and this would save him time commuting to and from work. Logan would like Tyler to live at the ranch, but insists that caring for Ben requires more than the two of them could provide.

3. Sustaining autonomy for all members of the family: Ben is struggling with the advances in his PD that he sees in himself; therefore, he continues to drive and tries to do some work on the ranch knowing that he is not safe. Logan is stressed to the maximum with role strain overload in the caregiver role.

4. Successfully grieve the loss incurred from the disability or chronic condition: All the family members present shared concerns about the "declining" status of Ben's health. The Current family is a close-knit family who are actively involved in Ben's life and care. Ben has held a strong patriarchal role for the family. Each family member is grieving the loss of Ben in this role and having to adjust to changes that are brought about by the progressive nature of PD.

The family discussed several options for seeking additional help and other interventions during the family meeting:

1. The family discussed having Ben move to an assisted-living facility that is about 30 miles from the ranch. Ben vetoed this option of care at this time. He insists that he will stay on the ranch as long as possible.

2. The second option was to hire a full-time caregiver who would either live at the ranch or in the town. This approach would mean that Logan would provide nighttime care for Ben. The cost of this avenue was considered too much at this time. All family members agreed that they would like to save financial resources for when Ben may need nursing home placement.

3. The third option considered by the family was to ask Ben's sister Grace if she would like to come live on the ranch where she grew up, and to help provide care for Ben. Grace, who was recently widowed and has no children, has a solid relationship with Ben. This option would relieve Logan, Kathleen, and Carole of many of the immediate daily caregiver responsibilities. Tyler could also move to the ranch and assume some of the caregiving tasks or home maintenance in

the evenings along with Logan. Carole mentioned that she had briefly brought up this idea with Grace. The family decided to have Aunt Grace come out for a trial run and determined that they would explore having a home health aide come to the ranch a couple of days a week to help with Ben's hygiene. The family also agreed that they would explore having a shower with a chair installed. The family genogram was updated to include Grace and to show Grace, Ben, Logan, and Tyler all living in the same household.

4. After a visit to the physical therapist during their time at the Movement Disorder Clinic in Portland, Logan was excited about the possibility of all the grandsons working together to build a flat walking trail not far from the ranch house for Ben that would incorporate many of the physical therapy exercise strategies that may help strengthen his muscles, improve agility, and help decrease the freezing episodes. They would put several logs at varying heights for him to practice high stepping. They could increase his stride by placing stepping stones across the creek. They would make the trail so that it had several direction changes and have Ben walk between two trees that were shoulder width. Logan agreed that he would spearhead this venture with all the cousins.

5. Julie worked with Logan and Ben on medication reconciliation. Together they designed a medication administration chart to help the family caregiver and Ben improve medication adherence. See the table below.

6. Julie made referrals to speech therapy to assist Ben with his soft voice (hypophonia). Kathleen agreed to accompany Ben to this part of the visit in an attempt alleviate Logan of some caregiving responsibilities.

7. Julie sent a written summary of the visit to the FNP, who is Ben's primary care provider. The summary included a suggestion to address Ben's sleep problems and repeat the study at the sleep clinic, perhaps fitting him with a different continuous positive airway pressure (CPAP) mask, as many more are available now.

8. Ben agreed to stop driving and surrender his license only if he could still drive on the ranch.

Presentation of Ben's mid-phase Parkinson Disease symptoms using some of the Unified Parkinson's Disease Rating Scale as format			
	Ben's Presentation and Score	*Family Concerns/Problems*	*Suggested Actions*
Mentation, behavior and mood			
IQ impairment	Score of 2: moderate memory loss with disorientation and moderate difficulty handling complex problems: needs prompting for some activities of daily living.	Ben wants to continue to drive during the day to do some errands, especially as Logan works during the day on the ranch. Ben is not driving safely especially with skills such as pulling out on the highway or turning left when traffic is present. In addition, Ben got lost on the ranch last week while trying to check on an area of fencing.	Discuss Ben surrendering his license. Allow him to continue to drive during daylight on the ranch as long as someone is with him.
Thought disorder	Score of 0: no problems.		
Depression	Score of 2: sustained depression (1 week or more). When asked, Ben reports feeling sad and depressed. He has made several statements of low self-esteem and how he is useless on the ranch anymore.	Family asks if Ben should be started back on an antidepressant medication. He was taking one right after Sarah, his wife, died 2 years ago, but he stopped quite a while ago.	Start on an SSRI medication. The prescription has been faxed to the local pharmacy in Joseph, OR, and will be there for the family to pick up when they get home. Need to build this into medication daily schedule.
Motivation-initiative	Score of 1: less assertive than usual; more passive. See above. Ben does report feelings of anxiety at times.	Logan reports that Ben repeatedly asks about the same aspect of work on the ranch; such as completing the corral repair.	Consider adding an anxiety medication but will hold off for now. Discuss next visit or during phone call with local FNP.
Activities of daily living			
Speech	Score of 2: when "on" and "off" or at end of dosing period as Ben has hypophonia due to his PD.	Family reports that Ben is hard to hear and they feel as though they are always asking him to repeat what he says.	Referral to speech therapist while here during this visit to review with family some simple vocal exercises that will help Ben speak louder.
Salivation	Score of 1: slight but definite excess of saliva in mouth; has nighttime drooling.	Ben says this is annoying but not a problem.	Suggest Ben chew gum or suck on hard candy if this bothers him as it will stimulate swallowing.
Handwriting	Score of 3: severely affected; not all words are legible.	Kathleen has assumed bookwork for the ranch.	No further interventions at this time.
Cutting food and handling utensils	Score of 2: can cut most food, although clumsy and slow; some help needed; this is becoming more of an issue and before Ben didn't need any assistance from Logan.	Logan and Ben eat breakfast and dinner together. Logan helps Ben when this is an issue. Logan has been doing all of the cooking.	Kathleen and Carole agreed to both bring home cooked meals for Logan to heat up. Kathleen and Carole take turns food shopping.
Dressing	Score of 2: occasional assistance with buttoning, getting arms in sleeves.	Logan helps Ben in the morning and at night with changing clothes. Ben struggles some at home in getting pants zipped and buttoned after toileting.	Suggest overalls that don't require buttons or pants with Velcro closures. Use slip-on shoes. Due to balance concerns, suggest Ben sit down when dressing.

Presentation of Ben's mid-phase Parkinson Disease symptoms using some of the Unified Parkinson's Disease Rating Scale as format—cont'd			
Hygiene	Score of 2: needs help to shower or is very slow in hygienic care.	This is new development. Logan is embarrassed by having to help his grandfather shower. In addition this adds increased caretaking time to Logan's day.	Discuss safety adaptations in the shower, i.e. chair, grab bars. Discuss not bathing every day. Refer to Occupational Therapy to see if there are assistive devices for brushing teeth.
Turning in bed and adjusting bed clothes	Score of 2: can turn alone or adjust sheets, but with great difficulty.	Logan was concerned as he didn't even think about this aspect of help his grandfather might need.	He will use silk PJ bottoms to decrease the friction of turning. Explore if a bed rail can be placed on the bed. Discuss the weight of the covers or blankets used at night.
Falling	Score is between a 2 and 3: Ben falls often but not daily. Sometimes he has fallen more than once in a day. Ben reports being dizzy when he stands (orthostatic hypotension).	All family members are very concerned about Ben falling and the difficulty he has getting up from the fall. Ben walks on a regular basis. He has not kept up with his physical therapy in the last year. Ben seems to be stiffer and has more abnormal movements even on his medications.	Family will increase fluids and get some support stockings to keep blood from pooling in his extremities. Have Kathleen and Carole complete a fall safety check in the home environment to help identify. Check to be sure Ben has cell phone on him or a cordless phone is within reach so he can call if he falls when alone.
Freezing when walking	Score of 3: Ben frequently freezes and occasionally falls from freezing.	See above. Explore more to see when Ben is freezing, such as, during a turn, going through doorways, at the start of walking, or when he is doing something that requires him to take a step back.	Review strategies with Ben to help him get going when he freezes while walking.
Walking	Score of 2: moderate difficulty. Ben refused to use a cane, but grandson Tyler made Ben a walking stick which he now uses. Ben has bradykinesia with a weak push off, reduced leg lift, small stride length, lack of right arm swing and a narrow stance.	See above. After much discussion Ben admitted that had trouble following his medication regimen during the day when Logan was at work. He also noted that he had been taking more Sinemet when he wanted to go out.	See above. Referral to PT for assistance in walking.
Pain	Score of 2: with complaints of numbness, tingling and frequent cramp and constant ache in calves and lower back.		Starting Ben on SSRI for depression may help decrease pain sensations. Stretching and heat may relieve pain in calves.

(continued)

Other complications

Sleep	Ben reports that he has insomnia. He has difficulty staying asleep. Before diagnosed with PD, Ben was assessed for sleep apnea in a sleep clinic. He reports that he dislikes the CPAP machine and the mask on his face, so he doesn't use it. He thinks he sleeps about 4 hours a night. He has daytime sleepiness.	Logan hears Ben up at all hours of the night, which interferes with his sleep. Ben has fallen at night too, which adds to Logan's vigilance of getting up to check on Ben.	Will discuss with FNP about having Ben reassessed for sleep at the sleep clinic in Pendleton, OR. Have Ben keep a simple sleep log if possible. Check on medications that Ben is taking and make sure that the timing is not affecting sleep.
Excessive sweating	Ben reports that has been having periods of excessive sweating . . . almost like he was caught in a rain storm.		Checking the timing of medications as these may be happening as the dosing is ending or the "off" periods.
Constipation	Ben has a long history of constipation, even before diagnosis.		As Ben is sweating excessively at times, consider he may be dehydrated . . . set up a plan so he drinks about 1500 mLs of fluids a day. Continue daily dose of Miralax.
Urinary Problems	Ben reports nocturia, which might contribute to his insomnia.	Note that Ben was given a diuretic for hypertension. Explore time of day he is taking this medication.	Be sure there is a nightlight in the bathroom and rugs in the bathroom.

See the Current family ecomap in Figure 9-5.

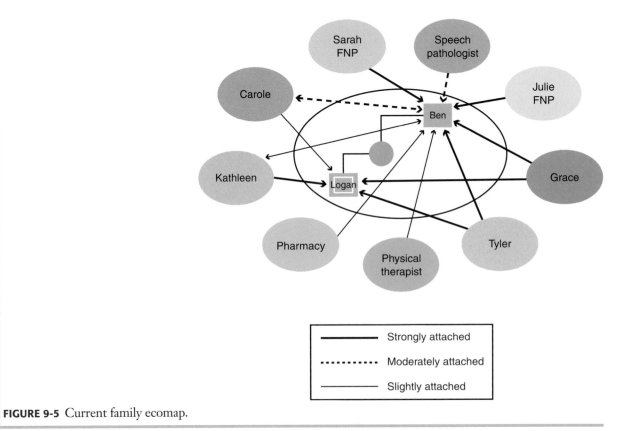

FIGURE 9-5 Current family ecomap.

SUMMARY

A family focus on care should not be considered optional when it comes to chronic illness. The long-term effects of chronic health conditions affect individuals and families differently than acute health events.

- Although the needs families experience may be similar initially, the duration of the illness alters the ways care is managed and perceived over a long life course.
- The severity, complexity, and longevity of care needs associated with chronic conditions can alter a desired or expected future into one that dramatically revolutionizes the lives of entire households.
- Financial costs and family resources are often highly taxed by years of debt and stress that would not be expected if a chronic condition had not occurred. Some conditions may worsen over time or require endless amounts of attention that can become especially burdensome as the chronically ill person ages and economic or family resources are exhausted.
- Some children with SHCN and adults may require extraordinary adaptations by parents, siblings, and others that strain relationships.
- Although the chronic illnesses of children may be primarily genetic or environmental in nature, many of the adult chronic conditions are linked with lifestyle behaviors.
- Healthier lifestyles can reduce risks for some chronic conditions and can prevent or delay many complications from these diseases.
- Family-focused care aimed at meeting family needs when a member or members have chronic illness requires nurses equipped with knowledge about families and their interactions.
- Optimal nursing care for those with chronic illness involves nurses who are knowledgeable about developmental alterations, willing to hear and listen to the voiced needs without judgment, and able to become collaborators that empower multiple household members to reorganize routines and manage existing resources.

REFERENCES

Administration for Community Living. (2013). Lifespan respite care program. Retrieved from http://acl.gov/Programs/Integrated_Programs/LifespanRespite/Index.aspx

Alwan, A., Maclean, D. R., Riley, L. M., d'Espaignet, E. T., Mathers, C. D., Stevens, G. A., & Bettcher, D. (2010). Monitoring and surveillance of chronic non-communicable diseases: Progress and capacity in high-burden countries. *Lancet*, *376*(9755), 1861–1868. doi:10.1016/S0140-6736(10)61853-3

American Academy of Pediatrics. (2011). Clinical report: Supporting the health care transition from adolescence to adulthood in the medical home. *Journal of the American Academy of Pediatrics*, *128*(1), 182–200.

American Association of Caregiving Youth. (2013). Retrieved from http://www.aacy.org

American Diabetes Association. (2008). Economic costs of diabetes in the U.S. in 2007. *Diabetes Care*, *31*(3), 1–20.

Arestedt, L., Persson, C., & Benzein, E. (2013). Living as a family in the midst of chronic illness. *Scandinavian Journal of Caring Sciences*. Advance online publication. doi:10.1111/scs.12023

Australian Bureau of Statistics. (2009). Disability, ageing and caregivers, Australia: Summary of findings, 2009. Retrieved from http://www.abs.gov.au/ausstats/abs@.nsf/mf/4430.0

Bandura, A. (1977). Self-efficacy: Toward a unifying theory of behavioral change. *Psychological Review*, *84*, 191–215.

Barlow, J. H., & Ellard, D. R. (2006). The psychosocial well-being of children with chronic disease, their parents and siblings: An overview of the research evidence base. *Child Care, Health & Development*, *32*(1), 19–31.

Bednar, V., Chadi, N., DeCourcey, M., Kuperman, A., Pillar, A., & Scott, B. (2013). Who cares about young caregivers? Raising awareness for an invisible population. Retrieved from http://www.actioncanada.ca/en/wp-content/uploads/2013/02/TF1-Report_Young-Careers_EN.pdf

Beeber, A. S., & Zimmerman, S. (2012). Adapting the family management style framework for families caring for older adults with dementia. *Journal of Family Nursing*, *18*(1), 123–145.

Behavioral Risk Factor Surveillance System. (2011). BRFSS annual survey data. Retrieved from http://www.cdc.gov/brfss/technical_infodata/surveydata.htm

Bellin, M. H., & Kovacs, P. (2006). Fostering resilience in siblings of youths with a chronic health condition: A review of the literature. *Health & Social Work*, *31*(3), 209–216.

Berge, J. M., Patterson, J. M., & Rueter, M. (2006). Marital satisfaction and mental health of couples with children with chronic health conditions. *Families, Systems, & Health*, *24*(3), 267–285.

Bloom, D. E., Cafiero, E. T., Jane-Llopis, E., Abrahams-Gessel, S., Bloom, L. R., Fathima, S., . . . Weinstein, C. (2011). The global economic burden of non-communicable diseases. Geneva: World Forum. Retrieved from http://www3.weforum.org/docs/WEF_Harvard_HE_GlobalEconomicBurdenNonCommunicableDiseases_2011.pdf

Bousso, R., Misko, M., Mendes-Castillo, A., & Rossato L. (2012). Family management style framework and its use with families who have a child undergoing palliative care at home. *Journal of Family Nursing*, *18*(1), 91–122.

Bowen, M., Henske, J., & Potter, A. (2010). Healthcare transition in adolescents and young adults with diabetes. *Clinical Diabetes, 28*(3), 99–106.

Bowden, V., & Greenberg, C. (2010). *Children and their families: The continuum of care* (2nd ed.). Philadelphia, PA: Lippincott Williams-Wilkins.

Bridgeland, J., DiIulio, J., & Morison, K. (2006). *The silent epidemic: Perspectives of high school dropouts. A report by Civic Enterprises in association with Peter D. Hart Research Associates for the Bill & Melinda Gates Foundation.* Washington, DC: Civic Enterprises.

Britto, M. T., Slap, G. B., DeVellis, R. F., Hornung, R. W., Atherton, H. D., Knopf, J. M., . . . DeFriese, G. H. (2007). Specialists' understanding of the health care preferences of chronically ill adolescents. *Journal of Adolescent Health, 40*(4), 334–341.

Canadian Diabetes Association. (2009). An economic tsunami: The cost of diabetes. Retrieved from http://www.diabetes.ca/documents/get-involved/FINAL_Economic_Report.pdf

Canadian Tobacco Use Monitoring Survey. (2010). Summary for annual results from 2010. Retrieved from http://www.hc-sc.gc.ca/hc-ps/tobac-tabac/research-recherche/stat/_ctums-esutc_2010/ann_summary-sommaire-eng.php

Caregivers Trust. (2012). Key facts about caregivers. Retrieved from http://www.caregivers.org/key-facts-about-caregivers

Centers for Disease Control and Prevention. (2008a). Chronic disease overview. Retrieved from http://www.cdc.gov/nccdphp/overview.htm#2

Centers for Disease Control and Prevention. (2008b). Chronic disease overview. Retrieved from http://www.cdc.gov/chronicdisease/overview/index.htm

Centers for Disease Control and Prevention. (2011). Tobacco-related mortality. Retrieved February 8, 2013, from http://www.cdc.gov/tobacco/data_statistics/fact_sheets/health_effects/tobacco_related_mortality

Centers for Disease Control and Prevention. (2012a). National diabetes fact sheet, 2011. Retrieved February 5, 2012, from http://www.cdc.gov/diabetes/pubs/pdf/ndfs_2011.pdf

Cohen, D., Greene, J. A., Toyinbo, P. A., & Siskowski, C. T. (2012). Impact of family caregiving by youth on their psychological well-being: A latent trait analysis. *Journal of Behavioral Health Services and Research, 39*(3), 245–256.

Cohen, D. M., Lumley, M. A., Naar-King, S., Partridge, T., & Cakan, N. (2004). Child behavior problems and family functioning as predictors of adherence and glycemic control in economically disadvantaged children with type 1 diabetes: A prospective study. *Journal of Pediatric Psychology, 29*(3), 171–184.

Collier, T. (2007). Dietary routines and diabetes: Instrument development. Unpublished master's thesis, Ohio University, College of Health and Human Services, Athens, OH.

Dall, T. M., Zhang, Y., Chen, Y. J., Quick, W. W., Yang, W. G., & Fogil, J. (2010). The economic burden of diabetes. *Health Affairs, 29*(2), 297–303.

Dashiff, C., Bartolucci, A., Wallander, J., & Abdullatif, H. (2005). The relationship of family structure, maternal employment, and family conflict with self-care adherence of adolescents with type 1 diabetes. *Families, Systems, & Health, 23*(1), 66–70.

Data Resource Center for Child and Adolescent Health. (2012). Prevalence profile of the National Survey for Children with Special Health Care Needs 2009–2010. Retrieved from http://www.childhealthdata.org/docs/nsch-docs/whoarecshcn_revised_07b-pdf.pdf

Deatrick, J. A., Knafl, K. A., & Murphy-Moore, C. (1999). Clarifying the concept of normalization. *Image: The Journal of Nursing Scholarship, 31*(3), 209–214.

Deatrick, J. A., Thibodeaux, A. G., Mooney, K., Schmus, C., Pollack, R., & Davey, B. H. (2006). Family management style framework: A new tool with potential to assess families who have children with brain tumors. *Journal of Pediatric Oncology Nurses, 23*(1), 19–27.

Denham, S. A. (1997). An ethnographic study of family health in Appalachian microsystems. Unpublished doctoral dissertation, University of Alabama at Birmingham, AL.

Denham, S. A. (1999a). The definition and practice of family health. *Journal of Family Nursing, 5*(2), 133–159.

Denham, S. A. (1999b). Family health: During and after death of a family member. *Journal of Family Nursing, 5*(2), 160–183.

Denham, S. A. (1999c). Family health in an economically disadvantaged population. *Journal of Family Nursing, 5*(2), 184–213.

Denham, S. A. (2003). *Family health: A framework for nursing.* Philadelphia, PA: F. A. Davis.

Denham, S. A., & Manoogian, M. (unpublished). Patterns of support: Type 2 diabetes and older rural families.

Denham, S. A., Manoogian, M., & Schuster, L. (2007). Managing family support and dietary routines: Type 2 diabetes in rural Appalachian families. *Families, Systems, & Health, 25*(1), 36–52.

DeVol, R. (2008). Center for health economics. Retrieved June 28, 2008, from http://www.milkeninstitute.org/research/research.taf?cat=health

DeVol, R., & Bedroussian, A. (2007). An unhealthy America: The economic burden of chronic disease charting a new course to save lives and increase productivity and economic growth. Milken Institute. Retrieved from www.milkeninstitute.org/pdf/chronic_disease_report.pdf

Dickinson, A. R., Smythe, E., & Spence, D. (2006). Within the web: The family-practitioner relationship in the context of chronic childhood illness. *Journal of Child Health Care, 10*(4), 309–325.

Drummond, A., Looman, W., & Phillips, A. (2012). Coping among parents of children with special health care needs with and without a health care home. *Journal of Pediatric Health Care, 26*(4), 266–275.

Feinberg, L., Reinhard, S., Houser, A., & Choula, R. (2011). Valuing the invaluable: 2011 update: The growing contributions and costs of family caregiving. AARP Public Policy Institute. Retrieved from http://assets.aarp.org/rgcenter/ppi/ltc/i51-caregiving.pdf

Fiese, B. H., & Everhart, R. S. (2006). Medical adherence and childhood chronic illness: Family daily management skills and emotional climate as emerging contributors. *Current Opinion in Pediatrics, 18*(5), 551–557.

Fiese, B. H., Tomcho, T. J., Douglas, M., Josephs, K., Poltrock, S., & Baker, T. (2002). A review of 50 years of research on naturally occurring family routines and rituals: Cause for celebration? *Journal of Family Psychology, 16*, 381–390.

Fiese, B. H., & Wambolt, F. (2000). Family routines and asthma management: A proposal for family-based strategies to increase treatment adherence. *Families, Systems, & Health, 18*, 405–418.

Framingham Heart Study. (2012). History of the Framingham Heart Study. Retrieved February 5, 2013, from http://www.framinghamheartstudy.org/about/history.html

Gibson, M. J., & Houser, A. (2007). AARP Policy Institute: Economic value of family caregivers brief. Retrieved from http://www.nfcacares.org/pdfs/NewLookattheeeconomic ValueofFamilyCaregivingIssueBrief.pdf

Glasdam, S., Timm, H., & Vittrup, R. (2012). Support efforts for caregivers of chronically ill persons. *Clinical Nursing Research*, *19*(3), 233–265.

Health Canada. (2009). About tobacco control. Retrieved from http://hc-sc.gc.ca/hc-ps/tobac-tabac/about-apropos/index-eng.php

Health Council of Canada. (2012). Self-management support for Canadians with chronic health conditions: A focus for primary care. Retrieved from http://healthcouncilcanada.ca/tree/ HCC_SelfManagementReport_FA.pdf

Henshaw, L. (2006). Empowerment, diabetes and the National Service Framework: A systematic review. *Journal of Diabetes Nursing*, *10*(4), 128, 130–135.

Hollander, M. J., Liu, G., & Chappell, N. (2009). Who cares and how much? *Health Care Quarterly*, *12*(2), 42–49.

House, J.A. (1981). *Work stress and social support*. Reading, MA: Addison-Wesley.

Hummel, F. I. (2013a). Uncertainty. In I. M. Lubkin & P. D. Larsen (Eds.), *Chronic illness: Impact and intervention* (8th ed., pp. 161–182). Burlington, MA: Jones & Bartlett Publishers.

Hummel, F. I. (2013). Powerlessness. In I. M. Lubkin & P. D. Larsen (Eds.), *Chronic illness: Impact and intervention* (8th ed., pp. 315–341). Burlington, MA: Jones and Bartlett Publishers.

Institute of Medicine. (2011). A nationwide framework for surveillance of cardiovascular and chronic lung diseases. Washington, DC: National Academy of Sciences. Retrieved January 22, 2013, from http://www.iom.edu/~/media/Files/Report% 20Files/2011/A-Nationwide-Framework-for-Surveillance-of-Cardiovascular-and-Chronic-Lung-Diseases/National% 20Surveillance%20Systems%202011%20Report%20Brief.pdf

Institute of Medicine. (2012). Living well with chronic illness: A call for public action. Washington, DC: National Academy of Sciences. Retrieved January 18, 2013, from http://iom.edu/ Reports/2012/Living-Well-with-Chronic-Illness

Jalkut, M., & Allen, P. (2009). Transition from pediatric to adult health care for adolescents with congenital heart disease: A review of the literature and clinical implications. *Pediatric Nursing*, *35*(6), 381–387.

Keefe, J. (2011). Supporting caregivers and caregiving in an aging Canada. IRPP Study 23. Montreal, Quebec, Canada: Institute for Research on Public Policy. Retrieved from http://www. irpp.org/pubs/irppstudy/irpp_study_no23.pdf

Kieckhefer, G., Trahms, C., Churchill, S., Kratz, L., Uding, N., & Villareale, N. (2013). A randomized clinical trial of the Building on Family Strengths Program: An education program for parents of children with chronic health conditions. *Maternal Child Health Journal*. Advance online publication. doi:10.1007/s10995-013-1273-2

Knafl, K., & Deatrick, J. (1990). Family management style: Concept analysis and development. *Journal of Pediatric Nursing*, *5*(1), 4–14.

Knafl, K., & Deatrick, J. (2003). Further refinement of the Family Management Style Framework. *Journal of Family Nursing*, *9*(3), 232–256.

Knafl, K. A., Deatrick, J. A., & Havill, N. L. (2012). Continued development of the Family Management Style Framework. *Journal of Family Nursing*, *18*(1), 11–24.

Kowal, S., Dall, T., Chakrabarti, R., Storm, M., & Jain, A. (2013). The current and projected economic burden of Parkinson's disease in the United States. *Movement Disorders*, *28*(3), 311–318.

Kralik, D., Visentin, K., & van Loon, A. (2011). Transition: A literature review. *Journal of Advanced Nursing*, *55*(3), 320–329.

Leonard, B., Jang, Y., Savik, K., & Plumbo, M. A. (2005). Adolescents with type 1 diabetes: Family functioning with metabolic control. *Journal of Family Nursing*, *11*(2), 102–121.

Lindley, L. C., & Mark, B. A. (2010). Children with special health care needs: Impact of health care expenditures on family financial burden. *Journal of Family Studies*, *19*(1), 79–89.

Lobato, D. J., & Kao, B. T. (2005). Brief report: Family-based group intervention for young siblings of children with chronic illness and developmental disability. *Journal of Pediatric Psychology*, *30*, 678–682.

Looman, W. S. (2006). Development and testing of the Social Capital Scale for families of children with chronic conditions. *Research in Nursing & Health*, *29*(4), 325–336.

Looman, W. S., O'Conner-Von, S. K., Ferski, G. J., & Hildenbrand, D. A. (2009). Financial and employment problems in families of children with special health care needs: Implications for research and practice. *Journal of Pediatric Health Care*, *23*(2), 117–125.

Lugasi, T., Achille, M., & Stevenson, M. (2011). Patients' perspective on factors that facilitate transition form child-centered to adult-centered health care: A theory integrated metasummary of quantitative and qualitative studies. *Journal of Adolescent Health*, *48*, 429–440.

Mack, J. W., Co, J. P., Goldmann, D. A., Weeks, J. C., & Cleary, P. D. (2007). Quality of health care for children: Role of health and chronic illness in inpatient care experiences. *Archives of Pediatrics & Adolescent Medicine*, *161*(9), 828–834.

Marshall, C., & Stainton, T. (2010). An overview of the demographics profiles and initial results from the British Columbia young caregivers project. *Relational Child and Youth Care Practice*, *23*(4), 65.

Mayberry, L. S., & Osborn, C. Y. O. (2012). Family support, medication adherence, and glycemic control among adults with type 2 diabetes. *Diabetes Care*, *35*, 1239–1245.

McClellan, C. B., & Cohen, L. L. (2007). Family functioning in children with chronic illness compared with healthy controls: A critical review. *Journal of Pediatrics*, *150*(3), 221–223.

Meltzer, L. J., & Mindell, J. A. (2006). Impact of a child's chronic illness on maternal sleep and daytime functioning. *Archives of Internal Medicine*, *166*(16), 1749–1755.

Miller, J. F. (2000). Client power resources. In J. F. Miller (Ed.), *Coping with chronic illness* (pp. 3–19). Philadelphia, PA: F. A. Davis.

Mirolla, M. (2004). *The cost of chronic disease in Canada*. Ottawa, ON: Chronic Disease Prevention Alliance of Canada.

Mitchell, M. J., Lemanek, K., Palermo, T. M., Crosby, L. E., Nichols, A., & Powers, S. W. (2007). Parent perspectives on pain management, coping, and family functioning in pediatric sickle cell disease. *Clinical Pediatrics*, *46*(4), 311–319.

Mussatto, K. (2006). Adaptation of the child and family to life with a chronic illness. *Cardiology in the Young*, *16*(Suppl 3), 110–116.

National Association for Down Syndrome. (2012). Facts about Down syndrome. Retrieved from http://www.nads.org/ pages_new/facts.html

National Health and Nutrition Education Survey (NHANES). (2011). NHANES 2009–2010. Retrieved from http://www.cdc.gov/nchs/nhanes/nhanes2009-2010/nhanes09_10.htm

National Institute of Alcohol Abuse and Alcoholism. (2004). NIAAA council approves definition of binge drinking. *NIAAA Newsletter 2004*, no. 3, p. 3.

Nuutila, L., & Salantera, S. (2006). Children with a long-term illness: Parents' experiences of care. *Journal of Pediatric Nursing, 21*(2), 153–160.

Osterkamp, E., Costanzo, A., Ehrhardt, B., & Gormley, D. (2013). Transition of care for adolescent patients with chronic illness: Education for nurses. *Journal of Continuing Education in Nursing, 44*(1), 38–42.

Patterson, J. (2002). Integrating family resilience and family stress theory. *Journal of Marriage and Family, 64*, 349–360.

Peter, N., Fork, C., Ginsburg, K., & Schwartz, D., (2009). Transition from pediatric to adult care: Internists' perspectives. *Pediatrics, 123*(4), 417–423.

Protudjer, J., Kozyrskyi, A., Becker, A., & Marchessault, G. (2009). Normalization strategies of children with asthma. *Qualitative Health Research, 19*, 94–104.

Putnam, R. (1996). Who killed civic America? *The American Prospect, 4*(13), 11–18.

Rabiee, P., Sloper, P., & Beresford, B. (2005). Desired outcomes for children and young people with complex health care needs, and children who do not use speech for communication. *Health & Social Care in the Community, 13*(5), 478–487.

Ray, L. D. (2003). The social and political conditions that shape special-needs parenting. *Journal of Family Nursing, 9*(3), 281–304.

Rehm, R. S., & Bradley, J. F. (2005). Normalization in families raising a child who is medically fragile/technology dependent and developmentally delayed. *Qualitative Health Research, 15*(6), 807–820.

Richard, A., & Shea, K. (2011). Delineation of self-care and associated concepts. *Journal of Nursing Scholarship, 43*(3), 255–264.

Rodrigues, N., & Patterson, J. M. (2007). Impact of severity of a child's chronic condition on the functioning of two-parent families. *Journal of Pediatric Psychology, 32*(4), 417–426.

Rolland, J. S. (1987). Chronic illness and the life cycle: A conceptual framework. *Family Process, 26*(2), 203–221.

Rosen, D., Blum, R., Britto, M., Sawyer, S., & Siegel, D. (2003). Transition to adult health care for adolescents and young adults with chronic conditions. Position paper of the Society for Adolescent Medicine. *Journal of Adolescent Health, 33*, 309–311.

Schuster, L. (2005). Family support in dietary routines in Appalachians with type 2 diabetes. Unpublished master's thesis, Ohio University, Athens, OH.

Sonneveld, H., Strating, M., van Staa, A., & Nieboer, A., (2013). Gaps in transitional care: What are the perceptions of adolescents, parents and providers. *Child Care, Health and Development, 39*(1), 69–80.

Spilkin, A., & Ballantyne, A. (2007). Behavior in children with a chronic illness: A descriptive study of child characteristics, family adjustment, and school issues in children with cystinosis. *Families, Systems, & Health, 25*(1), 68–84.

Steinbeck, K., Brodie, L., & Towns, S. (2007). Transition care for young people with chronic illness. *International Journal of Adolescent Medicine and Health, England, 19*(3), 295–303.

Steinbeck, K., Brodie, L., & Towns, S. (2008). Transition in chronic illness: Who is going where? *Journal of Paediatrics and Child Health, Australia, 44*(9), 478–482.

Strohm, K. (2001). Sibling project. *Youth Studies Australia, 20*(4), 48–53.

Sullivan-Bolyai, S., Knafl, K. A., Sadler, L., & Gilliss, C. L. (2004). Family matters. Great expectations: A position description for parents as caregivers: Part II. *Pediatric Nursing, 30*(1), 52–56.

Tang, T. S., Funnell, M. M., & Anderson, R. M. (2006). Group education strategies for diabetes self-management. *Diabetes Spectrum, 19*(2), 99–105.

Theriault, L., Hermus, G., Goldfarb, D., Stonebridge, S., & Bounajm, F. (2012). *Cost risk analysis for chronic lung disease in Canada.* Ottawa, Ontario, Canada: The Conference Board of Canada.

U.S. Department of Health and Human Services. (2012). National family caregiver support program (OAA: Title IIIE). Retrieved from http://www.aoa.gov/aoa_programs/hcltc/caregiver/index.aspx

U.S. Department of Health and Human Services, Health Resources and Services Administration, Maternal and Child Health Bureau. (2008). *The National Survey of Children with Special Health Care Needs Chartbook 2005–2006.* Rockville, MD: Author.

U.S. Department of Labor. (2013). Family and medical leave act. Retrieved from http://www.dol.gov/whd/fmla

Van Cleave, J., Heisler, M., Devries, J. M., Joiner, T. A., & Davis, M. M. (2007). Discussion of illness during well-child care visits with parents of children with and without special health care needs. *Archives of Pediatrics & Adolescent Medicine, 161*(12), 1170–1175.

van Staa, A., van der Stege, H., Jedeloo, S., Moll, H., & Hilberink, S. (2011). Readiness to transfer to adult care of adolescents with chronic conditions: Exploration of associated factors. *Journal of Adolescent Health, 48*(3), 295–302.

Wagner, E. H., Austin, B. T., Davis, C., Hindmarsh, M., Schaefer, J., & Bonomi, A. (2001). Improving chronic illness care: Translating evidence into action. *Health Affairs, 20*, 64–78.

Wennick, A., & Hallstrom, I. (2007). Families' lived experience one year after a child was diagnosed with type 1 diabetes. *Journal of Advanced Nursing, 60*, 299–307.

Wollenhaupt, J., Rodgers, B., & Sawin, K. J. (2011). Family management of a chronic health condition: Perspectives of adolescents. *Journal of Family Nursing, 181*, 65–90.

Wong, L., Chan, F., Wong, F., Wong, E., Huen, K., Yeoh, E., & Fok, T. (2010). Transition care for adolescents and families with chronic illness. *Journal of Adolescent Health, 47*, 540–546.

World Health Organization. (2013a). Chronic diseases. Retrieved from http://www.who.int/topics/chronic_diseases/en

World Health Organization. (2013b). Integrated chronic disease prevention and control. Retrieved from http://www.who.int/chp/about/integrated_cd/en

World Health Organization. (2013c). Cardiovascular diseases. Retrieved from http://www.who.int/mediacentre/factsheets/fs317/en/index.html

World Health Organization. (2013d). Cancer. Retrieved from http://www.who.int/mediacentre/factsheets/fs297/en/index.html

World Health Organization. (2013e). Diabetes. Retrieved from http://www.who.int/mediacentre/factsheets/fs312/en/index.html

World Health Organization. (2013f). Overweight and obesity. Retrieved from http://www.who.int/mediacentre/factsheets/fs311/en/index.html

chapter *10*

Families in Palliative and End-of-Life Care

Rose Steele, PhD, RN

Carole A. Robinson, PhD, RN

Kimberley A. Widger, PhD, RN

Critical Concepts

- Palliative care is both a philosophy and a type of care.

- Palliative care is "whole person" care that involves a focus on quality of life, or living well, for all family members when they are dealing with a life-limiting illness. It can start long before the end-of-life period, as early as at the diagnosis of a life-limiting illness, and extend beyond death to bereavement.

- The principles of palliative care are applicable in a sudden, acute event—such as an accident, suicide, or myocardial infarction—though the context is different because there is a shorter time span in which to work with a family. A palliative approach complements the disease orientation that is often the focus of acute care.

- The majority of palliative care is provided by family caregivers.

- Skilled nursing interventions and relationships between nurses and families are crucial in creating positive outcomes in palliative and end-of-life care.

- Interprofessional teamwork is essential in palliative and end-of-life care and the team is inclusive of family members.

- People who have advanced, life-limiting illnesses worry about being a burden on their families and about the consequences of their death on their families. Family members worry about burdening their ill member. Everyone involved is often afraid. This fear can lead to communication problems, isolation, and lack of support within the family.

- Perceived barriers to nurses providing quality end-of-life care may be ameliorated when the nurse understands palliative care principles.

- Nurses need strong patient and family assessment and intervention skills to provide optimal palliative and end-of-life care.

- End-of-life decision making is a process that involves all relevant family members identified by the ill person and evolves over time. Advance care planning is an important part of this process.

- A "good" death is one that happens in alignment with patient and family preferences.

Nurses encounter families who are facing end-of-life issues in virtually all settings of practice. From newborns to seniors in their nineties and older, people die, and their families are affected by the experience. Nurses are in an ideal position to influence a family's experience, either positively or negatively. Ideally, nurses facilitate a positive experience for families, one that will bring them comfort in the future as they recall what it was like when their loved one died. Unfortunately, not all families have a positive experience, and it is often because health care providers do not know how to work effectively with families at this challenging time (Andershed, 2006). Yet, palliative and end-of-life nursing can be extremely rewarding and professionally fulfilling. It offers an opportunity for personal growth in patients, families, and health care providers; interactions among all concerned are especially meaningful (Webster & Kristjanson, 2002).

This chapter details the key components to consider in providing palliative and end-of-life care, as well as families' most important concerns and needs when a family member experiences a life-threatening illness or is dying. It also presents some concrete strategies to assist nurses in providing optimal palliative and end-of-life care to all family members. More specifically, the chapter begins with a brief definition of palliative and end-of life care, including its focus on improving quality of life for patients and their families. The chapter then outlines principles of palliative care and ways to apply these principles across all settings and regardless of whether death results from chronic illness or a sudden or traumatic event. Two palliative care and end-of-life case studies follow.

PALLIATIVE AND END-OF-LIFE CARE DEFINED

Palliative care and *end-of-life care* are not synonymous terms. End-of-life care focuses exclusively on the immediate period around death, whereas palliative care includes end-of-life care but extends for many months, even years (especially in children), and can coexist with treatments aimed at curing an illness (World Health Organization [WHO], 2006). Palliative care focuses on improving the quality of life of patients and their families facing problems associated with life-limiting illness. Palliative care helps families in these situations live well by preventing and relieving suffering through early identification and excellent assessment and treatment of pain and other physical, psychosocial, or spiritual problems (WHO, 2006). Employing a team approach, palliative care offers a support system to help patients live as actively as possible, and to help families cope during the patient's illness and their own bereavement. Life is affirmed and dying is regarded as a normal process (WHO, 2006).

Focus on the family as a unit is a key principle in palliative care. Nowhere is this more evident than when a child is the patient. Support targets both individual family members and the family as a whole. The age range of patients receiving pediatric palliative care, typically 0 to 19 years of age, requires that children's developmental, social, educational, recreational, and relational needs be considered. The developmental stage of the family must also be considered, regardless of the patient's age.

Palliative care in adults developed primarily around care for patients with cancer. The current trend in palliative care, however, is an expanded focus on life-threatening illnesses beyond cancer. Patients and their families have similar needs for information, care, and support in a wide variety of chronic illnesses, including heart disease (Barnes et al., 2006), muscular dystrophy (Dawson & Kristjanson, 2003), motor neuron disease (Dawson & Kristjanson, 2003; Hughes, Sinha, Higginson, Down, & Leigh, 2005), dementia (Caron, Griffith, & Arcand, 2005), Parkinson's disease (Goy, Carter, & Ganzini, 2007), and neurodegenerative diseases (Kristjanson, Aoun, & Oldham, 2006), as well as when patients are simply of an advanced age (Forbes-Thompson & Gessert, 2005).

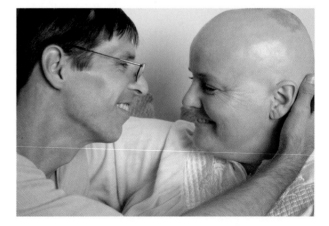

Palliative care is about nurturing and maintaining quality of life from diagnosis of life-limiting illness through bereavement. The approach encompassed by palliative care principles can be used in any setting with any family, regardless of how long a person has to live or how sudden the death is. Murray and Sheikh (2008) described three main trajectories of decline at the end of life. Awareness of these trajectories (Fig. 10-1) helps nurses recognize when palliative care may best be introduced. Palliative care can be offered alongside care that is curative in intent (Murray, Kendall, Boyd, & Sheikh, 2005). But at some point in the illness trajectory, the primary goal of care shifts from curative to palliative intent. This point often occurs when there are no available curative treatments, or treatments are no longer effective or are associated with burden that is no longer tolerable to the patient. It is well recognized that communication about the transition of care from curative to palliative intent is difficult but crucial (Marsella, 2009). It requires discussion about shifting the focus to quality of life rather than quantity of life. When a sudden or traumatic event occurs, there is little time to hold such discussions. But when someone has a protracted illness, this discussion can be introduced gradually and can be repeated over time.

Unfortunately, in many clinical settings, palliative care is raised only in the last few days or weeks of life, even when death has been anticipated. The introduction of palliative care is particularly challenging for health care providers when patients suffer from illnesses that are difficult to prognosticate, such as advanced lung, heart, and liver disease (Fox et al., 1999). Nevertheless, it is important to ensure that patients, family members, and health care providers are aligned in their goals for care (Thompson, McClement, & Daeninck, 2006) and have a common understanding of what quality of life means for the patient and family. Goals of care and the meaning of quality of life will be unique in each situation and care should be tailored to the needs of each particular family (Heyland, Dodek, et al., 2006).

Death occurs in many settings, from various causes, and across the life span. Some differences can be expected in families' experiences depending on the context, for example:

- Where the death takes place (e.g., home versus intensive care unit)
- The cause of death (e.g., natural progression of a chronic illness versus an unexpected, acute event)
- The dying trajectory (e.g., over a period of years versus sudden)
- The age of the family member who is dying (e.g., a 3-year-old child versus an 85-year-old person)
- The cultural and spiritual backgrounds of families (e.g., white versus Chinese; religious faith versus no faith)

No matter the context, the principles of palliative care should be consistent, with implementation tailored to address the particular family and the family's context. Consistent use of these principles contributes to high-quality palliative and end-of-life care. See Box 10-1 for some of the basic principles of palliative care.

Identifying Relevant Literature

The amount of research about the provision of palliative and end-of-life care to adults is growing. Research in pediatric palliative care is much more limited, but many of the reported issues for families are similar across the life span. An electronic search of the Cumulative Index to Nursing and Allied Health Literature (CINAHL) database from 2002 until summer 2012 uncovered more than 2000 articles that reported on some aspect of patient or family perceptions of the palliative,

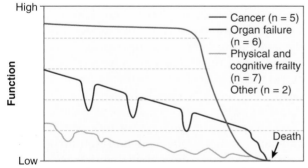

Number of Deaths in Each Trajectory, Out of Average 20 Deaths Each Year Per UK General Practice List of 2000 Patients

Cancer (n = 5)
Organ failure (n = 6)
Physical and cognitive frailty (n = 7)
Other (n = 2)

FIGURE 10-1 The three main trajectories of decline at the end of life. *(Reproduced from Murray, S. A., & Sheikh, A. [2008]. Care for all at the end of life.* British Medical Journal, *336[7650], 958–959, with permission from BMJ Publishing Group Ltd.)*

- Palliative care begins as soon as there is a diagnosis of life-limiting illness.
- Palliative care can occur concurrently with care that is curative in intent.
- The focus of palliative care is on supporting and enhancing quality of life.
- Patient and family are cared for as a unit.
- Attention is paid to physical, developmental, psychological, social, and spiritual needs and concerns.
- Education and support of patient and family are crucial.
- An interprofessional approach is required.
- Care extends across settings.
- Bereavement support is part of good palliative care.

end-of-life, or bereavement care provided to the family by health professionals. Despite the number of articles in existence, only about a third presented research findings or a systematic review of research findings and most of the research was published in the last 4 years. Virtually all areas of palliative care need more research to strengthen the evidence base. The studies included exploration of patient and family concerns and needs in relation to different diseases (cancer being the most common); causes of death (sudden deaths, deaths after illness); care settings (long-term care, acute hospital care, critical care, home, and hospice); ages (pediatric to elderly patients); countries; and cultures.

Often, great variation existed in beliefs and needs within a given cultural or other type of group, as well as within individual families (Aspinal, Hughes, Dunckley, & Addington Hall, 2006; Heyland, Dodek, et al., 2006; Torke, Garas, Sexson, & Branch, 2005). Therefore, one cannot determine from the literature what the exact needs of, for example, family members of an elderly African American person living with Alzheimer's disease in a long-term care setting will be. But the literature does highlight the key considerations in providing palliative and end-of-life care, important areas to assess for any family facing life-limiting illness, and interventions that may be helpful for many families or that can be adjusted to fit with a particular family's assessed needs. The literature found through this search, plus seminal articles, forms the evidence base for the remainder of this chapter.

KEY CONSIDERATIONS IN PALLIATIVE AND END-OF-LIFE CARE

In order to provide optimal palliative and end-of-life care, there are key areas that must be considered, such as the following: nurses' own personal assumptions and biases about death and dying; your personal assumptions about people and their backgrounds; the involvement of the family in all aspects of care; the involvement of the interprofessional team; the inclusion of bereavement care as part of palliative care; and potential barriers to optimal palliative and end-of-life nursing care.

Personal Assumptions and Biases About Death and Dying

To provide optimal palliative and end-of-life care, nurses need to be aware of their own assumptions and biases about death and dying. As a nurse, it is important to explore your own beliefs, attitudes, and personal and professional experiences to understand how they may influence your attitudes toward death, dying, and bereavement. For example, if you believe that a family member should be physically present with someone who is dying, you may find it difficult to work with family members who choose not to be present. It is neither possible nor wise to separate the "nurse as person" from the "nurse as professional," because if your personal reactions are ignored, you are less able to focus on meeting the needs of patients and their families (Davies & Oberle, 1990).

Many nurses do not know how to deal with dying and death. They are afraid, nervous, or anxious when faced with a dying patient and grieving family. But some nurses experience great satisfaction when working with dying patients. They have developed their palliative knowledge and skills, not simply through caring for many dying patients, but through reflecting on their experiences with those patients and in their personal lives, on the meaning of life and death, and on their own behavior. They are able, therefore, to provide competent physical care and also to be a welcome presence to those who are dying and their family members. All nurses, from novice to expert, need to develop basic competencies in the area of death and dying, from how to provide effective symptom management, using both pharmacological and nonpharmacological therapies, to being comfortable enough with death and dying that they can be present for family members. See Box 10-2 for

BOX 10-2

Key Areas of Focus for Education in Palliative and End-of-Life Care

The Registered Nurses' Association of Ontario (2011) recommends that entry to practice nursing programs and post-registration education should incorporate specialized end-of-life care content that includes the following areas:

- Dying as a normal process, including the social and cultural context of death and dying, dying trajectories, and signs of impending death
- Care of the family (including caregiver)
- Grief, bereavement, and mourning
- Principles and models of palliative care
- Assessment and management of pain and other symptoms (including pharmacological and nonpharmacological approaches)

- Suffering and spiritual/existential issues and care
- Decision making and advance care planning
- Ethical issues
- Effective and compassionate communication
- Advocacy and therapeutic relationship-building
- Interprofessional practice and competencies
- Self-care for nurses, including coping strategies and self-exploration of death and dying
- End-of-life issues in mental health, homelessness, and the incarcerated
- The roles of grief and bereavement educators, clergy, spiritual leaders, and funeral directors
- Knowledge of relevant legislation

Source: Registered Nurses' Association of Ontario. (2011). Best practice guidelines: End-of-life care during the last days and hours. Toronto, ON: Author. Retrieved from http://rnao.ca/sites/rnao-ca/files/End-of-Life_Care_During_the_Last_Days_and_Hours_0.pdf

some key areas of focus when seeking education about palliative and end-of-life care.

As a novice nurse, you can develop these competencies by building on your own strengths and learning ways to become more comfortable with death and dying. It is often helpful to begin with your own experiences around loss, death, and dying. Reflecting on your beliefs about life and death will help clarify your understanding of and appreciation for the human condition—the only thing certain in life is that everyone will die. This reflection will form the foundation for the inner strength that will enable you to provide optimal palliative and end-of-life care (Davies & Oberle, 1990). You may want to further your education on death, dying, and providing care at life's end through one of the many available resources, such as workshops, books, and conferences; best practice guidelines (Registered Nurses' Association of Ontario, 2011); or even popular movies (e.g., *Life as a House; One True Thing*). Gaining knowledge through formal education can help improve your comfort with providing care to patients facing a life-threatening illness and their families (Kwak, Salmon, Acquaviva, Brandt, & Egan, 2007).

Personal Assumptions and Biases About People and Their Backgrounds

An underlying principle in palliative care is respect for persons. As a nurse, it is helpful to be aware of the assumptions and stereotypes that you hold about the people you care for because assumptions and stereotypes get in the way of person- and family-centered care. Part of good palliative and end-of-life care is recognizing that each and every person is valuable in their own right; however, this is sometimes negatively influenced by judgments about a particular person's or family's worth. Valuing appreciates the possibility that every human being has the potential for actualization or optimal development (Davies & Oberle, 1990; Widger, Steele, Oberle, & Davies, 2009).

Sometimes, assumptions and biases about people relate to their cultural or spiritual background. Similar to exploring your assumptions and biases about death and dying, it is important to recognize your own cultural or spiritual background or previous experiences with other cultures and how they might influence your practice, as well as your expectations of others (Huang, Yates, & Prior, 2009). For example, if you do not understand the importance of an Aboriginal smudging ceremony to a family, you may be unwilling to create an environment that allows for such a ceremony within a hospital setting. The cultural and spiritual implications discussed elsewhere in this text also are relevant to quality palliative care. Effectively implementing the palliative care philosophy means that you must be sensitive to diversity and able to deal with issues that arise when caring for people with varied cultural and spiritual backgrounds (Davies & Oberle, 1990). Cultural beliefs, as well as spirituality, spiritual beliefs, or faith, may be important in how some patients and families cope with illness (Aspinal et al., 2006; Donovan, Williams, Stajduhar, Brazil, & Marshall, 2011; Ferrell, Ervin, Smith, Marek, & Melancon, 2002; Knapp et al., 2011; Perreault, Fothergill Bourbonnais, & Fiset, 2004; Robinson, Thiel, Backus, & Meyer, 2006; Sharman, Meert, & Sarnaik, 2005; Torke et al., 2005). Some may find strength and renewed connection to their cultural or spiritual background, whereas others may question previously held beliefs. It is very important that you do not impose your own beliefs on the patient and family; you need to determine what is most important to them. Although across cultures different needs may exist, there is likely more similarity than differences among cultures in terms of basic human needs for connections with others, physical care, dignity, and support (Kongsuwan, Chaipetch, & Matchim, 2012). On the other hand, it is important to remember that there may be a great deal of diversity *within* cultures or faiths. This means there will never be a single approach that is appropriate for all people from a particular culture or faith group, so one of the best strategies is to ask families about their beliefs and preferred way of doing things (Kleinman & Benson, 2006). From this place of understanding, nurses can negotiate care so that it aligns as closely as possible with the family's values and beliefs and demonstrates a fundamental respect for people.

Involvement of the Family

Life-threatening illness is often referred to by family members as "our" illness (Ferrell et al., 2002). When the ill person is having a "good" day, so is the family caregiver (Stajduhar, Martin, Barwich, & Fyles, 2008). If the ill person is in emotional or physical pain or has difficulty coping with the illness, the caregiver's suffering dramatically increases as well (Brajtman, 2005; Milberg & Strang, 2011; Sharman et al., 2005). Siblings too may suffer if parents are too focused on the ill child to meet sibling needs (de Cinque et al., 2006; Horsley & Patterson, 2006). Therefore, interventions directed at one family member can also be supportive to other family members, and this is the case whether the ill person is a child or an adult. Family members feel supported when they believe that professionals have the best interests of their loved one at heart. As a result, nurses need to ensure that the patient

is well cared for, but also keep in mind that interventions directed at family members as a group and individually have been found to be most effective in supporting families and achieving the best outcomes (Northouse, Katapodi, Song, Zhang, & Mood, 2010).

Among the top concerns of dying patients is the well-being of their family members in terms of caregiving burden and their ability to cope after the death (Aspinal et al., 2006; Fitzsimons et al., 2007; Jo, Brazil, Lohfeld, & Willison, 2007; Kristjanson, Aoun, & Yates, 2006; Kuhl, 2002; Perreault et al., 2004). Even ill children may make decisions based on what they believe is best for their family rather than what they particularly want (Hinds et al., 2005). Patients do not want to become a burden to their families (Fitzsimons et al., 2007; Heyland, Dodek, et al., 2006; Heyland et al., 2005). If patients know that their family is well supported, it may reduce their own suffering.

Family members provide the majority of care for persons with life-threatening illness, and a home death relies on their strong involvement (Grande et al., 2009; Stajduhar, Funk, Jakobsson, & Ohlen, 2010; Stajduhar, Funk, Toye, et al., 2010). Family members carry many burdens when a family member is dying, including ill health (e.g., depression, back pain, shingles, difficulty sleeping, and preexisting chronic illnesses), conflicting family responsibilities (e.g., caring for the ill parent or spouse plus their own children), little time to meet their own needs, cumulative losses, fear, anxiety, insecurity, financial concerns, loss of physical closeness with a spouse, and lack of support from other family members and health professionals (Corà, Partinico, Munafò, & Palomba, 2012; Ferrell et al., 2002; Funk et al., 2010; Grande et al., 2009; Jo et al., 2007; Kenny, Hall, Zapart, & Davis, 2010; Osse, Vernooij, Dassen, Schade, & Grol, 2006; Perreault et al., 2004; Proot et al., 2003; Riley & Fenton, 2007; Robinson, Pesut, & Bottorff, 2012; Sherwood, Given, Doorenbos, & Given, 2004; Wollin, Yates, & Kristjanson, 2006).

Moreover, the work of caregiving can be both physically and mentally exhausting (Riley & Fenton, 2007; Robinson et al., 2012; Sherwood et al., 2004). There also may be an ambivalent sense of waiting for the person to die but not wanting the person to die (Riley & Fenton, 2007). Family members may experience these issues whether their relative is mostly at home (Andershed, 2006) or in an institutional setting

(Abma, 2005). They often have increased responsibilities and may view the situation as burdensome (Andershed, 2006). Yet, family caregivers often are more concerned about the care of the dying person than about their own health (Robinson et al., 2012), so as not to burden the patient or take focus off the patient (Fridriksdottir, Sigurdardottir, & Gunnarsdottir, 2006; Grande et al., 2009; Konrad, 2008; Perreault et al., 2004; Proot et al., 2003; Riley & Fenton, 2007). A recent study found that one of the most effective ways of supporting family caregivers is to help them fulfill their caregiving role rather than focus on their personal needs (Robinson et al., 2012).

Although patients may want to remain at home, family members often have to assume extra responsibilities, such as administering medications, which can lead to a great deal of anxiety (Kazanowski, 2005). Further, when patients choose to receive care or die at home—perhaps to increase their quality of life through greater normalcy; increased contact with family, friends, and pets; and the familiar, comfortable surroundings (Hansson, Kjaergaard, Schmiegelow, & Hallström, 2012)—this location may not be the caregiver's first choice. For some families, a home death brings additional burdens, worry, and responsibility, and the home becomes more like an institution (Brazil, Howell, Bedard, Krueger, & Heidebrecht, 2005; Funk et al., 2010). Decisions related to care location must be made with family members because the course chosen has a profound impact on the well-being of both the patient and the family (Stajduhar, 2003; Tang, Liu, Lai, & McCorkle, 2005). Recognize too, however, that family caregivers often cannot express their preferences if they differ from those of the ill person and may need assistance from a nurse to navigate the competing demands and priorities (Robinson et al., 2012).

Family members may not be available or able to give care at home. Patients and family members may perceive that hospitals or hospices are able to provide a higher quality of end-of-life care than can be given at home, or the patient and family may feel a close connection to the health care providers in the institution (Tang et al., 2005). Some family members may experience profound guilt if they are not able to provide end-of-life care at home. Health care professionals can alleviate some of this guilt if they alert patients and families early on that plans for location of care may need to change as time goes on to ensure provision of the best possible care (Stajduhar, 2003).

Family caregivers may be vulnerable to burnout if they are not able to cope with the caregiving requirements (Proot et al., 2003). The burden may be increased by the physical and emotional demands of the patient; reduced opportunities for the caregiver to participate in usual activities; and feelings of fear, insecurity, and loneliness (Proot et al., 2003). Caregiver strain also may increase when patients need more assistance with activities of daily living or have greater levels of psychological and existential distress. Differences may exist in needs based on age and sex, with younger caregivers having more concerns about finances and maintaining social activities and relationships. Female caregivers may have more difficulties with their own health (lack of sleep and muscle pain), with transportation, coordinating care, and feeling underappreciated (Osse et al., 2006). When a child dies, from any cause, mothers in particular have a greater risk for psychiatric hospitalization and death from suicide or accidents shortly after their child's death, compared with those who have not experienced a child's death (Li, Laursen, Precht, Olsen, & Mortensen, 2005; Li, Precht, Mortensen, & Olsen, 2003). Bereaved mothers also have a greater risk for death from cancer and cardiovascular disease long after their child has died (Li, Johansen, Hansen, & Olsen, 2002; Li et al., 2003, 2005).

On the other hand, some people report positive aspects of caregiving, such as feelings of satisfaction, greater appreciation for life, greater purpose and meaning to life, increased closeness and intimacy, newfound personal strength and ability, and the opportunity to share special time together and show their love for their family member (Andershed, 2006; Ferrell et al., 2002; Grande et al., 2009; Hudson, 2006; Jo et al., 2007; Riley & Fenton, 2007; Sherwood et al., 2004; Steele 2005a, 2005b; Steele & Davies, 2006). Some family members may view care provision as an opportunity and a privilege (Hudson, 2006; Jo et al., 2007; Kazanowski, 2005; Sherwood et al., 2004). Hudson (2006) suggested a link between the caregiver's ability to see the positives in the situation and both better coping and less traumatic grief. It is important, therefore, to help families uncover the positive aspects and help families recognize the value in what they are doing because it may contribute to their overall well-being and may enhance their experience. Further, when high-quality care and optimal family support are provided, research indicates that adult family members who care for another adult family member live longer after the patient's death (Christakis & Iwashyna, 2003). Similarly, some researchers have found links between parents' satisfaction with care, or assessment of care quality, and their coping ability or emotional state in the years after the child's death (Kreicbergs et al., 2005; Rosenberg, Baker, Syrjala, & Wolfe, 2012; Surkan et al., 2006). Nurses are in an excellent position to identify and foster a family's strengths, as well as to identify, prevent, and alleviate many of the negative aspects of caregiving. Through provision of optimal palliative and end-of-life care, nurses can have a significant, lifelong effect on the well-being of family members.

Involvement of the Interprofessional Team

Although the focus of this chapter is on the role of the nurse, provision of care through an interprofessional team approach is one of the principles of palliative care. The composition of the team may look quite different depending on the care setting. For example, in a rural setting, the team may be comprised of a family physician and a nurse, whereas in a large urban setting there may be a team of palliative specialists including palliative physicians, advanced practice nurses, psychologists, spiritual care advisors, pharmacists, social workers, and volunteers. In all settings, nurses are core team members. The *interprofessional* team approach focuses on health professionals collaboratively working with each other and with a patient/family as members of the team to develop and achieve common goals (Oliver, Porock, Demiris, & Courtney, 2005). Despite sharing common goals, each team member will bring different ideas and skills to the team, which is both the strength and the challenge of the interprofessional approach. Multiple perspectives contribute to holistic care and the ability to meet the multiple complex patient and family needs that arise in palliative care. The challenge is how to make best use of each person's contributions while negotiating differences in perspective and respectfully managing tensions around professional boundaries and expertise. Palliative care is known for blurring of team member roles in order to meet the current needs of the patient and family members.

An interprofessional model of care is different from a multiprofessional model. In health care settings, traditional roles and expectations among the professions involved in providing care can raise barriers to integrated and effective teams. Traditional medical services have been based on a *multiprofessional* model that has tended to hinder the development of an effective team because a multiprofessional team is composed of individuals from different professional backgrounds who work with the same patient and family, but who may develop individual goals and work relatively independently. In contrast, the *interprofessional* team approach focuses on collaboratively working with a patient/family to develop and achieve common goals. See Box 10-3 for a summary of the

---

BOX 10-3
Interprofessional Versus Multiprofessional Teams

Multiprofessional Team	Interprofessional Team
■ Medical treatment model	■ Holistic, "patient-centered" approach to care
■ Fragmented approach to care	■ Group control
■ Centralized control	■ Facilitative team leader
■ Autocratic team leader	■ Decision making by consensus
■ Decision making by team leader	■ Leadership by team members
■ Vertical communication between professionals	■ Horizontal communication between professionals
■ Treatment geared toward *intra*professional goals	■ Treatment geared toward *inter*professional goals
■ Separate goals among professionals	■ Common goals among professionals
■ Professional goals are basis of plan	■ Patient goals are basis of care plan
■ Families are peripheral	■ Families are integral
■ Meetings/rounds involve individual professional reporting	■ Meetings/rounds involve group problem solving and decision making

differences between the interprofessional and multiprofessional approaches.

For nurses, being an effective member of an interprofessional team often means that they share information and consult with others on the team, mediate on behalf of patients and families when necessary, and act as a liaison between various members, institutions, and programs. As a novice nurse, one of the key things you can do is to learn and understand the patient's and family members' hopes, preferences, beliefs, fears, and goals and to share this understanding with the team. Knowledge about group dynamics is invaluable in learning how to become a successful team member. Everyone needs to know and accept that each member of the team is unique and valuable, and good communication skills are crucial so that supportive rather than defensive communication can be fostered. A lack of communication among health professionals is common and frustrating for families because they then receive conflicting information or need to repeat information and relay decisions that have been made already (Antle, Barrera, Beaune, D'Agostino, & Good, 2005; Hammes, Klevan, Kempf, & Williams, 2005; Hudson, 2006; Macdonald et al., 2005; Perreault et al., 2004; Widger & Picot, 2008; Wiegand, 2006).

Bereavement Care

One of the principles of palliative care is that care continues after the death and into bereavement. The need for follow-up with the family after the death by involved health professionals is considered by many families to be a crucial component of end-of-life care, but unfortunately one that is often missing (Cherlin, Schulman Green, McCorkle, Johnson Hurzeler, & Bradley, 2004; D'Agostino, Berlin-Romalis, Jovcevska, & Barrera, 2008; de Jong-Berg & Kane, 2006; Kreicbergs et al., 2005; Macdonald et al., 2005; Meyer, Ritholz, Burns, & Truog, 2006; Widger & Picot, 2008; Wisten & Zingmark, 2007; Woodgate, 2006). Families sometimes feel abandoned after the death, which adds to the grief they experience (D'Agostino et al., 2008; de Cinque et al., 2006; Heller & Solomon, 2005; Meert et al., 2007; Widger & Picot, 2008). Bereavement care is important because family caregivers may experience negative effects, such as feelings of loneliness, sadness, and physical exhaustion caused by difficulty sleeping, as well as the aftermath of the demands of caregiving (Funk et al., 2010). These feelings may be juxtaposed with feelings of relief that the patient's suffering has ended and that everything possible was done to keep the patient comfortable (Hudson, 2006; Sherwood et al., 2004; Wollin et al., 2006). After the death, some caregivers may feel "lost" because they now have "free" hours that were previously devoted to caregiving (Sherwood et al., 2004). Support for families after the death may help prevent or alleviate prolonged suffering. Specific interventions for bereavement care are highlighted later in the chapter and in the second case study.

Barriers to Optimal Palliative and End-of-Life Nursing Care

A major barrier to optimal palliative and end-of-life care for patients and their families arises from the limited formal education and training nurses receive (Espinosa, Young, & Walsh, 2008). Although some improvements have been made, historically little attention has been given to palliative and end-of-life care in nursing and other health care professionals' curricula. In particular, health professionals report being unprepared to treat pain and symptoms effectively, emotionally support the dying person and his or her family, or deal with the ethical issues that may be present at end of life (Contro, Larson, Scofield, Sourkes, & Cohen, 2004; Davies et al., 2008; Feudtner et al., 2007).

Another barrier is the availability and usage of palliative services. Specialist palliative care services may not be available in all care settings, particularly at home or in more rural and remote areas, to provide support to practicing health professionals in addressing learning needs or providing care to patients and families. Even when appropriate hospice and palliative care services are available, a lack of understanding of palliative care on the part of health professionals can lead to delayed, or even a lack of, referral to these services.

Involvement of the patient and family members in the interprofessional team is a critical component of palliative care, yet barriers may exist that limit this involvement. In many cases, the program setup and lines of communication do not allow for families to be included to the extent they could and should be, nor do they allow for provision of bereavement care by the health professionals who provided care before the death. Although work needs to be done to remove the identified barriers, it is possible for nurses to practice high standards within constraining contexts. It is important to seek out opportunities to improve your knowledge and skills in palliative and end-of-life care and to be an advocate for the needs and views of patients and families regardless of barriers that may present themselves.

A different type of barrier that can be even more challenging to manage is the moral distress that can arise for nurses when they provide end-of-life care to patients and their families (Elpern, Covert, & Kleinpell, 2005; Espinosa et al., 2008). Moral distress occurs when a person is powerless to carry out an action that he believes to be ethically appropriate. Some situations common to the provision of palliative care that may cause moral distress include the following:

- Patients receiving medical treatments that are believed to be inappropriate and/or contributing to patients' suffering (e.g., a ventilator, providing artificial nutrition and hydration via a gastrostomy tube)
- Inadequate management of pain or other symptoms
- Lack of communication with family members about prognosis
- Provision of false hope to family members (Epstein & Degado, 2010)

Moral distress can affect nurses' job satisfaction, physical and psychological well-being, self-image, spirituality, and decisions about their own health. Such distress may lead to burnout and leaving the work environment (Elpern et al., 2005).

FAMILY NURSING PRACTICE ASSESSMENT AND INTERVENTION

Nurses must possess strong patient and family assessment skills if they are going to provide optimal care (e.g., excellent pain and symptom management, psychosocial support), because the most appropriate interventions can be designed and implemented only once a family's needs and goals have been assessed accurately. Your assessment will help you determine what a specific family or family member needs, and you can then tailor your approach and the interventions you offer in consultation with the family. Assessment and intervention are, therefore, intertwined and are discussed together in the following sections.

Keep in mind that assessment should be ongoing and sequential, building on what is known about the family and shaping interventions to meet the family's changing needs and preferences throughout the palliative and end-of-life process. This section is organized around interventions that may be helpful to families. Unfortunately, definitive research with high-quality designs to identify the best interventions for promoting optimal long-term outcomes for family members is lacking (Grande et al., 2009; Harding, List, Epiphaniou, & Jones 2012; Hudson, Remedios, & Thomas, 2010; Rosenberg et al., 2012; Stajduhar, Funk, Toye, et al., 2010). The interventions discussed are informed by existing research evidence and have been used successfully in the authors' clinical practices. The most important thing to remember is that each family is unique. Although your practice should be evidence informed, do not try to apply theory and research uncritically. What works for one family or family member may not be right for another. You must not lose sight of the need to assess and critically analyze each situation on its own merits, and actively involve the family in the process. Because we can never know whether an intervention will be useful to a particular family, interventions should always be offered tentatively and then evaluated from the family perspective. An intervention is only helpful if a family or family member experiences it as helpful.

It is not possible to cover every potential scenario in palliative and end-of-life care; therefore, the focus is on discussing the main assessment and intervention concepts that are needed for palliative and end-of-life care. Most deaths you will encounter when providing end-of-life care occur as the result of chronic disease rather than an acute event. Therefore, these situations are the focus of the remaining discussion and the case studies.

Connections Between Families and Nurses

The relationships that families develop with health care professionals have a significant effect on how families manage palliative and end-of-life events (Robinson, 1996). In your nursing education, you may have learned about the characteristics of a helping or therapeutic relationship, but in practice, nurses often speak of their "connections" with families rather than their "relationships." Making a connection with family members helps uncover what is meaningful to them and builds a bridge between you as human beings.

Understanding the family's situation apart from the illness is important (Benzein & Britt-Inger, 2008; Contro, Larson, Scofield, Sourkes, & Cohen, 2002, 2004; Maynard, Rennie, Shirtliffe, & Vickers, 2005; Steele, 2002; Steele & Davies, 2006; Surkan et al., 2006; Tomlinson et al., 2006). Asking about their previous experiences with death, any recent or concurrent life changes (e.g., new job, new house, new baby), or work and school responsibilities (e.g., self-employed, supportive work environment, nearing final examinations) may allow you to gain a more in-depth perspective and appreciate the creativity and ingenuity of their efforts.

Connecting allows you to apply your general scientific knowledge in ways that are more likely to be successful for individual patients and their families, given their specific background, needs, and ways of being in the world. Connecting is a two-way process where both the nurse and the patient/family members get to know one another at a personal level and begin to establish trust. With trust comes a greater sense of comfort and ease for the family, and an increased ability for nurses to offer effective interventions and to act as advocates (Davies & Oberle, 1990; Robinson, 1996).

Communication and interpersonal skills can facilitate or hinder connecting with patients and families. Therefore, nurses need to be aware of how their personal styles of interaction and communication can make, sustain, and break connections. These connections need to be attended to and nourished over time. Families typically are not used to talking about death and dying (Andershed, 2006). The presence of a mutual, trusting relationship is foundational to palliative assessment and intervention (Davies & Oberle, 1990; Robinson, 1996; Widger et al., 2009) and is crucial in providing a safe environment for difficult and emotional conversations to occur.

Nursing interventions that promote connections and trusting relationships include the following: careful listening to the family's experience with illness and suffering, asking good questions that encourage family members' understanding of the differences in their perspectives, demonstrating compassion by showing that you are touched by the family's suffering, remaining nonjudgmental, offering a new perspective or information through open and honest communication, working *with* the family,

acknowledging family strengths, and being reliable and accessible (Aspinal et al., 2006; Heyland, Dodek, et al., 2006; Kristjanson, Aoun, & Oldham, 2006; Mok, Chan, Chan, & Yeung, 2002; Robinson, 1996; Shiozaki et al., 2005; Torke et al., 2005). It is important to show families through your attitude and behavior that you not only have the knowledge to assist them, but that you are willing and able to do so. The sense of security and trust a family experiences in relationships with health care professionals can add to and strengthen the family's resources (Andershed, 2006). Simple acts of addressing family members by name, smiling, making eye contact, showing emotion, and physical contact such as a hand on the shoulder can foster connections between family members and the health professional (Heller & Solomon, 2005; Macdonald et al., 2005; Pector, 2004a; Sharman et al., 2005).

It is the nurse's responsibility to take the lead in developing a trusting relationship with families and to provide an environment of openness where all family members feel comfortable asking questions. Completion of a brief family genogram is one effective way of learning family members' names, relationships, and level of involvement in care, including decision making. Getting to know each family member demonstrates respect for the patient's and family members' individuality, dignity, needs, concerns, and fears (Aspinal et al., 2006; Dwyer, Nordenfelt, & Ternestedt, 2008; Gordon et al., 2009; Hinds et al., 2009; Kristjanson, Aoun, & Oldham, 2006; Midson & Carter, 2010; Monterosso & Kristjanson, 2008; Riley & Fenton, 2007; Shiozaki et al., 2005). Further, it enables recognition of differences within the family. Box 10-4 provides some questions to help you open up communication and learn about family members' perspectives as you build your connections with a family.

Making a connection does not necessarily happen instantly, nor does it have to take a lot of time; however, it does require attention and cannot be taken for granted. Sometimes you will feel a connection easily exists between you and a family; other times, you may need to make an extra effort to get to know the family and to establish a relationship. You might feel as if you have to "prove" your trustworthiness to the family or set aside your own negative reaction to a particular family or family member. Developing your reflective practice and seeking the assistance of an experienced nurse may be helpful.

BOX 10-4

Key Questions to Ask Families to Open Up Communication and Obtain Family Members' Perspectives

Ideally, questions to open up communication and obtain family members' perspectives should be asked with all involved family members present, including the patient. Keep in mind, however, that family members may not want to burden their ill member with their emotions and concerns, so you may find that some of these questions need to be asked of family members when they are alone. You will need to finesse questioning depending on where the ill family member is in the palliative care experience.

Start by saying, "I'd like to understand what it has been like for your family to live with [illness]." Then, use the following key questions to open up communication and obtain family members' perspectives. It is often helpful to indicate that you expect different family members will have different views about things. So you may need to ask a question multiple times in order to have all family members' views.

- What is your understanding of what is happening with [ill family member]?
- What experience do you have as a family in dealing with serious health problems? With death and dying?
- If you were to think ahead a bit, how do you see things going in (the next few days, the next few weeks, the next few months [use the timeframe that is most appropriate])?
- How are you hoping this will go?
- What is most important for me to know about your family?
- What are you most concerned or worried about?
- When you think about your loved one getting really sick, what fears or worries do you have?
- I've found that many families caring for someone with this condition think about the possibility of their loved one dying. They have questions about this. Do you have questions?
- Who is suffering most?
- How do they show their suffering?

- How are you managing?
- I understand that different family members will have different talents or strengths: how do you most want to be involved?
- How can I be most helpful to you at this time?
- How does your family like to talk about challenging things?
- How have you been talking about the situation you find yourselves in? Who has been involved?
- Is there anyone involved who is important and who I haven't met?
- How are important decisions made in your family? How would you like important decision making to go now?
- Families often find it helpful to talk about the care they want at end of life. Have you been able to have a conversation about this? I wonder if I might be able to help you start this conversation.
- Do you have any cultural beliefs, rituals, or traditions around illness and end of life that I should be aware of?
- What have you found most helpful or useful to you as a family at this time?
- What do you most need to manage well?
- What has not been helpful?
- What sustains you in challenging times?
- What is going well?
- What do you most want to be doing at this time? What brings you joy (or helps you get out of bed in the morning)?
- If your loved one were to die tonight, is there anything you have not said or done that you would regret? If so, how can I help you do or say what you need to do? (Ask this of the patient as well, i.e., If you were to die suddenly, is there anything you would regret not doing or saying?)
- In families, often many things are happening apart from the illness that we do not know about. Is there anything going on that is adding to what you are already coping with?

Unfortunately, all too often, families report a lack of support and sense of connection that contributes to negative experiences and dissatisfaction with care (Andershed, 2006). Even single incidents related to poor communication and interpersonal skills on the part of health professionals can contribute to intense emotional distress, such as anxiety, depression, and guilt, long after the event (Contro et al., 2002, 2004; Gordon et al., 2009; Meert et al., 2007; Pector, 2004a; Rini & Loriz, 2007; Surkan et al., 2006; Widger & Picot, 2008). Understanding this leads some nurses to worry about saying the wrong thing. Listening carefully may assist you to know where to start and sometimes there are no "good" words to say, but simply being present and staying with the family can be helpful.

Humor may be one way to facilitate a connection with families, but it is important first to assess receptivity to humor (Dean & Gregory, 2005). Generally, when families use humor, it is fine to then enter into the humor with them, but it may be more difficult for the nurse to initiate humor. The use of humor can provide respite from thinking about the illness, relieve tension, and demonstrate respect for the patient and family members as people if it fits with their way of being. Some strategies that nurses can use to make a connection

between themselves and patients and families are provided in Box 10-5.

Relieving the Patient's Suffering

What do dying people want? They want adequate pain and symptom control, to avoid inappropriate prolongation of dying, to achieve a sense of control, to relieve burdens for their loved ones, and to

---

BOX 10-5
Establishing and Sustaining Connections With Families

■ Patients and families need to know who you are; when you meet a patient and family for the first time, make them feel welcome, introduce yourself by name, then find out who they are and learn about them as people as well. Ask them how they would like to be called (e.g., by full name or first name). Ask them about their relationship to one another (e.g., to find out whether they are partners, sisters, friends). This is a good time to begin a genogram, which can be supplemented over time.

■ Begin any interaction by clarifying your role and telling the patient and family about your "professional" self so you establish your credentials. For example, "Hello, Mr. Li. My name is Rose Steele. I'm a third-year student nurse. Sandyha Singh, the Registered Nurse supervising me, and I are taking care of your wife today. I'm working until 3:30 p.m. today and also will be here tomorrow, so I'll be her nurse then too. I have worked on this unit for the past three weeks, so I am pretty familiar with all the routines, but I'm really interested in finding out how we can fit in with what you and Mrs. Li want."

■ The best approach is not "This is how we do it here," but rather "How do you like to do this?" and "How can we find a way to do that in this context?" Sometimes we cannot do it exactly the way the patient and/or family would like, so then we need to ask about what the most important pieces are so that we can come as close as possible to the desired result.

■ Ensure a comfortable physical environment; let patients and families know the routines and how they can get help as needed, to provide a sense of familiarity and help you begin to make the connection.

■ Privacy is often an issue and it is critical to some of the sensitive discussions that occur in palliative and end-of-life care. Try to find a private location before broaching sensitive issues.

■ Describe who other team members are and what their roles are so families understand the context. Family members often do not know who to ask for what.

■ Attend to the patient's and family's immediate state of well-being; it is impossible to connect with someone when you have not attended to their basic needs first. If a patient is lying in a wet bed or is in pain, family members will not be open to a "connecting" conversation with the nurse. When you demonstrate good assessment and intervention skills that result in enhanced comfort, your practice invites trust.

■ Be sensitive to an individual's particular characteristics such as cultural or gender differences; making eye contact is a useful strategy for connecting in many cases, but a First Nations person, for instance, may be uncomfortable with direct eye contact. Touch is often welcome but is not universally experienced as supportive. You may need to ask about what provides comfort to the patient and family members.

■ Do not let your observations of particular characteristics limit your perception by stereotyping the person; be aware of your own assumptions and biases, guarding against "operationalizing" your biases—for example, do not assume that an elderly person is deaf.

■ Be sensitive to a person's way of being. Some people are outgoing and talkative; others are more withdrawn. It is a good idea to check out your observations rather than simply assuming that your interpretation of what you are seeing is correct. For example, some people become very quiet and stoic when in pain. This approach may be their way of managing pain, and not their usual "way of being." Humor may be appropriate for some people or situations, but not for others. Responding to people in ways that match their style enhances their comfort level. Another useful habit is to use the family's language. If you need to use medical terms, be sure to

Continued

BOX 10-5
Establishing and Sustaining Connections With Families—cont'd

explain them. Sometimes family members use incorrect words (e.g., prostrate instead of prostate). Generally, the best way to handle it is to use the correct word in a matter-of-fact way and say something like, "Oh yes, I understand that the problem is prostate cancer."

■ Not all people will want the same level of connection; you need to respect where the person is coming from and not try to force a deeper relationship. Families dealing with prolonged, life-threatening illness often have negative health care encounters that lead them to be wary of new health care professionals and make them careful in how much, and in whom, they trust. Sometimes it takes time and the repeated demonstration of trustworthy behaviors before they are willing to begin to trust a new health care professional.

■ Patients and families differ in their expectations of what health care workers should provide; some only want information, some expect only physical care, and still others expect more of a supportive relationship. The key here is in asking for expectations. This does not mean that you can meet the expectations and you may want to preface the request with a statement such as, "To be most helpful to you, I need to know what you would like. I may not be able to do things exactly as you prefer, but we can work together to get as close as possible."

■ Many times you will find that when you simply meet the patient's and family's expectations without imposing your own, further opportunities for connecting may evolve.

■ Once the connection has been made, it is important to pay attention to nurturing it so that it is sustained over time.

■ Sustaining the connection allows you to learn even more about the patient and family so you can continually adapt your care according to their needs; it is also a way of demonstrating your trustworthiness by inviting the patient and family to get to know and trust you. When you are well connected, you are more likely to offer useful interventions that the family will accept.

■ Ways of sustaining the connection include spending time with the patient and family, asking good questions, noticing what they are doing that is positive or helpful, and being available. Sometimes the only thing we can do is to stay with patients and families as a witness to their suffering.

■ Making and sustaining the connection is a two-way process that has to do with sharing parts of yourself with patients and families as you seek a common bond. This process may mean revealing some personal details about your life and there are a few circumstances when

it is appropriate, for example, when the patient or family ask you a direct question about yourself or when you have had an experience that helps you understand what the family may be experiencing. Revealing personal details can be helpful in inviting trust, but they should be brief and should not take the focus away from the patient and family.

■ Continuity of care, such as having the same nurse be in contact with the same patient over some period of time, is important. It is critical that team members effectively communicate with one another to support continuity of care.

■ It is not just the quantity but also the quality of time we spend with a family that makes the difference. For example, if you clear your mind before coming into the room, come to the bedside and are calmly attentive to the patient rather than doing multiple tasks while also talking, the encounter will seem longer and be more satisfying to the patient.

■ The "best" nurses are those who give the impression of "having all the time in the world," even when they are really busy. One way of doing this is to come into the room and sit or stand by the bedside, even if only briefly.

■ Taking the time to "be there" for patients and families instead of being in a rush maintains the connection. This requires you to be mindful and to let go momentarily of all the demands that compete for your attention.

■ Even when you are not actually with patients and families, it is important that they feel as if you will be available when they need you; simple things such as saying hello and good-bye at the beginning and end of shifts, and also at break times, help them know your availability. Let the patient and family know how long you are available and when you will be back (e.g., "I'm just popping in to see how your pain is and won't be able to stay long, but I'll be back in about half an hour and will be able to spend more time with you then").

■ Informing patients and families so they know what to expect and keeping your word, such as being there when you say you will be, also sustain the connection.

■ Instead of having your routine set for the day, adapt your routine to what the patient and family need at the time.

■ Be flexible because you are always working under constraints; share these constraints with patients and families, and tell them if you need to change the plan you have made with them.

■ Changing plans often requires the support of colleagues who can take over for you or help out as needed.

strengthen relationships with loved ones (Singer, Martin, & Kelner, 1999). Concern about becoming a burden to their family may keep dying people from talking to family members about their fears, and about dying (Kuhl, 2002). You can see that family figures prominently for dying people. At the same time, family members are worried about burdening the dying person. These worries, coupled with health professionals' avoidance of difficult discussions because of fear of disrupting hope (Robinson, 2012), can create a conspiracy of silence that contributes to a sense of isolation and aloneness for dying people and their loved ones. One of the ways nurses can be helpful is to assess who is talking to whom, who knows what, and what is holding people back from having conversations that nurture and strengthen the relationships that are often deeply desired within the family. Suffering can be alleviated by inviting and assisting families to come closer together and to engage in meaningful conversations.

This is not going to be possible, however, unless the dying person is physically comfortable. Adequate pain and symptom control is the first priority of dying people. It is also the first priority for family caregivers, who need to become skilled palliative care providers (Robinson et al., 2012). Witnessing the suffering of their dying family member when there is uncontrolled pain and symptoms is traumatic for family members. Therefore, foundational to good family palliative and end-of-life care is knowledge and skills in pain and symptom management. Nurses need to understand the variety of symptoms common to patients at the end of life so they can anticipate, prevent when possible, recognize, assess, and effectively manage pain and symptoms with both traditional and complementary therapies (see Chapter Web Sites later in this chapter for resources). Key to this is regular, systematic assessment using standardized assessment tools, such as the Edmonton Symptom Assessment System (ESAS; Cancer Care Ontario, 2005). Involving the dying person, as much as possible, in planning and treatment decisions supports the need for achieving a sense of control as more and more of life moves out of control.

Relieving suffering yields improved quality of life, but no single definition exists for the most important factors that contribute to a good quality of life (Johansson, Axelsson, & Danielson, 2006; Norris et al., 2007). This is because only the individual and family know what constitutes quality of life for them. Individual needs must be assessed. Norris and colleagues found higher patient quality of life ratings associated with a variety of activities, such as playing music that was meaningful to the patient, attending a place of worship, having a familiar health care team available at all times (for patients at home), and having individual preferences respected. Predictably, other components contributing to better quality of life include valuing everyday things, maintaining a positive attitude, having symptoms relieved, feeling in control, and feeling connected to and needed by family, friends, and health professionals (Aspinal et al., 2006; Johansson et al., 2006).

Empowering Families

Family palliative and end-of-life care is a strengths-based approach. It is about building and nurturing family strengths to ensure that quality of life, as defined by the family, can be achieved as closely as possible. Rather than solely focusing on deficits or areas that the nurse perceives as problematic, palliative care emphasizes empowering families to manage this challenging time in their own unique way by noticing and building on strengths, while at the same time effectively addressing problems. All of the empowering strategies require good communication skills. The focus should be on maximizing the patient's and family's capacity to use their own resources to meet their needs and respecting their ability to do so. Nurses empower patients and families by creating an environment in which their strengths and abilities are recognized, by encouraging them to consider various options, by assisting them in fulfilling their needs and desires through the provision of information and resources, and by supporting their choices. Several specific interventions that empower families are commending families, educating families about clinical options and constraints, and helping families to help themselves.

Family members appreciate recognition for their knowledge of the patient, their competencies, and their caring. Nurses can facilitate this appreciation by commending the work of the caregiver in the presence of the ill person. Commending families and family members is a very powerful intervention (Houger, Limacher, & Wright, 2003; Mok et al., 2002; Wright & Leahey, 2005), especially in the presence of the ill person. Caregivers may be better able to cope with caregiving when the ill person recognizes and appreciates their role (Hunstad & Svindseth, 2011; Stajduhar et al., 2008). Effective commendations involve making specific observations of patterns of family strengths that occur across time (Wright & Leahey, 2005). Similarly, parents appreciate recognition of their parenting role and skills. Nurses' commendations may help to strengthen parents' relationships with their child and their view of their parental role (Antle et al., 2005; Hinds et al., 2009; Steele, 2002).

Empowering also is about making patients and families aware of options and constraints about clinical care and available resources so they can make choices that are most appropriate for them. For example, families may be unaware of the possibility of having death occur outside the hospital, yet that may be a support for some families (Pector, 2004b). Home death is often the patient's desire and, typically, family caregivers are deeply committed to doing whatever it takes to honor this preference (Robinson et al., 2012). Yet there is growing evidence that family caregivers are unprepared to take on the job of providing care and they lack the necessary education and support along the journey (Robinson et al., 2012; Topf, Robinson, & Bottorff, 2013). Under these circumstances, family caregivers can suffer negative health consequences and are at risk for complicated bereavement (Topf et al., 2013). Engaging both the patient and involved family members in discussion about preferences for care, preferences for place of death, and available resources may assist negotiation of decisions that can be simply taken for granted when family members automatically step forward to take up the role of caregiver. Choice empowers families.

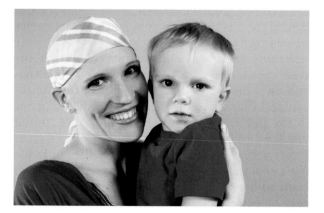

Strain on families may be reduced when families are more accepting of the patient's illness, feel more capable in their ability to provide and manage the patient's end-of-life care (Redinbaugh, Baum, Tarbell, & Arnold, 2003), and feel better able to attend to their own self-care needs and difficult emotions or interactions (Merluzzi, Philip, Vachon, & Heitzmann, 2011). Nurses need to assess families for their knowledge, skills, and concerns, and then offer appropriate interventions. Some interventions include providing information about the illness, its treatment and prognosis; teaching family members how to provide adequate care to their loved one; and encouraging family members to share their fears and other emotions, and then providing the needed support (e.g., in discussions, or referring to appropriate resources such as a social worker who can arrange for respite care). Facilitating hope for a longer life or for a peaceful death and providing adequate information and emotional and instrumental support also may help reduce the burden (Hunstad & Svindseth, 2011; Proot et al., 2003).

Empowering patients and families may include helping them to do what they themselves want and need to do, rather than professionals taking over and doing it for them. For example, although it may appear quicker and easier for the nurse to assist a patient out of bed, it may be important that the patient moves by herself or that a family member is taught to assist. Sometimes you will need to be creative in finding ways to empower patients and families. You might find that your abilities are stretched as you try to accommodate them, especially within the constraints of your clinical setting, so do not be afraid to talk with your clinical facilitator or other staff members about your struggles. They can be great resources for you. At the same time, you might have some innovative ideas to share that they will find useful in their practice.

It is important to assess the capacity of patients and families to do for themselves, and then find ways of supporting them when hopes and expectations exceed capacity. Careful assessment of the situation is central to knowing when to act on behalf of patients and families, and when to encourage them to manage themselves, because if you "do for" patients and families when they can care for themselves, you may diminish their sense of competency and disempower them. On the other hand, if you expect them to do everything on their own, you may inadvertently leave them feeling isolated and unsupported (Stajduhar, Funk, Jakobsson, et al., 2010).

Providing Information

Families often have a need for information, but may not know what questions to ask. A lack of knowledge and feeling uninformed can leave people feeling isolated, frustrated, and distressed (Andershed, 2006; Hunstad & Svindseth, 2011). Some families want a great deal of detailed information, whereas others feel overwhelmed and find that it interferes with their ability to live as normal a life as possible. Therefore, ongoing assessment of how much and what types of information families want is important (Maynard et al., 2005; Pector, 2004a; Steele, 2005a, 2005b). This assessment also needs to include how much information should be offered directly to the patient, especially a child (Hays et al., 2006; Hsiao, Evan, & Zeltzer, 2007; Mack et al., 2005). A wide variation exists in the age at which parents believe a child is old enough to be included in illness discussions (Mack et al., 2005). Even when the patient is an adult, some families may believe that not all information should be shared with the patient (Royak Schaler et al., 2006). These beliefs may be based on cultural norms. As a nurse, you need to be aware of your legal responsibilities and ensure that you do not withhold information inappropriately. You also must convey your responsibilities to the family and initiate an open dialogue about the importance of communication. As alluded to above, some families may hold a culturally based belief that an adult patient should not be told a life-limiting diagnosis. One way of approaching this is to ask the patient whether she wants information about her medical condition, and if not, who in the family should be given information, and whether this person should be considered her designate decision maker.

As a beginning family nurse, what information can you offer that may make a positive difference for family caregivers? You are in one of the best positions to understand and appreciate what it is like for family members to take up the job of caregiving. Most do not have a medical background and so they do not know what will be asked of them. They do not know how to provide basic care effectively, such as toileting, assisting the ill person to

move without causing more pain, and managing symptoms such as pain and breathlessness, or even safely working with an oxygen tank. They need knowledge and skills that they do not even know they need until they are alone in the midst of providing care. Noticing what the ill family member needs, anticipating future needs, listening to both the ill person and the family caregiver, assisting them to negotiate how care will be done at home, working directly with the family caregiver to provide knowledge and model essential skills, and determining available resources and gaps in services are some examples of interventions that may prove supportive. The key is listening carefully to both the ill person and the family caregiver and bringing your knowledge forward to support them in their mutual goals. At the same time, it is important to recognize and assist with strategies to maintain "normal" roles within a family, such as parent or spouse (Price, Jordan, Prior, & Parkes, 2011; Stajduhar, Funk, Jakobsson, et al., 2010; Weidner et al., 2011). Family caregivers have reported that interventions aimed at separating them from their dying family member, such as exhortations to leave the bedside and get some sleep, are often not helpful and can be experienced as disrespectful (Robinson et al., 2012). Family caregivers may see these interventions as evidence that nurses really do not understand their commitment to the dying person and to providing care. As previously mentioned, one intervention that is very powerful is the offering of situation-specific commendations.

When patients and family members are empowered with the amount and kind of information they want, at the time they need it, the result is more effective partnerships with professionals. Nurses are in a key position to act as a liaison between the professional team members and the family. Patients and families should be encouraged to ask questions, and these questions should be answered with full explanations and support. There is some evidence that family caregivers may be reluctant to reveal difficulties providing care because they are afraid that care will be taken away from them (Topf et al., 2013). Therefore, nurses need to create an environment that allows family members to speak openly and without fear.

Beginning nurses are sometimes reluctant to invite questions from families because an expectation exists that you will have an answer. Simply knowing the questions is valuable information, and many times the questions do not have answers. As a novice, you may not know the answer, and that is all right. If possible, however, you can show your trustworthiness by seeking the information and providing it in a timely fashion.

Overall, families need to have honest and understandable information about a variety of areas, including the following:

- The patient's condition
- The illness trajectory
- Prognosis (keeping in mind that prognosis is inherently uncertain because we cannot predict when death will occur)
- Symptoms to expect and treatment options
- How to provide physical care
- What to expect (including signs of impending death, which allows family members the opportunity to say final good-byes)
- Ways of coping (including helping families become aware of possible strategies, such as respite and mental pauses)
- The dying process
- How to access additional support
- What aids (e.g., wheelchairs, beds, lifts) may be helpful and where to get them
- The care system in which this all occurs

Provision of this type of information is linked to reduced caregiver burden, improved coping, self-efficacy, and enhanced quality of life (Northouse et al., 2010).

The way in which information is shared is as important as the content of the information. Critical components of the process of sharing information include timing, pacing, and both verbal and non-verbal conveyance of respect, empathy, and compassion (Gutierrez, 2012; Kirk, Kirk, & Kristjanson, 2004). The timing and pacing, in particular, are important to allow families to absorb the reality of the situation and to make informed decisions (Meert et al., 2007). Do not rush families to make decisions, and give information as early as possible to allow for ongoing discussions and decision making with a clearer mind rather than waiting for a crisis that may be fraught with emotion (Hammes et al., 2005; Macdonald, Liben, & Cohen, 2006; Sharman et al., 2005). The use of simple, jargon-free language is likely to be helpful. In emotionally intense situations, often little information is absorbed and it must be repeated over time, so nurses should be

willing to clarify repeatedly for family members without becoming impatient and ask questions of all family members to ensure that information is being understood. Nurses also need to attend to their own and family members' nonverbal language; at least three-quarters of a message is conveyed nonverbally. For instance, watch the person's face to determine if she looks confused, upset, or comprehending. Moreover, be aware of your own body language; stand close to a family member rather than standing in the doorway of a patient's room so you give the impression of having time to talk and listen. Moderate your tone of voice so that you sound respectful and empathetic rather than annoyed or without compassion.

Through learning about other families' experiences, patients and family members can better understand their own experience. Nurses can share insights gained from other families both from practice and research. For example, "Other families have told me that talking about what their child's death might be like was one of the hardest things they ever had to do, but once they knew there was a plan in place for how to handle the possible symptoms or issues that may happen, they were able to stop worrying about all the 'what-ifs' and just focus on having the best time possible with their child." Having information enables patients and family members to collaborate with health care providers from an informed position and is required for making decisions and planning for the future.

Balancing Hope and Preparation

A fair amount of ambiguity always exists when working with families at end of life, regardless of whether the situation is acute or chronic. Nurses need to become comfortable with the inherent uncertainty and help families live well within an uncertain context. One common ambiguity surrounds prognostic uncertainty. Given that we cannot predict when death will occur, families need to be encouraged to attend to what they view as important and to take advantage of the moment. When a patient or family member asks, "How long?" you might reply by asking, "What would you be doing differently now if you knew that the time was very short?" In response to their answer, you might suggest that they do whatever "it" is, and if they get to do "it" again next week or next month or even next year, then that would be a bonus.

As a patient's condition changes and deteriorates, the hopes and expectations of the patient and family may change as well. Hope often shifts from a more global perspective—such as hope for a cure—to a more focused or specific perspective, such as a hope to live long enough to see her grandchild who is due in a few months. Nurses can help facilitate this change in hope by asking powerful questions, such as, "If your loved one were to die tonight, is there anything you have not said or done that you would regret?" or "If you were to die suddenly, is there anything you would regret not doing or saying?" Such questions encourage patients and families to consider what is most meaningful to them and allow them to shift their hope to areas that may be more attainable. Nurses who participate in these discussions can help maintain hope for some things while not providing false hope. They also can offer to help patients and families do or say what they need to do.

For some families and in some cultures, a need is present to keep fighting for every chance at life, hoping for a miracle, until the last possible moment, even when they may know this is considered medically unrealistic (Kirk et al., 2004; Robinson, 2012; Shiozaki et al., 2005; Torke et al., 2005). As a nurse, it is important to find the balance between supporting families in their hopes and still being comfortable talking about death and preparing the patient and family for what is to come, including advance care planning (Hsiao et al., 2007; Rini & Loriz, 2007; Robinson, 2012; Robinson et al., 2006; Shiozaki et al., 2005; Steele, 2005a). Therefore, when preparing the family for what is to come, the information must be provided in a sensitive manner that acknowledges hope (Kirk et al., 2004; Robinson, 2012; Shiozaki et al., 2005). One way of doing this is to use a hypothetical question (Wright & Leahey, 2005), such as, "If things don't go as we hope, what is most important for you to have happen?" Another phrase that is sometimes helpful is suggesting that a family "hope for the best and plan for the worst."

Parents of dying children identify a need to balance hope and despair (Konrad, 2008; Moro et al., 2011) and appreciate when health professionals support hope without offering false hopes (Gordon et al., 2009; Monterosso & Kristjanson, 2008). Lack of discussions about the possibility of death are closely linked to parents' belief that health professionals sometimes give false hope that the child will survive the illness (Gordon et al., 2009; Monterosso & Kristjanson, 2008). False hope may be detrimental to parents' ability to prepare for the child's death, so nurses need to be mindful of what they say and how they say it. Honest acknowledgment of the severity of the situation is important.

Facilitating Choices

A major role for nurses is to be an advocate for patients and families and facilitate their choices. But to do so, nurses need to know what the patient and family want. One specific intervention is to encourage advance care planning so that everyone is clear about the patient's preferences regarding end-of-life care. Other interventions include assessing the extent of both the patient's and family members' desire for involvement in decision making, and then respecting that desire; assessing their awareness about the possibility of death, and opening lines of communication; and identifying and then building on the patient's and family's strengths in order to optimize choices.

Advance Care Planning

At the end of life, patients may be unable to participate in making decisions about their care, leaving family members to make decisions based on their understanding of what the patient would want if he were able to participate. One way in which families can prevent misunderstandings and can promote facilitation of choices is by discussing wishes and desires in advance. Advance care planning is a process that involves reflection and communication. It is a way of letting others know your future health and personal care preferences, so that if you become incapable of consenting to or refusing treatment, others—especially your substitute decision maker, the person who will speak for you when you cannot—will make decisions for you that reflect your values and wishes, regardless of their own desires. Advance care planning often involves not only discussions with family and friends, but also writing down your wishes; it may even involve talking with health care providers and financial and legal professionals. The Canadian Hospice Palliative Care

Association (n.d.), in collaboration with the National Advance Care Planning Task Group, provides a number of valuable online resources about advance care planning, including a workbook to guide writing the plan.

Less than 30% of adults have an advance directive, and even for those adults who do have them, they may not be available when needed or be specific enough (Dunn, Tolle, Moss, & Black, 2007). If someone has written advance directives, his or her substitute decision maker should also have a copy. It is important that health care providers are made aware of a patient's advance directives and, preferably, a copy kept with the patient's chart. Nurses need to make themselves familiar with such advance directives so they can advocate for the patient as needed when decisions are being made.

Advance care planning is a process that is best initiated early in the illness experience and revisited as the illness progresses because preferences can change over time (Robinson, 2011, 2012). These types of conversations are difficult to have among family members, and families may appreciate assistance to initiate and facilitate the conversation. Nurses can facilitate the process and empower both patients and families by encouraging them to talk about end-of-life issues and preferences long before they are faced with the situation and by initiating discussions about substitute decision making, including the legalities of representation. The process of substitute decision making can be a very demanding one for families (Meeker, 2004), and written advance directives can be helpful to family members (Robinson, 2011, 2012), particularly in reminding them of their loved one's wishes when there may be differences in what each thought would be best. In addition, when faced with actually making decisions, family members often appreciate acknowledgment of the difficulty of their role, and the nurse's attentive, respectful support throughout the process will be very helpful (Meeker, 2004).

Involvement in Decision Making

Families may be facing their first experience with death and dying, and they often depend on nurses to help them in their process. Families may not know what they need or what might be possible (Selman et al., 2007); they may expect health professionals to bring up issues when appropriate—that is, the family members may feel it is not their place to raise issues first (Robinson, 2011), so

nurses need to open the conversation. It is important first to assess and then respect the patient's and family's desired level of involvement in discussions about end of life and in decision making. Nurses should ask questions such as, "How are important decisions made in your family?" and "How would you like important decision making to go now?" so they understand the family's approach and can facilitate appropriate interactions that respect family choice.

Some patients and families may want full responsibility for decisions; some may want to be involved but not make final decisions; some may want the physician to take the initiative and make all decisions (Selman et al., 2007; Shiozaki et al., 2005); and some patients want their family members to make decisions (Torke et al., 2005). Some parents feel that making decisions for the child is inherently a parental role, but not all want to have complete responsibility for final decisions (Brosig, Pierucci, Kupst, & Leuthner, 2007; Contro et al., 2002, 2004; Hays et al., 2006; Meyer et al., 2006; Pector, 2004b; Sharman et al., 2005). Again, assessment of preferences about decision making is important. Nurses can use questions such as, "I understand that different family members will have different talents or strengths; how do you most want to be involved?" to uncover family members' preferences so they can work with the family in ways that facilitate choice.

Regardless of their actual role in the decision-making process, parents want to be recognized as the experts on their child and as the central, consistent figures in their child's life. As such, they want health professionals to seek out and respect their knowledge, opinions, observations, and concerns about their child (Kars, Grypdonck, & van Delden, 2011; Hsiao et al., 2007; Meyer et al., 2006; Steele, 2002, 2005a; Weidner et al., 2011; Widger & Picot, 2008; Woodgate, 2006). Therefore, nurses should verbally acknowledge that the parent's input is critical and they should be mindful of paying attention to facilitating the parent's choices, regardless of their own beliefs.

The involvement of family members in decision making can have a lifelong effect on the well-being of family members (Christakis & Iwashyna, 2003; Kreicbergs et al., 2005; Surkan et al., 2006). Nurses, therefore, must foster good communication to ensure that the patient's and family's needs and wishes are understood and supported within a caring relationship that is built on partnership between professionals and families (Robinson, 2011). Many times health care providers block families from participating because they feel they know what is best or because they are trying to protect families. But effective end-of-life care is not possible unless open and mutual communication occurs between families and professionals, and families participate in shared decision making to the extent they desire (Robinson, 2011). Questions such as, "If you were to think ahead a bit, how do you see things going in the next few weeks?" and "Families often find it helpful to talk about the care they want at end of life. Have you been able to have a conversation about this? I wonder if I might be able to help you start this conversation," can be used to learn what a patient and family want. See Box 10-4 for other questions that may help nurses become cognizant of a family's choices.

Awareness of Possibility of Death

Lack of early information about the possibility of death makes it difficult for family members to come to terms with decisions such as the withdrawal of life-sustaining therapy or the use of cardiopulmonary resuscitation (Heyland, Frank, et al., 2006). Families faced with these types of decisions usually place great value on open, honest, and timely information, but they also need to be listened to in terms of their intimate knowledge of the patient rather than just spoken to (Hunstad & Svindseth, 2011; McDonagh et al., 2004). Moreover, it is crucial to prepare the family for what to expect when life-sustaining therapy is withdrawn. For example, families need to be aware that death may occur very quickly, or may take hours or days (Wiegand, 2006). When decisions are made, such as withdrawal of life-sustaining therapy, any delays past the agreed-on time for implementing the decision may greatly increase the family's anxiety (Wiegand, 2006). Therefore, it is important for nurses to keep the family informed about the reasons for any changes to the plan and to be available to talk with family members when needed.

Building on Strengths

Nurses need to recognize the dying person's and family members' rights and abilities to make their own decisions and then make an effort to find out what is important to them. It is important to focus on what patients and families *can* do, rather than on what they cannot do. As a nurse, you can reinforce those aspects of the self that remain intact, and assist patients and families to recognize their own strengths and abilities. Once you identify and build on individual and family strengths, you can smooth the way for patients and families to meet their own needs. Nurses can work with patients and families by making suggestions, providing options, and planning strategies that will allow them to achieve their goals. Your professional knowledge may be invaluable in guiding families to consider options and possible routes of actions that they would not have thought of without your input, for example, the use of special equipment that allows a patient to have the bath that he thought was not possible because of his weakness. Furthermore, you may have a clearer sense of the consequences of certain choices, which again is extremely valuable information. At the very least, you can seek out answers to families' questions and be a resource for families.

Facilitating choices also means identifying and accepting a patient's and family's limitations, and finding ways to work with them so they achieve an outcome that is both positive and satisfactory to them. For example, you can suggest new activities that are appropriate for the patient's current capabilities. It is important that relationships remain mutual and reciprocal, and patients in particular need to experience their positive contribution to their family members. Thus, as patients get sicker, their contribution will look different and may focus on such things as words of wisdom rather than concrete actions.

Offering Resources

One nurse cannot be all things to every patient and family. It is important to be aware of other team members, such as spiritual or pastoral care providers (Wall, Engelberg, Gries, Glavan, & Curtis, 2007), social workers, and others who may be available to provide support to the family. Furthermore, the nurse should be knowledgeable about hospital- and community-based services, such as hospice, that may be available to support families both before and after the death (Casarett, Crowley, Stevenson, Xie, & Teno, 2005). You can offer these other resources and services to families, but each family will decide what will actually be helpful for them. For some families, using inpatient respite services during the last year of life may help relieve their burden, if only for a short time, whereas other caregivers may experience feelings of guilt and increased stress caused by worrying about the quality of care provided during respite (Skilbeck et al., 2005). Caregivers may be supported in their role simply by knowing there are other resources and support readily available, even if they do not make use of them (Stajduhar et al., 2008).

Encouraging Patients and Families

Patients and family members often seek approval and encouragement from professionals as they make decisions about how to meet their needs. Encouraging is an important strategy in empowering patients and families to do for themselves. It means verbally and nonverbally supporting patients and families in their choices, providing reinforcement for each individual's ideas, and demonstrating your support by finding ways to facilitate their choices. Encouraging does not necessarily mean that you *agree* with the choice, merely that you support the patient or family member in finding ways to enact the choice. At the same time, encouraging does not mean you abandon your expertise, which is complementary to the expertise of the family. Sharing your knowledge and perspective contributes to fully informed decision making.

It can sometimes be too easy to think that you know what is "best" for patients and their families. As a caring professional, you have their best interests at heart and you want to protect them as much as possible. Even as you value each person as a worthwhile individual who has the right and ability to make his or her own choices and decisions, you may find that the patient's and family's desires conflict with what you believe is "best" based on your professional experience and knowledge. Times such as these can cause you moral distress as you struggle with supporting the patient and family, while remaining "true" to the knowledge you have. Your negotiation skills may be severely tested in such situations, and sometimes you will be tempted to override a patient's wishes. Some nurses describe their bottom line as "ensuring patient safety," and unless the patient's physical safety is compromised they will support the patient's choice, even when they disagree with it. Encouraging supports families to figure out ways to do what is important for them in the best way possible.

Managing Negative Feelings

End-of-life care is not all encouragement and positive feelings. Many patients and family members also have negative feelings that influence their experiences. Talking with patients and family members (often individually) about those negative feelings gives them permission to have, experience, and deal with them. For many people, negative feelings, such as guilt or anger, are suppressed or internalized. Others openly express their anger but displace it onto someone else, often the nurse or other family members. The ability to diffuse a situation effectively requires nurses to learn how to accept someone else's negative feelings in an open and nondefensive manner. It means not taking their words as a personal attack, but realizing that patients and family members simply need a safe outlet for their frustrations and negative feelings. Your role is to listen in an accepting way and allow them to ventilate. It can be hard to face an angry tirade, but most people will calm down once they have said what they need to say and they realize that you value their feelings even if they are negative ones. Questions that are often useful include "How can I help?" or "What needs to be different?"

Sometimes, however, people will remain angry or guilty despite your best efforts. Diffusing will not always be as successful as you would like. Some people are so angry about what is happening to their loved one and their family that they cannot move to any other emotional state. You will need to accept that this is their reality and find ways to work with them. This is often a time when nurses need the support of colleagues, and a team approach may help to lessen the effects of working with these patients and families (Namasivayam, Orb, & O'Connor, 2005). Other interventions that may be helpful include referral to resources such as social work, pastoral care, psychology, and support groups.

Facilitating Healing Between Family Members

Negative feelings and misunderstandings can cause or expand rifts in families. If a nurse can facilitate healing between family members that unifies the family, the family can function better as a team and members are better equipped to move through the dying process. You can help mend relationships by interpreting family members' behaviors to one another and helping them to see each other's point of view. Sometimes an outsider can bring clarity to a situation that is impossible for those members who are enmeshed in it. An assessment question that may be useful is this: "Is there anything that is unsaid or undone in the family that needs your attention?" Be careful, though, that you do not try to "fix broken families." Many families that you might think are dysfunctional do not see themselves as having difficulties or needing to change. They will not invite you to fix them and, indeed, may find your concern about the family intrusive. Furthermore, relationships develop over many years and your interventions will occur in a relatively short period. Do not expect a huge change in family dynamics during the time you know a family, unless the family wants to change and makes an effort to do so. Sometimes all you can do is acknowledge to yourself that certain things cannot be fixed and your presence is all you have to offer. Levels of family functioning will need to be attended to carefully as you work with a family, and the expectation that a family will pull together to cope with the process of dying may be unrealistic. Noticing the family members' love for the ill member and acknowledging their mutual desire for the best for their ill member (even though there may be quite different ideas about what is best) is sometimes helpful.

Family Meetings

Family meetings typically involve the patient, those family members desired by the patient, and the relevant health professionals (Hudson, Quinn, O'Hanlon, & Aranda, 2008). They should routinely be offered on admission to a setting and further meetings may be called by the patient/family or health care professional on an "as needed" basis. Family meetings should be considered a proactive approach and not be held in reserve only for "crisis" situations. Family meetings are beneficial to facilitate consistency in everyone's understanding of the situation and the expected course for the illness (Hudson et al., 2008; Wiegand, 2006), as well as for negotiation of care. They enable patients, family members, and professionals to meet together to discuss any issue, but they are not family therapy (Fineberg, 2005, 2010).

Nurses are ideal partners to lead these end-of-life family conferences. In all settings, you can assist families in preparing for the meetings by helping them to write down questions that they want to raise at the meeting, informing the family about what to expect during the conference, and discussing what the patient values in life, the patient's and the family members' spiritual and religious needs, and what the patient may want if she is unable to participate in the conference (Curtis et al., 2001). It is helpful to begin by eliciting the family's understanding of the situation, as well as pressing concerns, before moving to the health professionals' perspectives. Different family members and professionals will have different ideas, so it is useful to request different perspectives. Afterward, you can talk with the family about how the conference went, what the changes in the patient's plan of care are and what they mean, and how the family feels about the conference and changed plan of care (Curtis et al., 2001; Hudson et al., 2008). You also should talk with the family about the decisions that were made and then support them in these decisions.

More than one family meeting may be necessary as the patient's condition changes or if the family needs time to think or further discuss issues before decisions are made (Hudson et al., 2008; Wiegand, 2006). The proportion of time the family spends talking during these conferences is more important than the total length of the conference in increasing family satisfaction and decreasing conflict between families and health professionals (McDonagh et al., 2004). Yet, on average, typical family conferences involve the health professional speaking for 70% of the time and listening for only 30% of the time (McDonagh et al., 2004). It is important that you pay careful attention to ensure that families do the majority of talking during family meetings. In addition, be mindful of your nonverbal communication, because it is often our main method of communication, and is particularly powerful when the topics are emotional. For example, wrapping your arms around yourself may indicate anxiety; interrupting may be a sign of impatience.

Finding Meaning

When recovery is impossible, nurses must consider their role in helping patients and families find meaning in the experience as they care for and assist families. Patients and families often struggle to understand why the patient is dying. They try to make sense of the experience, and they search for ways to make the patient's life and inevitable death meaningful. Their search for meaning may involve examining relationships within the family or with a higher power (Hexem, Mollen, Carroll, Lanctot, & Feudtner, 2011). Some people will be more successful at finding meaning than others or the process may not occur until long after the death (Widger et al., 2009).

As a nurse, you can assist in this process of finding meaning by truly listening and hearing what family members have to say. Engaging in relationship and dialogue will be empowering and can help families create meaning even in a difficult situation (Abma, 2005). But there are many different ways of finding meaning, and not all individuals will overtly search for meaning. As a nurse, you will accompany people as they try to make sense of their situation. You cannot find meaning for someone else, however (Robinson et al., 2006). Each individual will seek his own meaning in his own unique way. Some may be very articulate about their philosophical and spiritual beliefs and how they influence meaning making (Hexem et al., 2011; Knapp et al., 2011). Others may talk about these issues in more concrete terms, perhaps rarely having articulated their thoughts and feelings. Still others may "talk" through their actions. Finding meaning gives strength to people, and therefore, you will find that it is empowering for families. Nurses who examine the concepts of meaning of illness and dying with patients may gain a deepened understanding of the patients' experiences, which may lead to changes and improvements in the way care is provided (Gauthier, 2002). You might begin this examination by asking the patient: "Can you tell me what it is like to be at this point in your life?"

Care at the Time of Actively Dying

Patients who are dying are often most concerned about how they will die rather than that they are dying (Kuhl, 2002). Excellent pain and symptom management is critical as uncontrolled pain or symptoms such as nausea and breathlessness create suffering for *all* family members. A "good death" may contribute to family members feeling more at peace with the death (Mok et al., 2002), and also having a sense of satisfaction and accomplishment (Perreault et al., 2004). Parents often believe that their child's peaceful death means that they made the right choices and that they did all that they could for their child (Hinds et al., 2000). Thus, facilitating a good death is an imperative for nurses. What constitutes a

good death, however, is not well understood. From observations of patients, family members, and health care providers, six major components of a good death have been identified: pain and symptom management, clear decision making, preparation for death, completion, contributing to others, and affirmation of the whole person (Steinhauser et al., 2000). A bad death has been defined by a "lack of opportunity to plan ahead, arrange personal affairs, decrease family burden, or say good-bye" (Steinhauser et al., 2000, p. 829).

In the context of a palliative care approach, the language of care, quality of life, relief of suffering, and the principles of palliative care become important in helping families attain a "good death." When a cure is not possible, families often react to the news with a blanket statement: "We want everything done." But that may not be what they mean literally. Families may just believe that if they agree to palliative care, treatment will be withheld, and they will be abandoned because death is the expected outcome (Gillis, 2008). Delaying palliative care compromises the ability to achieve a good death. Clear discussions are needed about the continued provision of active care with a shift in emphasis to quality of life instead of prolongation of life. Such discussions will reassure families that, indeed, everything is being done and they are not being abandoned.

No matter the setting, family members are often afraid of the actual death event and have little or no understanding of what dying entails. You will find that sometimes the greatest gift you can give families as they prepare for the death is helping them release the dying person, to forgive themselves and their loved one so she can die in peace (Cooke, 1992). Nurses can help alleviate families' fears by finding out what they know and what they need. You can then prepare families for the death and help them recognize the signs of imminent death so they are aware of what will likely happen when the signs appear (see Box 10-6). This preparation may be even more crucial for families in the home, who may be alone at the time. It also is important in the intensive care unit (ICU) and emergency department to tailor your information to the situation. For example, a patient's breathing will not change if he is on a ventilator.

Generally, an illness begins to weaken the body when a person is nearing death. Some health conditions affect vital body systems, such as the brain and nervous system, lungs, heart and blood vessels, or the digestive system, including the liver and bowels. As illnesses progress, the body becomes unable to use the nutrients in food, resulting in weight loss and a decline in appetite, energy, and strength. More time is spent resting, and in the final few days before death, people usually sleep most of the time. If families are aware of this natural progression, they may be less distressed, for example, when their loved one stops eating. One sign of imminent death, terminal restlessness, can be distressing for family members to watch (Brajtman, 2005). Sedation at the end of life may be necessary to control severe symptoms such as terminal restlessness. Box 10-6 lists signs of imminent death that should be shared with families.

Communication and relationships continue to be important as death approaches (Munn & Zimmerman, 2006). Nurses can encourage family members to continue talking to their loved ones even if they are nonresponsive, because they may still be able to hear (Brajtman, 2005). You can model this type of interaction by continuing to speak to the patient and treating him with dignity throughout the dying process. You can demonstrate respect for the family and its intimate knowledge of the patient by seeking its advice on things that were soothing or calming to the patient in the past, such as particular music, foot rubs and back rubs, or a particular way of arranging the pillows, and then following these suggestions or encouraging the family to do so (Brajtman, 2005).

BOX 10-6
Signs of Imminent Death

Decline in physical capabilities
Decreased alertness and social interaction
Decreased intake of food and fluids
Difficulty swallowing medications, food, and fluids
Visual and auditory hallucinations
Confusion, restlessness, agitation
Physical changes as death nears include the following:
- Circulation gradually shuts down; hands and feet feel cool, and a patchy, purplish color called *mottling* appears on the skin; heart speeds up, but also weakens, so pulse is rapid but hard to feel.
- Bowel movements and urine production decrease as less food and fluid are taken in; may be no urine output in last day or two of life; constipation is not usually an issue to be managed in the last week of life; loss of bladder or bowel control can be managed with frequent skin care and the use of adult incontinence products, or even a urinary catheter if needed.
Changes in breathing often provide clues about how close someone is to death. As the automatic centers in the brain take over the regulation of breathing, changes generally occur in the following ways:
- The rate of breathing tends to be more rapid.
- The pattern or regularity in breathing becomes irregular, almost mechanical.
- How deep the breaths are (may be shallow, deep, or normal) tends to become more shallow. There may be periods of apnea where breathing pauses for a while. When the pauses in breathing appear, a noticeable pattern often develops: clusters of fairly rapid breathing that start with shallow breaths that become deeper and deeper, and then fade off, becoming shallower and shallower; may be 5 to 10 breaths in each cluster, and each cluster is separated by a pause that may last a few seconds or perhaps up to 30 seconds; called the Cheyne-Stokes pattern of breathing and is occasionally seen in healthy elderly people as well, especially during sleep.
- The kinds of muscles used in breathing may change; the person may start to use the neck muscles and the shoulders, but though it may look as if the person is struggling, unless he or she is agitated it is simply "automatic pilot."
- The amount of mucus or secretions that build up because the person is unable to cough can be noisy (rattling or gurgling) and sometimes upsets people at the bedside even though it is unlikely to be distressing to the dying person, who is usually unconscious; some people call it the "death rattle," and it can be treated by medication to dry up the secretions. Because the term *death rattle* may cause strong emotional reactions, the term *respiratory congestion* is now recommended.
- The pattern of breathing in the final minutes or perhaps hours of life: the breathing takes on an irregular pattern in which there is a breath, then a pause, then another breath or two, then another pause, and so forth. There may be periods of 15 to 30 seconds or so between final breaths.
- After the last breath very slight motions of breathing may happen irregularly for a few minutes. These are reflex actions and are not signs of distress.

Many family members want to be present when their loved one is imminently dying; it is often important that they have an opportunity to say good-bye (Andershed, 2006). Thus, you need to be aware ahead of time about a family's wishes and ensure that members are called if there is a change in the patient's condition so they can be present, if possible, at the time of death if that is what they want. The days, hours, and minutes leading up to a child's death are often seen by parents as their last opportunity to be a "good parent" to the child. Their ability to be physically present, emotionally supportive, and an effective advocate for their child is often key to viewing themselves as good parents in the years after their child's death (Meert et al., 2005; Rini & Loriz, 2007; Sharman et al., 2005; Woodgate, 2006). "Normal" parent activities such as bathing, feeding, or holding the child, even in the midst of technology that is being used to support the child's life, allow parents to develop or continue their bond with their child and sometimes to be able to say good-bye to their child (Brosig et al., 2007; Meert et al., 2005; Meyer et al., 2006; Pector, 2004a, 2004b; Rini & Loriz, 2007; Robinson et al., 2006; Sharman et al., 2005; Steele, Davies, Collins, & Cook, 2005). As a nurse, therefore, you need to facilitate parents' wishes at this time and provide an environment that allows for parents to fulfill their parental role.

We cannot know when a patient will die, and despite our best efforts, sometimes this happens when family members are not present. Sometimes the patient dies when the family member has nodded off to sleep or stepped out of the room for a cup of tea. When family members wish to be present, it is important to talk about the possibility that this may not happen.

Bereavement Care

Once the patient dies, the work of the nurse does not end (O'Connor, Peters, Lee, & Webster, 2005). A lot of family members may be present for the death, all of whom may need support, advice, information, and time to begin the grieving and healing process. Family members may wish to stay by the bedside and say whatever words seem appropriate. For some cultures, rituals may need to be conducted (O'Connor et al., 2005). Some families may want active involvement in caring for the

patient's body or at least to know the body will be cared for in a respectful manner (Pector, 2004a; Widger & Picot, 2008). There is no harm in touching the person's body, and there should be no rush to move the person until everyone has had a chance to say their final good-byes.

Family members who were not present for the death may need to be contacted and may wish to see the patient before she is taken to the morgue or a funeral home. As a nurse, you can encourage the family to be together if it wishes and to take as much time as needed after the death. Your presence as family members express their emotions may help them to create meaningful final memories and begin to process their experience (Hannan & Gibson, 2005; Meert et al., 2005; Pector, 2004a; Rini & Loriz, 2007; Steele et al., 2005; Wisten & Zingmark, 2007). You may need to contact pastoral care or other professionals to assist in supporting the family. Some families will appreciate your assistance with or information on arranging funerals (de Jong-Berg & Kane, 2006; Pector, 2004a; Rini & Loriz, 2007).

Particularly when the patient who has died is a child, families may appreciate you giving them a collection of mementos such as pictures, locks of hair, and handprints or footprints (de Jong-Berg & Kane, 2006; Meert et al., 2005; Pector, 2004b; Rini & Loriz, 2007; Tan, Docherty, Barfield, & Brandon, 2012; Widger & Picot, 2008). Some families later regret not taking mementos (de Jong-Berg & Kane, 2006), but others may be distressed if you take mementos, especially pictures, against their wishes (Skene, 1998); therefore, determining what each family wants and needs requires sensitivity and a careful approach.

In some cases, autopsy and organ or tissue donation may be possible. Nurses and other health professionals sometimes view such discussions as an intrusion and, thus, because of their own discomfort, they do not approach families. Parents in particular may have lingering regrets, however, if they miss an opportunity to help another child or to receive answers to some questions about their own child's death (Macdonald et al., 2006; Widger & Picot, 2008). Therefore, you should not be afraid to initiate these conversations should they be indicated, or at least ensure that someone initiates them. It is also important to make sure that when autopsies are done, families are given the results in a timely and compassionate manner

(Macdonald et al., 2006; Meert et al., 2007; Rini & Loriz, 2007; Wisten & Zingmark, 2007). Families may want to meet with health professionals to discuss autopsy results, clarify the events leading to and the circumstances of the death, and be reassured that everything possible was done and the right decisions were made (Kreicbergs et al., 2005; Macdonald et al., 2006; Milberg, Olsson, Jakobsson, Olsson, & Friedrichsen, 2008; Pector, 2004a; Wisten & Zingmark, 2007; Woodgate, 2006).

It was previously thought that healing meant a person got over their loss and severed ties with the deceased. It is now known that one does not "get over" the loss of a loved one; rather, families will forever have links with the person who has died (Moules, Simonson, Fleiszer, Prins, & Glasgow, 2007). The ways in which continuing bonds exist for different types of loss and their associations with positive and negative outcomes for bereaved individuals is only beginning to be explored (Foster et al., 2011). As a nurse, you can do much to facilitate a healthy start to their grieving journey and to help them find meaning in death. Your actions at the actual death event are critical. Family members vividly remember the moment of their loved one's death. They often remember who was present, what was said, what was done that was helpful, and what was not so helpful. Many remember that it was the nurse who was with them at the moment of death, or that the nurse was the first to respond to the family's call about a change in their loved one's condition. More often than not, families clearly recall the nurse's words and actions. What you do for and with family members at the time of their loved one's death can have a profound and long-lasting impact on them. It is important to remember that, although the death may be one of many for the nurse, it may be the first and only for the family; therefore, a person's death should never be treated as "just a job" on the part of the nurse (Shiozaki et al., 2005). Be cognizant too that clichés such as "this was meant to be," "he is in a better place," or referring to the deceased person as an angel may make families feel that you are minimizing the impact of the death on the family (Pector, 2004a, 2004b). Simple expressions, such as "I am sorry your husband is dying" (Tilden, Tolle, Garland, & Nelson, 1995, p. 637), are more often appreciated.

Nurses should have an understanding of loss, know how to support families in grief, and be able to provide quality bereavement care. Beginning nurses often worry about showing emotion, such as crying, in the presence of family members. Family members are often deeply touched when they see a nurse's genuine emotional response, but it is critical that the family not be put in the position of caring for the nurse.

Provision of bereavement care by the nurse offers the opportunity for continued contact with the family and signifies the importance of the family to the nurse (Collins-Tracey et al., 2009; Davies et al., 2007; de Cinque et al., 2006; de Jong-Berg & Kane, 2006; Kreicbergs et al., 2005; Macdonald et al., 2005; Meert et al., 2007; Rodger, Sherwood, O'-Connor, & Leslie, 2007). Follow-up activities that many families appreciate include calls, cards, attendance at the funeral, and offers to make referrals to additional sources of support as needed (Cherlin et al., 2004). Families may appreciate written information on practical issues, such as what to do next, and about grief or other sources of support (D'Agostino et al., 2008; de Cinque et al., 2006; de Jong-Berg & Kane, 2006; Pector, 2004a; Rini & Loriz, 2007; Rodger et al., 2007), as well as information to share with extended family and friends on how to offer effective support. Depending on the setting, bereavement care may continue for a period of time in the community. Sometimes health care professionals call or send a card to families on the first anniversary of the patient's death, especially if it was a child who died. This simple contact acknowledges that the grieving process takes time and can make families feel really cared for, once again highlighting the importance of the patient and family to the professional (Collins-Tracey et al., 2009).

Special Situations

There are some situations that can be challenging for nurses to consider and deserve additional attention. More specific assessment and intervention tools may be required in order to offer optimal care.

Facilitating Connections for Children When a Family Member Is Critically Ill

When a family member is critically ill, families and professionals may have a concern about the importance and impact of bringing children to visit, whether at home, in the ICU, or in any other setting. Yet, these visits may reduce feelings of separation, guilt, abandonment, fear, loneliness, and worry for the child (Nolbris & Hellstrom, 2005; Vint, 2005). Children can generally decide for themselves if they wish to visit and, where possible, families and health care professionals should respect their decision. Those younger than 10 visiting a relative may be most interested in the equipment, whereas older children may spend more time focused on the person they are visiting (Knutsson & Bergbom, 2007). The visit can also benefit the patient by acting as a diversion, offering hope, and bringing a sense of normalcy (Vint, 2005). Thus, nurses should offer families the option of bringing children in to visit loved ones.

Talking with the patient and family about previous experiences with children visiting can be helpful, for example, "Sometimes family members are afraid that a child will be very upset to see grandpa looking so sick. Are you worried about that possibility?" and "In my experience, children are very curious, as well as resilient. They often suspect that something bad is happening and they imagine terrible scenarios. Being truthful and also letting them see for themselves what is happening can be very beneficial." You can assist families to prepare children beforehand about what they will see and what to expect; you also can be present during the visit to support family members in answering questions and to make the child feel welcome and an important part of the family (Knutsson & Bergbom, 2007; Nolbris & Hellstrom, 2005; Vint, 2005). It is important that everyone realizes a child's reactions are somewhat unpredictable; one child may seem unaffected while another may be upset and crying. Nurses should acknowledge that every reaction is "normal" and work with the child in a way that meets his needs at the time. Though it may be difficult for a critically ill patient when a child chooses not to visit, you can help the patient understand by sharing your knowledge about how children need to make their own decisions and you can offer ways to assist in maintaining connections between the child and the ill family member through cards, calls, and frequent updates about how the patient is doing.

When Death Is Sudden or Traumatic

Unlike with chronic illness, a sudden or traumatic death leaves little time for families to come to terms with the situation. Further, the nature of a frequently chaotic environment when death is traumatic or sudden may contribute to a lack of communication between professionals and families. It is important that the information given to families include the big picture; otherwise, families often receive different pieces of information from each health professional and may have trouble putting it all together to understand that it actually means the patient is dying. This may be more of an issue in situations when there is a sudden illness or injury because the family has little experience and may be unprepared for what is happening (Meert, Thurston, & Briller, 2005; Rini & Loriz, 2007; Wiegand, 2006).

In critical care areas, nurses may be less apt to support patients and their families emotionally and psychologically (Nordgren & Olsson, 2004; Price, 2004) because they give more attention to managing the patient's physical symptoms systematically and efficiently. Family members may not be attended to as nurses deal with the acuity of evolving situations. Yet, research shows that family members of patients in ICUs often experience anxiety and depression (Pochard et al., 2001). Furthermore, insufficient information and death in the ICU have been associated with posttraumatic stress disorder in families of ICU patients (Azoulay et al., 2005). Therefore, it is necessary to offer psychological support, such as ongoing assessment of and information for families of patients who are cared for and who may ultimately die in ICUs (White & Luce, 2004).

Whether during a sudden or traumatic event that necessitates admission to the emergency department or the quickly shifting situations in ICU, nurses need to remember that amidst the technology are real people who need connections. You may need to take a breath and briefly step back so you can focus on the "bigger picture" before you are able to help the family, but it is critical that someone takes time for them. All of the ways that you can connect with families can work in ICU and emergency department settings, but you need to create some space for the family to ensure that the connections and communication happen. If family members are in the room, you need to talk with them, explain what is happening, and be available to answer their questions. If they are waiting outside, make sure they have somewhere comfortable and private to sit, and provide frequent updates about their loved one. If you yourself are too busy providing urgent care for the patient, make sure that someone is designated to care for the family members and to keep them involved as much as they want to be. It is especially important that after a sudden or traumatic death, nurses provide family members with information about what will happen (e.g., involvement of the coroner, how to contact a funeral home, and how to obtain support in the future). Nurses should also make sure that a family member has a companion before leaving the setting, so a friend or relative may need to be called to be with the family member.

Sudden life-threatening events also bring the possibility of administering cardiopulmonary resuscitation. Although some debate exists regarding the presence of family members during attempts at resuscitation, many settings do allow for it. Parents in particular may voice a strong belief that it is their right to be present during these events (McGahey-Oakland, Lieder, Young, & Jefferson, 2007; Meert et al., 2005; Rini & Loriz, 2007; Wisten & Zingmark, 2007), because they believe that their presence is a source of strength and support for the child and being present offers the opportunity to see for themselves that everything possible was done to assist their child. Families need frequent updates if they choose not to be present and must be given information about what is happening if they are present (McGahey-Oakland et al., 2007).

Dying at Home

Families need professional support, particularly in the area of symptom control, to make a home death "happen" (Brazil et al., 2005). Caring for a dying family member at home can be extremely demanding work—physically, emotionally, psychologically, and spiritually. The primary caregivers require support and resources to be successful. First and foremost, the family and the nurse need to discuss the dying process, existing resources, and present and future needs. Then together they can develop a plan that anticipates changes. For example, symptom crises, such as escalating pain, need to be anticipated and addressed in advance. When the family is committed to supporting death at home, it can be devastating when a symptom crisis results

in death in the middle of a busy emergency department. Box 10-7 provides some practical suggestions about what you need to consider and perhaps facilitate when someone is dying at home.

PALLIATIVE CARE AND END-OF-LIFE FAMILY CASE STUDIES

Two family case studies are presented in this section to demonstrate the art and science of family nursing in palliative and end-of-life care. The Jones family was introduced in Chapter 3 and is reintroduced here to demonstrate family care when the person who is dying is the mother. Please return to Chapter 3 and reacquaint yourself with the family and familiarize yourself with the Jones family genogram in Figure 10-2. The Garcia family case study illustrates how a student nurse working with a preceptor assists a young family with the death of an infant.

BOX 10-7
Practical Considerations When Someone Is Dying at Home

- Involvement of expert resources, such as hospice, and an interprofessional team, including volunteers.
- Symptom management plan, including anticipating changes such as inability to swallow and the need for parenteral medications, as well as management of breathlessness and agitation.
- Advance care planning, including the presence of a "Do Not Resuscitate" order if necessary.
- Equipment such as a hospital bed and commode.
- Identification of willing informal support persons (friends, church, extended family).
- Development of a list of things that willing people can do, for example, a calendar for preparation of meals, house cleaning, someone to visit so the caregiver can get out for a walk.
- Respite for the caregiver(s), which may be planned hospice admissions or the overnight placement of a paid professional.
- Financial implications and available support, for example, compassionate benefits program.
- Contact numbers of resources.
- Discussion of unfinished business to enable a peaceful death.
- Discussion of alternatives should dying and death at home become impossible for any reason.

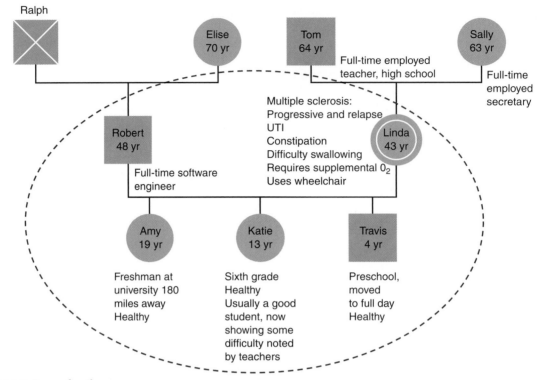

FIGURE 10-2 Jones family genogram.

Family Case Study: Jones Family

Linda, the mother in the Jones family, has been living with multiple sclerosis (MS) for 13 years. Early in the illness, Linda experienced relapses where her symptoms worsened, but these were followed by periods of remission where she recovered back to "normal." Since Travis's birth, her relapses became more frequent, and although her symptoms sometimes improved a little, her condition steadily worsened.

Before Linda's discharge from the hospital where she was treated with antibiotics for pneumonia after aspiration, the primary nurse, Catherine, initiated a family meeting with Linda, Robert, and Linda's physician. Catherine had noticed Robert's fatigue and his repeated questions about whether Linda was really ready to come home. Catherine had also noticed Linda's reluctance to take medications (particularly for pain), her determination to walk with her cane despite serious unsteadiness, and the deepening silence between the husband and wife.

Catherine began the conversation by asking Linda and Robert about their understanding of the MS at this point. Linda quickly responded, saying that the pneumonia was really an unusual "one-time" problem, and although it had set her back, it would not be long before she was back on

her feet. Robert worried out loud that it seemed things were getting progressively worse. He was concerned about how Linda would manage at home alone in the mornings and with Travis in the afternoon when he returned from preschool. Noticing the difference in perspective, Catherine acknowledged she could see how there might be differences because MS is, indeed, a "tricky" illness that is difficult to predict. She asked Linda and Robert to think back to how things were a year ago and to what had happened over the last year. Both noticed that the hospitalizations had become more frequent, the recoveries were more difficult, and overall, Linda was not doing as well. The physician, Dr. Brooks, who had been listening quietly, remarked that, although MS was often an unpredictable disease, it seemed that Linda's MS had changed into a different kind of illness than it had been at first. He agreed that now the MS was more steadily progressing, and that it seemed things were getting worse more quickly. Linda said she could see this but kept hoping that the situation would turn around.

Catherine then asked what the family's goals for care were. Linda was quick to answer, "Remission—I want full remission." Robert was slower to reply. He said, "I am so tired, and it hurts me so much to see you suffer. I want you to be comfortable, to be free of pain, to enjoy the kids rather than snapping at them..." Linda said, "I'm just trying so hard to get back to normal. I always thought that a wheelchair would be the end for me. And I'm just so tired." Catherine acknowledged that MS often creates profound fatigue in many family members and wondered which of the children might be most affected. Both Linda and Robert agreed that, of the children, Katie was suffering the most from tiredness. She picked up a lot of the pieces of Linda's work in the home, beginning supper preparations and looking after Travis. Often, she would be up late at night working on homework, but her grades had been slipping and she had been crying more. Linda worried that Amy was also tired as she spent a great deal of time driving home on weekends to care for the family.

Dr. Brooks interjected at this point saying that their primary goal for care during this hospitalization had been to cure the pneumonia. He noted that, although they were successful, they had not been able to assist Linda toward a remission of her MS. He remarked that with the change in the MS, it seemed that the hope for remission might not be possible. He then asked, "If things continue the way they are going, where do you think you will be in six months?" Linda began to cry and said she was thinking she might not be alive. The pneumonia scared her, and she was frightened about aspirating again, so she had been decreasing what she ate and drank. Robert was worried about how he could continue to work full time supporting the family and also care for Linda at home, especially as it seemed there was so little he did that was "right" for Linda.

Catherine replied that the "new" MS was clearly creating challenges for the family and wondered if it was time to shift the focus of care more toward comfort and quality of life for all family members, while at the same time working to prevent problems such as aspiration. She explained that as illness gets more demanding, additional supports are needed. She also explained that as illness gets intrusive, attention needs to be paid to what is most important to living well for all family members. Linda was getting tired at this point and having a lot of difficulty holding her head up, so Catherine asked if they could schedule another meeting. Robert and Linda readily agreed, saying they knew they needed to talk about these things but just did not know how. Catherine asked them to do some homework: to each identify their biggest concern, as well as what was most important to living well at this time. They were asked to find this out from the children too, and a meeting was scheduled for the next day. Dr. Brooks let them know that he wanted to speak with them about Linda's preferences for care should she have another experience with pneumonia.

The next day, Linda, Robert, Catherine, and Dr. Brooks all met again. Linda began the conversation, saying she had done a great deal of soul searching and was most worried about suffering from unmanageable pain and being a burden to her family. She was wondering if perhaps she should not go home but should be admitted into a care facility. Robert was most worried about burning out and not being able to support Linda and the children as he wanted. They had had a three-way conversation with each of the children last evening. Amy was most worried that her mother was going to die, and she let her parents know that she was planning on leaving university to move back home. Katie was most troubled by her lack of friends as her friends were no longer including her in their activities. Travis missed his mother, and wanted her to be able to read stories to him and play with him more.

The things that were most important to Linda's quality of life were reducing her pain, having Amy continue at university, being more involved in Katie's and Travis's everyday lives, being able to attend a service at her church on a weekly basis, and reconnecting with Robert. She said her greatest hope was to be at home as long as possible. Robert wanted to be able to sleep, to go to work without constantly worrying about Linda, and to reconnect to Linda. He too wanted her at home as long as possible. Both Linda and Robert agreed that for them to live well, they needed more help in their home. Options were discussed, including the possibility of Elise (Robert's mother) moving in to be of assistance, and preplanned, short stays in hospice for respite. Linda did not want Elise doing her personal care, so again, they discussed their options. Dr. Brooks and the family developed a systematic plan for pain management. During the assessment process, he learned that Linda was refusing her medications because she was concerned they were contributing to her irritability with Robert and the children. He was able to reassure her that this was not the case; in fact, her unmanaged pain was more likely a major negative influence. They devised a plan for long-acting pain medication so that Robert would be able to sleep through the night. They consulted a dietitian regarding ways to manage swallowing problems, and scheduled a home assessment by the team physiotherapist so as to safely maximize Linda's mobility.

Both Catherine and Dr. Brooks commended Linda and Robert on the deep love they saw between the couple and how effective they were at problem solving, systematically working their issues through until achieving a mutually satisfying outcome. Finally, Dr. Brooks raised the topic of what Linda's preferences for care would be if she should experience development of pneumonia again. He explained that

(continued)

this was a real possibility because Linda's respiratory muscles were weakening. Dr. Brooks understood that both Linda and Robert wanted her home as long as possible, so he was curious about whether she would want to come to the hospital to be treated with intravenous antibiotics as she had during this hospitalization. Linda stated this would be her preference, especially if she was likely to be able to go home again after the treatment. Dr. Brooks explained that as her muscles become weaker, she might need the assistance of a breathing machine (ventilator) to give the antibiotics time to work against the infection, and asked whether she would want that. Linda was not sure what her preference would be in this situation, but she was very clear that she did not want to be "kept alive on a machine." She and Robert wanted more time to discuss this question, and they wanted to consult with their pastor, so they agreed to continue the conversation at the next doctor's appointment. Robert and Linda agreed to visit the local hospice to explore respite opportunities, as well as end-of-life care, should staying at home prove too difficult.

Three weeks later at the scheduled appointment with Dr. Brooks, Linda let him know that many things were going better with Elise in the house and home visits from Catherine, as well as a personal care aide. Amy agreed to stay in college with the promise from her parents that she would be told immediately if Linda's health changed. All family members were feeling less tired. Linda stated that she was not ready to leave Robert and the children, but was in a dilemma about the use of a ventilator if she developed pneumonia. She continued to worry that she might be kept alive on the machine, which to her would not be considered living. Dr. Brooks explained that, if necessary, one possibility was a time-limited trial of a ventilator to determine whether the antibiotics would work. Both Linda and Robert agreed. This was a difficult discussion, and Linda expressed distress about her loss of independence and her deep sorrow about the possibility of leaving her children. She admitted to swinging between despair and anger, and that both made it hard for her to enjoy her days. This was new information to Robert, who had noticed her struggling but thought things would work out over time. Through assessment, it became apparent that Linda was experiencing depression. She agreed to try an antidepressant medication and to join a local MS support group.

Eight Months Later:

Linda experienced fever, congestion, and shortness of breath after aspiration. The health team initiated antibiotics and managed symptoms to relieve pain, breathlessness, fever, and constipation. Linda occasionally had periods of acute shortness of breath where she worried that she might not be able to take her next breath. The fear served to make the breathlessness worse, so the visiting nurse showed both Linda and the family how to slow and deepen breathing by consciously breathing together. Dr. Brooks made a home visit and asked Linda about admission to the hospital. When he could not assure her that she would get off the ventilator, Linda declined, saying she wanted to stay with her family. Robert agreed. A family meeting with Catherine and Dr. Brooks was held at Linda's bedside to discuss what the family would experience if the pneumonia progressed. They developed a family ecomap (Fig. 10-3) and they increased support services with more frequent visits from the nurse, care aide, and friends (particularly from Linda's support group). They discussed a move to hospice, but all agreed that home was the best place for Linda, and that death at home was their preference.

Linda engaged in one-on-one time with each of her children. They talked about their best memories together, what they most loved about each other, and their hopes and dreams for the future as the children grow up. Robert participated by videotaping the conversations. Each child was given a journal, and together with Linda, they drew pictures, wrote notes, and gathered mementos to capture these conversations. She organized gifts for their birthdays and for Christmas in the upcoming year. It was not that she knew she was dying, but she had been encouraged to plan for the worst and hope for the best, to do the things that needed doing. The family received the same encouragement so they were all able to have special time with Linda over the last few months. Linda died surrounded by her family.

Six Weeks Later:

Catherine visited the family six weeks after Linda's death and found them managing well. Pictures of Linda were everywhere. Elise continued to live with the family, and they thought this was the best plan for the time being. Robert had taken some time off work to be with the children after Linda's death, but shortly afterward all went back to work and school. Amy still came home on some weekends. Robert, Amy, and Katie talked of their sense of having done the very best they could to honor Linda's preferences. They took comfort in the fact that she died at home. They marked the 1-month anniversary of Linda's death with a visit to her grave site, taking flowers and a picture Travis had drawn of his mother. Family members drew support from different sources: each other, friends, their pastor, and some of the people from the MS support group who continued to visit. The children continued to read and reread the letters Linda had written; for Travis, this was part of his bedtime ritual. They were sad, and some days were better than others; they had a sense that the weight of their grief was lifting.

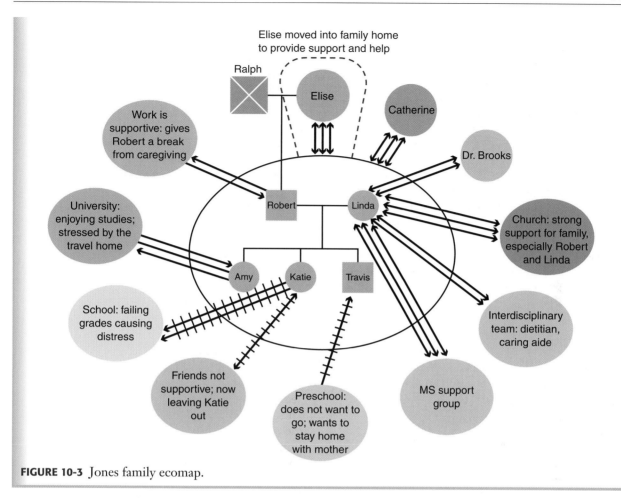

Elise moved into family home
to provide support and help

FIGURE 10-3 Jones family ecomap.

Family Case Study: Garcia Family—Living and Dying a Good Death; Saying Hello and Good-Bye

You are a nursing student in your final clinical placement. I am your preceptor, a clinical nurse specialist (CNS) on the palliative care team in a children's hospital. You asked for this placement as a final-year nursing student because you have come across a number of situations during your student experiences where you wished you knew how to talk and be with a patient and her family when the patient was dying. You realize that all nurses, from novice to expert and in all areas of nursing practice, need to develop skills in the area of death and dying. Please acquaint yourself with the Garcia family genogram in Figure 10-4. Consider

what it would be like if you were the student working with this family.

We have received a new consultation to meet with Emma and her parents, Eduardo and Karina Garcia. We learn that Emma is 7 days old and is a beautiful little baby with a perfect little face, big dark eyes, and lots of dark hair. Emma is on a ventilator because she has severe congenital muscular dystrophy and is unable to breathe on her own. Babies with severe disease, like Emma, have a very limited life expectancy, typically only a few weeks. Her severe muscle weakness means she is not able to breathe on her own for any length of time. We have been asked to meet with Emma and her family because they have decided, in consultation with their health care team, to withdraw ventilator support. As part of the palliative care team, we have been invited to assist

(continued)

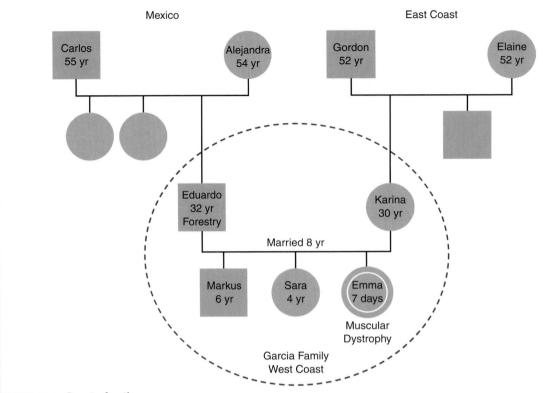

Mexico

East Coast

Carlos
55 yr

Alejandra
54 yr

Gordon
52 yr

Elaine
52 yr

Eduardo
32 yr
Forestry

Karina
30 yr

Married 8 yr

Markus
6 yr

Sara
4 yr

Emma
7 days

Muscular
Dystrophy

Garcia Family
West Coast

FIGURE 10-4 Garcia family genogram.

Eduardo and Karina to decide how, when, and where the withdrawal might occur.

Before meeting with this family for the first time, we realize how important it is to prepare ourselves. We know that we need to pause for a moment and consider how we might begin this conversation with Eduardo and Karina. We also want to ensure that we have in place whatever we might need to facilitate this first meeting.

We make arrangements to meet with Eduardo and Karina in a quiet, private room where we will not be interrupted. Pagers are turned off and other staff are covering for us so that we will have time to sit with the parents and really listen to what they have to say. Given that there will be several challenging things to discuss, we invite the neonatal intensive care unit (NICU) social worker, who already has a relationship with the family, to join us for this meeting.

Before meeting the family we spend some time talking about different ways to begin the conversation with the parents. There are as many ways to start this conversation as there are clinicians. This is the beginning of what we hope will be a therapeutic relationship during

one of the most difficult times a family can experience. Eduardo and Karina need to know who we are. It is often hard for parents to keep track of health care professionals—who we are, what we do, and how we can be helpful. This is especially true in highly emotionally charged situations. So typically we start with brief introductions. Sometimes, rather than starting the conversation by saying why we are here, it is helpful to gain an understanding of why the parents think we are meeting and then continue from there.

We start the meeting by each introducing ourselves. Then one of us says, "Tell us your understanding of why we are meeting today." To facilitate our connection with this family, we also ask Eduardo and Karina to tell us about Emma—*not* her medical condition, but what they have noticed about her or experienced in their relationship with her as parents. In answer to our query, one of the things Karina tells us is that she thinks Emma has Eduardo's eyes. Eduardo has noticed that she follows Karina with her eyes and he says, "She really knows her mom."

We learn that after talking with both sets of grandparents (mostly by telephone as Eduardo's family is in Mexico where he and Karina met and Karina's parents live across the country), the health care team, and their priest, Karina and Eduardo have indeed come to the decision that the most loving thing they can do as parents is to withdraw Emma's ventilator and allow natural death. We encourage them to discuss their concerns, fears, and hopes for the time they have now with Emma. There is much silence and tears as the parents try to put into words all the thoughts swirling in their heads. They tell us that their focus is on having Emma experience as much of normal newborn life as she can. And they want to touch her and care for her. They want her to spend time with her 4-year-old sister, Sara, and 6-year-old brother, Markus; to be in her car seat; to be bathed, cuddled, and have her diaper changed by both her mom and dad; to be baptized; and most of all to see the sun. We learn that it was the middle of the night when Emma was born and then immediately transferred from her small community to our tertiary urban hospital 3 hours away, so she had seen the moon but not the sun. Eduardo is a forestry worker and the family loves to be outdoors. They cannot believe that one of their children will never spend any time outdoors. Neither Karina nor Eduardo had been able to hold Emma before she was whisked away. Karina has held her in the NICU, but Eduardo has been reluctant because of all the tubes. He is feeling sad that her pervasive muscle weakness means she cannot grab onto his finger the way Sara and Markus did as babies and he is searching to find another way to connect with Emma. Both parents express worry about how to help Sara and Markus understand what is happening in a way that does not frighten them. Although both Karina and Eduardo are committed to their decision, they are afraid that Emma may suffer when the ventilator is withdrawn. They are worried about watching her struggle for breath. The parents ask us for a week to have these experiences with Emma; they also want time for additional family members to visit and to plan for withdrawal of the ventilator.

Following our meeting with Eduardo and Karina, we meet with the involved NICU staff members, who are quite concerned with the proposal that we wait a week to discontinue the ventilator. This is not the way it usually happens and they worry the family will only become more attached to Emma, finding it harder and harder to let her go, or that something will change in Emma's health status that may lead to an earlier death than what the parents expect. We provide further explanation and facilitate a meeting between the parents, Eduardo and Karina, and the NICU staff. At the meeting, NICU staff members are able to

express their concerns and the family is able to respond, as well as talk about their wishes. Hearing each others' fears and hopes is helpful and there is now agreement and support for the parents' request. Eduardo and Karina understand that it is possible something could happen unexpectedly with Emma and, although everything possible will be done to ensure that she is comfortable, the staff would not provide cardiopulmonary resuscitation (CPR) if her heart stopped.

Emma and her parents move into one of the private family rooms in the NICU. Karina's parents, Elaine and Gordon, who came to care for Sara and Markus in the family home, bring them to stay in a nearby hotel. This proximity enables them to visit often and to get to know the newest member of their family. Before their first visit, we spend time talking with Eduardo and Karina about how to prepare the siblings for seeing Emma, as well as explaining similarities and differences in how Sara and Markus may understand what is happening. Another member of the team, a child life therapist, spends time with Sara and Markus individually and together to assess and support their understanding and coping with Emma's illness. Eduardo and Karina join some of the discussions and have some of their own time with the child life therapist. They learn how young children come to understand serious illness and death and that Sara and Markus will likely have questions about Emma for many years. They are happy about the picture books and other resources on how to support their children over time.

During the week, even in the midst of the technology that is still needed to keep Emma breathing, Eduardo, Karina, Grandma Elaine, Grandpa Gordon, Sara, and Markus do all the things that families with newborns usually do. The family is given the opportunity to say hello and good-bye to their new family member all at the same time. Eduardo holds Emma for the first time and they take many, many pictures and videos. They give Emma her first haircut and each save a tiny lock of hair tied with a ribbon. Sara and Markus each create a memory box with drawings, the locks of hair, Emma's hand and foot prints, and copies of the photos. They also help the child life therapist make molds of Emma's hands and feet and of their own. Eduardo's parents arrive from Mexico and several close family members and friends come to meet Emma and witness her baptism in the hospital chapel. The list of hopes and dreams for this time gets ticked off. Eduardo and Karina also use this time to contact a funeral home

(continued)

in their home community and make arrangements with their priest for her wake and funeral.

One day we take Emma, her parents, her siblings, and her grandparents outside to the hospital's play garden where it is beautifully clear and sunny with a gentle breeze blowing. Hospital security has closed the garden to other families and staff so it is intimate and peaceful. Emma is able to feel the sun on her face for the first time. The child life therapist is there to support Sara and Markus. They both seem to enjoy this family outing; running over to see Emma, giving her a kiss, and then heading off to explore the sandbox and the swings before coming back again for a hug from their parents. Eduardo and Karina ask if we think that Sara and Markus really don't understand the situation and that is why they keep running off to play. The child life therapist reassures them that this is a typical way for children to cope and essentially they are just taking in what they can handle at their own pace. The child life therapist continues to follow the children's lead in supporting whatever they want to do and wherever they want to be in the garden. A nurse from NICU stays close to Emma to assist her to breathe while she is being held by her parents and grandparents. Everyone relaxes and shares stories about Karina's pregnancy, the labor and delivery, and the things they have learned about Emma the last few days. We take more family pictures and video to send to the rest of the extended family that night. To our surprise, the parents feel so comfortable in the garden that they ask if the ventilator can be discontinued in the garden. We set about making this request happen.

Eduardo, Karina, and Elaine meet with us, the neonatologist, the NICU CNS, and the NICU social worker; we explain how we will keep Emma comfortable when the ventilator is withdrawn. The family is reassured to learn that there are medications that will ensure that Emma does not struggle for breath and that we will not allow her to suffer. Eduardo asks what it will be like when the ventilator is taken away. We are able to help them understand that we do not know how long Emma will be able to breathe without assistance, but it could be minutes to hours; her breathing will slow, become irregular, and then stop. Her color will change and she will feel cool. Eduardo and Karina decide that they would like to be by themselves with Emma when she dies. Sara and Markus will stay at the hotel with their grandparents and then may come back to see Emma before she is taken to the funeral home.

Both parents seem to be coping fairly well with the situation, with Eduardo taking on the role of the "strong one" and Karina appearing more fragile. On the day of Emma's death, however, we are surprised at the reversal of roles, as Eduardo looks disheveled and distressed while Karina has done her hair and makeup; she's wearing a special outfit and seems "in control." We had hoped for sun, but somehow the weather seems more in keeping with the mood. You comment to her parents that Emma has seen the moon and the sun and now she is experiencing a true West Coast day—foggy and gloomy! Emma is given some medications so she won't experience any pain or distress and is settled with her parents in a secluded corner of the garden. The priest performs last rites. The nurse removes all of the tape and then the endotracheal tube while Emma remains peaceful in her parent's arms. We give the family private space to be together but, along with other members of the team (the priest, the NICU social worker, and the NICU nurse with additional medications ready in case Emma experiences any distress) are available in the play garden if needed.

The play garden is on a busy street and we are concerned that the level of traffic noise might be disturbing to the family. Our concerns are heightened when the siren starts at the nearby fire hall and the fire truck roars past; Emma's dad simply walks over to the fence and lifts her up to see her first fire truck. Emma and her parents walk the paths of the garden. Although there is still bustle and noise around them, it is clear that Emma and her family are in their own little world. Although they had opportunities to do "normal" family things over the last week, this is the first time Emma and her parents experience each other without interference of machines, tubes, wires, or other people.

Emma lives for another 2 hours. After she dies, her parents continue to hold her for another hour. Both sets of grandparents return with Sara and Markus to say good-bye to Emma. Although the children were both told what Emma would look and feel like after she died, Markus in particular has many questions about whether or not she is hungry, why she is cold, and if she is just sleeping. Karina responds gently to all of their questions to help them understand what has happened. When the family is ready, Sara and Markus spend some time with the child life therapist while a senior nurse, Patrick, partners with you to help Karina and Eduardo prepare Emma's body. Patrick asks the parents if they have any special rituals they would like to do and he also explains about what needs to be done to meet the hospital rules.

Everyone works together and though it is sad there is also a peacefulness as Karina and Eduardo talk about how happy they are to have done things the way they wanted to. They thank you and Patrick and say how grateful they are that the staff made it possible for Emma to die in peace in such a beautiful setting; Karina and Eduardo say that they will never forget what the staff did. With one last kiss on Emma's forehead, they leave for home with the rest of their family.

Patrick assists you to complete all of the charting and necessary paperwork related to Emma's death. As Eduardo and Karina decided against having an autopsy, Emma does not need to go to the hospital morgue. Patrick calls the funeral home and accompanies you as you carry Emma's body in a special softly colored and patterned bag to meet the funeral home director at the staff entrance to the hospital. You return to the unit and spend some time talking with Patrick and me. We make sure that you have a way home and a friend available to spend the evening with you. I also contact your clinical coordinator to let her know about the day's events to make sure that you have some ongoing support from the faculty. A few days later I invite you to attend a special debriefing session to be held with NICU staff.

As the funeral is held 3 hours away, you are unable to attend. I suggest that you may want to send a note to the family and offer to review it if needed (Box 10-8).

One Month Later:

That was not the end of our relationship with this family. We make a home visit a month after Emma's death where we learn about the funeral. Karina and Eduardo remark that they were very happy when two of their favorite NICU nurses came to Emma's funeral. They tell us about how moved they were when they received notes from you and some of the other nurses, as well as a card from NICU staff. They tell us that it helps them to know she touched the hearts of those who looked after her. We discuss how Karina and Eduardo are managing as a couple and as parents. Eduardo is back at work; Sara and Markus are back at preschool and school. Both sets of grandparents have gone home. At this point we draw an ecomap (Fig. 10-5) of the family's community connections, discuss their experiences of grief, and work together to map out avenues of support available locally.

BOX 10-8

Example Note to Family From Student Nurse

Dear Eduardo, Karina, Markus, and Sara,

It was my privilege to get to know all of you and to meet Emma. She had the most beautiful expressive eyes and so clearly looked at each of you when you spoke to her. It was amazing to watch all of you together and to see Emma experience so much life in such a short time. Your love for her and for each other was evident in everything that you did.

I learned so many things about how families can be together and live life to the fullest even in the midst of such difficult circumstances. I know my experience with your family will make me a better nurse with other families in the future. Emma and all of you will forever remain in my thoughts.

All my best,

_____, Student Nurse

We let Karina and Eduardo know that they will receive a letter with an appointment to see a geneticist in about 6 months. Because there was a genetic component to Emma's diagnosis, they may want to explore genetic testing and understand any possible risks for future pregnancies. A follow-up visit with the NICU neonatologist, CNS, and social worker will be coordinated to occur on the same day to respond to any questions the parents may have about Emma's illness and death, as well as to see how they are all coping. They are invited to bring Sara and Markus at that time to meet with the child life therapist.

We also let them know that the NICU has a formal program where, with the parents' permission, staff nurses are supported to contact families at regular intervals in the first year after the death and then send a plant on the 1-year anniversary. Karina and Eduardo express their appreciation for such a program and say they can only imagine how hard it will be on the anniversary of Emma's death; to know that the NICU staff who looked after her will be thinking of them gives them great comfort.

(continued)

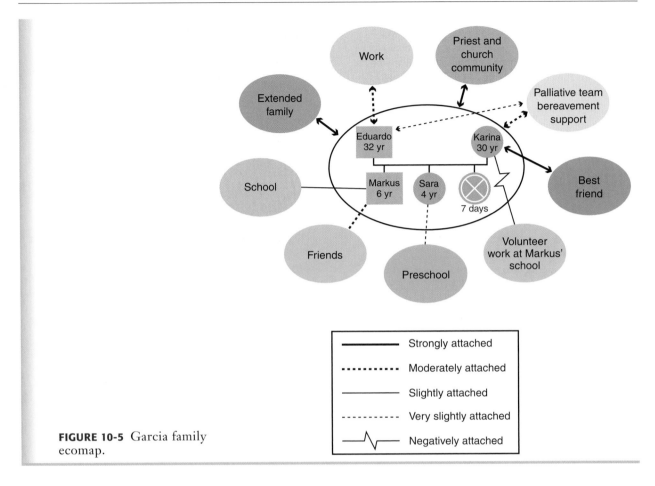

FIGURE 10-5 Garcia family ecomap.

Legend:
- ———— Strongly attached
- ·········· Moderately attached
- ——— Slightly attached
- - - - - - Very slightly attached
- —√√— Negatively attached

SUMMARY

Nurses are in a unique position to help families manage their lives when a loved one has a life-limiting illness or faces an acute or sudden death. Providing palliative and end-of-life nursing care as you accompany a family during this intense period is a privilege that should not be taken lightly. The importance of the nurse-family relationship in affecting and effecting positive outcomes cannot be overstated; this relationship can make the difference between a family who has good memories about their loved one's death and a family who experiences prolonged suffering because of a negative experience. Open and trusting communication; physical, psychological, and spiritual support; and respect for the families' right to make their own decisions, as well as support to facilitate these decisions, are essential components of quality palliative and end-of-life care. The following points highlight the concepts that are addressed in this chapter:

- Palliative and end-of-life care is inherently family focused.
- The principles of palliative care can be enacted effectively in any setting, regardless of whether death results from a chronic illness or a sudden/traumatic event.
- All nurses need to develop at least basic competencies in the area of death and dying.
- Therapeutic nurse-patient and nurse-family relationships are central to quality palliative and end-of-life care.
- Nurses who incorporate the principles of palliative care are more effective in tailoring their nursing practice and family interventions.

REFERENCES

Abma, T. A. (2005). Struggling with the fragility of life: A relational-narrative approach to ethics in palliative nursing. *Nursing Ethics, 12*(4), 337–348.

Andershed, B. (2006). Relatives in end-of-life care. Part 1: A systematic review of the literature the five past years, January 1999–February 2004. *Journal of Clinical Nursing, 15,* 1158–1169.

Antle, B. J., Barrera, M., Beaune, L., D'Agostino, N., & Good, B. (2005, Fall). Paediatric palliative care: What do parents want? *Rehab and Community Care Medicine,* 24–26.

Aspinal, F., Hughes, R., Dunckley, M., & Addington Hall, J. (2006). What is important to measure in the last months and weeks of life? A modified nominal group study. *International Journal of Nursing Studies, 43*(4), 393–403.

Azoulay, E., Pochard, F., Kentish-Barnes, N., Chevret, S., Aboab, J., Adrie, C.,...Schlemmer, B. (2005). Risk of post-traumatic stress symptoms in family members of intensive care unit patients. *American Journal of Respiratory and Critical Care Medicine, 171*(9), 987–994.

Barnes, S., Gott, M., Payne, S., Parker, C., Seamark, D., Gariballa, S., & Small, N. (2006). Characteristics and views of family carers of older people with heart failure. *International Journal of Palliative Nursing, 12*(8), 380–389.

Benzein, E. G., & Britt-Inger, S. (2008). Health-promoting conversations about hope and suffering with couples in palliative care. *International Journal of Palliative Nursing, 14*(9), 439–445.

Brajtman, S. (2005). Helping the family through the experience of terminal restlessness. *Journal of Hospice and Palliative Nursing, 7*(2), 73–81.

Brazil, K., Howell, D., Bedard, M., Krueger, P., & Heidebrecht, C. (2005). Preferences for place of care and place of death among informal caregivers of the terminally ill. *Palliative Medicine, 19*(6), 492–499.

Brosig, C. L., Pierucci, R. L., Kupst, M. J., & Leuthner, S. R. (2007). Infant end-of-life care: The parents' perspective. *Journal of Perinatology, 27,* 510–516.

Canadian Hospice Palliative Care Association. (n.d.). Start the conversation about end-of-life care. Retrieved from http://www.advancecareplanning.ca

Cancer Care Ontario. (2005). The Edmonton Symptom Assessment System (ESAS). Retrieved from https://www.cancercare.on.ca/common/pages/UserFile.aspx?fileId=13262

Caron, C. D., Griffith, J., & Arcand, M. (2005). End-of-life decision making in dementia: The perspective of family caregivers. *Dementia, 4*(1), 113–136.

Casarett, D., Crowley, R., Stevenson, C., Xie, S., & Teno, J. (2005). Making difficult decisions about hospice enrollment: What do patients and families want to know? *Journal of the American Geriatrics Society, 53*(2), 249–254.

Cherlin, E., Schulman-Green, D., McCorkle, R., Johnson-Hurzeler, R., & Bradley, E. (2004). Family perceptions of clinicians' outstanding practices in end-of-life care. *Journal of Palliative Care, 20*(2), 113–116.

Christakis, N. A., & Iwashyna, T. J. (2003). The health impact of health care on families: A matched cohort study of hospice use by decedents and mortality outcomes in surviving, widowed spouses. *Social Science & Medicine, 57,* 465–475.

Collins-Tracey, S., Clayton, J. M., Kirsten, L., Butow, P. N., Tattersall, M. H., & Chye, R. (2009). Contacting bereaved relatives: The views and practices of palliative care and oncology health care professionals. *Journal of Pain & Symptom Management, 37*(5), 807–822.

Contro, N., Larson, J., Scofield, S., Sourkes, B., & Cohen, H. (2002). Family perspectives on the quality of pediatric palliative care. *Archives of Pediatrics & Adolescent Medicine, 156*(1), 14–19.

Contro, N. A., Larson, J., Scofield, S., Sourkes, B., & Cohen, H. J. (2004). Hospital staff and family perspectives regarding quality of pediatric palliative care. *Pediatrics, 114*(5), 1248–1252.

Cooke, M. A. (1992). The challenge of hospice nursing in the 90's. *American Journal of Hospice & Palliative Care, 9*(1), 34–37.

Corà, A., Partinico, M., Munafò, M., & Palomba, D. (2012). Health risk factors in caregivers of terminal cancer patients: A pilot study. *Cancer Nursing, 35*(1), 38–47.

Curtis, J. R., Patrick, D. L., Shannon, S. E., Treece, P. D., Engelberg, R. A., & Rubenfeld, G. D. (2001). The family conference as a focus to improve communication about end-of-life care in the intensive care unit: Opportunities for improvement. *Critical Care Medicine, 29*(2 Suppl), N26–N33.

D'Agostino, N. M., Berlin-Romalis, D., Jovcevska, V., & Barrera, M. (2008). Bereaved parents' perspectives on their needs. *Palliative and Supportive Care, 6*(1), 33–41.

Davies, B., Collins, J., Steele, R., Cook, K., Distler, V., & Brenner, A. (2007). Parents' and children's perspectives of a children's hospice bereavement program. *Journal of Palliative Care, 23*(1), 14–23.

Davies, B., & Oberle, K. (1990). Dimensions of the supportive role of the nurse in palliative care. *Oncology Nursing Forum, 17*(1), 87–94.

Davies, B., Sehring, S. A., Partridge, J. C., Cooper, B. A., Hughes, A., Philp, J. C.,...Kramer, R. F. (2008). Barriers to palliative care for children: Perceptions of pediatric health care providers. *Pediatrics, 121*(2), 282–288.

Dawson, S., & Kristjanson, L. J. (2003). Mapping the journey: Family carers' perceptions of issues related to end-stage care of individuals with muscular dystrophy or motor neurone disease. *Journal of Palliative Care, 19*(1), 36–42.

Dean, R. A., & Gregory, D. M. (2005). More than trivial: Strategies for using humor in palliative care. *Cancer Nursing, 28*(4), 292–300.

de Cinque, N., Monterosso, L., Dadd, G., Sidhu, R., Macpherson, R., & Aoun, S. (2006). Bereavement support for families following the death of a child from cancer: Experience of bereaved parents. *Journal of Psychosocial Oncology, 24*(2), 65–83.

de Jong-Berg, M. A., & Kane, L. (2006). Bereavement care for families. Part 2: Evaluation of a paediatric follow-up programme. *International Journal of Palliative Nursing, 12*(10), 484–494.

Donovan, R., Williams, A., Stajduhar, K., Brazil, K., & Marshall, D. (2011). The influence of culture on home-based family caregiving at end-of-life: A case study of Dutch reformed family care givers in Ontario, Canada. *Social Science & Medicine, 72*(3), 338–346.

Dunn, P. M., Tolle, S. W., Moss, A. H., & Black, J. S. (2007). The POLST paradigm: Respecting the wishes of patients and families. *Annals of Long-Term Care, 15*(9), 33–40.

Dwyer, L., Nordenfelt, L., & Ternestedt, B. (2008). Three nursing home residents speak about meaning at the end of life. *Nursing Ethics, 15*(1), 97–109.

Elpern, E. H., Covert, B., & Kleinpell, R. (2005). Moral distress of staff nurses in a medical intensive care unit. *American Journal of Critical Care, 14*(6), 523–530.

Epstein, E. G., & Delgado, S. (2010). Understanding and addressing moral distress. *OJIN: Online Journal of Issues in Nursing, 15*(3), Manuscript 1.

Espinosa, L., Young, A., & Walsh, T. (2008). Barriers to intensive care unit nurses providing terminal care: An integrated literature review. *Critical Care Nursing Quarterly, 31*(1), 83–93.

Ferrell, B., Ervin, K., Smith, S., Marek, T., & Melancon, C. (2002). Family perspectives of ovarian cancer. *Cancer Practice: A Multidisciplinary Journal of Cancer Care, 10*(6), 269–276.

Feudtner, C., Santucci, G., Feinstein, J., Snyder, C., Rourke, M., & Kang, T. (2007). Hopeful thinking and level of comfort regarding providing pediatric palliative care: A survey of hospital nurses. *Pediatrics, 119*(1), e186–e192.

Fineberg, I. C. (2005). Preparing professionals for family conferences in palliative care: Evaluation results of an interdisciplinary approach. *Journal of Palliative Medicine, 8*(4), 857–866.

Fineberg, I. C. (2010). Social work perspectives on family communication and family conferences in palliative care. *Progress in Palliative Care, 18*(4), 213–220.

Fitzsimons, D., Mullan, D., Wilson, J. S., Conway, B., Corcoran, B., Dempster, M.,...Fogarty, D. (2007). The challenge of patients' unmet palliative care needs in the final stages of chronic illness. *Palliative Medicine, 21*(4), 313–322.

Forbes-Thompson, S., & Gessert, C. E. (2005). End of life in nursing homes: Connections between structure, process, and outcomes. *Journal of Palliative Medicine, 8*(3), 545–555.

Foster, T., Gilmer, M. J., Davies, B., Dietrich, M., Barrera, M., Fairclough, D.,...Gerhardt, C. (2011). Comparison of continuing bonds reported by parents and siblings after a child's death from cancer. *Death Studies, 35*(5), 420–440.

Fox, E., Landrum-McNiff, K., Zhong, Z., Dawson, N. V., Wu, A. W., & Lynn, J. (1999). Evaluation of prognostic criteria for determining hospice eligibility in patients with advanced lung, heart, or liver disease. *Journal of the American Medical Association, 282*(17), 1638–1645.

Fridriksdottir, N., Sigurdardottir, V., & Gunnarsdottir, S. (2006). Important needs of families in acute and palliative care settings assessed with the family inventory of needs. *Palliative Medicine, 20*(4), 425–432.

Funk, L., Stajduhar, K. I., Toye, C., Aoun, S., Grande, G. E., & Todd, C. J. (2010). Part 2: Home-based family caregiving at the end of life: A comprehensive review of published qualitative research (1998–2008). *Palliative Medicine, 24*(6), 507–607.

Gauthier, D. M. (2002). The meaning of healing near the end of life. *Journal of Hospice and Palliative Nursing, 4*(4), 220–227.

Gillis, J. (2008). "We want everything done." *Archives of Disease in Childhood, 93*(3), 192–193.

Gordon, C., Barton, E., Meert, K. L., Eggly, S., Pollacks, M., Zimmerman, J.,...Nicholson, C. (2009). Accounting for medical communication: Parents' perceptions of communicative roles and responsibilities in the pediatric intensive care unit. *Communication & Medicine, 6*(2), 177–188.

Goy, E. R., Carter, J. H., & Ganzini, L. (2007). Parkinson disease at the end of life: Caregiver perspectives. *Neurology, 69*(6), 611–612.

Grande, G., Stajduhar, K., Aoun, S., Toye, C., Funk, L., Addington-Hall, J., & Todd, C. (2009). Supporting lay carers in end of life care: Current gaps and future priorities. *Palliative Medicine, 23*(4), 339–344.

Gutierrez, K. M. (2012). Experiences and needs of families regarding prognostic communication in an intensive care unit: Supporting families at the end of life. *Critical Care Nursing Quarterly, 35*(3), 299–313.

Hammes, B. J., Klevan, J., Kempf, M., & Williams, M. S. (2005). Pediatric advance care planning. *Journal of Palliative Medicine, 8*(4), 766–773.

Hannan, J., & Gibson, F. (2005). Advanced cancer in children: How parents decide on final place of care for their dying child. *International Journal of Palliative Nursing, 11*(6), 284–291.

Hansson, H., Kjaergaard H., Schmiegelow, K., & Hallström I. (2012). Hospital-based home care for children with cancer: A qualitative exploration of family members' experiences in Denmark. *European Journal of Cancer Care, 21*(1), 59–66.

Harding, R., List, S., Epiphaniou, E., & Jones, H. (2012). How can informal caregivers in cancer and palliative care be supported? An updated systematic literature review of interventions and their effectiveness. *Palliative Medicine, 26*(1), 7–22.

Hays, R. M., Valentine, J., Haynes, G., Geyer, J. R., Villareale, N., McKinstry, B.,...Churchill, S. S. (2006). The Seattle pediatric palliative care project: Effects on family satisfaction and health-related quality of life. *Journal of Palliative Medicine, 9*(3), 716–728.

Heller, K. S., & Solomon, M. Z. (2005). Continuity of care and caring: What matters to parents of children with life-threatening conditions. *Journal of Pediatric Nursing, 20*(5), 335–346.

Hexem, K. R., Mollen, C. J., Carroll, K., Lanctot D. A., & Feudtner, C. (2011). How parents of children receiving pediatric palliative care use religion, spirituality, or life philosophy in tough times. *Journal of Palliative Medicine, 14*(1), 39–44.

Heyland, D. K., Dodek, P., Rocker, G., Groll, D., Gafni, A., Pichora, D.,...Lam, M. (2006). What matters most in end-of-life care: Perceptions of seriously ill patients and their family members. *Canadian Medical Association Journal, 174*(5), 627–633.

Heyland, D. K., Frank, C., Groll, D., Pichora, D., Dodek, P., Rocker, G., & Gafni, A. (2006). Understanding cardiopulmonary resuscitation decision making: Perspectives of seriously ill hospitalized patients and family members. *Chest, 130*(2), 419–428.

Heyland, D. K., Groll, D., Rocker, G., Dodek, P., Gafni, A., Tranmer, J.,...Lam, M. (2005). End-of-life care in acute care hospitals in Canada: A quality finish? *Journal of Palliative Care, 21*(3), 142–150.

Hinds, P. S., Drew, D., Oakes, L. L., Fouladi, M., Spunt, S. L., Church, C., & Furman, W. L. (2005). End-of-life care preferences of pediatric patients with cancer. *Journal of Clinical Oncology, 23*(36), 9146–9154.

Hinds, P., Oakes, L., Hicks, J., Powell, B., Srivastava, D., Spunt, S.,...Furman, W. L. (2009). "Trying to be a good parent" as defined by interviews with parents who made phase I, terminal care, and resuscitation decisions for their children. *Journal of Clinical Oncology, 27*(35), 5979–5985.

Hinds, P. S., Oakes, L., Quargnenti, A., Furman, W., Bowman, L., Gilger, E.,...Drew, D. (2000). An international feasibility study of parental decision making in pediatric oncology. *Oncology Nursing Forum, 27*(8), 1233–1243.

Horsley, H., & Patterson, T. (2006). The effects of a parent guidance intervention on communication among adolescents who have experienced the sudden death of a sibling. *American Journal of Family Therapy, 34*, 119–137.

Houger Limacher, L., & Wright, L. M. (2003). Commendations: Listening to the silent side of a family intervention. *Journal of Family Nursing, 9*(2), 130–135.

Hsiao, J. L., Evan, E. E., & Zeltzer, L. K. (2007). Parent and child perspectives on physician communication in pediatric palliative care. *Palliative & Supportive Care, 5*(4), 355–365.

Huang, Y. L., Yates, P., & Prior, D. (2009). Factors influencing oncology nurses' approaches to accommodating cultural needs in palliative care. *Journal of Clinical Nursing, 18*(24), 3421–3429.

Hudson, P. (2006). How well do family caregivers cope after caring for a relative with advanced disease and how can health professionals enhance their support? *Journal of Palliative Medicine, 9*(3), 694–703.

Hudson, P., Quinn, K., O'Hanlon, B., & Aranda, S. (2008). Family meetings in palliative care: Multidisciplinary clinical practice guidelines. *BCM Palliative Care, 7*, 12.

Hudson, P. L., Remedios, C., & Thomas, K. (2010). A systematic review of psychosocial interventions for family carers of palliative care patients. *BMC Palliative Care, 9*, 17.

Hughes, R. A., Sinha, A., Higginson, I., Down, K., & Leigh, P. N. (2005). Living with motor neurone disease: Lives, experiences of services and suggestions for change. *Health and Social Care in the Community, 13*(1), 64–74.

Hunstad, I., & Svindseth, M. F. (2011). Challenges in home-based palliative care in Norway: A qualitative study of spouses' experiences. *International Journal of Palliative Nursing, 17*(8), 398–404.

Jo, S., Brazil, K., Lohfeld, L., & Willison, K. (2007). Caregiving at the end of life: Perspectives from spousal caregivers and care recipients. *Palliative & Supportive Care, 5*(1), 11–17.

Johansson, C. M., Axelsson, B., & Danielson, E. (2006). Living with incurable cancer at the end of life—Patients' perceptions on quality of life. *Cancer Nursing, 29*(5), 391–399.

Kars, M. C., Grypdonck, M. H. F., & van Delden, J. J. M. (2011). Being a parent of a child with cancer throughout the end-of-life course. *Oncology Nursing Forum, 38*(4), E260–E271.

Kazanowski, M. (2005). Family caregivers' medication management of symptoms in patients with cancer near death. *Journal of Hospice and Palliative Nursing, 7*(3), 174–181.

Kenny, P., Hall, J., Zapart, S., & Davis, P. R. (2010). Informal care and home-based palliative care: The health-related quality of life of carers. *Journal of Pain and Symptom Management, 40*(1), 35–48.

Kirk, P., Kirk, I., & Kristjanson, L. J. (2004). What do patients receiving palliative care for cancer and their families want to be told? A Canadian and Australian qualitative study. *British Medical Journal, 328*(7452), 1343–1347.

Kleinman, A., & Benson, P. (2006). Anthropology in the clinic: The problem of cultural competency and how to fix it. *PLoS Medicine, 3*(10), e294.

Knapp, C., Madden, V., Wang, H., Curtis, C., Sloyer, P., & Shenkman, E. (2011). Spirituality of parents of children in palliative care. *Journal of Palliative Medicine, 14*(4), 437–443.

Knutsson, S. E., & Bergbom, I. L. (2007). Custodians' viewpoints and experiences from their child's visit to an ill or injured nearest being cared for at an adult intensive care unit. *Journal of Clinical Nursing, 16*(2), 362–371.

Kongsuwan, W., Chaipetch, O., & Matchim, Y. (2012). Thai Buddhist families' perspective of a peaceful death. *Nursing in Critical Care, 17*(3), 151–159.

Konrad, S. (2008). Mothers' perspectives on qualities of care in their relationships with health care professionals: The influence of relational and communicative competencies. *Journal of Social Work in End-of-Life & Palliative Care, 4*(1), 38–56.

Kreicbergs, U. C., Lannen, P., Onelov, E., & Wolfe, J. (2007). Parental grief after losing a child to cancer: Impact of professional and social support on long-term outcomes. *Journal of Clinical Oncology, 25*(22), 3307–3312.

Kreicbergs, U., Valdimarsdottir, U., Onelov, E., Bjork, O., Steineck, G., & Henter, J. I. (2005). Care-related distress: A nationwide study of parents who lost their child to cancer. *Journal of Clinical Oncology, 23*(36), 9162–9171.

Kristjanson, L. J., Aoun, S. M., & Oldham, L. (2006). Palliative care and support for people with neurodegenerative conditions and their carers. *International Journal of Palliative Nursing, 12*(8), 368–377.

Kristjanson, L. J., Aoun, S. M., & Yates, P. (2006). Are supportive services meeting the needs of Australians with neurodegenerative conditions and their families? *Journal of Palliative Care, 22*(3), 151–157.

Kuhl, D. (2002). *What dying people want: Practical wisdom for the end of life.* Toronto, ON: Doubleday.

Kwak, J., Salmon, J. R., Acquaviva, K. D., Brandt, K., & Egan, K. A. (2007). Benefits of training family caregivers on experiences of closure during end-of-life care. *Journal of Pain and Symptom Management, 33*(4), 434–445.

Li, J., Johansen, C., Hansen, D., & Olsen, J. (2002). Cancer incidence in parents who lost a child: A nationwide study in Denmark. *Cancer, 95*(10), 2237–2242.

Li, J., Laursen, T. M., Precht, D. H., Olsen, J., & Mortensen, P. B. (2005). Hospitalization for mental illness among parents after the death of a child. *New England Journal of Medicine, 352*(12), 1190–1196.

Li, J., Precht, D. H., Mortensen, P. B., & Olsen J. (2003). Mortality in parents after death of a child in Denmark: A nationwide follow-up study. *Lancet, 361*(9355), 363–367.

Macdonald, M. E., Liben, S., Carnevale, F. A., Rennick, J. E., Wolf, S. L., Meloche, D., & Cohen, S. R. (2005). Parental perspectives on hospital staff members' acts of kindness and commemoration after a child's death. *Pediatrics, 116*(4), 884–890.

Macdonald, M. E., Liben, S., & Cohen, S. R. (2006). Truth and consequences: Parental perspectives on autopsy after the death of a child. *Pediatric Intensive Care Nursing, 7*(1), 6–15.

Mack, J. W., Hilden, J. M., Watterson, J., Moore, C., Turner, B., Grier, H. E.,...Wolfe, J. (2005). Parent and physician perspectives on quality of care at the end of life in children with cancer. *Journal of Clinical Oncology, 23*(36), 9155–9161.

Marsella, A. (2009). Exploring the literature surrounding the transition into palliative care: A scoping review. *International Journal of Palliative Nursing, 15*(4), 186–189.

Maynard, L., Rennie, T., Shirtliffe, J., & Vickers, D. (2005). Seeking and using families' views to shape children's hospice services. *International Journal of Palliative Nursing, 11*(12), 624–630.

McDonagh, J. R., Elliott, T. R., Engelberg, R. A., Treece, P. D., Shannon, S. E., Rubenfeld, G. D.,...Curtis, J. R. (2004). Family satisfaction with family conferences about end-of-life care in the intensive care unit: Increased proportion of family speech is associated with increased satisfaction. *Critical Care Medicine, 32*(7), 1484–1488.

McGahey-Oakland, P. R., Lieder, H. S., Young, A., & Jefferson, L. S. (2007). Family experiences during resuscitation at a children's hospital emergency department. *Journal of Pediatric Health Care, 21*(4), 217–225.

Meeker, J. (2004). A voice for the dying. *Clinical Nursing Research, 13*(4), 326–342.

Meert, K. L., Eggly, S., Pollack, M., Anand, K. J., Zimmerman, J., Carcillo, J.,...Nicholson, C. (2007). Parents' perspectives regarding a physician-parent conference after their child's death in the pediatric intensive care unit. *Journal of Pediatrics, 151*(1), 50–55, 55.e1–55.e2.

Meert, K. L., Thurston, C. S., & Briller, S. H. (2005). The spiritual needs of parents at the time of their child's death in the pediatric intensive care unit and during bereavement: A qualitative study article. *Pediatric Critical Care Medicine, 6*(4), 420–427.

Merluzzi, T. V., Philip, E. J., Vachon, D. O., & Heitzmann, C. A. (2011). Assessment of self-efficacy for caregiving: The critical role of self-care in caregiver stress and burden. *Palliative and Supportive Care, 9*, 15–24.

Meyer, E. C., Ritholz, M. D., Burns, J. P., & Truog, R. (2006). Improving the quality of end-of-life care in the pediatric intensive care unit: Parents' priorities and recommendations. *Pediatrics, 117*(3), 649–657.

Midson, R., & Carter, B. (2010). Addressing end of life care issues in a tertiary treatment centre: Lessons learned from surveying parents' experiences. *Journal of Child Health Care, 14*(1), 52–66.

Milberg, A., Olsson, E. C., Jakobsson, M., Olsson, M., & Friedrichsen, M. (2008). Family members' perceived needs for bereavement follow-up. *Journal of Pain & Symptom Management, 35*(1), 58–69.

Milberg, A., & Strang, P. (2011). Protection against perceptions of powerlessness and helplessness during palliative care: The family members' perspective. *Palliative & Supportive Care, 9*(3), 251–262.

Mok, E., Chan, F., Chan, V., & Yeung, E. (2002). Perception of empowerment by family caregivers of patients with a terminal illness in Hong Kong. *International Journal of Palliative Nursing, 8*(3), 137–145.

Monterosso, L., & Kristjanson, L. (2008). Supportive and palliative care needs of families of children who die from cancer: An Australian study. *Palliative Medicine, 22*, 59–69.

Moro, T., Kavanaugh, K., Savage, T., Reyes, M., Kimura, R., & Bhat, R. (2011). Parent decision making for life support for extremely premature infants: From the prenatal through end-of-life period. *Journal of Perinatal & Neonatal Nursing, 25*(1), 52–60.

Moules, N. J., Simonson, K., Fleiszer, A. R., Prins, M., & Glasgow, B. (2007). The soul of sorrow work: Grief and therapeutic interventions with families. *Journal of Family Nursing, 13*(1), 117–141.

Munn, J. C., & Zimmerman, S. (2006). A good death for residents of long-term care: Family members speak. *Journal of Social Work in End-of-Life & Palliative Care, 2*(3), 45–59.

Murray, S. A., Kendall, M., Boyd, K., & Sheikh, A. (2005). Illness trajectories and palliative care. *British Medical Journal, 330*(7498), 1007–1011.

Murray, S. A., & Sheikh, A. (2008). Care for all at the end of life. *British Medical Journal, 336*(7650), 958–959.

Namasivayam, P., Orb, A., & O'Connor, M. (2005). The challenges of caring for families of the terminally ill: Nurses' lived experience. *Contemporary Nurse, 19*(1-2), 169–180.

Nolbris, M., & Hellstrom, A. (2005). Siblings' needs and issues when a brother or sister dies of cancer. *Journal of Pediatric Oncology Nursing, 22*(4), 227–233.

Nordgren, L., & Olsson, H. (2004). Palliative care in a coronary care unit: A qualitative study of physicians' and nurses' perceptions. *Journal of Clinical Nursing, 13*(2), 185–193.

Norris, K., Merriman, M. P., Curtis, J. R., Asp, C., Tuholske, L., & Byock, I. R. (2007). Next of kin perspectives on the experience of end-of-life care in a community setting. *Journal of Palliative Medicine, 10*(5), 1101–1115.

Northouse, L. L., Katapodi, M. C., Song, L., Zhang, L., & Mood, D. W. (2010). Interventions with family caregivers of cancer patients: Meta-analysis of randomized trials. *CA: A Cancer Journal for Clinicians, 60*, 317–339.

O'Connor, M., Peters, L., Lee, S., & Webster, C. (2005). Palliative care work, between death and discharge. *Journal of Palliative Care, 21*(2), 97–102.

Oliver, D., Porock, D., Demiris, G., & Courtney, K. (2005). Patient and family involvement in hospice interdisciplinary teams. *Journal of Palliative Care, 21*(4), 270–276.

Osse, B. H., Vernooij Dassen, M. J., Schade, E., & Grol, R. P. (2006). Problems experienced by the informal caregivers of cancer patients and their needs for support. *Cancer Nursing, 29*(5), 378–390.

Pector, E. A. (2004a). How bereaved multiple-birth parents cope with hospitalization, homecoming, disposition for deceased, and attachment to survivors. *Journal of Perinatology, 24,* 714–772.

Pector, E. A. (2004b). Views of bereaved multiple-birth parents on life support decisions, the dying process, and discussions surrounding death. *Journal of Perinatology, 24,* 4–10.

Perreault, A., Fothergill Bourbonnais, F., & Fiset, V. (2004). The experience of family members caring for a dying loved one. *International Journal of Palliative Nursing, 10*(3), 133–143.

Pochard, F., Azoulay, E., Chevret, S., Lemaire, F., Hubert, P., Canoui, P.,...Schlemmer, B. (2001). Symptoms of anxiety and depression in family members of intensive care unit patients: Ethical hypothesis regarding decision-making capacity. *Critical Care Medicine, 29*(10), 1893–1897.

Price, A. M. (2004). Intensive care nurses' experiences of assessing and dealing with patients' psychological needs. *Nursing in Critical Care, 9*(3), 134–142.

Price, J., Jordan, J., Prior, L., & Parkes, J. (2011). Living through the death of a child: A qualitative study of bereaved parents' experiences. *International Journal of Nursing Studies, 48*(11), 1384–1392.

Proot, I. M., AbuSaad, H. H., Crebolder, H. F., Goldsteen, M., Luker, K. A., & Widdershoven, G. A. (2003). Vulnerability of family caregivers in terminal palliative care at home; balancing between burden and capacity. *Scandinavian Journal of Caring Sciences, 17*(2), 113–121.

Redinbaugh, E. M., Baum, A., Tarbell, S., & Arnold, R. (2003). End-of-life caregiving: What helps family caregivers cope? *Journal of Palliative Medicine, 6*(6), 901–909.

Registered Nurses' Association of Ontario. (2011). Best practice guidelines: End-of-life care during the last days and hours. Toronto, ON: Author. Retrieved from http://rnao.ca/sites/rnao-ca/files/End-of-Life_Care_During_the_Last_Days_and_Hours_0.pdf

Riley, J., & Fenton, G. (2007). A terminal diagnosis: The carers' perspective. *CPR, 7*(2), 86–91.

Rini, A., & Loriz, L. (2007). Anticipatory mourning in parents with a child who dies while hospitalized. *Journal of Pediatric Nursing, 22*(4), 272–282.

Robinson, C. A. (1996). Health care relationships revisited. *Journal of Family Nursing, 2*(2), 152–173.

Robinson, C. A. (2011). Advance care planning: Re-visioning our ethical approach. *Canadian Journal of Nursing Research, 43*(2), 18–37.

Robinson, C. A. (2012). "Our best hope is a cure." Hope in the context of advance care planning. *Palliative & Supportive Care, 10,* 75–82.

Robinson, C. A., Pesut, B., & Bottorff, J. L. (2012). Supporting rural family palliative caregivers. *Journal of Family Nursing, 18*(4), 467–490.

Robinson, M. R., Thiel, M. M., Backus, M. M., & Meyer, E. C. (2006). Matters of spirituality at the end of life in the pediatric intensive care unit. *Pediatrics, 118*(3), e719–e729.

Rodger, M. L., Sherwood, P., O'Connor, M., & Leslie, G. (2007). Living beyond the unanticipated sudden death of a partner: A phenomenological study. *Omega: Journal of Death and Dying, 54*(2), 107–133.

Rosenberg, A. R., Baker, K. S., Syrjala, K., & Wolfe, J. (2012). Systematic review of psychosocial morbidities among bereaved parents of children with cancer. *Pediatric Blood & Cancer, 58*(4), 503–512.

Royak-Schaler, R., Gadalla, S. M., Lemkau, J. P., Ross, D. D., Alexander, C., & Scott, D. (2006). Journal club. Family perspectives on communication with healthcare providers during end-of-life cancer care. *Oncology Nursing Forum, 33*(4), 753–760.

Selman, L., Harding, R., Beynon, T., Hodson, F., Coady, E., Hazeldine, C.,...Higginson, I. J. (2007). Improving end-of-life care for patients with chronic heart failure: "Let's hope it'll get better, when I know in my heart of hearts it won't." *Heart, 93*(8), 963–967.

Sharman, M., Meert, K. L., & Sarnaik, A. P. (2005). What influences parents' decisions to limit or withdraw life support? *Pediatric Critical Care Medicine, 6*(5), 513–518.

Sherwood, P. R., Given, B., Doorenbos, A. Z., & Given, C. W. (2004). Forgotten voices: Lessons from bereaved caregivers of persons with a brain tumour...including commentary by Krishnasamy M. *International Journal of Palliative Nursing, 10*(2), 67–75.

Shiozaki, M., Morita, T., Hirai, K., Sakaguchi, Y., Tsuneto, S., & Shima, Y. (2005). Why are bereaved family members dissatisfied with specialised inpatient palliative care service? A nationwide qualitative study. *Palliative Medicine, 19*(4), 319–327.

Singer, P., Martin, D. K., & Kelner, M. (1999). Quality end-of-life care: Patients' perspectives. *Journal of the American Medical Association, 281*(2), 163–168.

Skene, C. (1998). Individualised bereavement care. *Paediatric Nursing, 10*(10), 13–16.

Skilbeck, J. K., Payne, S. A., Ingleton, M. C., Nolan, M., Carey, I., & Hanson, A. (2005). An exploration of family carers' experience of respite services in one specialist palliative care unit. *Palliative Medicine, 19*(8), 610–618.

Stajduhar, K. I. (2003). Examining the perspectives of family members involved in the delivery of palliative care at home. *Journal of Palliative Care, 19*(1), 27–35.

Stajduhar, K., Funk, L., Jakobsson, E., & Ohlen, J. (2010). A critical analysis of health promotion and "empowerment" in the context of palliative family care-giving. *Nursing Inquiry, 17*(3), 221–230.

Stajduhar, K Funk, L., Toye, C., Grande, G. E., Soun, S., & Todd, C. J. (2010). Part 1: Home based family caregiving at the end of life: A comprehensive review of published quantitative research (1998–2008). *Palliative Medicine, 24*(6), 573–593.

Stajduhar, K. I., Martin, W. L., Barwich, D., & Fyles, G. (2008). Factors influencing family caregivers' ability to cope with providing end-of-life cancer care at home. *Cancer Nursing, 31*(1), 77–85.

Steele, R. (2002). Experiences of families in which a child has a prolonged terminal illness: Modifying factors. *International Journal of Palliative Nursing, 8*(9), 418–434.

Steele, R. (2005a). Navigating uncharted territory: Experiences of families when a child is dying. *Journal of Palliative Care, 21*(1), 35–43.

Steele, R. (2005b). Strategies used by families to navigate uncharted territory when a child is dying. *Journal of Palliative Care, 21*(2), 103–110.

Steele, R., & Davies, B. (2006). Impact on parents when a child has a progressive, life-threatening illness. *International Journal of Palliative Nursing, 12*(12), 576–585.

Steele, R., Davies, B., Collins, J. B., & Cook, K. (2005). End-of-life care in a children's hospice program. *Journal of Palliative Care, 21*(1), 5–11.

Steinhauser, K. E., Clipp, E. C., McNeilly, M., Christakis, N. A., McIntyre, L. M., & Tulsky, J. A. (2000). In search of a good death: Observations of patients, families, and providers. *Annals of Internal Medicine, 132*(10), 825–832.

Surkan, P. J., Kreicbergs, U., Valdimarsdottir, U., Nyberg, U., Onelov, E., Dickman, P. W., & Steineck, G. (2006). Perceptions of inadequate health care and feelings of guilt in parents after the death of a child to a malignancy: A population-based long-term follow-up. *Journal of Palliative Medicine, 9*(2), 317–331.

Tan, J. S., Docherty, S. L., Barfield, R., & Brandon, D. H. (2012). Addressing parental bereavement support needs at the end of life for infants with complex chronic conditions. *Journal of Palliative Medicine, 15*(5), 579–584.

Tang, S. T., Liu, T., Lai, M., & McCorkle, R. (2005). Discrepancy in the preferences of place of death between terminally ill cancer patients and their primary family caregivers in Taiwan. *Social Science & Medicine, 61*(7), 1560–1566.

Thompson, G. N., McClement, S. E., & Daeninck, P. J. (2006). "Changing lanes": Facilitating the transition from curative to palliative care. *Journal of Palliative Care, 22*(2), 91–98.

Tilden, V. P., Tolle, S. W., Garland, M. J., & Nelson, C. A. (1995). Decisions about life-sustaining treatment. *Archives of Internal Medicine, 155*(6), 633–638.

Tomlinson, D., Capra, M., Gammon, J., Volpe, J., Barrera, M., Hinds, P. S.,...Sung, L. (2006). Parental decision making in pediatric cancer end-of-life care: Using focus group methodology as a prephase to seek participant design input. *European Journal of Oncology Nursing, 10*(3), 198–206.

Topf, L., Robinson, C. A., & Bottorff, J. L. (2013). When a desired home death does not occur: The consequences of broken promises. *Journal of Palliative Medicine, 16*(8), 875-880.

Torke, A. M., Garas, N. S., Sexson, W., & Branch, W. T., Jr. (2005). Medical care at the end of life: Views of African American patients in an urban hospital. *Journal of Palliative Medicine, 8*(3), 593–602.

Vint, P. E. (2005). An exploration of the support available to children who may wish to visit a critically adult [sic] in ITU. *Intensive & Critical Care Nursing, 21*(3), 149–159.

Wall, R. J., Engelberg, R. A., Gries, C. J., Glavan, B., & Curtis, J. R. (2007). Spiritual care of families in the intensive care unit. *Critical Care Medicine, 35*(4), 1084–1090.

Webster, J., & Kristjanson, L. (2002). "But isn't it depressing?" The vitality of palliative care. *Journal of Palliative Care, 18*(1), 15–24.

Weidner, N. J., Cameron, M., Lee, R. C., McBride, J., Mathias, E. J., & Byczkowski, T. L. (2011). End-of-life care for the dying child: What matters most to parents. *Journal of Palliative Care, 27*(4), 279–286.

White, D. B., & Luce, J. M. (2004). Palliative care in the intensive care unit: Barriers, advances, and unmet needs. *Critical Care Clinics, 20*(3), 329–343.

Widger, K., & Picot, C. (2008). Parents' perceptions of the quality of pediatric and perinatal end-of-life care. *Pediatric Nursing, 34*(1), 53–58.

Widger, K., Steele, R., Oberle, K., & Davies, B. (2009). Exploring the Supportive Care Model as a framework for pediatric palliative care. *Journal of Hospice and Palliative Nursing, 11*(4), 209–216.

Wiegand, D. L. (2006). Withdrawal of life-sustaining therapy after sudden, unexpected life-threatening illness or injury: Interactions between patients' families, healthcare providers, and the healthcare system. *American Journal of Critical Care, 15*(2), 178–187.

Wisten, A., & Zingmark, K. (2007). Supportive needs of parents confronted with sudden cardiac death: A qualitative study. *Resuscitation, 74*(1), 68–74.

Wollin, J. A., Yates, P. M., & Kristjanson, L. J. (2006). Supportive and palliative care needs identified by multiple sclerosis patients and their families. *International Journal of Palliative Nursing, 12*(1), 20–26.

Woodgate, R. L. (2006). Living in a world without closure: Reality for parents who have experienced the death of a child. *Journal of Palliative Care, 22*(2), 75–82.

World Health Organization. (2006). WHO definition of palliative care. Retrieved from http://www.who.int/cancer/palliative/definition/en

Wright, L. M., & Leahey, M. (2005). *Nurses and families: A guide to family assessment and intervention* (4th ed.). Philadelphia: F. A. Davis.

Chapter Web Sites

- *American Academy of Hospice and Palliative Medicine:* http://www.aahpm.org
- *American Association of Colleges of Nursing End-of-Life Nursing Education Consortium (ELNEC) Project:* http://www.aacn.nche.edu/elnec
- *The American Geriatrics Society:* http://www.americangeriatrics.org
- *The Association for Children's Palliative Care:* http://www.act.org.uk
- *Association for Death Education and Counseling:* http://www.adec.org
- *Canadian Hospice Palliative Care Association:* http://www.chpca.net
- *Canadian Organization for Rare Disorders:* http://www.cord.ca
- *Canadian Network of Palliative Care for Children:* http://cnpcc.ca
- *Canadian Virtual Hospice:* http://www.virtualhospice.ca
- *The Compassionate Friends of Canada Resource Links:* http://www.tcfcanada.net
- *Complementary Medicine Education and Outcomes (CAMEO) Program:* http://www.bccancer.bc.ca/RES/ResearchPrograms/cameo/default.htm
- *Education on Palliative and End-of-Life Care EPEC Project:* http://www.epec.net
- *End of Life/Palliative Education Resource Center:* http://www.eperc.mcw.edu
- *European Organization for Rare Diseases:* http://www.eurordis.org
- *GriefNet.org:* http://griefnet.org
- *Hospice and Palliative Nurses Association:* http://www.hpna.org
- *Institute of Medicine of the National Academies:* http://www.iom.edu
- *National Hospice and Palliative Care Association:* http://www.nhpco.org
- *National Organization for Rare Disorders:* http://www.rarediseases.org
- *Promoting Excellence in End-of-Life Care (tools):* http://www.promotingexcellence.org
- *Registered Nurses' Association of Ontario (Best Practice Guidelines):* http://rnao.ca/bpg
- *World Health Organization:* http://www.who.int/cancer/palliative/definition/en

chapter 11

Trauma and Family Nursing

Deborah Padgett Coehlo, PhD, C-PNP, PMHS, CFLE

Critical Concepts

- Trauma is a key experience affecting the family system.

- The threat or fear of death or serious injury is a salient feature of trauma.

- Post-traumatic stress disorder (PTSD), which is a response to trauma, is more likely to develop when resiliency traits are lacking.

- PTSD can be acute or chronic and can occur months, even years, after a disaster or traumatic event such as war.

- The Ecological Systems Theory can guide nursing assessment and interventions to help families dealing with trauma.

- When one or more family members are traumatized by an experience, all family members and family relationships can be affected.

- The more severe the trauma an individual family member suffers, the more likely the other members of the family are to suffer secondary trauma.

- The family response to trauma of one or more of its members cannot be understood or treated by focusing on individual family members alone. Family members can provide key contextual information about past traumatic events and experiences that help explain current responses.

- Community systems can prevent, treat, and measure negative outcomes to traumatic events. If community agencies are not well trained and prepared, communities will suffer.

- Larger political and social systems can influence and be influenced by individual, family, and community trauma. If nations experience severe trauma, they, as a whole, show signs of PTSD.

- Nursing focuses on the individual, family, community, and societal reactions to trauma in order to optimize positive outcomes and prevent or treat negative implications.

Trauma has been an increasing area of attention across the field of mental health for the past two decades. Between the advanced understanding of brain function and general physiology, and the mind and body response to severe and/or prolonged stress; and the increase in trauma experienced by families through war, natural disasters, and family violence, the need to understand, prevent, treat, and monitor the effects of trauma on individuals and families has never been more vital. Further, the effects of trauma transcend individuals and families, but also affect communities, and the broader society. Trauma influences future generations as the effects influence individual family genetics, and community and societal cultures. The negative effects of trauma are most profound during early childhood development, touching every domain of development, with the potential of negative developmental outcomes in adulthood, such as higher rates of mental illness, unemployment, and failed relationships. The diagnosis of post-traumatic stress disorder (PTSD) has grown significantly over the past decade, as well as the understanding of differences in symptoms across developmental ages and stages. Whereas the key symptoms of reexperiencing the trauma through painful memories and nightmares, hypervigilance, and emotional instability are common to adults, children are more likely to react with withdrawal and mood irregularity. These symptoms cross ethnic groups and time. The number of individuals with PTSD in turn affects communities. Larger cultures and societies shift as the number of trauma victims grows, adding other negative consequences, including poor health, higher rates of other mental health disorders, and an increase in family violence. The care of trauma in families, therefore, centers around preventing trauma when possible, and when not preventable, working toward positive rather than negative outcomes, building resiliency traits in individuals and families, and helping individuals and families work toward understanding the positive meaning traumatic events can have on all of us. For example, families who experience trauma together, such as those experiencing natural disasters or terrorism together, have a stronger connection to each other than those who never had these experiences (Ozer, Best, Lipsey, & Weiss, 2003). This chapter considers developing knowledge about trauma and nurses' key role in the field of trauma and emphasizes the importance of preventing, treating early, and encouraging resilience and the ability to make meaning out of negative events. This chapter also stresses an understanding of secondary trauma, or the negative effects of witnessing trauma of others, whether that other person is a stranger, family, or a patient of a nurse. This discussion is particularly salient for nurses, because they are some of the most likely professionals to encounter traumatized victims in their everyday practice.

The American Psychological Association began to categorize symptoms of PTSD in 1980. Since that time, researchers and clinicians have identified the complexity of this disorder, and the lifelong, intergenerational impact of repeated and prolonged trauma experienced by individuals, families, communities, and societies. PTSD was a diagnosis first recognized in 1980. Since this publication, research has attempted to clarify and expand the diagnosis to cover different categories of trauma, such as combat, horrific accidents, and child abuse; different content, such as domestic violence, natural disasters, and war; and different cultures, such as genocide victims (Dyregrov, Gupta, Gjestad, & Mukanoheli, 2000) and victims of natural disasters across cultures and across time. The DSM-IV and DSM-IV-TR included PTSD as a subcategory under anxiety disorders, including three categories of symptoms (APA, 2000; McNally, 2004):

1. Reexperiencing the trauma
2. Avoidance and numbing
3. Increased arousal

The DSM-5 has taken PTSD out of the category of anxiety and developed a separate category titled Trauma and Stressor Related Disorders (Friedman, Resick, Bryant, Strain, Horowitz, & Spiegel, 2011; Schmid, Petermann, & Fegert, 2013). The scope has been expanded to include both experiencing a traumatic event and witnessing or repeatedly hearing about a traumatic event. Further, the DSM-5 has included four categories of symptoms (APA, 2013):

1. Intrusion of thoughts about the trauma
2. Avoidance of discussion or other stimulus reminding the person of the trauma
3. Increased arousal or sensory sensitivity
4. Negative cognitions and moods

Today, it is estimated that up to 10% of the general population across the world meets the criteria for a diagnosis of PTSD, with areas experiencing war or severe natural disasters experiencing the highest rates. When further divided between geographical areas, ages, and genders, the prevalence rates vary with risks higher for women and adolescents, and lower in Asian countries (U.S. Department of Veterans Affairs, 2007). These rates, however, are lower when veterans are separated out of the general population. The National Vietnam Readjustment Study of 30,000 veterans of this war found that 31% of men and 27% of women who participated in the Vietnam War had a lifetime prevalence of PTSD (Kulka et al., 1990). When evaluating 11,441 veterans from the Gulf War, only 10% were found to have symptoms consistent with PTSD (Kang, Natelson, Mahan, Lee, & Murphy, 2003). Veterans returning from Iraq and Afghanistan appear to be following this pattern, with a current prevalence rate for PTSD of 13% (Tanielian & Jaycox, 2008). When considering children and adolescents, it is important to note that most PTSD is caused by (1) abuse and neglect across time, (2) witnessing violence within the home and/or neighborhood, and (3) experiencing traumatic events such as motor vehicle accidents and natural disasters (Salmon, Meiser-Stedman, Glucksmann, Thompson, Dalgleish, & Smith, 2011).

The number of studies on individual trauma and outcomes has increased in the past decade, as has awareness that PTSD is not limited to individuals, but rather affects individuals, families, communities, and societies. The understanding of the political and societal influences on the diagnosis and treatment, and continued research in this area, explains in part the continued need to explore trauma and the relationship to family health. The extent of damage to physical and mental health caused by trauma has now been realized. This chapter uses the Ecological Systems Model (Bronfenbrenner, 2005) to explore current understanding of risk and protective factors of PTSD, identify those experiencing symptoms, and discuss treatment strategies to reduce symptoms and enhance recovery. Family nurses are in a key position to understand, recognize, prevent, and treat trauma at multiple levels. Case studies at the conclusion of this chapter illustrate the complexities of trauma and its effect on all family members.

THEORY APPLIED TO PTSD

Trauma is treated differently now than it was in the past. Historically, health care practitioners considered trauma to be a form of hysteria, meriting ineffective treatments such as hysterectomies. Currently, the approach recognizes the modern understanding of trauma as a complex stress disorder with a number of underlying theories applicable. For purposes of this book, we delve into PTSD using the Ecological Theory (Bronfenbrenner, 1984, 1995: Bronfenbrenner & Lerner, 2004) as the underlying model to guide practice. The Family Systems Theory likewise is helpful.

Ecological Theory

In this model, Bronfenbrenner identifies four systems that interact together: the *microsystem*, *mesosystem*, *macrosystem*, and *exosystem*. He later added the system of time, or the *chronosystem* (Bronfenbrenner, 1996), to describe the impact of history and time on individuals, families, communities, and societies. Time is integrated as a concept within each of the four other ecological systems. The understanding of the impact of trauma on a micro to exosystem level helps practitioners and policy makers understand the interconnections between trauma and abuse to individuals, families, communities, and societies, and the impact of that trauma across time, geographical and cultural systems, and generations. Trauma tends to repeat itself if nothing intervenes to stop the pattern. Interventions intended to stop and/or alter these patterns are much more effective when chosen and implemented with the complexity and interconnections between systems in mind. See Figure 11-1 for a visual portrayal of Bronfenbrenner's Ecological Theory.

Microsystem

The *microsystem* describes the individual and the systems within that individual, including physiological (i.e., respiratory, cardiovascular), developmental, and psychological (i.e., sensory perceptions, memory). The role of trauma in violating and damaging physical and mental well-being and negatively affecting development of children and adults is no longer questioned. The negative impact of trauma on individuals ranges from interference with healthy development of attachment to physical and mental illness across the life span (Afifi, Boman, Fleisher, & Sareen, 2009). Although understanding the impact of trauma on individuals is important to understanding family trauma, care of these individuals in isolation is less effective than providing care within the context of the family. The *microsystem* provides a beginning knowledge to family trauma, but the *mesosystem* adds a deeper understanding.

Mesosystem

The effect of trauma on any one individual within the family has a significant impact on family development and family functioning. As mentioned earlier, the DSM-IV-TR (APA, 2000) expanded its definition of trauma from an individual perspective to a broader definition that included experiencing, witnessing, being confronted, or being informed about an act of violence against others (APA, 2000). This broader definition has been supported by the

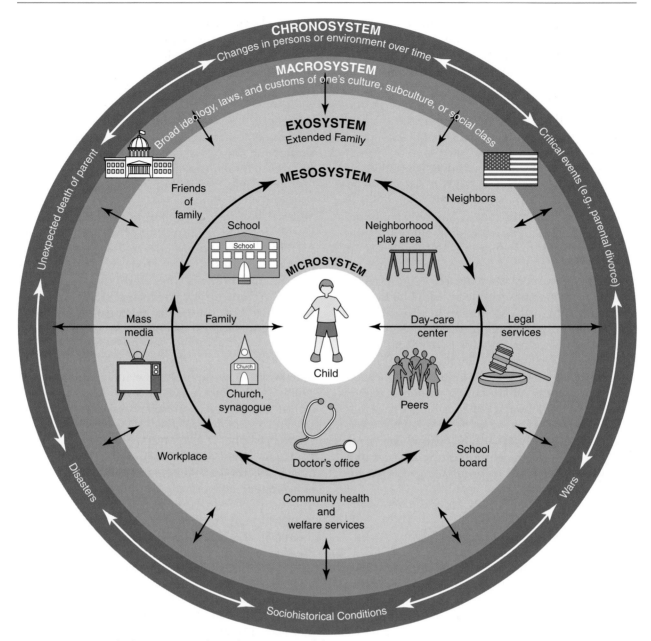

FIGURE 11-1 Bronfenbrenner's Ecological Systems Model.

DSM-5, with increased separation between developmental stages and reactions to trauma (APA, 2013). This definition includes trauma experienced by families directly or witnessed by other family members, expanding the experience beyond the *micro* level to the *meso* level of reaction. For example, children's reactions to trauma and their resiliency against PTSD are shaped in part by family experiences and reactions. Family members witnessing trauma can and do experience symptoms of PTSD. The act of witnessing includes direct observation and hearing about traumatic events repeatedly from family members. Further, family members' reactions to a traumatic event have a direct impact on whether or not other family members will experience symptoms of PTSD. For example, if parents cannot regulate their own reactions and cannot support the child because of their own PTSD, the child is at higher risk for developing symptoms of PTSD. Likewise, if a parent lacks support and positive coping strategies, he is less likely to be able to provide support to the child.

Macrosystem

Trauma at the macro level includes all trauma within a community. This level of trauma not only influences individuals (micro) and families (meso), but has an impact on how a community reacts and recovers from trauma. Over the past two decades, the growing disparity between mental health and access to mental health services within a community has been well documented (National Institute of Mental Health, 2008). Traumatic events within schools, for example, have increased the awareness of the need for more in-depth and comprehensive mental health services to prevent these events and to be available to treat the victims following these events. Schools have been identified as key community systems that can provide both prevention and treatment services. Over 60% of schools already attempt to address trauma at a community, or *macrosystem*, level through prevention services, and community preparedness such as town meetings and educational programs, provision of temporary food and shelter following a disaster, counseling services, and/or behavioral programs (Taylor, Weist, & DeLoach, 2012). Working with schools when it comes to trauma care improves outcomes, especially for traumatized youth (Cohen et al., 2009).

Exosystem

The exosystem includes the larger culture and government or laws and justice within a culture. The exosystem is touched by and touches on individuals, families, and communities. For example, the cultural reactions and legal responses to a natural disaster have grave implications for individuals, families, and communities. Consider the response by the government to Hurricane Katrina in 2005, with the delays and the disorganization during and after the disaster. These gaps in services were believed to be a contributing factor to the high rates of PTSD in survivors (Mills, Edmondson, & Park, 2007). Researchers have explored the dysregulation and hyperarousal of individuals during this time, and have found that similar processes can and do occur at a larger, systemic level. Judith Warner, in a 2010 *New York Times* article (Warner, 2010),

observed that the large-scale dysfunction of federal regulatory systems, including the banking meltdown, collapse of the housing market, and the failure of levees during Hurricane Katrina, resulted in the United States as a *country* struggling with symptoms of PTSD for several months after the hurricane hit the shores of Louisiana.

Family Systems Theory

The Family Systems Theory focuses on the interaction between family members, and the impact of an individual's health and behavioral responses on other family members, as well as other family members' reaction and health impact on individuals. The metaphor of a wind chime is commonly used to describe the Family Systems Theory, with one chime being struck by other chimes to make music or cacophony. The wind flowing through the wind chimes represents the stressors that flow through every family. The wind can be a gentle breeze, or low stress level, or higher winds, similar to high stress and less controlled stress levels. The Family Systems Theory, when considered through an ecological looking glass, can help explain the impact of trauma within and surrounding families. The remainder of the chapter describes the types of trauma that individuals, families, communities, and societies at large face currently, along with implications for family nurses.

EARLY TRAUMA

Early trauma shapes early attachment to others, developmental progress, and early brain development. In the context of the Ecological Model, the impact of trauma in the individual child (micro) is strongly influenced by the responses of the parent(s) (macro) level.

Attachment

Because early trauma has been shown to interfere with healthy development of attachment, attachment theories are used as a basis of research and understanding. Early attachment disorders are commonly linked to later issues with developmental success and physical and mental well-being. Bowlby, an early researcher and theorist in the area of attachment, identified the importance of early attachment and the effect on later personality development, interpersonal relationships, self-esteem, and self-regulation of emotions, daily function, and behavior (Bowlby, 1973). Normally, an infant trusts caregivers to provide a safe environment to explore. When trauma occurs, such as abuse and severe neglect from caregivers, and when that trauma is repeated and/or severe, an infant loses the basic coping and adaptation skills of compartmentalizing threats to self, therefore becoming disorganized, disconnected, dysregulated, isolated, and later struggling with separation between reality and fantasy.

Heller and LaPierre (2012), in describing their developmental trauma theory, categorized this early traumatic interference with attachment by describing five core areas of concern: (1) interference with connection to others, (2) lack of attunement or ability to recognize physical and emotional needs, (3) lack of trust in caregivers and the environment, (4) difficulty with boundaries between self and others, and (5) difficulty developing a sense of love and healthy sexuality. Table 11-1 illustrates the Neuroaffective Relational Model with the Five Core Needs developed by Heller and LaPierre. More specific symptoms of trauma-induced attachment disorder include the following:

- Absence of self-regulation—inconsistent and unpredictable patterns of eating and sleeping
- Lack of response to caregivers—poor eye contact, lack of response to consoling measures
- Lack of response to the environment—inability to pretend play, interact with toys, and/or

Table 11-1	Neuroaffective Relational Model Five Core Needs
Core Need	**Description**
Connection	Lack of ability to form healthy connection with caregivers or significant support people
Attunement	Lack of ability to recognize physical and emotional needs
Trust	Lack of ability to trust others
Boundaries	Difficulty setting healthy boundaries
Deep sense of love and sexuality	Inability to form deep loving relationships, and, as adults, connect deep love with healthy sexuality

Source: Heller & LaPierre, 2012.

experience shared pleasure with others (Heller & LaPierre, 2012; Joubert, Webster, & Hackett, 2012)

If untreated, children experiencing trauma struggle in cognitive, emotional, and social development (Heller & LaPierre, 2012; Joubert et al., 2012; Perry & Pollard, 1998).

Developmental Trauma Theory

The developmental trauma theory (Heller & LaPierre, 2012) describes the survival strategies individuals (micro level) learn to cope with trauma; it expands the understanding of the negative impact of trauma on attachment. These coping strategies interfere with healthy development. For example, whenever an individual experiences a severe threat, a fight-or-flight response is activated. When repeated trauma occurs, a state of constant fear develops causing distinct physiological and psychological changes. At the core, stress hormones from the adrenal glands are released stimulating the sympathetic nervous system. The neurological system, in response, alerts the brain to stay in survival mode. Because this system is activated continuously when repeated trauma occurs, the individual's ability to feel safe is threatened, resulting in a state of constant hyperarousal. The sympathetic nervous system eventually becomes overwhelmed, leading to an abrupt shift to the parasympathetic system, and the individual shuts down, withdraws, becomes numb, disassociates, or falls into sleep. Sleep, eating, and digestive patterns are affected, and excitable behavior builds again with the next remembered or experienced trauma. Emotions range from hyperstimulated (i.e., hysteria or excessive, inconsolable crying) to numbness (no reaction to the environment). Without resolution, the individual develops a state of fear, and gradually loses the ability to regulate emotional and autonomic reactions. If uninterrupted, the young child will develop secondary complications, including anxiety, shame, isolation, mood dysregulation, and uncontrolled anger or explosive outbursts (Alisic, Jongmaks, Van Wesel, & Kleber, 2011; Salmond, Meiser-Stedman, Glucksmann, Thompson, Dalgleish, & Smith, 2011).

As a child develops into adulthood, he may try to adapt to those feelings by abusing substances or avoiding emotions (Dansky, Byrne, & Brady, 1999;

Heller & LaPierre, 2012). The underlying fear remains; the threat to self and to the ability to survive is not over. Symptoms emerge over time, including the following (Dansky et al., 1999; Glaser, 2000; Heller & LaPierre, 2012; Perry & Pollard, 1998):

- Lack of affect
- Feelings of shame
- Separation from others
- Avoidance of emotionally disturbing situations or people
- Overintellectualizing and avoiding of emotions
- Lack of attunement or awareness of bodily and related needs
- Fear of being alone while at the same time feeling overwhelmed by others
- Fear of death and illness
- Fear of their own anger
- Fear of intimacy
- Strong need to control
- Desire for altered states and disassociation
- Cognitive impairments, including difficulty with auditory processing, memory, and attention
- Feelings of helplessness
- Hypovigilance or hypervigilance

Physical symptoms of prolonged and repeated trauma in childhood include the following:

- Disrupted sleep
- Eating disorders
- Panic disorders
- Obsessive-compulsive disorders
- Rage
- Depression
- Addiction
- Cardiovascular disorders
- Autoimmune disorders

A pattern emerges across time. Figure 11-2 illustrates the developmental pattern of maladaptation to early trauma.

Studies on the impact of war, terror, and unexpected natural disasters on children have resulted in the identification of the term *disaster syndrome* (Smith, 2013). This syndrome is described as a combination of symptoms of PTSD—including anxiety, dissociation, depression—and grief from loss of people, support, routines, and assumptions regarding safety and regularity, and parental response. Parental response is influenced by parents' prior diagnosis of mental illness, prior coping

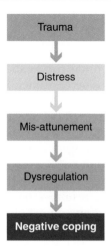

FIGURE 11-2 *Developmental pattern of maladaptation to early trauma.*

strategies, and number of past traumatic experiences. Children respond to their family members' emotional and physical changes related to trauma. When an individual (micro level) experiences trauma over time, his interaction with others (meso level) and his ability to interact in a functional manner with his community (macro level) are altered.

The human desire for regulation of the autonomic nervous system, with a return to balance, is strong. Individuals are highly motivated to find this balance, and will pursue strategies to achieve this goal through either positive measures (e.g., healthy patterns of sleep, eating, exercise, meditation or yoga, and spiritual connection), or negative measures (e.g., drug-seeking behavior, obsessive thinking patterns, or avoidance patterns) (Dansky et al., 1999). These negative patterns interfere with every stage of development, primarily altering cognitive, emotional, communication, and social domains. Although young infants cannot consciously think about their reactions to trauma, their emotions and related autonomic reactions are affected in a measurable way (Heller & LaPierre, 2012). Infants have bottom-up responses, or responses starting with brainstem or autonomic reactions to external threat, moving up toward emotional responses. Adults, in contrast, experience trauma initially from thought, or the cortex of the brain, and move down to emotional response, and finally autonomic or brainstem reaction. This is considered top-down reaction. Another important differentiation between infants and adults is that infants tend to have a broad interpretation of experiences, whereas adults are able to separate experiences and feelings between experiences. The difference in reaction is caused by the difference in development of pathways from the frontal cortex to the brainstem as the brain develops across time. The pathways are reinforced by experiences and interactions in the environment. Figure 11-3 illustrates bottom-up and top-down responses to trauma.

This variance in response to trauma is important to understand: adults who experience trauma can make a distinction between different experiences in their lives, and as a result *feel* badly about a specific experience; infants and young children cannot differentiate between experiences and therefore when they experience trauma, they tend to think *they are* bad (Heller & LaPierre, 2012). Young children and adults, however, if left untreated following a trauma, can regress back to thinking and feeling they are bad as a global response to trauma.

Early Trauma and Brain Development

The understanding of the impact of early trauma on brain development has led to detailed study of the impact on brain development and plasticity, or the ability of the brain to recover from injury. When considering trauma or major stress, the body is governed by two main systems: the neurological system and the endocrine system. These two systems ensure survival of the individual through stimulation of the sympathetic nervous system when the individual is threatened, and the parasympathetic nervous system when the individual is safe and relaxed. Hans Selye, a renowned theorist on stress, identified the connection between the hypothalamus, the pituitary gland, and the adrenal glands, now commonly referred to

as the HPA axis (Selye, 1976). To summarize this process, the hypothalamus links the nervous system to the pituitary system, which secretes hormones that regulate homeostasis. If homeostasis is not reached, the adrenal glands secrete the stress hormones, epinephrine and norepinephrine. These hormones stimulate the sympathetic nervous system, and the result is increased heart rate, dilation of pupils, relaxation of bronchial tubes, increased tension and circulation of blood to large muscles, and initial stimulation of the frontal cortex through a surge of dopamine, followed by bypassing the frontal cortex to the amygdala.

This bypass process encourages rapid action based on the previous experience of threats, and the assumption that the same threat has occurred and the same action for survival is needed. When this process is stimulated repeatedly and without resolution, the connection between the limbic system—where automatic actions based on emotions and repeated actions rather than thought occur—and the cortex—or the thinking part of the brain that includes judgment, creativity, and prediction of action on future consequences—is pruned. When the connection is pruned, sensory perception becomes scattered and disorganized. By bypassing the frontal cortex, the individual exchanges accuracy, judgment, and the ability to learn, for speed. The bypassed frontal cortex provides the individual with the executive functions of detailed assessment, regulation of emotion or thought, inhibition of inappropriate responses, internal speech, and problem-solving skills. Over time, an individual constantly facing threat through trauma develops a fearful identity, avoids relationships due to previous threats, has uncontrolled emotional outbursts

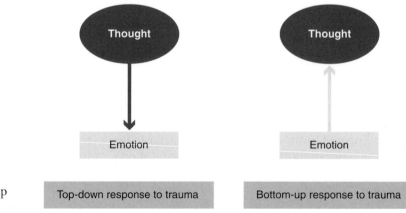

FIGURE 11-3 Top-down and Bottom-up reaction.

or withdrawal, disassociates from the present, and/or experiences depression. The hippocampus, which is key in neuroplasticity or the ability to generate new neurons and new neuron pathways (known as neurogenesis), is impaired. This process explains why many who experience prolonged and repeated trauma struggle with cognitive impairments, such as poor short-term memory, difficulty with concentration, difficulty learning new skills, and poor sensory integration, especially auditory processing (Anda et al., 2006). This process has been found to be more severe in both children and adults experiencing relational trauma, or trauma inflicted by relatives (meso level), than those experiencing trauma from inanimate objects (e.g., motor vehicle accidents) (Heller and LaPierre, 2012). This process is most damaging when the trauma experienced occurs early in life, and continues throughout childhood, causing an initial and prolonged damage to normal brain development (Alisic, Jongmaks, Van Wesel, & Kleber, 2011; Anda et al., 2006). For family nurses, it is important to assess the start and duration of any family trauma occurring to a child or young adult.

Early Childhood Trauma Creates Understanding of Adult Trauma

The impact of early trauma and the negative long-term outcomes has led to further study of the impact of childhood trauma on adult health. The Adverse Childhood Experiences Study (1996) provided landmark evidence that early trauma does indeed have negative consequences for adult health. This study was conducted as a collaboration between Kaiser Permanente and the Centers for Disease Control and Prevention (CDC), and entailed surveying 11,000 individuals across a decade, linking adverse childhood experiences with adult physical and mental health variables. The results revealed a relationship between the number of adverse childhood experiences and the number of comorbid outcomes, including adulthood depression, panic disorder, substance abuse, sexual promiscuity, relationship problems, and domestic violence (Anda et al., 2006). Figure 11-4 illustrates the relationship between adverse childhood experiences and adult comorbid conditions. The findings of this hallmark study led to a more in-depth understanding of the cumulative effect of repeated and numerous

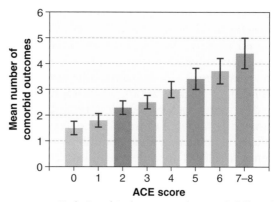

FIGURE 11-4 Relationship between adverse childhood experiences and comorbid conditions. Adverse childhood experiences include verbal, physical, or sexual abuse, as well as family dysfunction (e.g., an incarcerated, mentally ill, or substance-abusing family member; domestic violence; or absence of a parent because of divorce or separation). *(Source: Anda, Felitti, Bremner, Walker, Whitfield, Perry,...Giles [2006]. The enduring effects of abuse and related adverse experiences in childhood: A convergence of evidence from neurobiology and epidemiology. European Archives of Psychiatry & Clinical Neuroscience, 256, 174–186.)*

traumas experienced during childhood, and the effect on brain development.

Clearly, understanding early trauma and the negative impact on children and development allows professionals to grasp better the impact of traumatic events on adults. Studies have found that resiliency is one factor that determines which adults will continue to suffer from childhood trauma. Of interest is that the number of traumatic events is found to be consistently higher in men, but women have a higher incidence of PTSD following trauma. This is consistently true for civilian populations across geographical locations (Terleggen, Strebe, & Kleber, 2001). One theory is that women experience sexual assault and traumatic abuse from male partners, supporting the idea that relational trauma is more traumatic and more difficult to cope with than inanimate or nonrelational trauma (Seedat, Stein, & Carey, 2005).

Resiliency

Through the improved understanding of childhood trauma and related reactions, we now understand more fully the concept of resiliency, or why some who experience the same or similar event will adapt without any measure of physical or emotional damage, while others become severely and chronically disabled. The term *resilience* for purposes of this chapter refers to individuals who (1) have been exposed to a significant threat or adversity, and (2) manifest positive adaptation, or absence of poor adaptation, in spite of the adversity (Luthar, Cicchetti, & Becker, 2000). Research has focused on identifying factors or characteristics that are consistently found in those individuals found to be resilient. The factors most commonly cited as resiliency qualities include the following (Rutler, 1987; Williams, Lindsey, Kurtz, & Jarvis, 2001; Overland, 2011):

- Social connectedness and positive supportive relationships
- Competent parenting
- Absence of mental illness in caregiver(s)
- Easy to moderate temperament
- High intelligence
- Ego-resiliency, or the acquisition of a strong sense of self across the life span with or without trauma (Philippe, Laventure, Beaulieu-Pelletier, LeCours, & Lekes, 2011)
- Compassion
- Optimism
- Gratitude
- Determination
- Meaning and purpose in life
- Caring for self and attuning to own needs
- Trusting others to help
- Internal locus of control
- High self-esteem
- Strong self-efficacy
- Vicarious resiliency (Hernández, Gangsei, & Engstrom, 2007)

Research on resiliency continues. For example, Philippe et al. (2011) investigated 118 clients from an outpatient clinic in Canada, and found that if ego-resiliency traits were present before a traumatic event, then negative outcomes, including anxiety, depression, and self-harm, decreased by as much as 30%. While resiliency characteristics often precede the traumatic experience, this is not always the case. The question remains as to how to build resiliency in individuals facing trauma. Williams et al. (2001) completed an in-depth qualitative case study to explore why some high-risk teens who had run away from traumatic homes fared well, whereas others fared poorly. These authors found that those individuals who developed resiliency traits after the trauma recovered faster

and shifted to a positive, goal-directed life. Resiliency traits therefore should be assessed by family nurses to determine those that were present before the trauma, and reinforced, versus those that are lacking and need to be taught and supported. Resiliency can buffer the negative impacts of trauma on the individual's brain development.

FAMILY TRAUMA

Families experience trauma as a family and through individual members. This section discusses both (1) family trauma through disasters and war; and (2) individual experiences of trauma and their effect on family members. Each member of the family experiences trauma differently, with different symptoms, reactions, and needs for recovery. For example, both parents and children experience similar symptoms of PTSD, but adults are more likely to experience reexperiencing the event through nightmares and flashbacks, whereas children are more likely to avoid similar experiences (e.g., riding in a car after a car accident) or talking about the event. Both children and adults experience hyperarousal, or the HPA axis response to stress (Heller & LaPierre, 2012). When this occurs, parenting often becomes overwhelming as children overreact to environmental stimuli, and parents overreact to the stressors of parenting. Each family member in turn can easily be misdiagnosed as depressed, anxious, or having attention-deficit hyperactivity disorder (ADHD) and the opportunity for effective and comprehensive treatment is therefore lost. The National Center for PTSD (2010) has identified seven key areas that affect family functioning when one or more members are diagnosed with PTSD:

1. Increased sympathy by family members, which may provide support for the family member with PTSD or prolong feelings of victimization.
2. Increased negative feelings about the person with PTSD. These feelings are often triggered by changes in the person with PTSD, from changes in mood regulation, to depression, to explosive outbursts.
3. Avoidance is a common reaction by individuals with PTSD and by family members. Family members often circumvent talking about anything related to the trauma, and

may dodge other topics hoping to avoid angry outbursts. Individuals with PTSD tend to avoid social situations due to fear of not fitting in or being questioned about the trauma. This, in turn, leads to social isolation of all family members as they try to support the individual with PTSD.

4. Depression is common among individuals with PTSD and their family members. The longer the symptoms of PTSD last, the higher the risk for depression in family members.

5. Anger is common among family members, as they struggle to cope with changes in the person with PTSD and anger that expectations are not being met.

6. Guilt is common for family members as they feel helpless to change negative family functioning and find themselves feeling angry about the individual's illness.

7. Health problems increase in individuals with PTSD and their family members, including substance abuse, reduction in healthy immune response, and negative effects of poor eating habits, poor sleep, smoking, and lack of healthy exercise.

These outcomes can leave parents feeling inadequate, and spouses feeling angry, guilty, and disillusioned. Nurses are often at the forefront of trauma care, as they encounter family members during traumatic events from war, natural disasters, family violence and abuse, and severe illness or unanticipated accidents.

Families Affected by War

Since the turn of the century, the nature of war has changed dramatically. Warfare in the 21st century rarely involves confrontations between professional armies. Instead, wars typically are fought as grinding struggles between military personnel and civilians, or groups of armed civilians in the same country in a city environment rather than in distant battlefields. As a result, civilian fatalities from battles fought in towns and cities have increased to 90% of the casualties of war in the 21st century, as compared to only 5% in the early 1900s. Worldwide, the caseload of refugee children has grown from 2.4 million in 1974 to 7.2 million in the past decade (Bridging Refugee Youth and Children's Services,

2013). In the United States, the impact of war on families, other than for refugees, is limited to wartime separation and reunion.

Over time, serving in one of the branches of the U.S. military has become far less common. Since 2001, only 1.6 million veterans (or less than 0.05% of the population) have served in Afghanistan or Iraq, compared to the 16 million or 12% of the population that served in World War II (Meagher, 2007). Still, the consequences for family members of military personnel are often dire and long lasting. Death, injury, and short- and long-term disability of the veteran are stressors that can make life difficult for families (Cozza, Chun, & Polo, 2005; Rosenheck & Fontana, 1994). An increase in traumatic brain injury sustained during war is associated with physical health problems that are made worse by PTSD and depression (Hoge et al., 2008). Alarmingly, one out of every four people in the United States who commits suicide is a veteran (Glauber, 2007).

The deployment of thousands of family members during Operation Iraq has opened eyes to the effects of the traumas of war on families. This war resulted in 6,364 casualities and 48,296 wounded U.S. troops. Two million children were affected by separation from parents, changes in health status of parents, and/or loss of parents as a result of this war. Forty-four percent of these children were under 6 years of age, so were particularly prone to the effects of trauma from co-experiencing family trauma (Smith, 2013). As evidence of the difficulty these families face, the telephone calls to the 24-hour helpline *Military OneSource*, which provides counseling to veterans and their families, numbered over 100,000 in the first 10 months of 2005; the calls increased by 20% in 2006. More than 200,000 antidepressant prescriptions were written for military families/service members over a 14-month period in 2005–2006.

Moreover, unidentified and untreated PTSD presented special risks for family reintegration and put the veterans and their families at higher danger for maladaptive responses to stress, such as alcoholism, depression, and family violence (Black et al., 2004; Bremner, Southwick, Darnell, & Charney, 1996; Dansky et al., 1999; Davis & Wood, 1999). Most soldiers, in particular, have transient symptoms of PTSD. These symptoms resolve for most when stability and routine is restored. This is the same pattern for children. But the risk for trauma-related symptoms in children from their parents' traumatic experiences increases with prolonged separation from parent(s), and decreased time between recovery from one traumatic event and to onset of another (i.e., repeated deployment, or repeated terror associated with war) (Smith, 2013). Because of the increased understanding of the risk of PTSD in family members, the military has funded numerous studies to identify effective strategies to prevent PTSD in soldiers and their family members. One program, entitled Building Resilience and Valuing Empowered Families (BRAVE Families), employs strategies used for families experiencing urban violence, Hurricane Katrina, and the World Trade Center terrorist attack. These strategies include individual and family education and support about PTSD, art and play therapy for children, parenting guidance, and group therapy and support (Smith, 2013). The goal of programs designed to reach PTSD at the *meso* level is to reach more families in a nonintrusive manner rather than waiting for families to experience pathology first.

Family Violence and PTSD

Family violence is generally divided into three categories: physical violence, emotional violence, and sexual abuse. The cause of family violence is well studied and is considered multifaceted, with influences ranging from multigenerational trauma (Hulette, Kaehler, & Freyd, 2011), social and cultural learning, mental disorders, and oppression (Abbassi & Aslinia, 2010).

Family violence is often both a cause and an outcome of PTSD in family members. Orcutt, King, and King (2003) examined the impact of early-life stressors, war-zone stressors, and PTSD symptom severity on partner's reports of recent male-perpetrated intimate partner violence (IPV) among 376 Vietnam veteran couples. The results indicated that several factors are directly associated with family violence, including relationship quality among the spouses, war-zone experiences of stress, and PTSD symptom severity. Experiencing PTSD symptoms as a result of previous trauma appears to increase an individual's risk for perpetrating family violence. Risk for partner violence is considerably higher among veterans with PTSD when both low marital satisfaction and alcohol abuse-dependence are present (Fonseca et al., 2006; Taft et al., 2005).

Domestic violence also increases the risk for PTSD and is a cause for PTSD for both the victims and witnesses of the violence. The incidence of witnessing domestic violence and related trauma continues to be a major public health problem. In 2006, it was estimated that 29.4% of children in dual-parent homes lived in a home where partner violence was present. The risk to children is great, including physical injury from getting in the "cross-fire" to psychological distress similar to children experiencing direct abuse (Kitzmann, 2012). In a meta-analysis of 118 studies from 1978 to 2000 on witnesses of domestic violence, Kitzmann, Gaylord, Holt, and Kenny (2003) found that children experiencing parental domestic violence fared poorly in the areas of both internalized (i.e., withdrawal) and externalized (i.e., aggression) behaviors compared to controls 63% of the time, and had similar outcomes to those children experiencing direct abuse. Of interest is that the age of the child did not predict the degree of psychological distress, indicating that witnessing parental domestic violence is as dangerous for young children as it is for adolescents.

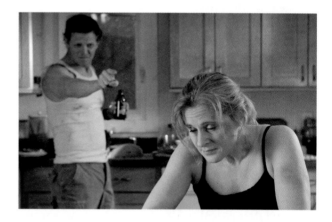

Other family trauma also negatively affects the individuals within the family. For example, children experiencing divorce and abuse are at particular risk for later adult mental health disorders, including PTSD and depression. In a study of 5,877 individuals ages 15 to 54 years from the National Co-morbidity Study, Affi et al. (2009) found that children exposed to both divorce and abuse had the highest rates of mental health disorders as adults, particularly PTSD. A meta-analysis of 124 articles on long-term outcomes of children experiencing physical abuse or neglect found more depression, suicide risks, family violence, and substance abuse when compared with those not exposed to abuse and neglect (Norman et al., 2012). The experience of trauma, especially repeated traumas, increases the risk of long-term negative outcomes for children and adults. Each family member exposed to abuse, neglect, and major transitions and loss, such as divorce, is at risk for PTSD, as well as continuing the cycle of violence within families (Hulette, Kaehler, & Freyd, 2011). These findings clearly support the need for family care and interventions by nurses and other health professionals to prevent family-centered trauma.

Families Affected by Disasters

Disasters are events that cause widespread destruction of property, dislocation of people, and immediate suffering through death or injury. Disasters interrupt meeting basic daily needs for an extended time, causing suffering that cannot be addressed easily by those affected and making recovery difficult (American Red Cross, 2003) for families. Disasters are classified as either natural or human caused. Natural disasters include weather and seismic events such as floods, hurricanes, and earthquakes. Human-caused disasters include events such as fires, building collapse, explosions, acts of terrorism, or war. Acts of terrorism or violence include the use of chemical, radioactive, nuclear, biological, or explosive weapons that can cause great harm and stress.

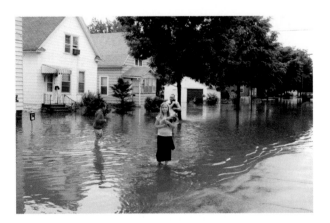

Natural disasters are the most frequently occurring type of disaster. In the last 10 years, the International Red Cross reported that 1.1 million people across the world were killed by natural disasters (e.g. hurricanes, tornadoes, earthquakes, storms, tsunamis, and volcanic eruptions) (International Federation of Red Cross and Red Crescent Societies, 2012). An additional 100,000 people were killed worldwide from technological disasters, ranging from industrial accidents to transportation accidents (International Federation of Red Cross and Red Crescent Societies, 2012). During the years 2004–2005, natural disasters killed 336,540 people in the world and further, over 300 million people were directly or indirectly affected by those disasters (International Strategy for Disaster Reduction, 2006). In the United States alone during 2007, tornadoes killed 80 people, and thunderstorms and accompanying floods, lightning, winds, and hail caused another 157 deaths (National Severe Storms Laboratory, 2007). In 2011 the Disaster Relief Fund requested $1.95 billion in aid for families and individuals affected by such disasters (U.S. Department of Homeland Security, 2011).

Regardless of the type of event, families are affected in multiple ways when disasters strike. Some of the many stressors that occur include loss of significant others, injuries to self or family, separation from family, or extensive loss of property (Norris, 2007). These losses result in heightened feelings of stress, with many families experiencing symptoms of acute and chronic PTSD.

Family Functioning and PTSD

Trauma-related reactions leading to PTSD have a negative impact on family functioning. In a study of current relationship functioning among World War II ex-prisoners of war, over 30% of those with PTSD reported relationship problems compared with only 11% of those without PTSD (Cook, Riggs, Thompson, Coyne, & Sheikh, 2004). In Vietnam veterans, PTSD symptoms have been significantly associated with poor family functioning (Evans, McHugh, Hopwood, & Watt, 2003), and problems with marital adjustment, parenting satisfaction, and psychological abuse (Gold et al., 2007). The PTSD symptoms of avoidance and emotional numbing in particular have deleterious effects on parent-child relationship satisfaction (Samper, Taft, King, & King, 2004). Among Iraq and Afghanistan veterans, trauma symptoms such as sleep problems, dissociation, and severe sexual problems predicted lower marital satisfaction for both the veteran and his partner (Goff, Crow, Reisbig, & Hamilton, 2007). In their review of the literature on secondary trauma in the United States, Galovski and Lyons (2004) identified that veterans' numbing and hyperarousal symptoms were especially predictive of family distress.

Secondary Traumatization and PTSD

The impact of PTSD is not limited to the traumatized persons themselves. Spouses of the injured persons seem particularly susceptible to a phenomenon called *secondary traumatization* (Dirkzwager, Bramsen, Ader, & van der Ploeg, 2005). Secondary traumatization has only recently been described and is not yet a diagnostic category in the DSM-IV (APA, 2000). In a study of Dutch peacekeeping soldiers and their families (Dirkzwager et al., 2005), it was found that partners of peacekeepers with PTSD symptoms reported more sleeping and somatic problems, more negative social support, and judged the marital relationship as less favorable when compared to the general population. Another study in Israel found that spouses of veterans with PTSD suffered from higher levels of emotional distress and a lower level of marital adjustment than the general population (Dekel, Solomon, & Bleich, 2005). In a qualitative study of wives of Israeli veterans with PTSD, Dekel et al. (2005) noted that the wives were carrying a heavy burden supporting and caring for their husbands and families; all of them identified personal symptoms of PTSD from hearing about their partner's trauma and experiencing the negative affects on their partner's health. Partners of veterans with combat-related PTSD experience significant levels of emotional distress (Manguno-Mire et al., 2007).

This pattern is not limited to family members caring for veterans with PTSD (Devilly, Wright & Varker, 2009). Other studies have looked at non–family members. Thomas and Wilson (2004) reported that 7% of professionals working with traumatized victims experience symptoms consistent with PTSD. Other researchers have attempted to define this phenomenon, using terms including compassion fatigue, professional burnout, and secondary traumatic stress (Meadors, Lamson, Swanson, White, & Sira, 2009; Newell & MacNeil, 2010). Each definition describes the psychological and physical response to caring for victims but not directly experiencing trauma. Meadors et al. (2009)

studied 167 professionals working in pediatric intensive care units. They found a significant correlation between compassion fatigue, or secondary traumatization, and symptoms of PTSD. Nurses, physicians, social workers, and chaplains described the difficulty of caring for families who had a child severely ill, injured, or dying. These professionals not only heard about the traumatic event repeatedly from families, but witnessed the traumatic events over and over as they cared for families across time. This witnessing of trauma led to secondary traumatization.

Prevention is the goal with primary treatment of potential PTSD; several programs start interventions at the time of the traumatic event within a family rather than waiting for symptoms to develop (Skelton, Loveland, & Yeagley, 1996). Outcomes improve with a combination of individual and family therapy, along with appropriate medication management of symptoms when needed. In a study of seven children following a bus accident, the combination of individual and family therapy with selective serotonin reuptake inhibitors (SSRIs) resulted in a remission of PTSD symptoms, whereas the control group who only received medication still had symptoms 3 months later (Stankovi_ et al., 2013). In the cases where medication and family therapy was used, researchers used Systematic Family Therapy (SFT), a structured family therapy protocol, to facilitate family involvement and family directed interventions. It proved effective in preventing chronic PTSD in victims.

COMMUNITY AND TRAUMA

The community response to trauma can have a major impact on the degree of PTSD experienced by individuals, families, and the community as a whole. The community has a key role in the prevention and treatment of trauma. Child welfare services often respond to threats of trauma from abuse and neglect, and police services often respond to threats of domestic or community violence. Hospitals are critical in the immediate treatment of physical and psychological trauma, and private and community or county mental health services are at the forefront in leading every community through prevention and treatment of trauma (Gard & Ruzek, 2006). These agencies each have a responsibility to be trained for their role in trauma care. For example, if child welfare workers are not properly trained on trauma, they may not support foster parents in appropriate reactions to children with trauma-related behaviors. This lack of support may lead to placement failure, and result in children being retraumatized by multiple interruptions in attachment, initiating a dangerous cycle (Richardson, Coryn, Henry, Black-Pond, & Unrau, 2012). Table 11-2 presents responses to questions regarding exposure to trauma, as a training guide for health care professionals.

Consider the following scenario: A 13-year-old child, who is recovering from PTSD resulting from sexual abuse by her father, is placed into foster care. During counseling, she is encouraged to retreat to a quiet place when stimulation from the crowded foster care becomes too much. Due to lack of training, however, her foster mother punishes her for "being too isolated." When she goes to school, she becomes overwhelmed by fear, and retreats to the library to regain her homeostasis. Because her teachers are untrained and unaware of her needs, she is again punished. She begins to distrust her counselor, foster parent, and teachers, and relapses into fear, disconnection, and dysregulation. She retreats back into rigid boundaries. This short vignette illustrates the importance of educating community-based service providers to understand trauma, and to integrate and collaborate services to promote positive rather than dangerous and negative outcomes.

SYSTEMIC TRAUMA

The symptoms of PTSD cross individual, family, and community boundaries. Many argue that the United States of America is suffering from PTSD from repeated traumatic events such as wars, natural disasters, and economic traumas across time without resolution or intervention. This has resulted in a nation with PTSD symptoms, including depression, intrusion of unwanted and negative thinking patterns, hyperarousal especially to perceived threats from others, and related health decline. One clear symptom of this premise is the decline in the general health of U.S. citizens, not unlike the health of individuals suffering from PTSD. We possess the shortest life span of any industrialized nation, with almost half of American adults struggling with hypertension, high cholesterol, diabetes, or all three. Further, more than one-third of adults and children are obese (U.S. Department of Health and Human Services, 2012). We are seeing increasing numbers of individuals with stress-related disorders, stemming from or causing mental illness, substance abuse, and domestic violence. Infant mortality is dismally high, with the United States rate ranking highest among the top seven industrialized countries of the world (U.S. Department of Health and Human Services, 2012). Child abuse rates are equally high when compared with other nations (U.S. Department of Health and Human Services, 2012). One-quarter of our nation's children take prescription medications. One-fifth of our nation's children have been diagnosed with a mental health disorder (Hensley, 2010). Twenty-six percent of all children in the United States will experience or witness a traumatic event before they reach age 4 years (Substance Abuse and Mental Health Services Administration, 2011). These statistics show symptoms of a country experiencing dysregulation and systemic trauma.

The high obesity rates in the United States are a clear example of a nation experiencing dysregulation and fear. Obesity is growing the fastest in our poor and crowded neighborhoods. The lack of healthy foods, safe neighborhoods that support outdoor activity, high levels of stress, and presence of early and repeated trauma are key factors in

Table 11-2	Responses to Questions Regarding Exposure to Western Trauma Discourse
Have you ever attended workshops or trainings about how people are affected by extremely frightening or traumatic events?	
Never: 85.9%	
<1 day: 7.7%	
<2 days: 1.3%	
2 days: 1.3%	
2+ days: 3.8%	
Have you ever listened to radio programs/read literature about how people are affected by extremely frightening or violent events?	
Never: 19.2%	
1–2 times: 16.7%	
3–4 times: 39.7%	
4+ times: 15.4%	
7+ times: 9.0%	

causing obesity and related chronic health conditions (Karr-Morse & Wiley, 2012). Yet, the response to obesity is not centered on trauma-related interventions, but instead on unsuccessful dieting and major surgeries.

Another indicator that the United States as a nation is struggling with PTSD is the increasing rate of substance abuse. Although nicotine addiction is at an all-time low, addiction to other substances, such as alcohol and opiates, is increasing at an alarming rate (National Institute on Drug Abuse, 2012). Researchers have found that those struggling with food cravings leading to obesity, and those struggling with drug addiction, both exhibit decreased dopamine levels. Overeating and drug use temporarily raises dopamine levels. A lack of dopamine, particularly in the frontal cortex, is caused by early trauma more often than genetics (Karr-Morse & Wiley, 2012). A country experiencing repeated trauma without resolution quickly fills with individuals, families, and communities highly stressed and traumatized, with resulting increase in stress-related disorders. Chronic stress is toxic stress. *Toxic stress*, as defined by the Center on the Developing Child at Harvard University, is when an individual experiences strong, frequent, and prolonged stress such as chronic child abuse or neglect, without adequate support (Center on the Developing Child, 2012). Toxic stress interferes with the ability to learn, be creative, stay healthy, and have joy. Countries that experience toxic stress through natural disasters, war, or dysregulation of major systems also experience a drop in the ability to learn, be creative, have healthy citizens, and have joyous outcomes. Robin Karr-Morse and Meredith Wiley, the authors of *Scared Sick: The Roles of Childhood Trauma in Adult Disease* (2012), compared our body's response to stress to the U.S. Department of Homeland Security. Both systems are aimed at a complex and integrated system that maintains safety. When part of that system is overtaxed or disconnected, safety is threatened. Threats to the larger system, whether real or imagined, can further overwhelm the system and lead to disease.

The greater culture and societal laws and policies can influence the incidence and the treatment of trauma. Countries riddled with war, poverty, and disease have higher incidents of PTSD, whereas countries that support policies that decrease violent solutions to problems, provide broad access to preventive and primary health care, and decrease

poverty have lower incidences of PTSD. For example, the incident of PTSD in New Zealand is estimated to be 6.1% of the population (U.S. Department of Veterans Affairs, 2007), whereas the incident of PTSD in the Gaza Strip was found to be 70.1% of 9- to 18-year-olds exposed to the ongoing Israeli-Palestinian conflict (Thabet & Vostanis, 2000). The extent that countries can prevent and/or treat the causes of PTSD early clearly influences the health of the citizens in every country.

Many argue that the traumatic events experienced over the course of the last two decades in the United States were too rapid to resolve and caused a chronic state of fear in the country. For example, in 2005 the United States experienced Hurricane Katrina, continued involvement in the Iraq war, economic collapse, raging wildfires in California, a severe snowstorm in New England, and a school shooting. U.S. citizens watched these disasters unfold with little support or education on how to process these events to avoid symptoms of PTSD. Today, many talk about feeling numb to the disasters watched on television, and have increased fear related to travel, economics, and routine activities, such as attending school. The treatment of PTSD needs to expand beyond individuals, families, and communities, and include national and international traumas and the impact on a nation as a whole.

NURSES AND TRAUMA

Nurses are key in helping with the diagnosis and treatment of PTSD in individuals and families. Their presence at the forefront of emergency care of victims of trauma, and their help throughout the healing process renders nurses important members of the interdisciplinary team that prevents, treats, and evaluates care for PTSD. This section outlines the nurse's role in the prevention, identification, and treatment of PTSD as part of an interdisciplinary team.

PTSD Nursing Assessment and Intervention

PTSD can develop after a traumatic event or events at any age. To be diagnosed with PTSD, certain conditions must exist. The person has to have been exposed to a traumatic event; experience intense feelings of fear, helplessness, or horror (for preverbal children, the feelings of helplessness are commonly seen as withdrawal, and feelings of fear are commonly seen as intense emotional arousal); reexperience the event through flashbacks, dreams, or disturbing memories; avoid any stimuli associated with the event, avoiding any reminders, thoughts, or feelings about the event; be hypervigilant; have difficulties falling or staying asleep; have an exaggerated startle response; and the symptoms must have lasted longer than 1 month and must cause significant distress or impairment in functioning (National Center for PTSD, 2010).

It is the role of nurses to assess for symptoms of PTSD. There are simple methods to screen patients who may have undetected PTSD. One easy to use tool is the Primary Care PTSD Screen (Prins et al., 2004), which consists of four questions preceded by the following introduction:

"In your life, have you ever had any experience that was so frightening, horrible, or upsetting that, in the past month, you...

1. Have had nightmares about it or thought about it when you did not want to?

2. Tried hard not to think about it or went out of your way to avoid situations that reminded you of it?

3. Were constantly on guard, watchful, or easily startled?

4. Felt numb or detached from others, activities, or your surroundings?"

The screen is positive if the patient answers *yes to any three items.*

It is also important for nurses to assess risk factors and provide families with protector factors, or positive coping strategies and enhancement of resiliency characteristics (Friedman, 2006; Warner, 2010). See Box 11-1 on vicarious trauma.

Risks Associated With PTSD

There are a number of risks and risk factors associated with both adult and child PTSD of which nurses should be conversant:

- Suicidal risk—due to feelings of numbness, disconnect with support people, chronic fear and anxiety, and feelings of hopelessness and helplessness.
- Danger to others—ask about firearms or weapons, aggressive intentions, feelings of persecution.

BOX 11-1
Vicarious Trauma

Trauma clearly transcends individuals, families, communities, and greater societies across time and across cultures. Nurses are often the front-line professionals to identify and intervene when acute and chronic trauma occurs. A real risk for nurses is the development of the attunement survival style described by Heller & LaPierre (2012). This style of coping is characterized by attuning to other's needs and neglecting one's own needs, which is an apt description of the lived experiences of many nurses. If nurses identify themselves as givers, yet neglect their own needs, they are at a high risk for vicarious trauma, or the development of PTSD symptoms from caring for or witnessing trauma in others. This condition is also referred to as *compassion fatigue* and *secondary trauma* in the literature (Afifi et al., 2009). This term has evolved as helping professionals were identified as being at high risk for negative psychological reactions to their job, with early descriptions of burnout. Symptoms of burnout include feeling overwhelmed, hopeless, helpless, and unappreciated. Motivation is lost, and if unrecognized and untreated, it may lead to depression, loss of job, and, in the long term, early death (Smith, Segal, & Segal, 2012). Although burnout can be caused by repetitious and uninspiring work, it can also be caused by vicarious trauma. Prevention of vicarious trauma is possible through education, avoiding professional burn-out, and professional and peer support during and after caring for traumatized patients (Trippany, White Kress, & Wilcoxon, 2004).

- Ongoing stressors—such as changes that have occurred at home, marital discord, problems at work.
- Risky behaviors—such as risky sexual adventures, nonadherence to medical treatment, substance use and misuse.
- Personal characteristics—past trauma history, coping skills, relationship attachment.
- Limited social support—the individual's lack of willingness to accept help and inclination to isolate.
- Comorbidity—coexisting psychiatric or medical problems such as depression and chronic widespread pain (CWP).

Child risks associated with PTSD include the following:

- Dysregulation—unpredictable or irregular sleep and eating patterns, and difficulty regulating moods and emotional responses.

- Poor connection—difficulty forming or maintaining relationships, with a tendency to be alone, have poor eye contact, and resist connection with others.
- Poor cognitive development—difficulty with attention, short-term memory, problem solving, creativity, and play. High incidence of learning disabilities, particularly auditory processing disability.
- Poor attunement skills—difficulty recognizing and asking for needs.
- Inability to trust—difficulty forming relationships, oppositional behavior, sleep problems.
- Hyperarousal—increased response to environmental stressors or memories, with rage, anger, or severe anxiety.

The best evidence-based nursing treatments for the individual with PTSD include both psychotherapeutic interventions—such as cognitive-behavioral therapy and family therapy—and medications, primarily SSRIs (Friedman, 2006; Herbert & Forman, in press; Herbert & Sageman, 2004). Partner and family engagement in PTSD treatment has been shown to improve the treatment outcomes. Predictors of partner engagement include higher income, patient-partner connection, and lower partner caregiver burden (Sautter et al., 2006).

Secondary Family Traumatization Assessment and Intervention

To help the traumatized family, the nurse should first realize that traumatized families rarely seek family-focused intervention. Instead, they often present with problems that are not immediately related to the traumatic events they have experienced (Figley & Barnes, 2005). Nurses should learn the parallel processes of individual and systemic stress reactions that follow a traumatic event. Figley and Barnes (2005) offer suggestions to help clinicians recognize family responses to traumatic events and offer some interventions to help patients and families affected by these events. For example, families are affected by the individual's symptoms of PTSD. They know the story of the trauma, witness the symptoms, and want to help in some way. As a result, the family spends more and more time caring for the traumatized member. Moreover, while the traumatic event is being persistently reexperienced by the exposed family member, the other family members are responding to this individual's increased demands for support. As the primary

affected family member tries to avoid stimuli and reminders of the trauma, the other family members must devote increased time, energy, and problem solving to avoid conversations, people, places, and things that might stimulate memories. They have to tolerate the withdrawal and numbing that goes along with the primary affected family member's diminished interest in usual activities, refusals to see friends, and inability to express love and caring. The family becomes increasingly more isolated. The other family members have to manage problems with sleep, outbursts of anger and rage, exaggerated startle responses, and hypervigilance about safety. These factors increase the risk of secondary traumatization, or symptoms of PTSD in family members from witnessing the traumatic stories and the negative impact on their family member. Secondary traumatization is considered acute if the duration is less than 3 months, chronic if the duration is 3 months or more, and delayed if the onset is at least 6 months after the stressor.

Nurses Applying the Ecological Systems Theory Approach to Trauma Treatment

Treatment of trauma begins with the treatment of interrupted trust and attachment (Heller & LaPierre, 2012). Infants and young children who experience rejection and abuse early in life often expect that same experience from present and future caregivers. A trusting and therapeutic relationship must form. This process is slow, as the child or adult who has learned to avoid feelings and relationships will first resist, and then struggle with moderating those feelings and relationships, and then, if successful, learn to trust. The initial steps of treatment are as follows:

1. Move slowly: building connections can be terrifying to a traumatized individual.
2. Build trust: building a therapeutic relationship depends on being predictable and trustworthy.
3. Be empathetic: you may be the first kind person in their lives.
4. Help children and adults listen to and explore their new skills at identifying emotions, organizing thoughts and emotions, and learning different reactions and responses to their emotions.
5. Help build self-esteem through teaching top-down thinking. For example, if an adult has always felt he was bad because of

traumatic events in his life, help him rethink about the events being bad instead.

6. Gradually support and encourage connection with their own feelings, then their body responses and reactions, and finally connection to other people. The connection to other people should also be gradual, starting with close caregivers or family members, and advancing as tolerated to outside peers and associates.

7. Be available to help the child or adult explore feelings of rejection, anger, abandonment, and fear. Many individuals who have experienced trauma have survived by becoming numb. As this numbness fades, survival feels threatened. During this transition from numbness to feeling, many may withdraw for varying periods of time. A therapeutic nurse will recognize this pattern and avoid judging the traumatized individual during these phases.

The nurse working with a traumatized family needs to explore each family member's perception of what happened both before and after the event (Figley & Barnes, 2005). The family may block the telling of trauma if the family was the cause of that trauma. Listening to individuals and observing for signs of secondary trauma can be critical to getting help for all family members. The nurse needs to recognize that the family's worldview will have been altered by the traumatizing events and that its attitudes and beliefs may shift from safety to suspicious, distrustful attribution regarding the motivations of others, including helping professionals. Hypervigilance and controlling behaviors may actually interfere with the family getting the help it needs. In addition, if the stressors impinging on the family go unattended, a pattern of triangulation and blaming may become the central family dynamic. Also, the roles in the family may shift, with some members becoming more enmeshed with the traumatized member, and others withdrawing from the family system. Children may have to take on the role of emotional caretaker for the parents and thus be compelled to hide their own feelings and fears, while other siblings act out to express anger, leading to more parenting stress. Most emerging trauma treatment has as its main shortcoming the focus on the individual rather than the family system. Careful implementation of interviewing techniques and the exploration of the family life experience through ecomaps will assist nurses to access the complex relationships and characteristics of families living with trauma or post-traumatic complications.

The nursing role also includes looking at community actions and societal responses to trauma at a personal, family, community, and societal level, and how that trauma affects health. Becoming involved with prevention strategies, such as community preparedness for disaster, can lead to improved community health. Working with national organizations to provide organized community-based interventions for traumas can be an important step to preventing negative long-term consequences. Participating in research and implementing research findings that demonstrate the impact of trauma on all ecological levels can help improve treatment plans and outcomes. Finally, shaping policies at the national level that support families in need, by decreasing poverty, improving access to health care, supporting parents with improved child care options and improved parenting education and support, and reducing environmental stress, can be an important step to reducing PTSD in children, adults, families, communities, and nations.

Case Study: Knoll Family—An Ecological Approach

This case study offers an example of a family that experienced trauma, and the impact of individual trauma and family trauma on all family members. The events that occurred within this family illustrate the complexities of prolonged stress, pile-up of stressors, risk factors, and resiliency characteristics touching the individual, family, community, and nation.

Family Members:

- Mother: Emma (age 45)
- Father: Peter (age 46)
- Oldest daughter: Ignes (deceased at age 11 years)
- Oldest son: Jason (age 14)
- Youngest son: Bradley (age 12)

Figure 11-5 shows the Knoll family genogram.

The Knoll family has experienced a number of losses and trauma over the past 5 years. This family lives in a low-income trailer within a trailer park. The neighborhood is run-down, but considered safe. The parents are currently divorced, and the father visits once a week for 2 to 3 hours.

(continued)

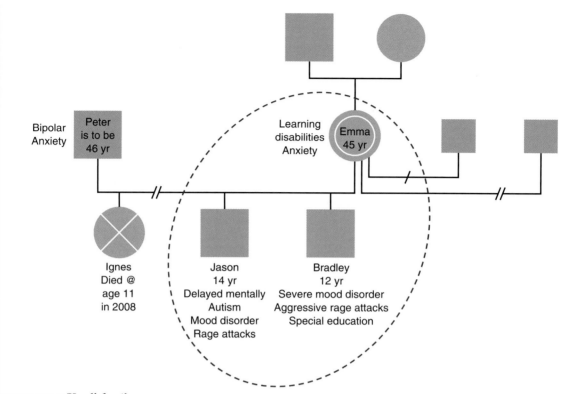

FIGURE 11-5 Knoll family genogram.

The family is white, non-Hispanic and the religion is Seventh Day Adventist. Because of the family's low income, family members have state-provided health care insurance, limiting access to mental health care to 30 minutes per week. Although county mental health care services are available in the community, the waitlist is over 6 months, and experts on family trauma are not currently available. Because of this, the family has sought mental health care and medication management for family members at a private family care clinic specializing in trauma.

Family Development:

The mother Emma has a history of learning disabilities and anxiety. Although she denies any stress in her childhood, and describes her parents as stable and loving, she experienced a series of traumas starting 5 years ago. The first trauma was the diagnosis of a severe anemia (Diamond Blackfan anemia) in her 11-year-old daughter. Although the doctors felt her daughter's prognosis was good, she died from complications following a bone marrow transplant. Because of the intense and traumatic nature of this event, the father left the hospital before his daughter died, and did not return to the family for 2 years. He stated he could not handle his grief at her death, and just wanted to "run

away" and not think about it. His abandonment led to the family losing their home to foreclosure, as the mother had never held a job outside of the home, and she was left with severe grief and the responsibility of caring for her two other children. Her two sons both had the diagnosis of autism, moderate mental retardation, and severe mood disorder. She felt immediately overwhelmed, and felt she had to find a partner to help her.

She met a man at her church. Unfortunately, he raped her during their third date. Her symptoms of PTSD started after this sexual assault, including flashbacks, severe anxiety, hyperarousal, and avoidance of friends and family members. Three months after the rape, she started dating a second man, whom she met on-line. This relationship was unstable, with episodes of verbal abuse, and frequent abandonment from weeks to months. In spite of this instability, the mother married this man. She divorced him 9 months later due to his abandonment back to the East Coast. She then met a third man on-line, and started dating him. The relationship went well for several months, leading to her decision that she would allow this new man to move into her home. He was initially very helpful with her sons. Soon, however, he revealed that he had been diagnosed with bipolar disorder, and could not afford his medications. He had a manic episode, which included domestic violence and "rage attacks" toward the mother and her two sons. She kicked him out, and has now remained single for several months.

The oldest son (14) is developmentally at the first-grade (6-year) level in all areas except art, at which he excels. He struggles with dysregulation of moods, inattention, poor short-term memory, impulsivity, and intermittent rage attacks resulting in aggression toward his mother and destruction of property. These rages occurred up to three times per day without medication, but less than once per month on medication. He is currently taking Abilify 15 mg, Straterra 25 mg, and Zoloft 75 mg. He also takes hydroxyzine up to 50 mg as needed for severe agitation and anxiety. He currently receives special education services through the school district and is placed in the Life Skills Program. He can read simple books, write three- to four-word sentences, and participate in age-level choir and art classes. He currently states that he has no friends at school or in his neighborhood. He spends his free time drawing, watching television, or playing video games.

The younger son (12) is developmentally at the fifth-grade (10-year) level in all areas. He struggles with dysregulation of moods, inattention, poor short-term memory, impulsivity, and intermittent rage attacks resulting in aggression toward his mother and brother, and has in the past threatened his mother and brother with a knife. These rages occurred up to three times per day without medication, but less than once per month on medication. He is currently taking Abilify 15 mg, Topamax 50 mg twice daily, Straterra 18 mg, and Zoloft 50 mg. He also takes hydroxyzine up to 50 mg as needed for severe agitation and anxiety. He currently receives special education services through the school district and is placed in the Life Skills Program. He can read chapter books, write three- to four-paragraph stories, and participate in age-level choir and music classes. He currently states that he has no friends at school or in his neighborhood. He spends his free time reading, watching television, or playing video games.

The father currently works full-time at a grocery store as a clerk. He has been diagnosed with bipolar disorder and anxiety. He does not take any medication, resulting in manic episodes an average of once every 2 years, evidenced by increased interest in pornography, insomnia, and running from his current situation. In between these manic attacks, he is functional and well regarded at work and at church. He currently has a girlfriend who lives 200 miles away. He visits her every weekend. He pays $350 per month for child support.

Function:

Emma assumes the role of primary caregiver of her two children. Her mother, an 83-year-old woman in good health, however, provides daily support, including caring for the two boys and helping with housecleaning. The grandparents also provide regular financial assistance, as child support payments are sporadic. Emma makes all decisions regarding finances, parenting, and leisure activities. Peter has very few roles within the family, as he inconsistently assists with finances, and only participates in parenting 3 hours per week. He allows Emma to make all decisions. The two boys are expected to participate in school and to help with chores within the home. Both boys neglect their chores, and the mother also dislikes housework, leading to the home being messy and disorganized. Child Welfare Services has been called due to the disarray of the house, which led to some community support, including assistance with painting, fixing the bathroom, and cleaning and replacement of the carpet.

Communication within the family started out as distant and emotionally abusive. Through intensive counseling and parent coaching within the clinic and through home visits, the family now participates in healthier communication patterns, nonviolent problem solving, and shared positive experiences. Each family member, however, continues to show signs of chronic PTSD, due to repeated and severe traumas within the family. When asked about adverse events, the mother summarized the events as follows:

- The diagnosis of autism in her oldest son.
- The diagnosis of autism in her youngest son.
- The diagnosis of Diamond Blackfan anemia in her daughter, with resulting death of her daughter.
- The loss of her husband and divorce.
- The loss of her home and the dependence on her parents for financial support.
- The sexual assault during a date (i.e., "date rape").
- The difficulty finding adequate health care for herself and her children.
- The difficulty finding adequate educational services for her sons.
- The abandonment by her second husband.
- The domestic violence by her domestic partner.

Emma was asked about resiliency skills for both herself and her sons. She felt she had positive support through her parents, a strong religious affiliation including daily prayer, the absence of any substance abuse, and the ability to adapt to the many changes and traumatic events occurring in the last 5 years. She noted that her sons were her support as well as her burden. She stated that they both were very adaptable at times to big changes, but could not

(continued)

tolerate small changes, such as changes in the schedule. Resiliency areas where this family lacked included: optimism, self-efficacy, low cognitive function for all family members except the grandmother, ability to participate in healthy self-care (i.e., the family had poor nutrition, never exercised, and had limited social support), and lack of trust of helping professionals due to negative involvement of Child Welfare Services.

Nursing Interventions:

Microsystem: The individuals within this family needed a thorough and comprehensive assessment of symptoms of PTSD given the history of repeated and prolonged trauma and caregiving overload. The mechanism of prolonged stress for the two sons could have started in early childhood, given their symptoms of mood dysregulation, attention-deficit disorder, rage, and cognitive impairment. Through a careful assessment, it was determined that both boys had experienced neglect during the first 4 years of their life, as mother described feeling depressed and overwhelmed by parenting responsibilities. She admitted that she would leave both boys alone for hours while she slept, with this pattern going on for days. She was not evaluated for or diagnosed with depression, but she stated that she lacked energy, motivation, or ability to care for her sons, and often felt resentful toward their care. While her 11-year-old daughter helped at times, she was at school or with friends a majority of the time until her illness was diagnosed. After this point, the mother devoted all of her available energy to her daughter's care. After the death of her daughter, she once again retreated to bed most days until she started counseling.

The understanding of each of the individual's experiences and related traumas helps the nurse identify the need for individual care for each family member. The boys started with individual counseling utilizing play and art therapy. They soon built a trusting relationship with the therapist, and learned across time to become more attuned to their own needs, learned to ask for their needs appropriately, and to regulate their responses to emotions. Their cognitive abilities improved from being years behind grade level to being considered "low normal" in their academic skills. Medications were adjusted to help both boys regulate moods, concentrate when needed, and to have regular sleep, eating, and digestive patterns. Meanwhile, the mother and father received individual counseling and medication management to address their symptoms of PTSD, and both received parent counseling and coaching.

Mesosystem: Family-centered care was instituted immediately to improve family development and functioning. Family self-care strategies were initially implemented to stabilize and organize the family, followed by family meetings to address communication skills, problem-solving skills, and to build positive connections between and among family members. During the family meetings, the family also discussed grief, including the loss of the daughter/sister, loss of the marriage, and loss of the family home and related stability.

Macrosystem: This family struggled with finding supportive community resources. See Figure 11-6, the Knoll family ecomap, which depicts the subsystems. While family members were devoted to their religion and sought support through this community service, the church would not allow the family to attend services due to the boys' disruptive behavior. When the church refused to baptize the youngest son due to his autism, the family left this church. They are currently seeking a new church to join. The mental health care services were at first difficult to find because of the long waitlist and lack of appropriate specialist to manage this family's care at the county mental health clinic. Private services were found, however, and these services helped this family gain the support it needed to thrive. Private services were funded through the state insurance program, ensuring health care for all children. The school system was equally frustrating, as it struggled to communicate with the mother about approaches to the boys' behavior and learning deficits. Supplemental services, including the use of an autism specialist, occupational therapist, counselor, and speech therapist, helped improve the boys' academic and cognitive abilities. Child Welfare Services, while trying to improve the home environment, ended up increasing mistrust of helping professionals through their unneeded threats. This outcome is consistent with studies showing that if community agencies are not well trained in trauma, the interventions may cause more harm than good (Richardson et al., 2012).

Exosystem: This family was affected by societal rules, culture, and policies. The availability of health care through the state allowed services to this family, but limited those services to brief weekly contacts. The system also allowed for free public education for the boys, which assisted in their cognitive and social gains. The exosystem also resulted in the family being part of a culture of trauma, with an inability to escape poverty and poor housing, and, because of lack of access to healthy foods

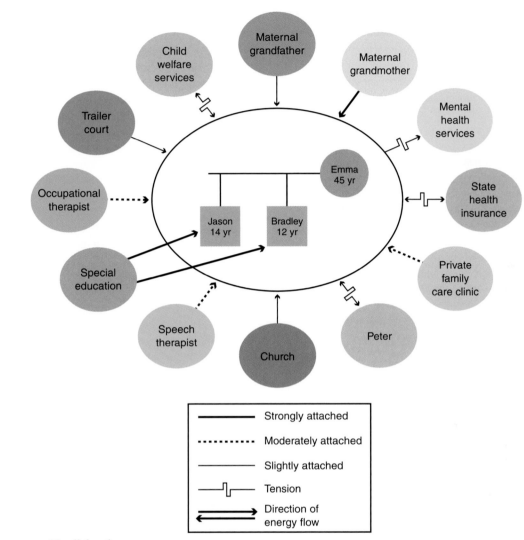

FIGURE 11-6 Knoll family ecomap.

and poor preventive health care, an increase in trauma-related health problems, including obesity, high cholesterol, and hypertension in all family members. The exosystem problems were addressed by increased awareness of risks, increased support of prevention behaviors, and referral to services that counteracted negative exosystem practices and policies.

Outcome Following Treatment:
Following 5 years of treatment, this family is no longer demonstrating symptoms of PTSD. Each family member is experiencing positive connections within and outside the family, stable housing, and improved nutrition, with resulting improved health, and improved cognitive functioning. The family is better connected to the community, and less resentful regarding social policies and practices that were unhelpful. During this 5-year time period, the family worked with the same nurse and interventions focused on ongoing family assessments, care coordination to facilitate better relationships across the family care–provider ecology, improving family communication and closeness through the use of rituals and routines, and individually targeted development of resiliency characteristics based on trauma-related care evidence.

Case Study: Caldwell Family

Mr. Caldwell, a 47-year-old National Guard soldier, in the hospital for a hernia repair, had returned home from a 12-month deployment to Iraq, where he had his first exposure to combat in his 18 years of National Guard duty. Before deployment, he worked successfully as a fireman paramedic and was a happily married father with two children. He and his wife were socially outgoing with a large circle of friends from the same rural area in which they both grew up. They have been married since high school. See a genogram and ecomap for the Caldwell family in Figures 11-7 and 11-8.

While in Iraq recently, Mr. Caldwell had extensive exposure to other soldiers' combat injuries as the noncommissioned officer in charge of the battlefield medical aide station. His unit treated the severe, crippling injuries of soldiers en route to the trauma hospital. The aide station was often overrun with multiple casualties. He treated soldiers from patrols and convoys in which improvised exploding devices destroyed vehicles and wounded or killed people. Although he did not have to kill enemy combatants, he agonized that he may also have been responsible for the deaths of some soldiers because he simply did not have enough men or resources to treat all of the casualties adequately. When asked about the worst moment during his deployment, he readily stated it was when he was unable to intercede, while a Humvee with a bleeding soldier draped over the hood and several wounded soldiers in the back drove by the aide station, because the driver's view was blocked by blood gushing on the windshield and could not see him waving the Humvee to safety.

When he first returned home, things seemed to be okay. But more than 2 years after coming home, he has had more and more difficulty relating to his wife. He reports feeling angry all the time, that no one will listen to him. Sleep has become difficult. He has to sleep on the recliner in the living room because his back hurts so badly that he cannot lay flat. When he does sleep, he has a recurring, vivid nightmare about turning a corner outside of a building in Baghdad where he encounters an insurgent with a rifle who shoots him. His daughter complains that he has become so overprotective that he will not let her go out with any friends, much less any boys. His wife reported that he has been emotionally distant since his return. His employer, who initially supported him, has reported that his work at the fire department has suffered dramatically. During a recent burning motor vehicle extradition drill, one of the car's tires exploded. The unexpected explosion rattled him so much that he became unable to go to work anymore. Mr. Caldwell says that since his deployment, he no longer has an identity—he cannot work, and he no longer feels like he can fulfill his obligations as a husband and a father. He reports that he sometimes experiences strong surges of anger, panic, guilt, and despair and that at other times he has felt emotionally dead, unable to return the love and warmth of family and friends. He does not want to get a divorce, but fears this will happen. Although he has not been actively suicidal, he reported that he sometimes

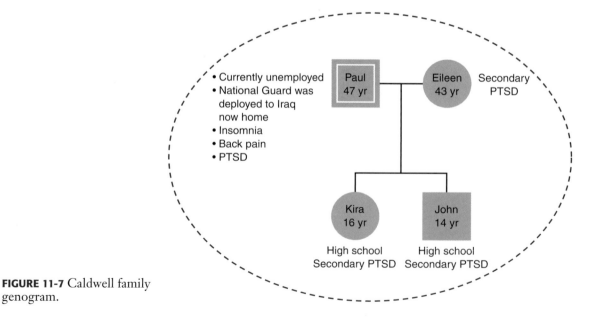

FIGURE 11-7 Caldwell family genogram.

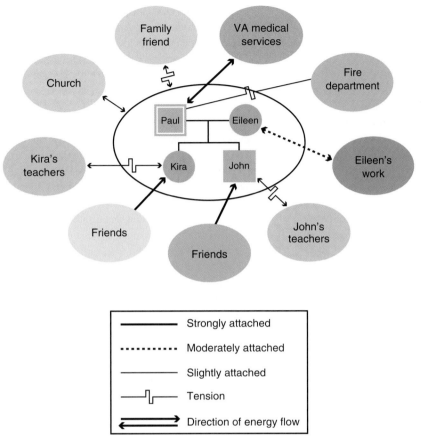

————————	Strongly attached
··············	Moderately attached
—————	Slightly attached
—⎍—	Tension
⇐⇒	Direction of energy flow

FIGURE 11-8 Caldwell family ecomap.

thinks everyone would be better off if he had not survived his tour in Iraq. He is currently on a number of medications for back pain from his on-the-job injury at the fire department. He is complaining of a lot of postoperative pain.

This composite case illustrates several kinds of war-zone stressors. Mr. Caldwell felt helpless to prevent several deaths. In addition to that feeling of helplessness, he had to witness the horror of many people dying, and had to respond to emergencies on a very unpredictable basis. Nurses, who are taking care of patients who have had a difficult return to civilian life, need to be aware of the complicated nature of readjustment. As this case illustrates, the prevalence of PTSD may increase considerably during the 2 years after veterans have returned from combat duty (Wolfe, Erickson, Sharkansky, King, & King, 1999).

This family is dealing with the chronic problems that occur when a veteran returns home with significant PTSD. The care for this family, when delivered from a Family Systems Theory perspective, will need to address Mr. Caldwell's PTSD, as well as the family's ever increasing secondary traumatization from his stress responses.

Theoretical Perspective:

Using a family systems theoretical approach, plan care for Mr. Caldwell that includes referral for his PTSD, and provides the family members with education and resources about what they can do to address their own secondary trauma, as well as support his recovery. As part of the plan, the nurse can help the Caldwell family by drawing a family ecomap that shows resources currently being used.

Because Mr. Caldwell has been traumatized by his experience with war, ultimately all of his family members and family relationships are affected. Mr. Caldwell's war experience was his alone, but his wife is being affected by the symptoms he is experiencing, symptoms that will get worse as she takes on even more of a caregiving role following his surgery. The children are baffled by the changes in their father, and do not know quite what to do. Because Mrs. Caldwell is so involved with caring for him, the children do not feel like they can go to her with their problems. In addition to their parents not being available to them

(continued)

emotionally, both children have had to take on family roles that their parents used to manage. For example, the daughter, Kira, now must do more of the family meal preparation and house cleaning. The son, John, has to do all of the yard work, which has made it harder to spend time with his friends. Both teenagers are starting not to do as well in school because of the constant tension in the home and their fears that their parents may divorce. Because Mr. Caldwell's trauma is so severe, it is highly likely the other members of the family will suffer secondary traumatization.

This family's response to the trauma of Mr. Caldwell from war cannot be understood or treated by focusing on just his care *(microsystem)*. His family members *(mesosystem)* can provide key contextual information about past traumatic events and experiences that can explain current responses. In fact, they are a central reason why Mr. Caldwell wants to get better and resume more of his leadership roles within the family. As he has been spiraling downward, the rest of the family has followed and all now report deteriorating mental health.

The boundaries or borders for this family may both be protective and act as a barrier to seeking help. It may be that Mrs. Caldwell feels it is disloyal to talk about her husband's problems with an outsider. Mr. Caldwell has many fears about admitting his difficulties and feels ashamed about how his problems have affected his wife. Mrs. Caldwell is afraid to ask for help because she does not want her husband to feel any more embarrassment than he does already. They are both suffering in silence, reluctant to talk to each other, or to anyone else. The nurse will have to create a trusting relationship to overcome this natural reluctance to share family secrets. One of the things that may help is to explain how providing this information may enhance the medical team's ability to provide quality care.

In this case, the spousal relationship has suffered because of Mr. Caldwell's trauma. Wartime separation and reunion, and then later problems with PTSD from combat, have created some marital dysfunction that was not there before. In this situation, the marital relationship as a subset within this family is the most problematic area. By helping this family improve this one area of its family functioning through appropriate referral, the nurse could have a great impact on the rest of the family subsystems. Because this is a new experience for Mr. and Mrs. Caldwell, they are not quite sure how to deal with it, plus they are reluctant to seek outside help at this time.

Assessment and Intervention Considerations:

The assessment and intervention for the Caldwell family focuses on PTSD and secondary trauma. As we can see clearly from this case, although Mr. Caldwell's traumatic exposure occurred some time ago, undiagnosed or inadequately treated PTSD could complicate his surgical recovery. PTSD is associated with more physical health problems and somatic symptom severity (Hoge, Terhakopian, Castro, Messer, & Engel, 2007). Although chronic widespread pain (CWP)—defined as pain in various parts of the body and fatigue that lasts for 3 months or longer—has thus far been documented only in veterans from the first Gulf War, the potential for this phenomenon to emerge in current combat veterans is high. CWP is associated with greater health care utilization and a lower quality of life (Forman-Hoffman et al., 2007). Researchers working for the Veterans Administration have documented that a substantial percentage of Iraq and Afghanistan veterans experience ongoing or new pain, of which 28% report is severe (Gironda, Clark, Massengale, & Walker, 2006).

In this instance, postoperatively Mr. Caldwell may be having more problems with pain perception, pain tolerance, and other kinds of untreated chronic pain. In addition, PTSD symptoms may make it difficult for the nurse to communicate with the patient, may reduce the patient's active collaboration in evaluation and treatment, and reduce patient adherence to medical regimens.

Assessment:

Because trauma is underrecognized, patients with PTSD are not properly identified and are not offered education, counseling, or referrals for mental health evaluation. There are simple methods to screen patients who may have undetected PTSD. As noted, one easy to use tool is the Primary Care PTSD Screen (Prins et al., 2004), consisting of four questions preceded by the following introduction:

"In your life, have you ever had any experience that was so frightening, horrible, or upsetting that, in the past month, you...

1. Have had nightmares about it or thought about it when you did not want to?
2. Tried hard not to think about it or went out of your way to avoid situations that reminded you of it?
3. Were constantly on guard, watchful, or easily startled?
4. Felt numb or detached from others, activities or your surroundings?"

The screen is positive if the patient answers *yes to any three items.*

Next, assess the family for possible symptoms of secondary traumatization. How are Mr. Caldwell's wife and children responding to his symptoms? What symptoms are they experiencing as a result of his difficulties? Identify how roles may have shifted for this family given Mr. Caldwell's current circumstances. Is the family still functioning as a strong cohesive unit? How have things changed? How open is this family to working with the nurse? What might help facilitate this?

Intervention:

Provide education about PTSD and secondary trauma. Because the family's participation is essential in identifying symptoms of PTSD and planning treatment, the nurse must create an environment that is supportive and inclusive of family members in order to work in partnership with the family. There are several sites on the Internet that can help the nurse develop educational fact sheets that can be shared with patients and families. The Veterans Affairs National Center for PTSD and the Defense Department's Walter Reed Army Medical Center collaborated to develop the Iraq War Clinician Guide (available at www.ncptsd.org/topics/war.html). The next step that the nurse should take in intervening with the Caldwell family is referring all family members for further care. Set up a plan for referring to a PTSD specialist those patients who show signs of potential PTSD and who are amenable to receiving additional evaluation or counseling. In this instance, the nurse could provide the family with a list of possible options. Many local areas have lists of returning veteran's counseling services that include counseling for couples and families. Involve the family in the plan of follow-up care.

SUMMARY

- Trauma affects the entire family system.
- Post-traumatic stress disorder (PTSD), which is a response to trauma, is more likely to develop when resiliency traits are lacking either before or after the trauma.
- PTSD can be acute or chronic and can occur months, even years, after a disaster or traumatic event such as war. PTSD affects both children and adults, with adults more likely to have flashbacks of the incident, and children more likely to develop hypersensitivity and avoidance of similar situations (e.g., avoiding cars after a motor vehicle accident).
- The Ecological Systems Theory can guide nursing assessment and interventions to help families cope effectively with trauma.
- When one or more family members are traumatized by an experience, all family members and family relationships are affected.

- The more severe the trauma an individual family member suffers, the more likely the other members of the family are at risk for secondary trauma.
- The family response to trauma of one or more of its members cannot be understood or treated by focusing on individual family members alone. Family members can provide key contextual information about past traumatic events and experiences that help explain current responses.
- Community systems can prevent, treat, and measure negative outcomes to traumatic events. If community agencies are not well trained and prepared, the risks for undetected and untreated PTSD increase.
- Larger political and social systems can influence and be influenced by individual, family, and community trauma. If nations experience severe trauma, they, as a whole, show signs of PTSD.
- Nursing focuses on the individual, family, community, and societal reactions to trauma in order to optimize positive outcomes and prevent or treat negative implications.

REFERENCES

Abbassi, A., & Aslinia, S. (2010). Family violence, trauma and social learning theory. *Journal of Professional Counseling: Practice, Theory & Research, 38*(1), 16–27.

Afifi, T. O., Boman, J., Fleisher, W., & Sareen, J. (2009). The relationship between child abuse, parental divorce, and lifetime mental disorders and suicidality in a nationally representative adult sample. *Child Abuse & Neglect, 33*(3), 139–147.

Alisic, E., Jongmans, M. J., van Wesel, F., & Kleber, R. J. (2011). Building child trauma theory from longitudinal studies: A meta-analysis. *Clinical Psychology Review, 31*(5), 736–747.

American Psychiatric Association. (2000). *Diagnostic and statistical manual of mental disorders—TR* (4th ed.) Washington, DC: American Psychiatric Association.

American Psychiatric Association. (2013). *Diagnostic and statistical manual of mental disorders* (5th ed.) Washington, DC: American Psychiatric Association.

American Red Cross. (2003). Disaster services. Retrieved June 18, 2008, from http://209.85.141.104/search?q=cache:P5RANQchefAJ:dutchesscounty.redcross.org/Documents/182%2520Community%2520Emergency.pdf+RED+CROSS+DEFINITION+OF+DISASTER&hl=en&ct=clnk&cd=3&gl=us&client=firefox-a

Anda, Felitti, Bremner, Walker, Whitfield, Perry,...Giles (2006). The enduring effects of abuse and related adverse experiences in childhood: A convergence of evidence from neurobiology and epidemiology. *European Archives of Psychiatry & Clinical Neurosciene, 256*, 174–186.

Black, D. W., Carney, D. P., Peloso, P. M., Woolson, R.F., Schwarts, D.A., Vollker, M.S. Barrett, D.H., & Doebbeling, B.N. (2004). Depression in veterans of the first Gulf War and comparable military controls. *Annual of Clinical Psychiatry*, *16*(2), 53–61.

Bowlby. J. (1973). *Attachment and loss: Volume 2, Separation: Anxiety and loss.* New York, NY: Basic Books.

Bremner, J. D., Southwick, S. M., Darnell, A., & Charney, D. S. (1996). Chronic PTSD in Vietnam combat veterans: Course of illness and substance abuse. *American Journal of Psychiatry*, *153*, 369–375.

Bridging Refugee Youth and Children's Services. (2013). Refugee 101. Retrieved July 2, 2013, from http://www.brycs.org/aboutRefugees/refugee101.cfm

Bronfenbrenner, U. (1984). The changing family in a changing world: America first? *Peabody Journal of Education*, *61*(3), 52–70.

Bronfenbrenner, U. (1995). Developmental ecology through space and time: A future perspective. In P. Moen, G.H. Elder, JR., & K. Luscher (Eds.). *Exmining lives in context:Perspectives in the ecology of human development* (pp. 619–647). Washington DC, American Psychological Association.

Bronfenbrenner, U. (1996). *The state of Americans: This generation and the next.* New York, NY: Free Press Bronfenbrenner, U., Lermer, R. M. (Eds.). (2004). *Making human beings human: Bioecological perspectives on human development.* Thousand Oaks, CA: Sage.

Bronfenbrenner, U. (2005). *Making human beings human: Bioecological perspectives on human development.* Thousand Oaks, CA: Sage Publications.

Center on the Developing Child. (2012). Toxic stress: The facts. Harvard University. Retrieved from http://developingchild.harvard.edu/topics/science_of_early_childhood/toxic_stress_response

Cohen, Jacox, Walker, Mannarino, Langley, & DuClos. (2009). Treating traumatized children after Hurrican Katrina: Project Fleur-de lis [TM], *Clinical Child and Family Psychology Review*, *12*, 55–64.

Cook, J. M., Riggs, D. S., Thompson, R., Coyne, J. C., & Sheikh, J. I. (2004). Posttraumatic stress disorder and current relationship functioning among World War II ex-prisoners of war. *Journal of Family Psychology*, *18*(1), 36–45.

Cozza, S. J., Chun, R. S., & Polo, J. A. (2005). Military familes and children during operation Iraqi Freedom, *Psychiatric Quarterly*, *76*(4), 371–378.

Crawford, A. (2010). If "the body keeps the score": Mapping the dissociated body in trauma narrative, intervention, and theory. *University of Toronto Quarterly: A Canadian Journal of the Humanities*, *79*(2), 702–719.

Dansky, B. S., Byrne, C. A., & Brady, K. T. (1999). Intimate violence and post-traumatic stress disorder among individuals with cocaine dependence. *American Journal of Drug & Alcohol Abuse*, *25*(2), 257.

Davis, T. M., & Wood, P. S. (1999). Substance abuse and sexual trauma in a female veteran population, *Journal of Substance Abuse Treatment*, *16*, 123–127.

Dekel, R., Solomon, Z., & Bleich, A. (2005). "Emotional distress and marital adjustment of caregivers: Contribution of level of impairment and appraised burden": Erratum. *Anxiety, Stress & Coping: An International Journal*, *18*(2), 157–159.

Devilly, G. J., Wright, R., & Varker, T. (2009). Vicarious trauma, secondary traumatic stress or simply burnout? Effect of trauma therapy on mental health professionals. *Australian & New Zealand Journal of Psychiatry*, *43*(4), 373–385.

Dirkzwager, A. J., Bramsen, I., Ader, H., & van der Ploeg, H. M. (2005). Secondary traumatization in partners and parents of Dutch peacekeeping soldiers. *Journal of Family Psychology*, *19*(2), 211–226.

Dyregrov, A., Gupta, L., Gjestad, R., & Mukanoheli, E. (2000). Trauma exposure and psychological reactions to genocide among Rwandan children. *Journal of Traumatic Stress*, *13*, 3–21.

Evans, L., McHugh, T., Hopwood, M., & Watt, C. (2003). Chronic posttraumatic stress disorder and family functioning of Vietnam veterans and their partners. *Australian & New Zealand Journal of Psychiatry*, *37*(6), 765–772.

Figley, C. R., & Barnes, M. (2005). External trauma and families. In P.C. McKenry & S. J. Price (Eds.). *Families and change: Coping with stressful events and transitions.* (3rd ed., pp. 379–399.). Thousand Oaks, CA: Sage.

Fonseca, C. A., Schmaling, K. B., Stoever, C., Gutierrez, C., Blume, A. W., & Russell, M. L. (2006). Variables associated with intimate partner violence in a deploying military sample. *Military Medicine*, *111*(7), 627–631.

Forman-Hoffman, V. L., Peloso, P.M., Black, D. W., Woolson, R. E., Letuchy, E. M., & Doebbeling, B. N. (2007). Chronic widespread pain in veterans of the First Guilf War: Impact of deployment status and associated health effects. *Journal of Pain*, *8*(12), 954–961.

Friedman, M. J. (2006). Posttraumatic stress disorder among military retunees from Afgahanistan and Iraq. *American Journal of Psychiatry*, *163*, 586–593.

Friedman, M. J., Resick, P. A., Bryant, R. A., Strain, J., Horowitz, M., & Spiegel, D. (2011). Classification of trauma and stressor-related disorders in DSM-5. *Depression & Anxiety*, *28*(9), 737–749.

Galovski, T., & Lyons, J. A. (2004). Psychological sequelae of combat violence: A review of the impact of PTSD on the veteran's family and possible interventions. *Aggression and Violent Behavior*, *9*(5), 477–501.

Gard, B. A., & Ruzek, J. I. (2006). Community mental health response to crisis. *Journal of Clinical Psychology*, *62*(8), 1029–1041. Gironda, R. J., Clark, M. E., Massengale, J. P., & Walker, R. L. (2006). Pain among veterans of operations Enduring Freedom and Iraqi Freedom. *Pain Medicine*, *7*(4), 339–343.

Glaser D. (2000). Child abuse and neglect and the brain—A review. *Journal of Child Psychology and Psychiatry*, *41*(1), 97–116.

Glauber, B. (2007). Experts tackle suicide prevention among combat veterans: Doctors, social workers here join VA's drive for awareness. Retrieved from http://www.jsonline.com/news/milwaukee/29249659.html

Goff, B. S., Crow, J. R., Reisbig, A. M., & Hamilton, S. (2007). The impact of individual trauma symptoms of deployed soldiers on relationship satisfaction. *Journal of Family Psychology*, *21*(3), 344–353.

Gold, J. I., Taft, C. T., Keehn, M. G., King, D. W., King, L. A., & Samper, R. E. (2007). PTSD symptom severity and family adjustment among female Vietnam veterans. *Military Psychology*, *19*(2), 71–81.

Heller, L., & LaPierre, A. (2012). *Healing developmental trauma: How early trauma affects self-regulation, self-image, and the capacity for relationship.* Berkeley, CA: North Atlantic Books.

Hensley, S. (2010). Kids become prime growth market for prescription drugs. National Public Radio. Retrieved from

http://www.npr.org/blogs/health/2010/05/19/126975784/
kids-become-prime-market-for-presention-drugs?sc=11&f=1001

Herbert, J. D., & Forman, E. M. (in press). Posttraumatic stress
disorder. In J. E. Fisher & W. O'Donohue (Eds.), *Practice guidelines for evidence based psychotherapy*. New York, NY: Springer.

Herbert, J. D., & Sageman, M. (2004). "First Do No Harm:"
Emerging guidelines for the treatment of posttraumatic reactions. In G. M. Rosen (Ed.), *Posttraumatic stress disorder: issues
and controversy* (pp. 213–232). Sussex, England: Wiley & Sons.

Hernández, P., Gangsei, D., & Engstrom, D. (2007). Vicarious
resilience: A new concept in work with those who survive
trauma. *Family Process, 46*(2), 229–241.

Hoge, C. W., McGurk, D., Thomas, J., Cox, A. L., Engel, C. C.,
& Castro, C. A. (2008). Mild traumatic brain injury in U.S.
soldiers returning from Iraq. *New England Journal of Medicine,
358*(5), 453–463.

Hoge, C. W., Terhakopian, A., Castro, C. A., Messer, S. C., &
Engel, C. C. (2007). Association of posttraumatic stress disorder with somatic symptoms, health care visits, and absenteeism
among Iraq War veterans, *American Journal of Psychiatry,
164*(4), 150–153.

Hulette, A., Kaehler, L., & Freyd, J. (2011). Intergenerational associations between trauma and dissociation. *Journal of Family
Violence, 26*(3), 211–225. International Federation of Red
Cross and Red Crescent Societies. (2012). World disasters report 2012—Disaster data. In *World Disasters Report*. Retrieved
from http://www.ifrc.org/en/publications-and-reports/

International Strategy for Disaster Reduction. (2006, July).
Disaster statistics. Retrieved January 23, 2008, from http://
www.unisdr.org/disaster-statistics/introduction.htm

Joubert, D., Webster, L., & Hackett, R. (2012). Unresolved
attachment status and trauma-related symptomatology in
maltreated adolescents: An examination of cognitive mediators. *Child Psychiatry and Human Development, 43*(3), 471–483.

Kang, H. K., Natelson, B. H., Mahan, C. M., Lee, K. Y., &
Murphy, F. M. (2003). Post-traumatic stress disorder and
chronic fatigue syndrome–like illness among Gulf War veterans: A population-based survey of 30,000 veterans. *American
Journal of Epidemiology, 157*(2), 141–148.

Karr-Morse, R., & Wiley, M. (2012). *Scared sick: The roles of
childhood trauma in adult disease*. New York, NY: Basic Books.

Kitzmann, K. M. (2012). Domestic violence and its impact on the
social and emotional development of young children. In H.
MacMillan et al. (Eds.), *Encyclopedia on early childhood development* (3rd ed.). Retrieved from http://www.child-encyclopedia.
com/document/KitzmannANGxp3.pdf

Kitzmann, K. M., Gaylord, N. K., Holt, A. R., & Kenny, E. D.
(2003). Child witnesses to domestic violence: A meta-analytic
review. *Journal of Consulting & Clinical Psychology, 71*(2), 339.

Kulka, R. A., Schlenger, W. A., Fairbanks, J. A., Hough, R. L.,
Jordan, B. K., Marmar, C. R., & Cranston, A. S. (1990).
*Trauma and the Vietnam War generation: Report of findings from
the National Vietnam Veterans Readjustment Study*. New York,
NY: Brunner/Mazel.

Luthar, S. S., & Cicchetti, D., & Becker, B. (2000). The construct of resilience: A critical evaluation and guidelines for
future work. *Child Development, 71*(3), 543–562.

Manguno-Mire, G., Sautter, F., Lyons, J., Myers, L., Perry, D.,
Sherman, M.,...Sullivan, G. (2007). Psychological distress and
burden among female partners of combat veterans with
PTSD. *Journal of Nervous and Mental Disease, 195*(2), 144–151.

McNally, R. J. (2004). Conceptual problems with the DSM-IV
criteria for posttraumatic stress disorder. In G. M. Rosen
(Ed.), *Posttraumatic stress disorder: Issues and controversy*
(pp. 1–14). Sussex, England: Wiley & Sons.

Meadors, P., Lamson, A., Swanson, M., White, M., & Sira, N.
(2009). Secondary traumatization in pediatric healthcare
providers: Compassion fatigue, burnout, and secondary traumatic stress. *Omega: Journal of Death & Dying, 60*(2), 103–128.

Meagher, I. (2007). *The war list: OEF/OIF statistics*. Retrieved
from http://www.ptsdcombat.com/documents/ptsdcombat_
war-list_oef-oif-statistics.pdf

Miehls, D. (2010). Contemporary trends in supervision theory: A
shift from parallel process to relational and trauma theory.
Clinical Social Work Journal, 38(4), 370–378. Mills, M. A.,
Edmondson, D., & Park, C. L. (2007). Trauma and stress
response among Hurricane Katrina evacuees. *American Journal
of Public Health, 97*(Suppl 1), S116–S123.

National Center for PTSD. (2010, June). Effects of PTSD on
family. Retrieved July, 2013, from http://www.ptsd.va.gov/
public/pages/effects-ptsd-family.asp

National Institute of Mental Health. (2008, August). The
National Institute of Mental Health Strategic Plan. NIMH
RSS. Retrieved July 2, 2013, from http://www.nimh.nih.gov/
about/strategic-planning-reports/index.shtml

National Institute on Drug Abuse. (2012, December). DrugFacts:
Nationwide trends. Retrieved July 2, 2013, from http://www.
drugabuse.gov/publications/drugfacts/nationwide-trends

National Severe Storms Laboratory. (2007). Retrieved June 9,
2008, from http://www.nssl.noaa.gov

Newell, J. M., & MacNeil, G. A. (2010). Professional burnout,
vicarious trauma, secondary traumatic stress, and compassion
fatigue: A review of theoretical terms, risk factors, and preventive methods for clinicians and researchers. *Best Practice in
Mental Health, 6*(2), 57–68.

Norman, R. E., Byambaa, M., De, R., Butchart, A., Scott, J., &
Vos, T. (2012). The long-term health consequences of child
physical abuse, emotional abuse, and neglect: A systematic
review and meta-analysis. *Plos Medicine, 9*(11), 1–31.

Norris, F. H. (2007, May 22). Psychosocial consequences of
natural disasters in developing countries: What does past research tell us about the potential effects of the 2004 tsunami?
Retrieved January 27, 2008, from http://www.ncptsd.va.
gov/ncmain/ncdocs/fact_shts/fs_tsunami_research.html

Orcutt, H. K., King, L. A., & King, D. W. (2003). Male-perpetrated
violence among Vietnam veteran couples: relationships with
veteran's early life characteristics, trauma history, and PTSD
symptomatology. *Journal of Traumatic Stress, 16*(4), 381–390.

Overland, G. (2011). Generating theory, biographical accounts
and translation: A study of trauma and resilience. *International
Journal of Social Research Methodology, 14*(1), 61–75. Ozer, E. J.,
Best, S. R., Lipsey, T. L., & Weiss, D. S. (2003). Predictors
of posttraumatic stress disorder and symptoms in adults: A
meta-analysis. *Psychological Bulletin, 129*, 52–73.

Perry, B. D., & Pollard, R. (1998). Review: Homeostasis, stress,
trauma, and adaptation. A neurodevelopmental view of
childhood trauma. *Child and Adolescent Psychiatric Clinics of
North America, 7*(1):33–51, viii.

Philippe, F. L., Laventure, S., Beaulieu-Pelletier, G., Lecours, S.,
& Lekes, N. (2011). Ego-Resiliency as a Mediator Between
Childhood Trauma and Psychological Symptoms. *Journal of
Social and Clinical Psychology 30*(6), 583–598.

Prins, A., Ouimette, P. C., Kimerling, R., Cameron, R. P., Hugelshofer, D. S., Shaw-Hegwer, J.,...Sheikh, J. I. (2004). The Primary Care PTSD Screen (PC-PTSD): Development and operating characteristics. *Primary Care Psychiatry.*, *9*, 9–14

Radstone, S. (2007). Trauma theory: Contexts, politics, ethics. *Paragraph: A Journal of Modern Critical Theory, 30*(1), 9–29.

Richardson, M., Coryn, C., Henry, J., Black-Pond, C., & Unrau, Y. (2012). Development and evaluation of the Trauma-Informed System Change Instrument: Factorial validity and implications for use. *Child & Adolescent Social Work Journal, 29*(3), 167–184.

Rosenheck, R., & Fontana, A. (1994). Long-term sequelae of combat in World War II, Korea and Vietnam: A comparative study. In R. J. Ursano, B. G. McCaughey, & C. S. Fullerton (Eds.), *Individual and community responses to trauma and disaster: The structure of human chaos* (pp. 330–359). New York, NY: Cambridge University Press.

Rutler, M. (1987). Psychosocial resilience and protective mechanisms, *American Journal of Orthopsychiatry, 57*, 316–331.

Salmond, C. H., Meiser-Stedman, R. R., Glucksman, E. E., Thompson, P. P., Dalgleish, T. T., & Smith, P. P. (2011). The nature of trauma memories in acute stress disorder in children and adolescents. *Journal of Child Psychology & Psychiatry, 52*(5), 560–570.

Samper, R. E., Taft, C. T., King, D. W., & King, L. A. (2004). Posttraumatic stress disorder symptoms and parenting satisfaction among a national sample of male Vietnam veterans. *Journal of Traumatic Stress, 11*(4), 311–315.

Sautter, F., Lyons, J. A., Manguno-Mire, G., Perry, D., Han, S., Sherman, M.,...Sullivan, G. (2006). Predictions of partner engagement in PTSD treatment. *Journal of Psychopathology and Behavioral Assessment, 28*(2), 123–130.

Schmid, M., Petermann, F., & Fegert, J. M. (2013). Developmental trauma disorder: Pros and cons of including formal criteria in the psychiatric diagnostic systems. *BMC Psychiatry, 13*(1), 1–12.

Seedat, S., Stein, D. J., & Carey, P. D. (2005). Post-traumatic stress disorder in women: Epidemiological and treatment issues. *CNS Drugs, 19*(5), 411–427.

Selye, H. (1976). *Stress in health and disease.* Reading, MA: Butterworth.

Skelton, J. A., Loveland, J. E., & Yeagley, J. L. (1996). Recalling symptom episodes affects reports of immediately-experienced symptoms: Inducing symptom suggestibility. *Psychology & Health, 11*, 183–201.

Smith, M., Segal, J., & Segal, R. (2012). Preventing burnout. Retrieved from http://www.helpguide.org/mental/burnout_ signs_symptoms.htm

Smith, R. J. (2013). Operation BRAVE Families: A preventive approach to lessening the impact of war on military families through preclinical engagement. *Military Medicine, 118*(2), 114–119.

Stankovi_, M., Grbe_a, G., Kosti_, J., Simonovi_, M., Milenkovi_, T., & Vi_nji, A. (2013). A preview of the efficiency of systemic family therapy in treatment of children with posttraumatic stress disorder developed after car accident. *Vojnosanitetski Pregled: Military Medical & Pharmaceutical Journal of Serbia & Montenegro, 70*(2), 149–154.

Substance Abuse and Mental Health Services Administration. (2011). Helping children and adolescents who have experienced traumatic events. Retrieved from http://digitallibraries. macrointernational.com/gsdl/collect/cmhsdigi/index/assoc/ HASH01f9.dir/doc.pdf

Taft, C. T., Pless, A. P., Stalans, L. J., Koenen, K. C., King, L. A., & King, D. W. (2005). Risk factors for partner violence among a national sample of combat veterans. *Journal of Consulting and Clinical psychology, 73*(1), 151–159.

Tanielian, T., & Jaycox, L. (Eds.). (2008). Invisible wounds of war: Psychological and cognitive injuries, their consequences, and services to assist recovery. Santa Monica, CA: Rand Corporation.

Taylor, L., Weist, M., & DeLoach, K. (2012). Exploring the use of the interactive systems framework to guide school mental health services in post-disaster contexts: Building community capacity for trauma-focused interventions. *American Journal of Community Psychology, 50*(3/4), 530–540.

Terleggen, M., Stroebe, M., & Kleber R. (2001). Western conceptualization and Eastern experience: A cross-cultural study of traumatic stress reactions among Tibetan refugees in India. *Journal of Traumatic Stress, 14*, 391–403.

Thabet, A. A., & Vostanis, P. (2000). Post traumatic stress disorder reactions in children of war: A longitudinal study. *Child Abuse and Neglect, 24*, 291–298.

Thomas, R., & Wilson, J. (2004). Issues and controversies in the understanding and diagnosis of compassion fatigue, vicarious traumatization and secondary traumatic stress disorder. *International Journal of Emergency Mental Health, 6*, 81–92.

Trippany, R. L., White Kress, V. E., & Wilcoxon, S. (2004). Preventing vicarious trauma: What counselors should know when working with trauma survivors. *Journal of Counseling & Development, 82*(1), 31–37.

U.S. Department of Health and Human Services, Administration for Children and Families, Administration on Children, Youth and Families, Children's Bureau. (2012). Child maltreatment 2011. Retrieved from http://www.acf.hhs.gov

U.S. Department of Homeland Security. (2011). Budget in brief: 2011. Retrieved from http://www.dhs.gov/xlibrary/assets/ budget_bib_fy2011.pdf

U.S. Department of Veterans Affairs. (2007). Epidemiology of PTSD. Retrieved from http://www.ptsd.va.gov/professional/ pages/epidemiological-facts-ptsd.asp

Van De Voorde, P., Sabbe, M., Tsonaka, R., Rizopoulos, D., Calle, P., De Jaeger, A., & Matthys, D. (2011). The long-term outcome after severe trauma of children in Flanders (Belgium): A population-based cohort study using the International Classification of Functioning–related outcome score. *European Journal of Pediatrics, 110*(1), 65–73.

Warner, J. (2010). Disregulation nation. Retrieved from http://www.nytimes.com/2010/06/20/magazine/20fFOB-WWLN-t.htm

Williams, N. R., Lindsey, E. W., Kurtz, P. D., & Jarvis, S. (2001). From trauma to resiliency: Lessons from former runaway and homeless youth. *Journal of Youth Studies, 4*(2), 233–253.

Wolfe, J., Erickson, D. J., Sharkansky, E. J., King, D. W., & King, L. A. (1999). Course and predictors of posttraumatic stress disorder among Gulf War veterans; A prospective analysis. *Journal of Consulting Clinical Psychology, 67*, 520–528.

Nursing Care of Families in Clinical Areas

chapter 12

Family Nursing With Childbearing Families

Linda Veltri, PhD, RN

Karline Wilson-Mitchell, RM, CNM, RN, MSN

Kathleen Bell, RN, MSN, CNM, AHN-BC

Critical Concepts

- Childbearing family nursing is not synonymous with obstetrical nursing, which only considers the woman as the client and as the family as context for care. In contrast, childbearing family nursing considers the family as client, the family as context for the care of its members, or both. Childbearing family nursing primarily focuses on health and wellness rather than on procedures and medical treatment.

- Nurses must understand and utilize multiple theories to plan and guide nursing care for childbearing families.

- Nurses must understand the impact that social policy, available resources, and geographical location have on child-bearing families.

- The holistic care of these families is best provided with an approach that acknowledges the social determinants of health and the integration of all of the members of the health care team and community resources.

- Nurses need to be aware of stressors childbearing families encounter before, during, and after reproductive events so they can anticipate, identify, and respond to needs appropriately.

- The family constellation and the definition of family depend on the culture, worldview, sexual orientation, and perspective of the family. Consequently, childbearing family nursing necessitates demonstrating respect and cultural competence.

- Nursing care for adoptive families should be provided in a manner similar to that which is provided to biological families. Nurses should recognize and meet these families' special needs, regardless of the family constellation.

- Nurses caring for childbearing families experiencing infertility must consider, understand, and address the family's emotional and physical needs.

- Understanding the many ways families experience grief and loss allows nurses to advocate for practices that best facilitate childbearing as a transitional event in the life of the family.

- A process of bereavement should be anticipated with perinatal loss, adverse perinatal outcome, diagnosis of congenital or genetic disorders, palliative care, or the birth of a special needs child.

(continued)

Before the onset of professional nursing in North America during the late 19th century, caregivers for childbearing families were women. Female family members, in-laws, neighbors, friends, and midwives came to the home to encourage, support, and nurture a woman during and after childbirth (Burst, 2004; Mander, 2004; Varney, Kriebs, & Gregor, 2004). During this time, many of these women midwives were settlers who followed the European colonists and were African slaves, or First Nations/Native Americans. Similarly, in Canada, Canadian pioneer and Aboriginal midwives also attended births up through the 1940s. It was these women caregivers who maintained family functions of the household, tended to new babies and mothers' other children, and provided postpartum physical care. During these same years, the father's role in childbirth was limited to announcing labor had begun and seeking assistance from other women (Mander, 2004). Although male obstetricians emerged as primary clinical providers of birth management and influenced both maternity education and health care policy in the 1860s, male family members, friends, and children were excluded from the childbirth experience until the 1970s. This practice was justified by the belief that nonmedical participants increased the risk of introducing infection into the perinatal setting.

Beginning in the late 1960s, families became increasingly knowledgeable about childbearing and desirous of a more satisfying birth experience as a family event. The families became savvy health care consumers who found hospital routines and policies too restrictive if they required strict adherence to newborn feeding and sleeping schedules, kept fathers and siblings out of the delivery room, or separated parents from their newborns. In response, informed families lobbied for changes in childbearing practices; they used evidence to support not separating mothers and babies immediately after delivery, as well as other hallmark findings demonstrating improved parent-child attachment with immediate and frequent contact between mothers, fathers, and siblings and their newborns (de Chateau, 1976, 1977; Klaus et al., 1972; Martell, 2006). Largely as a result of the women's rights and health reproductive movement (Morgan, 2002), families presented compelling arguments for hospitals to support exclusive breastfeeding, kangaroo-care or "skin-to-skin" baby carrying, and delayed cord clamping (Britton, McCormick, Renfrew, Wade, & King, 2007; Gray, Miller, Philipp, & Blass, 2002; Gray, Watt, & Blass, 2000; Hutton & Hassan, 2007; Mercer et al., 2006).

In time, nurses, hospitals, and other health care providers for women began to recognize the effect reproductive events have on all family members, as well as the reciprocal influence of the family on the parents and infants. This recognition has resulted in inclusion of family concepts into nursing care of childbearing families. With the trend for increased family education about reproductive events, increased responsibility for family members to plan for care during pregnancy and delivery, and shorter hospital stays after birth, postpartum care is returning to family care within the context of the home with nursing guidance, rather than being medically based in a hospital. This shift in focus from caring for the individual woman as client toward consideration and inclusion of the family in care from preconception to the postpartum period is known as *childbearing family nursing*. The historical perspective is outlined in Box 12-1.

Notably, the practice of childbearing family nursing is not synonymous with obstetrical nursing. Obstetrical nursing considers the woman as the client and views the family as the context for care. Childbearing family nursing, by contrast, considers the family as the client and the family as context for the care of its members. It is a health and wellness, rather than an illness, model of care. Similarly, childbearing family nurses take

a holistic approach to care; they consider the woman and her family's physical, mental, emotional, spiritual, social, and cultural indicators of health. Although the woman, as an individual, is most affected by the event of childbirth, the family unit is intimately involved in that event. For example, the addition of a new human being into the world involves caring for the minds, bodies, and spirits of all those who will be entrusted to nurture the newborn. Becoming a part of this transitional time through engagement in the

---

BOX 12-1
Historical Perspective of Childbearing Family Nursing

Historical Perspective

Late 1800s: Industrialization

- Families moved to more urban areas; household size and functions diminished.
- Traditional networks of women were not always available, and mothers needed to replace care previously carried out in the home.
- Childbearing still occurred at home for many middle-class families (Leavitt, 1986; Wertz & Wertz, 1989).
- European colonists, African slaves, and First Nations/Native Americans served as midwives.

First Third of the 20th Century

- The hospital became the place for labor, birth, and early postpartum recovery for middle-class families.
- Many immigrant and working-class urban families continued to have newborns at home with their traditional care providers.
- An impetus to the development of public health nursing was concern for the health of urban mothers and babies.
- Realizing that the health needs of all the family members were intertwined, early public health nurses considered families, not individuals, as their clients.

1930s Through the "Baby Boom" of the 1950s

- In Canada, Canadian pioneer and Aboriginal midwives attended births up through the 1940s.
- With the dramatic shift of births to hospitals, family involvement with childbearing diminished (Leavitt, 1986).
- Concerns about infection control contributed to separation of family members.
- Family members, especially males, were forbidden to be with women in the hospital.
- Babies were segregated into nurseries and brought out to their mothers only for brief feeding sessions.
- Nurses focused on the smooth operation of postpartum wards and nurseries through the use of routine and order.

- Despite these inflexible conditions, families tolerated them because they believed that hospital births were safer for mothers and newborns.

1960s to 1970s

- Families and health care professionals questioned the need for heavy sedation and analgesia for childbearing and embraced natural childbirth.
- A feature of natural childbirth was the close relationship between the laboring woman and a supportive person serving as a coach; in North America, husbands assumed this supportive role (Wertz & Wertz, 1989).
- Expectant parents actively sought out physicians and hospitals that would best meet their expectations for father involvement and the control over childbearing began to shift from health care professionals to families.
- Some nurses were skeptical about the changes families demanded, but others were enthusiastic about increased family participation.
- Many hospital-based maternity nurses began to consider themselves to be mother-baby nurses rather than nursery or postpartum nurses, and labor and delivery nurses often collaborated with family members in helping women cope with the discomforts of labor.

1980s to the Present

- Klaus and Kennel's research (1976) served as the impetus for the growth of family-centered care (American College of Obstetricians and Gynecologists and the Interprofessional Task Force on Health Care of Women and Children, 1978).
- Today, promotion of family contact is becoming the hallmark of childbearing care.
- Many hospitals have renamed their obstetrical services, using names such as Family Birth Center to convey the importance of family members in childbearing health care even though obstetrical care is becoming more dependent on technology.

woman and family's lived experience throughout its entirety versus remaining at a functional level by "doing for" the client is an emerging role for childbearing family nurses. As a result, nurses and families are being challenged by societal and health care system changes to adapt and expand their perspectives regarding family health. This new emphasis requires nurses to move away from a linear model of interventions aimed at moving clients from a state of disease/illness to wellness, toward a shared experience of controlling or transcending a threat to health and helping the client/family integrate their experience as one with purpose and meaning (LeVasseur, 2002). In other words, childbearing family nurses are changing their focus from "caring for" to "caring about" families (Cronqvist, Theorell, Burns, & Lutzen, 2004). Using a holistic and transpersonal approach to understanding the woman's entire mind/body/soul during times of health threats offers one of the most fulfilling roles for the nurse and it may be one of the first experiences of empowered caring for the client (Ward & Hisley, 2009).

Family nursing with childbearing families covers the period before conception, pregnancy, labor, birth, and the postpartum period. Childbearing family nursing traditionally begins with a family's decision to start having children and continues until parents have achieved a degree of relative comfort in their roles as parents of infants and/or have ceased the addition of new children to their families. Often, childbearing family nursing is expanded to include the periods between pregnancies and includes other aspects of reproductive care such as family planning, infertility, perinatal loss, sexuality, adoption, foster care, and parenting grandchildren. Decisions and changes surrounding childbearing vary for families throughout the reproductive cycle. Factors driving these decisions or changes include prevailing health policies and the family's cultural, socioeconomic, and psychological needs. As a result, the beginning and end points of the reproductive period may be different for each family.

Childbearing family nursing practice offers nurses the opportunity to engage in transpersonal care by applying the nursing process of assessment, diagnosis, planning, implementation, and evaluation in a new way to orient knowledge and direct care

activities to the entire childbearing family. It is through this process that nurses assess a family's knowledge and confidence to manage the health concerns, diagnose alterations in health from the client's viewpoint, conceptualize the outcome as the client and family sees it, and support the client in making the changes needed either to restore health or transcend the threat, concern, or event. The final step of this process is evaluation of ongoing maintenance of health and wellness as it is lived by the client and family (Ward & Hisley, 2009). When childbearing family nurses incorporate transpersonal care in this way, the essence of family-centered care, which involves placing family relationships, coping mechanisms, values, priorities, and perceptions at the center of the health event or concern, is maintained.

The focus of childbearing family nurses is centered on family relationships and the health of all family members. Therefore, nurses involved with childbearing families use family concepts and theories as part of developing the plan of nursing care. This chapter starts by presenting theoretical perspectives that guide nursing practice with childbearing families. It continues with an exploration of family nursing with childbearing families before conception through the postpartum period. The chapter concludes with implications for nursing practice, research, and policy, along with two case studies that explore family adaptations to stressors and changing roles related to childbearing.

THEORY-GUIDED, EVIDENCE-BASED CHILDBEARING NURSING

Application of theory to family health situations during childbearing can guide family nurses in making more complete assessments and planning interventions congruent with the pattern of events during childbearing. Several of the theories discussed in Chapter 3 contribute to nurses' understanding of how families grow, develop, function, and change during childbearing. Two of these theories in particular, Family Systems Theory and Family Developmental and Life Cycle Theory, are especially applicable to childbearing families. A brief summary of these theories and their application to childbearing families follows.

Family Systems Theory

Family Systems Theory provides a framework for viewing the family as a system: as an organized whole and/or as individuals within the family who form interactive and interdependent systems. Four main concepts underlie this theory: (1) all parts of the system are interconnected, (2) the whole is more than the sum of the parts, (3) all systems have some form of boundaries or borders between the system and its environment, and (4) systems can be further organized into subsystems. Family systems are primarily designed to maintain stability, and a change in one member of the family affects all of the family.

Becoming parents or adding a child brings stress to a family by challenging family stability, not only for the nuclear and extended family systems themselves but also for the individual members and subsystems of the family. As new subsystems are created or modified by pregnancy and childbirth, a sense of disequilibrium exists until a family adapts to its new member and re-achieves stability. For example, changes in the husband-wife subsystem occur as a response to development of the new parent-child subsystems.

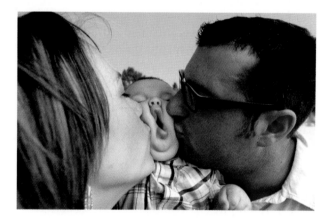

Imbalance, or disequilibrium, occurs while adjustments are still needed and new roles are being learned. Families with greater flexibility in role expectations and behaviors tend to experience these periods of disequilibrium with less discomfort. The greater the range or number of coping strategies available to the family, and the greater the ability and support available to engage in various family roles, the more effective the family's response will be to both internal strains and external stress associated with childbearing. External stresses, such as concerns about outside employment, child care, and lack of health insurance, may be important in predicting family disequilibrium. Internal strains such as an ill or special needs child or unhealthy habits, such as substance abuse, may tax family coping mechanisms to the breaking point. Therefore, it is imperative that nurses identify both present and potential family stressors and assess the effect of stressors on family stability.

Family Systems Theory is especially effective for use by childbearing family nurses because following childbirth, families who are in a state of change and readjustment tend to have more permeable boundaries and are more likely to be open to the outside environment. This openness stems from the need for additional resources beyond what the family can supply for itself. Consequently, a family in transition is apt to be engaged in more interactions with systems outside the family and may become more receptive to interventions such as health teaching than it would be at other times in the family life cycle (Martell, 2005). This openness of family boundaries allows nurses more access to the family for assessment, diagnosis, and health promotion.

On the other hand, childbearing family nurses should be aware of very closed or enmeshed families who may have nonpermeable boundaries and reject outside influences, including nursing care. Families can become closed because they interpret the outside environment and systems as hostile, threatening, or difficult to cope with. These families are challenging for nurses because they are less readily accessible or responsive to family nurses.

Nurses working with childbearing families from a systems perspective view the family as the client and aim to assist families to maintain and regain stability. Therefore, assessment questions should be focused on the family as a whole. At the same time, it is important to remember that family nurses also work with the individuals and the subsystems within the family. Interventions need to be directed at the various systems and levels of subsystems within the family. For example, a family ecomap will help the nurse see how individual members and the family as a whole relate to one another and to the community around them. Understanding the family process and functioning through careful assessment of the family as a whole and the individual family members allows the nurse to offer intervention strategies that will help provide stability in the family's everyday functioning.

Family Developmental and Life Cycle Theory

Duvall's (1977) Family Developmental and Life Cycle Theory described a process of developing over time that is predictable and yet individual, based on unique life circumstances and family interactions. Although the life cycle of most families around the world follows a universal sequence of family development, it is important for childbearing family nurses to recognize that wide variations exist in the timing and sequencing of family life cycle phases (Berk, 2007; Carter & McGoldrick, 2005; Duvall, 1977). Many present-day childbearing families in North America do not fit into the classic sequence and timing of family developmental stages and tasks originally described by Duvall and Miller (1985). For example, families may be blended, with one or both partners having children from a previous relationship. Other types of nontraditional family structures include adoptive families; communal or multigenerational families; and parents who may be cohabitating, unmarried, single, of the same sex, or have children born later in life (Berk, 2007; McKinney, James, Murray, Nelson, & Ashwill, 2013). As a result, nontraditional and high-risk families such as those experiencing unusual levels of stress from marital conflict and divorce, violence, substance abuse, having a child with special needs, or being an adolescent parent require care that is different from that needed by traditional families (McKinney et al., 2013).

Despite how diverse the family is today, Family Developmental and Life Cycle Theory remains a helpful guide for childbearing family nurses because it addresses the patterns of adaptation to parenthood that are typical for many families. This theory has relevance for family nurses regardless of how families are structured, because the essential tasks families must perform to survive as healthy units are generally present to some extent in all families (Pillitteri, 2003).

According to Duvall's (1977) Family Developmental and Life Cycle Theory, family changes occur in stages during which there is upheaval while adjustments are being made. What occurs during these stages is generally referred to as a developmental task. The "Childbearing Family With Infants" stage is pertinent to childbearing family nursing practice because it is during this stage that childbearing families must accomplish nine specific tasks in order to grow and achieve family well-being. These nine tasks for childbearing families and nursing interventions are explained in the following subsections.

Task One: Arranging Space (Territory) for a Child

Arranging space (territory) involves families making space preparations for their infants. Families often accommodate newborns by moving to a new residence during pregnancy or the first year after birth or by modifying their living quarters and furnishings. Families may delay or avoid space preparations for a new baby for several reasons. For example, busy families, those who fear or have experienced prior fetal loss, and families involved with adoption or foster placement may delay or avoid space preparations. For some groups, such as Orthodox Jews, preparation for a baby's material needs, such as blankets and diapers during pregnancy, is not acceptable; it may mean bad luck or misfortune for the baby (Cassar, 2006). The lack of space preparation may also result from the parents not having accepted the reality of the coming baby (denial). It may also emerge from various social risks or health disparities, including expensive health care needs incurred by other family members; inadequate, unsafe housing arrangements or homelessness; underemployment or poverty; recent immigration; and incarceration. Adolescent parents may not make space arrangements because of denial of the pregnancy or fear of repercussions from their families if pregnancy is revealed.

Family Nursing Interventions
- Inquire about the safety and health of the family's home environment, food, security (including freedom from domestic violence), space arrangements made for baby, and other child care resources, community resources, or other support systems.
- Refer families who are homeless or live in inadequate or unsafe housing to appropriate resources for obtaining safer housing.
- Inquire about the families' thoughts, values, beliefs, and possible fears about making preparations for the anticipated arrival of the baby.
- Assist families to explore and manage their fear about survival or loss of the baby and

then mobilize resources to help them cope so that family development can continue.

- Assist adolescents to find ways to communicate with their families and make plans for the future placement and well-being of the infant and the adolescent parents.
- Work with prisoners, interested stakeholders, and state/federal penal systems to establish units where newborns and mothers can stay together to encourage bonding and breastfeeding while the mother is incarcerated.

Task Two: Financing Childbearing and Child Rearing

Childbearing results in additional expenses and lower family income. American families, having experienced two economic downturns since the start of the 21st century, are finding the decision to bear and the ability to raise children increasingly financially difficult (Guttmacher Institute, 2009; Oberg, 2011). Low-income families and children, especially African Americans and those of Hispanic descent, have been disproportionally burdened by these recessions and continue to struggle just to make ends meet (Bruening, MacLehose, Loth, Story, & Neumark-Sztainer, 2012; Oberg, 2011). Financial stresses can be even harder for mothers without partners, women who provide most of the income for their families, mothers who are fleeing domestic violence, or mothers experiencing unplanned pregnancy. Families with precarious immigration status (including refugee claimants or migrant workers) may likewise experience severe financial stress due to lack of health insurance coverage (Simich, Hamilton, & Baya, 2006). These populations are particularly vulnerable to fiscally restrictive social policies aimed at limiting systemic health care costs. For example, the Canadian Immigration Bill C-31 reduces accessibility to Interim Federal Health Program (IFHP) coverage and limits eligibility for immigration and refugee status, thus producing increases in uninsured newcomers as a consequence (Parliament of Canada, 2012).

Health care surrounding childbirth can add another layer of financial stress on a family as the proportion of Americans with employer-sponsored health insurance has declined in the past 10 years, particularly for adults (Holahan, 2011). Additionally, health care providers may not be able to accept patients who are uninsured, insured by federal or state programs, or cannot pay out of pocket for

obstetrical services, further increasing the financial strain on families. The recently passed Affordable Care Act (H.R. 3590) will help alleviate some of the financial stressors childbearing families face by reducing the number of uninsured Americans and increasing accessibility for maternal-child health care services (U.S. Department of Human and Health Services, 2013). Canadians are eligible to be insured by a publicly funded universal health care plan, which reduces a portion of financial stress experienced by childbearing families.

While most employed women miss some employment during childbearing, many return to the labor force or increase the number of hours worked following childbirth (Mattingly & Smith, 2010). Others, especially those of high socioeconomic status or with a college/university education, may choose to delay reentry into the workforce or forego possible career advancement during childbearing (Mattingly & Smith, 2010). Regardless of the reason, there are many consequences of missed employment for woman beyond loss of earnings during the childbearing years. Other consequences are detailed in Box 12-2.

Men traditionally have been more likely to take on additional paid work, leaving them less time for family matters, which may be a source of more anxiety and stress for the family (Martell, 2005; Mennino & Brayfield, 2002). The family's ability to supplement income in this manner has been severely restricted following the second collapse of the U.S.

BOX 12-2

Consequences of Maternal Unemployment During the Childbearing Years

- Earnings lost during the times of unemployment.
- Loss of on-the-job training opportunities and opportunities for advancement in career.
- Depreciation of skills and experience, often followed by a loss of confidence about returning to work.
- Loss of work-related benefits if job is subsequently lost.
- Leave taken before childbirth may reduce the leave time available postpartum.
- Reinforcement of traditional roles and responsibilities in two-parent, heterosexual families where the father takes the breadwinner role.

Source: Adapted from Galtry, J., & Callister, P. (2005). Assessing the optimal length of parental leave for child and parental well-being. How can research inform policy? *Journal of Family Issues, 26*(2), 219–246.

economy in 2007. Since that time, unemployment levels have remained high particularly for men and low-income families, which creates added strain on families (Bruening et al., 2012; Mattingly & Smith, 2010). Though less severe in Canada, higher than usual unemployment levels have presented challenges within this country too. In response, women are entering the workforce or increasing the number of hours worked and families may fall back onto savings, increase their debt, or alter their lifestyles to match changing levels of income. Financial stresses are even harder for mothers without partners or for women who provide most of the income for their families. Adolescent mothers are especially prone to financial difficulties because childbearing may disrupt their education, which increases their risk for future poverty (McKinney et al., 2013).

Family Nursing Interventions

- Assist families to find high-quality resources, such as nutrition programs, food banks, family shelters, counseling or settlement services, and government-funded prenatal clinics, including midwifery clinics, community health centers, or public health clinics that support families with limited socioeconomic resources.
- Identify barriers to prenatal care, such as cultural differences, lack of transportation or insurance coverage, child care, hours of service that conflict with family employment, and difficulty obtaining or using health care benefits.
- Assist families to find safe and appropriate child care by providing culturally appropriate information and resources in their preferred language.
- Fully inform families about changes in their health care options resulting from reform and redesign of the health care system.

Task Three: Assuming Mutual Responsibility for Child Care and Nurturing

The care and nurturing of infants bring sleep disruptions, demands on time and physical and emotional energy, additional household tasks, and personal discomfort for caretakers. New parents spend most of their time caring for children, thus decreasing both leisure and downtime, both of which are important to maintain balance in the family. Parents can experience role strain and role overload from combining the increased work within the family with employment demands, or they may face difficulty arranging and affording child care.

The first decision parents make regarding their infant's nutrition is whether to breastfeed or bottle feed. With the exception of decreased feeding costs, the benefits of breastfeeding have traditionally been viewed in North America as being primarily for the child. For example, breastfed babies are less likely to develop diarrhea or ear infections and their rate of sudden infant death syndrome (SIDS) is reduced (Galtry & Callister, 2005; Godfrey & Lawrence, 2010). An association between breastfeeding and enhanced cognitive development has also been reported (Galtry & Callister, 2005). Worldwide, the consensus is that "at least 6 months of exclusive breastfeeding is best for both mother and child" and that "the duration of breastfeeding that is best must be individualized to the family unit" (Godfrey & Lawrence, 2010, p. 1598). Breastfeeding likewise benefits the mothers. Sufficient evidence confirms that mothers who breastfeed for 1 year or longer experience multiple physiological and emotional benefits. These benefits include reduced risk for breast and ovarian cancer, osteoporosis, type 2 diabetes, cardiovascular disease, rheumatoid arthritis, and postpartum depression (Galtry &Callister, 2005; Godfrey & Lawrence, 2010). Nurses must be aware that the father's role in the newborn feeding decision and his level of support and encouragement are important factors in the success of the breastfeeding relationship (Datta, Graham, & Wellings, 2012).

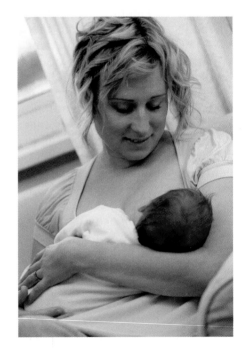

In both the United States and Canada, the rate at which women initiate breastfeeding is very high. The rate at which women in North American are exclusively breastfeeding at 6 months following birth falls dramatically (Chalmers et al., 2009; Godfrey & Lawrence, 2010). While the rate of breastfeeding has increased in all demographic groups, certain populations are less likely to breastfeed, including lower income; first-time mothers; blacks; women participating in the Special Supplemental Nutrition Program for Women, Infants, and Children (WIC); those with high-school education or less; and those employed full-time outside the home (Godfrey & Lawrence, 2010; Johnston & Esposito, 2007). It is crucial for childbearing family nurses to understand the relationship between maternal employment and breastfeeding practices, including the phenomenon of infant feeding with breast milk that has been pumped while the mother is away from the home.

For both mothers and fathers, one of the benefits of having a period of time off from work following childbirth is the increased ability for parents and their newborn to establish a relationship through the process of bonding and attachment. A vast body of research on bonding and attachment, beginning with Bowlby (1952), continued by Ainsworth (1967), and popularized by Klaus and Kennel (1976), supports the premise that optimum child development and well-being is achieved through early and ongoing contact between mothers, fathers, and their newborn. Mothers may automatically bond with their newborns throughout pregnancy and early contact within minutes of the child's birth. By contrast, fathers must work to establish a bond by being involved in the delivery, as well as being available to the infant to strengthen paternal attachment through early contact with the infant in the months following birth (Klaus, Kennell, & Klaus, 1995). St. John, Cameron, and McVeigh (2005) have documented the benefits of early and ongoing contact between fathers and infants. Additionally, Riley and Glass (2002) found that more than half of women who returned to paid employment within the first year postpartum preferred father care over other forms of nonrelative care. When this child care option is available to families, it can provide additional opportunity for father-child attachment.

If an infant must be separated from the parents due to prematurity or for medical or surgical interventions, interruptions in bonding may occur. To promote optimal bonding in these special circumstances, the nurse must allow parents early and frequent access to the baby and should encourage parents to practice skin-to-skin contact, as well as speaking to and holding their newborn. If these actions are not possible, photographs of the infant should be sent to parents as soon as possible and information updated frequently about the newborn's status. It is very important to reassure parents that this disruption will not interfere with the development of a positive, normal, and loving relationship within the family (Ward & Hisley, 2009). The affectionate bond (or attachment) that develops between parents and their children may be one of the motivational driving forces for engaging in infant care and nurturing even under difficult circumstances.

Family Nursing Interventions

- Educate parents about the realities of parenting, such as interrupted sleep and changes in time management and family roles.
- Teach the family to alternate who responds to the baby's needs, including feeding, changing, and comforting.
- Assist parents to develop new skills in caregiving and ways of interacting with their babies, such as baby carrying, smiling, talking to their infant, or making eye contact.
- Observe for signs of attachment by listening to what parents say about their babies and by observing parent behaviors. Box 12-3 outlines parental behaviors that facilitate attachment.
- Refer families who do not demonstrate nurturing behaviors to other professionals, such as local counselors, psychologists, social workers, or childhood development experts, who can provide more intensive intervention.
- Promote culturally competent perceptions of parenting behavior in minority cultures by building partnerships in the ethnic community of the families in care. Respected elders, doulas, or community members may act as translators and cultural brokers for the health care team (Wilson-Mitchell, 2008).
- Provide information about and support for breastfeeding, including how to manage lactation problems, feeding expressed breast milk when appropriate, and referral for lactation consultation as necessary (Lawrence, 2010; Newman & Pitman, 2009).

BOX 12-3

Parental Behaviors That Facilitate Attachment

- Arranges self or the newborn so as to have face-to-face and eye-to-eye contact with infant.
- Directs attention to the infant; maintains contact with infant physically and emotionally.
- Identifies infant as a separate, unique individual with independent needs.
- Identifies characteristics of family members in infant.
- Names infant; calls infant by name.
- Smiles, coos, talks to, or sings to infant.
- Verbalizes pride in the infant.
- Responds to sounds made by the infant, such as crying, sneezing, or grunting.
- Assigns meaning to the infant's actions; interprets infant's needs sensitively.
- Has a positive view of infant's behaviors and appearance.

Sources: Adapted from Davidson, M. R., London, M. L., & Ladewig, P. A. (2008). *Olds' maternal-newborn nursing and women's health across the lifespan* (8th ed.). Upper Saddle River, NJ: Pearson Prentice Hall; Lowdermilk, D. L., & Perry, S. E. (2004). *Maternity and women's health care* (8th ed.). St. Louis, MO: Mosby; and Schenk, L. K., Kelley, J. H., & Schenk, M. P. (2005). Models of maternal-infant attachment: A role for nurses. *Pediatric Nursing, 31*(6), 514–517.

Task Four: Facilitating Role Learning of Family Members

Learning roles is particularly important for childbearing families, including those families that depart from traditional heterosexual structures. For many couples, taking on the role of parents is a dramatic shift in their lives. Difficulty with adaptation to parenthood may be related to the stress of learning new roles. Role learning involves coming to understand the expectations about the role, developing the ability to assume the role, and taking on the role. Women are most likely to feel the demands of a parental role because they remain the primary caretakers in child rearing (Nomaguchi & Milke, 2003). Another important demand that children create, which affects women in particular, is increased housework. Household chores associated with children (laundry, cleaning, cooking, child care) can lead to increased levels of distress for women and can affect relationships between partners. The relationship between gay men is also affected when the couple takes on the parenting role. For example, parenting can result in differing

energy levels between partners, especially if one partner has assumed primary responsibility for child rearing. The toll parenting has on their ability to be good partners to each other influences their relationship (Giesler, 2012, p. 132).

The stress of parenting depends in large part on whether the parents are married or identify as heterosexual or gay. For example, heterosexual single mothers report higher levels of stress than married mothers, due to fewer resources that limit coping strategies (Nomaguchi & Milke, 2003). Moreover, gay couples who decided to become parents revealed that sacrificing lifestyle goals and desires—such as travel and changes to the quality of their sex life—was a source of stress in their partner relationship (Giesler, 2012).

Family Nursing Interventions

- Encourage expectant women to bring their partners into the experience by sharing their physical sensations and emotions of being pregnant and restating the value of their role as parents.
- Assist and encourage pregnant couples to explore their attitudes and expectations about the role(s) of their partner within the household and family after the baby arrives.
- Encourage contact with others who are in the process of taking on the parenting role, especially if the parents are isolated, adolescent, same sex, or culturally diverse and living apart from traditional networks. Respect culturally prescribed roles that resist (or require) change from the prevailing Western cultural worldview.
- Provide opportunities for fathers and other partners or significant others in the family to become skilled infant caregivers.
- Empower parents by assisting them to recognize their own strengths.

Task Five: Adjusting to Changed Communication Patterns

Childbearing families experience changes in their overall communication patterns in order for the family to accommodate newborn and young children. The role of "new parents" also requires changes in communication patterns. As parents and infants learn to interpret and respond to each other's communication cues, they develop effective, reciprocal communication patterns. Infant cues may be so subtle, however, that parents may not be sensitive to cues until nurses point them out (Martell, 2005; Schiffman, Omar, & McKelvey, 2003). For example, many babies respond to being held by cuddling and nuzzling, but others respond by back arching and stiffening. Parents may interpret the latter as rejecting and unloving responses, and these negative interpretations may adversely affect the parent-infant relationship.

The most extreme example of an inability to adapt to changed communication patterns with an infant is shaken baby syndrome. Whether intentional or unintentional, shaking a baby as a form of communication, in frustration or in an attempt to accomplish discipline, will result in traumatic brain injury. Most victims of shaken baby syndrome are under 6 months of age, with the source of abuse usually the father or a male acquaintance of the mother (Ward & Hisley, 2009).

Communication between parents also changes with the transition to parenthood. During the years of childbearing, many couples devote considerable time to career development. The time demands of work coupled with parenting may affect a couple's relationship. While taking on the everyday aspects of rearing children, parents often do not give their couple relationship the attention needed to sustain it (Martell, 2005). A marriage relationship faces tremendous changes with the arrival of the first child (Demo & Cox, 2000), and communication can either fall to the wayside or be the key way to make the new family structure function effectively.

Family Nursing Interventions

- Educate parents about different infant temperaments so they are able to interpret their baby's unique style of communication.
- Teach parents how to recognize and respond to their baby's cues.
- Encourage parents to talk to and engage in eye contact with their baby.
- Educate parents and infant caretakers that it is never appropriate or safe to shake a baby.
- Incorporate couple communication techniques into education of expectant parents.
- Promote effective couple communication by encouraging the partners to listen to each other actively using "I" phrases instead of blaming one another.

- Encourage couples to set aside a regular time to talk and to enjoy each other as loving partners.

Task Six: Planning for Subsequent Children

After the birth, some couples will have definite, mutually agreed-on plans with each other for additional children, whereas others may have decided against future children or be ambivalent about family plans. The nurse should be aware that many couples resume sexual intimacy before the routine 6-week postpartum checkup. It is important for the nurse to inform the woman and her partner that ovulation can resume as early as 2 weeks after childbirth, and pregnancy can occur (Ward & Hisley, 2009). Further teaching should be done regarding the safety of when to resume intercourse after childbirth. Additionally, childbearing family nurses are a valuable resource for those desiring information or demonstrating a willingness to discuss family planning options.

Family Nursing Interventions

- Identify the power structure and locus of decision-making control in the family when discussing reproductive matters.
- Consider a family's cultural and religious background before initiating a discussion about contraceptive choices because these factors often dictate whether the discussion is appropriate.
- Explore previously used methods of contraception for appropriateness after childbirth.
- Provide current, evidence-based information about family planning options either during pregnancy or in the immediate postpartum period.
- Debunk myths about breastfeeding as a method of family planning.
- When appropriate, refer to a nurse genetic specialist for assessment and counseling if there is a positive family history of hereditary diseases.

Task Seven: Realigning Intergenerational Patterns

The first baby adds a new generation in the family lineage that carries the family into the future. Expectant parents change roles from being their parents' children to becoming parents themselves. Childbearing may signify the onset of taking on an adult role for adolescent parents and for some cultural groups. Childbearing changes relationships within extended families as parents' siblings become aunts and uncles, children from previous relationships become stepsiblings, and parents become grandparents.

Siblings typically experience many emotional changes with the arrival of a new family member. Feelings of confusion, hurt, anger, resentment, jealousy, and sibling rivalry are common among younger siblings, as is behavioral regression. Parents should be prepared for these emotional upheavals with strategies that will help the sibling(s) adjust to and accept the new baby.

Grandparents often provide the greatest amount of support to families when a child is born. The degree of their involvement may be linked to cultural expectations. Hispanics, Asians (Zhao, Esposito, & Wang, 2010), Africans, and many other cultures highly value the extended family. The nurse should be aware that in these cultures grandparents are a strong influence on child-rearing practices and are often intimately involved in daily family dynamics (Lewallen, 2011).

Family Nursing Interventions

- Assist new parents to seek support from friends, family members, organized parent groups, and work colleagues as a way to cope with the demands of parenting.
- Work with families to develop strategies that maintain their couple activities, adult interests, and friendships.
- Facilitate partner discussions about perceptions of extended family involvement in care of the new child.
- Facilitate new parents' participation in the decision-making process when health care decisions are required for their child, such as infant nutrition decisions.
- Provide learning opportunities to help move new parents from dependence to independence and self-reliance.
- Offer sibling classes during childbirth education for young children (2 to 8 years) and provide parents with information on how to help ease the transition.
- Offer classes for grandparents during childbirth education with topics varying from assistance with household management to current recommendations on infant positioning, feeding, and clothing, as well as positive

strategies to help them assume a supportive (nonparenting) role.

Task Eight: Maintaining Family Members' Motivation and Morale

After the initial excitement that often surrounds the arrival of a new baby, families must learn to adjust to and cope with the demands that caring for the baby will have on their time, energy, sexual relationship, and personal resources. Many new moms experience postpartum fatigue, which is a feeling of exhaustion and decreased ability to engage in physical and mental work (Davidson, London, & Ladewig, 2008). Women may be fatigued for months due to many reasons: the blood loss associated with birth, breastfeeding, sleep difficulties, depression, the demands of multiple roles, or returning to work outside the home, all of which are compounded by the demands of infant care (Davidson et al., 2008; Martell, 2005; Troy, 2003). In addition, a relationship exists between maternal fatigue and postpartum depression (PPD), both of which affect family processes (Davidson et al., 2008). The first 3 months after childbirth are recognized as the most vulnerable emotional period for mothers (Ward & Hisley, 2009) and, by extension, for their families. During this time and up through 1 year postpartum, nurses must be alert for cues of depression from the new mother and other family members.

In the months following childbirth, families must be realistic about infant sleep patterns and crying behaviors, the potential to experience loneliness, and changes in their sexual relationship. For example, many young families, especially single mothers, experience loneliness in the postpartum period because they live in communities far from their extended families. Some families have recently moved into a new neighborhood and may not have established friendships or a sense of community. Many ethnically diverse groups had special support and recognition of the postpartum period in their countries of origin, but in North America replacements may not exist for traditional postpartum care (Martell, 2005). One way mothers have found to overcome this lack of connectedness is through social networking. For many, Mommy blogs are satisfying and affirming of their experiences, as well as distinct from the dominant culture in which they live (Friedman, 2010).

Family Nursing Interventions

- Inform family members about ways to promote comfort, rest, and sleep, which will make it easier for them to cope with fatigue.
- Promote parental rest while a baby needs nighttime feedings by encouraging parents to alternate who responds to the baby.
- Teach parents ways to cope with a crying infant, which will boost family morale, increase confidence, and allow family members to get additional sleep.
- Provide information on ways parents can reduce isolation and loneliness by seeking support from friends, family members, organized parent groups, work colleagues, and community support groups such as La Leche League.
- Encourage parents to articulate their needs and to find help in ways that support their self-esteem as new parents.
- Counsel couples about changes in sexuality after birth and help them develop mutually satisfying sexual expression.
- Help families to develop strategies that maintain their couple activities, adult interests, and friendships.
- Take a proactive approach to prepare and educate women and their families about signs of postpartum depression.

Task Nine: Establishing Family Rituals and Routines

Family rituals and routines consist of activities that the family performs and teaches its members for continuity and stability (Ward & Hisley, 2009). The predictability of rituals helps babies develop trust. Family rituals have been described as celebrations, traditions, religious observances, and other symbolic events. Routines are those behaviors associated with daily activities pertinent to health (Denham, 2003). Family rituals include the observance of celebrations such as birthdays while family routines center on meal, bedtime, and bathing; greeting and dismissal routines (a kiss goodbye or goodnight); children's special possessions such as a treasured blanket; and nicknames for body functions. For some families, rituals have special cultural meanings that nurses should respect. When families are disrupted or separated during childbearing, nurses can help them deal with stress by encouraging them to carry out their usual routines and established rituals related to their babies and other children.

Family Nursing Interventions

- Determine the special cultural meaning each ritual has for the family and respect those meanings.
- Assess through observation and/or questioning, or as guided by an assessment survey tool, how families observe or acknowledge important days.
- Encourage families to carry out their usual routines and established rituals related to their babies and other children.
- Create a supportive environment that encourages parental knowledge and confidence in caring for themselves and their infants.
- Facilitate couple discussion of bedtime and bathing routines, a baby's special possessions such as a treasured blanket, nicknames, language for body functions, and welcoming rituals such as announcements, baptisms, circumcision, or other celebrations.

Family Transitions

Though it is not another task, transition is a major concept in the Family Developmental Theory (Duvall, 1977). Inherent in transition from one developmental stage to the next is a period of upheaval as the family moves from one state to another. Historically, "transition to parenthood" was thought by early family researchers to be a crisis (LeMasters, 1957; Steffensmeier, 1982). The idea of transition to parenthood as a crisis is being abandoned. More recent work focuses on the transition processes associated with change in families. In a more contemporary approach, transition to parenthood has been defined as a long-term process that results in qualitative reorganization of both inner life and external behavior (Carter & McGoldrick, 2005). In other words, changes occur within the family and also in how the family interacts with the external world. Current discourse on family development is tempered by acknowledgement that the definition of family is dynamic, with intersections of race, class, and poverty influencing how families address challenges such as disabled children, disparity, discrimination, and illness (Conger et al., 2012).

Nurse researchers have mostly focused on transition to motherhood. Even though other family members experience the transition when a newborn joins the family, concepts related to motherhood give nurses insight into family transition. For example,

Nelson (2003) described the primary process of transition as "engagement," or opening one's self to the opportunity to grow and be transformed. Opening of self relates to making a commitment to mothering, experiencing the presence of a child, and caring for the child. The notion of family transition gives foundation to nursing interventions that promote parenting because opening of self involves the real experience of being with and caring for the child. Nurses who understand the stressors that families experience as they transition from one state to another can use this theoretical concept to realize that a mother or father may be frustrated over not being able to cope in old ways.

Just as no one theory covers all aspects of nursing, no single theory will work for every situation involving childbearing families. Therefore, nurses must understand and utilize multiple theories to plan and guide nursing care for childbearing families. Major concepts from Family Systems Theory and Family Developmental and Life Cycle Theory help nurses organize assessments and manage the predictable and unpredictable experiences childbearing families encounter.

CHILDBEARING FAMILY STRESSORS

Childbearing family nursing begins when a couple anticipates and plans for pregnancy, has already conceived, or is planning to adopt a child. Reproductive life planning is an emotional task all types of families—traditional nuclear, blended, gay or lesbian, adoptive, heterosexual cohabiting couples—must negotiate (Pillitteri, 2003). Any pregnancy-related event such as infertility, adoption, pregnancy loss, or an unplanned pregnancy may be enough to disrupt the delicately formed bonds of the family in this stage. Nurses need to be aware of problems childbearing families might encounter before, during, and after reproductive events so that they can anticipate, identify, and respond to needs appropriately.

Infertility

The ability to conceive is a major milestone in a couple's life (Wong, Pang, Tan, Soh, & Lim, 2012). Both men and women perceive fertility to be a sign of competence as reproductive human beings. Therefore, the experience of infertility can be a life crisis that disrupts a couple's marital and/or sexual relationship. Infertility, a common stress-producing event, occurs when couples are unable to achieve a successful pregnancy after 12 or more months of unprotected, regular intercourse (American Society for Reproductive Medicine, 2008; Steuber & Solomon, 2008; Wong et al., 2012). It is a medical and social problem that is of concern to childbearing family nurses, especially in cultures where the expectation of motherhood is strong and because of the increasing trend of delayed childbearing in Western societies (Balasch & Gratacos, 2012; Day, 2005; Sherrod, 2006; Wong et al., 2012).

Nurses should anticipate that infertile couples will experience several different physical, emotional, and psychological symptoms. Couples dealing with infertility struggle between feelings of hope and hopelessness, report feelings of being on a roller-coaster ride, feel a sense of despair, and feel that time is running out (Day, 2005; Eggertson, 2011; Sherrod, 2004). Problems with infertility change a couple's social relationships and support, which may result in increased levels of depression and psychological distress (Box 12-4).

The experience of infertility is stressful for both men and women. Yet the way in which men and women respond varies (Peterson, Newton, & Rosen, 2003). For example, many men believe their central role during fertility treatment is to be a source of strength and support for their partner (Malik &

BOX 12-4

Common Symptoms and Stressors Infertile Couples May Experience

- Irritability
- Insomnia
- Tension
- Depression
- Increased anxiety
- Anger toward each other, God, friends, and other fertile women
- Feelings of rejection, alienation, stigmatization, isolation, and estrangement

Sources: Adapted from Sherrod, R. A. (2004). Understanding the emotional aspects of infertility. Implications for nursing practice. *Journal of Psychosocial Nursing, 42*(3), 42–47; and Day, R. D. (2005). Relationship stress in couples. In P. C. McKenry & S. J. Price (Eds.), *Families and changes: Coping with stressful events and transition* (3rd ed., pp. 332–353). Thousand Oaks, CA: Sage.

Coulson, 2008). In contrast, women typically experience a higher risk for emotional distress than men. Feelings of anger, anxiety, shame, loss of self-esteem, grief, and depression are just some emotions that infertile woman report experiencing (Wong et al., 2012). Women want to spend time talking about their infertility experience, whereas men report that talking about it only increases their anxiety. As a result, men dealing with infertility tend to talk, communicate, and listen less than do women. Additionally, men cope with infertility through avoidance and they may disguise their feelings to protect themselves, their partners, or both (Sherrod, 2006; Wong et al., 2012).

Testing and treatment for infertility is expensive. Assisted reproductive therapy services provided in the United States and Canada, for the most part, are not covered under most health insurance plans or by provincial health insurance. Two Canadian provinces, Quebec and Ontario, have made provision for in vitro fertilization, a type of advanced assisted reproductive therapy, to be a covered treatment under certain conditions only.

Infertility testing and treatment is also painful, time consuming, and inconvenient. It can lead to a loss of spontaneity and privacy in sexual activities, which only compounds the stress and strain couples are experiencing. Although every test or treatment is another painful reminder of the inability to reproduce, it is nurses' lack of knowledge and understanding of the emotional aspects of infertility that really frustrates infertile couples. As a result, couples interpret nursing care to be insensitive and uncompassionate when nurses focus primarily on physiological or technical aspects of infertility rather than on emotional needs (Lutter, 2008; Sherrod, 2004). Therefore, it is vital that nurses caring for childbearing families experiencing infertility understand, consider, and address the emotional needs of couples undergoing assessment, diagnosis, and treatment for infertility. Families experiencing the crisis of infertility are in as much need of a personal touch as they are of technical competence and accurate, evidence-based information about testing and treatment options. See Box 12-5 for specific nursing interventions to help couples deal with infertility.

Adoption

Adoption is one of the many ways women, alternative couples, and those experiencing infertility or other issues may become parents (Giesler, 2012;

> ### BOX 12-5
> ### Nursing Interventions That Are Helpful to Couples Dealing With Infertility
>
> - Avoid assigning blame to one partner or the other.
> - Encourage social support from friends, spouse, or significant other.
> - Assess couples' coping strategies, encourage open discussion between couples, suggest different coping strategies.
> - Facilitate communication between couples in order to give men, in particular, the opportunity to acknowledge and express their feelings and process their response to the infertility experience.
> - Provide information related to cost and insurance coverage for treatment.
> - Suggest appropriate stress-relieving activities, such as acupuncture or other complementary and alternative therapies.
> - Refer to support groups and/or other professionals for counseling.

Sources: Adapted from Sherrod, R. A. (2004). Understanding the emotional aspects of infertility. Implications for nursing practice. *Journal of Psychosocial Nursing, 42*(3), 42–47; Sherrod, R. A. (2006). Male infertility: The element of disguise. *Journal of Psychosocial Nursing, 44*(10), 31–37; Smith, C., Ussher, J., Perz, J., Carmady, B., & de Lacey, S. (2001). The effect of acupuncture on psychosocial outcomes for women experiencing infertility: A pilot randomized controlled trial. *Journal of Alternative and Complementary Medicine, 17*(10), 923–930; and Wong, C., Pang, J., Tan, G., Soh, W., & Lim J. (2012). The impact of fertility on women's psychological health: A literature review. *Singapore Nursing Journal, 39*(3), 11–17.

London, Ladewig, Ball, & Bindler, 2007; Sherrod, 2004). Many different types of families adopt (U.S. Department of Health and Human Services, n.d.), including single parents, families formed by second parents or with stepparents, transracial, transcultural, relative, and lesbian, gay, bisexual, or transgendered (LGBT) families. While adoptive mothers and families may not experience the physical context of pregnancy, they will have many of the same feelings and fears as biological families (Fontenot, 2007). Childbearing family nurses must be aware that all parents react to the strong intense feelings and emotions, ranging from happiness to distress, in the first moments they meet their child, regardless of the way in which a family is formed. Even though the child is not biological or the parental relationship may not be established immediately at birth, bonding can be just as strong and immediate for adoptive parents and children (Hockenberry, Wilson, Winkelstein,

& Kline, 2006; Rykkje, 2007). Therefore, nurses caring for women in the preadoptive and early postadoptive period must recognize and provide care in a manner similar to that provided to biological mothers during the prenatal and postpartum periods (Fontenot, 2007).

Once families decide to adopt a child, they may pursue several routes, such as international adoption (also known as intercountry), public domestic adoption, or private domestic adoption. In the United States, domestic adoption can be a difficult, lengthy, bureaucratic, and costly process that takes anywhere from 12 months to 5 or 6 years (Fontenot, 2007; London et al., 2007; Pillitteri, 2003). The laws favoring birth mothers also complicate domestic adoption. This long waiting period, and fear of the court system, resulted in many families turning to international/intercountry adoptions, which used to provide a child in a much shorter amount of time. In the current climate, however, international adoptions have become much more difficult; in some situations, such adoptions may no longer be an option for parents. One drawback to an international adoption is that little to no information about the child's birth parents' background, prenatal health care, or medical history may be available to the adopting family (Gunnar & Pollak, 2007; Smit, 2010). The lack of birth history places families at risk for adopting a child who may have experienced a significant number of threats to physical health as well as normal brain and behavioral development, which can contribute to future struggles as families cope with the consequences of these problems (Gunnar & Pollak, 2007; Smit, 2010). Box 12-6 lists other issues and challenges related to international and transracial adoption.

In Canada, approximately 20% of families are affected by adoption, either through the public child welfare (foster care) system or private adoption agencies. A prerequisite for all Canadian adoption is successful completion of the Parent Resource for Information Development and Education (PRIDE) course. In addition, private Canadian adoptions agencies are required to provide birth parents with counseling before the birth, to offer emotional support for adoptive parents, and to organize the court and legal services involved.

Private adoption is another alternative for families considering adoption. Private adoptions can range from being strictly anonymous to very open, where the adopting couple and birth mother get to

---

BOX 12-6

International and Transracial Adoption: Issues and Challenges

Issues and Challenges to Families Before International and Transracial Adoption

- Ability to travel on short notice to pick up a child.
- Changing political conditions may stop the adoption process at any time.
- Ways family will maintain the adopted child's natural heritage.
- Ways family will deal with racial and other types of prejudice.
- The many rules and conditions sometimes prevent families from adopting a child from a particular country.

Issues and Challenges to Families After International Adoption

- Limited postadoption resources such as pediatricians trained in international adoption or international adoption clinics for families seeking help for a child's developmental and behavioral problems.
- Child's emotional and developmental issues can be exhausting and financially tax the family.
- Limited or no information about child's maternal or paternal medical history can be a source of uncertainty and adoptive parental stress.

Issues and Challenges to Families After Transracial Adoption

- Need to redefine the family as multiracial and multiethnic when white families adopt nonwhite children.
- Extra attention and comments about the child's looks from strangers in public places.
- Neighbors, family members, and others may express prejudice toward the child.

Sources: Adapted from Gunnar, M., & Pollak, S. D. (2007). Supporting parents so that they can support their internationally adopted children: The larger challenge lurking behind the fatality statistics. *Child Maltreatment, 12*(4), 381–382; Pillitteri, A. (2003). *Maternal and child health nursing* (4th ed.). Philadelphia: Lippincott Williams & Wilkins; Rykkje, L. (2007). Intercountry adoption and nursing care. *Scandinavian Journal of Caring Sciences, 21*(4), 507–514; and Smit, E. (2010). International adoption families: A unique health care journey. *Pediatric Nursing, 36*(5), 253–258.

---

know each other extremely well. Often, the Internet is a place where women wanting to place babies for adoption and families seeking to adopt connect. Canadian families wishing to adopt should be aware that some provinces do not allow for direct advertising on the Internet or in newspaper classifieds (Canada Adopts, 2001). Regardless of how North American families connect or interact with the birth mother, it is paramount that families pursuing private adoption retain professional legal advice and counsel to ensure that everyone involved, including the birth father, understands the legal ramifications and to work out all aspects related to the adoption before the baby's birth. In Canada, adoption falls under provincial jurisdiction and, therefore, laws are highly variable between provinces. For example, some provinces allow families themselves to find a child to adopt rather than having an agency choose one for them. Nurses should encourage Canadian families working with private agencies to understand any adoption restrictions or limitations set by the province in which they reside (Canada Adopts, 2001).

Nurses should be aware that when a private adoption has been negotiated, one of the important points is whether the adopting family will be present at the child's birth. Nurses must also be prepared and ready to intervene should a birth mother reverse her decision to give the baby up for adoption, or a birth father who has not relinquished his legal right to the baby asserts his rights (McKinney et al., 2013; Pillitteri, 2003). See Box 12-7 for appropriate nursing interventions when caring for adoptive families.

Perinatal Loss

Perinatal loss is not uncommon and it is a traumatic event for families (Armstrong, Hutti, & Myers, 2009; Callister, 2006). Losing a child during pregnancy, after birth, or in the early postpartum period is one of the hardest things a family can experience. The loss may be anticipated and voluntary, such as with abortion or relinquishing parental rights for adoption, or unanticipated, such as death or loss of custody to the state. An adoptive family may lose their intended child if a birth mother changes her mind about giving up a baby for adoption. Box 12-8 lists other types of perinatal loss that families may experience.

Loss of a child is a unique and profound experience for parents. When parents lose a child, they lose a part of their hoped-for identity, including all hopes and dreams held for the child they anticipated and loved; they also often experience a lack of social recognition regarding the significance of their loss (Armstrong et al., 2009; Callister, 2006; O'Leary & Thorwick, 2006). Societal invisibility of infant loss contributes to parental frustration,

---

BOX 12-7
Nurse Interventions for Adoptive Families

- Encourage families to seek help from adoption experts and agencies.
- Encourage families to understand and follow any legal and provincial limitations or restrictions related to adoption.
- Refer families to adoption specialists, such as social workers, counselors, and lawyers.
- Recommend families speak with and secure pediatric providers during the preadoptive process.
- Recommend adoptive parents attend parenting classes and include them in prenatal and infant care classes.
- Incorporate adoptive-sensitive material into classes and other educational resources.
- Keep lines of communication open between nurses and adoptive families as a way to alleviate fears about being judged or undermined.
- Address other siblings' response to the adopted child because a biological child's feelings of inferiority or superiority to an adopted child can interfere with relationships within the family.
- Address family concerns about attachment issues.

Sources: Adapted from Canada Adopts! (2001). Adopting in Canada. Retrieved from http://www.canadaadopts.com/canada/domestic_private.shtml; Fontenot, H. (2007). Transition and adaptation to adoptive motherhood. *Journal of Obstetrics, Gynecologic and Neonatal Nursing, 36*(2), 175–182; Pillitteri, A. (2003). *Maternal and child health nursing* (4th ed.). Philadelphia: Lippincott Williams & Wilkins; and Smit, E. (2010). International adoption families: A unique health care journey. *Pediatric Nursing, 36*(5), 253–258.

---

especially when they are denied time to mourn or are asked why they are not yet over their loss (Callister, 2006; Chichester, 2005). One mother put it this way when describing her loss experience during the second trimester of pregnancy: "When I lost my baby there was no memorial service, no outpouring of sympathy, no evidence that I gave birth and lost a baby" (Callister, 2006, p. 228). Therefore, nurses caring for childbearing families must engage in ongoing assessment and interventions related to potential, previous, or current loss. Grief and a process of bereavement should also be anticipated secondary to perinatal loss, an adverse perinatal outcome, diagnosis of congenital or genetic disorders, palliative care, or the birth of a special needs child.

Nurses providing care to childbearing families should anticipate that each family member will

Types of Perinatal Loss Families May Experience

- Miscarriage
- Elective abortion
- Ectopic pregnancy
- Selective reduction after in vitro implantation of multiple fertilized eggs
- Stillbirth
- Death of a child after a live birth
- Recurrent pregnancy loss
- Loss of a "perfect" child because of anomalies or malformations
- Death of a twin during pregnancy, labor, birth, or after birth
- Termination of pregnancy for identified fetal anomalies, which is increasing because of technological advances in prenatal diagnosis of such anomalies

Sources: Adapted from Callister, L. C. (2006). Perinatal loss: A family perspective. *Journal of Perinatal Neonatal Nursing, 20*(3), 227–234; and Robson, F. (2002). Yes! A chance to tell my side of the story: A case study of a male partner of a woman undergoing termination of pregnancy for foetal abnormality. *Journal of Health Psychology, 7*(2), 183–193.

experience loss differently. For example, mothers are more apt to grieve visibly by emotional expression, sharing of feelings and participation in grief support groups. Fathers, in contrast, tend to feel a sense of loneliness and isolation and have feelings of helplessness. Fathers, who often see their role as primarily supportive of their partner, may feel the need to "act as men" by being strong and may hold back their own feelings of grief and pain (Armstrong et al., 2009; Callister, 2006; McKinney et al., 2013; O'Leary & Thorwick, 2006; Robson, 2002). Siblings may describe their grief experience as "hurting inside" as a way to express feelings of sadness, frustration, loneliness, fear, and anger (Davies, 2006). Grandparents experience a triple measure of grief and sorrow when a grandchild dies: their own personal grief as a human being suffering the death of a loved one; the pain over the loss of a grandchild, which carries with it the loss of their dreams and expectations for their relationship with that child; and seeing their own children suffer (Lemon, 2002).

Considering the effect of perinatal loss on all family members, nurses must work to support and strengthen the familial bond in the face of such loss (Callister, 2006). Nurses can support families' experience of perinatal loss by being present and listening attentively, expressing emotions, gathering memorabilia, and helping the family make meaning of the experience. Referral to support groups or provision of a list of available resources may be helpful depending on the needs of the grieving couple or family (Callister, 2006; McKinney et al., 2013). Compassionate Friends is one of many groups to which nurses might refer grieving parents, siblings, and grandparents for support.

Culture influences how families respond to perinatal loss. Therefore, it is essential for nurses to understand several different culturally diverse practices and rituals associated with loss, as well as provide culturally competent care. Nurses demonstrate cultural sensitivity when they validate what families perceive to be the "right way" to grieve (Callister, 2006; Chichester, 2005). Box 12-9 lists cultural perinatal loss practices and rituals of select cultural groups.

Pregnancy Following Perinatal Loss

Psychological distress is higher in parents who have experienced a prior perinatal loss, with maternal anxiety about a child's well-being extending a year or more after birth of another child (Armstrong et al., 2009). Women may not perceive pregnancy as normal after experiencing perinatal loss but rather may be plagued with a sense of anxiety, insecurity, ambivalence, doubt, and concern that another loss may occur (Callister, 2006; Davidson et al., 2008). They also experience higher levels of anxiety than fathers (Armstrong et al., 2009). Fathers may shut down their feelings when pregnancy occurs after loss because of unresolved feelings related to prior pregnancy loss. They may even be too frightened to share or may not be conscious of their feelings. Nurses caring for childbearing families during pregnancy after perinatal loss are in a prime position to help mothers and fathers open doors of communication that may have been closed because of fear. One strategy nurses could use to encourage communication is to ask fathers "How are you doing?" in front of the mothers, which provides an opportunity to share what they are feeling (Davidson et al., 2008; O'Leary & Thorwick, 2006).

BOX 12-9
Perinatal Loss Cultural Practices and Rituals

- Hmong families may request the placenta following birth due to their belief that burying it prevents problems of the soul.
- Jewish families may request to remain with the body at all times out of respect. Newborns are named and circumcised at burial so they can be included in family records.
- Muslim babies born after more than 4 months' gestation are to be named, bathed, wrapped in a seamless white sheet, and buried within 24 hours. Bodies are buried intact, so taking locks of hair is not permitted.
- Puerto Rican families may call on faith healers and spiritualists to assist the baby on his or her journey into the next life.
- Roma (gypsy) families want to avoid any association with death and bad luck/impurity (mahrime), so they may leave the hospital suddenly and shift responsibility for burial to the hospital.
- American Indians/Alaskan Natives may request to remain with the baby until death to pray.

Sources: Adapted from Callister, L. C. (2006). Perinatal loss: A family perspective. *Journal of Perinatal Neonatal Nursing, 20*(3), 227–234; Chichester, M. (2005). Multicultural issues in perinatal loss. *Lifelines, 9*(4), 314–320; Palacios, J., Butterfly, R., & Strickland, C. J. (2005). American Indians/Alaskan Natives. In J. G. Lipson & S. L. Dibble (Eds.), *Cultural and clinical care* (pp. 27–41). San Francisco, CA: The Regents University of California; and Sutherland, A. H. (2005). Roma (Gypsies). In J. G. Lipson & S. L. Dibble (Eds.), *Cultural and clinical care* (pp. 404–414). San Francisco, CA: The Regents University of California.

THREATS TO HEALTH DURING CHILDBEARING

For the majority of families, childbearing is a physically healthy experience. For some families, health during childbearing is threatened, and the childbearing experience becomes an illness experience. In such cases, concern for the physical health of the mother and the fetus tends to outweigh other aspects of pregnancy; rather than eagerly anticipating the birth and baby, family members experience fear and apprehension. Moreover, the family's functioning and developmental tasks are disrupted as the family focuses its attention on the health of the mother and survival of the fetus or baby. Childbearing nurses must be aware that families with threats to health have additional needs for maintaining and preserving family health.

Acute and Chronic Illness During Childbearing

This chapter defines "acute" as health threats that come on suddenly and may have life-threatening implications. Examples of acute health threats childbearing families may encounter are fetal distress during labor and pulmonary embolism for postpartum women. In contrast, "chronic" comprises conditions occurring during pregnancy that persist, linger, need control, or have no cure and that require careful monitoring and treatment to avoid becoming an acute threat to maternal or infant health. Pregnancy-induced hypertension, gestational and preexisting diabetes, and postpartum depression are some examples of chronic health threats. Some threats to health during childbearing vacillate between acute and chronic. For example, preterm labor can be an acute health threat that results in a preterm birth. If preterm labor contractions are suppressed, it becomes a "chronic" health threat requiring adherence to prescribed regimens to keep contractions from recurring.

Effect of Threats to Health on Childbearing Families

Chronic threats to childbearing health are disruptive to childbearing families. Knowledge of the family as a dynamic system explains why the effects of these chronic conditions extend to the entire family and result in the upset of family functioning, development, and structure that normally keep the family system stable (Denham & Looman, 2010; Maloni, Brezinski-Tomasi, & Johnson, 2001). When childbearing health is threatened, all family members experience stress as families strive to regain balance. For example, three sources of stress that alter family processes when the mother or infant experiences a chronic health threat are (1) assuming household tasks, (2) managing changes in income and resources, and (3) facing uncertainty and separation.

Assuming Household Tasks

When women experience chronic threats to childbearing health, other members of the family must assume responsibility for household tasks and functioning, regardless of whether the condition is managed at the hospital or at home. Assumption of household tasks by others creates family stress, especially for partners who must take on the role of caring for the family, as well as caring for the expectant mother and/or infant (Bomar, 2004; Maloni, 2010). Expectant fathers especially may find that all their time and energy are consumed by employment and household management, tasks that previously were shared or done solely by their partners. Children's lives change when mothers have to limit activities. Toddlers do not understand why their mothers cannot pick them up or run after them. The resulting frustration for children can manifest itself in behavioral changes, such as tantrums and regression in developmental tasks (e.g., toilet training).

Managing Changes in Income and Resources

An at-risk pregnancy is stressful in terms of the family's finances and other resources. For example, if a mother is placed on bedrest because of risk for preterm labor, she may miss time away from paid employment. Or a mother may not have the ability to seek employment, which also results in loss of income. At the same time, medical expenses may increase because of the need for increased care, including possible neonatal intensive care and maintaining multiple health care provider visits or hospital stays. Personal expenses associated with the cost of specialized diets, medications, and hiring personnel to assist with household tasks may also increase; such costs are not usually covered by health care systems in Canada or the United States. For families already in debt or struggling with unemployment or other financial challenges, these threats to health serve to increase the burden of debt.

Although resources, such as energy and social networks, cannot be measured as easily as money, family nurses are in a position to help families consider and manage changes in their nonmonetary resources. Some of the nonmonetary changes that family nurses should anticipate families will encounter include the following: that others outside of the nuclear family may need to assume various household tasks such as meal preparation, laundry, and cleaning; that all families may not have social networks or extended families in the immediate vicinity; that changes in employment may cause separation from persons and activities that were

stimulating; and that isolation, regardless of the cause, can increase a family's burden.

Facing Uncertainty and Separation or Loss

The unpredictable nature of high-risk childbearing makes planning for the future difficult for childbearing families because it leaves them facing uncertainty and possible separation. For example, expectant parents, especially employed women, face uncertainty with pending preterm birth because they may not be able to determine accurately when to begin and end parental leave because of the need to cope with sudden hospitalization. Separation can occur when mothers are suddenly hospitalized or when families living in remote rural areas are transferred to a distant perinatal center for days or weeks. When families are separated, it becomes difficult for them to maintain and develop family relationships. Separation from the family and concerns about family status are two of the greatest stressors experienced by women hospitalized for chronic threats to childbearing health (Maloni, Margevicius, & Damato, 2006). In addition, small children experience extreme anxiety over the sudden departure of their mother, especially if they are unprepared or unable to comprehend what is happening to their mother and the new baby.

Even if the logistical problems related to separation are solved and a family can be together, coping with basic tasks of living is challenging in new settings. For instance, a family may not know where to stay, how to find reasonably priced meals, how to obtain transportation, or where to park a car. Box 12-10 presents nursing interventions related to childbearing families who are experiencing chronic threats to health.

FAMILY NURSING OF POSTPARTUM FAMILIES

All family members experience household upheaval during the first few days and weeks a newborn is in the home. Throughout the childbearing cycle, nurses assist families to understand, prepare, and respond to the effect of a new baby on the family. Assisting parents to be realistic in their expectations about themselves, each other, and their children helps them to plan ahead by identifying appropriate support and resources. This section

BOX 12-10

Family Nursing Interventions for Childbearing Families Experiencing Chronic Threats to Health

Assuming Household Tasks

- Help families find ways to streamline and prioritize household tasks to reduce stress and increase adherence to medical regimens.
- Assist adults to list household management tasks and determine who does what when so that the family can be more efficient and effective in managing these tasks.
- Educate families about the impact of parents' health difficulties on children.
- Provide practical, age-appropriate suggestions for managing children, such as hiring a teenager after school for active play with young children.
- Encourage parents to provide ways for young children to have some quiet one-on-one time with their mothers as a way to reduce stress for both mothers and children.

Managing Changes in Income and Resources

- Refer families to an appropriate counselor who can explore with family members ways to manage financial problems.
- Assist families to identify others outside of the nuclear family who can assume various household tasks, such as meal preparation, laundry, and cleaning.
- Help families identify and use resources, such as home-health agencies and parents' groups in the community, to assist with household management.
- Encourage families with necessary resources to use a computer to connect with each other, friends, coworkers, and other at-risk families to prevent or decrease feelings of isolation.

- Direct families to appropriate Internet sites, such as the ones listed in the Selected Resources section at the end of this chapter.

Facing Uncertainty and Separation and Loss

- Acknowledge the difficulties of uncertainties associated with difficult perinatal situations.
- Be honest and informative about the condition and prognosis of both the mother and fetus.
- Use terms understood by all family members to provide accurate and thorough explanations tailored to families' anxiety levels.
- Assist families to cope with basic tasks of living in high-tech settings such as the neonatal intensive care unit.
- Investigate and reduce the barriers families may encounter at a distant perinatal center, such as lack of transportation, employment, and the threatening environment of a strange setting.
- Provide families with information on where to stay, how to find reasonably priced meals, how to obtain transportation, and where to park a car.
- Encourage use of electronic communication, such as e-mail, to facilitate contact between family members and health care professionals.
- Encourage calling families about their members' progress and sending photographs as a way to help families cope with uncertainty and enhance relationships of physically separated family members.
- Encourage family members to participate in care of their infants to promote development of parenting skills.

Source: Adapted from Martell, L. K. (2005). Family nursing with childbearing families. In S. M. H. Hanson, V. Gedaly-Duff, & J. R. Kaakinen (Eds.), *Family health care nursing: Theory, practice and research* (3rd ed., pp. 291–323.) Philadelphia: F. A. Davis.

discusses appropriate nursing assessments and interventions family nurses should incorporate into their practice when caring for families during the postpartum period.

Feeding Management

Success in feeding their babies induces feelings of competency in mothers. A family's comfort with its infant feeding method is as crucial for physical, emotional, and social well-being of the infant as is the food itself. Regardless of the parents' choice of feeding method, nurses' instructions need to emphasize the development of relationships between infant and parent through feeding. Being held during feeding enhances social development whether

a baby is being breastfed or bottle fed. Parents should take the time during feedings to enjoy interacting with their babies. When the infant is adopted, social interaction with feeding is a special opportunity for developing attachment.

Even though the act of breastfeeding is a strictly female function, fathers need not be excluded from the feeding experience. Nurses can promote paternal-infant attachment by encouraging fathers to be involved with feeding. For example, the father can burp the baby during or after feedings, as well as hold and comfort the infant once feeding has been completed. Another way to involve fathers is to have them give the breastfed baby an occasional bottle of expressed breast milk once breastfeeding is well established (Davidson et al., 2008; McKinney et al., 2013). Early involvement of fathers in feeding is beneficial later when infants are being weaned from the breast or mothers are preparing to return to employment.

Many people assume that breastfeeding is "natural" and so should not present any difficulties. Nevertheless, many women initially may experience breastfeeding difficulties, especially if the baby has difficulty latching or milk takes longer than expected to come in. It is important that nurses assess a mother's breastfeeding technique early and provide hands-on teaching so mothers can learn how to breastfeed successfully. Referral to a lactation consultant may be necessary before the new family leaves the hospital. Nurses should also ensure that the family is given resource information about breastfeeding, including how to obtain assistance at postdischarge clinics when breastfeeding challenges arise.

Attachment

Positive parent-infant attachment must take place to foster optimal growth and development of infants, as well as to encourage the parent-infant love relationship. The attachment process requires early involvement and physical contact between parents and their infant for a strong link to develop (Schenk et al., 2005). Extreme stress, health risk factors, and illness can interfere with the physical contact and early parent-infant involvement needed for the development of attachment. Stressful conditions that pull parents' energies and attention away from their newborns can be detrimental to attachment. Adoption can be another factor influencing attachment, especially if the child had multiple caretakers or frequently changed living location. Children who were adopted from more stable environments may also have attachment difficulties if they struggle to transfer their attachment from a previous caretaker to their adoptive parents (Smit, 2010).

Nurses should be alert for families who are likely to have difficulty with attachment, especially if family history indicates a parent has suffered abuse, neglect, or abandonment during childhood. In addition, nurses may identify families at risk for poor attachment through listening to what parents say about their babies and by observing parent behaviors. Families at risk for poor attachment may have misconceptions about infant behavior, such as believing that infants cry just to annoy their parents.

Hence, family nurses must address verbal expressions of dissatisfaction with the infant, comparison of the infant with disliked family members, failure to respond to the infant's crying, lack of spontaneity in touching the infant, and stiffness or discomfort in holding the infant after the first week. Although isolated incidences of these behaviors are probably not detrimental to attachment, persistent trends and patterns could be an indicator of future relationship difficulties.

Another signal of attachment difficulty is inconsistent maternal behaviors, such as a mother who exhibits intense concern at times interspersed with apathy at other times without any predictable cause or pattern. Therefore, an important step when assessing attachment behaviors is to evaluate whether the parent-infant relationship is progressing positively and if the enjoyment and love of the child is growing over time. If the parents' enjoyment of the baby as a unique individual and their commitment to the baby are not progressing, the nurse needs to help the family understand what attachment is and also needs to identify factors that might be interfering with attachment to the infant. For example, mothers struggling with PPD need treatment for their depression before they can address attachment to the infant. Childbearing family nurses may need to refer families who do not demonstrate nurturing behaviors to other professionals such as social workers, psychotherapists, and developmental specialists who can provide more intensive interventions that will help parents care for and nurture their children.

Siblings

No matter what age siblings are, the addition of a new baby affects the position, role, and power of older children, thereby creating stress for both parents and children. Teaching parents to emphasize the positive aspects of adding a family member helps them focus on sibling "relationships" rather than "rivalry." Parents need help to address *all* of the children's needs, not just those of the new baby. Parents may be concerned about whether they have "enough" energy, time, and love for additional children. Practical ideas for time and task management can alleviate some of their concerns, as can helping parents delegate nonparenting tasks, such as housecleaning and meal preparation, to friends and relatives when possible.

Postpartum Depression

The period after childbirth can be a stressful time for women because of their need to face the new tasks of the maternal role. Changes in relationships, economic demands, and social support also take place during this time and can result in postpartum stress (Hung, 2005). PPD, one type of postpartum mood disorder, has been described as "a dangerous thief that robs women of precious time together with their infants that they had been dreaming of throughout pregnancy" (Beck, 2001, p. 275). Although "baby blues" are a predictable and temporary mood shift that occurs during the first 2 weeks after childbirth, symptoms of stress that take hold and persist during the first year are of concern to family nurses because they can adversely affect maternal health and the ability of mothers to function in their new role (Blass, 2005; Hung, 2005). The effects of maternal depression are not limited to the mother herself but spread to family, friends, and coworkers alike (Grantmakers in Health, 2004). Left unidentified and untreated, PPD leads to serious consequences for families, such as maternal suicide, poor attachment to the infant, altered family dynamics, and lowered cognitive development in children. Considering these consequences, it becomes imperative that family nurses educate woman and their families about potential causes and symptoms of PPD, as well as immediately identify and appropriately refer women experiencing this mood disorder so that early treatment can begin (Doucet, Dennis, Letourneau, & Blackmore, 2009; Driscoll, 2006; Ross, Dennis, Blackmore, & Stewart, 2005). Box 12-11 lists signs of PPD.

Usually women do not volunteer information about their depression out of shame, fear, lack of understanding about the seriousness of their illness and available access to appropriate health care services (Doucet et al., 2009; Driscoll, 2006). Therefore, it is left to the nurse to identify its existence by understanding and recognizing the signs and symptoms, even if they are subtle. If the new mother is making negative comments about herself, the baby, or her partner; if she is ignoring her other children's needs; if her physical appearance shows signs of neglect; or if family members report a change in the woman's mood or behavior, it is time to screen for PPD. Childbearing family nurses might consider incorporating the two-question screening measure that Jesse and Graham (2005)

BOX 12-11
Signs of Postpartum Depression

- Sadness
- Frequent crying
- Insomnia or excessive sleeping
- Lack of interest or pleasure in usual activities, including sexual relations
- Difficulty thinking, concentrating, or making decisions
- Lack of concern about personal appearance
- Feelings of worthlessness
- Fatigue or loss of energy
- Depressed mood
- Thoughts of death: suicidal ideation without a plan; suicide plan or attempt

Sources: Adapted from Davidson, M. R., London, M. L., & Ladewig, P. A. (2008). *Olds' maternal-newborn nursing and women's health across the lifespan* (8th ed.). Upper Saddle River, NJ: Pearson Prentice Hall; and Driscoll, J. W. (2006). Postpartum depression: How nurses can identify and care for women grappling with this disorder. *Lifelines, 10*(5), 399–409.

---

developed as a rapid way to begin the identification of women at risk for PPD. Use of this scale simply involves nurses asking women two questions: "Are you sad or depressed?" and "Have you experienced a loss in pleasurable activities?" Women who answer yes to both of these questions should be referred to a mental health provider (Driscoll, 2006).

Family nurses caring for childbearing families might also consider using one of many readily available and easy-to-use depression scales, such the Edinburgh Postnatal Depression Scale or the Postpartum Depression Predictors Inventory—Revised, as a routine screening tool for PPD (Davidson et al., 2008; McKinney et al., 2013). In particular, the Edinburgh Postnatal Depression Scale has been found to be valid for several cultures, has been translated into several different languages, and has been used with men (Driscoll, 2006; Eberhard-Gran, Eskild, Tambs, Opjordsmoen, & Samuelsen, 2001; Goodman, 2004). Regardless of which screening tool is used to identify women at risk for PPD, childbearing family nurses have a professional responsibility to assess for the disorder, recommend women be referred for treatment, and provide self-care strategies and support to the woman and her family (Driscoll, 2006; Doucet et al., 2009).

Although much attention has been given to maternal PPD, shifting gender roles and paternal involvement in child care require adjustments for men as well, which puts them at risk for experiencing depression after the birth of a child, especially if the mother is depressed. This consequence makes sense to nurses who understand Family Systems Theory because anything that affects one family member directly or indirectly affects other family members. Viewed from this theoretical perspective, it is easy to see how maternal or paternal depression affects all family members and relationships within the family and results in serious implications for family health and well-being. Therefore, family nurses must recognize PPD in fathers just as in mothers, because when both parents are depressed, the risk to infants and children increases (Goodman, 2004). As with mothers, recommendation of a referral for fathers to mental health care providers should be made in an effort to initiate early treatment and reduce negative effects on the family system (Goodman, 2004). Box 12-12 lists additional nursing interventions for PPD.

POLICY IMPLICATIONS FOR FAMILY NURSING

The concerns of childbearing family nursing go beyond care of the individual family. Nurses are participants in understanding, developing, and implementing policy as it relates to childbearing families. Much of Chapter 5 addresses important issues for childbearing families. The legal definitions of family, official recognition of the diversity of families, access to health care, alternatives to traditional childbearing such as cross-cultural adoption, and growing needs of poverty-stricken and other disenfranchised families are just a few of the policy areas vital to childbearing family nursing.

Nurses need to be aware of the effect of legislation on childbearing families. One example is family leave for childbirth, which can profoundly affect the health and development of childbearing families. In the United States, the Family and Medical Leave Act (FMLA), a federal law enacted in 1993, entitles family members to take *unpaid* time away from employment without penalty to care for a family member, such as a newborn, with health care needs. Unfortunately, many families cannot take advantage of the benefits of this act because it applies only to certain size businesses and employers are not obligated to pay on-leave employees. Further, the FMLA only allows for 3 months of

---

BOX 12-12

Nursing Interventions for Postpartum Depression

- Help women differentiate between myths of the mother role—which imply that at 6 weeks after birth, women are ready to resume all their previous activities—and the reality of motherhood, where prepregnancy clothes do not fit, infants periodically become demanding malcontents, and houses are messy because family members are too exhausted to clean.
- Encourage women with postpartum depression to share feelings as they grieve the loss of who they were and begin to build on who they are becoming. Solicit input from family members about changes in mood or behavior.
- Encourage women to seek help with symptoms of anxiety, anger, obsessive thinking, fear, guilt, and/or suicidal thoughts.
- Assist women to re-create, restructure, and integrate changes that new motherhood brings into their daily lives.
- Develop standard protocols for screening men whose partners are depressed after childbirth.

Sources: Adapted from Driscoll, J. W. (2006). Postpartum depression: How nurses can identify and care for women grappling with this disorder. *Lifelines, 10*(5), 399–409; Goodman, J. H. (2004). Paternal postpartum depression, its relationship to maternal postpartum depression, and implications for family health. *Journal of Advanced Nursing, 45*(10), 26–35; and Martell, L. K. (2005). Family nursing with childbearing families. In S. M. H. Hanson, V. Gedaly-Duff, & J. R. Kaakinen (Eds.), *Family health care nursing: Theory, practice and care* (3rd ed., pp. 267–289). Philadelphia: F. A. Davis.

---

unpaid parental leave. Although the intent of the FMLA is commendable, it must be noted that eligibility criteria are quite restrictive and thus can rule out many workers (Galtry & Callister, 2005). Unlike the citizens of many developed nations, parents in the United States are not entitled to government benefits for childbearing except for tax deductions and other incentives. Many European countries, by contrast, offer paid paternity leave.

In Canada, some social policies have been put into place in an effort to assist both parents to balance work-life issues and manage the care of newborns. All families in every Canadian province and territory are entitled to "maternity leave" or "parental leave" following childbirth and adoption. A federally funded Employment Insurance (EI) program, except in Quebec, provides 15 weeks of paid maternity/parental leave at 55% of the mother's usual salary (to a maximum amount, currently $485 per week) providing she worked 600 hours in the 52 weeks prior to the onset of maternity leave; medical documentation of her expected or actual date of delivery is required. In the event of a premature birth, this benefit may be extended anywhere from 17 to 52 weeks for every week that a newborn remains in the hospital because of prematurity. In Quebec, similar maternity leave coverage is available for 18 weeks under the provisions of the Quebec Parental Insurance Plan (QPIP). Some employers, particularly in the province of Quebec, opt to "top up" this payment for part of the maternity leave period; that is, they pay the difference between the maternity payment and the employee's usual salary (Marshall, 2010).

All types of policies affect family nursing every day. Health policy has far-reaching ethical and practical implications for childbearing family nursing. For instance, genetic screening during pregnancy and hearing screens for the newborn have become compulsory for health care providers in some Canadian provinces. Moreover, cystic fibrosis screening in pregnancy and newborn screening for metabolic and genetic diseases have become mandatory for maternity providers in many American states. The informed decision-making models that are the impetus for these policies are not replicated in European health care systems; by contrast, they often are negatively viewed as eugenic solutions to reduce the incidence of disability. European systems, unlike in North America, heavily fund services for disabled children and their families.

Hospitals also have policies affecting families that should be of concern to family nurses, especially considering how varied the family of today is. For example, increasing numbers of nontraditional families, such as lesbian couples, are having children through donor insemination or adoption (Roberts, 2006). Yet policies that guide perinatal practices—from the visual images hanging on the wall to if or how well partners are welcomed in prenatal groups, the delivery room, or other hospital environments—may be a barrier to these particular families' welfare and relationships (Goldberg, 2005; Roberts, 2006). In these situations, family nurses have an obligation to speak out on behalf of families. Often, nurses think of policies as entities beyond their control. In actuality, nurses have a voice and power in forming and changing policies. Beginning steps include close scrutiny of their practice settings for issues related to the welfare of families and their members.

FAMILY CASE STUDIES

This section illustrates the art and science of nursing with childbearing families. The Sanders family demonstrates family nursing care when unexpected health problems occur during pregnancy. The Housah-Ibrahim family case study reveals how a nurse provides culturally sensitive care to young parents who are quite new in the country.

Family Case Study: Sanders Family—A Family Experiencing a Preterm Birth

Tom and Mary Sanders have been married to each other for 6 years. Tom, age 28, and Mary, age 28, have one child named Jenny who was born at full term 2 years ago. Mary did not experience any health problems with her first pregnancy. At that time, the Sanders lived in a large city in the western part of the United States, near their parents, siblings, and childhood friends. Two years later, the Sanders had moved to a small town 500 miles away from their friends and families to find better professional opportunities for Tom, a software engineer, and more affordable housing. A month after the move, they discovered that Mary was about 3 months pregnant. Although Tom's new job provided medical insurance for the family, Mary was concerned about finding and obtaining obstetrical care in their new community. Even though it would strain family finances, Mary decided to postpone seeking employment as a secretary until after the birth and to concentrate instead on fixing up the older two-story house they had bought.

Unexpectedly, Mary had health problems with this pregnancy. At 27 weeks' gestation, her obstetrician diagnosed gestational diabetes, which required Mary to modify her diet to keep her blood glucose under control. At 29 weeks, she began to have preterm labor. To stop the contractions, her physician insisted that Mary stay on bedrest around the clock except for a very brief daily shower and use of the bathroom. Tom had to take over meal preparation, house cleaning, and caring for Jenny. He arranged the living room so Mary could lie on the couch and Jenny could play near her mother while he

(continued)

was at work. Because he had not yet accrued vacation or sick time, Tom could not take time off from his job to help Mary and take care of Jenny without sacrificing pay. Mary found it difficult to follow her diet and stay on bedrest. She was frustrated because she had to stop her house renovation, and Tom's cooking and housecleaning were not up to her standards. She was tempted to run the vacuum cleaner, wash dishes, and eat sweets while Tom was at work. The medication to suppress contractions made her so anxious and tremulous that she could not amuse herself with crafts, sewing, or puzzles. She was lonely for her mother and the support of friends who were 500 miles away; she longed for companionship, but found herself complaining and nagging Tom when he was home. Jenny frequently had tantrums because she could not play outside with her mother and began to have lapses in toilet training.

At 32 weeks of pregnancy, Mary's membranes ruptured; her physician sent her to a perinatal center 100 miles away from home because it had better facilities to care for preterm babies. Jenny went with her parents to the perinatal center to wait until one of her grandmothers could come and take care of her. Jason was born 28 hours after the Sanders arrived at the perinatal center hospital. Figure 12-1 presents a Sanders family genogram.

Mary was discharged from the perinatal center within 24 hours after Jason's birth. At home, she felt extremely weak and was overwhelmed by household tasks and caring for Jenny. She was disappointed that she was unable to breastfeed the baby. Two weeks later, she was weeping frequently, felt very sad, had no appetite, and had difficulty sleeping. Being with their new son was difficult because each visit required a 200-mile round-trip, Tom had a full-time job, and Mary cared for Jenny during the day. Jason, the new baby, remained at the perinatal center in the special care nursery until he was mature and stable enough to go home 4 weeks later. At her 6-week postpartum checkup, Mary told the office nurse that she did not enjoy caring for her new baby and she had difficulty with her sleep. Based on this information the office nurse asked Mary to complete the Edinburgh Postnatal Depression Scale. Figure 12-2 presents the Sanders family ecomap and how the nurse mobilized resources to help this family.

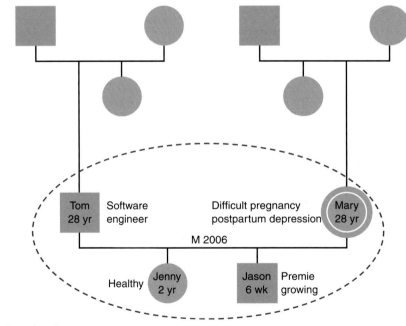

FIGURE 12-1 Sanders family genogram.

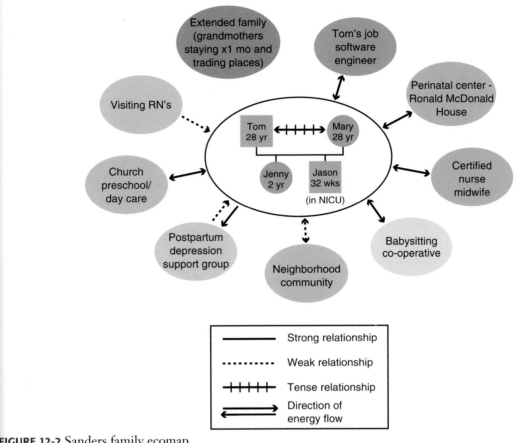

FIGURE 12-2 Sanders family ecomap.

Case Study: Housah-Ibrahim Family—A Somalian Family in Canada Experiencing Childbirth

Fatima Housah, age 21, and Abdi Ibrahim, age 28, have been married for 3 years and are excited that Fatima is expecting their first baby. Abdi grew up in Somalia and was trained as an engineer in South Africa. He currently works as a taxicab driver in a large urban city in Canada while attending night school to obtain credentials in engineering. Abdi's mother and father live and work 1 hour away in an adjacent city. Following a wait of 3 years, Abdi was relieved when Fatima's application for permanent residence was finally accepted so that she could remain in Canada. She had arrived 1 year earlier as a refugee claimant who had experienced much hardship and ethnic persecution in Somalia and then in the refugee camp in Uganda. Her experience of frequent moving between refugee camps and fleeing rebel-led violence has left her with post-traumatic stress disorder. She is receiving emotional support from the women at the local mosque. Fatima has two sisters, a brother, and an aunt who reside in another Canadian province and she feels lonely for them at times. Talking by computer on Skype only causes her to miss them more. Fortunately, many of the women from the local Muslim Community Centre have offered her friendship. They are teaching her how to take the bus and subway and how to find ethnic foods in the local markets. She is grateful that they taught her how to use the kitchen appliances safely. She had never used a stove before coming Canada. Figure 12-3 presents a family genogram for Fatima and Abdi's family.

Fatima is concerned about her prenatal care. Even though the Imam at the mosque says that a male physician could provide emergency care for her, she believes that a female provider might be more understanding. Finding a female maternity care provider has been a challenge in this community despite being insured by

(continued)

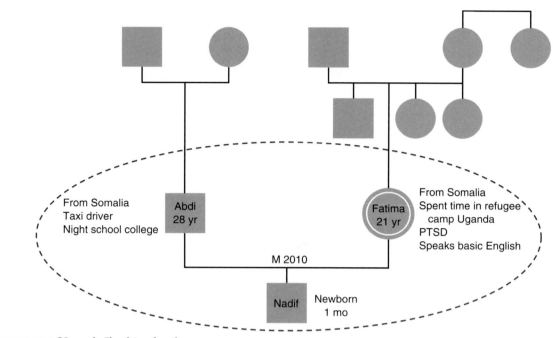

FIGURE 12-3 Housah-Ibrahim family genogram.

Canada's universal health care plan. To date, Fatima has had sporadic prenatal care at the walk-in center. By 32 weeks, however, she was able to find a female midwife with whom she has had five prenatal visits so far. At one of these visits Fatima reveals that she is worried about how her first-degree circumcision as an infant (which involved only a clitorectomy, thus leaving the labia and urethra intact) will affect the birth.

At 41 weeks' gestation, Fatima starts to feel lower abdominal cramps that continue over 2 hours and proceed to include lower back pain. The couple does not own an automobile, so they rush to the closest hospital by ambulance. Fatima notes that the nurse who greets them in the Labour Floor Triage room is a female; she is very kind and speaks slowly and gently. This approach is helpful because Fatima's English is still fairly basic. She defers to Abdi who answers all of the medical history questions. Further assessment reveals that her cervix has not started to change and that she is contracting regularly. Fatima is admitted to the hospital after 22 hours of prodromal labor and her female midwife consults the attending obstetrician regarding the need for oxytocin augmentation. A Somali interpreter is called to the bedside so the midwife

and female consulting obstetrician can obtain consent to start medication to augment labor. Because of her past experiences, Fatima is resistant to medication and distrustful of medical authorities. In halting English, Fatima asks why the midwife wants to interfere with the natural processes of labor. Although she is not crying, her face appears to be drawn and frightened under her hijab (head scarf).

Twenty-four hours following vaginal delivery of a healthy baby boy named Nadif, Fatima is discharged home. Abdi is eager to participate in infant care although this is not the traditional father's role in Somali culture. He has learned how to change Nadif's diapers and to bathe him. Abdi stays up late surfing the Internet to learn more about fatherhood and about how to cook iron-rich foods for Fatima because she is too exhausted most evenings to cook. Abdi's parents are able to visit on weekends to help with the baby and thus provide much-needed support for this family. In addition, this couple has several community supports in place, as well as a follow-up appointment with a pediatrician at the public health center for the baby. Figure 12-4 presents Fatima and Abdi's family and how the nurse mobilized resources to help this family.

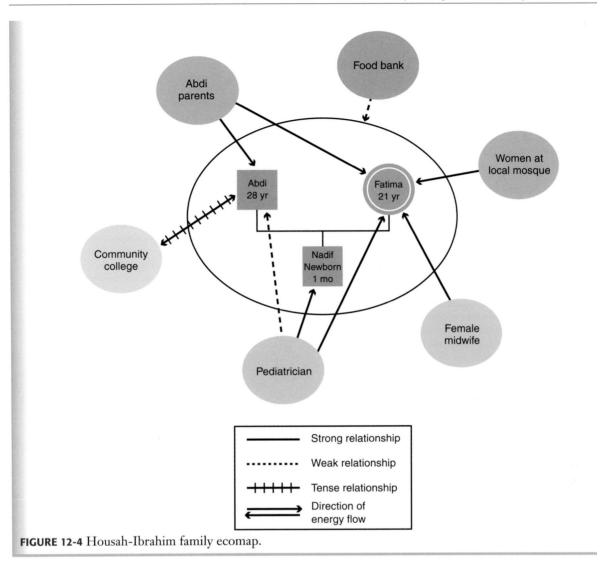

FIGURE 12-4 Housah-Ibrahim family ecomap.

SUMMARY

Childbearing family nursing focuses on family relationships and the health of all members of the childbearing family, even during times of extreme threats to maternal health. Several different theories available to nurses encountering families during childbearing can help guide their assessment of the family, their plan of care, and interventions for the family. Nurses are also in a position to have a powerful influence on the development of family-friendly policies at both the federal and practice setting levels.

■ Several theories, including Family Systems Theory and Family Developmental Theory,

are helpful to guide nurses' understanding of childbearing families and to structure nursing care.

■ Stress-producing pregnancy-related events disrupt family functioning regardless of how the family is structured (traditional or nontraditional).

■ While giving direct physical care, teaching patients, or performing other traditional modes of childbearing nursing, family nurses focus on family relationships and health of all members of the childbearing family.

■ Acute and chronic health conditions can develop during pregnancy and, thus, disrupt family functioning, development, and structure. When health threats arise, all family members experience stress as they strive to regain balance.

■ Childbearing family nurses can assist families to understand, prepare for, and respond to the effect each newborn has on the family.

■ Nurses must participate in policy development and implementation as it relates to childbearing families.

■ Nurses need to be aware of the effect of legislation on childbearing families.

REFERENCES

Ainsworth, M. (1967). *Infancy in Uganda: Infant care and the growth of love.* Baltimore, MD: Johns Hopkins.

American College of Obstetricians and Gynecologists and the Interprofessional Task Force on Health Care of Women and Children. (1978). *Joint statement on the development of family centered maternity/newborn care in hospitals.* Chicago, IL: American College of Obstetricians and Gynecologists.

American Society for Reproductive Medicine. (2008). Definitions of infertility and recurrent pregnancy loss. Retrieved from http://www.asrm.org/uploadedFiles/ASRM_Content/News_and_Publications/Practice_Guidelines/Committee_Opinions/Definitions_of_infertility_and_recurrent.pdf

Armstrong, D. S., Hutti, M. H., & Myers, J. (2009). The influence of prior perinatal loss on parent's psychological distress after the birth of a subsequent healthy infant. *Journal of Obstetric, Gynecologic, and Neonatal Nursing, 38*(6), 654–666.

Balasch, J., & Gratacos, E. (2012). Delayed childbearing: Effects on fertility and the outcome of pregnancy. *Current Opinions in Obstetrics and Gynecology, 24*(3), 187–193.

Beck, C. T. (2001). Predictors of postpartum depression: An update. *Nursing Research, 50*(5), 275–285.

Berk, L. (2007). *Development through the lifespan* (4th ed.). Boston, MA: Allyn & Bacon.

Blass, D. (2005). *Riding the emotional roller coaster.* Washington, DC: American College of Obstetricians and Gynecologists.

Bomar, P. (Ed.). (2004). *Promoting health in families: Applying family research and theory in nursing practice* (2nd ed.). Philadelphia: Saunders.

Bowlby, J. (1952). *Maternal care and mental health.* (Report prepared on behalf of the WHO as a contribution to the UN program for the welfare of homeless children). Geneva, Switzerland: World Health Organization.

Britton, C., McCormick, F., Renfrew, M., Wade, A., & King, S. (2007). Support for breastfeeding mothers. *Cochrane Database of Systematic Reviews*, Issue 1. Art. No.: CD001141. Retrieved from http://apps.who.int/rhl/reviews/CD001141.pdf

Bruening, M., MacLehose, R., Loth, K., Story, M., & Neumark-Sztainer, D. (2012). Feeding a family in a recession: Food insecurity among Minnesota parents. *American Journal of Public Health, 102*(3), 520–526.

Burst, H. V. (2004). The history of nurse-midwifery/midwifery education. *Journal of Midwifery & Women's Health, 50*(2), 129–137.

Callister, L. C. (2006). Perinatal loss: A family perspective. *Journal of Perinatal Neonatal Nursing, 20*(3), 227–234.

Canada Adopts! (2001). Adopting in Canada. Retrieved from http://www.canadaadopts.com/canada/domestic_private.shtml

Carter, B., & McGoldrick, M. (2005). *The expanded family life cycle: Individual, family and social perspectives* (3rd ed.). New York: Allyn & Bacon, Pearson Education.

Cassar, L. (2006). Cultural expectations of Muslims and Orthodox Jews in regard to pregnancy and the postpartum period: A study in comparison and contrast. *International Journal of Childbirth Education, 21*(2), 27–30.

Chalmers, B., Levitt, C., Heaman, M., O'Brien, B., Sauve, R., & Kaczorowski, J. (2009). Maternity experiences study group of the Canadian perinatal surveillance system, public health agency of Canada. *Birth, 36*(2), 122–132.

Chichester, M. (2005). Multicultural issues in perinatal loss. *AWHONN Lifelines, 9*(4), 314–320.

Conger, R. D., Song, H., Stockdale, G. D., Ferrer, E., Widaman, K. F., & Cauce, A. M. (2012). Resilience and vulnerability of Mexican origin youth and their families: A test of a culturally-informed model of Family Economic Stress. In P. Kerig, M. S. Schulz, & S. T. Hauser (Eds.), *Adolescence and beyond: Family processes and development* (pp. 270–273). New York, NY: Oxford University Press.

Cronqvist, A., Theorell, T., Burns, T., & Lutzen, K. (2004). Caring about-caring for: Moral obligations and work responsibilities in intensive care nursing. *Nursing Ethics, 11*(1), 63–76.

Datta, J., Graham, B., & Wellings, K. (2012). The role of fathers in breastfeeding: Decision-making and support. *British Journal of Midwifery, 20*(3), 159–167.

Davidson, M. R., London, M. L., & Ladewig, P. A. (2008). *Olds' maternal-newborn nursing and women's health across the lifespan* (8th ed.). Upper Saddle River, NJ: Pearson Prentice Hall.

Davies, B. (2006). Sibling grief throughout childhood. *The Forum, 32*(1), 5. Retrieved from http://www.adec.org/AM/Template.cfm?Section=The_Forum&Template=/CM/ContentDisplay.cfm&ContentID=1543

Day, R. D. (2005). Relationship stress in couples. In P. C. McKenry & S. J. Price (Eds.), *Families and changes: Coping with stressful events and transition* (3rd ed., pp. 332–353). Thousand Oaks, CA: Sage.

de Chateau, P. (1976). Influence of early contact on maternal and infant behavior in primiparae. *Birth Family Journal, 6,* 149–155.

de Chateau, P. (1977). Importance of the neonatal period for the development of synchrony in the mother-infant dyad. *Birth Family Journal, 4*(1), 10–22.

Demo, D. H., & Cox, M. J. (2000). Families with young children: A review of research in the 1990s. *Journal of Marriage and the Family, 62*(4), 876–895.

Denham, S. A. (2003). Relationships between family rituals, family routines, and health. *Journal of Family Nursing, 9*(3), 305–330.

Denham, S. A., & Looman, W. (2010). Families with chronic illness. In J. R. Kaakinen, V. Gedaly-Duff, D. P. Coehlo, & S. M. Harmon-Hanson (Eds.), *Family health care nursing: Theory, practice and care* (4th ed., pp. 235–272). Philadelphia, PA: F. A. Davis.

Doucet, S., Dennis, C., Letourneau, N., & Blackmore, E. (2009). Differentiation and clinical implications of postpartum depression and postpartum psychosis. *Journal of Obstetric, Gynecologic and Neonatal Nursing, 38*(3), 269–279.

Driscoll, J. W. (2006). Postpartum depression: How nurses can identify and care for women grappling with this disorder. *Lifelines, 10*(5), 399–409.

Duvall, E. M. (1977). *Marriage and family development* (5th ed.). Philadelphia, PA: J. B. Lippincott.

Duvall, E. M., & Miller, B. C. (1985). *Marriage and family development* (6th ed.). New York, NY: Harper & Row.

Eberhard-Gran, M., Eskild, A., Tambs, K., Opjordsmoen, S., & Samuelsen, S. O. (2001). Review of validation studies of the Edinburgh Postnatal Depression Scale. *Acta Psychiatrica Scandinavica, 104*(4), 243–249.

Eggertson, L. (2011). Giving mother nature a helping hand. *Fertility Nurses, 107*(3), 32–36.

Fontenot, H. (2007). Transition and adaptation to adoptive motherhood. *Journal of Obstetrics, Gynecologic and Neonatal Nursing, 36*(2), 175–182.

Friedman, M. (2010). On mommyblogging: Notes to a future feminist historian. *Journal of Women's History, 22*(4), 197–208.

Galtry, J., & Callister, P. (2005). Assessing the optimal length of parental leave for child and parental well-being. How can research inform policy? *Journal of Family Issues, 26*(2), 219–246.

Giesler, M. (2012). Gay fathers' negotiation of gender role strain. A qualitative inquiry. *Fathering, 10*(2), 119–139.

Godfrey, J. R., & Lawrence, R. A. (2010). Toward optimal health: The maternal benefits of breastfeeding. *Journal of Women's Health, 19*(9), 1597–1602.

Goldberg, L. (2005). Understanding lesbian experience: What perinatal nurses should know to promote women's health. *AWHONN Lifelines, 9*(6), 463–467.

Goodman, J. H. (2004). Paternal postpartum depression, its relationship to maternal postpartum depression, and implications for family health. *Journal of Advanced Nursing, 45*(10), 26–35.

Grantmakers in Health. (2004). *Fact sheet. Addressing maternal depression*. Washington, DC: Author.

Gray, L., Miller, L. W., Philipp, B. L., & Blass, E. M. (2002). Breastfeeding is analgesic in healthy newborns. *Pediatrics,109*, 590–593.

Gray, L., Watt, L., & Blass, E. M. (2000). Skin-to-skin contact is analgesic in healthy newborns. *Pediatrics, 105*, 1–6.

Gunnar, M., & Pollak, S. D. (2007). Supporting parents so that they can support their internationally adopted children: The larger challenge lurking behind the fatality statistics. *Child Maltreatment, 12*(4), 381–382.

Guttmacher Institute. (2009). *A real-time look at the impact of the recession on women's family planning and pregnancy decisions*. New York, NY: Author.

Hockenberry, M. I., Wilson, D., Winkelstein, M. L., & Kline, N. E. (2006). *Wong's nursing care of infants and children* (7th ed.). St. Louis, MO: Mosby.

Holahan, J. (2011). The 2007–09 recession and health insurance coverage. *Health Affairs, 30*(1), 145–152.

Hung, C. H. (2005). Women's postpartum stress, social support and health status. *Western Journal of Nursing Research, 27*(2), 148–159.

Hutton, E. K., & Hassan, E. S. (2007). Late vs. early clamping of the umbilical cord in full-term neonates. *Journal of the American Medical Association, 297*(11), 1241–1252.

Jesse, D. E., & Graham, M. (2005). Are you often sad and depressed? Brief measures to identify women at risk for depression in pregnancy. *American Journal of Maternal Child Nursing, 30*(1), 40–45.

Johnston, M. L., & Esposito, N. (2007). Barriers and facilitators for breastfeeding among working women in the United States. *Journal of Obstetric, Gynecologic, and Neonatal Nursing, 36*(1) 9–20.

Klaus, M. H., Jerauld, R., Kreger, N. C., McAlpine, W., Steffa, M., & Kennel, J. H. (1972). Maternal attachment: Importance of the first postpartum days. *New England Journal of Medicine, 286*(9), 460–463.

Klaus, M. H., & Kennel, J. H. (1976). *Maternal-infant bonding*. St. Louis, MO: Mosby.

Klaus, M. H., Kennell, J. H., & Klaus, P. H. (1995). *Bonding*. Boston, MA: Addison-Wesley.

Lawrence, A. (2010). *Breastfeeding: A guide for the medical profession* (7th ed.). St. Louis, MO: Mosby.

Leavitt, J. W. (1986). *Brought to bed: Childbearing in America 1750–1950*. New York: Oxford University Press.

LeMasters, E. E. (1957). Parenthood as crisis. *Marriage and the Family, 31*, 352–355.

Lemon, B. S. (2002). Experiencing grandparent grief: A piece of my heart died twice. *AWHONN Lifelines, 6*(5), 470–472.

LeVasseur, L. P. (2002). A phenomenological study of the art of nursing: Experiencing the turn. *Advances in Nursing Science, 24*(4), 14–26.

Lewallen, L. P. (2011). The importance of culture in childbearing. *Journal of Obstetric, Gynecologic and Neonatal Nursing, 40*(1), 4–7.

London, M. L., Ladewig, P. W., Ball, J. W., & Bindler, R. C. (2007). *Maternal and child nursing care* (2nd ed.). Upper Saddle River, NJ: Pearson.

Lowdermilk, D. L., & Perry, S. E. (2004). *Maternity and women's health care* (8th ed.). St. Louis, MO: Mosby.

Lutter, S. L. (2008). Psychosocial impact of infertility. *Advance for Nurses, 10*(13), 29. Retrieved from www.nursing.advanceweb.com

Malik, S., & Coulson, N. (2008). The male experience of infertility: A thematic analysis of an online infertility support group bulletin board. *Journal of Reproductive and Infant Psychology, 26*(1), 18–30.

Maloni, J. (2010). Antepartum bedrest for pregnancy complications: Efficacy and safety for preventing preterm birth. *Biological Research for Nursing, 12*(2), 102–124.

Maloni, J. A., Brezinski-Tomasi, J. E., & Johnson, L. A. (2001). Antepartum bed rest: Effect upon the family. *Journal of Obstetric, Gynecologic, and Neonatal Nursing, 30*(2), 165–172.

Maloni, J. A., Margevicius, S. P., & Damato, E. G. (2006). Multiple gestation: Side effects of antepartum bed rest. *Biological Research for Nursing, 8*(2), 115–128.

Mander, R. (2004). *Men and maternity*. New York: Routledge.

Marshall, K. (2010). Employer top-ups. *Perspectives*, February. Statistics Canada Catalogue no. 75-001-X. Retrieved from http://www.statcan.gc.ca/pub/75-001-x/2010102/pdf/11120-eng.pdf

Martell, L. K. (2003). Postpartum women's perceptions of the hospital environment. *Journal of Obstetric, Gynecologic, and Neonatal Nursing, 32*(4), 478–485.

Martell, L. K. (2005). Family nursing with childbearing families. In S. M. Hanson, V. Gedaly-Duff, & J. R. Kaakinen (Eds.), *Family health care nursing: Theory, practice and care* (3rd ed., pp. 267–289). Philadelphia, PA: F. A. Davis.

Martell, L. K. (2006). From innovation to common practice: Perinatal nursing pre-1970 to 2005. *Journal of Perinatal and Neonatal Nursing, 20*(1), 8–16.

Mattingly, M., & Smith, K. (2010). Changes in wives' employment when husbands stop working: A recession-prosperity comparison. *Family Relations, 59*(4), 343–357.

McKinney, E. S., James, S. R, Murray, S. S., Nelson, K. A., & Ashwill, J. W. (2013). *Maternal-child nursing* (4th ed.). St. Louis, MO: Saunders.

Mennino, S. F., & Brayfield, A. (2002). Job-family trade-offs: The multidimensional effects of gender. *Work and Occupations, 29*(2), 226–256.

Mercer, J. S., Vohr, B. R., McGrath, M. M., Padbury, J. F., Wallach M., & Oh, W. (2006). Delayed cord clamping in very preterm infants reduces the incidence of intraventricular hemorrhage and late-onset sepsis: A randomized, controlled trial. *Pediatrics, 117*(4), 1235–1242.

Morgan, S. (2002). *In our own hands: The women's health movement 1969–1990.* Piscataway, NJ: Rutgers University Press.

Nelson, A. M. (2003). Transition to motherhood. *Journal of Obstetric, Gynecologic, and Neonatal Nursing, 32*(4), 465–477.

Newman, J., & Pitman, T. (2009). *Dr. Jack Newman's guide to breastfeeding* (1st rev. ed.). Toronto, ON: HarperCollins Canada.

Nomaguchi, K., & Milke, M. A. (2003). Costs and rewards of children: The effects of becoming a parent on adults' lives. *Journal of Marriage and Family, 65*(2), 356–374.

Oberg, C. N. (2011). The great recession's impact on children. *Maternal Child Health Journal, 15*(5), 553–554.

O'Leary, J., & Thorwick, C. (2006). Fathers' perspectives during pregnancy, postperinatal loss. *Journal of Obstetrics, Gynecology and Neonatal Nursing, 35*(1), 78–86.

Palacios, J., Butterfly, R., & Strickland, C. J. (2005). American Indians/Alaskan Natives. In J. G. Lipson & S. L. Dibble (Eds.), *Cultural and clinical care* (pp. 27–41). San Francisco, CA: The Regents University of California.

Parliament of Canada. (2012). House Government Bill C-31: An act to amend the Immigration and Refugee Protection Act, the Balanced Refugee Reform Act, the Marine Transportation Security Act and the Department of Citizenship an Immigration Act. Retrieved from http://www.parl.gc.ca/HousePublications/ Publication.aspx?Language=E&Mode=1&DocId=5581460

Peterson, B. D., Newton, C. R., & Rosen, K. H. (2003). Examining congruence between partners' perceived infertility-related stress and its relationship to marital adjustment and depression in infertile couples. *Family Process, 42*(1), 59–70.

Pillitteri, A. (2003). *Maternal and child health nursing* (4th ed.). Philadelphia, PA: Lippincott Williams & Wilkins.

Riley, L. A., & Glass, J. (2002). You can't always get what you want: Infant care preferences and use among employed mothers. *Journal of Marriage and Family, 64*, 2–15.

Roberts, S. J. (2006). Healthcare recommendations for lesbian women. *Journal of Obstetrics, Gynecology and Neonatal Nursing, 35*(5), 583–591.

Robson, F. (2002). Yes! A chance to tell my side of the story: A case study of a male partner of a woman undergoing termination of pregnancy for foetal abnormality. *Journal of Health Psychology, 7*(2), 183–193.

Ross, L. E., Dennis, C. L., Blackmore, E. R., & Stewart, D. (2005). *Postpartum depression: A guide for front line health and social service providers.* Toronto, ON: Centre for Addiction and Mental Health.

Rykkje, L. (2007). Intercountry adoption and nursing care. *Scandinavian Journal of Caring Sciences, 21*(4), 507–514.

Schenk, L. K., Kelley, J. H., & Schenk, M. P. (2005). Models of maternal-infant attachment: A role for nurses. *Pediatric Nursing, 31*(6), 514–517.

Schiffman, R. F., Omar, M. A., & McKelvey, L. M. (2003). Mother-infant interaction in low-income families. *MCN: American Journal of Maternal/Child Nursing, 28*(4), 246–251.

Sherrod, R. A. (2004). Understanding the emotional aspects of infertility. Implications for nursing practice. *Journal of Psychosocial Nursing, 42*(3), 42–47.

Sherrod, R. A. (2006). Male infertility: The element of disguise. *Journal of Psychosocial Nursing, 44*(10), 31–37.

Simich, L., Hamilton, H., & Baya, B. K. (2006). Mental distress, economic hardship and expectations of life in Canada among Sudanese newcomers. *Transcultural Psychiatry, 43*(3), 418–444.

Smit, E. (2010). International adoption families: A unique health care journey. *Pediatric Nursing, 36*(5), 253–258.

Smith, C., Ussher, J., Perz, J., Carmady, B., & de Lacey, S. (2001). The effect of acupuncture on psychosocial outcomes for women experiencing infertility: A pilot randomized controlled trial. *Journal of Alternative and Complementary Medicine, 17*(10), 923–930.

Steffensmeier, T. H. (1982). A role model of the transition to parenthood. *Journal of Marriage and the Family, 44*(2), 319–334.

Steuber, K. R., & Solomon, D. H. (2008). Relational uncertainty, partner interference, and infertility: A qualitative study of discourse within online forums. *Journal of Social and Personal Relationships, 25*(5), 831–855.

St. John, W., Cameron, C., & McVeigh, C. (2005). Meeting the challenge of new fatherhood during the early weeks. *Journal of Obstetric, Gynecologic, and Neonatal Nursing, 34*(2), 180–189.

Sutherland, A. H. (2005). Roma (Gypsies). In J. G. Lipson & S. L. Dibble (Eds.), *Cultural and clinical care* (pp. 404–414). San Francisco, CA: The Regents University of California.

Troy, N. W. (2003). Is the significance of postpartum fatigue being overlooked in the lives of women? *MCN: American Journal of Maternal/Child Nursing, 28*(4), 252–257.

U.S. Department of Health and Human Services (n.d.). Adoption by family type. Retrieved from http://www.childwelfare.gov/ adoption/adoptive/family_type.cfm

U.S. Department of Health and Human Services. (2013). Affordable Care Act (HR3590). Washington, DC: Author. Retrieved from http://www.healthcare.gov/law/full/index.html

Varney, H., Kriebs, J. M., & Gregor, C. L. (2004). *Varney's midwifery* (4th ed.) Sudbury, MA: Jones & Bartlett.

Ward, S. L., & Hisley, S. M. (2009). *Maternal-child nursing care: Optimizing outcomes for mothers, children, and families.* Philadelphia, PA: F. A. Davis.

Wertz, R. W., & Wertz, D. C. (1989). *Lying-in: A history of childbirth in America.* New Haven, CT: Yale University Press.

Wilson-Mitchell, K. (2008). Mental illness in refugee and immigrant women: A midwife's perspective on culturally competent care. *Canadian Journal of Midwifery Research and Practice, 7*(3), 9–18.

Wong, C., Pang, J., Tan, G., Soh, W., & Lim J. (2012). The impact of fertility on women's psychological health: A literature review. *Singapore Nursing Journal, 39*(3), 11–17.

Zhao, M., Esposito, N., & Wang, K. (2010). Cultural beliefs and attitudes toward health and health care among Asian born women in the United States. *Journal of Obstetric, Gynecologic and Neonatal Nurses, 39*(4), 370–385.

SELECTED RESOURCES

Organizations

- *The Association of Women's Health, Obstetric, and Neonatal Nurses (AWHONN):* http://www.awhonn.org
- *Depression After Delivery, Inc.:* http://www.depressionafterdelivery.com
- *The Compassionate Friends, Inc.:* www.compassionatefriends.org
- *International Childbirth Education Association (ICEA):* http://www.icea.org
- *The International Lactation Consultant Association (ILCA):* http://www.ilca.org
- *La Leche League International:* http://www.lalecheleague.org
- *National Council on Family Relations (NCFR):* http://www.ncfr.org
- *NCAST-AVENEW (University of Washington):* http://www.ncast.org

Journals

- *Birth*
- *Family Relations*
- *Journal of Obstetric, Gynecologic, and Neonatal Nursing (JOGNN)*
- *Journal of Perinatal and Neonatal Nursing*
- *Nursing for Women's Health (formally AWHONN Lifelines)*
- *MCN: American Journal of Maternal Child Nursing*

chapter 13

Family Child Health Nursing

Deborah Padgett Coehlo, PhD, C-PNP, PMHS, CFLE

Critical Concepts

- A major task of families is to nurture children to become healthy, responsible, and creative adults.

- Families are the major determinant of children's health and well-being.

- Most parents learn the parenting role "on the job," relying on experiences from their own childhood in their families of origin to guide them.

- Parents are charged with keeping children healthy, as well as caring for them during illness.

- Common health promotion challenges of children and their families are experienced during transitions as individual members and their families grow and change.

- Because the leading causes of morbidity and mortality among youth are substance use, sexual activity, and violence (both suicidal and homicidal), there is need for increased attention to health promotion and prevention in these areas.

- Abuse and neglect may be defined differently across cultures, but nurses must be alert to helping families understand when child-rearing practices harm rather than nurture children.

- Families with children will experience challenges related to specific chronic health conditions, and will have challenges related to transitions associated with all health conditions, including acute, chronic, and end-of-life phases.

- The Family-Centered Care Model can be used by family child health nurses to facilitate and teach healthful activities for growth, prevention of injury and disease, and management of illness conditions in families.

- The aim of nurses is to help families develop appropriate ways to carry out family tasks necessary to promote health and to prevent or positively cope with illness and disease.

- While most child-rearing families experience acute illnesses and become familiar with managing these crises, families do not anticipate that their children may have chronic illness.

- With their knowledge of family and child development, nurses can collaborate with families with chronically ill children to help them strive toward developmental landmarks.

- Family child health nursing must be practiced in collaboration and cooperation with families, as well as other health professionals, according to principles of family-centered care.

A major task of families is to nurture children to become healthy, responsible, and creative adults who can develop meaningful relationships across the life span. An important job of all parents is to keep children healthy and care for them during illness. Yet most mothers and fathers have little formal education for health care of children. In fact, most parents learn the role "on the job," relying on their childhood experiences in their families of origin to help guide them. Advice from other parents and professionals augment information from families of origin, but this advice is generally implemented only when questions or problems arise.

Family nurses help families promote health, prevent disease, and cope with illness. The importance of family life for children's health and illness care is often invisible, because families' everyday routines are commonplace and lie below the level of awareness. Family daily life, however, influences many aspects of children's health, including the promotion of health and the experience of illness in children. In turn, family daily life is influenced by the children's health and illness. Families are groups with unique characteristics, including specific family experiences, memories, and related intergenerational relationships; structure and membership; family rules and routines; aspirations and achievements; and ethnic or cultural patterns (Burr, Herrin, Beutler, & Leigh, 1988). Family structure and function interact with and are influenced by these family characteristics. Healthy outcomes for children—such as tripling their birth weight by 1 year of age, or successfully completing high school—are partially attributable to the intangible, invisible daily interactions among family members. Nurses, in partnership with families, examine how the characteristics of families influence health.

Family child health nursing entails employing nursing actions that consider the relationship between family tasks and health care and their effects on family well-being and children's health. Nurses care for children within the context of their family, and they care for children by treating the family as a whole. Nurses keep in mind that families affect their children's health, while children's health affects their families. Family child nurses care for children in a variety of clinical settings and care situations.

This chapter provides a brief history of family-centered care of children and then presents foundational concepts that will guide nursing practice with families with children. The chapter goes on to describe nursing care of well children and families with an emphasis on health promotion, nursing care of children and families in acute care settings, nursing care of children with chronic illness and their families, and nursing care of children and their families during end of life. The case study illustrates the application of family-centered care across settings.

ELEMENTS OF FAMILY-CENTERED CARE

Family-centered care is a system-wide approach to child health care. It is based on the assumption that families are children's primary source of nurturance, education, and health care. Family-centered care has emerged, in part, in response to increasing family responsibilities for health care. The general principles of family-centered care include the following:

1. Recognizing families as "the constants" in children's lives while the personnel in other systems, including the health care system, fluctuate
2. Openly sharing information about alternative treatments, ethical concerns, and uncertainties with families to guide decision-making processes
3. Forming partnerships between families and health professionals to decide jointly what is important for families
4. Respecting the racial, ethnic, cultural, and socioeconomic diversity of families and their ways of coping
5. Supporting and strengthening families' abilities to grow and develop (Lewandowski & Tesler, 2003)

See Table 13-1 for more detail on the elements of family-centered care.

Families are the key health care providers for children. Families determine the culture of health care, including establishing healthy living patterns, care for acute illnesses, and care for chronic illnesses. Health care providers have recently acknowledged the importance of families in developing a comprehensive and holistic treatment plan for those children who need health care services. Families acknowledge the uncertainty that surrounds their child's health, and they want to be informed partners of the health team's decision making and valued

Table 13-1	**Elements of Family-Centered Care**
Elements	**Definition**
1. The Family Is at the Center	The family is the constant in the child's life.
2. Family-Professional Collaboration	Collaboration includes the care of the individual child, program development, policy formation at all levels of care—hospital, home, and community.
3. Family-Professional Communication	Information exchange is complete, unbiased, and occurs in a supportive manner at all times.
4. Cultural Diversity of Families	Honors diversity (ethnic, racial, spiritual, social, economic, educational, and geographical), strengths, and individuality within and across all families.
5. Coping Differences and Support	Recognizes and respects family coping, supporting families with developmental, educational, emotional, spiritual, environmental, and financial resources to meet diverse needs.
6. Family-Centered Peer Support	Families are encouraged to network and support each other.
7. Specialized Service and Support Systems	Support systems for children with special health and developmental needs in the hospital, home, and community are accessible, flexible, and comprehensive.
8. Holistic Perspective of Family-Centered Care	Families are viewed as families, and children are viewed as children, recognizing their strengths, concerns, emotions, and aspirations beyond their specific health needs.

Source: Lewandowski, L., & Tesler, M. (Eds.). (2003). *Family-centered care: Putting it into action. The SPN/ANA guide to family-centered care.* Washington, DC: Society of Pediatric Nurses/American Nurses Association.

collaborators in the care of their child (Griffin, 2003). In societies that respect diverse opinions, a health team that includes the family is preferable to a hierarchical team with physicians at the top, nurses in between, and families at the bottom. Family-centered care attends to the importance of families in health care.

Starting in 1987, Surgeon General Koop began the initiative to include families on the team that provided care for children with special needs. Although the ideas presented were initiated with children with special health care needs, the elements apply to all families with children, and both well-child care and care for children with diagnosed illnesses. The Association for the Care of Children's Health further defined the specific key elements to family-centered care in 1994. These elements are now widely accepted and used by professionals and families with children with health care needs (Conway et al., 2006):

1. Recognize that the family is the constant in the child's life, while the service systems and personnel within those systems fluctuate.
2. Share complete and unbiased information with parents about their child's health on an ongoing basis. Do so in an appropriate and supportive manner.
3. Recognize family strengths and individuality. Respect different methods of coping.
4. Encourage and make referrals to parent-to-parent support, such as parent support groups.
5. Facilitate parent/professional collaboration at all levels of health care—care of an individual child, program development, implementation, and evaluation policy formation.
6. Ensure that the design of health care delivery systems is flexible, accessible, and responsive to families.
7. Implement appropriate policies and programs that provide emotional and financial support to families.
8. Understand and incorporate the developmental needs of children and families into the health care delivery systems.

Although family-centered care is recognized as being key in the care of children, the term itself is not consistently defined (Shields, Pratt, & Hunter, 2006) or practiced (Corlett & Twycross, 2006; Power &

Franck, 2008). There have been conflicting assumptions between nurses and parents about the degree of parent participation during hospitalization, for instance. Rather than a direct discussion about what caregiving parents wanted and could do, nurses and parents indirectly worked out their roles during their interactions surrounding the care of the child (Corlett & Twycross, 2006). In an integrative review of 11 qualitative studies about family-centered care, Shields et al. (2006) found that care was a negotiation between families and staff; some parents felt imposed on when nurses made the assumption that they would do their children's basic care while in the hospital without discussing it with them first.

CONCEPTS OF FAMILY CHILD HEALTH NURSING

Several foundational concepts guide nursing care of families with children: family development or career, including tasks, communication, development of support, transitions, and understanding and working together with family routines; individual development; and transitions (e.g., developmental, situational, and health/illness). Family developmental theories assume that families and individuals change over time. Not only do families experience the various developmental stages of each member, but they also progress through a series of family developmental stages. Nurses, by comparing their observations of particular families to expected family and individual developmental stages, can plan appropriate care (Table 13-2).

Family Career

Family career is the dynamic process of change that occurs during the life span of the unique group called the family. Family career incorporates stages, tasks, and transitions, and is similar to family development theory in that it takes into account family tasks and raising children. They differ, however, in that family development theory views the family in standard sequential steps, progressing from the birth of the first child, to raising and launching children, to experiencing the death of a parent figure in old age (Duvall & Miller, 1985). By contrast, family career takes

into account the diverse experiences of American families (Aldous, 1996). The family career includes both the expected developmental changes of the family life cycle, and the unexpected changes of situational crises, such as divorce, remarriage, and death.

The notion of family career involves the many paths that families can take during their life span. Changes do not necessarily occur in a linear fashion. For example, family career takes into account the possibility that a person without children may marry a partner who already has adolescent children, resulting in starting parenting with adolescent children. This new parent does not build on parenting skills experienced across time, but rather starts his career at the end of his child's childhood career. Family career is a useful concept because it reminds us that families are dynamic. Table 13-3 summarizes the definitions of family career, individual development, and patterns of health/disease/illness in families. Nurses working with child-rearing families need to know that family careers are inclusive of family development stages, transitions, and diversity because these dynamics affect family health.

Family Stages

Duvall's eight stages of family development, based on the oldest child, describes expected developmental changes in families that are raising children (Duvall & Miller, 1985). According to Duvall, family careers start with marriage without children, then proceed to childbearing, preschool children, school children, adolescents, the launching of young adults (i.e., first child gone to last child leaving home), middle age of parents (i.e., empty nest to retirement), and aging of family members (i.e., retirement to death of both parents). This theory has been challenged recently with the understanding that families experience several developmental stages at one time as they care for children of different ages and stages, as well as accommodate changes and transitions in family structure through separation, divorce, and remarriage. Knowledge of family stages helps nurses anticipate the reorganization necessary to accommodate the expected growth and development of family members. For example, families with school-age children expect children to be able to take care of their own hygiene, whereas families with infants expect to do all the hygiene care. Likewise, family activities shift with the developmental needs of the individual family members. Families with preschoolers may enjoy a day at the playground, whereas families with adolescents would likely not choose this outing. Nurses can serve families better if they understand and work with families at different stages of family development. Nurses can also help families understand competing developmental tasks and transitions across family members and across time.

Family Tasks

Across all family stages, there are basic family functions and tasks essential to survival and continuity (Duvall & Miller, 1985): (1) to secure shelter, food, and clothing; (2) to develop emotionally healthy individuals who can manage crisis and experience nonmonetary achievement; (3) to ensure each individual's socialization in school, work, spiritual, and community life; (4) to contribute to the next generation by giving birth, adopting a child, or fostering a child; and (5) to promote the health of family members and care for them during illness. The aim of nurses is to help families develop appropriate ways to carry out the tasks necessary to prevent or handle illness and disease, and to promote health.

Transitions

Transitions are central to nursing practice because they have profound health-related effects on families and family members (Meleis, Sawyer, Im, Hilfinger Messias, & Schumacher, 2000). Family transitions are events that signal a reorganization of family roles and tasks. The literature supports the idea that how families transition early in their family careers strongly influences future transitions (Meleis et al., 2000). Further, support from health professionals and other agencies has a positive impact on transitions through time, from early infancy to transition to adulthood (Rous, Myers, & Stricklin, 2007). The transitions can be developmental, situational, or health and illness. Developmental transitions are predictable changes that occur in an expected timeline congruent with movement through the eight family stages (e.g., the addition of a family member by birth). Because they are typical and expected, developmental transitions are also called normative transitions. Thus, family members expect and learn to interact differently as children grow. Sometimes

families may not make the transition to an expected family stage. For example, families with children who have disabilities and are not capable of independent living have difficulty launching their children because of lack of residential living facilities and caregivers.

Situational transitions include changes in personal relationships, roles and status, the environment, physical and mental capabilities, and the loss of possessions (Rankin, 1989; Rankin & Weekes, 2000). Situational transitions are also called nonnormative transitions. Not all families experience each situational transition and they can occur irrespective of time. For example, changes occur in personal relationships when a stepchild is integrated into the family group, when one becomes a new stepparent after divorce and remarriage. Changes in role and status also happen when an only child becomes a sibling after the family adopts another child. This is different than the normative process of having a second child through birth, as the preparation during pregnancy is absent, and the adopted child is often older than an infant, and can even be older than the biological child. Changes in the environment occur when working parents move to a new job and family members adjust to a new house, school, friends, and community. Even greater changes occur when families immigrate to a new country, learn a new language and a new culture, and perhaps have to work at a lower-status job. A natural disaster can destroy family possessions and heirlooms, resulting in stress, fear, a sense of loss, and problems with family members' ways of being and interacting (Schumacher & Meleis, 1994). For nursing care of families dealing with trauma, see Chapter 11.

(Text continued on page 396)

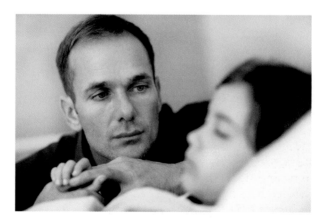

Table 13-2	Social-Emotional, Cognitive, and Physical Dimensions of Individual Development		
Period	**Social-Emotional Stages/ Significant Relationships**	**Stage-Sensitive Family Development Tasks**	**Values Orientation**
Infancy Birth–1 year	Trust vs. mistrust (I am what I am given.) Primary parent	Having, adjusting to, and encouraging the development of infants Establishing a satisfying home for both parents and infant(s) Establishing well-child health care	Undifferentiated
Toddlerhood 1–3 years	Autonomy vs. shame or doubt (I am what I "will.") Parental persons	Parenting role development. Learning to parent toddler. Developing approaches to discipline. Understanding child's increasing autonomy. Family planning. Providing safe environment. Maintaining well-child health care.	Punishment and obedience

Cognitive Stages of Development	Developmental Landmarks	Physical Maturation	Developmental Steps
Sensory-Motor Ages—Birth–2 years Infants move from neonatal reflex level of complete self world undifferentiation to relatively coherent organization of sensory-motor actions. They learn that certain actions have specific effects on the environment.	Gazes at complete patterns Social smile (2 mo) 180° visual pursuit (2 mo) Rolls over (5 mo) Ranking grasp (7 mo) Crude purposeful release (9 mo) Inferior pincer grasp Walks unassisted (10–14 mo)	*Rapid (Skeletal)* Transitory reflexes present (3 mo) (i.e., Moro reflex, sucking, grasp, tonic neck reflex) Muscle constitutes 25% of total body weight Birth weight doubles (6 mo) Eruption of deciduous central incisors (5–10 mo) Birth weight triples (1 yr) Anterior fontanel closes (10–14 mo) Transitory reflexes disappear (10 mo) Eruption of deciduous first molars (11–18 mo)	Anticipation of feeding Symbiosis (4–18 mo) Stranger anxiety (6–10 mo) Separation anxiety (8–24 mo) Self-feeding
Recognition of the constancy of external objects and primitive internal representation of the world begins. Uses memory to act. Can solve basic problems.	Words: 3–4 (13 mo) Builds tower of 2 cubes (15 mo) Scribbles with crayon (18 mo) Words: 10 (18 mo) Builds tower of 5–6 cubes (21 mo) Uses 3-word sentences (24 mo) Names 6 body parts (30 mo) Uses appropriate personal pronouns, i.e., I, you, me (30 mo) Rides tricycle (36 mo) Copies circle (36 mo) Matches 4 colors (36 mo) Talks to self and others (42 mo) Takes turns (42 mo)	Babinski reflex extinguished (18 mo) Bowel and bladder nerves myelinated (18 mo) Increase in lymphoid tissue Weight gain 2 kg per year (12–36 mo)	Oppositional behavior Messiness Exploratory behavior Parallel play Pleasure in looking at or being looked at Beginning self-concept Orderliness Curiosity

(continued)

Table 13-2	Social-Emotional, Cognitive, and Physical Dimensions of Individual Development—cont'd		
Period	**Social-Emotional Stages/ Significant Relationships**	**Stage-Sensitive Family Development Tasks**	**Values Orientation**
Pre–school-age 3–5 years	Initiative vs. guilt (I am what I imagine I can be.) Basic family	Adapting to the critical needs and interests of preschool children in stimulating, growth-promoting ways. Monitoring child development. Seek developmental screening as needed. Coping with energy depletion and lack of privacy as parents. Socializing children. Providing safe environment/accident prevention. Maintenance of couple relationship. Fostering sibling relationships.	Punishment and obedience moves to meeting own needs and doing for others if that person will do something for the child.
School-Age 6–12 years	Industry vs. inferiority (I am what I learn.) Neighborhood and school	Fitting into the community of school-age families in constructive ways. Letting children go, as they become increasingly independent. Encouraging child's education achievement. Balancing parental needs with children's needs.	Moves from instrumental exchange: "If you scratch my back, I'll scratch yours" into wanting to follow rules to be "good." Then to rule orientation for maintenance of social order.

Cognitive Stages of Development	Developmental Landmarks	Physical Maturation	Developmental Steps
Preoperational Thought (Prelogical)—Ages 2–7 years Begins to use symbols. Thinking tends to be egocentric and intuitive. Conclusions are based on what they feel or what they would like to believe.	Uses 4-word sentences (48 mo) Copies cross (48 mo) Throws ball overhand (48 mo) Copies square (54 mo) Copies triangle (60 mo) Prints name Rides two-wheel bike	Weight gain 2 kg per year (4–6 yr) Eruption of permanent teeth (5.5–8 yr) Body image solidifying	Cooperative play Fantasy play Imaginary companions Masturbation Task completion Rivalry with parents of same sex Games and rules Problem solving Achievement Voluntary hygiene Competes with partners Hobbies Ritualistic play Rational attitudes about food Companionship (same sex) Invests in community leaders, teachers, impersonal ideals
Concrete Operational Thought—Ages 7–12 years Conceptual organization increasingly stable. Children begin to seem rational and well organized. Increasingly systematic in approach to the world. Weight and volume are now viewed as constant, despite changes in shape and size.	As child moves through stage: Copies diamond, knows simple opposite analogies, names days of the week, repeats 5 digits forward, defines "brave" and "nonsense," knows seasons of the year, able to rhyme words, repeats 5 digits in reverse, understands pity, grief, surprise, knows where sun sets, can define "nitrogen" and "microscope"	Weight gain 2–4 kg per year (7–11 yr) Uterus begins to grow Budding of nipples in girls Increased vascularity of penis and scrotum Pubic hair appears in girls Menarche (9–11 yr)	Task completion Rivalry with parents of the same sex Games and rules Problem solving Achievement Voluntary hygiene Competes with partners Has hobbies Ritualistic play Rational attitudes about food Values companionship Invest in community leaders, teachers, impersonal ideals

(continued)

Table 13-2	Social-Emotional, Cognitive, and Physical Dimensions of Individual Development—cont'd		
Period	**Social-Emotional Stages/ Significant Relationships**	**Stage-Sensitive Family Development Tasks**	**Values Orientation**
Adolescence 13–20 years	Identity vs. role confusion (I know who I am.) Peer in-groups and out-groups Adult models of leadership	Balancing freedom with responsibility as teenagers mature and emancipate themselves. Maintaining communication with teen. Establishing post-parental interests and careers as growing parents.	Increasing internalization of ethical standards; can use to make decisions.
Early Adulthood	Intimacy vs. isolation Partners in friendship, sex, completion	Releasing young adults into work, military service, college, marriage, and so on with appropriate rituals and assistance. Maintaining a supportive home base.	Principled social contract
Middle Adulthood	Generativitiy vs. self-absorption or stagnation Divided labor and shared household	Refocusing on the marriage relationship. Maintaining kin ties with older and younger generations.	Self-actualization—doing what one is capable of.
Late Adulthood	Integrity vs. despair, disgust "Humankind" "My kind"	Coping with bereavement and living alone. Closing the family home in adapting to aging. Adjusting to retirement.	Universal ethical principles

Adapted from Duvall, E. M., & Miller, B. C. (1985). In *Marriage and family development* (6th ed., p. 62). New York, NY: Harper and Collins; Prugh, D. (1983). *The psychological aspects of pediatrics.* Philadelphia, PA: Lea & Febiger; Thomas, R.M. (2005), *Comparing theories of child development* (6th ed.). Belmont, CA: Wadsworth; and Duvall, E. M., & Miller, B. C. (1985). Developmental tasks: Individual and family. In E. M. Duvall & B. C. Miller (Eds.), *Marriage and family development.* New York, NY: Harper & Row.

Health-illness transitions are changes in the meaning and behavior of families as they experience an illness over time. Even though there are different diseases and conditions, the illness experience follows a pattern of prediagnosis signs and symptoms, crisis of diagnosis, daily management of the condition called the "long haul," and resolved or terminal phase (Rolland, 2005). Knowing the trajectory of a condition helps nurses and families recognize transition points and learn new ways of coping. For example, a family that has learned to manage its child's asthma requires new coping strategies when hospitalization occurs after the child's asthma symptoms are complicated by an upper respiratory illness and become too severe to manage at home. The family will need to reorganize itself to deal with the child's hospitalization and possibly learn to implement different asthma management approaches after hospitalization.

Transition events are signals to nurses that families may be at risk for health problems. Although families work to create and implement strategies to

Cognitive Stages of Development	Developmental Landmarks	Physical Maturation	Developmental Steps
Formal Operational Thought Abstract thought and awareness of the world of possibility develop. Adolescents use deductive reasoning and can evaluate the logic and quality of their own thinking. Increased abstract power allows them to work with laws and principles.	Knows why oil floats on water. Can divide 72 by 4 without pencil or paper. Understands "espionage." Can repeat six digits forward and five digits in reverse.	*Spurt (Skeletal)* Girls 1.5 years ahead of boys. Pubic hair appears in boys. Rapid growth of testes and penis. Axillary hair starts to grow. Down on upper lip appears. Voice changes. Mature spermatozoa (11–17 yr). Acne may appear. Cessation of skeletal growth Involution of lymphoid tissue Muscle constitutes 43% total body weight Permanent teeth calcified Eruption of permanent third molars (17–30 years)	"Revolt" Loosens tie to family Cliques Responsible independence Work habits solidifying Heterosexual interests Recreational activities Preparation for occupational choice Occupational commitment Elaboration of recreational outlets Marriage readiness Parenthood readiness

keep their children safe, these safety measures often fall behind during times of transition as parents find themselves coping with the stress of transition while continuing to cope with parenting stress. A developmental example is placing a crawling infant in a playpen to decrease the risk of falling while the parent is temporarily busy. When the infant transitions from crawling to pulling up to standing and walking, the family needs to allow the child to expand her environment by allowing her out of the security of the playpen and by modifying the environment to make it safe for her. A situational example occurs when a married family transitions to a divorced family. Parents will need to think about new routines for caring for the children. In a two-parent family, one parent may have gotten breakfast ready while the other parent attended to the child. Now one parent will be doing both. An example of a health and illness transition would be when a child is diagnosed with type 1 diabetes mellitus. The family will make major changes in family tasks to accommodate the nutrition and medication needs of one member. Nurses, by

Term	Definition
Family career	The dynamic process of change that occurs during the life span of the unique group called the family. Whereas family development views the family in standard sequential steps or stages, family career takes into account the diverse experiences of American families that do not occur in anticipated stages.
Individual development	Physical and maturational change of the individual over time. Some theories perceive change as stages, and others are interactional change.
Health and illness Families and their members experience dimensions of health while managing illness among members.	Health is behavior that promotes optimal dimensions of well-being. Family and individual health is multidimensional; therefore, a family and/or member can have a disease and be "healthy" in another dimension of health. Illness is a disease (and family management of the disease) that may be acute (time-limited), chronic (live with over time), or terminal (end-of-life).

Table 13-3 Definitions of Family Career, Individual Development, and Patterns of Health/Disease/Illness

assessing families for anticipated changes related to family and child developmental transitions, as well as situational and health-illness transitions, can help families plan for changes.

Individual Development

It is important to consider the individual development of all the family members in nursing care of families with children. Child-raising families are complex groups of adults and children at different stages of development. A schematic overview of human development highlights the stages of individual experiences over time. Adult developmental needs may complement or conflict with children's developmental needs.

When nurses review with families the individual family member's developmental stages that are occurring concurrently among children and adults, they validate the complexity of family interactions. Through this review process, nurses can assist families to accommodate to children's and adults' changing needs, abilities, and thought processes across time. Table 13-2 presents three dimensions of individual development: social-emotional, cognitive, and physical. The table is meant to be a guide and is not all-inclusive; it may not be representative of all cultures or socioeconomic statuses. Nurses can use these dimensions to identify expected developmental progression and potential areas of concern for families. This table can also be used to help understand when parents of children with developmental disabilities may feel recurrent sorrow, as they watch their child miss expected milestones (Blaska, 1998).

NURSING INTERVENTIONS TO SUPPORT CARE OF WELL CHILDREN AND FAMILIES

Families are the context for health promotion and illness care for all family members, including children. Family beliefs, rituals, and routines affect the health of all family members, including, for instance, traditional health practices around food, eating, and types of food served at meals; physical activity and rest; use of alcohol and other substances; and providing care and connection for family members (Novilla, Barnes, De La Cruz, Williams, & Rogers, 2006). Christensen (2004) concluded that the role of families in health promotion of children goes beyond protecting their health, well-being, development, and decreasing risk behavior, to teaching children to be "health promoting actors" by encouraging their active participation in health care and providing information and having them make their own healthy life choices. Families are, of course, linked to and interact with their larger environments. See Chapter 3 for a discussion on the bioecological theory (Bronfenbrenner, 1997).

In well-child care, families are considered the care environment for their children. Proposed nursing outcomes of current well-child care focus on family functioning and capacity, or the ability to care and nurture children while providing a safe and developmentally stimulating environment. Specific outcomes include that parents: (a) are knowledgeable about their children's physical health status and needs; (b) feel valued and supported as their children's primary caregiver and teacher, and function in partnership with their children's health care providers and teachers; (c) are screened for maternal depression, family violence, and family substance abuse and referred to specialists when needed; (d) understand and are able to use well-child care services; (e) understand and can implement developmental monitoring, stimulation, and regulation such as reading regularly to their children; (f) are skilled in anticipating and meeting their children's developmental needs; and (g) have access to consistent sources of emotional support and are linked to appropriate community services (Schor, 2007). In promoting child and family well-being, nurses support families in care of their children using the following skills and interventions:

- Communicating with families
- Supporting development of parenting skills and healthy family functioning
- Understanding and working with family routines
- Identifying health risks and teaching prevention strategies
- Supporting health promotion in families with children

Communication With Families

Therapeutic communication with family groups is the foundation of nursing care of families with children. One important feature of communication with families with children is including all of the family members in a discussion or interaction (Wright & Leahey, 1999). In initial communication, Cooklin (2001) recommends that each family member be asked to introduce himself or herself, beginning with the parent or adults of the family, and proceeding with each family member in order of age from oldest to youngest. North American children are often valued as autonomous beings. Research supports that children want to be consulted about decisions concerning their health care and want their opinions to be respected (Coyne, 2006). Nurses can assure children that they have a "real voice" by inviting them to speak, conveying that their opinion really matters, and demonstrating genuine interest in their point of view. Because the role of children in social situations is influenced by family culture, it is important to confirm that the children feel that they have permission to choose how they want to participate and that the parents confirm that they will allow the children to participate freely in the discussion (Cooklin, 2001).

Another important feature of communication with families is considering and adjusting communication style, content of message, and vocabulary for developmental appropriateness for each family member (Barnes et al., 2002; Cooklin, 2001; McKinney, James, Murray, & Ashwill, 2005). Engaging children in a casual conversation initiates a beginning relationship. Coyne's study (2006) found that children wanted to "chat" with the nurse, to know a little about the nurse as a person, and wanted the nurse to know about them. Instead of starting the conversation with the reasons behind the hospital visit, children wanted to start the conversation with questions they were familiar with and were used to answering, such as their age, grade, and where they live. Asking children what they are good at, followed by asking about personal experiences, can enhance the start of a therapeutic relationship. Playfulness may assist in establishing communication with children. Children's temperament influences how they engage with new experiences and new people. A quiet, shy child, for example, often wants to watch and see what others are doing before interacting with new people. Instead of asking questions, a nurse may elicit more conversation by inviting the shy child to color together and chat during an activity instead of putting the focus on what the child is saying. "Draw and tell" helps nurses learn what children are thinking (Driessnack, 2005). Asking children to draw their family and tell the nurse about the picture starts a meaningful conversation. As a child becomes more comfortable with the nurse, the nurse can ask the child to draw the clinic or hospital and tell about the picture. Another strategy to use to communicate with children is play. Similar to drawing, playing a developmentally appropriate game with children helps them to relax and share their thoughts and feelings.

Cognitively, children developmentally move from concrete to abstract thought. Careful explanation of abstract concepts using real objects is especially important when working with children younger than middle-school age. If explaining surgery, for example, children will understand more if shown what the incision and bandage will look like on a doll or stuffed animal with a drawn incision and bandage on the appropriate body part rather than just explaining the process verbally (Li & Lopez, 2008). See Box 13-1 for examples of discussing surgery with children. It is important to validate or confirm with all family members that the message conveyed is understood and to explain medical words fully. Use of clichés, such as "this won't hurt" or "it will be over before you know it," are rarely appropriate when communicating with children and adolescents. The amount

BOX 13-1
Preparing Children and Their Families for Surgery Using Hospital Play

Children learn by doing and playing. Using dolls and real equipment helps children know what to expect and act out their fears. Having parents observe helps them learn how to help their child using play.

Before starting, consult with the physician and parent to learn what information the child has been given. Decide the appropriate explanation for age and emotional maturity. For young children use neutral words such as *opening, drainage,* and *oozing* instead of *cut* and *bleed.* Gather the visual aids (e.g., pictures, doll) and equipment to be used. Do not give too much information because the child may be overwhelmed. Plan for three sessions: why she needs surgery, what the operating room is like, and what she will feel and do after surgery.

If a child has never been in the hospital, have toys familiar to the child such as blocks, doll houses, and stuffed animals available along with "real" equipment such as a doll with bandages similar to what child will have, operating room masks, scrubs that nurses and doctors wear, and IV poles. The child may play with the familiar toys. As the child observes the nurse, tell the story of what will happen to the doll using the "real" equipment on the doll, and the child will learn that the equipment is safe.

Session 1: How Will the Surgery Make You Better?

Ask the child what she thinks is going to happen. A child may be silent or say, "I do not know," when talking to a stranger. You can repeat a simple explanation reinforcing what she knows.

Reassure the child that no one is to blame for her condition; make it clear that nothing she did is responsible.

Using the doll, show where the surgery will take place and what the surgery will do to make her better.

Session 2: What Will the Operating Room Be Like and What Will Happen Before the Surgery?

Review why surgery will make the child better.

Talk about the steps of getting ready for surgery, such as not eating or drinking the night before and

what the operation room will smell like (alcohol), feel like (cold), and look like (big lights, a clock, people in special clothes).

Child will wear special clothes (hospital gown). Note: Toddlers' body image includes keeping on their underwear, because they have just finished learning toilet training.

Put a mask on the face and talk about a "funny smell." Use a real anesthesia mask on the doll and have the child do this too. This gives the child some control.

Play with the thermometer, blood pressure cuff, and stethoscope for taking temperatures and listening to heartbeats and breathing on the doll and nurse and parent.

Show pictures of an operating room. Point out the "big lights," the clock, the nurses, and doctors dressed in blue (or whatever color your hospital personnel wear in the operating room suites) clothes and wearing "masks." Talk about the ride on a bed with wheels and doors that open like grocery store doors. These are things the child is familiar with and will notice.

Reaffirm that parents will walk with them to the operating room and be with them when they wake up from the surgery. Play with a mommy doll walking with the toy doll going to the operating room. Children need to know that their parents know where they are and will be there for them.

Session 3: Postoperative Expectations

Using dolls, act out what will happen after surgery:

- Soreness at the site of surgery
- Pain and medication
- Positioning (how to turn after surgery, deep breathe, and cough)
- Bandages (the word "dressing" may be understood as "turkey dressing" at Thanksgiving, or playing "dress-up")
- No eating and drinking right away

---

of information given also varies across cultures and across individuals. Nurses should be careful not to overwhelm family members with information they do not want or understand. Many cultures rely and trust health professionals to make health decisions, and when too much information is given, they question that trust. Other cultures and individuals, in contrast, want as much information as possible, and feel uncomfortable when they perceive information is not being shared. Each culture tends to have an identified

adult that accepts and conveys information to other family members. These differences should be considered during all teaching opportunities.

Supporting Development of Parenting Skills and Healthy Family Functioning

Providing support for the development of parenting skills is an important nursing intervention. Beginning at birth, children have a need for warm, affectionate relationships with parents. One of the earliest parenting skills found to establish healthy caregiving behavior is a parent's responsiveness to the infant's cues. Responsiveness is noticing and interpreting the infant's cues, then acting promptly in response to those cues. For example, if an infant looks away from a parent, a responsive parent will decrease stimulation until the infant turns back and reestablishes eye contact. An integrative research review about responsive parenting concluded that in developed countries maternal responsiveness in early childhood was positively correlated with increased intelligence quotient (IQ), whereas unresponsiveness was associated with lower IQs and higher childhood behavior problems. In developing countries, maternal responsiveness was associated with increased IQ, as well as with increased survival and growth, thought to be related to improved nutrition through positive interaction during meal times (Eshel, Daelmans, de Mello, & Martines, 2006). A more recent study of 40 European American mothers confirmed these results, revealed a strong relationship between mother's interaction with toddlers and preschoolers and the children's rate of development (Bornstein, Tamis-LeMonda, Hahn, & Haynes, 2008).

After the infancy period, parents begin to develop a "style" of nurturing and caring for their children. The parenting style of either two-parent or one-parent families influences outcomes in children, including health, academic achievement, and social development (Baumrind, 1991, 2005; Richaud de Minzi, 2006). An authoritative parenting style is characterized by reciprocity, mutual understanding, shared decision making, and flexibility (Sorkhabi, 2005). While parents using this style convey clear expectations and "demands" of their children, those expectations take into consideration their children's developmental level and individual strengths, weaknesses, and personality traits, and parents provide rationale for and support to meet those characteristics, as well as warmth in their relationship with the children (Baumrind, 2005). This parenting style promotes feelings of competence in the children. The ultimate goal is to promote positive self-esteem and autonomy in their children. Authoritative parenting styles influence health by providing the ongoing message that the children have some control over good health and healthy lifestyle choices and have a positive responsibility to care for their own health through these life choices (Luther, 2007). The outcomes of this parenting style are positive across time and across cultures. While behaviors may be more difficult during preschool years as children are given more chances to negotiate with parents than other parenting styles, long-term outcomes tend to be better (Underwood, Beron, & Rosen, 2009). Variables studied include self-reliance, self-competence, academic performance, socially accepted behavior, and social acceptance. Williams, Ciarrochi, and Heaven (2011) illustrated that authoritative parenting styles increased flexible problem-solving skills of adolescents across 6 years compared to other parenting styles. Other family characteristics associated with healthy authoritative parenting and well-child health outcomes include parent engagement, closeness, communication, positive discipline techniques, and healthy role modeling. These positive qualities have correlated with increased adolescent social competence and self-esteem, health-promoting behaviors, and less drug abuse, as well as fewer externalizing (e.g., aggression and anger) and internalizing behaviors (e.g., depression).

Authoritarian parenting style, in contrast, is an inflexible and unilateral style in which parents have clear expectations and demands of their children, but insist on compliance with the parental perception of what is best for their children, with limited explanation and rationale or acceptance of their children's perceptions (Sorkhabi, 2005). The authoritarian style promotes the belief that children should not control their own behavior and cannot contribute to decisions about their own health care because they do not have the knowledge or experience needed to make good decisions (Luther, 2007). Several studies have shown short- and long-term negative effects of authoritarian parenting styles across ethnic groups and cultures. For example, children raised by authoritarian parents tend to be less socially accepted and less self-reliant and have poorer academic outcomes across the United States, India, and China (Chen, Dong, & Zhou, 1997; Rao, McHale, & Pearson, 2003; Steinberg, Dornbusch, & Brown, 1992; Steinberg, Lamborn, Dornbusch, & Darling, 1992). When asking adults to recall parenting styles used by their parents, those who recalled authoritarian parents have a higher rate of depressive symptoms and poor psychological adjustment across time (Rothrauff,

Cooney, & An, 2009). Family aggression and parental aggravation commonly found in authoritarian parenting were associated with less social competence, less health-promoting behavior, and lower self-esteem scores (Youngblade et al., 2007). The long-held consensus is that children fare better when praised than when criticized or punished (Schmittmann, Visser, & Raijmakers, 2006).

Permissive parenting style allows children to pursue child-determined goals with little guidance from the parents. Parents using this style tend to ignore behavior problems and may not provide the organizational support needed to assist children in reaching goals (Sorkhabi, 2005). Children raised in the permissive style are less assertive and achievement oriented, and are more likely to develop ineffective and possibly dangerous coping strategies such as using drugs, compared with authoritative and authoritarian parenting styles (Baumrind, 1991; Washington and Dunham, 2011). Permissive parents can be nurturing and warm, but too passive to establish healthy boundaries. Or they may be rejecting or neglecting in their parenting style, in which case, along with having limited expectations and responsiveness, these parents can also be punitive and have a negative reaction to parent-child interactions, as well as lack of parental involvement with the children. This passive, but negative, parenting style is also associated with generally poor academic and social-emotional outcomes (Baumrind, 1991; Williams et al., 2012).

The fourth parenting style studied is the uninvolved parent. This parenting style is similar to the permissive parenting style, except the parent(s) not only lacks clear boundaries and expectations, but also lacks any nurturing, warmth, and responsiveness (Maccoby & Martin, 1983). The outcomes of these children are considered far worse than the first three parenting styles, with children being at risk for negative coping strategies, including poor academic performance, drug abuse, criminal behavior, and poor social acceptance across time (Steinberg, 2001).

The findings regarding parenting style and childhood outcomes span cultures and geographical locations. One review paper, for example, concluded that in collectivist or interdependent cultures, authoritarian and authoritative styles had similar outcomes as found in individualist cultures (Sorkhabi, 2005). The effects not only cross cultures, but also cross time, as studies showing similar outcomes across cultures have been consistent from the early studies in the 1980s to more recent studies into the 2000s (Rao et al., 2003).

Nurses can teach about parenting styles and help parents adopt authoritative parenting strategies when doing health promotion and illness care with child-raising families (Bond & Burns, 2006). Numerous studies have revealed that increasing knowledge about parenting increases authoritative parenting practices. Likewise, authoritative parents often seek out parenting knowledge from the moment they discover they will be parents (Washington & Dunham, 2011). Early interest in parenting leads to early positive attachment practices, and later warm and involved parenting strategies. Differing parenting styles between the two parents in one family can cause conflict in both stable and divorced families. Using counseling and education with parents can help them recognize and reflect on their differences, which can lead to a united change toward more authoritative practices.

Nursing interventions for family-focused well-child care include identification of teachable moments to discuss child development, explore parental feelings, model positive interactions with children, and reframe parents' negative attributions about their children's behavior. For example, a nurse may help a parent to see that a child's temper tantrum may be a sign of independence and a need to communicate new thoughts and feelings without the language to do so, rather than a deliberate behavior to embarrass or disobey the parent. The positive health outcomes from parents learning more appropriate parenting include using less physical and harsh discipline approaches, increasing use of safety strategies such as placing newborns on their backs to sleep, increasing likelihood that children will have up-to-date vaccines, and increasing family time spent in pleasurable interactions and experiences. Nursing actions to reduce negative outcomes in child-raising families are to identify parental risk factors associated with abuse/neglect such as depression, family violence, drug and alcohol use, and cigarette smoking (Zuckerman, Parker, Kaplan-Sanoff, Augustyn, & Barth, 2004). In contrast, children's readiness for school has been found to be related to identifying and supporting parental strengths, promoting strong parent-child relationships, teaching parents about child development, and involving parents in activities that encourage learning (Zigler, Pfannenstiel, & Seitz, 2008).

Understanding and Working With Family Routines

Establishing daily routines and family rituals is an important health promotion strategy. These predictable patterns influence the physical, mental, and social health of children, as well as the health of the family itself (Denham, 2002). Nurses help families integrate physical, social-emotional, and cognitive health promotion into family routines; and in doing so, they affirm positive patterns of health or provide alternative ones (Greening, Stoppelbein, Konishi, Jordan, & Moll, 2007). Discussing or observing family routines and rituals offers the potential, in a nonthreatening way, to gain entrée and understand family dynamics to a greater depth (Denham, 2003). Routines are important to all families in all settings. For instance, predictable and familiar routines were used by parents in homeless shelters to preserve family bonds and their connection with their community (Schultz-Krohn, 2004). Conversely, because routines and rituals have great meaning and stability for families, it is important to recognize that they are potential threats and barriers when implementing new prevention or treatment interventions, as these changes will change the stability and predictability of a family's routines and rituals (Segal, 2004). Nurses can help families understand the importance of maintaining healthy routines, especially during times of transition such as divorce or hospitalization.

Child Care, After-School Activities, and Children's Health Promotion

Child-raising families nurture children through partnerships with siblings, extended family members, nonrelated child care providers, teachers, and other adults within the community. These relationships help to establish and maintain the family routines that are so important to health and child development. An important trend of American families today is the increasing number of women with children in the workforce requiring assistance with child care. This trend is partly due to economic changes, increases in family instability and divorce, and the continued increase in the number of single-headed households, primarily women. In 1975, 47% of women with children under age 18 years were in the labor force; by 1990, that figure was 52%

(Bianchi, 1995). In 2012, close to 75% of mothers were in the labor force, with three out of four working full time (Child Care Aware of America, 2013). Sixty-one percent of working mothers had children under the age of 3 years (U.S. Department of Labor, Bureau of Labor Statistics, 2011).

Another important trend is the speed at which mothers return to work after the birth of their babies. In 1960, only 10% of mothers worked within 3 months of giving birth. In 2009, that percentage rose to 42% (Bianchi, 1995), and by 2010 that percentage rose to 57% (Bureau of Labor Statistics, 2013). This trend continues to grow in spite of mounting evidence that children fare better when parents provide care for the first year of life (Offer & Schneider, 2012). Another important trend is the decreased birth rate for women with higher education levels. This trend is international, and highest among Japanese women. The societal impact is a growing number of low-educated mothers raising a majority of children. Meanwhile, low-educated men are choosing not to marry or have children. This trend has caused, in part, the growing number of low-educated single women raising children, while highly educated professional couples are choosing careers over child rearing. Family care policies are changing internationally to address this trend, with increased paid time off, increased support of early childhood education, and increased pressure on employers to secure parents' jobs and job opportunities regardless of family leave.

Many families search for the best routines to balance family and work. Care for children while mothers are at work is divided between fathers, grandparents, other relatives, friends, neighbors, other nonpaid care, lay professional care (e.g., nannies and unlicensed providers), licensed home care providers, or licensed and certified center care providers. In 2005, the trend for care while parent(s) worked continued to be split between relatives and paid nonrelative employees. Thirty percent of the 11.3 million children less than 5 years whose mothers were employed were cared for by a grandparent during their mother's working hours. A slightly higher percentage was cared for in a home-based or center-based child care facility or preschool. Fathers cared for 25% of children, while siblings cared for 3%, and other relatives cared for 8% during mothers' working hours (U.S. Census Bureau, 2008). Today, that trend continues with 51% of children being cared for by their parents up until age 3, and 31% being cared for in formal child care centers (Offer & Schneider, 2011). Some parents strive to work nontraditional hours, flexible hours, and work while caring for their children to avoid the risks and costs of formal child care. Studies, reveal, however, that parents working either nontraditional hours or trying to work while caring for their infant spend less quality time with their infant than other mothers, and struggle to find consistent and high-quality care for their children during nontraditional hours (Moss, 2009). Moss (2009) found, in a qualitative study of parents in New Zealand, that when given a choice, most parents would choose to work fewer hours when caring for young children, but feel they cannot make that choice because of the effect on family finances and job opportunities. Similar results have been found in studies in the United States across socioeconomic classes (Hertz & Fergusen, 1996).

The quality of early childhood education and support for children is an ongoing concern for parents and societies. Multiple studies have documented the importance of education and training of early childhood teachers, developmentally appropriate environments, activities and equipment, and a recommended safe and effective teacher. Things to consider include child/teacher ratio, culturally appropriate learning strategies, family involvement, and nurturing and caring interactions between the teacher and the children. Nevertheless, most families are forced to choose child care based on cost rather than quality. Not surprisingly, families in poverty who paid for child care in 2005 spent a greater proportion of their monthly income on child care than did families at or above the poverty level (i.e., 29% compared with 6%) (U.S. Census Bureau, 2008). Nurses can assist with this concern by educating families about employers providing stipends or pretax payments of child care, or about use of government stipends and tax credits for child care, by referring families to Child Care Resource and Referral Services (Child Care Resource and Referral Network, n.d.), and by discussing with them the possibility of flex hours to share child care responsibilities between mothers and fathers. Families composed of minority groups and families with children with disabilities require special consideration when choosing child care and after-school options (U.S. Census Bureau, 2008).

School-age children often attend before- and after-school care programs. Some children care for

themselves and that number increases with the age of the child. Six percent of children ages 5 to 11 care for themselves, and 33% of children ages 12 to 14 regularly care for themselves (U.S. Census Bureau, 2008). It is important that families whose children care for themselves understand safety measures, such as having a contact person the child can call in an emergency; concealing the house key during the school day so that it is not readily apparent that the child will be going home alone; and setting rules about safety, allowing friends in the house when parents are not present, and screen time (e.g., television, video games, and computer). Nurses can educate parents on the risks for children being alone at home during afternoon and early evening hours, including loneliness, increased fears, increased criminal activity, and increased adolescent sexual activity and teen pregnancy.

Nurses, parents, teachers, governmental agencies, and other invested community members must work together to develop before- and after-school programs at schools, homework telephone services with teachers and teachers' aides during the school year, and community center programs during the summer months, holidays, and other times when school is not in session and parents continue to work. Nurses can help families review the types of child care and after-school options available and examine the site for health protection features. They can also participate on community boards that advocate for and regulate these facilities. By supporting working parents and care of children during working hours, healthy and predictable family routines are better maintained. Lack of reliable, predictable, and safe care for children during work hours is a significant threat to family health.

Identifying Health Risks and Teaching Prevention Strategies

Because of the relationship between health behaviors and illness or death, increased attention to unhealthy social-emotional behaviors is an important part of nursing practice in families with children. Specifically, nurses assess for, identify, and provide interventions to reduce risk factors associated with morbidity (sickness) and mortality (death). Specific risk factors include safety concerns for unintentional and intentional injuries and death; patterns leading to overweight and obese children and adolescents; lack of parenting knowledge and support associated with family violence and child maltreatment; health concerns more common to families living in poverty, including higher rates of violence, drug use, and teen pregnancy; and mental health.

Unintentional and Intentional Injuries

The leading cause of death among children and youth is unintentional injuries from accidents. In 2003, more than 4,000 children, ages 1 to 14 years, died from unintentional injuries (National Center for Injury Prevention and Control, 2006). The leading cause of unintentional injuries is motor vehicle crashes, causing the death of an average of six children per day ages 1 to 14 years (NHTSA.dot.gov, National Center for Statistics and Analysis, 2003). The risk for motor vehicle crashes is higher among youth ages 16 to 19 years than for any other group and substance abuse, primarily alcohol, is considered a contributing factor in a majority of these accidents (National Center for Injury Prevention and Control, 2006). It is crucial that children of all ages be properly restrained for their age and body size in motor vehicles, and that all adolescents participate in traffic education and receive repeated information on the risks of driving under the influence of drugs and/or alcohol.

Intentional injuries are the second highest cause of death in children, particularly adolescents. Homicide and suicide are the second and third leading cause of death for children ages 12 to 19 (National Center for Injury Prevention and Control, 2006). Suicide rates increase for minority groups throughout the United States. For example, Native Alaskan and Native American youth between the ages of 10 and 18 years have a suicide rate of 10.37 per 100,000, compared with an overall rate of 3.95 per 100,000 (Centers for Disease Control and Prevention [CDC], 2012). The access to firearms, especially in high-risk groups, increases this risk.

Family child health care nurses can teach and support families in prevention of unintentional and intentional injuries. For example, nurses can teach appropriate car seat restraints and water safety. They can educate parents on child proofing the home to prevent poisoning and electrical burns from uncovered electrical outlets in toddlers. Teaching the importance of bicycle helmet use and helping families locate resources when they have limited financial means for purchasing helmets can help to minimize head trauma from bike accidents.

Nurses, either in an informal role as a next-door neighbor or a formal role as working at community or clinic programs, can help parents understand the importance of and access approved safety devices, such as car seats, helmets, and door/cabinet locks. Nurses can be key educators in recognizing signs and symptoms of suicide in adolescents, and can support friends and family members in getting help when these signs and symptoms are identified. Family nurses can also be key professionals to teach gun safety to families to prevent unintentional and intentional injury from firearms. Many communities are adopting suicide prevention strategies to reduce suicide rates, including decreasing risk factors (e.g., bullying, exposure to violence, access to firearms, and substance abuse), and increasing protective factors (e.g., cultural connectiveness, improved access and awareness of mental health care, and development of crisis response teams to major family and community traumas) (CDC, 2012). Nurses are important to these efforts from the individual and family level of education and support, to the community level of advocacy and participation in identifying and supporting needed change.

Obesity and Overweight in Families With Children

Nurses help families recognize the harm and offer methods to intervene for one of the leading public health problems, obesity. Although obesity rates in children have reached a plateau over the past decade, the rates continue to be a major concern for children's health. Studies across the past 5 years indicate that up to 27% of all children ages 2 to 5 years were overweight (Ogden, 2012). Between 1980 and 2010, the percentage of children ages 6 to 11 years who were obese increased from 7% to 32.6%; for adolescents, it increased from 5% to 33.6% (Ogden, Carroll, Kit, & Flegal, 2012). Overweight and obese family members, including children, are at increased risk for type 2 diabetes, hypertension, hyperlipidemia, cancer, asthma, joint problems, social rejection, and depression (Jeffreys, Smith, Martin, Frankel, & Gunnell, 2004; Miller, Rosenbloom, & Silverstein, 2004; Ogden et al., 2012; Urrutia-Rojas et al., 2006). Prevention and treatment are crucial to the child and family's well-being.

The causes of childhood obesity and overweight are complex, involving the environment (e.g., home and society), genetics, family attitudes and beliefs, cultural practices, nutritional practices, and family activities (Baughcum, Burklow, Deeks, Powers, & Whitaker, 1998; Bruss, Morris, & Dannison, 2003; Ritchie, Welk, Styne, Gerstein, & Crawford, 2005). Family beliefs, mediated by cultural and family traditions, are thought to affect family eating behaviors (Baughcum et al., 1998; Bruss et al., 2003). Societal and environmental changes that include decreased physical activity, perceived threats to safety resulting in children playing indoors rather than outdoors, increased screen time, and greater consumption of high-calorie fast foods in the community and schools has contributed to the rise in obesity around the world.

Research about obesity is also increasing, but effective strategies to address the problem have remained elusive. Because it is difficult to lose weight, prevention of overweight—particularly in the preschool years, a time when children are prone to become overweight or obese—is seen as one important approach (Wofford, 2008). A combined approach of education for families and children, support for changes in policies, such as building safe bike trails, offering better meals at schools, and reducing fast food access while replacing access to healthier foods will likely have the greatest influence on reducing overweight in families. Parental involvement as role models for physical activity and healthy eating has been found to be essential in prevention of obesity in children (Floriani & Kennedy, 2007; Wofford, 2008).

Supporting families in use of an authoritative approach to parenting, helping them to develop sensitive but clear parental expectations regarding self-care and food and activity choices are important nursing interventions (Luther, 2007). Specifically, childhood overweight management in families includes providing children with nutrient-dense foods; reducing children's access to high-calorie, nutrient-poor beverages and food; avoiding excessive restriction of food and use of food as a reward; encouraging children to eat breakfast; finding ways to make physical activity fun; reducing children's TV, computer, and video time; and teaching parents to model healthful eating practices for children (Hodges, 2003; Ritchie et al., 2005). The American Medical Association (AMA) recommends encouraging families to eat meals at home, limit meals outside the home, and give children no sugar-sweetened beverages; the AMA also specifies that children should get 1 hour or more of physical activity per day (AMA, 2007). Nurses can influence weight not only by helping families consider their eating and exercise activities, but also by contributing to community actions that will work in concert with family health behavioral changes.

Child Maltreatment

Nurses recognize situations in which children are in danger because of child maltreatment. In 2010, an estimated 3.1 million cases of child abuse and neglect occurred and approximately five children died each day from abuse or neglect (U.S. Department of Health and Human Services, Administration for Children and Families, 2011). Children ages birth to 1 year had the highest rate of victimization of maltreatment at 24.4 per 1,000 cases. Physical abuse is generally defined as a non-accidental physical injury to the child and can include striking, kicking, burning, or biting the child by a parent, sibling, child care provider, or other caregiver. Physical abuse represents 17.6% of child maltreatment. Child neglect is defined as not providing for a child's basic physical, educational or emotional needs and represents 78.3% of child maltreatment (U.S. Department of Health and Human Services, Administration for Children and Families, 2011). In 2010, almost 9.2% of all cases of child maltreatment involved sexual abuse, and psychological maltreatment accounted for 8.1%. Psychological maltreatment is defined as child exploitation (i.e., child prostitution), threats (i.e., threat to kill child), and isolation. Approximately 2% of the cases involved medical neglect. Some children were victims of more than one type of abuse. Children with disabilities are especially vulnerable. Nearly 8% of victims had a reported disability, a figure that is thought to be underreported. Abuse can also lead to permanent disabilities, ranging from physical injury to lifelong mental illness. Also at higher risk for maltreatment are children of unwanted pregnancies, living in substance abuse homes, living with a parent with a mental health disorder, and with difficult temperaments. Nearly 80% of perpetrators of maltreatment were parents, and most victims know their perpetrators. More than half of all reports of abuse came from professionals involved with the children and families, including health care providers and teachers (U.S. Department of Health and Human Services, Administration for Children and Families, Administration on Children, 2011).

Child maltreatment represents a problem in family behaviors that demands immediate assessment and action/intervention. In most states, nurses are mandatory reporters and are required by law to report to authorities when they suspect that a child is being maltreated. It is important for nurses who work with children and families to understand their legal and ethical responsibilities. The Child Welfare Information Gateway (2014) provides specific information about mandatory reporting laws per state.

Nurses screen families for domestic violence by asking questions regarding the safety of the home and the incidence of family violence within the home. See Box 13-2 (Gedaly-Duff, Stoeger, & Shelton, 2000) for pertinent questions regarding family violence that affects families with children. Inquiring about family violence can be uncomfortable for nurses and other health professions. Family violence occurs across social, economic, and ethnic groups. The standard of practice is to ask all families these questions so that the stigma becomes standardized. Families frequently will seek help if given the opportunity to talk about their situations (Hibbard, Desch, Committee on Child Abuse Neglect, & Council on Children With Disabilities, 2007). By screening for family violence, nurses can assess families and children for dangerous situations, teach safety, and make a referral as necessary.

Prevention is the preferred approach for intervening with families for child maltreatment. Nurses identify situations that might foster child maltreatment and intervene accordingly. Risk factors thought to contribute to abuse are categorized into four domains: parent or caregiver factors, family factors, child factors, and environmental factors. Parent or caregiver factors include personality characteristics (e.g., low self-esteem, depression, poor impulse control), a history of abuse in the parent's own childhood, substance abuse, attitudes about child behavior, inaccurate knowledge about child development, inappropriate expectations of the child, and younger maternal age. Family factors include marital conflict, domestic violence, single parenthood, unemployment, financial stress, and social isolation. Child factors include age, with younger children and infants being the most vulnerable, presence of disabilities or chronic illness, and difficult temperaments. Environmental factors include poverty, unemployment, and social isolation. In all cases it is important to remember that the presence of risk factors is not an indication that the parents or family members are, in fact, abusive (U.S. Department of Health and Human Services, Administration on Children, Youth and Families, 2005). Rather, when the nurse identifies the presence of various stressors and risks, it may be appropriate to evaluate and implement interventions that may decrease the potential for abuse.

Nurses should also keep in mind the following protective factors against child abuse and neglect: parental resilience, social connections, knowledge of child development, concrete support in times of need, increased social and emotional competence of children, and non-acceptance of abuse by the community and larger society (Moxley, Squires, & Lindstrom, 2012). Strategies thought to help families are those that facilitate friendships and mutual support, strengthen parenting by teaching and modeling appropriate behavior with children, respond to family crises, link families to services, facilitate children's social and emotional development, and value supporting parents (Horton, 2003; Moxley et al., 2012). For example, social support from peers and professionals has been shown to be positively related to health promotion efforts in adolescent mothers (Black & Ford-Gilboe, 2004). The difference between discipline and abuse may be unclear because of different cultural

---

BOX 13-2
Family Violence Screening Questions

Right now, who is living at home with you and your child?

- Is everyone getting along well at home or is there a lot of stress, arguing, or fighting?
- Has anybody ever been hit or hurt, pushed, or shoved in a fight or argument at your house?
- Has anybody in the family been in trouble with the police or in jail?
- Is anybody worried that your children have been disciplined too harshly?
- Is anybody worried that your children have been touched inappropriately or sexually abused?
- Is there anybody living with you or close to you who drinks a lot or uses drugs?
- Are there guns or knives or weapons at your house?
- Has anything major (e.g., people dying, losing jobs, disasters or accidents) happened recently in your family?
- What is the best part and the worst part of life for you right now?

traditions, but nurses must be alert to helping families learn appropriate discipline measures (Stein & Perrin, 1998). Children's early nurturing experiences and attachment relationships with their caring adults affect their future relationships and well-being.

Specific Adolescent Risks

Adolescents as a group are especially vulnerable to high-risk behaviors that can lead to illness and death. Data on the prevalence of risk behaviors among adolescents is collected by the Youth Risk Behavior Surveillance System (YRBS), using a national probability sample of 9th to 12th graders, state and local school-based surveys, and a national household-based survey (CDC, 2011). In 2010-2011 in the United States, 21% of all deaths among persons age 10 to 24 years resulted from four causes: motor-vehicle crashes (26%), other unintentional injuries or accidents (17%), homicide (16%) and suicide (13%) (CDC, 2011). Health behaviors that contributed to unintentional injury or to violence were the use of alcohol and other substances, nonuse of seatbelts, and availability of weapons. Other health behaviors that contributed to illness and death were tobacco use, poor nutrition, sedentary lifestyle, and sexual behaviors that led to pregnancies and sexually transmitted infections.

The 2011 YRBS report revealed that adolescents engaged in behaviors associated with significant morbidity and mortality. Nationwide, 70.8% reported drinking alcohol, with 38% reporting having alcohol within 30 days of taking the survey (a decrease from 45% in 2007), 24.1% had ridden with a driver who had been drinking alcohol, 8% had rarely or never worn a seat belt, and 23.1% had used marijuana. Twenty-six percent of all adolescents in school currently used tobacco. Thirty-three percent of high school students had experienced sexual intercourse within 3 months prior to the survey. Among students who were sexually active, 60.2% reported using a condom at their last intercourse (CDC, 2011).

Violence is a significant risk for morbidity and mortality for adolescents. In 2010, the second and third leading causes of death for young people ages 15 to 34 were homicide and suicide (CDC, 2010). In 2010, there were 2,711 infant, child, and teen firearm deaths. On average there were seven such fatalities daily and 52 weekly (National Association of School Psychologists, 2012. In 2011, 5% of high school students carried a gun on school property, and 7% were threatened or

injured by a weapon (e.g., gun, knife, or club) on school property (National Association of School Psychologists, 2012). Child and youth access to firearms is part of the problem. A significant percentage of adults who have minor children living in their homes report their firearms are not safely stored (Johnson, Miller, Vriniotis, Azrael, & Hemenway, 2006). Children's reports often contradict parental reports about their children's access to firearms, with children reporting knowing the location of firearms and handling firearms when parents said they did not. This is true whether or not parents lock firearms and discuss firearm safety with their children (Baxley & Miller, 2006; Grossman et al., 2005).

The American Academy of Pediatrics (2012) takes a public health position to prevent firearm injuries by removal of guns from families' homes and communities, however it is crucial that education in gun use also occur. In 2011, the Emergency Nurses Association, one of the few nursing organizations, made a public statement that safety for children by removing firearms in the home is a crucial step in decreasing injury and death from firearms. Nurses should include screening for guns in the home and incorporate a discussion and information about gun safety with parents. Specific results from the 2011 National Youth Risk Behavior Survey follow:

> Many high school students are engaged in priority health-risk behaviors associated with the leading causes of death among persons aged 10–24 years in the United States. During the 30 days before the survey, 32.8% of high school students nationwide had texted or e-mailed while driving, 38.7% had drunk alcohol, and 23.1% had used marijuana. During the 12 months before the survey, 32.8% of students had been in a physical fight, 20.1% had ever been bullied on school property, and 7.8% had attempted suicide. Many high school students nationwide are engaged in sexual risk behaviors associated with unintended pregnancies and STDs, including HIV infection. Nearly half (47.4%) of students had ever had sexual intercourse, 33.7% had had sexual intercourse during the 3 months before the survey (i.e., currently sexually active), and 15.3% had had sexual intercourse with four or more people during their life. Among currently sexually active students, 60.2% had used a condom during their last

sexual intercourse. Results from the 2011 national YRBS also indicate many high school students are engaged in behaviors associated with the leading causes of death among adults aged ≥25 years in the United States. During the 30 days before the survey, 18.1% of high school students had smoked cigarettes and 7.7% had used smokeless tobacco. (CDC, 2011, p.1)

Family nurses in school-based health clinics are especially well placed to participate in health prevention programs directed at high-risk behaviors leading to sexually transmitted disease and early pregnancy, depression, injuries, substance use, suicidal ideation, and violence. In addition, nurses have a crucial role in educating parents, especially those of adolescents how to address safety and risk behaviors.

An alternate approach to risk assessment is to support what young people need to facilitate positive development. The America's Promise Alliance program (2013) lists the assets believed to be protective for children and predictive of positive outcomes and behaviors: violence avoidance, thriving (i.e., having a special talent or interest that gives them joy), good school grades, and volunteering. The program's five "Promises," or goals for positive outcomes, are (1) presence of caring adults, (2) safe places and constructive use of time, (3) a healthy start, (4) effective education, and (5) opportunities to make a difference. One large study demonstrated that the presence of four to five Promises resulted in positive adolescent development outcomes. Still, the same study found that only a minority of youth experienced enough of the Promises that were related to positive outcomes. Furthermore, non-Hispanic white youth were much more likely to experience the Promises than were Hispanic and African American youth (Scales et al., 2008). The primary goal in 2013 of the America's Promise Alliance program is to increase the nation's high school graduation rates.

The Influence of Poverty

Socioeconomic factors, such as poverty, lack of education, little or no health insurance, and immigrant status, are strong risk factors related to poor health (Hardy, 2002). There is evidence that behavioral symptoms of child psychiatric disorders are associated with poverty and that those symptoms can be reduced as the family moves out of poverty (Costello, Compton, Keeler, & Angold, 2003). Programs that provide families with employment, adequate income,

day care, and health insurance have been shown to have positive effects on academic achievement, classroom behavior, and aspirations (Huston et al., 2001). Children from families from ethnic minority backgrounds are more likely to live below the poverty line (Annie E. Casey Foundation, 2007) and thus they are at risk for health problems.

Families with limited financial resources and those who do not have health insurance have more difficulty with health promotion than families with insurance or other methods of payment. In the United States in 2010, 22% of children (16 million) were poor, meaning that they lived in households where the income was below $22,350 for a family of two adults and two children (National Center for Children in Poverty, 2012). In the United States in 2010, 9% of all children (6.8 million) were uninsured. Thirteen percent of children who lived in families with incomes at or below 100% of the federal poverty level were uninsured (National Center for Children in Poverty, 2012). Minority families are consistently found to be less likely to have health insurance than are white non-Hispanic families. Nearly 9% of children with special health care needs or 2 out of every 5 children with special health care needs are uninsured for all or part of the year and of those covered many do not have adequate insurance coverage (Szilagyi, 2012). The federal government has stepped up to decrease health disparities for all children and especially children with special health care needs by implementing the Children's Health Insurance Program (CHIP). These state-run programs are designed to ensure that all children have health insurance. The criteria expanded health insurance to low-income families with children who would not qualify for state-funded health insurance (e.g., MediCal or Oregon Health Plan).

The *Affordable Care Act of 2010* maintained CHIP funding and increased the percentage of federal matching dollars from 50% to 65% to an average of 93% per state, maintained until 2015. Each state designs state-funded CHIP programs, with 28 states using a combination of expanded Medicaid services with separate child health programs, 15 states using only separate child health programs, and 7 states only using Medicaid expansion plans. The differences in design determine whether all children are entitled to CHIP benefits, or only those that qualify for Medicaid. The cost of this program has been debated, with many states concerned about the increased cost based on enrollment. The cost of health care is actually reduced, however, when children have a medical home and receive routine well-child care. The number of children now getting health care is notable, as Oregon and Washington lead the nation in increasing the number of children with health insurance by over 20% (Medicaid.gov, 2013). Although this program has had positive effects on the health of children, there are still 7.8 million children uninsured, with 5.4 million of those children living in poverty. Further, when investigating barriers to children enrolling in state and federal programs, the most likely reason given by parents is that if the parents cannot obtain insurance, they are less likely to enroll their children. Although uninsured children pose a major risk to the health of any nation, non-elderly adults are four times more likely not to have insurance than children. In the United States, 36 million parents are uninsured. New initiatives are being proposed to combine programs to insure children and parents rather than just children alone (Kenny & Dorn, 2009).

Strategies to Support Health Promotion in Families With Children

Families are the major determinant of children's well-being. Nurses and other health professionals collaborate with parents, and do not view parents as secondary and apart from nurses (Bruns & McCollum, 2002). Health promotion and illness prevention can occur using a variety of strategies across settings, including the following:

1. Writing or providing health information for school or community newsletters, e-mail, or online messaging.
2. Demonstrating and teaching health promotion activities, such as games or physical activities that promote health.
3. Cultivating attributes of healthy families that include accountability, self-reliance, informed decision making, access to supportive social networks, and nurturing relationships.
4. Encouraging family councils or family nights that provide venues for communications among all the family members.
5. Providing anticipatory guidance about high-risk periods in child and youth development. For example, childproofing the home before the infant begins to crawl or walk or providing assistance with appropriate limit setting as an adolescent gets his driver's license. The

use of a contract for teen driving has reduced teen reports of risky behaviors such as driving under the influence of alcohol or riding with someone who has been drinking (Haggerty, Fleming, Catalano, Harachi, & Abbott, 2006; Novilla et al., 2006).
6. Providing connections with school and community services. For example, children learn meanings, responses to, and values about health through their interactions in their school communities. Nurses can refer families to community resources, such as the federally funded Head Start programs that serve families of children who are economically disadvantaged and children who have disabilities (American Academy of Pediatrics, 1973). Head Start has increased high-school graduation rates and lowered rates of juvenile arrests and school dropout rates (Gray & McCormick, 2005).

CARE OF CHILDREN WITH CHRONIC ILLNESS AND THEIR FAMILIES

While most families raising children experience acute illnesses and become familiar with managing these crises, families do not anticipate that their children may have a chronic illness. They are often unprepared for the unknowns and uncertainties of the course of the disease, the effect on their children's development and adulthood, or the effect on each family member and family life.

Defining Chronic Illness in Families With Sick Children

Families of children with chronic illness are diverse and represent all racial and ethnic groups and income levels. Chronic health problems, long-term conditions, disability, and children with a special health care need (CSHCN) are phrases used to describe children with a health problem that cannot be cured. These heterogeneous conditions include, but are not limited to, the following:

- Medical problems—allergies, asthma, diabetes, congenital heart disease, joint problems, blood disease, spina bifida
- Disabilities related to developmental delay and rare genetic syndromes—Down syndrome, cerebral palsy, mental retardation, autism

- Health-related behavioral and educational problems—attention-deficit hyperactivity disorder, learning disability
- Social-emotional conditions—depression and anxiety
- Consequences of unintended injuries or acute illness—head trauma and paralysis.

Many children have more than one problem.

The phrase "children with special health care needs" (CSHCN) is used for families whose children "have or are at increased risk for a chronic physical, developmental, behavioral, or emotional condition and who also require health and related services of a type or amount beyond that required by children generally" (McPherson et al., 1998). According to the 2011–2012 National Survey of Children with Special Health Care needs approximately 14.6 million between 0–17 years of age in the United States have a special health care need (Data Resource Center for Child and Adolescent Health, 2012). Of these special needs children, 78.4% reported having one disorder and 41.4% report having 2 or health conditions. The most common health conditions are as follows:

- Attention-deficit disorder (32.2%)
- Asthma (35.3%)
- Learning disability (27.2%)
- Speech problem (15.6%)
- Development disability (14.7)
- Behavioral problem (13.6%)
- Anxiety disorder (13.4%)

Of these children, 65% have complex health care needs beyond a medication prescription. The functional impact of these special health needs is significant for the children and families. Approximately 92% of these children have at least one functional deficit, 72% have two functional deficits and 46% have 4 or more functional deficits.

All families fare better when they have knowledge of the trajectory and management of the specific disease or chronic illness. The trajectory of the disease or condition, according to Rolland's model of chronic illness, includes the following categories:

1. Sudden or gradual onset: Sudden onset of a chronic illness can be from an acute illness, such as meningitis or an acute accident, whereas gradual onset can be from genetic conditions such as muscular dystrophy.
2. Prognosis of chronicity, relapse, or death: Chronic conditions include cystic fibrosis,

learning disabilities, or cerebral palsy; relapsing conditions include arthritis, certain mental health disorders such as depression, and asthma; and death or fatal disorders include certain types of cancer or genetic disorders.
3. A stable or degenerative course over time: A stable course over time includes disorders such as well-managed asthma, whereas a degenerative condition includes certain types of cancer, and multiple sclerosis.
4. The degree of incapacitation and amount of uncertainty: The degree of incapacitation varies by illness and within illnesses, such as cerebral palsy ranging from mild and non-incapacitating to severely incapacitating. The amount of uncertainty also varies, such that children diagnosed with certain types of cancer can receive effective treatment, or follow a course of uncertainty and instability over many years.

These categories are helpful to review with families as the specifics of disease management (Rolland, 2005). Nurses and other health professionals tend to reteach the disease and medicine management when it is really the social-emotional and behavioral responses that are troubling families. It may be the degree of unpredictability and lack of role models that interfere with children and their families' abilities to cope, rather than the degree of severity of the illness or disease management (Rodrigues & Patterson, 2007). If nurses spend time with the family carefully assessing their knowledge versus social and emotional responses to their child's illness, the plan of care will be more appropriate and effective.

Families with children who have chronic illnesses vary greatly in their needs, ranging from families who are rarely affected by their children's condition, such as mild asthma, to those who are significantly affected, such as children who are ventilator dependent. But to varying degrees, all families of children with chronic conditions bear consequences of their children's conditions. A noncategorical approach, or the understanding by health care providers and parents that care across different diagnoses has similar needs and qualities, directs attention to the consequences that several different chronic conditions have on the children, their families, their communities, and health care systems (Perrin et al., 1993; Stein, Bauman, Westbrook, Coupey, & Ireys, 1993).

The intent is to manage the symptoms so that the children and families can maintain their well-being and move toward each member's and the family's goals. The 2001 CSHCN survey provided questions to help nurses and families understand the impact of chronic illness on the family. To gain a family perspective, nurses can ask similar questions as the 2001 CSHCN survey (U.S. Department of Health and Human Services et al., 2008):

- Does the condition limit the child's ability to dress and learn self-care?
- Does the condition interfere with the child's daily activities, such as playing and going to school?
- Does the condition require special assistance or technology and/or medication management?
- Does the condition cause family members to cut back or stop working?
- Can the family access and get a referral for special services for the child, as well as family support services?
- Is health care insurance adequate for the child and other family members?
- In the case of adolescence, has the young person's health care begun to be transferred to adult providers?

Parenting a Child With Chronic Illness

Parenting is the nurturance of children to become healthy, responsible, and creative adults. The interdependencies among child, parents, and the whole family within their community are like a set of nesting dolls. Children with chronic illnesses are cared for by their families, who share a household and family history, are nested in communities, and use local and national health care systems. The complex, changing interactions among child, family, and community provide the context of parenting a child with chronic illness into adulthood. Tasks specific to health care are integrated with nurturance during their caregiving. Caregiving burden involves both the amount of time spent and the degree of difficulty in caregiving activities; however, parents have objected to the word "burden" to describe the care they willingly give to their children (Wells et al., 2002). Sullivan-Bolyai, Sadler, Knafl, and Gilliss (2003) described the parenting responsibilities as taking care of the illness, nurturing and caring for their child, maintaining family life, and taking care of oneself.

Taking Care of the Illness

Direct care of their children's illness involves the time, knowledge, and skills to do technical and nontechnical management, while simultaneously caring for the child's developmental and emotional needs (Moskowitz et al., 2007). Technical care and time involves doing procedures and monitoring for changes in their children's illness. This includes specialized care, such as administering medications and cleaning indwelling tubes. It accounts for crisis care (e.g., unanticipated seizure, elevated temperature), which may involve complex first aid or emergent transportation to the hospital. Nontechnical care is the time and skills needed for feeding, bathing, dressing, grooming, bowel and bladder care, transferring from the bed to a chair, and toileting, along with the necessary extra laundry and house cleaning.

Complex illness care, such as suctioning tracheotomy tubes or diet and insulin regulation, sometimes frightens relatives (e.g., grandparents) who may normally help with child care (Nelson, 2002). Finding qualified caregivers that parents trust is more difficult than finding care for healthy children (Macdonald & Callery, 2008). Parents cut back or quit work in order to provide care (U.S. Department of Health and Human Services et al., 2008) or decide against taking a new job if the health insurance benefits will not cover their children's health care needs.

Parents also coordinate resources for their children with special health care needs. Illness needs involve clinic visits, specialized therapy, community pharmacy stocking medications, and medical equipment delivered to the home. Children with special health care needs (CSHCN) also need wellness care. The American Academy of Pediatrics (AAP) recommends a "medical home" in pediatric offices in order to provide disease prevention through immunizations, promote wellness through anticipatory guidance, address illness questions, and ideally serve as a coordination center for families of CSHCN (Sadof & Nazarian, 2007; Van Cleave, Heisler, Devries, Joiner, & Davis, 2007). Not all pediatrician offices have the resources or training to provide coordination of care and specialized consideration of well-child care for children with special health care needs.

Besides health care, parents advocate for special educational services. The Individuals with Disabilities Education Act (IDEA), passed in 1975 and renewed by the Disabilities Educational Improvement

Act of 2004 (U.S. Department of Education, 2004), requires free public education to all eligible children. For children with disabilities, this involves an individual family service plan (IFSP) for children birth to 5 years, and an individual education program (IEP) for children 5 to 21 years. The 504 Plans mandated from the Rehabilitation Act of 1973 can also be used for children with health impairments to provide appropriate accommodations and adaptations to curriculum, daily instruction and test taking, and standardized local and state level testing. Local school system budgets are challenged to meet all the educational and special needs of their students. Some families may move to another school district if a school has reduced special needs services. Families living in rural areas seem to struggle the most with finding appropriate and available special educational services for their children. Families add time to an already stretched schedule to advocate for their child's educational needs.

Nurturing the Child

The care of a child with chronic illness does not exclude nurturing the child as the foundation to care. Parents often feel overwhelmed with the tasks involved with illness care and management, and may need support and encouragement to maintain optimum nurturing. The common aspects of positive nurturing—including regular touch and rocking; encouragement of social connections, such as mutual eye contact; shared positive experiences; shared discoveries; shared communication; and response to physical, emotional, and spiritual needs—can be pushed aside as medical treatments, procedures, and appointments take precedence. While other parents are enjoying play dates, parents of children with chronic illnesses are often transporting their child to appointments with professionals, or providing medical care and therapies at home. Nurses can be key in helping parents reprioritize nurturing their child by explaining the importance of nurturing to health and optimum brain development, and by modeling nurturing actions while providing medical care. Nurses can also help to alleviate parents' guilt of wanting to nurture and play with their child rather than provide medical care, and help parents delegate medical care to professionals when possible.

Maintaining Family Life

Nurturing the family as a whole and keeping each member moving toward family and individual goals are as important as illness management (Sullivan-Bolyai, Sadler, Knafl, & Gilliss, 2003). Parents, as the leaders, help the family find meaning in the situation and find ways to include caregiving into daily life. The meaning of the child's illness and the family's identity can change over time. Families may define themselves by the illness, such as a "diabetic family." Illness patterns that are chaotic challenge efforts to create family life. For example, children with attention-deficit hyperactivity disorder (ADHD) can exhibit poor impulse control, learning difficulties, and hyperactivity. Families are constantly adjusting to their child's behavior. As children with ADHD mature and learn ways to be successful with the help of teachers and health professionals (National Institute of Mental Health, 2006), the family identity may become "a family" with a child with special health care needs rather than an "ADHD family."

Parents maintain the household and financial security (Sullivan-Bolyai et al., 2003). Mothers tend to do the immediate household activities and care of the children. Fathers continue to focus on instrumental activities, such as financial security and home repairs. Both parents grieve and worry about their children's future and struggle balancing work and time with their family (Chesler & Parry, 2001; Feudtner, 2002). Single-parent households are faced with the demands of caregiving, household management, and maintaining financial security (Ganong, Doty, & Gayer, 2003).

A common concern for parents of children with special health care needs is the healthy development and care of siblings. Parents want the siblings not to be forgotten or overshadowed by the child with the chronic illness (Hallstrom & Elander, 2007). Siblings may assume the responsibilities of the parent, such as the 5-year-old who shares a bedroom with the sick sibling alerting his parents that his baby sister needs suctioning (Coffey, 2006). Siblings often try to do well in school to gain parent approval and alleviate parent concern for them because they see their parents working so hard to care for their ill sibling (Hutson & Alter, 2007). They take pride in being able to help their sibling, simultaneously complaining of doing more than their share of chores and noticing differential treatment from their parents and other relatives. Sibling research has mixed findings that show increased risks for behavior and academic problems on one hand, with improved empathy and independence skills on the other (Sharpe & Rossiter,

2002). Sibling adjustment improved when parents provided problem-solving skills, established open communication about current and future concerns, and supported resiliency characteristics, including support outside the home, establishing positive experiences and interests, and supporting positive meaning to challenging experiences (Giallo & Gavidia-Payne, 2006).

A strong husband-wife relationship is important in any family, but creating opportunities for being a couple is even more challenging for families with children with special health care needs. A ritual such as "date night" fosters closeness and provides an opportunity for open communication and problem solving without the distractions of parenting (Imber-Black, 2005). Another challenge is deciding roles and responsibilities between parents to avoid caregiver burnout. Some parents agree to divide activities, while some trade, so that each can learn the other's skills. Agreement and support of each other's parenting is the anchor for the family. Also, accepting the need for time away from parenting for both parents is important. Finding safe and appropriate respite care for families with CSHCN is a barrier to partners and marital couples, especially in rural areas. Coordinated care between health clinics, specialty clinics, educational services, and social services can increase the resources for parents and increase the chances of finding appropriate respite care.

Parents also have to manage social stigma, most common for families of children who have visible disabilities, such as limb deformities or morbid obesity; are technology dependent; have developmental/behavioral disabilities; or have a fear-based disease, such as HIV infection. Managing stigma means finding safe environments where families can relax and participate, such as Special Olympics or organizations designed to bring similar families together (e.g., National Autism Association). Without a feeling of trust and safety, families are likely to limit social activities or split the family so that the child with the disability is cared for while other family members participate in social events (Rehm & Bradley, 2005a; Sandelowski & Barroso, 2003). A major risk for families with CSHCN is social isolation and lack of social support (Wang & Barnard, 2004).

Parental Self-care

It is difficult for parents to take care of themselves when they are balancing illness care and the ongoing demands of family life (Hallstrom & Elander, 2007;

Sullivan-Bolyai et al., 2003). Mothers and fathers, each in their own way, grieve the lost dream of a healthy child. The busy-ness of daily care can distract parents from thinking that their child is not normal. The differences, however, become more evident when the condition worsens or at family events, making distraction a more difficult coping strategy to use. For example, the "first day of school" is celebrated when boarding the school bus, but using the wheelchair lift or watching other children board the regular bus while a child with special health care needs waits for the special education bus makes the child's difference visible. Validating their sadness is a nursing action that gives parents and children the opportunity to grieve what might have been and celebrate what is and has been accomplished. Their sadness, called "chronic sorrow," is a normal grief response (Gordan, 2009). Evidence-based nursing intervention strategies for families experiencing chronic sorrow (Gordan, 2009) are divided into two areas: (1) internal management methods and (2) external management methods. Internal management builds on interventions initiated by an individual such as: reading literature about their child's or sibling's condition, engaging in a personal stress reduction activity, or joining a support group. Nurses can provide these individuals local, regional, and national resources; Internet resources that are vetted as evidenced-based; or other credible resources. External management strategies are those provided by health care professionals, such as: counseling, medications for insomnia or anxiety, pastoral or spiritual care, and referrals to organization or resources to assist with financial concerns created by their child's health condition.

Conditions that were fatal in the past (e.g., premature birth, leukemia, cystic fibrosis) are now considered chronic, and are now managed in outpatient clinics and in the home (Eiser, 1994). Parents may struggle and not be able to care for their child, especially if needs are complex or behavior is so difficult that injury to the child or other family members is a risk. These parents may seek out-of-home placement, but feel guilty about it. They may see themselves as being a "bad parent" (Nelson, 2002; Wang & Barnard, 2004). Finding appropriate community resources for specialized care is difficult. Respite services and home care are fragmented. Parents move between hope and despair, and are at risk for caregiver burnout and depression if appropriate support is not available (Wong & Heriot, 2008). Nurses have a key role in assessing the family's ability to maintain care, the need for increased support or home care, and the need for out-of-home placement when needed.

"Living worried" was found to be part of the day-to-day parenting of children with chronic illness (Coffey, 2006). Parents worried about their judgment. When should they call the doctor or go to the emergency department? They worried about their family. Did their in-laws blame their side of the family for the illness (Seligman & Darling, 1997)? They worried that the neighbors would report them for child abuse, as their toddler screamed, "Don't do it, Mommy . . . please don't hurt me anymore," during an insulin injection. They worried their child was parenting them, after saying "It's alright Mommy, don't be sad. It doesn't hurt too bad." Parents continue to worry even after the child transitioned from home to an adult independent living situation, with concerns about financial stability, exploitation of the adult child by others, and general happiness (Coffey, 2006). Nurses can help families to decrease their worry by connecting parents to support groups to discuss their worries. Connecting a family with another similarly situated family is an important nursing intervention (Gallo & Knafl, 1998).

Normalization and Family Management Styles in Childhood Chronic Illness

Families are expected to take their children home, master complex treatments, and do it in such a way as to not dominate the child's life, but to integrate the care into daily family life (Knafl, Deatrick, & Kirby, 2001). Interestingly, nurses use the language of sickness or disability, such as "families of children with chronic illness" and "families of children with special health care needs." In contrast, families use the phrase, "my child is normal except for . . . [fill in the condition]." Families tend to focus on the entire child, and work continuously to normalize their child, whereas nurses continue to focus on the illness. An important stage for families, after the crisis of a chronic illness diagnosis, is to act to normalize their situation. The characteristics of normalization are as follows:

1. Acknowledging the condition and its potential to threaten family life
2. Adapting a normalcy lens for defining child and family

3. Engaging in parenting behaviors and family routines that are consistent with normalcy
4. Developing management of the condition that is consistent with normalcy (e.g., schedule preschool for afternoon session so that physical therapy and medications can be done in the morning)
5. Interacting with others based on view of the child and family as normal (Knafl et al., 2001; Knafl, Deatrick & Havill, 2012)

Striving for normalcy is not the same as denial. Parents in denial refuse to adjust schedules to meet the needs of their child's health needs in hopes of the child being viewed as normal by others, whereas parents who strive for normalcy alter schedules to allow their child to participate in as many normal activities as possible.

Families are stressed but not all are adversely affected and some report being stronger from the experience of having a child with a chronic illness (Hayes, 1997; McClellan & Cohen, 2007; Miles, 2003; Mussatto, 2006; Rodrigues & Patterson, 2007). Nurses knowledgeable about disease, illness, and family interactions can assess the complexity of a family's situation and adaptation to the chronic illness over time. Nurses can help families benefit from identifying individual and group family strengths and thinking about their goals as individuals and as a family (Tapp, 2000). Other nursing interventions to help normalize include matching support to the family's developmental stage and addressing areas assessed for individual care planning. Challenges of families whose children have disabilities and chronic conditions are listed in Table 13-4.

CONSENT IN FAMILY CHILD HEALTH NURSING

Families with children experiencing acute or chronic illness or injury may be asked to make difficult decisions regarding health care. In most instances, when young children are involved, health care providers collaborate with parents to obtain informed consent, except in emergency situations when parents are absent. As children grow and develop, it is important for them to take on more responsibility as primary guardians of personal health and decision making (American Academy of Pediatrics, 2007; American Academy of Pediatrics Committee on Bioethics,

Table 13-4	Stages, Tasks, and Situational Needs of Families of Children With Disabilities and Chronic Conditions	
Stages	**Tasks**	**Situational Needs that Alter Transitions**
1. Beginning family: *Married couple without children.*	a. Establish mutually satisfying relationship. b. Relate to kin network. c. Family planning.	a. Unprepared for birth of children with disabilities; prenatal testing or visible anomalies at birth begins process. b. In the United States, parents usually want to know their infants' diagnosis as early as possible.
2. Early childbearing: *First birth, up to 36 months.*	a. Integrate new baby into family. b. Reconcile conflicting needs of various family members. c. Parental role development. d. Accommodate to marital couple changes. e. Expand relationships with extended family, adding grandparent and aunt/uncle roles.	a. Learn the meaning of infants' behavior, symptoms, and treatments. b. Hampered nurturing and parenting, if children are not able to respond to parents' efforts to interact with them (e.g., not smiling or returning sounds in response to parental cooing). c. Search for adequate health care. d. Establish early intervention programs (speech and physical therapist, specially trained teachers).
3. Family with preschool children: *First child developmental age 3–5 years.*	a. Foster development of children. b. Parental privacy. c. Increased competence of child. d. Socializing children. e. Maintenance of couple relationship.	a. Formal education of disabled children starts at birth with early intervention programs. Families may not find adequate programs even into preschool years. b. Failure to achieve developmental milestones (toilet training, self-feeding, language) signals chronic sorrow. c. Families try to establish routines for themselves and their children.
4. Family with school-age children: *Oldest child developmental age 6–13 years.*	a. Letting children go. b. Parental needs balanced with children's needs. c. Promoting school achievement. d. Prepare for high-risk behavior related to drugs and sexual experimentation.	a. Move children from family care to community care requires creating new routines and relationships. b. Explain to school officials and others the needs of the children. c. Negotiate appropriate school services and curriculum. d. Behavioral problems may isolate families.
5. Family with adolescents: *Oldest child developmental age 13 years until leaves home.*	a. Loosening family ties. b. Couple relationship. c. Parent-teen communication. d. Maintenance of family moral and ethical standards. e. Promote safe sexual development.	a. Continued dependency may mean children never achieve leaving home. b. Family examines how to continue family life with increasing physical growth but ongoing dependence of children. c. High-risk behavior related to sexual activity and drugs.
6. Launching center family: *First through last child to leave home.*	a. Promote independence of children while maintaining relationship. b. Couple relationship, build new life together. c. Midlife developmental crisis for adults.	a. Financial costs do not decrease because children still require dependent-type care.

Table 13-4	Stages, Tasks, and Situational Needs of Families of Children With Disabilities and Chronic Conditions—cont'd		
Stages	**Tasks**	**Situational Needs that Alter Transitions**
7. Families in middle years: *Empty nest to retirement.*	a. Redefine activity and goals. b. Provide healthy environment. c. Meaningful relationships with aging parents. d. Strengthen couple relationship.	a. Redefine relationships with grown children and child with special health care needs.
8. Retirement to old age: *Retirement to death of both parents.*	a. Deal with losses. b. Living place may change. c. Role changes. d. Adjust to less income. e. Chronic illness. f. Mate loss. g. Aware of death. h. Life review.	a. Arrangements for children with special health care needs.

Source: Gedaly-Duff, V., Stoeger, S., & Shelton, K. (2000). Working with families. In R. E. Nickel & L. W. Desch (Eds.), *The physician's guide to caring for children with disabilities and chronic conditions* (1st ed., pp. 31–76). Baltimore, MD: Paul H. Brookes.

1995). Some family members and health care providers may feel uncomfortable with the inclusion of children in health care decision making. Some authorities believe that children may not make rational decisions, and yet adults are not held to the same standard of being rational when they make personal health care decisions (Zawistowski & Frader, 2003). Each child's decision-making capacities should be assessed and given serious consideration using Piaget's cognitive developmental stages as a guide (American Academy of Pediatrics, 2007; American Academy of Pediatrics Committee on Bioethics, 1995).

The wishes and concerns of children should be taken into account during decision making and the assent of children undergoing treatment and procedures should be solicited. Even when the child's desires cannot be met, the discussion of the situation with the child may help to build child-health provider trust. Regardless of the outcome of any decision, it should be a dialogue, versus a "top-down" conversation, with honest and developmentally appropriate answers provided to the child (American Academy of Pediatrics, 2007; American Academy of Pediatrics Committee on Bioethics, 1995).

Laws regarding informed consent of minors vary from state to state. It is important that health care providers be knowledgeable of individual state statues. In Virginia, for example, Abraham's Law resulted from a case where an adolescent refused to comply with physician-recommended treatment (*Starchild Abraham Cherrix v. Commonwealth of Virginia*, for the County of Accomack, 2006). This 2007 law allows minors 14 years of age or older to refuse medical treatment for a life-threatening condition. Even with this law, most adolescents make these decisions in collaboration with parents and health care professionals when able.

Some states consider some minors "emancipated," and give these individuals the authority to make personal health care decisions. The age of minors is decided by each individual state, and varies depending on the decision being considered. For example, whereas consuming alcohol is limited to those 21 years and older, most states allow for specific medical decisions to be made by individuals over the age of 18 years. These minors may be self-supporting, live outside of the parental home, be married, pregnant, a parent, in the military, or declared emancipated by the courts. Some states also have statutes related to "mature minors." These persons are not emancipated but still have the authority to make health care decisions in certain situations, such as addiction, pregnancy, and sexually transmitted disease care (American Academy of Pediatrics, 2007; American Academy of Pediatrics Committee on Bioethics, 1995).

On occasion, the wishes of children, families, and health care providers may differ. It is assumed that all parties will act in the best interest of the child, but best interests are in the eye of the beholder when it comes down to personally held values, such as "what makes a life worth living" (Kon, 2006). Although it is uncommon for parents to be overruled, there are circumstances where the courts will invoke the Child Abuse Prevention and Treatment Act, which gives the state's interest in protecting minors greater weight than the rights of parents in decision making (Holder, 1983; Kon, 2006; U.S. Code of Federal Regulations, 2006). In a 2006 case, a mother was charged with second-degree kidnapping when she smuggled her child out of a children's hospital to explore alternative treatments. In situations such as these, health care providers should respect the fact that some patients may need time to understand the situation or come to terms with concerns regarding proposed care (American Academy of Pediatrics, 2007; American Academy of Pediatrics Committee on Bioethics, 1995). Legal intervention should be the last resort, and should only occur when there is a substantial risk to the child, as state intervention can cause serious harm itself (Ostrom, 2006).

CARE OF CHILDREN AND FAMILIES IN THE HOSPITAL

Another issue that family nurses experience when caring for families with children is the admission of a child to the hospital. Hospital admission is a stressful event for families. Nurses and health care providers have the opportunity to take this crisis situation and make it the best it can be for the child and family by decreasing stressors whenever possible. Applying the principles of partnering, setting mutual goals with the family, enhancing family connectedness to the child, valuing the family's areas of expertise, and assisting the family to understand health care processes and procedures are all ways to help alleviate some of the stress of a hospital stay (Curley & Meyer, 2001). Family and child attendance at interdisciplinary team rounds is an ideal place to set mutual goals, and such rounds have been shown to increase patient and family satisfaction. In fact, positive feelings from the family can improve health outcomes. For example, including family as valued team members has been shown to

decrease intensive care unit length of stay of ill children (Dutton et al., 2003; Vazirani, Hays, Shapiro, & Cowan, 2005). Latta, Dick, Parry, and Tamura (2008) identified communication as the most important aspect of rounds for families. Family members expressed a need to be included in rounds and found comfort in the fact that they were respected members of the team with an important perspective to share. Family-centered rounds hold a potential to create a patient-centered environment, enhance medical and nursing education, and improve patient outcomes (Cypress, 2012).

Nurses often take on the role of coordinating and maintaining communication with family members throughout a hospitalization. Identifying one or two point people to provide communication to the family helps build trust and decreases the risk for communication errors and related conflict. It opens and strengthens communication, builds trust, and lessens anxiety if a consistent, limited number of health care providers are assigned to care for the child and family, and maintain regular communication with family members (Mullen & Pate, 2006).

Referring to family members as "visitors" diminishes the significance of the family relationship (Slota, Shearn, Potersnak, & Haas, 2003) and may even be perceived as insulting; it is the health care providers who are the "visitors" or temporary caregivers for the hospitalized child. Ensuring that "family" is broadly defined can make available a wide base of support from loved ones. Close friends and family members are seen as sources of security for children, and extended family members can also provide parents or guardians time for self-care and opportunities to address work and home responsibilities. The family, rather than hospital administrators, should determine individuals allowed to be part of the care of the child.

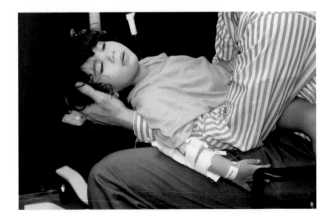

Health care providers, especially those working with critically ill children, need to be aware that parents may have increased stress due to the severity of illness their child is experiencing and about their ability to parent and serve as the child's caretaker and protector during hospitalization. This may be especially true if health care providers do not communicate with family members and if they take over traditional activities the parents are used to performing. Family members may feel uncomfortable with this ambiguity, as they face uncertainties about who performs which roles and tasks (Boss & Greenberg, 1984). Health care providers can allay much of this stress by assisting the family to maintain parenting and caretaking as much as possible during the child's stay. Nurses can assist families to know "how to be" at the bedside with unfamiliar hospital equipment, unit routines, and limitations to activity. Families need to be oriented to the child's room on admission and all potentially unfamiliar sights and sounds described. For instance, family members unfamiliar with alarms may mistake one that signifies the completion of a medication for something more life threatening (Board & Ryan-Wenger, 2003). Nurses caring for patients and their families should anticipate issues such as the one just described. Orientation can provide a time for education and encouragement to be an active part of the child's care (Mullen & Pate, 2006). Nurses should acknowledge parents' expertise in care and monitoring, especially for children using technology at home. Parents should also be given the opportunity to take a break from care if they need that break. On admission, nurses should also assess the child's usual routine and follow it as closely as possible (Mullen, 2008).

The needs of siblings should also be addressed during hospitalization. Younger siblings have vivid imaginations and may believe that they caused a brother or sister to become ill or injured, or that the hospitalized child is at risk of dying. Nurses are equipped to provide parents with information, guidance, and reassurance about the appropriateness of sibling visitation for individual situations and to support these visits with appropriate preparation and support that is developmentally appropriate. Child life therapists may be available to prepare siblings for visits to the hospital and assess their readiness to visit (Mullen & Pate, 2006). In a study of critically ill children, it was found that best friends had some of the same concerns and needs

as siblings (Lewandowski & Frosch, 2003). Screening siblings and young friends for contagious illnesses before visits can theoretically prevent the spread to hospitalized patients and families. There is no evidence, however, to support that sibling visits increase infection rates, even in the neonatal population (Moore, Coker, DuBuisson, Swett, & Edwards, 2003). Rather, hospital-acquired and endogenous infections pose a greater risk to the hospitalized child (Rozdilsky, 2005). Siblings do provide support to the hospitalized family member, and visits by siblings help to reduce anxiety about being separated from a family member during times of illness and stress.

Avoiding family separation from the hospitalized child is a priority. Separation increases stress for children and families and does not encourage a partnership philosophy. The Society of Pediatric Nurses and the American Nurses Association (Lewandowski & Tesler, 2003) support 24-hour parental access to hospitalized children. This access includes giving families the option to remain with their children during procedures, treatments, and resuscitation attempts, including in the emergency department (American Academy of Pediatrics Committee on Pediatric Emergency & American College of Emergency Physicians Pediatric Emergency Medicine, 2006; American Association of Critical Care Nurses, 2010; Emergency Nurses Association, 2010). Families benefit from presence because it removes doubt about the child's condition, and they can rest assured that "everything" was done for the child. In the event of death, families may be comforted by the fact that the child did not die alone with strangers; the togetherness may foster a sense of closure (Bauchner, Waring, & Vinci, 1991; Halm, 2005; Mangurten et al., 2006). Nurses can assist families by supporting the decision to be present or not, assessing family reactions as needed, answering questions, helping family members to find "a place" in the room, providing instructions of what they can and cannot do, contacting spiritual support as requested, and providing comfort items such as tissues, beverages, and seating. See Box 13-3, describing a family's experience during their child's resuscitation.

Transitions during a hospital stay can become added stressors for families. For example, those who have been accustomed to one-to-one nursing care for a child in an intensive care unit (ICU) may find it stressful when transferred to an acute care pediatric unit where the nurses have more patients

---

BOX 13-3

Research Brief: Family Experiences During Resuscitation at a Children's Hospital Emergency Department

Introduction: Family presence during cardiopulmonary resuscitation has been recommended by national professional organizations, which include the American Association of Critical Care Nurses, the Emergency Nurses Association, and the American Academy of Pediatrics.

Purpose of Study: In an effort to improve the care of families during resuscitation events, the authors of this study examined the experiences of family members whose children underwent resuscitation and their health and mental health following the episode.

Methodology: Ten family members participated in a 1-hour audiotaped interview in this descriptive, retrospective study. Data collection included both quantitative and qualitative instruments, which contained previously validated and investigator-developed items.

Seven family members were present during resuscitation and three were not.

Results: Analysis of interview data revealed that families felt that: (a) they had the right to be present during resuscitation; (b) their child wanted them present during resuscitation and that they were sources of strength for the child; (c) they were reassured by seeing that all possible options to help their child were exhausted; and (d) a facilitator for information-giving would be helpful during the event, as no one was prepared to face resuscitation.

Nursing Implications: Whether present or not, all family members in this study expressed the importance of the option to be present during resuscitation. There was no indication of post-traumatic stress to family members following the event.

Source: McGahey-Oakland, P. R., Lieder, H. S., Young, A., & Jefferson, L. S. (2007). Family experiences during resuscitation at a children's hospital emergency department. *Journal of Pediatric Health Care, 21*(4), 217–225.

---

to attend. Preparation of the families for the differences between units by use of a transfer protocol may help to prevent undue stress and increase family satisfaction (Van Waning, Kleiber, & Freyenberger, 2005).

Although families are glad to have their children discharged from the hospital, there are stressors that can accompany this transition as well. This is especially true for parents of children who have been in the ICU. Evidence shows that these individuals can experience feelings of uncertainty and unpreparedness as caregivers following discharge home (Bent, Keeling, & Routson, 1996). Adequate time for planning and preparation with families can make the transition easier. Some patient discharge situations may require collaboration with multidisciplinary team members, such as social workers, discharge planners, pharmacists, and home health providers, to ensure that the resources needed following discharge are available.

Family Case Study: Comantan Family

The following case study of the Comantan family demonstrates family nursing approaches to providing health care to a family with children. The primary patient is Carl,

although other family members have health care issues as well. The focus of this case study is his health and the health of his family. See the genogram and environmental ecomap of the Comantan family in Figures 13-1 and 13-2.

Setting:

Carl Comantan is a 9-year-old boy who lives with his family in a wood-frame house in a coastal, rural area of the northwest region of the Alaska. He has chronic respiratory illnesses and has been diagnosed by his physician as having asthma.

Family Members:

Carl's ethnicity is Alaskan Native, or Inuit. Many people call these people Eskimos. Their nationality is American, as they were all born in the United States of America. His father and mother, and maternal and paternal grandfathers and grandmothers, are also Alaskan Native. His maternal grandfather and grandmother both passed away several years ago from pneumonia. The remaining family members have light brown skin and dark brown or black hair. The family speaks English and the elders also speak their native language, Inuktitut.

Carl's family consists of his mother, Carine, age 32; his father, Big Frank, age 33; and his two brothers, Sam, age 7, and little Frankie, age 2½. Carine is approximately 4 months pregnant. Big Frank's sister, Leena, age 30, helps with child care. Grandfather Harry and Grandmother Relah are very involved with their children and grandchildren.

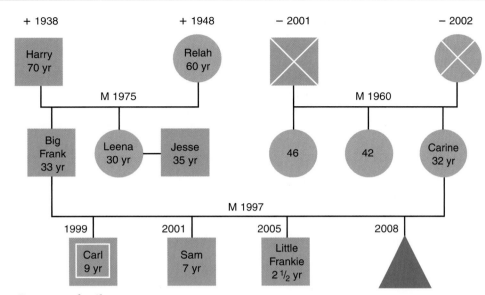

FIGURE 13-1 Comantan family genogram.

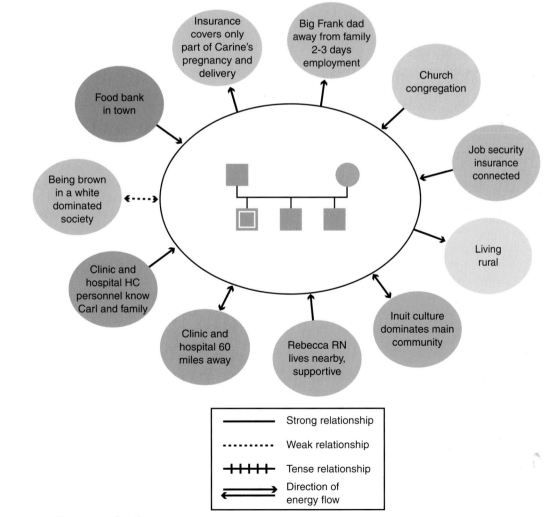

FIGURE 13-2 Comantan family ecomap.

The Family Story:

Big Frank and Carine have been married for over 11 years. The children are their biological children from this marriage. Neither has been married before. They went to high school together and met when Big Frank did business at the gas station where Carine worked. They both attend the same church.

Big Frank works part-time as a professional truck driver for a trucking corporation in the region. He is often gone from home for 2 to 3 days at a time for his work. The company offers limited major medical insurance for Big Frank and his family. Office visits and care under $800 are not covered. Carine's pregnancy care and births are covered at 60% of the cost. She receives no paid maternity leave benefit from her employer.

Carine works at a local gas station that has a small grocery store attached. She manages the grocery store. The store is five miles from their home in the nearby village of Anokiviac. Big Frank and Carine are worried that they cannot make enough money to save, let alone pay the ongoing bills for electricity, gasoline for their vehicles, heating oil for their home, and clothing. They feel fortunate to be members of a cohesive community of family and friends, and to have jobs. Many people in their area do not have full-time employment. There are no family aid programs in the area. Monthly, they travel to the town an hour's drive away to go to the local food bank. They get a box of staples that includes flour, rice, canned vegetables, and dried milk. The food bank requires that they show bills and pay statements to prove that they qualify for the food. Sometimes the food bank has a very limited number of items.

Big Frank and Carine strongly believe in making and keeping strong relationships with the people in their family and community circles. They talk about how people have helped each other in the past and how they are always on the lookout for someone who needs help. From one conversation with a teacher, Carine learned about a summer program for first graders. She was able to enroll Sam in that 2-week-long program in the town, where he stayed with a cousin's family. In exchange for the cost of the program, she helped several evenings in their local school program during the school year.

These evening programs during the school year were also helpful for Carl, since he missed several days during the school year due to his coughing and respiratory illnesses. As a result of the extra time and attention, he has been able to keep up with his classmates at his school. Carine and Big Frank help the children's Aunt Leena understand how to help Carl with his studies, since she cares for the children while the parents are working. Carine and Big Frank believe that if they and a few other people, such as

Aunt Leena and the school teachers, know Carl well, they will notice when he starts to become ill. They believe that they have been able to avert many serious illnesses for Carl because they and the adults he is around know him well. They do not get overly worried if he wheezes a little, which they consider normal for Carl. If he gets more short of breath, however, or if his appetite wanes, then they know he is getting sick. Even his brother, Sam, knows about Carl being "fever hot" as he calls it, and worries openly about his brother when he is ill. Sam and little Frankie will bring Carl water and crackers when he is sick. The younger children also know about Carl's inhaler and will bring it to him when he is wheezing.

The physicians and nurses at the clinic in the town know that, when Carine, Big Frank, Aunt Leena, or other family members call saying Carl is ill, the situation is serious. They listen with high regard.

Big Frank is a partially disabled veteran of the U.S. Army. He served in an international war overseas and was injured in a tank attack. His disability involves his left leg and left arm, both of which are severely scarred from burns. He has decreased range of motion and sensation in both of these limbs. His left chest and face are also scarred; however, he did not lose vision or function of his shoulder or face. He is not overweight and is physically strong and fit.

Carine has good health but knows there is a family history of coughing spells. She is not overweight and is physically strong and fit. Both Carine and Big Frank work hard to eat well and feed their children healthy food. They eat frozen vegetables and fruits, and bread made by various family members. Their protein sources include fish that they catch and either elk or caribou from the annual fall family hunt. Occasionally they have seal, obtained as a result of traditional hunts by Big Frank and the extended family.

Carine and Big Frank will drink an occasional beer but do not drink any other alcoholic beverages. Many of their extended family members and folks in their community drink beer, sometimes to excess, resulting in drunken behavior. Carine and Big Frank worry that their children may drink excessively as adolescents and adults. They do not allow their children to drink any beer or other alcoholic beverage. The extended family members and the folks in the community practice the same behavior. Group disapproval occurs when drunken behavior occurs and those persons are taken home.

Carl is generally healthy except for his asthma and frequent episodes of upper respiratory infections. These often progress into lengthy bouts of wheezing and coughing. He frequently wheezes in the morning on awakening and when he plays outside. He misses all or parts of days from school due to his illnesses approximately 25% of the time.

He has an inhaler, but he occasionally forgets to bring it with him to school and church or out to play. He takes his antibiotics and other medications well. He says out loud, "This is for my breathing!" He also says to little Frankie, "This is not for you, this is my medicine! It is icky, you should never eat it!" Carl knows that his mother, Aunt Leena, school teacher, and Sunday school teacher know about each of his medicines. Carine and Big Frank are considering sending Carl to asthma camp for 2 weeks in the city during the summer. The physician at the hospital has recommended Carl receive a foundation-funded scholarship at the camp because they note that he learns quickly and likes to be with other children. Also, the physician told Carine and Frank that they think Carl could benefit from the time to focus on learning more about managing his own condition.

Sam and little Frankie are both healthy. They have had occasional respiratory illnesses. Sam and Carl both had the chickenpox, as the varicella vaccine was not available in their area at the time. Carine and the children are up-to-date on their vaccines. Big Frank has not had an influenza vaccine and does not recall when he had other immunizations since he left the military.

While Carine is at work, all three children go to their Aunt Leena's home either all day or after school, depending on their age. Aunt Leena's home is a 5-minute walk from the school. Aunt Leena has a car and has driven Carl to the emergency department several times during the last year when he has had severe bouts of wheezing and a fever. Aunt Leena lives with her husband, Uncle Jesse, who works as a truck driver and bush plane pilot in the area. Aunt Leena does not work outside her home. She is involved in the care of her brother's children and is looking forward to the next child. She occasionally takes a little gas money when her brother, Big Frank, offers. She is committed to helping her brother and his family in any way she can. She and her husband want children but have been unable to conceive.

Grandparents Harry and Relah, who are a 5-minute walk from Big Frank and his family, are also involved in watching, guiding, and helping their three grandchildren. Grandmother Relah has learned many treatments for illnesses over her lifetime. She studied for a while with one of the tribal shamans many years ago and maintains contact with the shaman. She makes mint and berry teas for Carl, makes steam for him in the kitchen, and feeds him dried fish for strength and healing. She talks to Carl and his brothers about the herbs she makes from various berries, bark, and leaves in their environment. She also encourages them to think about being strong and quick, wise and caring in their world. She talks to Big Frank about taking Carl to

visit the shaman. They have not yet decided if they will follow through with this recommendation.

Big Frank and Carine consult extended family members, particularly the elderly parents and other elders in the area regarding health and family matters of all kinds, including seeking advice regarding Carl's respiratory infections and wheezing. As the nearest clinic, hospital, or health care facility is more than 60 miles away, they are careful about taking the time and gasoline to drive there. Big Frank and Carine consider themselves equal decision makers with regard to family health matters and will consult providers and family members. Both are held in high esteem in their family and surrounding community. They are supported through congregational prayer in their church, particularly when Carl is ill. Church members, especially direct relatives, often bring food to the Comantan family home when Carl is ill or when Big Frank is gone for several days on his job.

One of the Comantan family's neighbors is a registered nurse, Rebecca, who lives about 5 miles away. She works at one of the clinics associated with the hospital that is in the town 60 miles away. One time she took Carl with her to the clinic so that he could see his physician and get a renewal on an anti-inflammatory medication. She often laughs and says she is another "Auntie" for Carl and his siblings. She says she is, at least, their cousin, even though she is Salish and not Inuit.

Health Care Goals for the Comantan Family:
- Reduce the frequency and severity of Carl's respiratory illnesses.
- Reduce the number of Carl's missed school days. Maintain age-appropriate academic success.
- Increase the number of developmentally appropriate responsibilities and decision-making processes for Carl as he learns to manage his own illness.
- Prevent Carl's daily wheezing by improving management of asthma.
- Promote Carine's health during her pregnancy.
- Promote Big Frank's healthy coping with the pain and discomfort of his injuries.
- Enhance health resources for the family in its community.
- Reduce the family's barriers to health and increase its strengths for health.

Goals for Nurses Working With the Comantan Family Across Health Care Settings:
- Build a therapeutic and collaborative health-focused relationship with Carl and the Comantan family.
- Explore ways to reduce the frequency and severity of Carl's respiratory symptoms.
- Explore with Carl and his family ways to mediate and adapt to the overall impact of his illness on him and his family.

(continued)

- Explore the health care resources for the Comantan family.
- Explore the main strengths and stressors for Carl and his family.
- Commend the Comantan family for its current health efforts and outcomes.
- Focus on maintaining stability in the Comantan family.

Family Systems Theory in Relation to the Comantan Family:

The use of Family Systems Theory addresses the complex needs of each individual within the family, and the family as a whole. The individual concepts from the Family Systems Theory apply as follows:

Concept 1—All Parts of the System Are Connected:

Carl and his family are deeply and actively embedded in their family life and their community. Each family and community member contributes to the health of Carl and his family. When Carl is ill, connections are activated to become supportive in a focused manner, according to the needs identified.

One assumption of family systems is that the features of the system are designed to maintain stability of the system, using both adaptive and maladaptive means. The Comantan family is adaptive to Carl's illnesses in its frequent, focused interactions with family and friends. The family members realize that their situation may change quickly, for example, with finances, and that they may suddenly find themselves in financial stress. Family members also recognize that Carl's health may change quickly, and they know several people should know how to monitor Carl's health and know what to do if he shows signs of respiratory distress. Their connections with Aunt Leena are part of that adaptation. They realize that with an intentional increase in the number of people who know Carl well, there is a greater likelihood that no matter where he is, he can be quickly and accurately assessed for severity and risk.

Each family member has many roles, each affecting one another. Big Frank, for instance, is a provider of financial resources, a responsible adult in his social community, a caring son to his parents, a guardian of the culture, and a caring father. These roles influence many aspects of his family. Carine is a provider of financial resources, a responsible adult in her social community, including the school, and a caring mother. These roles influence many aspects of her family.

Concept 2—The Whole Is More Than the Sum of Its Parts:

The family members consistently support each other, recognizing the strength of the whole. The Comantan family believes individuals doing their part contribute to the overall health of all and the ability of each to help at various times. The Comantan family adults focus on increasing health of all members in the long term while adapting to Carl's illness. For example, because Carl misses school due to his illness, they plan for Aunt Leena to help him. They also arrange for Sam and Carl to be in summer programs. The family adapts to health needs of one member while taking care not to compromise the health of the other members.

The Comantan family is a cohesive unit with a lot of interdependence. This is consistent with its societal beliefs of helping each other survive and thrive. Family members believe that each person has value, yet each has responsibilities to the others in the group. They take great pride in teaching each other necessary and helpful things. This is especially true of the elders to the younger members. The elders do listen to the new ideas of the younger members, however, realizing that all ideas are worth consideration.

The entire family is happily anticipating the arrival of the new baby. They hope it is a girl, but they will be happy whether the baby is a boy or a girl. This normative, expected event may require the three boys, Carl, Sam, and little Frankie, to stay with Aunt Leena and Uncle Jesse during the birth and early postpartum stage. This will depend on the circumstances, and the aunt and uncle are prepared.

Concept 3—All Systems Have Some Form of Boundaries or Border Between the System and Its Environment:

The Comantan family stays close to family and friends, yet is mindful of the amount and types of contributions made between families. For example, if Carl needs to go to the hospital, Aunt Leena will strive to be the one who takes him, rather than asking Rebecca to do so.

The family has fairly open boundaries within its local community, and does reach out to a few resources in the town 60 miles away. The family likes the idea of Sam going to the summer program and staying with his cousins because they knew the teacher and the supervisors.

The grandparents help Carl and his brothers find the boundaries of their heritage within the larger white American culture. They are teaching Carl about these boundaries and expect Carl to model these for his two younger brothers, as well as for other children in the community.

Rebecca, the nurse, who is Salish (not Inuit), is trusted and the family is open with her. The family is also open with the members of the congregation of their church.

Concept 4—Systems Can Be Further Organized Into Subsystems:

The Comantan family and the family of Aunt Leena and Uncle Jesse are an important subsystem in the Comantan family's overall functioning. Aunt Leena and Uncle Jesse contribute a lot while gaining contact with their beloved nephews. The grandparents, Harry and Relah, are also an important subsystem of the Comantan family, as are the children versus the adults.

Nursing Plan Using the Family Systems Approach:

The nursing plan for this family is more holistic if the Family Systems Approach is used.

Nurse Assessment—Noticing/Data Gathering and Interpretation:

- Explore in detail the expectations the family—including parents, grandparents, and aunt and uncle—has for Carl in relation to managing his health. Use affirmations, clarifications, respect, salutations, and honesty.
- Ask the family to share details of its health practices, including any herbal or practice treatments used by Grandparents Harry and Relah.
- Learn the history and what the family expects about the future of Carl's chronic illness.
- Explore triggers and factors that worsen his condition.
- Assess Carl's overall growth and development, his medications, what substances he has used or been given for his health, his health-related behaviors, and his interpretations of all of these items. For example, determine the level of growth and development impairment the family has noticed as a result of his respiratory illnesses and treatment.
- Discuss the concept of illness trajectory for the Comantan family.
- Explore what the family thinks is helpful, what might be helpful, and what is not helpful.
- Explore the main adaptive features the family identifies.
- Explore additional health and health cost resources for the family, particularly for the occasions of Carl's potential hospitalizations in the future, for Carine's pregnancy and delivery, and for Big Frank's pain management.
- Explore any health care disparities the family has experienced or perceived.
- Assess the entire family's immunization status.
- Explore the impact of Big Frank's absence for 3 days at a time when he is driving his truck for work.
- Ensure that various family members have Carl's medications handy at their homes.
- Assess the boundaries of care and involvement for Aunt Leena and Grandparents Harry and Relah.

- Look for trends, health patterns, illness patterns, and disease patterns for Carl's management behaviors and outcomes.

Interpretations:

- The Comantan family strengths include their health behaviors, health actions, and beliefs. They reportedly practice health behaviors that help all members without the expense of hurting another family member.
- The Comantan family has coordinated care for Carl within its family and community. They are strong advocates for his health and well-being.
- Many members of the extended family are integral to Carl's health and the health of the entire Comantan family.
- Realize that the data so far do not support any major stressors when Big Frank is gone for 3 days at a time. This may change with Carine's advancing pregnancy and birth.
- The Comantan family career has multiple concurrent developmental needs, tasks, and transitions. For example, consider the dynamics of the transition of the new baby coming via Carine's pregnancy, Carl's chronic illness, and developmental needs of all the family's children.

Nursing Actions/Interventions:

- After assessing parents' interest and ability to read written material, bring appropriate written materials to Carl and his family about treatment and management of asthma.
- Review with Carl how to use an inhaler and talk with Carl and his family about recognizing and reducing respiratory triggers.
- Counsel and educate family members on appropriate treatment and management of asthma, reviewing treatment goals and objectives.
- Commend the family on its management of each illness episode and its overall management of family members' health.
- Explore with the family members what they believe will be risky times for Carl's health, such as spring, when plants are blooming and his asthma symptoms increase.
- Support the various roles of family members and subsystems within the family, such as Carl interacting with his uncle and grandfather as adult male role models when his father is away on the road.
- Recognize the principle of honoring cultural diversity and incorporate the roles of Aunt Leena and Uncle Jesse.
- Recognize the role of the grandparents in Carl's cultural upbringing, especially learning about his Inuit culture and history.

(continued)

- Recognize the strengths in the family, for example, its efforts to keep Carl successful at his grade level in school.
- Work collaboratively with the family in identifying and evaluating sources of help and support they already use.
- Discuss with the Comantan family the advantages and disadvantages of sending Carl to a 2-week residential camp for children with asthma.

Evaluation:
- Noticing how the family has coordinated many people for Carl's care: the nurse, Rebecca, Aunt Leena, and the grandparents.
- Assessing how the family is doing with reducing triggers for Carl's asthma, as well as helping him when he wheezes.
- Monitoring the presence or absence of wheezing, number and duration of respiratory infections, and number of school days attended.

- Considering the impact on the family if Carl is hospitalized for a severe attack, infection, or both.
- Considering the question of the projected impact of Carl's illnesses on the new baby. For example, the risks of Carl's infections on a newborn infant.
- Considering types and potential impact of health-illness transitions for the Comantan family.
- Considering additional developmental challenges the family may face in the future, such as the increased mobility of little Frankie and the increased activity needs of Sam.
- Asking if there are any additional foci for the family that have not been addressed.
- Considering asking the family about their plans for financial resources during Carine's maternity leave.
- Asking what additional family strengths could be engaged to assist them in the future.

Web Sites of Interest to Family Child Health Nurses

Organization	Web Site Address
Adolescent Health Resources	http://www.ama-assn.org/ama/pub/category/1981.html
American Academy of Pediatrics	http://www.aap.org
American Cancer Society	http://www.cancer.org
American Obesity Association	http://obesity1.tempdomainname.com/subs/childhood
Assets Approach to Promoting Healthy Child Development	http://www.search-institute.org/assets
Bright Futures at Georgetown University	http:///www.brightfutures.org
Census Bureau Minority Links for Media, American Indians, and Alaskan Natives Minorities	http://www.census.gov/pubinfo/www/NEWamindML1.html
Child and Adolescent Health Measurement Initiative	http://www.cahmi.org/pages/Home.aspx
Child maltreatment	http://www.childwelfare.gov/index.cfm
Childhood Asthma	http://www.aaaai.org/patients/publicedmat/tips/childhoodasthma.stm
Children's Defense Fund	http://childrensdefense.org
Cultural Competence Resources for Health Care Providers	http://www11.georgetown.edu/research/gucchd/nccc
Family Voices	http://www.familyvoices.org
Grandparents Raising Grandchildren	http://www.usa.gov/Topics/Grandparents.shtml
Healthy People 2010	http://www.health.gov/healthypeople
Institute for Patient- and Family-Centered Care	http://www.ipfcc.org
Kids-N-Crisis	http://www.geocities.com/Heartland/Bluffs/5400/sickkid.html
National Center for Cultural Competence	http://www11.georgetown.edu/research/gucchd/nccc
Parents Without Partners	http://www.parentswithoutpartners.org
Together for Short Lives	http://www.togetherforshortlives.org.uk

SUMMARY

- Family child health nurses focus on the relationships between family life and children's health and illness, and they assist families and family members to achieve and maintain well-being.

- Through family-centered care, family child health nurses enhance family life and the development of family members to their fullest potential.

- The family child health concepts incorporate relevant components of family life and interaction, family careers, family development and transitions, family tasks, family communication, family routines, and family health and illness, and help nurses to take a comprehensive and collaborative approach to families.

- The family child health concepts enable nurses to screen for potentially harmful situations (e.g., risk for unintentional and intentional injury and death); instruct families about health issues and healthy lifestyles; and help families to cope with acute illness, chronic illness, and life-threatening conditions.

- The family child nurse addresses the needs of individuals within the family and the family as a whole to reach developmental and health potential. For example, siblings of children with special needs can fair well if given the guidance and support they need to develop understanding and empathy, and if included in the care of their sibling.

REFERENCES

Aldous, J. (1996). *Family careers: Rethinking the developmental perspective.* Thousand Oaks, CA: Sage.

America's Alliance Program. (2013). Our work. Retrieved from http://www.americaspromise.org/Our-Work.aspx

American Academy of Pediatrics. (1973). Day care for handicapped children. *Pediatrics, 51,* 948.

American Academy of Pediatrics. (2004). Writer bytes . . . childhood injury: It's no accident. Retrieved February 1, 2004, from http://www.aap.org/mrt/ciaccidents.htm

American Academy of Pediatrics. (2007). AAP publications retired or reaffirmed, October 2006. *Pediatrics, 119*(2), 405.

American Academy of Pediatrics Committee on Bioethics. (1995). Informed consent, parental permission, and assent in pediatric practice. *Pediatrics, 95*(2), 314–317.

American Academy of Pediatrics Committee on Hospital Care. (2003). Family-centered care and the pediatrician's role. *Pediatrics, 112*(3 pt 1), 691–697.

American Academy of Pediatrics Committee on Pediatric Emergency & American College of Emergency Physicians Pediatric Emergency Medicine. (2006). Patient- and family-centered care and the role of the emergency physician providing care to a child in the emergency department. *Pediatrics, 118*(5), 2242–2244.

American Academy of Pediatrics. (2012). Preventing firearm-related injuries in the pediatric population. Retrieved from http://www.aap.org/en-us/advocacy-and-policy/federal-advocacy/Documents/AAPGunViolencePreventionPolicy Recommendations_Jan2013.pdf

American Association of Critical Care Nurses. (2010). Practice alert: Family presence during CPR and invasive procedures. Retrieved from http://www.aacn.org/wd/practice/docs/practicealerts/family%20presence%2004-2010%20final.pdf

American Medical Association. (2007, January 25). Expert committee recommendations on the assessment, prevention, and treatment of child and adolescent overweight and obesity. Retrieved January 2008 from http://www.ama-assn.org/ama1/pub/upload/mm/433/ped_obesity_recs.pdf

Annie E. Casey Foundation. (2007). Kids count data book on-line. Retrieved http://www.kidscount.org/datacenter/summary07

Barnes, J., Kroll, L., Lee, J., Burke, O., Jones, A., & Stein, A. (2002). Factors predicting communication about the diagnosis of maternal breast cancer to children. *Journal of Psychosomatic Research, 52*(4), 209–214.

Bauchner, H., Waring, C., & Vinci, R. (1991). Parental presence during procedures in an emergency room: Results from 50 observations. *Pediatrics, 87*(4), 544–548.

Baughcum, A. E., Burklow, K. A., Deeks, C., Powers, S. W., & Whitaker, R. C. (1998). Maternal feeding practices and childhood obesity: A focus group study of low-income mothers. *Archives of Pediatrics & Adolescent Medicine, 152*(10), 1010–1014.

Baumrind, D. (1991). The influence of parenting style on adolescent competence and substance use. *Journal of Adolescence, 11,* 56–95.

Baumrind, D. (2005). Patterns of parental authority and adolescent autonomy. In J. Smetana (Ed.), *New directions for child development: Changes in parental authority during adolescence* (pp. 61–69). San Francisco, CA: Jossey-Bass.

Baxley, F., & Miller, M. (2006). Parental misperceptions about children and firearms. *Archives of Pediatric and Adolescent Medicine, 160,* 542–547.

Bent, K. N., Keeling, A., & Routson, J. (1996). Home from the PICU: Are parents ready? *Maternal Child Nursing, 21,* 80–84.

Bianchi, S. M. (1995). The changing demographic and socioeconomic character of single-parent families. *Marriage and Family Review, 20,* 71–98.

Black, C., & Ford-Gilboe, M. (2004). Adolescent mothers: Resilience, family health work and health-promoting practices. *Journal of Advanced Nursing, 48*(4), 351–360.

Blaska, J. K. (1998). Cyclical grieving: Reoccuring [sic] emotions experienced by parents who have children with disabilities. Retrieved from http://www.eric.ed.gov/contentdelivery/servlet/ERICServlet?accno=ED419349

Board, R., & Ryan-Wenger, N. (2003). Stressors and stress symptoms of mothers with children in the PICU. *Journal of Pediatric Nursing, 18*(3), 195–202.

Bond, L. A., & Burns, C. E. (2006). Mothers' beliefs about knowledge, child development, and parenting strategies: Expanding the goals of parenting programs. *Journal of Primary Prevention, 27*(6), 555–571.

Bornstein, M. H., Tamis-LeMonda, C. S., Hahn, C., & Haynes, M. (2008). Maternal responsiveness to young children at three ages: Longitudinal analysis of a multidimensional, modular, and specific parenting construct. *Developmental Psychology, 44*(3), 867–874.

Boss, P., & Greenberg, J. (1984). Family boundary ambiguity: A new variable in family stress theory. *Family Process, 23*(4), 535–546.

Bronfenbrenner, U. (1997). Ecology of the family as a context for human development: Research perspectives. In J. L. Paul et al. (Eds.), *Foundations of special education* (pp. 49–83). Pacific Grove, CA: Brooks/Cole.

Bruns, D. A., & McCollum, J. A. (2002). Partnerships between mothers and professionals in the NICU: Caregiving, information exchange, and relationships [comment]. *Neonatal Network—Journal of Neonatal Nursing, 21*(7), 15–23.

Bruss, M. B., Morris, J., & Dannison, L. (2003). Prevention of childhood obesity: Sociocultural and familial factors. *Journal of the American Dietetic Association, 103*(8), 1042–1045.

Bureau of Labor Statistics. (2013). Employment characteristics of families—2010. Retrieved from http://www.bls.gov/news.release/famee.nr0.htm

Burr, W. R., Herrin, D. A., Beutler, I. F., & Leigh, G. K. (1988). Epistemologies that lead to primary explanations in family science. *Family Science Review, 1*(3), 185–210.

Centers for Disease Control and Prevention. (2010). 10 leading causes of death by age group in the United States–2010. Retrieved from http://www.cdc.gov/injury/wisqars/pdf/10LCID_All_Deaths_By_Age_Group_2010-a.pdf

Centers for Disease Control and Prevention. (2011). Youth risk behavior surveillance. *MMWR Morbidity and Mortality Weekly Report, 61*(4), 1–162. Retrieved from http://www.cdc.gov/mmwr/pdf/ss/ss6104.pdf

Centers for Disease Control and Prevention. (2012). *Suicide: Facts at a glance.* Retrieved from http://www.cdc.gov/violenceprevention/pdf/Suicide_DataSheet-a.pdf

Chen, X., Dong, Q., & Zhou, H. (1997). Authoritative and authoritarian parenting practices and social and school performance in Chinese children. *International Journal of Behavioral Development, 21*(4), 855–873.

Chesler, M. A., & Parry, C. (2001). Gender roles and/or styles in crisis: An integrative analysis of the experiences of fathers of children with cancer. *Qualitative Health Research, 11*(3), 363–384.

Child Care Resource and Referral Network. (n.d.). Child Care Resource and Referral Network. Retrieved from http://www.ccrrn.com

Child Care Aware of America. (2013). *Child care in America: 2013 state fact sheets.* Retrieved from http://www.naccrra.org/sites/default/files/default_site_pages/2013/2013_state_fact_sheets_082013.pdf

Child Welfare Information Gateway. (2014). State child abuse reporting numbers. Retrieved from https://www.childwelfare.gov/pubs/reslist/printer_friendly.cfm?rs_id=5&rate_chno=W-00082

Christensen, P. (2004). The health-promoting family: A conceptual framework for future research. *Social Science & Medicine, 59*(2), 377–387.

Coffey, J. S. (2006). Parenting a child with chronic illness: A metasynthesis. *Pediatric Nursing, 32*(1), 51–59.

Conway, J., Johnson, B., Edgman-Levitan, S., Schlucter, J., Ford, D., Sodomka, P. & Simmons, L. (2006). Partnering with patients and families to design a patient- and family-centered health care system: A roadmap for the future. A work in progress. Institute for Patient- and Family-Centered Care. Retrieved from http://www.ipfcc.org/pdf/Roadmap.pdf

Cooklin, A. (2001). Eliciting children's thinking in families and family therapy. *Family Process, 40*(3), 293–312.

Corlett, J., & Twycross, A. (2006). Negotiation of parental roles within family-centred care: A review of the research. *Journal of Clinical Nursing, 15*(10), 1308–1316.

Costello, E. J., Compton, S. N., Keeler, G., & Angold, A. (2003). Relationships between poverty and psychopathology: A natural experiment. *Journal of the American Medical Association, 290*(15), 2023–2029.

Coyne, I. (2006). Consultation with children in hospital: Children, parents' and nurses' perspectives [see comment]. *Journal of Clinical Nursing, 15*(1), 61–71.

Curley, M. A. Q., & Meyer, E. C. (2001). Caring practices: The impact of the critical care experience on the family. In M. A. Q. Curley & P. A. Moloney-Harmon (Eds.), *Critical care nursing of infants and children* (2nd ed., pp. 47–67). Philadelphia, PA: W. B. Saunders.

Cypress, B. (2012). Family presence on rounds: A systematic review of literature. *Dimensions of Critical Care Nursing, 31*(1), 53–64.

Data Resource Center for Child and Adolescent Health. (2012). Who are children with special health care needs? Retrieved from http://childhealthdata.org/docs/nsch-docs/whoarec-shcn_revised_07b-pdf.pdf

Denham, S. A. (2002). Family routines: A structural perspective for viewing family health. *Advances in Nursing Science, 24*(4), 60–74.

Denham, S. A. (2003). Relationships between family rituals, family routines, and health. *Journal of Family Nursing, 9*(3), 305–330.

Driessnack, M. (2005). Children's drawings as facilitators of communication: A meta-analysis. *Journal of Pediatric Nursing: Nursing Care of Children and Families, 20*(6), 415–423.

Dutton, R. P., Cooper, C., Jones, A., Leone, S., Kramer, M. E., & Scalea, T. M. (2003). Daily multidisciplinary rounds shorten length of stay for trauma patients. *Journal of Trauma-Injury Infection & Critical Care, 55*(5), 913–919.

Duvall, E. M., & Miller, B. C. (1985). Developmental tasks: Individual and family. In E. M. Duvall & B. C. Miller (Eds.), *Marriage and family development.* New York, NY: Harper & Row.

Eiser, C. (1994). Making sense of chronic disease. The eleventh Jack Tizard Memorial Lecture. *Journal of Child Psychology and Psychiatry, 35*(8), 1373–1389.

Elliott, G. R., & Smiga, S. (2003). Depression in the child and adolescent. *Pediatric Clinics of North America, 50*(5), 1093–1106.

Emergency Nurses Association. (2010). *Position statement: Family presence at the bedside during invasive procedures and cardiopulmonary resuscitation.* Retrieved from https://www.ena.org/SiteCollectionDocuments/Position%20Statements/FamilyPresence.pdf

Emergency Nurses Association. (2011). Firearm safety and injury prevention: Position statement. Retrieved from http://www.ena.org/SiteCollectionDocuments/Position%20Statements/FirearmInjuryPrevention.pdf

Eshel, N., Daelmans, B., de Mello, M. C., & Martines, J. (2006). Responsive parenting: Interventions and outcomes. *Bulletin of the World Health Organization, 84*(12), 991–998.

Feudtner, C. (2002). Grief-love: Contradictions in the lives of fathers of children with disabilities. *Archives of Pediatrics & Adolescent Medicine, 156*(7), 643.

Floriani, V., & Kennedy, C. (2007). Promotion of physical activity in primary care for obesity treatment/prevention in children. *Current Opinion in Pediatrics, 19*(1), 99–103.

Gallo, A. M., & Knafl, K. A. (1998). Parents' reports of "tricks of the trade" for managing childhood chronic illness. *Journal of the Society of Pediatric Nurses, 3*(3), 93–102.

Ganong, L., Doty, M. E., & Gayer, D. (2003). Mothers in post-divorce families caring for a child with cystic fibrosis. *Journal of Pediatric Nursing, 18*(5), 332–343.

Gedaly-Duff, V., Stoeger, S., & Shelton, K. (2000). Working with families. In R. E. Nickel & L. W. Desch (Eds.), *The physician's guide to caring for children with disabilities and chronic conditions* (pp. 31–76). Baltimore, MD: Paul H. Brookes.

Giallo, R., & Gavidia-Payne, S. (2006). Child, parent and family factors as predictors of adjustment for siblings of children with a disability. *Journal of Intellectual Disability Research, 50*(pt 12), 937–948.

Gordan, J. (2009). An evidence-based approach for supporting parents experiencing chronic sorrow. *Pediatric Nursing, 35*(2), 115–119.

Gray, R., & McCormick, M. C. (2005). Early childhood intervention programs in the US: Recent advances and future recommendations. *Journal of Primary Prevention, 26*(3), 259–275.

Greening, L., Stoppelbein, L., Konishi, C., Jordan, S. S., & Moll, G. (2007). Child routines and youths' adherence to treatment for type 1 diabetes. *Journal of Pediatric Psychology, 32*(4), 437–447.

Griffin, T. (2003). Facing challenges to family-centered care. II: Anger in the clinical setting. *Pediatric Nursing, 29*(3), 212–214.

Grossman, D. C., Mueller, B. A., Riedy, D., Dowd, D. M., Villaveces, A., Prodzinski J, . . . Harruff, R. (2005). Gun storage practices and risk of youth suicide and unintentional firearm injuries. *JAMA, 293*, 707–714.

Grunbaum, J. A., Kann, L., Kinchen, S., Ross, J., Hawkins, J., Lowry, R., . . . Collins, J. (2004). Youth risk behavior surveillance—United States, 2003 (abridged). *Journal of School Health, 74*(8), 307–324.

Grunbaum, J. A., Kann, L., Kinchen, S. A., Williams, B., Ross, J. G., Lowry, R., & Kolbe, L. (2002). Youth risk behavior surveillance—United States, 2001. *Journal of School Health, 72*(8), 313–328.

Haggerty, K. P., Fleming, C. B., Catalano, R. F., Harachi, T. W., & Abbott, R. D. (2006). Raising healthy children: Examining the impact of promoting healthy driving behavior within a social development intervention. *Prevention Science, 7*(3), 257–267.

Hallstrom, I., & Elander, G. (2007). Families' needs when a child is long-term ill: A literature review with reference to nursing research. *International Journal of Nursing Practice, 13*(3), 193–200.

Halm, M. A. (2005). Family presence during resuscitation: A critical review of the literature. *American Journal of Critical Care, 14*(6), 494–511.

Hardy, M. S. (2002). Behavior-oriented approaches to reducing youth gun violence. In K. Reich (Ed.), *Children, youth, and gun violence* (vol. 12, pp. 100–117). Los Altos, CA: David and Lucile Packard Foundation.

Hayes, V. E. (1997). Families and children's chronic conditions: Knowledge development and methodological considerations. *Scholarly Inquiry for Nursing Practice, 11*(4), 259–290. Hertz, R., & Ferguson, F. I. (1996). Childcare choice and constraints in the United States: Social class, race and influence of family views. *Journal of Comparative Family Studies, 27*(2), 249–280.

Hibbard, R. A., Desch, L. W., Committee on Child Abuse Neglect, & Council on Children With Disabilities. (2007). Maltreatment of children with disabilities. *Pediatrics, 119*(5), 1018–1025.

Hodges, E. A. (2003). A primer on early childhood obesity and parental influence. *Pediatric Nursing, 29*(1), 13.

Holder, A. R. (1983). Parents, courts, and refusal of treatment. *Journal of Pediatrics, 103*(4), 515–521.

Horton, L. (2003). Protective factors literature review: Early care and education programs and the prevention of child abuse and neglect. Center for the Study of Social Policy. Retrieved June 2008 from http://www.cssp.org/uploadFiles/horton.pdf

Houck, G. M., Darnell, S., & Lussman, S. (2002). A support group intervention for at-risk female high school students. *Journal of School Nursing, 18*(4), 212–218.

Huston, A. C., Duncan, G. J., Granger, R., Bos, J., McLoyd, V., Mistry, R., . . . Ventura, A. (2001). Work-based antipoverty programs for parents can enhance the school performance and social behavior of children. *Child Development, 72*(1), 318–336.

Hutson, S. P., & Alter, B. P. (2007). Experiences of siblings of patients with Fanconi anemia. *Pediatric Blood & Cancer, 48*(1), 72–79.

Imber-Black, E. (2005). Creating meaningful rituals for new life cycle transitions. In B. Carter & M. McGoldrick (Eds.), *The expanded family life cycle: Individuals, family, and social perspectives* (3rd ed., pp. 202–214). Boston: Allyn & Bacon.

Jeffreys, M., Smith, G. D., Martin, R. M., Frankel, S., & Gunnell, D. (2004). Childhood body mass index and later cancer risk: A 50-year follow-up of the Boyd Orr study. *International Journal of Cancer, 112*(2), 348–351.

Johnson, R. M., Miller, M., Vriniotis, M., Azrael, D., & Hemenway, D. (2006). Are household firearms stored less safely in homes with adolescents? Analysis of a national random sample of parents. Archives of Pediatric and Adolescent Medicine, 160, 788–792.

Kenny, G. M., & Dorn, S. (2009). Health care reform for children with public coverage: How can policymakers maximize gains and prevent harm? Timely analysis of immediate health policy issues. Retrieved from http://www.urban.org/UploadedPDF/411899_children_healthcare_reform.pdf

Knafl, K. A., Deatrick, J., & Havill, N. L. (2012). Continued development of the family management style framework. *Journal of Family Nursing, 18*(1), 11–34.

Knafl, K. A., Deatrick, J., & Kirby, A. (2001). Normalization promotion. In M. Craft-Rosenberg & J. Denehy (Eds.), *Nursing interventions for infants, children, and families* (pp. 373–388). Thousand Oaks, CA: Sage.

Kon, A. A. (2006). When parents refuse treatment for their child. *JONA's Healthcare Law, Ethics, & Regulation, 8*(1), 5–9.

Latta, L. C., Dick, R., Parry, C., & Tamura, G. S. (2008). Parental responses to involvement in rounds on a pediatric inpatient unit at a teaching hospital: A qualitative study. *Academic Medicine, 83*(3), 292–297.

Lewandowski, L., & Frosch, E. (2003). Psychosocial aspects of pediatric trauma. In P. Moloney-Harmon & S. Czerwinski (Eds.), *Nursing care of the pediatric trauma patient* (pp. 340–354). Philadelphia: W. B. Saunders.

Lewandowski, L., & Tesler, M. (Eds.). (2003). *Family-centered care: Putting it into action. The SPN/ANA guide to family-centered care.* Washington, DC: Society of Pediatric Nurses/American Nurses Association.

Li, H. C., & Lopez, V. (2008). Effectiveness and appropriateness of therapeutic play intervention in preparing children for surgery: A randomized controlled trial study. *Journal for Specialists in Pediatric Nursing, 13*(2), 63–73.

Luther, B. (2007). Looking at childhood obesity through the lens of Baumrind's parenting typologies. *Orthopaedic Nursing, 26*(5), 270–278; quiz 279–280.

Maccoby, E. E., & Martin, J. A. (1983). Socialization in the context of the family: Parent–child interaction. In P. H. Mussen (Ed.) & E. M. Hetherington (Vol. Ed.), *Handbook of child psychology: Vol. 4. Socialization, personality, and social development* (4th ed., pp. 1–101). New York: Wiley.

Macdonald, H., & Callery, P. (2008). Parenting children requiring complex care: A journey through time. *Child: Care, Health & Development, 34*(2), 207–213.

Mangurten, J., Scott, S. H., Guzzetta, C. E., Clark, A. P., Vinson, L., Sperry, J., . . . Voelmeck W. (2006). Effects of family presence during resuscitation and invasive procedures in a pediatric emergency department. *Journal of Emergency Nursing, 32,* 225–233.

McClellan, C. B., & Cohen, L. L. (2007). Family functioning in children with chronic illness compared with healthy controls: A critical review. *Journal of Pediatrics, 150*(3), 221–223.

McKinney, E., James, S., Murray, S., & Ashwill, J. (2005). *Maternal-child nursing* (2nd ed., pp. 795–801). St. Louis, MO: Elsevier Sanders.

McPherson, M., Arango, P., Fox, H., Lauver, C., McManus, M., Newacheck, P. W., . . . Strickland, B. (1998). A new definition of children with special health care needs. *Pediatrics, 102* (1 pt 1), 137–140.

Medicaid.gov. (2013). Children's Health Insurance Program. Retrieved from http://www.medicaid.gov/CHIP/CHIP-Program-Information.html

Meleis, A. I., Sawyer, L. M., Im, E. O., Hilfinger Messias, D. K., & Schumacher, K. (2000). Experiencing transitions: An emerging middle-range theory. *Advances in Nursing Science, 23*(1), 12–38.

Miles, M. S. (2003). Parents of children with chronic health problems: Programs of nursing research and their relationship to developmental science. *Annual Review of Nursing Research, 21,* 247–277.

Miller, J., Rosenbloom, A., & Silverstein, J. (2004). Childhood obesity. *Journal of Clinical Endocrinology & Metabolism, 89*(9), 4211–4218.

Moore, K. A., Coker, K., DuBuisson, A. B., Swett, B., & Edwards, W. H. (2003). Implementing potentially better practices for improving family-centered care in neonatal intensive care units: Successes and challenges. *Pediatrics, 111*(4 pt 2), e450–e460.

Moskowitz, J. T., Butensky, E., Harmatz, P., Vichinsky, E., Heyman, M. B., Acree, M., . . . Folkman, S. (2007). Caregiving time in sickle cell disease: Psychological effects in maternal caregivers. *Pediatric Blood & Cancer, 48*(1), 64–71.

Moss, J. (2009). Juggling acts: How parents working non-standard hours arrange care for their pre-school children. *Social Policy Journal of New Zealand, 35,* 68–77.

Moxley, K. M., Squires, J., & Lindstrom, L. (2012). Early intervention and maltreated children: A current look at the Child Abuse Prevention and Treatment Act and Part C. *Infants and Young Children, 25*(1), 3–18.

Mullen, J. E. (2008). Supporting families of technology-dependent patients hospitalized in pediatric intensive care unit. *AACN Advanced Critical Care, 19*(2), 125–129.

Mullen, J. E., & Pate, M. (2006). Caring for critically ill children and their families. In M. Slota (Ed.), *AAC Core curriculum for pediatric critical care nursing* (2nd ed., pp. 1–39). Philadelphia, PA: W.B. Saunders.

Mussatto, K. (2006). Adaptation of the child and family to life with a chronic illness. *Cardiology in the Young, 16*(Suppl 3), 110–116.

National Association of School Psychologists. (2012).Youth gun violence fact sheet. Retrieved from http://www.nasponline. org/resources/crisis_safety/Youth_Gun_Violence_Fact_ Sheet.pdf

National Center for Children in Poverty. (2012). Child poverty. Retrieved from http://www.nccp.org/topics/childpoverty.html

National Data Resource Center for Child and Adolescent Health. (2007). Who are children with special health care needs? Retrieved May 26, 2008, from http://nschdata.org/ viewdocument.aspx?item=256

National Institute of Mental Health. (2006, last revised). The family and the ADHD child. Attention deficit hyperactivity disorder. U.S. Department of Health and Human Services. Retrieved July 31, 2008, 2008, from http://www.nimh. nih.gov/health/publications/adhd/summary.shtml

National Survey of Children With Special Health Care Needs. (2010). NS-CSHCN 2009/10. Data query from the Child and Adolescent Health Measurement Initiative, Data Resource Center for Child and Adolescent Health Web site. Retrieved from www.childhealthdata.org

Nelson, A. M. (2002). A metasynthesis: Mothering other-than-normal children [see comment]. *Qualitative Health Research, 12*(4), 515–530.

NHTSA.dot.gov, National Center for Statistics and Analysis. (2003). Traffic safety facts 2003 data. Retrieved June 16, 2013, from http://www-nrd.nhtsa.dot.gov/Pubs/809762.pdf

Northington, L. (2000). Chronic sorrow in caregivers of school age children with sickle cell disease: A grounded theory approach. *Issues in Comprehensive Pediatric Nursing, 23*(3), 141–154.

Novilla, M. L., Barnes, M. D., De La Cruz, N. G., Williams, P. N., & Rogers, J. (2006). Public health perspectives on the family: An ecological approach to promoting health in the family and community. *Family & Community Health, 29*(1), 28–42.

Offer, S., & Schneider, B. (2011). Revisiting the gender gap in time use patterns: Multitasking and well-being among mothers and fathers in dual earner families. *American Sociological Review, 76*(6), 809–833.

Ogden, C. L., Carroll, M. D., Kit, B. K., & Flegal, K. M. (2012). Prevalence of obesity and trends in body mass index among U.S. children and adolescents, 1999–2010. *Journal of the American Medical Association, 307*(5), 483–490.

Ostrom, C. M. (2006, June 27). Is mom a criminal for not allowing surgery on her son? Retrieved from http://community.seattletimes.nwsource.com/archive/?date=20060627&slug=rileyrogers27m

Parsons, C. (2003). Caring for adolescents and families in crisis. *Nursing Clinics of North America, 38*(1), 111–122.

Perrin, E. C., Newacheck, P., Pless, I. B., Drotar, D., Gortmaker, S. L., Leventhal, J., . . . Weitzman, M. (1993). Issues involved in the definition and classification of chronic health conditions. *Pediatrics, 91*(4), 787–793.

Power, N., & Franck, L. (2008). Parent participation in the care of hospitalized children: A systematic review. *Journal of Advanced Nursing, 62*(6), 622–641.

Prugh, D. (1983). In *The psychological aspects of pediatrics.* Philadelphia, PA: Lea & Febiger.

Rankin, S. H. (1989). Family transitions. In C. L. Gilliss, B. L. Highley, B. M. Roberts, & I. M. Martinson (Eds.), *Toward a science of family nursing* (pp. 173–186). Menlo Park, CA: Addison-Wesley.

Rankin, S. H., & Weekes, D. P. (2000). Life-span development: A review of theory and practice for families with chronically ill members. *Scholarly Inquiry for Nursing Practice, 14*(4), 355–373; discussion, 375–358.

Rao, N., McHale, J. P., & Pearson, E. (2003). Links between socialization goals and child-rearing practices in Chinese and Indian mothers. *Infant & Child Development, 12*(5), 475–492.

Rehm, R. S., & Bradley, J. F. (2005a). The search for social safety and comfort in families raising children with complex chronic conditions. *Journal of Family Nursing, 11*(1), 59–78.

Richaud de Minzi, M. C. (2006). Loneliness and depression in middle and late childhood: The relationship to attachment and parental styles. *Journal of Genetic Psychology, 167*(2), 189–210.

Ritchie, L. D., Welk, G., Styne, D., Gerstein, D. E., & Crawford, P. B. (2005). Family environment and pediatric overweight: What is a parent to do? *Journal of the American Dietetic Association, 105*(5 Suppl 1), S70–S79.

Rodrigues, N., & Patterson, J. M. (2007). Impact of severity of a child's chronic condition on the functioning of two-parent families. *Journal of Pediatric Psychology, 32*(4), 417–426.

Rolland, J. S. (2005). Chronic illness and the family life cycle. In B. Carter & M. McGoldrick (Eds.), *The expanded family life cycle: Individual, family and social perspectives* (3rd ed., pp. 492–511). Boston: Allyn & Bacon.

Rothrauff, T. C., Cooney, T. M., & An, J. S. (2009). Remembered parenting styles and adjustment in middle and late adulthood. *Journals of Gerontology Series B: Psychological Sciences & Social Sciences, 64*(1), 137–146.

Rous, B., Myers, C., & Stricklin, S. (2007). Strategies for supporting transitions of young children with special needs and their families. *Journal of Early Intervention, 30*(1), 1–18.

Rozdilsky, J. R. (2005). Enhancing sibling presence in pediatric ICU. *Critical Care Nursing Clinics of North America, 17*(4), 451–461.

Sadof, M. D., & Nazarian, B. L. (2007). Caring for children who have special health-care needs: A practical guide for the primary care practitioner. *Pediatrics in Review, 28*(7), e36–e42.

Sandelowski, M., & Barroso, J. (2003). Motherhood in the context of maternal HIV infection. *Research in Nursing & Health, 26*(6), 470–482.

Scales, P. C., Benson, P. L., Moore, K. A., Lippman, L., Brown, B., & Zaff, J. F. (2008). Promoting equal developmental opportunity and outcomes among America's children and youth: Results from the National Promises Study. *Journal of Primary Prevention, 29*(2), 121–144.

Schmittmann, V. D., Visser, I., & Raijmakers, M. E. J. (2006). Multiple learning modes in the development of performance on a rule-based category learning task. *Neuropsychologia, 44,* 2079–2091.

Schor, E. L. (2007). The future pediatrician: Promoting children's health and development. *Journal of Pediatrics, 151*(5 Suppl), S11–S16.

Schultz-Krohn, W. (2004). The meaning of family routines in a homeless shelter. *American Journal of Occupational Therapy, 58*(5), 531–542.

Schumacher, K. L., & Meleis, A. I. (1994). Transitions: A central concept in nursing. *Image: Journal of Nursing Scholarship, 26*(2), 119–127.

Segal, R. (2004). Family routines and rituals: A context for occupational therapy interventions. *American Journal of Occupational Therapy, 58*(5), 499–508.

Seligman, M., & Darling, R. B. (1997). *Ordinary families, special children. A systems approach to childhood disability* (2nd ed.). New York, NY: Guilford Press.

Sharpe, D., & Rossiter, L. (2002). Siblings of children with a chronic illness: A meta-analysis. *Journal of Pediatric Psychology, 27*(8), 699–710.

Shields, L., Pratt, J., & Hunter, J. (2006). Family centred care: A review of qualitative studies. *Journal of Clinical Nursing, 15*(10), 1317–1323.

Slota, M., Shearn, D., Potersnak, K., & Haas, L. (2003). Perspectives on family-centered, flexible visitation in the intensive care unit setting. *Critical Care Medicine, 31*(5 Suppl), S362–S366.

Sorkhabi, N. (2005). Applicability of Baumrind's parent typology to collective cultures: Analysis of cultural explanations of parent socialization effects. *International Journal of Behavioral Development, 29,* 552–563.

Starchild Abraham Cherrix v. Commonwealth of Virginia, for the County of Accomack. (2006). Juvenile and Domestic Relations District Court. Retrieved July 28, 2008, from http://www.oag.state.va.us/LEGAL_LEGIS/CourtFilings/AbrahamCherrixAmicusJuly252006.pdf

Stein, M. T., & Perrin, E. L. (1998). Guidance for effective discipline. American Academy of Pediatrics. Committee on psychosocial aspects of child and family health. *Pediatrics, 101*(4 pt 1), 723–728.

Stein, R. E., Bauman, L. J., Westbrook, L. E., Coupey, S. M., & Ireys, H. T. (1993). Framework for identifying children who have chronic conditions: The case for a new definition. *Journal of Pediatrics, 122*(3), 342–347.

Steinberg, L. (2001). We know some things: Parent-adolescent relationships in retrospect and prospect. *Journal of Research on Adolescence, 11*(1), 1–19.

Steinberg, L., Dornbusch, S. M., & Brown, B. B. (1992). Ethnic differences in adolescent achievement. An ecological perspective. *American Psychologist, 47*(6), 723–729.

Steinberg, L., Lamborn, S. D., Dornbusch, S. M., & Darling, N. (1992). Impact of parenting practices on adolescent achievement: Authoritative parenting, school involvement, and encouragement to succeed. *Child Development, 63*(5), 1266–1281.

Sullivan-Bolyai, S., Sadler, L., Knafl, K. A., & Gilliss, C. L. (2003). Great expectations: A position description for parents as caregivers: Part I. *Pediatric Nursing, 29*(6), 457–461.

Szilagyi, P. (2012). Health insurance and children with disabilities. *The Future of Children, 22*(1). 123–148.

Tapp, D. M. (2000). The ethics of relational stance in family nursing: Resisting the view of "nurse as expert." *Journal of Family Nursing, 6*(1), 69–91.

Thomas, R. M. (2005), *Comparing theories of child development* (6th ed.). Belmont, CA: Wadsworth.

Underwood, M. K., Beron, K. J., & Rosen, L. H. (2009). Continuity and change in social and physical aggression from middle childhood through early adolescence. *Aggressive Behavior, 35*(5), 357–375.

Urrutia-Rojas, X., Egbuchunam, C. U., Bae, S., Menchaca, J., Bayona, M., Rivers, P. A., & Singh, K. P. (2006). High blood pressure in school children: Prevalence and risk factors. *BMC Pediatrics, 6,* 32.

U.S. Census Bureau. (2008). Nearly half of children receive care from relatives. [Press release, February 28]. Retrieved July 2008 from http://www.census.gov/population/www/socdemo/childcare.html and http://www.census.gov/Press-Release/www/releases/archives/children/011574.html

U.S. Code of Federal Regulations. (2006). Title 42—The Public Health and Welfare, Chapter 67: Child abuse prevention and treatment and adoption reform. Last amended 2006. Retrieved July 24, 2008, from http://www4.law.cornell.edu/uscode/html/uscode42/usc_sup_01_42_10_67.html

U.S. Department of Education. (2004). Individuals with Disabilities Education Improvement Act of 2004. Retrieved June 2008 from http://www.nichcy.org/reauth/PL108-446.pdf

U.S. Department of Health and Human Services, Administration for Children and Families, Administration on Children. (2011). Child maltreatment 2011: Key summary findings. Retrieved from https://www.childwelfare.gov/pubs/factsheets/canstats.pdf

U.S. Department of Health and Human Services, Administration on Children, Youth and Families. (2005). *Child maltreatment 2003.* Washington, DC: U.S. Government Printing Office. Retrieved July 31, 2008, from http://nccanch.acf.hhs.gov/index.cfm

U.S. Department of Labor, Bureau of Labor Statistics. (2011). Women in the labor force: A databook (2010 edition). Retrieved from http://www.bls.gov/cps/wlf-databook- 2011.pdf

Van Cleave, J., Heisler, M., Devries, J. M., Joiner, T. A., & Davis, M. M. (2007). Discussion of illness during well-child care visits with parents of children with and without special health care needs [see comment]. *Archives of Pediatrics & Adolescent Medicine, 161*(12), 1170–1175.

Van Waning, N. R., Kleiber, C., & Freyenberger, B. (2005). Pediatric care. Development and implementation of a protocol for transfers out of the pediatric intensive care unit. *Critical Care Nurse, 25*(3), 50–55.

Vazirani, S., Hays, R. D., Shapiro, M. F., & Cowan, M. (2005). Effect of a multidisciplinary intervention on communication and collaboration among physicians and nurses [see comment]. *American Journal of Critical Care, 14*(1), 71–77.

Wang, K. K., & Barnard, A. (2004). Technology-dependent children and their families: A review. *Journal of Advanced Nursing, 45*(1), 36–46.

Washington, A., & Dunham, M. (2011). Early parenting practices and outcomes for adolescents. *Educational Research Quarterly, 35*(2), 43–75.

Wells, D. K., James, K., Stewart, J. L., Moore, I. M., Kelly, K. P., Moore, B., . . . Speckhart, B. (2002). The care of my child with cancer: A new instrument to measure caregiving demand in parents of children with cancer. *Journal of Pediatric Nursing, 17*(3), 201–210.

Williams, K. E., Ciarrochi, J., & Heaven, P. C. (2012). Inflexible parents, inflexible kids: A 6-year longitudinal study of parenting style and the development of psychological flexibility in adolescents. *Journal of Youth and Adolescence, 41,* 1053–1066.

Wofford, L. G. (2008). Systematic review of childhood obesity prevention. *Journal of Pediatric Nursing, 23*(1), 5–19.

Wong, M. G., & Heriot, S. A. (2008). Parents of children with cystic fibrosis: How they hope, cope and despair. *Child: Care, Health and Development, 34*(3), 344–354.

Wright, L. M., & Leahey, M. (1999). Maximizing time, minimizing suffering: The 15-minute (or less) family interview. *Journal of Family Nursing, 5*(3), 259–274.

Youngblade, L. M., Theokas, C., Schulenberg, J., Curry, L., Huang, I. C., & Novak, M. (2007). Risk and promotive factors in families, schools, and communities: A contextual model of positive youth development in adolescence. *Pediatrics, 119*(Suppl 1), S47–S53.

Zawistowski, C. A., & Frader, J. E. (2003). Ethical problems in pediatric critical care: Consent. *Critical Care Medicine, 31* (5 Suppl), S407–S410.

Zigler, E., Pfannenstiel, J., & Seitz, V. (2008). The parents as teachers program and school success. A replication and extension. *Journal of Primary Prevention, 29,* 103–120.

Zuckerman, B., Parker, S., Kaplan-Sanoff, M., Augustyn, M., & Barth, M. C. (2004). Healthy Steps: A case study of innovation in pediatric practice. *Pediatrics, 114*(3), 820–826.

chapter 14

Family Nursing in Acute Care Adult Settings

Vivian Tong, PhD, RN

Joanna Rowe Kaakinen, PhD, RN

Critical Concepts

- Families who are viewed as part of the health care team are empowered to deal with the stressors of a family member's hospitalization, and are prepared to provide support, aid in recovery, or facilitate a comfortable death.

- Supportive actions by family members, as well as conflict and criticism, have an effect on the patients' health behaviors, emotional well-being, immune function, and illness exacerbations.

- During the acute illness phase, nursing interventions should focus on patients and their families by providing physical care and emotional support, facilitating family communication, providing timely information, and establishing a collaborative, trusting partnership.

- Family nursing is the provision of care to the entire family unit and is an integral aspect of care provided by nurses in adult acute care settings.

- Unit or hospital policies need to be updated so that patient-identified family members are not excluded. Restricted, nonflexible visitation policies add stress and trauma for both the patient and the patient's loved ones.

- Transferring loved ones from critical care units to the medical-surgical units is stressful for families because it creates a sense of conflict. On one hand, families are glad their loved ones are better, but they also worry that their family members may not be ready to be moved out of such intensive nurse watchfulness.

- The family member who advocates for a loved one in the hospital assumes a difficult, time-consuming, and fatiguing role: he or she often travels long distances to get to the hospital, takes time off work to be there, often stays all night in the hospital, manages the informational needs of the patient and the family, and works through a complex health care system.

- Effective communication with patients, families, and interdisciplinary health care providers improves client satisfaction, promotes positive response to care, reduces length of stay in care settings, and results in decreased overall cost and resource utilization.

- Compassionate communication provides crucial care to families as they are asked to make multiple decisions as their loved one dies in the hospital.

The family is the core of the social environment for most individuals and serves as the foundation for social support during health and illness (Gallant, Spitz, & Prohaska, 2007). Family nursing is the provision of care to the entire family unit and is an integral aspect of care provided by nurses in adult acute care settings. Hospitalization for an acute illness, injury, or exacerbation of a chronic illness is stressful for patients and their families. The ill adult enters the hospital usually in a physiological crisis, and the family most often accompanies the ill or injured family members into the hospital; both the patient and the family are usually in an emotional crisis (Kosco & Warren, 2000). Hospitalized family members worry about the effects of their illness and their potentially changed capabilities on the rest of their family members (Perry, Lynam, & Anderson, 2006). The family members also worry about their loved ones, sometimes to the extent of being neglectful of their own needs (Perry et al., 2006). When nurses provide care for the whole family, this allows families to be more supportive of their ill members, to experience less anxiety, and to have less disruption in the family system (Davidson, 2009; Nelms & Eggenberger, 2010). Involving family members in intervention strategies strengthens family relationships and enhances the effects of the interventions (Cypress, 2011; Gooding, Pierce, & Flaherty, 2012; Gutierrez, 2012; Nelms & Eggenberger, 2010; Shelton, Moore, Socaris, Gao, & Dowling, 2010). Close social relationships, especially family relationships, affect physical and psychological well-being, and promote adherence to disease management plans that involve changes in health behavior. When families are involved in the care of the loved one in the hospital, the patient has an increased likelihood of positive health outcomes (Gooding et al., 2012; Martire, Lustig, Schulz, Helgeson, & Miller, 2007).

Since the late 1970s, progress to move to a more family-centered care model in adult critical care and medical-surgical nursing has been slow but steady (Latour & Haines, 2007). Families with members who are acutely or critically ill are seen in adult medical-surgical units, intensive care or cardiac care units, or emergency departments. The acute phase of illness or injury refers to the period immediately after the onset of the illness or the injury. During this time, family members want to be able to ask the following questions about their family members who are ill or injured: Are they doing as well as can be expected? Are they getting any better? Are they in any pain? Has there been any change? What can I expect in the future? These questions may be expressed in thousands of different ways but stem from the common concern that they fear for their loved one's well-being. Having loved ones in today's acute care hospital can be an upsetting experience at any time, but when a stay in an adult critical care unit occurs (anticipated or not), it can be especially traumatic (Alvarez & Kirby, 2006; Kentish-Barnes & Azoulay, 2012). Family members and significant others of critically ill patients are integral to the recovery of their loved ones (Molter, 1979, 1994; Pearce, 2005).

The purpose of this chapter is to describe family nursing in acute care settings, including families in the critical care units and medical-surgical units. A review of literature captures the major stressors families face during hospitalization of an adult family member: the transfer from one unit to another, being discharged home, participation in cardiopulmonary resuscitation (CPR), withdrawing life support therapy, and organ donation. This chapter concludes with a family case study that (1) highlights the issues families experience and adapt to when an adult member is ill; and (2) applies the Family Assessment and Intervention Model in order to demonstrate one theoretical approach for working with families.

FAMILIES IN CRITICAL CARE UNITS

The American College of Critical Care Medicine Task Force (2004–2005) developed 43 evidence-based practice guidelines for supporting and involving family in intensive care units (ICUs) (Davidson et al., 2007). These guidelines address topics such as the "endorsement of a shared decision-making model, early and repeated care conferencing to reduce family stress and improve consistency in communication, honoring culturally appropriate requests for truth-telling and informed refusal, spiritual support, staff education and debriefing to minimize the impact of family interactions on staff health, family presence at both rounds and resuscitation, open flexible visitation, way-finding and family-friendly signage, and family support before, during, and after a death" (Davidson et al., 2007, p. 605). This section presents evidence-based practice on family nursing in critical care units, specifically addressing family needs when a member is in the ICU: visiting policies, waiting rooms, family interventions in the ICU, and ways to work with families to decrease family relocation stress and transfer anxiety.

Family Needs in the ICU

Family visitors in ICUs report and demonstrate symptoms of anxiety or depression after having their family members in the ICU for a few days (Pouchard et al., 2005). In addition, family members were at significant risk for development of post-traumatic stress disorder (PTSD) when they had family members in the ICU (Azoulay et al., 2005). The needs of family members with loved ones in the ICU have long been studied (Paul & Rattray, 2008). The classic work of Molter in 1974 first identified the following 10 family needs in the intensive care unit, listed in descending order:

1. Hope
2. Health care provider caring about the patient
3. Having a waiting room near the patient
4. Being called at home for a change in patient condition
5. Knowing about the prognosis
6. Having questions answered honestly
7. Knowing specific facts about prognosis
8. Receiving information about patient once a day
9. Having explanations in understandable terms
10. Seeing patient frequently

Warren developed the Critical Care Family Needs Inventory (CCFNI) based on this work by Molter. The CCFNI has been demonstrated to be a valid and reliable instrument to assess family needs (Paul & Rattray, 2008). It collapsed family needs into three categories: assurance, proximity, and information.

What is crucial for nurses to know about this research is that health care settings have been only partially responsive to the needs of families for information or assurance. Table 14-1 illustrates that, although nurses are providing more information to family members and that families can see their loved ones more frequently, nurses are not providing reassurance to family members or meeting the needs that families identify as important to their own health and well-being (Browning & Warren, 2006).

Kinrade, Jackson, and Tomnay (2009) used the CCFNI in an ICU with no restriction on visiting hours to determine family needs and found that the most important family need was to have questions answered honestly and for information to be shared in a timely manner. A study by Douglas, Daly, and Lipson (2012) found that patient quality of life

Table 14-1	**Family Needs in the Intensive Care Unit**

Family Needs Always/Usually Met	**Family Needs Never/Sometimes Met**
• Informed about medical treatments	• Need explanations in lay terminology
• Aware of why and what care is being provided	• Need to have access to quality food in the hospital
• Knows somewhat about the prognosis	• Assured it is okay to leave the hospital for a while
• Allowed to visit in the intensive care unit (ICU) frequently	• To be prepared for the ICU environment before entering the unit the first time
• Understands different types of staff caring for family member	• Talk to the same nurse every day
• Knows who to call in the ICU for information	• Have feeling of hope supported
• Given directions for things to do at bedside while visiting	• Share feelings, especially those of guilt, anger, or fear
• Called at home for condition changes	• Feel accepted by the hospital staff
• Has support of friends and family	• Discuss the possibility that family member may die
• Knows what is being done for their family member	• Visit anytime

Adapted from Browning, G., & Warren, N. (2006). Unmet needs of family members in the medical intensive care waiting room. *Critical Care Nursing Quarterly, 29*(1), 86–95.

rarely was discussed with families when a loved one had a long stay in the ICU. Families with a member who had unexpected admissions to the ICU were noted to have different needs than families who had planned admissions. When a patient has an uncertain prognosis from a stay in the critical care unit, family needs were found to be different than when the prognosis was favorable (Prachar et al., 2010). Family members who were dealing with a poor prognosis expressed a need to talk about their feelings of what happened and wanted a pastor to visit (Prachar et al., 2010).

Overall, families reported that they had two different sets of feelings when a family member was in the ICU (Eriksson, Bergbom, & Lindahl, 2011). First, families expressed that they fluctuated between hope and despair. They felt that information was a way to help them manage these feelings (Eriksson et al., 2011). Second, families reported that they hungered for information to help them make sense of what was happening and described themselves as being hypervigilant to even the smallest information. The most helpful aspect of the whole experience was their interaction with the staff (Eriksson et al., 2011). Families want authentic connection with nurses who are caring for their loved ones (Nelms & Eggenberger, 2010), and communication is the center of family experiences in the critical care unit. The family depends on the whole critical care team to provide care and keep it informed so it can make crucial decisions for loved ones (Kentish-Barnes & Azoulay, 2012).

Families are the primary support for loved ones in the ICU (Verhaeghe, Defloor, Van Zuuren, Duijnstee, & Grypdonck, 2005; Williams, 2005). Patients reported knowing that their family was at their bedside and this supported their desire to get well (Eriksson et al., 2011). Families have been found to experience cognitive, emotional, and social stress when family members are in the ICU. These worries include:

- Information ambiguity
- Uncertain prognosis
- Fear of death
- Role changes
- Financial concerns
- Disruption of normal routines

Nursing Role Ambiguity and Conflict

ICU nurses are in the best position to support these families because they see them often, know the patient intimately, and are called to practice holistically instead of based on a biomedical model. Yet, many ICU nurses continue to view families as obstacles to care and consistently underestimate their professional role in meeting the needs of these families (Verhaeghe et al., 2005). What ICU nurses believe families need does not always match what families identify as their needs (Kinrade et al., 2009; Maxwell, Stuenkel, & Saylor, 2007; Prachar et al., 2010). Therefore, it is important to explore why this dichotomy continues to exist given the evidence that has been known since Molter's work was published in 1974.

Stayt (2007) investigated nurses' perceptions of their ability to practice family nursing in the ICU. Two important findings in this research offer an insight into understanding these nurses' experiences: nurses express role ambiguity and role conflict. Role ambiguity is when nurses find themselves with an unrealistic role expectation. The nurses were found to believe that it was their responsibility to "make it right" or to "take away the family members' worries" rather than to provide emotional support for families dealing with the uncertainty of outcome for a family member in the ICU. The nurses expressed that they felt guilty for not helping families. The nurses undervalued their contribution to meeting the family needs during this stressful time. Nurses identified that they felt they lacked training in how to work with families.

Moreover, ICU nurses identified two types of role conflict (Stayt, 2007). The first role conflict was difficulty in balancing the biomedical technical model of care with the holistic nursing model of care. Chesla (1997) reports a similar role conflict for ICU nurses between technical care and social-emotional care. Nurses are torn between caring for the medically unstable patient, who is their priority, yet recognizing that they are responsible for caring for the entire family. The second type of role conflict was the balance of their professional relationship and the more personal relationship the family seeks with the nurse (Stayt, 2007). The nurse-family relationship is established during an intense emotional time for the family. After a period of time, the family was described as seeking too much self-disclosure from the nurses. Nurses found keeping professional boundaries fatiguing and time-consuming. Therefore, the nurses described that they used detachment strategies to keep their relationship professional. For example, they would ask for a different patient assignment. Or nurses would physically distance themselves by focusing only on tasks when they entered the patient's room. They found ways to limit conversation with the family. They found themselves emotionally distancing themselves from the family so they would not engage on a personal level.

Nurses recognized the importance of families and wanted to work with them in the ICU, but they found it difficult to provide for the emotional needs of family members. Hospital educational programs are needed to support nurses in providing family-centered care versus patient-centered care. Communication with families can be learned and practiced in the ICU environment (White & Curtis, 2006).

Visiting Policy

Most ICUs (70%) have visitation policies to the ICU that restrict visitors (American Association of Critical Care Nurses [AACN] Practice Alerts, 2012). Yet the evidence is clear that unrestricted visitation decreases patient anxiety, confusion, and agitation; reduces cardiovascular complications; decreases ICU length of stays; makes patients feel more secure; increases patient satisfaction; and enhances quality and safety (AACN Practice Alerts, 2012, p. 76). Moreover, evidence suggests that unrestricted visitation increases family satisfaction, decreases family member anxiety, promotes better communication, contributes to better understanding of the patient, allows more opportunities for patient/family teaching as the family becomes more involved in care, and is not associated with longer family visits (AACN Practice Alerts, 2012, p. 76). The AACN suggests that there are times when family visits should be restricted: documented legal reasons, when a visitor has a communicable disease, or if the behavior of a visitor is a direct risk to the patient. AACN (2012) recommends that children supervised by an adult family member should be welcome in the ICU and should not be restricted by age alone.

Unit or hospital policies may need to be updated so that patient-identified family members are not excluded (Harvey, 2004; Rushton, Reina, & Reina, 2007). Such administrative revisions need to take into consideration evidence-based data so that both nursing staff and families can be confident that patient care systems reflect these visionary professional standards even when patients cannot speak for themselves (Latour & Haines, 2007; Verhaeghe et al., 2005).

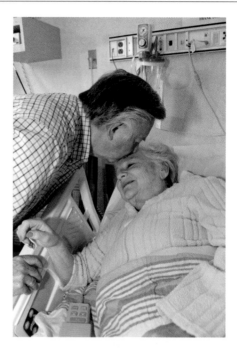

Debate over the "correct" quantity and frequency of visits in adult critical care units continues into the 21st century (Day, 2006; Miracle, 2005). Policies that have been tried and often revisited have included 10 minutes every hour, 30 minutes several times a day, two visitors at a time, immediate family only, open visiting, closed visiting with rare exceptions, and many more versions of all of the above. These restrictions often are in place because health professionals feel that having visitors interrupts patient care and also may affect the patient's well-being. But research has shown otherwise. Here are some specifics. Fumagalli et al. (2006) found that when cardiac patients had unrestricted visiting hours, these patients had fewer cardiovascular complications compared to those patients who were restricted to visitors twice a day. Liberal visiting hours not only helped patients, but benefited the staff. Family members served as historians, participated in daily rounds, and assisted with care. In addition, allowing visitors decreased unexpected calls, increased participation and engagement with staff, and increased patient and family satisfaction (Jacobowski, Girard, Mulder, & Ely, 2010). More important, unrestricted visitation reduced anxiety among patients and families (Garrouste-Orgeas et al., 2008; Gooding et al., 2012).

Professional nursing organizations, such as the American Association of Critical Care Nurses

(AACN) (mentioned above) and the American Nurses Association (ANA), have supported the position that, despite being in critical condition, patients cannot receive adequate care when they are isolated from their families (Bice-Stephens, 2006; Latour & Haines, 2007). The Joint Commission of Hospitals likewise recognizes the importance of visitation. In 2011, the Commission added an element to the Patient Rights Standard, which states that hospitals should permit friends and family members to be present during hospitalization in order to provide emotional support to the patient (Joint Commission on Accreditation of Healthcare Organizations, 2010). Based on scientific evidence, the American College of Critical Care Medicine also endorses more flexible visiting hours in the intensive care unit (Davidson et al., 2007). Families are foundational to the comprehensive care of all patients, so it is the responsibility of every nurse and every health care agency to implement and regularly evaluate visitation policies and procedures that reflect this philosophy (Pearce, 2005).

Cell Phones

Cell phones are an integral tool of our lives. Family members rely heavily on cell phones to remain connected to others (Eriksson et al., 2011). In many intensive care units, cells phones are banned because there is concern that these devices may emit electromagnetic radiation that interferes with the functioning of medical devices (Makic, VonRueden, Rauen, & Chadwick, 2011). But newer data and voice phones do not present these issues. Hospitals should consider assessing their policies on banning cell phones. Limiting the use of cell phones requires family members to leave and locate a designated cell phone area, which may be a challenge. Given that visiting hours and the number of guests allowed in the intensive care unit are restricted, family members may hesitate to leave the ICU to make phone calls considering the barriers for reentry. Reevaluating and updating cell phone policies is vital in promoting patient and family satisfaction.

Waiting Rooms

When families of critically ill patients are not in the unit with their loved ones, they are more than likely spending a significant amount of time in the unit's waiting room (Deitrick et al., 2005). Attention to the details that may help relieve family stress is critical. Little research has focused on family comfort and amenities provided in the waiting rooms adjacent to critical care units (Alvarez & Kirby, 2006). But families have consistently voiced desires to have better access to healthy food and drinks, a variety of comfortable seating options to account for all people, available computer access, and nearby rooms for private meetings with physicians, nurses, or other care providers. Families have expressed issues with the lack of privacy, since the waiting room is often shared with other families (Engstrom, Anderson, & Soderberg, 2008; Karlsson, Tissell, Engstrom, & Andershed, 2011). A room that is quiet and comfortable improves the well-being of family members (Karlsson et al., 2011). Many ICUs have been responsive to these expressed needs of families by providing a clean, organized waiting room area with several small seating sections for family conversations, adequate soft lighting, a section for computer work, private meeting rooms, and a special play area with age-appropriate toys for various children's ages. Some ICUs have dedicated sleeping rooms for family members. Providing a beeper system for the family to carry when they leave the unit or waiting room was found to be helpful to families (Deitrick et al., 2005). Receptionists in family waiting room areas are gaining in popularity (Alvarez & Kirby, 2006).

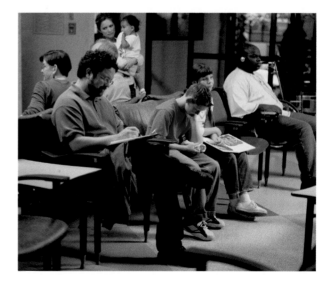

Family Interventions

Aside from open visitation policies, revisited cell phone policies, and improved waiting rooms, family intervention strategies that support both nurses and families include the following: helping family members feel as comfortable as possible while in the room with the patient, including families in the nurse-to-nurse shift change bedside report, including family members in the physician rounds when they discuss the progress of the patient, involving families in shared decision making, facilitating family conferences, offering families the opportunity to keep progress journals, and creating a family nurse specialist in the ICU (Gooding et al., 2012).

Families are often overwhelmed and intimidated with the fast-paced, noisy, and highly technological environments that surround their loved ones in the ICU (Pikka & Beaulieu, 2004). Patients appear "lost" among all the equipment, tubes, lines, beeping, and bonging sounds, especially when interventions such as dressings or indwelling tubes around the face and head distort facial features (Maxwell et al., 2007). ICU nurses who practice from a family perspective realize how their everyday world in this fast-paced, emotionally charged setting is stressful for families. After the patient is initially stabilized on admission to the ICU, the nurses should spend time explaining the equipment and the immediate goals of nursing care, and role modeling how family members can support their loved one, including how to touch the person. Nurses should address fear of all the equipment used in this setting. This approach is helpful to decrease family stress and builds on the knowledge that family members have a strong desire to be by their loved one, particularly when there is a change in the patient's condition. They want to be an integral part of the patient's care. Allowing families to participate in the actual care of their family members likewise has been found to offer reassurance, as well as a way for family members to contribute to their loved one's recovery (Alvarez & Kirby, 2006). Family members believe that being close to the patient is their obligation and is a sign of their commitment to the patient (Eggenberger & Nelms, 2007). Fear of "not being there" if something goes wrong reinforces family members' desire to be with the patient (Eggenberger & Nelms, 2007). Therefore, nurses must see and include families as an integral part of the patient's care.

Supporting the family is another important nursing intervention. Although the nurses' priority is to the patient, families also need support. Emotional stress rises when a family member is acutely ill and families suffer with the patient during illness and treatment. They have feelings of helplessness, sadness, and fear (Eggenberger & Nelms, 2007). Some express that their emotions fluctuate like a "roller coaster" (Linnarsson, Bubini, & Perseius, 2010, p. 3102). They attempt to control these emotions in order to be supportive to the patient and other members of the family. In addition, many families feel the need to be watchful and protective of the patient in order to shield the patient from the emotions of the illness (Eggenberger & Nelms, 2007; Karlsson et al., 2011). Families are gatekeepers of information as they protect and shield their loved ones from emotional turmoil related to the care and the illness (Burr, 1998). It is important that the nurse support the family members by connecting with them. Nurses should spend time, provide information (good and bad), be honest, share themselves, involve families in care, and acknowledge the emotional stress they are undergoing. Families do want and depend on nurses for social support (Eggenberger & Nelms, 2007; Engstrom & Soderberg, 2007; Fry & Warren, 2007; Karlsson et al., 2011). Because nurses provide 24-hour care, they are in the best position to identify and support families.

Families often say waiting in the ICU creates tremendous physical strain. Families stay long hours in the ICU just waiting. They wait for information, to see their loved ones, and for the next thing to happen. They try to manage their personal affairs from the hospital, commute back to their homes after a long day, and take care of the patient (Eggenberger & Nelms, 2007; Higgins, Joyce, Parker, Fitzgerald, & McMillan, 2007). Family members of patients in the ICU also have been found to be at increased risk for experiencing anxiety, depression, and PTSD (Azoulay et al., 2005; Pouchard et al., 2005). Nurses can reduce some of the strain by providing and seeking information for the family members, asking how they are doing, providing a quiet place for them to rest or sleep, and determining each day how much they wish to be involved in the patient's care (Cioffi, 2006).

Timed daily family rounds with nurses and physicians decreased family anxiety and increased communication (Cypress, 2012; Gooding et al., 2012; Mangram et al., 2005). Careful and consistent information can help mitigate fears. Patients and families gain a better understanding of the plan of care when they have the opportunity to verify information, ask questions, and share concerns when they are involved in nursing end-of-shift reports (Reinbeck & Fitzsimmons, 2013; Tobiano, Chaboyer, & McMurray, 2013). Involving families and patients fosters an environment of trust, mutual respect, and understanding (Reinbeck & Fitzsimmons, 2013). When away from the bedside and the stimulation of the ICU environment, family members are able to hear more clearly and accurately the explanations and answers to their questions and concerns. Therefore, nurses should plan to spend time (e.g., a short 10-minute conference) with families away from the patient's bedside on every shift. Plans for language interpreters should be made in advance.

Shared decision making is a collaborative process in which patients and providers make health care decisions together, weighing the medical evidence of various options and considering the patient's values. Shared decision making is crucial in the ICU because patients often cannot speak for themselves and many of the treatment options are highly invasive and may have a high mortality or morbidity component to them; therefore, most treatment decisions should be made from a family perspective (Douglas et al., 2012). Refer to Chapter 4 for detailed information on family shared decision making. Ahmann and Dokken (2012) outline the following strategies nurses could use to invite families into partnership and shared decision making:

■ Use "we" language that demonstrates a team approach.
■ Request specific help from a family member.
■ Encourage the family members to let the nurse know when they are confused by test results or what they are seeing or hearing.
■ Use whiteboards in the patient rooms that include who is in the room, phone numbers, and a place for family questions.
■ Give the family a journal in which to keep notes or write experiences.
■ Invite the family on rounds.

Family meetings or conferences help keep all members of the health care team, including the family, focused on the needs of the loved one and the family. In addition, family meetings help health care providers communicate among team members (Nelson, Walker, Luhrs, Cortez, & Pronovost, 2009). Unfortunately, family conferences that are not well planned in advance have hindered family learning where too many people were included, the agenda was too full, and there were time constraints (Paterson, Kieloch, & Gmiterek, 2001). The most important point made was that the health care providers should be sure not to dominate the discussion and should allow adequate time for the family to voice concerns and pose their questions. Nelson et al. (2009) designed a toolkit for family meetings in the ICU. The toolkit helps ensure that the meetings are efficient, effective, and give all parties time to be heard in directing client care. The guide for families includes the following elements (p. 626.e13):

1. Review what you know:
   ■ Are you clear about why the person was brought to the ICU and what the current medical problems are?
   ■ What is the plan for your loved one?
   ■ What treatment choices are available?
   ■ What medical decisions need to be made?
2. Concerns or worries
   ■ List what concerns you have about the current situation.
   ■ Identify what you are worried about the most given the current situation.
   ■ If the team could answer one thing for you today, what would that be?
3. If the patient can't talk to you or the team now, what would the patient say about what is happening now in her care? Bring any documents or papers such as a health care proxy or living will.

Encouraging families to keep a family progress journal (Kloos & Daly, 2008) or a computer family blog for extended family and friends decreased family anxiety. In their analysis of family progress journals, Kloos and Daly (2008) found the following top three family issues addressed: the family experiencing negative emotions about the physical appearance of their loved one in the ICU, the need for more regular communication about what was going on, and the worry about the pain their loved one was experiencing. The journals illustrated that families coped with their stress through their faith in God, support of family and friends, and seeing their loved one get better physically. Families wrote that the characteristics of the health care providers that were the most helpful to them were kindness, compassion, watchfulness over their loved one, and availability to answer questions.

To meet family needs, one idea was to design a specific nursing position to work with families. This approach allowed the ICU nurses to focus on providing care to the ill person and relieved some stress of providing care to the family client. Having this clinical nurse specialist in the ICU resulted in increased family satisfaction. These nurses assessed family unmet needs and relayed information that increased family understanding, especially about tests, treatments, and condition (Nelson & Poist, 2008; Shelton et al., 2010). Interestingly, the ICU nurses reported that they felt this position somewhat interfered with their work, and said that not working as much with the family was not as satisfying for them in the long run.

As patients improve to the point that they are stable enough to transfer out of the ICU, families experience different stressors related to relocation stress and anxiety (Chaboyer, Kendall, Kendall, & Foster, 2005).

Family Relocation Stress and Transfer Anxiety

Moving ill family members from the critical care unit to the medical-surgical unit is stressful for families. Even though families report relief that their loved ones are able to transfer out of the ICU, they also fear that the loss of one-to-one nurse-patient vigilance will lead to failure to detect important changes in condition (Chaboyer et al., 2005; Latour & Haines, 2007). Some families feel they were unprepared for the transfer and that they were given little information about what to expect (Hughes, Bryan, & Robbins, 2005). Families may interpret the transfer as someone throwing them out of the ICU (Engstrom & Soderberg, 2004).

Once the patient is transferred, families found that the nursing care on the medical-surgical unit is not as predictable as the ICU and families did not understand the different ratio of nurse-to-patient staffing patterns (Carr, 2002). Families also found the relocation stressful because they missed their relationship with the ICU nurses, and they struggled with changes in the environment, and the changes in the amount of information they received (Streator et al., 2001).

Chaboyer et al. (2005) classified the families' emotions with relocation stress into four emotions or feelings: abandonment, vulnerability, unimportance, and ambivalence. Families feel *abandonment* when the transfer is abrupt and not planned. Families describe experiencing *vulnerability* when they had to accept their new responsibility as a different kind of family caregiver within the hospital setting. For example, rather than be supportive family members from the background, they now had to provide more actual physical care for their loved one as physical status improved. Their sense of vulnerability was found to be the most intense of these family emotions. The families reported having a feeling of *unimportance* because of the different staffing ratio on the medical-surgical unit. The last feeling identified was *ambivalence*. The families expressed being caught between the extremes of feeling relieved and happy their loved ones were better, and their fears and doubts that they were well enough to leave the ICU.

Involving families in the transfer process effectively contributed to less relocation stress (Eldredge, 2004; Latour & Haines, 2007, McKinley, Nagy, Stein-Parbury, Bramwell, & Hudson, 2002). Family conferences scheduled with the health care team are a perfect opportunity for family members to express these concerns, and for team members to respond to all concerns with factual, straightforward information. Ideally, both the nurse manager and supervisor of the sending and receiving hospital units should participate in this transition. A detailed and comprehensive written patient care plan helps to smooth out this important phase of the patient and family journey (Day, 2006). Family input into this care plan empowers and reassures families during this transition to the medical-surgical unit.

FAMILIES IN MEDICAL-SURGICAL UNITS

It is clear that families who have adult members in acute medical surgical areas are stressed by hospitalization, yet this is one of the least studied areas of family nursing. In this section, family visitation, family communication needs, and family needs are explored. Family interventions relative to discharge are discussed.

Families in acute care settings reported numerous stressors and changes in their family environment, and are often desperately in need of support. Nurses are in a position to provide support in the following ways:

■ Use effective communication: listen to family's concerns, feelings, and questions; answer all questions or assist the family in finding the answers.
■ Respect and support family coping mechanisms and caregiving behaviors.
■ Recognize the uniqueness of each family.
■ Assist family in decision making by providing information about options.
■ Permit the family to make decisions about patient care when appropriate.
■ Provide adequate time to visit privately, when possible.
■ Facilitate family conferences to allow open sharing of family feelings.
■ Clarify information and share resources regarding support groups.
■ Foster positive nurse-family relationships through all phases of care.

Family Visitation and Caregiving in the Hospital

Visitation helps to promote family cohesion and unity (Van Horn & Kautz, 2007). Many of the same issues about family visitation in the intensive care unit described previously in the chapter hold true for family visitation on a medical-surgical inpatient setting.

Many families enact a bedside vigilance that provides a close protective function (Carr & Fogarty, 1999). Families displayed both *directive* behaviors and *supportive* behaviors as family caregivers in the hospital, especially when the hospitalized family member was older (Jacelon, 2006). Family *directive* behaviors were described as follows:

■ Acting in place of the ill family member by making decisions about care without consulting the ill family members, talking to health care providers, and being the organizer of care
■ Acting as an advisor to the ill family member by working collaboratively with him on decisions
■ Not acting in some cases; some family members were found to be available but did not become involved in any decision making

Family *supportive* behaviors identified by Jacelon (2006) were as follows:

■ Keeping the older family members going and active: families brought items from home, visited daily, and sometimes brought the family pet in for a visit.
■ Keeping the older family member's life going: they did many things "behind the scenes" such as running errands, paying bills, keeping up homes, and keeping friends informed.
■ Staying in the background: some family members were available but not actively involved in daily caregiving.

More specifically, families help their loved ones in the hospital in many ways that enhanced their care in hospitals (MacLeod, Chesson, Blackledge, Hutchison, & Ruta, 2005). On the other hand, health care providers on medical-surgical units did not always see families as partners in patient care in either the United States or the United Kingdom (MacLeod et al., 2005). As a result, families reported feeling unwelcome. Families have stated that gaining access to see their loved ones was a privilege, which was extended to them by the nurses, and that they were careful not to abuse the visiting rules. While in the patient's room, they were fearful of annoying the nurses by their constant presence (Cioffi, 2006). They avoided asking any personal or emotional questions (Soderstrom, Saveman, & Benzein, 2006). For them, they were guests of the patient, not partners in the care of the patient.

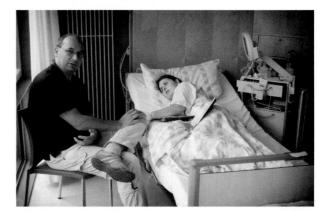

The work environment can be an obstacle to allowing medical-surgical nurses to provide family-centered care. The floor nurses often carry a heavy nurse-patient caseload. Many of these patients are of high acuity, which challenges these nurses with the same role conflict mentioned earlier: balancing technical needs of their patients and practicing holistic family-centered care. As a result of these work challenges, nurses may convey their stress to families and patients in unintended ways (Astedt-Kurki, Paavilainen, Tammentie, & Paunonen-Ilmonen, 2001; McQueen, 2000). Nurses may send unintended messages by saying something in casual conversation about how busy they were tonight, moving quickly and being in a hurry when they enter the room, and not addressing the family when they enter the room but instead being very procedure focused. Nurses can work on being sure their nonverbal, inadvertent communications match their concern and caring for the client. Taking a few moments to center oneself before entering the client's room allows the nurses to slow down and focus on the client and family in the room and not on what needs to be done in the busy day.

Communication with the family is crucial for the nurses, the patients, and the families in order to improve the patients' health outcomes. The placement of whiteboards in patient rooms is an increasingly common strategy used in hospital settings to improve communication. These boards, typically placed on a wall near a patient's hospital bed, allow any number of providers to communicate a wide range of information such as date of the day, the name of the nurse, aide, doctors on that shift, notes from loved ones to the ill person, phone numbers of the family to call in case of condition changes, patient-identified outcome goals for that specific day, questions for providers, and expected date of discharge (Sehgal, Green, Vidyarthi, Blegen, & Wachter, 2010). Including families in patient rounds with physicians and nurses helps to keep communication clear between providers and family members. Limiting the number of interruptions to the nurse while working with the patient and family would improve communication and send messages of importance to the family and patient (Darc, Lennon, & Sanders, 2013). Hospitals have moved to limited number of overhead pagers so that patients and families are not bombarded with noise and the workings of the facility. Proactively providing information to patients' families will reduce the number of interruptions for nurses. Some hospitals text families with updates on a family member that do not contain intimate details but are updated status reports (Darc et al., 2013).

Family Communication Needs

Effective communication between and with patients, families, and interdisciplinary health care providers improves client satisfaction, promotes positive response to care, reduces length of stay in care settings, and results in decreased overall cost and resource utilization (Ahrens, Yancey, & Kollef, 2003). Nurses believe that conveying information to families is essential when caring for both acute and chronically ill patients; at the same time, however, they reported refraining from doing so because they do not want to be "in the middle" or cause conflict between the family and the attending physician (Zaforteza, Gastaldo, de Pedro, Sánchez-Cuenca, & Lastra, 2005). It was found that nurses provide only basic information to family members and rarely attend to the families awaiting news in waiting rooms (Zaforteza et al., 2005). Nurses underestimate the needs of families, particularly the need for information and the need of family to be close to the patient (Higgins & Cadd, 1999; Kleinpell & Powers, 1992).

Nurses identified additional barriers to family communication that included the lack of perceived permission to share information and lack of knowledge regarding what information has already been shared with family members by the physician (Zaforteza et al., 2005). Nurses did not want to contradict physician information and expressed being worried about creating false hopes in the family. Nurses were concerned about families misinterpreting what was said because the nurses lacked training in managing family's emotional responses, especially when the family shared negative emotions. Thus, nurses as part of the interdisciplinary team were found to avoid communication needs of the patients and the families. Rather, nurses focused their communication efforts on the needs of the institution, other health professionals, and themselves (Hardicre, 2003; Zaforteza et al., 2005). Nurses must advocate more readily for sharing information with families. One way for nurses to advocate is to be sure to be present in the room and participate in physician family conferences. Nurses are in a position to help families understand what the physician means and they serve as a sounding board for the family. Nurses must learn to facilitate patient-family interaction and communication that will increase family support of patients at the bedside (Zaforteza et al., 2005). Clear, concise, timely information has been found to reduce family anxiety and have a calming effect (Mitchell, 2009; Zaforteza et al., 2005).

Assessment of patient care needs is integral to nursing and to providing optimal care at the bedside. It is essential to complete a thorough psychosocial and emotional evaluation to communicate effectively with patients and their families. In particular, nurses should explore each family's feelings about the uncertainty of the situation, anxiety, frustration, and fear of losing a family member (Chien, Chiu, Lam, & Ip, 2006; Zaforteza et al., 2005).

Communicating with families in an empathetic, timely, and sensitive manner is particularly effective to decrease tension, uncertainty, and distress (Zaforteza et al., 2005). Offering systematic, integrated, relevant information provides guidance to family members. Relevant information includes the nature of the illness, prognosis, treatment options, potential complications, care needs after discharge, and alternatives to continued treatment (Nelson, Kinjo, Meier, Ahmad, & Morrison, 2005). In addition, Chien et al. (2006) note the importance of communicating specific facts regarding a client's progress and expected outcomes, exploring family feelings including guilt and anger, informing family members of what was to be done for the client and why, and providing suggestions to families about actual care they could provide at the bedside to support the patient and help reduce family anxiety (Chien et al., 2006).

Family members find communication from a variety of providers to be worthwhile when health care providers are perceived as sensitive, unhurried, and honest, and use understandable language (Nelson et al., 2005). Furthermore, follow-up with written verification of information that was shared verbally at patient care conferences was found to be effective in promoting family coping (Kleiber, Davenport, & Freyenberger, 2006; Lautrette et al., 2007). Chien et al. (2006) have determined that conducting a family needs assessment and subsequent systematic education in response to identified issues is an effective means by which to facilitate both patient and family health.

Family-nurse communication is crucial during the hospital stay. Because families are key members of the health care team and will be the primary provider of care once the patient leaves the acute setting, addressing the family's educational and information needs is a critical part of the discharge process.

Family Needs During Discharge

Families and patients are excited about leaving the hospital. For some, however, it is a time when anxieties and uncertainties are high; families worry about their loved one not receiving the round-the-clock care available in the hospital. Adverse and poor outcomes are associated with poor transitions, specifically, with problems in continuity of care and caregiver burden (Coleman, Parry, Chalmers, & Minn, 2006). Readmission rates to hospitals were at an all time high, but have been noted in the last 2 years to have decreased slightly from 19% to 18.4% nationally. It is not clear what the cause of this improvement is (American Hospital Association, 2013). It is believed that approximately 75% of these readmissions may have been preventable (Medicare Payment Advisory Commission, 2009). Clearly, involving family in discharge planning is crucial for a smooth transition of care.

Families worry about adding the home caregiver role to their already overburdened load of family responsibilities. In fact, families coping with members with traumatic brain injuries reported forgetting what they were taught about what to expect, what resources were available to them, and experienced confusion in the home setting (Paterson et al., 2001). These families actually participated in extensive discharge planning and teaching, yet their severe anxiety inhibited their learning. The families told of not being able to hear the conversations during the care conferences, because they were so worried about how they were going to manage at home. Other families shared that they were so overwhelmed with the complexity of the situation and the health care system that they could not pay attention in the conferences (Paterson et al., 2001).

Nurses should facilitate discharge care conferences and help families transition smoothly to providing care in the home environment. In today's health care environment, families are often caring for very ill family members at home before they are fully recovered and ready to assume their normal family roles (Bjornsdottir, 2002; DesRoches, Blendon, Young, Scoles, & Kim, 2002). Families are providing nursing care at home that is traditionally done by nurses in the hospital, such as assisting with ambulation, transfer, wound care, medication administration, and, in some cases, operating high-tech equipment. Hooyman and Gonyea (1999) call this the "informalization of health care."

The importance in providing a comprehensive discharge plan cannot be overemphasized. Discharge planning should begin when the person is admitted to the acute care setting by anticipating and identifying the patient's continuing needs. A comprehensive plan should include, at minimum, the following: what to do when the person gets home, how to do it, and what to look for and do when a problem develops. In addition, the plan should include instructions about who will follow the care of the client in the outpatient setting and a follow-up appointment, if possible. The plan should also contain referrals to other care providers in advance of discharge. Review client management plans with families daily and update progress toward discharge with the family. Discuss possible needs the family will need to address in the home once the family members arrive there.

Given today's concern over health care costs, nurses can play a key role in helping patients maintain optimal health, and discharge planning is one key component. Interestingly, a study published in the *New England Journal of Medicine* (Jencks, Williams, & Coleman, 2012) found that about one-fifth (19.6%) of Medicare beneficiaries were readmitted to the hospital within 30 days of discharge and over one-third (34%) were readmitted within 90 days. About one-half (50.2%) of nonsurgical hospital patients who were readmitted within 30 days did not visit a physician. The study also found that when readmitted to the hospital, these patients stayed an average of 0.6 days (13.2%) longer than those patients admitted the first time for the same problem.

As the coordinator of care, nurses can facilitate the planning of care before the patient is discharged. Establishing guidelines so that every patient has a medical appointment before discharge is essential. Nurses can make sure that patients have the correct discharge medications and receive a sufficient amount to last them for a few days. Comparing discharge medications to those medications the patients normally take at home should be part of the discharge planning. It is not unusual for a patient's medication list at discharge to be different from the medication list before admission. Unfortunately, these changes often are not conveyed to the patient's primary doctors. Sometimes patients end up taking medications from both lists or they take duplicate medications because these medications have different brand names (Alonso-Zaldivar, 2012).

Recently, hospitals have been using transition coaches to help reduce hospital readmission by targeting population groups that have a higher hospital readmission rate. These programs vary but the central tenet is to begin discharge planning while the patient is hospitalized and continue with intensive postdischarge care. Often, nurses assume the role of the transition/hospital coach. Research has demonstrated that a multicomponent intervention program—which includes early assessment of the patient's discharge needs, enhanced patient education and counseling, and early postdischarge follow-up care—is associated with reduced readmissions, particularly among older patients and those with heart failure (Coleman et al., 2006; Osborne, 2011).

Family Interventions at Discharge

Follow-up conversations with families indicate that discharge by a nurse who has been trained in transition care helps support families (Coleman et al., 2004). One in four Medicare patients returns home with an unmet need for an existing or new activity of daily living (DePlama et al., 2012), which is known to increase readmission rates. Therefore, it is crucial that nurses work with patients and families not only to address the medical discharge regimen, but also to include education or resources for how to manage the new or existing activity of daily living need, such as dressing, cooking, toileting, transportation, eating, or mobility.

In fact, patient discharge is an area that has been studied for decades. It has come more into the spotlight with the current focus in the United States on reducing health care costs and client morbidity and mortality rates by reducing hospital readmission rates. Health care systems are creating transition care programs. As a part of these programs, one intervention is to have family care transition conferences, which entail discussion on the physical care of the patient, ways to assist the family to adjust to having an ill or recuperating family member at home, and barriers to providing care at home. Concepts to include in this discharge family conference are listed in Box 14-1. Other interventions include interprofessional follow-up teams, nurse navigators, and less formalized telephone and e-mail tracking.

In a concerted effort to reduce hospital readmission rates of high-risk adults—defined as ones being discharged on 10 or more medications, having three

---

BOX 14-1

Addressing Family Needs During Discharge Conference

It is important to talk about the physical care of the family member who is being discharged home and to work with the family on its specific needs. The following points are examples of items to cover with family at discharge:

- Discuss when the family member can be left alone and for how long.
- Help family set up an emergency call system.
- Discuss concerns about modifying the home environment.
- Facilitate setting up a family routine of care.
- Be sure the family knows when to call for help.
- Help the family learn to handle visitors, especially children.
- Talk about the balance of sleep and rest for the family caregivers.
- Provide names and numbers for personnel in the billing department for the family members to call when they start to receive insurance forms and hospital bills.

---

chronic illnesses, and having been hospitalized at least twice in the last year—researchers designed an intervention, that begins even before discharge, with a follow-up interprofessional team (Hospital Case Management, 2013a). The team discusses the case and different members work to ensure that by discharge, clients and family members understand their medications, have follow-up appointments, and order any post–acute care services. The team makes follow-up phone calls to discuss care and any concerns for up to 30 days after discharge. Outcomes of this intensive program are still being determined; it is a future step in helping families care for loved ones in the home.

Specifically, nurses conducting a follow-up care phone call should address the following information:

- The client's health status since discharge and any changes that may have occurred
- Whether or not the client is taking medications correctly or following the recommendations for care correctly
- The need for, or the status of, follow-up visits
- What to do when or if a problem arises

The nurse should thoroughly document the call.
Another intervention to help adults and families in the acute care setting is the creation of a position

termed *nurse navigator*. Nurse navigators are educated in a specific area of nursing and in the hospital system, such as working with clients who have heart failure or working with clients who have cancer. They meet with patients and families, conduct client and family education, advocate on their behalf by helping ensure clear communication between the client/family and their health care team, conduct medication reconciliation, and help them transition from one setting to another, such as arranging for home visits with community health nurses (Aston, 2013). Some nurse navigators work closely with families and clients in clinic or physician offices and follow clients and families into inpatient settings and back home (Case Management Advisor, 2013).

The San Francisco Medical Center experienced a 46% drop in its readmission rates for heart failure patients over 3 years when it instituted a multipronged approach to working closely with patients and family during hospitalization and follow-up after discharge (Hospital Case Management, 2013b). Two nurse coordinators (navigators) met with clients and families for approximately 15 to 20 minutes each day during hospitalization to ensure that they understood their care needs and to work on discharge education. They followed up with families and clients via phone calls. In addition, they redesigned their patient educational materials from a health literacy perspective.

Telephone and e-mail follow-up care provided by nurses have been found to improve treatment and outcomes by developing communication and education, improving symptom management, and assisting with early recognition of complications (Mistianen & Poot, 2006). A Cochrane systematic review of follow-up phone calls or e-mails to clients recommends that these interventions should, at a minimum, include knowledge about the illness; postoperative or medical complications; self-care, including behavioral and lifestyle changes; and psychosocial evaluation and emotional support (Furuya et al., 2013).

END-OF-LIFE FAMILY CARE IN THE HOSPITAL

A different type of transition that occurs in the hospital is from life to the death of a loved one. Regardless of whether the death occurs in the ICU, the emergency department, or on the medical-surgical unit, families are challenged by the death of a family member. For a detailed discussion of how to work with families in palliative and end-of-life care, refer to Chapter 10. This section is specific to working with adult patients and their families at the end of life in the acute hospital setting and includes discussion of advance directives, family-witnessed CPR, do not resuscitate orders and situations, withholding or withdrawing life sustaining procedures, and organ donation.

One main component of patient and family experience—and one with which many families have expressed dissatisfaction—of hospital end-of-life care is management of care before death. Factors contributing to dissatisfaction included patient suffering and pain and lack of communication with the family (Clark et al., 2003). Part of the reason for this dissatisfaction is that health care professionals, particularly nurses, are uncomfortable caring for and communicating with the dying patients. Nurses expressed discomfort when speaking with families and patients about death and felt ill-prepared in this task (Lloyd-Williams, Morton, & Peters, 2009). As a result, nurses tend to distance themselves from the patients and engage only in practical tasks, where they are most comfortable (Shorter & Stayt, 2010), thereby missing opportunities to facilitate interactions with the family (Curtis et al., 2005). Hospitals need to provide educational opportunities for nurses so they will have the knowledge and skills to plan and deliver end-of-life care (Efstathiou & Clifford, 2011).

Mixed messages pertaining to end-of-life issues commonly arise in the acute care setting. Patients and families hear and see numerous health care professionals. They receive conflicting and divergent information and opinions so that it is challenging for them to understand the care plan, thus compromising the quality of end-of-life care (Beckstrand & Kirchhoff, 2005). Because nurses spend the most time with the patient, they are instrumental in gathering the team players together to provide clarity for the patient and the family (Puntillo & McAdam, 2006). Identifying the needs of the patient and the family can help nurses direct end-of-life care. Researchers (Heyland et al., 2006) have found that patients and families have a number of similar needs, along with their own

individual needs. Both patients and families ranked three most common needs:

1. Trust and confidence in the doctors
2. Not to be kept alive on life support when there is little hope for a meaningful recovery
3. Information about the disease communicated by the doctor in an honest manner

Following these three common needs, the dying patients hoped to resolve conflicts and say goodbye to friends and family. For the family, the fourth major need was to find and obtain services to help them with patient care following discharge should the patient be allowed to go home to die (Heyland et al., 2006).

Informing family members about what is most important to the dying patient requires communication between these two groups, and nurses can be instrumental in facilitating these discussions. For example, families sometimes prefer not to tell the patient she is dying because they fear that the patient will lose hope. Yet patients want to resolve personal issues before they die (Heyland et al., 2006). Therefore, it is important to assess the personal wishes of the dying patient and to facilitate open discussion between the patient and the family members. Compassionate communication provides crucial care to families as they are asked to make multiple decisions during the dying of their loved ones in the hospital. The more the nurse knows about the family, the better. The way a family deals with death is affected by cultural background, stage in the family life cycle, values and beliefs, and nature of the illness. Whether the loss is sudden or expected, the role played by the dying person in the family and the emotional functioning of the family before the illness also influence the family needs and reactions to the situation (Artinian, 2005).

Offering and providing emotional support to families of dying patients is one way of meeting the needs of the family. Being at the bedside, providing comfort, and offering a listening ear demonstrate that families are not dealing with the grieving process alone (Bach, Ploeg, & Black, 2009). Providing for privacy allows families emotional and physical intimacy. Of utmost concern to family members is to be reassured that the nurse is keeping their loved one comfortable, as pain free as possible, and is continuing to provide comfort nursing care (Artinian, 2005). Keeping the family informed through anticipatory guidance of the physical signs and symptoms they are likely to see is important. Giving family members the option to be present or excused during the actual death is compassionate caring. Ask the family members whether they have any special spiritual or religious rituals and ceremonies that need to be conducted at this time. For many families, spirituality provides immense comfort while for the patient, it is an essential element in creating a peaceful death (Kruse, Ruder, & Martin, 2007). Most hospitals have various religious services available that can be called in to help the dying patient and their family. After the death, it is important to allow enough time for questions, allow the family the opportunity to view the body, and describe the events at the time of death (Artinian, 2005). Offering families the choice to participate in after-life preparations, such as bathing the body, is providing culturally sensitive care.

Caring for families when a member is dying is not easy. It is challenging for nurses to help families cope. Rarely do nurses in most acute care settings feel comfortable and confident discussing death with patients or families. Several issues are especially difficult for nurses and families, and are covered in more detail below.

Advance Directives

The Patient Self-Determination Act passed in 1991 in the United States requires hospitals to ensure that patients have been informed of their right to decide whether or not, and to what degree, to participate in life-preserving measures (Artinian, 2005). This legislation stimulated a host of documents related to end-of-life choices, such as advance directives, living wills, durable power of attorney for health care, do not resuscitate (DNR) orders, and physician orders for life-sustaining treatment (POLST). Box 14-2 defines each of these documents. Despite this legislation, the actual completion rate of such directives among the U.S. population remains low, with an average completion rate of 20% (Duke, Thompson, & Hastie, 2007; Ko & Lee, 2013).

When queried as to why people did not complete advance directives either before or at the beginning of a hospital stay, many state that they find talking about their own mortality difficult (Golden, Corvea, Dang, Llorente, & Silverman, 2009). The barriers to completion that have been identified by individuals and families also include lack of knowledge, confusing language, complexity of process, and procrastination (Butterworth, 2003). Moreover, the timing of completion of

---

BOX 14-2
Documents Related to End-of-Life Choices

Advance directive: A legal document that a competent person completes. It specifies instructions regarding medical care preferences regarding interventions or medical treatments, such as termination of life support or organ donation, the individual would like in the event he or she is incompetent to make such decisions. The purpose is to reduce confusion and disagreement. Typically, the advance directive includes the name of the person who is the durable power of attorney for health care.

Living will: A legal document that specifically outlines medical treatments and interventions that the person does or does not want administered when the person is terminally ill or in a coma and is unable to communicate personal desires.

Durable power of attorney for health care: A legal document that designates an individual to act as a health care proxy or agent, to make medical decisions in the event that a person is not able to communicate his or her own choices or make his or her own decisions.

Do not resuscitate (DNR) order: A request not to have cardiopulmonary resuscitation in the event one's heart stops. This order may or may not be part of an advance directive or living will. A physician can put this order in a client's chart for that person.

Physician orders for life-sustaining treatment (POLST): A form (not a legal document) that states what kind of medical treatment patients want toward the end of their life. It is signed by both the patient and the doctor or nurse practitioner. This form documents the end-of-life conversation between the patient and his or her health care provider. POLST gives seriously ill patients more control over their end-of-life care. It is typically written on bright-colored (pink) paper.

advance directives on admission to the hospital is fraught with emotion and distraction (Johnson, Zhao, Newby, Granger, & Granger, 2012). In addition, culture has been found to be a barrier to the completion of advance directives (Volandes, Ariza, Abbo, & Paasche-Orlow, 2008).

Of those individuals who completed advance directives, they reported doing so because they did not want to be a burden on their family at the time of death and because they had significant health problems over which they wanted to exercise some control (Duke et al., 2007). A signed advance directive implies that families have engaged in discussions about end-of-life choices. These families reported experiencing less of a burden when faced with making end-of-life decisions (Kaufman, 2002). Patients who have family members involved in their care in the hospital were found to be more likely to have a DNR order written (Tschann, Kaufman, & Micco, 2003).

Although the ANA's Code of Ethics for Nurses contains provisions about every patient's right to self-determination (American Nurses Association, 2001), many nurses fail to discuss advance directives with their patients (Duke & Thompson, 2007). There could be several reasons for this failure. First, nurses have expressed that they need more education about the state laws that govern advance directives and both legal and ethical issues that surround advance directives (Duke & Thompson, 2007; Jezewski, Meeker, & Robillard, 2005). Jarr, Henderson, and Henley (1998) noted that there was a relationship between nurses' level of knowledge on advance directives and their comfort level in discussing this topic with their patients. Nurses who lacked knowledge were more likely to state that they did not discuss advance directives with their patients and that they did not view this task as part of their professional role. Second, nurses generally feel uncomfortable discussing death and dying with their patients. This can affect nurses' willingness to talk to patients about subject matters that relate to dying (Duke & Thompson, 2007; Stoeckle, Doorley, & McArdle, 1998). And third, many nurses in the acute care setting witnessed patients with advance directives having their expressed wishes overridden by physicians and/or family members (Duke & Thompson, 2007; Tammelleo, 2000). For these nurses, having an advance directive did not even guarantee that patients' wishes were going to be followed.

The studies above have implications for the nurse and the patient. Evidence-based practice requires that nurses assist patients in end-of-life decisions (Browning, 2006). Nurses can play a key role in providing information about advance directives and encouraging discussion between patients and families about end-of-life care (Kelley, Lipson, Daly, & Douglas, 2006). Sometimes a patient may not be willing to talk about death, but the nurse can broach this topic by asking the patient her thoughts about the future. This may help the patient talk about her wishes (Gamble, 2008).

Nurses can also clarify and review treatment options as well as discuss when these may be initiated and when they could be discontinued. Other possible topics that may be a concern for the patient include feeding, hydration, ventilator support, pain management, and resuscitation measures (Ryan & Jezewski, 2012). The nurse should encourage other members of the health team to provide clarity in finalizing patients' advance directives (Haras, 2008). These team members may include the social worker, the chaplain, the psychologist, and/or the physician.

Family Presence During Cardiopulmonary Resuscitation

For many years it was standard practice of both ICUs and emergency departments that family members be removed from the bedside during periods of cardiac arrest, and emergent and invasive procedures. That trend is gradually changing. An increasing number of critical care units and emergency departments allow (but do not put pressure on) family members to remain present at the patient's bedside no matter what. This changing trend is due in large part to the work of clinical researchers who, after 20 years of research, have found that family presence does not disrupt patient care and actually results in positive outcomes for both family members and patients (Compton et al., 2011; Tweibell et al., 2008). The Emergency Nurses Association (2005) and the American Association of Critical Care Nurses (2004) have issued position papers calling for the establishment of written hospital policies and standards allowing for the option of family presence during invasive and resuscitation procedures in critical care units.

If family members wish to remain at or return to the bedside while resuscitation efforts are still ongoing, a nurse should be assigned who counsels and coaches families members, so that each person can anticipate exactly what he or she will see and hear (MacLean et al., 2003). It is possible to allow family members to be physically close to their loved one, so they can speak into an ear, as well as touch the person. Careful and often repeated explanations are necessary by the health care providers, because these are stressful and busy times for all present. Nurses need to be assessing continually how family members are coping and be prepared to intervene as necessary. Research has demonstrated that nurses are learning to provide more information and comfort to families and patients during times of invasive procedures, including resuscitation efforts (MacLean et al., 2003; Rushton et al., 2007).

Family Involvement in Do Not Resuscitate Orders

Handy, Sulmasy, Merkel, and Ury (2008) investigated the experience of surrogate decision makers—durable power of attorney or next of legal kin—who are involved in authorizing DNR orders. These individuals described this experience as a process, as a cascade of decisions and negotiations, not just a single decision not to resuscitate. One of the essential elements of this process was honest, sensitive, ongoing communication with the health care team. The surrogates reported a dichotomy of emotions about feeling guilty if they authorized the order and guilty if they did not authorize the order. In the end, the surrogates reported that knowing they were alleviating their loved one's pain was crucial in their decision making. The decision-making process of determining to authorize a DNR order has some similarity to the family decision whether to withdraw or withhold life-sustaining therapies.

A study of 122 women with gynecological cancers uncovered preferences for end-of-life choices. This study indicates that these women would like end-of-life discussions to occur as a routine part of their care, but they would like the discussion to be initiated by their providers (Díaz-Montes, Johnson, Giuntoli, & Brown, 2013). Patients report that they would like these discussions as they desire to have an opportunity to prepare for the end of their lives (Steinhauser et al., 2000). These end-of-life preparations included assigning someone to make decisions, arranging financial matters,

knowing what to expect as their health status declines, and preparing written preferences for management of their end-of-life care. The most important factors regarding end-of-life care to patients included trust in the treating physician, avoidance of unwanted life support, effective communication from the physician regarding disease status, and the ability to prepare for the end of life (Heyland et al., 2006).

Family Experiences of Withdrawing or Withholding Life-Sustaining Therapies

Families are intricately involved in the decisions to withdraw or withhold life-sustaining therapies (LSTs). These types of decisions are complex and occur in phases (Tilden, Tolle, Nelson, & Fields, 2001): (1) recognition of futility (that the survival was unlikely to occur), (2) coming to terms (that the person was likely going to die), (3) shouldering the surrogate role (accepting the responsibility for making decisions for their loved one), and (4) facing the question to withdraw or not withdraw LSTs (discussing and thinking about all the options surrounding stopping interventions that are sustaining their loved one's life). Factors that influenced families to withdraw LSTs were poor quality of life, poor overall prognosis, and current level of the family members' suffering (Wiegand, 2006). In families where there was a signed advance directive of some type or where previous conversations occurred about end-of-life choices, this difficult family decision was less of a burden.

Wiegand, Deatrick, and Knafl (2008) conducted research to describe the different family management styles when faced with making decisions about withdrawing or withholding LSTs. The five family management styles described are progressing, accommodating, maintaining, struggling, and floundering. Table 14-2 illustrates how families differ in their approach to making this crucial family decision. Families were found to vary in the following areas:

- Their level of understanding of the severity of their loved one's illness
- Their level of hope for recovery
- The tense (past, present, or future) with which they talked about their family member
- Their willingness to engage in a discussion about possibly withdrawing LSTs
- The overall family communication

Table 14-2   Family Management Styles for Family Decision to Withhold Life-Sustaining Therapies

Family Management Style	Severity of Condition Understood	Hope of Recovery	Verb Tense Used to Talk About Family Member	Willingness to Engage in Discussion of Withdrawal	Family Communication	Primary Factors Used in Decision Making	Family Made the Decision to Sustain Treatments
Progressing family type	Yes	No/minimal	More past tense used	Willing	Good communication with each other and extended family	Mostly used facts and supported wishes of family member	Planned date and time of withdrawal
Accommodating family type	Yes	No/minimal	More past tense used	Somewhat willing	Fairly good communication	Mostly facts used, mixed with some emotions	Yes, with little-to-moderate conflict
Maintaining family type	Yes	Very hopeful of recovery	Present and past tense used	Undecided	Varied communication, good at times and not good at times	Mixed some facts with emotions	Yes, with moderate-to-extreme difficulty
Struggling family type	Uncertain if understood	Very hopeful of recovery	Present tense used	Not willing	Most family conflict of all styles	Mostly emotions	Some unable to decide, family not in agreement
Floundering family type	No	Believe full recovery was going to happen	Present and future tense used	Not willing	Little family discussion with each other	Emotions only and not follow family member's wishes	Decided when dying was active and made with extreme family conflict

Adapted from Wiegand, D. L., Deatrick, J. A., & Knafl, K. (2008). Family management styles related to withdrawal of life-sustaining therapy from adults who are acutely ill or injured. *Journal of Family Nursing, 14*(1), 16–32.

- The prevalence of facts or emotions in making the decision
- The actual decision to withdraw LSTs

Culture has also been shown to influence family consideration of withdrawing LSTs. For example, African Americans are more likely to continue futile therapies (Hopp & Duffy, 2000).

Family presence during CPR also influences decisions to withdraw LSTs. Tschann et al. (2003) compared the prevalence of decisions to withdraw LSTs when families were present and when families were not present. Over a set period of time where withdrawal was considered by the health care team to be appropriate, they found that patients were more likely to be removed from mechanical ventilation if the family was present than if the family was not present. Furthermore, when families were involved in their loved one's care and present during the dying process, patients were more likely to have their health care provider order medications that would alleviate their suffering, such as narcotics or an antianxiety medication. In all situations, families work collaboratively with the health care team to determine when and how to withdraw LSTs.

It is important for families to be informed early about death, well before the final decision is made to withdraw life support. Doctors were found to prolong the withdrawal of life support systems to accommodate the needs of the families, which resulted in families' higher level of satisfaction (Gerstel, Engelberg, Koepsell, & Curtis, 2008). But in doing so, physicians felt that patients did not benefit from this prolongation because it caused nonbeneficial and sometimes painful therapies. In fact, the lack of communication between physicians and families caused slower decision making by families. If families are alerted to the possibility of the patient's death earlier in the hospital stay, when the indication for withdrawal is finally made by the physician, the families will be better prepared. Given that most deaths in critical care occur within 4 hours of withdrawal of treatment, this short time period does not allow for families to prepare for death. This short time frame puts an enormous demand on nurses as they attempt to provide palliative care for the patient and the bereaved family (Efstathiou & Clifford, 2011; Neuberger, 2003).

Hsieh, Shannon, and Curtis (2006) analyzed 51 family conferences with the health care team in the decision-making process to withdraw LSTs. Their insight into this emotional process for these families offers nurses ideas about how to help support families during this difficult time. They identified five contradictory arguments that families often talked about during these family conferences:

- If the family believed that its decision to remove LSTs was actually killing the loved one versus allowing him to die a natural death
- If the family's decision was viewed as a benefit by alleviating suffering or by eliminating a burden on the family
- If the family was honoring its loved one's end-of-life choices or following its own personal wishes
- If the ill family member expressed several differing end-of-life choices, the family had to work through which one to follow
- Determining whether one family member would be responsible for making the final decision or the family as a whole would make the decision

Regardless of which of these contradictions families discussed during the conference, information-seeking strategies used by the health care team members were found to facilitate these difficult emotional discussions. Some of these information-seeking strategies included acknowledging the contradictions, clarifying views of each person including the patient who was not present, bringing the conversation back to the point that all family members wanted to help their loved one, and reaffirming their choices even if the health care team did not agree with them.

Once a family has reached a decision to withdraw LSTs, nurses work closely with family members to guide them through this difficult procedure. A trusting nurse-family relationship is crucial to the family (Wiegand, 2006). The following nursing actions help prepare the family (Kirchhoff, Palzkill, Kowalkowski, Mork, & Gretarsdottir, 2008):

- Telling the family that the exact time of death cannot be anticipated, but that the nurse will be monitoring the situation and informing them when death appears more imminent.
- Assuring the family that the nurse will continue to provide compassionate comfort care.
- Giving each family member a choice to watch the actual withdrawal of the therapies.

- Providing for physical and emotional intimacy needs of the family.
- Informing the family of expected signs and symptoms it may see during the active dying process.
- Encouraging or giving permission for the family to hold, touch, caress, lie with, talk to, and show emotion to the dying family member.

Nurses need to make every effort to keep families involved and informed as death approaches. Providing the ideal level of privacy is not always possible in ICU environments, but every effort needs to be made to allow for families to be with their loved ones, and to remain with their hospitalized family members in a private, unhurried, and quiet environment. Many families and cultures have rituals or spiritual beliefs and procedures that need to be honored. Resources such as Chaplaincy Services and Social Work can offer assistance, especially when death is approaching. Nurse managers need to relieve bedside nurses from responsibilities of caring for other patients, so that they can remain with families and patients who are dying.

Offering the Option of Organ Donation

The number of people who need organs far exceeds the number of donors. In the United States, 121, 278 people are waiting for a donor organ (Organ Donor, 2014). Each day 79 people receive an organ transplant and 18 people die because an organ was unavailable (Organ Donor, 2014). Between January and November of 2013 there were 26,517 transplants from 12,994 donors (United Network for Organ Sharing, 2014). It has been shown that when the family knows of a loved one's intent to donate his or her organs, there are higher rates of donation than when the family is not aware of the loved one's intent (Smith, Lindsey, Kopfman, Yoo, & Morrison, 2008).

Discussing organ donation with a family whose loved one has suddenly died or with whom the decision has been made to withdraw LSTs is difficult. The discussion about organ donation should take place separately from the notification of the family member's death, and it should be done by someone who has been specifically trained in asking for organ and tissue donation (Artinian, 2005). Federal regulations now stipulate that hospitals are required to contact their local Organ Procurement Organization (OPO) concerning any death or impending death (Truog et al., 2001). Once contacted, the OPO sends a representative, or a local hospital representative will approach the family at the appropriate time about the option of organ donation and answer questions.

If organ donation is viewed as a consoling act, the option to elect organ donation is easier for the family (Artinian, 2005). Organ donation benefits the donor family, as well as the recipients and their families. Families reported that knowing that the organ of their loved one helped someone else, that a positive came out of a negative, and their family member lives on in someone else helped them cope with their loss (Artinian, 2005).

Many families worry that donation is disfiguring or will delay the funeral, but neither of these worries is valid and nurses should reassure families on these points. The body is not disfigured in the process of removing the organs. If the body parts that are removed have the potential to disfigure the person, replacement plastic or wooden parts are inserted in the place of those removed so that the person is not disfigured. The organ donation team has a rapid response; therefore, the funeral arrangements are not delayed.

The donor family does not pay for the medical expenses once death has been declared; the costs are paid by the OPO and the recipients. The donor family receives a letter from the OPO informing it of the number of people who received organs from the deceased family member. After time, the donor family can contact the OPO to find out whether the recipient of the organs is interested in corresponding and meeting.

Case Study: Howe Family

This case study presents a family dealing with an acute exacerbation of a longstanding chronic illness and hospitalization of one of its members. The Family Assessment and Intervention Model is used as the theoretical approach to the Howe family (refer to Chapter 3 for specific details of this family nursing theory and model). The Howe family genogram and ecomap are presented in Figures 14-1 and 14-2.

Glenn Howe, a 64-year-old married white male, had his first major myocardial infarction at age 41. Since that time,

(continued)

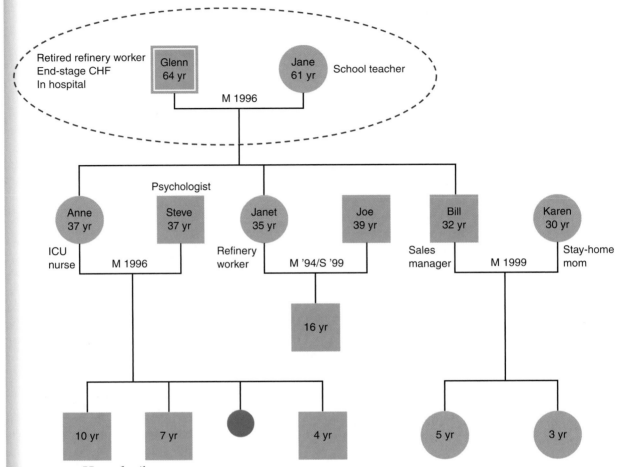

FIGURE 14-1 Howe family genogram.

he dutifully embraced numerous lifestyle changes, including smoking cessation, diet modifications, and the establishment of a regular exercise regimen. In addition, he began to take numerous cardiovascular medications to control his blood pressure and enhance his cardiac function. Despite his adherence to his chronic disease management program, Glenn's cardiovascular disease worsened, and he underwent coronary artery bypass surgery 10 years ago. Initial results of the surgery were positive, and Glenn continued to manage his chronic illness well. Recently, however, he experienced another small myocardial infarction, after which his cardiac function declined drastically. As a result, physicians increased his medications, recommended more severe lifestyle modifications, and dashed his hopes for recovery.

Glenn's immediate family consists of his wife, Jane, three children—Anne, age 37; Janet, age 35; and Bill, age 32—and six young grandchildren. Glenn is currently retired while Jane continues to work as a special education teacher. All family members are upper middle class and attend an Episcopal Church regularly. All family members are geographically and emotionally close to Glenn, and are quite concerned that he may not survive much longer. Since his first myocardial infarction, the family members have lived their lives in a state of anxiety, feeling as if their time with Glenn is likely to be limited, as if they are on "borrowed time." This anxiety has resulted in a number of benefits for the family: numerous family vacations, all holidays together, and the perspective that every chance to be together is special. After Glenn's most recent decline in cardiac function, the family experienced a heightened sense of preciousness, wanting to spend as much time as possible together and wanting every moment with Glenn to be perfect.

Before his first myocardial infarction, Glenn was a healthy, robust, active man with many interests and hobbies. After his cardiac surgery, many of his hobbies,

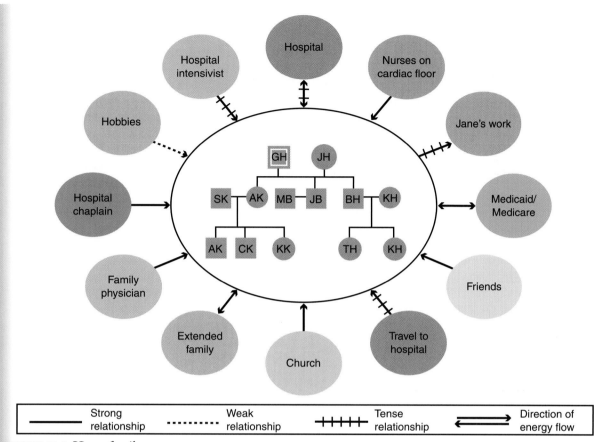

FIGURE 14-2 Howe family ecomap.

including golf, fell by the wayside. He became increasingly short of breath with exertion and resorted to armchair hobbies, such as coin collecting, crossword puzzles, and world history. Family activities changed as well. Family vacations necessarily became sedate and wheelchair oriented, rather than activity-oriented hiking, fishing, and camping trips. The family endeavored, however, to have at least one very special trip every year, the last two being a trip to Disney World with Glenn in a wheelchair and a cruise that required very little exertion.

Glenn became more and more debilitated. His cardiac function was so poor he could not eat without becoming short of breath and tachycardic. His appetite decreased dramatically, and he lost more than 60 pounds. He began to suffer from orthopnea and often tried to sleep upright in his recliner all night. As he and Jane tried to cope with his acute and chronic health care needs, their relationship changed. She became a full-time caretaker, trying anything she could to get him to eat and to make him comfortable. A normally unflappable individual, she found herself expressing her

frustration at his refusal to eat more than a few bites at a time. Her outbursts were distressing to her and her children because they were so out of character. Glenn, usually a more demanding individual, became compliant and resigned as his health deteriorated. The children became hypervigilant and attentive to their parents, making frequent visits on weekends and calling every day. Family roles changed as the stressors affecting the family intensified.

Glenn had been hospitalized on numerous occasions, and he approached the impending admission to a medical-surgical unit with his usual calm and trust in his caregivers. He was being admitted for tests because his ventricular function had decreased, his weight had decreased from 200 to 140 pounds, and his urine output was declining. He called his oldest daughter, Anne, a cardiovascular intensive care nurse, the morning of his scheduled admission and asked her to meet him at the hospital. She replied that she had to travel out of town for an important meeting but would drive up later that night and be with him for the

(continued)

tests the next day. The other children counted on the old-est child to take care of health care needs, and because of her education and experience, it was a role she gladly assumed.

Given the chronic nature of Glenn's cardiovascular disease and the life-threatening potential for acute exacer-bations requiring frequent hospitalizations, Jane and Glenn had discussed advance directives openly and honestly. Jane was well aware that Glenn did not wish for any heroic measures, especially CPR. He felt that his two cardiac surgeries were trauma enough and that his heart condition was irreparable. Jane was terrified of losing her husband, best friend, and companion, and was very concerned about having to make the decision that would honor Glenn's wishes.

During this hospital stay, Glenn and Jane renewed their close and trusting relationship with the nurses at their small community hospital. While awaiting his tests and the arrival of their daughters, Glenn experienced a lapse in consciousness with Jane at his bedside. Jane called for help, and two nurses entered the room and quickly assessed the situation. Glenn was in full cardiac arrest. One of the nurses turned to Jane and said, "Do you want us to bring him back? We can bring him back." Jane hesitated, then shook her head no. The nurse asked again, "Are you sure? Do you want us to bring him back?" Once again, Jane answered, "No." She immediately realized the consequences of her decision to deny CPR. Glenn, her husband of 45 years, was gone; her children did not expect this hospitalization to result in his death; and she was alone at his bedside.

Jane experienced regret for her decision not to "bring him back." Her decision was so very final. She also regret-ted the times that she had felt frustrated at his disinterest in eating and his hobbies. Though never an angry person, she had experienced anger at her husband on more than one occasion. The children all felt a measure of guilt as well: Anne for going to a meeting instead of being with her dad, Janet for being at work instead of at her dad's bed-side, and Bill for living so far away. Everyone wished they had more time together as a family.

Jane became a grieving widow, very dependent, sad, and indecisive—a person her children barely recognized. At a time when they needed a strong, supportive mother, that person was absent. The individuals best able to pro-vide support to Jane and her children were the grandchil-dren and spouses. Having never experienced the death of someone so dear to them, all family members struggled with daily life for several weeks after Glenn's death.

Family Assessment and Intervention Model and the Family Systems Stressor-Strength Inventory Applied to the Howe Family:

The Family Systems Stressor-Strength Inventory (FS³I) was used to assess stressors (problems) and the strengths (resources) that the Howe family had in coping with its situation soon after Glenn's admission to the medical-surgical unit. The patient and his wife, Glenn and Jane, were interviewed together by the nurse, but they each completed their own FS³I. Both Glenn's and Jane's individual scores were tallied using the scoring guide for the FS³I. Anne, the eldest daughter (37 years old), Jan, the middle child (35 years old), and Bill (32 years old) were all present, and all completed the assessment instrument (FS³I).

The general stressors were viewed similarly by both Glenn and Jane, and these stressors were assessed as slightly less serious by the nurse than by the couple. Glenn, Jane, and the nurse concurred that the general stress level was high, which was consistent with their experience. The specific stressors were perceived slightly differently by Glenn and Jane. Figures 14-3 through 14-7 summarize the information gained from the Howe family: (1) Figure 14-3 presents their FS³Is; (2) Figure 14-4 provides the Howe family Quantitative Summary of Family Systems Stressors Form: General and Specific; (3) Figure 14-5 lists the Howe family and clinician summary on family strength; (4) Figure 14-6 shows the Howe family Qualitative Summary and Clinician Remarks; (5) and Figure 14-7 presents the Howe Family Care Plan.

The Qualitative Summary and Clinician Remarks form in Figure 14-6 serves as the groundwork for the Family Care Plan in Figure 14-7. This form synthesizes informa-tion pertaining to general stressors, specific stressors, family strengths, and the overall functioning and physical and mental health of the family members. The nurse completed this form using her assessment skills with information obtained from the conversation with the family and the data obtained from the written FS³I.

The family members and the nurse perceived that the worsening of Glenn's physical condition because of his chronic heart disease was the major general stressor. Glenn's specific stressors included his growing inability to function as a husband, father, and grandfather, as well as a fear of the unknown. Specific stressors for Jane included concerns regarding the financial impact of Glenn's illness and her inability to provide care for Glenn. The strengths of the family were seen as commu-nication between all family members, religious faith, and

INSTRUCTIONS FOR ADMINISTRATION

The Family Systems Stressor-Strength Inventory (FS³I) is an assessment and measurement instrument intended for use with families. It focuses on identifying stressful situations occurring in families and the strengths families use to maintain healthy family functioning. Each family member is asked to complete the instrument on an individual form before an interview with the clinician. Questions can be read to members unable to read.

After completion of the instrument, the clinician evaluates the family on each of the stressful situations (general and specific) and the strengths they possess. This evaluation is recorded on the family member form.

The clinician records the individual family member's score and the clinician perception score on the Quantitative Summary. A different color code is used for each family member. The clinician also completes the Qualitative Summary, synthesizing the information gleaned from all participants. Clinicians can use the Family Care Plan to prioritize diagnoses, set goals, develop prevention and intervention activities, and evaluate outcomes.

Family Name _Howe_   **Date** _6/10/14_

Family Member(s) Completing Assessment _Glenn, Jane Anne_

Ethnic Background(s) _Caucasian-German-English_

Religious Background(s) _Protestant_

Referral Source _Family Physician_

Interviewer _CCU RN_

Family Members	Relationship in Family	Age	Marital Status	Education (highest degree)	Occupation
1. _Glenn_	_Father_	_64_	_Married_	_BS_	_Refinery Worker_
2. _Jane_	_Mother_	_61_	_Married_	_MA_	_Teacher_
3. _Anne_	_Daughter_	_37_	_Married_	_BSN_	_RN_
4. _Janet_	_Daughter_	_35_	_Divorced_	_AA_	_Refinery Worker_
5. _Bill_	_Son_	_32_	_Married_	_PhD_	_Psychologist_
6. _____					

Family's current reasons for seeking assistance:

Glenn's heart disease is worsening, requiring sudden hospitalization for stabilization

Source: Hanson, S. M. H. (2001). *Family health care nursing: Theory, practice, and research* (2nd ed.),
    pp. 425–437. Philadelphia: F.A. Davis.

FIGURE 14-3 Summary for Howe case study on Introduction Form for the Family Systems Stressor-Strength Inventory.

(continued)

Part I: Family Systems Stressors (General)

DIRECTIONS: Each of 25 situations/stressors listed here deals with some aspect of normal family life. They have the potential for creating stress within families or between families and the world in which they live. We are interested in your overall impression of how these situations affect your family life. Please circle a number (0 through 5) that best describes the amount of stress or tension they create for you.

STRESSORS	DOES NOT APPLY	LITTLE STRESS		MEDIUM STRESS		HIGH STRESS	CLINICIAN PERCEPTION SCORE
1. Family member(s) feel unappreciated	0	①	2	3	4	5	1
2. Guilt for not accomplishing more	0	1	2	3	4	⑤	4
3. Insufficient "me" time	0	1	2	3	4	⑤	4
4. Self-Image/self-esteem/ feelings of unattractiveness	0	1	2	3	④	5	3
5. Perfectionism	0	1	2	3	④	5	3
6. Dieting	0	①	2	3	4	5	1
7. Health/Illness	0	1	2	3	4	⑤	4
8. Communication with children	0	1	2	3	④	5	4
9. Housekeeping standards	0	1	2	③	4	5	4
10. Insufficient couple time	0	1	2	3	④	5	3
11. Insufficient family playtime	0	1	2	3	4	⑤	4
12. Children's behavior/discipline/ sibling fighting	⓪	1	2	3	4	5	1
13. Television	0	①	2	3	4	5	1
14. Overscheduled family calendar	0	1	2	③	4	5	3
15. Lack of shared responsibility in the family	0	1	2	3	4	⑤	5
16. Moving	⓪	1	2	3	4	5	0
17. Spousal relationship (communication, friendship, sex)	0	1	2	3	4	⑤	4
18. Holidays	⓪	1	2	3	4	5	0
19. In-laws	⓪	1	2	3	4	5	0
20. Teen behaviors (communication, music, friends, school)	⓪	1	2	3	4	5	0
21. New baby	⓪	1	2	3	4	5	0
22. Economics/finances/budgets	0	1	2	3	4	⑤	5
23. Unhappiness with work situation	0	1	2	3	④	5	4
24. Overvolunteerism	⓪	1	2	3	4	5	0
25. Neighbors	0	1	②	3	4	5	2

$66 \div 18 = 3.6$ (Family Perception Score)

$60 \div 18 = 3.3$ (Clinician Perception Score)

FIGURE 14-3—cont'd

Additional Stressors: _Uncertainty about the future, spiritual issues_

Family Remarks: _Feeling a sense of urgency related to Glenn's physical condition_

Clinician: Clarification of stressful situations/concerns with family members.

Prioritize in order of importance to family members: _Impact of physical illness on all family activities and interactions_

Part II: Family Systems Stressors (Specific)

DIRECTIONS: The following 12 questions are designed to provide information about your specific stress-producing situation/problem or area of concern influencing your family's health. Please circle a number (1 through 5) that best describes the influence this situation has on your family's life and how well you perceive your family's overall functioning.

The specific stress-producing situation/problem or area of concern at this time is: _Glenn's worsening physical condition, uncertain future and inability to maintain usual family activities_

STRESSORS	FAMILY PERCEPTION SCORE			CLINICIAN PERCEPTION
	LITTLE	MEDIUM	HIGH	SCORE
1. To what extent is your family bothered by this problem or stressful situation? (e.g., effects on family interactions, communication among members, emotional and social relationships)	1 2 3 4		⑤	_5_

Family Remarks: _"This is huge for our family." "We love Grandpa — we want him to get better."_

Clinician Remarks: _All family members affected by Glenn's physical condition._

2. How much of an effect does this stressful situation have on your family's usual pattern of living? (e.g., effects on lifestyle patterns and family developmental task)	1 2 3 4		⑤	_5_

Family Remarks: _"We haven't been able to vacation together this year."_

Clinician Remarks: _Normal family activities severely limited by Glenn's illness_

FIGURE 14-3—cont'd

(continued)

STRESSORS	FAMILY PERCEPTION SCORE			CLINICIAN PERCEPTION
	LITTLE	MEDIUM	HIGH	SCORE
3. How much has this situation affected your family's ability to work together as a family unit? (e.g., alteration in family roles, completion of family tasks, following through with responsibilities)	1 2 3	④	5	4

Family Remarks: _"Dad cannot do anything anymore – Mom has to do everything"_

Clinician Remarks: _All family members helpful to Glenn and Jane_

Has your family ever experienced a similar concern in the past?

   YES If YES, complete question 4

   (NO) If NO, complete question 5

4. How successful was your family in dealing with this situation/problem/concern in the past? (e.g., workable coping strategies developed, adaptive measures useful, situation improved)	1 2 3	4	5	

Family Remarks: _No experience, with critical illness "Nothing like this has ever happened to us"_

Clinician Remarks: _New territory for this family._

5. How strongly do you feel this current situation/ problem/concern will affect your family's future? (e.g., anticipated consequences)	1 2 3	4	⑤	4

Family Remarks: _Impending loss of head of family will be devastating to entire family_

Clinician Remarks: _Openly discussing future and ways to be together now_

6. To what extent are family members able to help themselves in this present situation/ problem/ concern? (e.g., self-assistive efforts, family expectations, spiritual influence, family resources)	1 2 3	④	5	4

Family Remarks: _Rely heavily on one another, friends, clergy and health care workers_

Clinician Remarks: _Well informed, knowledgeable, eager to provide care_

FIGURE 14-3—cont'd

STRESSORS		FAMILY PERCEPTION SCORE			CLINICIAN PERCEPTION SCORE
	LITTLE	MEDIUM		HIGH	SCORE
7. To what extent do you expect others to help your family with this situation/ problem/concern? (e.g., what roles would helpers play; how available are extra-family resources)	1 2	3	④	5	3

Family Remarks: _Neighbors, coworkers, and health care personnel_

Clinician Remarks: _Very trusting, open and cooperative with visitors and nurses_

STRESSORS	POOR	SATISFACTORY	EXCELLENT	SCORE
8. How would you rate the way your family functions overall? (e.g., how your family members relate to each other and to larger family and community)	1 2	3 ④	5	4

Family Remarks: _Recent worsening of physical problems has frightened family members_

Clinician Remarks: _Anxious, asking frequent questions regarding prognosis_

9. How would you rate the overall physical health status of each family member by name? (Include yourself as a family member; record additional names on back.)

a. _Glenn_	①	2	3	4	5	1
b. _Jane_	1	2	3	④	5	4
c. _Anne_	1	2	3	4	⑤	5
d. _Janet_	1	2	3	④	5	5
e. _Bill_	1	2	3	4	⑤	5

10. How would you rate the overall physical health status of your family as a whole?   1   2   3   ④   5   4

Family Remarks: _Glenn's deteriorating health is affecting the activities of the entire family_

Clinician Remarks: _Healthy family members are curtailing their usual activities due to Glenn's illness_

11. How would you rate the overall mental health status of each family member by name? (Include yourself as a family member; record additional names on back.)

a. _Glenn_	1	②	3	4	5	2
b. _Jane_	1	2	③	4	5	4
c. _Anne_	1	2	3	④	5	4
d. _Janet_	1	2	③	4	5	3
e. _Bill_	1	2	3	④	5	3

FIGURE 14-3—cont'd

(continued)

STRESSORS		FAMILY PERCEPTION SCORE			CLINICIAN PERCEPTION SCORE
	LITTLE		MEDIUM	HIGH	SCORE
12. How would you rate the overall mental health status of your family as a whole?	1　　2		③	4　　5	3

Family Remarks: _Glenn is feeling guilty, both Glenn and Jane are anxious, Janet is depressed_

Clinician Remarks: _Glenn's anxiety & fear of the unknown is affecting the entire family_

Glenn 3.6　　　　Clinician 3.3

Part III: Family Systems Strengths

DIRECTIONS: Each of the 16 traits/attributes listed below deals with some aspect of family life and its overall functioning. Each one contributes to the health and well-being of family members as individuals and to the family as a whole. Please circle a number (0 through 5) that best describes the extent to which the trait applies to your family.

MY FAMILY	DOES NOT APPLY	SELDOM	FAMILY PERCEPTION SCORE			CLINICIAN PERCEPTION SCORE
			USUALLY	ALWAYS		SCORE
1. Communicates and listens to one another	0	1　　2	3	④　　5		5

Family Remarks: _All family members feel they are communicating openly about everything except Glenn's health_

Clinician Remarks: _Need to talk more about Glenn's prognosis and future financial concerns_

| 2. Affirms and supports one another | 0 | 1　　2 | 3 | 4 | ⑤ | 4 |

Family Remarks: _All members feel supported especially by Jane_

Clinician Remarks: _Very supportive family_

| 3. Teaches respect for others | 0 | 1　　2 | 3 | 4 | ⑤ | 4 |

Family Remarks: _Very respectful of one another_

Clinician Remarks: _Respectful of health care team_

FIGURE 14-3—cont'd

MY FAMILY	DOES NOT APPLY	SELDOM	FAMILY PERCEPTION SCORE			CLINICIAN PERCEPTION
			USUALLY		ALWAYS	SCORE
4. Develops a sense of trust in members	0	1	2	3	4	⑤ 4

Family Remarks: *Trust each other and the health care team*

Clinician Remarks: *Work very well with nurses and health care workers*

MY FAMILY	DOES NOT APPLY	SELDOM	USUALLY		ALWAYS	SCORE
5. Displays a sense of play and humor	0	1	2	3	④	5 3

Family Remarks: *Less often now as very anxious about Glenn's health*

Clinician Remarks: *Rarely demonstrated*

MY FAMILY	DOES NOT APPLY	SELDOM	USUALLY		ALWAYS	SCORE
6. Exhibits a sense of shared responsibility	0	1	2	· 3	④	5 4

Family Remarks: *Depend on one another*

Clinician Remarks: *Take turns at the bedside*

MY FAMILY	DOES NOT APPLY	SELDOM	USUALLY		ALWAYS	SCORE
7. Teaches a sense of right and wrong	0	1	2	3	4	⑤ 4

Family Remarks: *"Of course!"*

Clinician Remarks:

MY FAMILY	DOES NOT APPLY	SELDOM	USUALLY		ALWAYS	SCORE
8. Has a strong sense of family in which rituals and traditions abound	0	1	2	③	4	5 3

Family Remarks: *Holidays very important missing the opportunity for family dinners*

Clinician Remarks:

FIGURE 14-3—cont'd

(continued)

MY FAMILY	DOES NOT APPLY	SELDOM		FAMILY PERCEPTION SCORE USUALLY		ALWAYS	CLINICIAN PERCEPTION SCORE
9. Has a balance of interaction among members	0	1	2	3	④	5	3

Family Remarks: *Balanced responsibilities overall though all very interactive with Jane*

Clinician Remarks: *Anne appears to take the lead interacting with nurses and physicians*

10. Has a shared religious core	0	1	2	3	④	5	3

Family Remarks: *Regular church attenders*

Clinician Remarks:

11. Respects the privacy of one another	0	1	2	3	④	5	4

Family Remarks: *Not a problem*

Clinician Remarks: *Not observed to be an issue*

12. Values service to others	0	1	2	3	4	⑤	4

Family Remarks: *Most in helping professions*

Clinician Remarks: *Very helpful and appreciative of nursing care provided.*

13. Fosters family table time and conversation	0	1	2	3	④	5	4

Family Remarks: *Missing those opportunities*

Clinician Remarks: *Hospital cafeteria offers some together time*

14. Shares leisure time	0	1	2	3	4	⑤	4

Family Remarks: *Usually spend all vacations together*

Clinician Remarks: *Seem to enjoy one another*

FIGURE 14-3—cont'd

MY FAMILY	DOES NOT APPLY	SELDOM	FAMILY PERCEPTION SCORE			CLINICIAN PERCEPTION SCORE
			USUALLY		ALWAYS	
15. Admits to and seeks help with problems	0	1	2	3	④ 5	5

Family Remarks: _Rely on family physician and nurses_

Clinician Remarks: _Back help appropriately_

16a. How would you rate the overall strengths that exist in your family?	0	1	2	3	④ 5	4

Family Remarks: _Excellent, though tested at the moment_

Clinician Remarks: _Very strong_

16b. Additional Family Strengths: _Love and enjoyment of grandchildren_

16c. Clinician: Clarification of family strengths with individual members: _____
       Anne - RN
       Bill - Psychologist

FIGURE 14-3—cont'd

(continued)

Family Systems Stressor-Strength inventory (FS³I) Scoring Summary
Section 1: Family Perception Scores

INSTRUCTIONS FOR ADMINISTRATION

The Family Systems Stressor-Strength Inventory (FS³I) Scoring Summary is divided into two sections: Section 1, Family Perception Scores, and Section 2, Clinician Perception Scores. These two sections are further divided into three parts: Part I, Family Systems Stressors (General); Part II, Family Systems Stressors (Specific); and Part III, Family Systems Strengths. Each part contains a Quantitative Summary and a Qualitative Summary.

Quantifiable family and clinician perception scores are both graphed on the Quantitative Summary. Each family member has a designated color code. Family and clinician remarks are both recorded on the Quantitative Summary. Quantitative Summary scores, when graphed, suggest a level for initiation of prevention/intervention modes: Primary, Secondary, and Tertiary. Qualitative Summary information, when synthesized, contributes to the development and channeling of the Family Care Plan.

Part 1 Family Systems Stressors (General)

Add scores from questions 1 to 25 and calculate an overall numerical score for Family Systems Stressors (General). Ratings are from 1 (most positive) to 5 (most negative). The Does Not Apply (0) responses are omitted from the calculations. Total scores range from 25 to 125.
Family Systems Stressor Score (General)

$(_{25}) \times 1 =$

Graph score on Quantitative Summary, Family Systems Stressors (General), Family Member Perception Score. Color-code to differentiate family members. Record additional stressors and family remarks in Part I, Qualitative Summary: Family and Clinician Remarks.

Part II Family Systems Stressors (Specific)

Add scores from questions 1 through 8, 10, and 12 and calculate a numerical score for Family Systems Stressors (Specific). Ratings are from 1 (most positive) to 5 (most negative). Questions 4, 6, 7, 8, 10 and 12

are reverse scored.* Total scores range from 10 through 50. Family Systems Stressor Score (Specific)

$(_{10}) \times 1 =$

Graph score on Quantitative Summary, Family Systems Stressors (Specific) Family Member Perception Score. Color-code to differentiate family members. Summarize data from questions 9 and 11 (reverse scored) and record family remarks in Part II, Qualitative Summary: Family and Clinician Remarks.

Part III Family Systems Strengths

Add scores from questions 1 through 16 and calculate a numerical score for Family Systems Strengths. Ratings are from 1 (seldom) to 5 (always). The Does Not Apply (0) responses are omitted from the calculations. Total Scores range from 16 to 80.

$(_{16}) \times 1 =$

Graph score on Quantitative Summary: Family Systems Strengths, Family Member Perception Score. Record additional family strengths and family remarks in Part III, Qualitative Summary: Family and Clinician Remarks.

Source: Mischke-Berkey, K., & Hanson, S. M. H. (1991). *Pocket guide to family assessment and intervention.* St. Louis, MO: Mosby.
*Reverse scoring:
Question answered as (1) is scored 5 points.
Question answered as (2) is scored 4 points.
Question answered as (3) is scored 3 points.
Question answered as (4) is scored 2 points.
Question answered as (5) is scored 1 point.

FIGURE 14-3—cont'd

SECTION 2: CLINICIAN PERCEPTION SCORES

Part I Family Systems Stressors (General)*

Add scores from questions 1 through 25 and calculate an overall numerical score for Family Systems Stressors (General). Ratings are from 1 (most positive) to 5 (most negative). The Does Not Apply (0) responses are omitted from the calculations. Total scores range from 25 to 125.
Family systems Stressor Score (General)

$(_{25}) \times 1 =$

Graph score on Quantitative Summary, Family Systems Stressors (General) Clinician Perception Score. Record clinicians' clarification of general stressors in Part I, Qualitative Summary: Family and Clinician Remarks.

Part II Family Systems Stressors (Specific)

Add scores from questions 1 through 8, 10, 12 and calculate a numerical score for Family Systems Stressors (Specific). Ratings are from 1 (most positive) to

5 (most negative). Questions 4, 6, 7, 8, 10, 12 are reverse scored.* Total scores range from 10 to 50.
Family Systems Stressor Score (Specific)

$(_{10}) \times 1 =$

Graph score on Quantitative Summary, Family Systems Stressors (Specific), Clinician Perception Score. Summarize data from questions 9 and 11 (reverse scored) and record clinician remarks in Part II, Qualitative Summary: Family and Clinician Remarks.

Part III Family Systems Strengths

Add scores from questions 1 through 16 and calculate a numerical score for Family Systems Strengths. Ratings are from 1 (seldom) to 5 (always). The Does Not Apply (0) responses are omitted from the calculations. Total scores range from 16 to 80.

$(_{16}) \times 1 =$

Graph score on Quantitative Summary, Family Systems Strengths, Clinician Perception Score. Record clinician's clarification of family strengths in Part III, Qualitative Summary: Family and Clinician Remarks.

---

*Reverse scoring:
Question answered as (1) is scored 5 points.
Question answered as (2) is scored 4 points.
Question answered as (3) is scored 3 points.
Question answered as (4) is scored 2 points.
Question answered as (5) is scored 1 point.

FIGURE 14-3—cont'd

(continued)

QUANTITATIVE SUMMARY OF FAMILY SYSTEMS STRESSORS: GENERAL AND SPECIFIC FAMILY AND CLINICIAN PERCEPTION SCORES

DIRECTIONS: Graph the scores from each family member inventory by placing an "X" at the appropriate location. (Use first name initial for each different entry and different color code for each family member.)

SCORES FOR WELLNESS AND STABILITY	FAMILY SYSTEMS STRESSORS (GENERAL)		SCORES FOR WELLNESS AND STABILITY	FAMILY SYSTEMS STRESSORS (SPECIFIC)	
	FAMILY MEMBER PERCEPTION SCORE	CLINICIAN PERCEPTION SCORE		FAMILY MEMBER PERCEPTION SCORE	CLINICIAN PERCEPTION SCORE
5.0			5.0		
4.8	X√4		4.8		
4.6			4.6		
4.4	X√2		4.4	X√4	
4.2	X√3		4.2		
4.0			4.0	X√3	
3.8			3.8	X√5	
3.6	X√1		3.6		
3.4	X√5	X	3.4		X
3.2			3.2	X√2	
3.0			3.0	X√1	
2.8			2.8		
2.6			2.6		
2.4			2.4		
2.2			2.2		
2.0			2.0		
1.8			1.8		
1.6			1.6		
1.4			1.4		
1.2			1.2		
1.0			1.0		

*PRIMARY Prevention/Intervention Mode: Flexible Line   1.0–2.3
*SECONDARY Prevention/Intervention Mode: Normal Line   2.4–3.6
*TERTIARY Prevention/Intervention Mode: Resistance Lines   3.7–5.0
*Breakdowns of numerical scores for stressor penetration are suggested values.
√1 = Glenn √3 = Anne √5 = Bill
√2 = Jane √4 = Janet

FIGURE 14-4 Howe family Quantitative Summary of Family Systems Stressors Form: General and Specific.

FAMILY SYSTEMS STRENGTHS FAMILY AND CLINICIAN PERCEPTION SCORES

DIRECTIONS: Graph the scores from the inventory by placing an "X" at the appropriate location and connect with a line. (Use first name initial for each different entry and different color code for each family member.)

SUM OF STRENGTHS AVAILABLE FOR PREVENTION/ INTERVENTION MODE	FAMILY SYSTEMS STRENGTHS	
	FAMILY MEMBER PERCEPTION SCORE	CLINICIAN PERCEPTION SCORE
5.0		
4.8		
4.6		
	√3	
4.4	√2	
	√1	
4.2		
4.0		
	√5	X
3.8		
	√4	
3.6		
3.4		
3.2		
3.0		
2.8		
2.6		
2.4		
2.2		
2.0		
1.8		
1.6		
1.4		
1.2		
1.0		

*PRIMARY Prevention/Intervention Mode: Flexible Line　1.0–2.3
*SECONDARY Prevention/Intervention Mode: Normal Line　2.4–3.6
*TERTIARY Prevention/Intervention Mode: Resistance Lines　3.7–5.0
*Breakdowns of numerical scores for stressor penetration are suggested values.

√1 = Glenn　　√3 = Anne　　√5 = Bill
√2 = Jane　　√4 = Janet

FIGURE 14-5 Howe family and clinician summary on family strengths.

QUALITATIVE SUMMARY FAMILY AND CLINICIAN REMARKS
PART I: FAMILY SYSTEMS STRESSORS (GENERAL)

Summarize general stressors and remarks of family and clinician. Prioritize stressors according to importance to family members.

The major general stressors of the family is the worsening heart disease and the impact of the disabling stress on the entire family

PART II: FAMILY SYSTEMS STRESSORS (SPECIFIC)

A. Summarize specific stressors and remarks of family and clinician.

Glenn's specific stressors: growing inability to function as a husband, father & grandfather, fear of the unknown

B. Summarize differences (if discrepancies exist) between how family members and clinicians view effects of stressful situation on family.

Concerns regarding financial impact of illness not shared with all family members

C. Summarize overall family functioning.

Functioning fairly well but uncertainty regarding physical health taking a toll on mental health of three family members

D. Summarize overall significant physical health status for family members.

The differences between Glenn's physical health and the physical health of all other family members are significant and problematic for planning family activities

E. Summarize overall significant mental health status for family members.

Glenn's anxieties and Jane's anxiety and Janet's depression are affecting all other family members

PART III: FAMILY SYSTEMS STRENGTHS

Summarize family systems strengths and family and clinician remarks that facilitate family health and stability.

Open communications, supportive family members, religious faith, trust in health care providers, having relationships

FIGURE 14-6 Howe family Qualitative Summary and clinician remarks.

Family Care Plan*

DIAGNOSIS AND GENERAL AND SPECIFIC FAMILY SYSTEM STRESSORS	FAMILY SYSTEMS STRENGTHS SUPPORTING FAMILY CARE PLAN	GOALS FOR FAMILY AND CLINICIAN	PREVENTION/INTERVENTION MODE		
			PRIMARY, SECONDARY, OR TERTIARY	PREVENTION/ INTERVENTION ACTIVITIES	OUTCOMES EVALUATION AND REPLANNING
Diagnosis of cardiac disease with sudden worsening of symptoms necessitating curtailment of family activities and uncertainty about the future	Family communication, social support, religious faith, good medical care, knowledgeable family members	Restoration of stable cardiac status sufficient to return home Family members will continue to support Glenn and each other	Education regarding new medications and activity restrictions Home health care & discharge O$_2$ therapy	Family counseling to deal with anxiety and uncertain future Financial counseling	Evaluation to be done once plan is implemented

*Prioritize the three most significant diagnoses.

FIGURE 14-7 Howe family care plan.

the availability of a supportive health care team. The overall family functioning was considered to be as good as could be expected under the circumstances. Whereas Glenn's physical health was compromised, Jane's physical health was good. Both Glenn and Jane expressed mental health concerns, including anxiety, guilt, depression, and fear of the unknown. Overall, the nurse perceived that the family had the strengths they needed to deal with both the general and specific stressors present when Glenn was hospitalized.

The Howe Family Care Plan (see Fig. 14-7) was developed by the nurse in collaboration with the family members who completed the FS³I. The Family Care Plan includes the diagnosis of general/specific family systems stressors and family systems strengths supporting the family care plan and the goals of the family, primary, secondary, and tertiary interventions and outcomes/evaluation. The goals of this Family Care Plan included restoring stable cardiac status sufficient to return home from the hospital, and all family members continuing to support Glenn and each other.

SUMMARY

When medical-surgical nurses view families as partners in the care provided to patients, they are providing unfragmented, holistic, humane, and sensitively delivered health care. When nurses practice family-centered care in acute care settings, families are empowered to manage the stressors of being in the hospital environment, which is foreign territory to most people. Families are better prepared to support their loved ones, aid in their recovery, or facilitate a comfortable death. Families are called on to support their ill family member in the hospital, make important life decisions on behalf of or in partnership with the patient, serve

as caregivers, and advocate for the patient in the complex health care system.

- The stress families experience when family members are in the hospital is significant. Family members are at risk for depression, anxiety, and PTSD.
- The role of families in the hospital setting is crucial because patients have been shown to have more positive outcomes when families are involved in their loved one's care while in the hospital.
- The benefits of practicing family nursing or family-centered care in the hospital setting have been well documented. Yet health care providers in the hospital environment continue

to practice individual patient-centered rather than family-centered care (family nursing).

■ Nurses in medical-surgical environments recognize and feel responsible to practice family-centered or family nursing. Yet they struggle with role ambiguity and role conflict, as they continue to practice in settings that reward the biomedical model of health care and not a holistic nursing model of care.

■ The environment for providing family-centered nursing care (family nursing) in acute care settings is dependent on hospital policies and procedures that consider the needs of families.

■ Transferring loved ones from critical care units to the medical-surgical units is stressful for families because it creates a sense of conflict. On one hand, families are glad their loved ones are better, but they also worry that their family members may not be ready to be moved out of such intensive nurse watchfulness.

■ The family member who advocates for his loved one in the hospital assumes a difficult, time-consuming, and fatiguing role as he often travels long distances to get to the hospital, takes time off work to be there, often stays all night in the hospital, manages the informational needs of the patient and the family, and works through a complex health care system.

■ Effective communication with patients, families, and interdisciplinary health care providers improves client satisfaction, promotes positive response to care, reduces length of stay in care settings, and results in decreased overall cost and resource utilization.

■ Compassionate communication provides crucial care to families as they are asked to make multiple decisions as their loved one dies in the hospital.

REFERENCES

AACN Practice Alerts. (2012). Family presence: Visitation in the adult ICU. *Critical Care Nurse, 32*(4), 76–78.

Ahmann, E., & Dokken, D. (2012). Strategies for encouraging patient/family member partnerships with the health care team. *Pediatric Nursing, 38*(4), 232–235.

Ahrens, T., Yancey, V., & Kollef, M. (2003). Improving family communications at the end-of-life: Implications for length of stay in the ICU and resource use. *American Journal of Critical Care, 12*(4), 317–323.

Alonso-Zaldivar, R. (2012). Hospital face Medicare penalties over readmitted patients. *StarTribune*. Retrieved from www.startribune.com/printarticle/?id=172130691

Alvarez, G., & Kirby, A. (2006). The perspective of families of the critically ill patient: Their needs. *Current Opinions in Critical Care, 12*(6), 614–618.

American Association of Critical Care Nurses. (2004). Practice alert: Family presence during CPR and invasive procedures. Retrieved from www.aacn.org

American Hospital Association. (2013). Hospital readmission rates decline in 2012. Retrieved from http://www.ahanews.com/ahanews/jsp/display.jsp?dcrpath=AHANEWS/AHANewsNowArticle/data/ann_052913_readmissions

American Nurses Association. (2001). *Code of ethics for nurses with interpretive statements*. Washington, DC: ANA.

Artinian, N. T. (2005). Family-focused medical-surgical nursing. In S. M. H. Hanson, V. Gedaly-Duff, & J. R. Kaakinen (Eds.), *Family health care nursing: Theory, practice and research* (3rd ed., pp. 323–346). Philadelphia: F. A. Davis.

Aston, G. (2013). A focus on heart failure. *Hospital & Health Networks, 87*(5), 40–50.

Astedt-Kurki, P., Paavilainen, E., Tammentie, T., & Paunonen-Ilmonen, M. (2001). Interaction between family members and health care providers in acute care settings in Finland. *Journal of Family Nursing, 7*(4), 371–390.

Azoulay, E., Pouchard, F., Kentish-Barnes, N., Chevret, S., Aboab, J., Adrie, C., . . . Schlemmer, B. (2005). Risk of post traumatic stress symptoms in family members in the intensive care unit patients. *American Journal of Respiratory and Critical Care Medicine, 171*(9), 987–994.

Bach, V., Ploeg, J., & Black, M. (2009). Nursing roles in end-of-life decision making in critical care settings. *Western Journal of Nursing Research, 31*, 496–512.

Beckstrand, R. L., & Kirchhoff, K. T. (2005). Providing end-of-life care to patients: Critical care nurses' perceived obstacles and supportive behaviours. *American Journal of Critical Care, 14*(5), 395–403.

Bice-Stephens, W. (2006). Ownership in the intensive care unit. *Critical Care Nurse, 26*(4), 10–11.

Bjornsdottir, K. (2002). From the state to the family: Reconfiguring the responsibility for long term nursing care at home. *Nursing Inquiry, 9*, 3–11.

Browning, A. M. (2006). Exploring advance directives. *Journal of Christian Nursing, 23*(1), 34–39.

Browning, G., & Warren, N. (2006). Unmet needs of family members in the medical intensive care waiting room. *Critical Care Nursing Quarterly, 29*(1), 86–95.

Burr, G. (1998). Contextualizing critical care family needs through triangulation: An Australian study. *Intensive and Critical Care Nursing, 14*(4), 161–169.

Butterworth, A. M. (2003). Reality check: 10 barriers to advanced planning. *Nurse Practitioner, 28*(5), 42–43.

Carr, J. M., & Fogarty, J. P. (1999). Families at the bedside: An ethnographic study of vigilance. *Journal of Family Practice, 48*(6), 433–438.

Carr, K. (2002). Ward visits after intensive care discharge: Why. In R. Griffiths & C. Jones (Eds.), *Intensive care aftercare*. Oxford: Butterworth Heinemann.

Case Management Advisor. (2013). Navigators help patients manage their health. *Case Management Advisor, 24*(4), 41–42.

Chaboyer, W., Kendall, E., Kendall, M., & Foster, M. (2005). Transfer out of intensive care: A qualitative exploration of patient and family perceptions. *Australian Critical Care, 18*(4), 138–145.

Chesla, C. A. (1997). Reconciling technologic and family care in critical care nursing. *Image: Journal of Nursing Scholarship, 28*(3), 199–203.

Chien, W. T., Chiu, Y. L., Lam, L. W., & Ip, W. Y. (2006). Effects of a needs-based education programme for family carers with a relative in an intensive care unit: A quasi-experimental study. *International Journal of Nursing Studies, 43,* 39–50.

Cioffi, J. (2006). Culturally diverse family members and their hospitalized relatives in acute care wards: A qualitative study. *Australian Journal of Advanced Nursing, 24*(1), 15–20.

Clarke, E. B., Curtis, J. R., Luce, J. M., Levy, M., Danis, M., Nelson, J., & Solomon, M. Z. (2003). Quality indicators for end-of-life care in the intensive care unit. *Critical Care Medicine, 31*(9), 2255–2262.

Coleman, E. A., Parry, C., Chalmer, S., & Minn, S. J. (2006). The care transitions interventions: Results of a randomized controlled trial. *Archives of Internal Medicine, 166,* 1822–1828.

Coleman, E. A., Smith, J. D., Frank, J. C., Min, S., Parry, C., & Kramer, A. M. (2004). Preparing patients and caregivers to participate in care delivered across settings: The care transition intervention. *Journal of the American Geriatric Society, 52,* 1817–1825.

Compton, S., Levy, P., Griffin, M., Waselewsky, D., Mango, L., & Zalenski, R. (2011). Family-witnessed resuscitation: Bereavement outcomes in an urban environment. *Journal of Palliative Medicine, 14*(6), 715–721.

Curtis, J. R., Engelberg, R. A., Wenrich, M. D., Shannon, S. E., Treece, P. D., & Rubenfeld, G. D. (2005). Missed opportunities during family conferences about end-of-life care in the intensive care unit. *American Journal of Respiratory Critical Care Medicine, 171,* 844–849.

Cypress, B. S. (2011). Family conference in the intensive care unit: A systematic review. *Dimensions of Critical Care Nursing, 30*(5), 246–255.

Cypress, B. S. (2012). Family presence in rounds: An evidence-based review. *Dimensions of Critical Care Nursing, 31*(1), 53–63.

Darc, F., Lennon, K., & Sanders, M. (2013). A call to action: Overcoming communication challenges in hospitals. Accenture Health. Retrieved from http://www.accenture.com/SiteCollectionDocuments/PDF/Accenture-Overcoming-Communication-Challenges-in-Hospitals.pdf

Davidson, J. E. (2009). Family-centered care: Meeting the needs of patients' families and helping families adapt to critical illness. *Critical Care Nurse, 29*(3), 28–34.

Davidson, J. E., Powers, K., Hedayat, K. M., Tieszen, M., Kon, A. A., Shepard, E., . . . Armstrong, D. (2007). Clinical practice guidelines for support of the family in the patient-centered ICU: American College of Critical Care Task Force 2004–2005. *Critical Care Medicine, 35*(2), 605–622.

Day, L. (2006). Family involvement in critical care: Shortcomings of a utilitarian justification. *American Journal of Critical Care, 15*(2), 223–225.

Deitrick, L., Ray, D., Stern, G., Fuhrman, C., Masiado, T., Yaich, S. L., & Wasser, T. (2005). Evaluation and recommendations from a study of critical-care waiting rooms. *Journal for Healthcare Quality, 27*(4), 17–25.

DePalma, G., Xu, H., Covinsky, K., Craig, B. A., Stallard, E., Thomas, J., & Sands, L. P. (2012). Hospital readmissions among older adults who return home with unmet need for ADL disability. *The Gerontologist, 53*(3), 454–461.

DesRoches, C., Blendon, R., Young, J., Scoles, K., & Kim, M. (2002). Caregiving in the post-hospitalization period: Findings from a national survey. *Nurse Economist, 20,* 221–224.

Díaz-Montes, T., Johnson, M., Giuntoli, R., & Brown, A. (2013). Importance and timing of end-of-life care discussions among gynecologic oncology patients. *American Journal of Hospice and Palliative Care Medicine, 30*(1), 50–67.

Douglas, S., Daly, B., & Lipson, A. R. (2012). Neglect of quality-of-life considerations in intensive care unit family meetings for long-stay intensive care unit patients. *Critical Care Medicine, 40*(2), 461–467.

Duke, G., & Thompson, S. (2007). Knowledge, attitudes and practices of nursing personnel regarding advance directives. *International Journal of Palliative Nursing, 13*(3), 109–115.

Duke, G., Thompson, S., & Hastie, M. (2007). Factors influencing completion of advanced directive in hospitalized patients. *International Journal of Palliative Nursing, 13*(1), 39–43.

Efstathiou, N., & Clifford, C. (2011). The critical care nurse's role in end-of-life care: Issues and challenges. *Nursing in Critical Care, 16*(3), 116–123.

Eggenberger, S. K., & Nelms, T. P. (2007). Being family: The family experience when an adult member is hospitalized with a critical illness. *Journal of Clinical Nursing, 16,* 1618–1628.

Eldredge, D. (2004). Helping at the bedside: Spouses' preferences for helping critically ill patients. *Research in Nursing and Health, 27,* 307–321.

Emergency Nurses Association. (2005). *Presenting the option for family presence* (3rd ed.). Des Plaines, IL: Emergency Nurses Association.

Engstrom, A., Anderson, S., & Soderberg, S. (2008). Re-visiting the ICU experiences of follow-up visits to an ICU after discharge: A qualitative study. *Intensive and Critical Care Nursing, 24*(4), 233–241.

Engstrom, A., & Soderberg, S. (2004). The experiences of partners of critically ill persons in an intensive care unit. *Intensive and Critical Care Nursing, 20*(5), 299–308.

Engstrom, A., & Soderberg, S. (2007). Close relatives in intensive care from the perspective of critical care nurses. *Journal of Clinical Nursing, 16,* 1651–1659.

Eriksson, T., Bergbom, I., & Lindahl, B. (2011). The experiences of patients and their families of visiting whilst in an intensive care unit—A hermeneutic interview study. *Intensive and Critical Care Nursing, 27,* 60–66.

Fry, S., & Warren, N. A. (2007). Perceived needs of critical care family members: A phenomenological discourse. *Critical Care Nursing Quarterly, 30*(2), 181–188.

Fumagalli, S., Boncinelli, L., Lo Nostro, A., Valoti, P., Baldereschi, G., Di Bari, M., Ungar, A., . . . Marchionni, N. (2006). Reduced cardiocirculatory complications with unrestrictive visiting policy in an ICU: Results from a pilot, randomized trial. *Circulation, 113*(7), 946–952.

Furuya, R., Mata, L., Veras, V., Appoloni, A., Dantas, R., Silveira, R., & Rossi, L. (2013). Telephone follow-up for patients after myocardial revascularization: A systematic review. *American Journal of Nursing, 113*(5), 28–40.

Gallant, M., Spitz, G., & Prohaska, T. (2007). Help or hindrance? How family and friends influence chronic illness self-management among older adults. *Research on Aging, 29,* 375–409.

Gamble, M. A. (2008). Ethically speaking: The nurses' role in end of life issues. *Minnesota Nursing Accent, 80*(3), 14–17.

Garrouste-Orgeas, M., Philippart, F., Timsit, J., Diaw, F., Williems, V., Tabah, A., . . . Carlet, J. (2008). Perception of a 24-hour visiting policy in the intensive care unit. *Critical Care Medicine, 36*(1), 30–35.

Gelling, L., Streator, C., Golledge, J., Sutherland, H., Easton, J., McNamara, R., & MacDonald, R. (2001). The relocation experiences of relatives leaving a neurosciences critical care unit: A phenomenological study. *Nursing in Critical Care, 6,* 163–170.

Gerstel, E., Engelberg, R. A., Koepsell, T., & Curtis, J. R. (2008). Duration of withdrawal of life support in the intensive care unit and association with family satisfaction. *American Journal of Respiratory and Critical Care Medicine, 178*(8), 798–804.

Golden, A. G., Corvea, M. H., Dang, S., Llorente, M., & Silverman, M. A. (2009). Assessing advanced directives in the homebound elderly. *American Journal of Hospice & Palliative Care, 26*(1), 13–17.

Gooding, T., Pierce, B., & Flaherty, K. (2012). Partnering with family members to improve the intensive care unit experience. *Critical Care Nursing Quarterly, 35*(3), 216–222.

Gutierrez, K. M. (2012). Experiences and needs of families regarding prognostic communication in an intensive care unit: Supporting families at end of life. *Critical Care Nursing Quarterly, 35*(3), 299–313.

Handy, C. M., Sulmasy, D. P., Merkel, C. K., & Ury, W. A. (2008). The surrogate's experience in authorizing a do not resuscitate order. *Palliative & Supportive Care, 6*(1), 13–19.

Haras, M. S. (2008). Planning for a good death: A neglected but essential part of ESRD care. *Nephrology Nursing Journal, 35*(5), 451–458, 483.

Hardicre, J. (2003). Nurses' experiences of caring for the relatives of patients in ICU. *Nursing Times, 99*(29), 34–37.

Harvey, M. (2004). Evidence-based approach to family care in the intensive care unit: Why can't we just be decent? *Critical Care Medicine, 32*(9), 1975–1976.

Heyland, D. K., Dodek, P., Rocker, G., Groll, D., Gafni, A., Pichora, D., Shortt, S., . . . Lam, M. (2006). What matters most in end-of-life-care: Perceptions of seriously ill patients and their family members. *Canadian Medical Association Journal, 174*(5), 627–633.

Higgins, I., & Cadd, A. (1999). The needs of relatives of the hospitalized elderly and nurses' perceptions of those needs. *Geriaction, 17*(2), 18–22.

Higgins, I., Joyce, T., Parker, V., Fitzgerald, M., & McMillan, M. (2007). The immediate needs of relatives during hospitalization of acutely ill older relatives. *Contemporary Nurse: A Journal for the Australian Nursing Profession, 26*(2), 208–220.

Hooyman, N. R., & Gonyea, J. G. (1999). A feminist model of family care: Practice and policy directions. *Journal of Women and Aging, 11,* 149–169.

Hopp, F. P., & Duffy, S. A. (2000). Racial variations in end-of-life care. *Journal of the American Geriatric Society, 48,* 658–663.

Hospital Case Management. (2013a). Team follows at-risk patients after discharge. *Hospital Case Management, 6,* 83–85.

Hospital Case Management. (2013b). Initiative leads to an 11% drop in heart failure readmissions. *Hospital Case Management, 21*(4), 48–49.

Hsieh, H., Shannon, S. E., & Curtis, J. R. (2006). Contradictions and communication strategies during end-of-life decision making in the intensive care unit. *Journal of Critical Care, 21*(4), 294–304.

Hughes, F., Bryan, K., & Robbins, I. (2005). Relatives' experiences of critical care. *Nursing in Critical Care, 10*(1), 23–30.

Jacelon, C. S. (2006). Directive and supportive behaviors used by families of hospitalized older adults to affect the process of hospitalization. *Journal of Family Nursing, 12,* 234–250.

Jacobowski, N. L., Girard, T. D., Mulder, J. A., & Ely, C. W. (2010). Communication in critical care: Family rounds in the intensive care. *American Journal of Critical Care, 19*(5), 421–430.

Jarr, S., Henderson, M. L., & Henley, C. (1998). The registered nurse: Perceptions about advance directives. *Journal of Nursing Care Quality, 12*(6), 26–36.

Jencks, S., Williams, M. V., & Coleman, E. A. (2012). Rehospitalizations among patients in the Medicare fee-for-service program. *New England Journal of Medicine, 360*(14), 1418–1428.

Jezewski, M. A., Meeker, M. A., & Robillard, I. (2005). What is needed to assist patients with advance directives from the perspective of emergency nurses. *Journal of Emergency Nursing, 31*(2), 150–155.

Johnson, R., Zhao, Y., Newby, L. K., Granger, C., & Granger, B. (2012). Reasons for noncompletion of advanced directives in a cardiac intensive care unit. *American Journal of Critical Care, 21*(5), 311–319.

Joint Commission on Accreditation of Healthcare Organizations. (2010). Approved: New and revised hospital EPs to improve patient-provider communication. *Joint Commission Perspectives, 30*(1), 5–6.

Karlsson, C., Tisell, A., Engstrom, A., & Andershed, B. (2011). Family members' satisfaction with critical care: A pilot study. *Nursing in Critical Care, 16*(1), 11–18.

Kaufman, S. R. (2002). A commentary: Hospital experience and meaning at the end-of-life. *Gerontologist, 42*(3), 449–457.

Kelley, C. G., Lipson, A. R., Daly, B. J., & Douglas, S. L. (2006). Use of advance directives in the chronically critically ill. *JONA's Healthcare Law, Ethics & Regulation, 8*(2), 42–47.

Kentish-Barnes, N., & Azoulay, E. (2012). The vulnerable family. *Critical Care Medicine, 40*(5), 1667–1668.

Kinrade, T., Jackson, A. C., & Tomnay, J. E. (2009). The psychosocial needs of families during critical illness: Comparison of nurses' and family members' perspectives. *Australian Journal of Advanced Nursing, 27*(1), 82–88.

Kirchhoff, K. R., Palzkill, J., Kowalkowski, J., Mork, A., & Gretarsdottir, E. (2008). Preparing families for intensive care patients for withdrawal of life support: A pilot study. *American Journal of Critical Care, 17*(2), 113–121, quiz 122.

Kleiber, C., Davenport, T., & Freyenberger, B. (2006). Open bedside rounds for families with children in pediatric intensive care units. *American Journal of Critical Care, 15*(5), 492–496.

Kleinpell, R. M., & Powers, M. J. (1992). Needs of family members of intensive care unit patients. *Applied Nursing Research, 5*(1), 2–8.

Kloos, J. A., & Daly, B. J. (2008). Effect of family-maintained progress journal on anxiety of families of critically ill patients. *Critical Care Nursing Quarterly, 31*(2), 96–107.

Ko, E., & Lee, J. (2013). Completion of advance directives among low-income older adults: Does race/ethnicity matter? *American Journal of Hospice & Palliative Medicine.* Advanced online publication. doi:10.1177/1049909113486170

Kosco, M., & Warren, N. A. (2000). Critical care nurses' perceptions of family needs as met. *Critical Care Nursing Quarterly, 23,* 60–72.

Kruse, B. G., Ruder, S., & Martin, L. (2007). Spirituality and coping at the end of life. *Journal of Hospice and Palliative Nursing, 9*(6), 296–304.

Latour, J., & Haines, C. (2007). Families in the ICU: Do we truly consider their needs, experiences, and satisfaction? *Nursing in Critical Care, 12*(4), 173–174.

Lautrette, A., Darmon, M., Megarbane, B., Joly, L. M., Chevret, S., Adrie, C., Barnould, D., . . . Azoulay, E. (2007). *New England Journal of Medicine, 356*(5), 469–478, 537–540.

Linnarsson, J. R., Bubini, J., & Perseius, K. I. (2010). Review: A meta-synthesis of qualitative research into needs and experiences of significant others to critically ill or injured patients. *Journal of Clinical Nursing, 19*(21–22), 3102–3111.

Lloyd-Williams, M., Morton, J., & Peters, S. (2009). The end-of-life experiences of relatives of brain dead intensive care patients. *Journal of Pain and Symptom Management, 37*(4), 659–664.

MacLean, S., Guzzeta, C., White, C., Fontaine, D., Eichorn, D., Meyers, T., & Desy, P. (2003). Family presence during cardiopulmonary resuscitation and invasive procedures: Practices of critical care and emergency nurses. *American Journal of Critical Care, 12*(3), 246–257.

MacLeod, M., Chesson, R. A., Blackledge, P., Hutchison, J. D., & Ruta, N. (2005). To what extent are carers involved in the care and rehabilitation of patients with hip fracture? *Disability and Rehabilitation, 27*(18–19), 1117–1122.

Makic, M. B., VonRueden, K. T., Rauen, C. A., & Chadwick, J. (2011). Evidence-based practice habits: Putting more sacred cows out to pasture. *Critical Care Nurse, 31*(2), 38–61.

Mangram, A. J., McCauley, T., Villarreal, D., Howard, D., Dolly A., & Norwood, S. (2005). Families' perception of the value of timed daily "family rounds" in a trauma ICU. *American Surgeon, 71*(10), 886–891.

Martire, L. M., Lustig, A. P., Schulz, R., Helgeson, V. S., & Miller, G. E. (2007). Is it beneficial to involve a family member? A meta-analysis of psychosocial interventions for chronic illness. *Health Psychology, 23*(6), 599–611.

Maxwell, K., Stuenkel, D., & Saylor, C. (2007). Needs of family members of critically ill patients: A comparison of nurse and family perceptions. *Heart & Lung, 36,* 367–376.

McKinley, S., Nagy, S., Stein-Parbury, J., Bramwell, M., & Hudson, J. (2002). Vulnerability and security in seriously ill patients in intensive care. *Intensive Critical Care Nursing, 18,* 27–36.

McQueen, A. (2000). Nurse-patient relationships and partnership in hospital care. *Journal of Clinical Nursing, 9*(5), 723–731.

Medicare Payment Advisory Commission. (2009). *Report to Congress: Improving incentives in the Medicare program.* Washington, DC: MedPAC. Retrieved from http://www.medpac.gov/documents/Jun09_EntireReport.pdf

Miracle, V. (2005). Critical care visitation. *Dimensions of Critical Care Nursing, 24*(1), 48–49.

Mistianen, P., & Poot, E. (2006). Telephone follow-up, initiated by a hospital-based health professional, for postdischarge problems in patients discharged from hospital to home. *Cochrane Database of Systematic Reviews, 6*(4), CD004510.

Mitchell, M. (2009). Positive effects of a nursing intervention on family-centered care in adult critical care. *American Journal of Critical Care, 18*(6), 543–552.

Molter, N. (1979). Needs of relatives of critically ill patients: A descriptive study. *Heart & Lung, 8*(2), 332–339.

Molter, N. (1994). Families are not visitors in the critical care unit. *Dimensions of Critical Care Nursing, 13*(1), 2–3.

Nelms, T. P., & Eggenberger, S. K. (2010). The essences of the family critical illness experiences and nurse-family meetings. *Journal of Family Nursing, 16*(4), 462–486.

Nelson, D. P., & Poist, G. (2008). An interdisciplinary team approach to evidence-based improvement in family-centered care. *Critical Care Nursing Quarterly, 31*(2), 110–118.

Nelson, J. E., Kinjo, K., Meier, D. E., Ahmad, K., & Morrison, R. S. (2005). When critical illness becomes chronic: Information needs of patients and families. *Journal of Critical Care, 20*(1), 79–89.

Nelson, J. E., Walker, A. S., Luhrs, C. A., Cortez, T. B., & Pronovost, P. J. (2009). Family meetings made simpler: A toolkit for the intensive care unit. *Journal of Critical Care, 24,* 626.e7–626.e14.

Neuberger, J. (2003). Commentary: A good death is possible in the NHS. *British Medical Journal, 326,* 30–34.

Organ Donor. (2014). Donation statistics. Retrieved July 5, 2008, from www.organdonor.gov

Osborne, M. (2011). Coaching helps cut readmissions. *Hospital Case Management, 19*(10), 155–156.

Paterson, B., Kieloch, B., & Gmiterek, J. (2001). "They never told us anything": Postdischarge instruction for families of persons with brain injuries. *Rehabilitation Nursing, 26*(2), 48–53.

Paul, F., & Rattray, J. (2008). Short and long-term impact of critical illness on relatives: Literature review. *Journal of Advanced Nursing, 62*(3), 276–292.

Pearce, L. (2005). Family matters—Liaison nurse offering support to families. *Nursing Standard, 20*(12), 22–24.

Perry, J., Lynam, J., & Anderson, J. M. (2006). Resisting vulnerability: The experiences of families who have kin in the hospital—a feminist ethnography. *International Journal of Nursing Studies, 43*(2), 173–184.

Pikka, L., & Beaulieu, M. (2004). Experiences of families in the neurological ICU: A "bedside phenomenon." *Journal of Neuroscience Nursing, 36*(3), 142–155.

Pouchard, F., Darmon, M., Fassier, T., Bollaert, P., Cheval, C., Coloigner, M., . . . Azoulay, E. (2005). Symptoms of anxiety and depression in family members of intensive care unit patients before discharge or death: A prospective multicenter study. *Journal of Critical Care, 20*(1), 90–96.

Prachar, T. L., Mahanes, D., Arceneaux, A., Moss, B. L., Jones, S., Conaway, M., & Burns, S. M. (2010). Recognizing the needs of family members of neuroscience patients in an intensive care setting. *Journal of Neuroscience Nursing, 4*(5), 274–279.

Puntillo, K. A., & McAdam, J. L. (2006). Communication between physicians and nurses as a target for improving end-of-life care in the intensive care unit: Challenges and opportunities for moving forward. *Critical Care Medicine, 34*(11 Suppl), S332–S340.

Reinbeck, D., & Fitzsimmons, V. (2013). Improving the patient experience through bedside shift report. *Nursing Management, 44*(2), 16–17.

Rushton, C., Reina, M., & Reina, D. (2007). Building trustworthy relationships with critically ill patients and families. *AACN Advances in Critical Care, 18*(1), 19.

Ryan, D., & Jezewski, M. A. (2012). Knowledge, attitudes, experiences, and confidence of nurses in completing advance directives: A systematic synthesis of three studies. *Journal of Nursing Research, 20*(2), 131–140.

Sehgal, N., Green, M., Vidyarthi, M., Blegen, A., & Wachter, R. (2010). Patient whiteboards as a communication tool in the hospital setting: A survey of practices and recommendations. *Journal of Hospital Medicine, 5*(4), 234–239.

Shelton, W., Moore, C. D., Socaris, S., Gao, J., & Dowling, J. (2010). The effect of family support intervention on family satisfaction, length-of-stay, and cost of care in the intensive care unit. *Critical Care Medicine, 38*(5), 1315–1320.

Shorter, M., & Stayt, L. C. (2010). Critical care nurses' experiences of grief in an adult intensive care unit. *Journal of Advanced Nursing, 66*(1), 159–167.

Smith, S. W., Lindsey, L. L., Kopfman, J. E., Yoo, J., & Morrison, K. (2008). Predictors of engaging in family discussion about organ donation and getting organ donor cards witnessed. *Health Communication, 23*(2), 142–152.

Soderstrom, I. M., Saveman, B. I., & Benzein, E. (2006). Interactions between family members and staff in intensive care units: An observation and interview study. *International Journal of Nursing Studies, 43*(6), 707–716.

Stayt, L. (2007). Nurses' experiences of caring for families with relatives in intensive care units. *Journal of Advanced Nursing, 57*(6), 623–630.

Steinhauser, K., Christakis, N., Clipp, E., McNeilly, M., McIntyre, L., & Tulsky, J. (2000). Factors considered important at the end of life by patients, family, physicians and other care providers. *Journal of the American Medical Association, 284*(19), 2476–2482.

Stoeckle, M., Doorley, J. E., & McArdle, R. M. (1998). Identifying compliance with end-of-life care decision protocols. *Dimensions of Critical Care Nursing, 17*(6), 314–321.

Tammelleo, A. D. (2000). Protecting patients' end-of-life choices. *RN, 63*(8), 75–79.

Tilden, V. P., Tolle, S. W., Nelson, C. A., & Fields, J. (2001). Family decision-making to withdraw life-sustaining therapies from hospitalized patients. *Nursing Research, 50*(2), 105–115.

Tobiano, G., Chaboyer, W., & McMurray, A. (2013). Family members' perceptions of the nursing bedside handover. *Journal of Clinical Nursing, 22*, 192–200.

Truog, R. D., Cist, A. F. M., Bracket, S. E., Burns, J. P., Curley, M. A. Q., Danis, M., . . . Hurford, W. E. (2001). Recommendations for end-of-life care in the intensive care unit: The Ethics Committee of the Society of Critical Care Medicine. *Critical Care Medicine, 29*(12), 2332–2348.

Tschann, J. M., Kaufman, S. R., & Micco, G. P. (2003). Family involvement in end-of-life hospital care. *Journal of the American Geriatrics Society, 51*(6), 835–840.

Tweibell, R. S., Siela, D., Riwitis, C., Wheatley, J., Riegle, T., Bouseman, D., . . . Neal, A. (2008). Nurses' perceptions of their self-confidence and the benefits and risks of family presence during resuscitation. *American Journal of Critical Care, 17*(2), 101–111.

United Network for Organ Sharing. (2014). Transplant trends. Retrieved from http://www.unos.org

Van Horn, E., & Kautz, D. (2007). Promotion of family integrity in the acute care setting. *Dimensions of Critical Care Nursing, 26*(3), 101–107.

Verhaeghe, S., Defloor, T., Van Zuuren, F., Duijnstee, M., & Grypdonck, M. (2005). The needs and experiences of family members of adult patients in an intensive care unit: A review of the literature. *Journal of Clinical Nursing, 14*, 501–509.

Volandes, A. E., Ariza, M., Abbo, E. D., & Paasche-Orlow, M. (2008). Overcoming educational barriers for advance care planning in Latinos with video images. *Journal of Palliative Medicine, 11*(5), 700–706.

White, D., & Curtis, J. R. (2006). Establishing an evidence base for physician-family communication and shared-decision making in the intensive care unit. *Critical Care Medicine, 34*(9), 2500–2501.

Wiegand, D. L. (2006). Families and withdrawal of life-sustaining therapy: State of the science. *Journal of Family Nursing, 12*(2), 165–184.

Wiegand, D. L., Deatrick, J. A., & Knafl, K. (2008). Family management styles related to withdrawal of life-sustaining therapy from adults who are acutely ill or injured. *Journal of Family Nursing, 14*(1), 16–32.

Williams, C. M. A. (2005). The identification of family members' contribution to patients' care in the intensive care unit: A naturalistic inquiry. *Nursing in Critical Care, 10*(1), 6–14.

Zaforteza, C., Gastaldo, D., de Pedro, J. E., Sánchez-Cuenca, P., & Lastra, P. (2005). The process of giving information to families of critically ill patients: A field of tension. *International Journal of Nursing Studies, 42*(2), 135–145.

chapter 15

Family Health in Mid and Later Life

Diana L. White, PhD

Jeannette O'Brien, PhD, RN

Critical Concepts

- In most care settings, a majority of those receiving care are older than 65 years.

- Although most older adults are healthy and independent, as a result of chronic illnesses, many become more limited in activities of daily living with advanced age.

- Most older adults have family ties that are positive, meaningful, and supportive. It is rare for older adults to be neglected or uncared for by their families.

- Like all families, families of older adults are diverse. This diversity is influenced by history, race, class, and gender, as well as by individual family history and traditions. These factors influence family composition, health status, health beliefs, and capacity to support each other during times of illness or stress.

- Older adults in families are givers of care, as well as receivers. Until very old age, older family members provide more economic, social, and emotional support to adult children than they receive; they step in to assist families members in crisis, and most caregivers of older adults are spouses.

- Families provide most of the care to older adults, regardless of the care setting. The ways families organize and structure care varies. Nursing care is most effective when done in partnership with families.

- All families experience transitions over the life course. Some are expected and some are not. Each transition is influenced by health status, culture, financial security, and social supports.

- Gerontological nursing takes place in all care settings, although the specific needs of older adults and their families vary. Most older adults live and receive care in community settings.

When we think about aging clients and their families, we often think of individuals or couples who are older than 65 years. These individuals, however, are embedded within a larger family system that includes different and intersecting generations. For example, a 75-year-old couple today may be newlyweds and have living parents. They may be completely healthy with no chronic conditions and spend some of their family time supporting themselves and others. In contrast, a 75-year-old person may be widowed and isolated from other social support, may have multiple chronic conditions, experience several limitations in activities of daily living (ADLs), and require significant help from others. In either case, if the 75-year-olds have children, they are likely to be grandparents and even great-grandparents, and they may be the primary caregivers to one or more of those grandchildren.

If these individuals need help, in any generation, it will come most often from family members. When older adults need care, whether at home, in the hospital, or in a range of long-term care (LTC) settings, families will be participating in that care in most circumstances. Some family members will be active leaders in that care, whereas others will require substantial support from nurses and other professionals. A minority of older adults will have weak social ties and may be isolated from family and friends in old age. These individuals will rely heavily on formal services.

LIFE COURSE PERSPECTIVE

The aging population is diverse, and family systems are complex. Family gerontologists (those who study aging) often use a life course perspective as a way to understand this complexity (Settersten, 2006). The life course perspective recognizes that individuals are embedded in a family system, and that individuals and the family as a whole develop and change over time. This outlook is compatible with many family and social science theories, and is often used in conjunction with other theories, including the theories that guide this book. This chapter discusses the life course perspective in relation to family systems theory, family life cycle theory, and the ecology model of family development. This section describes ways the life course perspective enhances these family theories in contributing to greater understanding of the diversity of family experiences in mid and later life.

Family Systems Theories

Family systems theories emphasize connections among family members. When something happens to or is experienced by one family member, others are affected in some way. The life course perspective encourages us to consider family systems broadly. Connidis (2010), for example, describes family relationships in terms of "family ties," which helps us think about families that extend beyond households

and the nuclear family. Family ties include extended family members and fictive kin—those who are "like family" but are not connected through blood or marriage. As described throughout this chapter, and as is evident in Chapter 3, the character of family ties varies within and between families. Responses to life events among family members are influenced by a history of family rules and traditions that have developed over time (Hanson, 1995) and the quality and characteristics of family ties within the family system. Family breakdown may occur when rules and traditions are not adequate to cover a particular situation. For example, in some families, breakdown may occur when siblings disagree strongly on how to provide support to frail, cognitively impaired parents. One may stress the importance of a parent remaining in her own home, whereas another may feel that the parent's unique health and safety needs demand nursing home care. At the same time, neither can agree on how to spend scarce resources to make either option workable. These disagreements are likely consistent with previous patterns and relationships.

Family Life Cycle Theory

The family life cycle model helps to predict when normative or expected changes will occur. For example, many middle-aged and older adults experience their children leaving home and establishing their own households, a normative change. Adult children form partnerships through marriage or cohabitation. They also begin to achieve financial independence through work. Middle-aged adults who are parents can expect to become grandparents. Retirement is an expected and often desired transition for those with an adequate income and retirement savings. These transitions have been considered normative and represent "on-time" events. For a variety of reasons, however, the timing and even the occurrence of these expected milestones are changing and becoming less predictable. The life course perspective, like the family life cycle theory, focuses on transitions, but also examines the timing of transitions, and the social circumstances, historical events, and the series of decisions that shape individual and family experiences over time.

Bioecological Model

The life course perspective in conjunction with the bioecological model helps explore how societal changes are influencing the timing and context of transitions within and across families, and how societal changes both shape and are influenced by individual and family decisions. For example, it is increasingly common for young adults to leave home and then return due in part to difficulties finding jobs in the current economic climate. Women and men go to college in midlife to begin new careers either voluntarily (e.g., a desire for more meaningful work or a better work-family balance) or involuntarily (e.g., needing new skills after a layoff). Many couples in middle age are beginning their families, not "launching them," reflecting changes in family planning norms, particularly for women pursuing professional careers. Some couples in their fifties adopt young children, sometimes their own grandchildren. Those in their seventies may seek paid employment because of a desire to work or because of financial necessity. According to Quadagno (2008), after several years of declining labor force participation by those older than 60, trends now for both women and men are to remain in the labor force longer. More than 30% of men and about 22% of women 65 to 69 years continue to work full-time or part-time. Past age 70, 10% of men and 8% of women are working. Thus, attitudes and expectations about what is normative or nonnormative, and what is on-time or off-time, are changing, resulting in much greater flexibility and diversity in family experiences. In addition, some transitions, although common, may not be expected and often cause difficulties for families. These include divorce, involuntary job loss, declining health or disability, providing care for ill or dependent family members, and death of a family member.

The life course perspective is particularly helpful in understanding the complexity and diversity of family life revealed in these examples, providing a dynamic understanding of family life across generations (Bengtson & Allen, 1993; Bianchi & Casper, 2005). As with bioecological models, the life course perspective emphasizes context, including the societal conditions in which individuals and families function, as well as the actions individuals take in shaping their relationships and the trajectories of their lives (Alwin, 2012). Individuals and families are influenced by the historical times in which they live. For example, those who are currently in their eighties and nineties and lived in the United States experienced the Great Depression as young

children and many men served in World War II. Later, these children of the Great Depression were parents of the baby boom generation. The baby boom represented a reversal in the trend toward smaller families, resulting in a population bulge that has dominated family life and public policy in the United States ever since. Baby boomers had a different set of challenges and opportunities than their parents and are now entering old age. Their worldview was shaped by the Vietnam war, the civil rights movement, assassinations of U.S. leaders, and the sexual revolution.

Young adults now in their twenties have grown up in a technological and global age quite different from either their parents or grandparents. They have experienced households in which both parents were more likely to work outside the home and divorce was more common. Compared to earlier generations, young adults are marrying later or choosing not to marry. Most are postponing or even forgoing childbearing regardless of marital status (Cherlin, 2010). They have also seen a growth in health and economic disparities among various segments of the population, come of age during the Great Recession, and, to varying degrees, experienced the Iraq and Afghanistan wars. Those pursuing higher education are incurring a huge amount of personal debt. These experiences will influence middle and late life for these individuals.

In all phases of history, societal issues related to race, class, gender, abilities, and immigration have influenced the kinds of opportunities and barriers individuals experience throughout their lives. This combination of historical events and social context must be considered in understanding how changing environments, cultural norms, economic conditions, and political circumstances affect families in mid and later life. Such influences can be seen in work and family decisions, access to health care, and educational opportunities. Many advantages or disadvantages accumulate over a lifetime and across generations (Dannefer, 2003; Hungerford, 2007). For example, children raised in poverty are more likely to have poorer health, less likely to attend college, and more likely to experience hardships in middle and old age (Hungerford, 2007). They are also more likely to marry young, have children before age 30, and divorce (Cherlin, 2010). In contrast, those with more privileged childhoods experience better health and education, are more likely to have higher-paying jobs as adults, have adequate health care, and enter old age with adequate retirement resources. In turn, they are likely to provide their own children with a relatively privileged upbringing.

Even as we emphasize the importance of social and historical context in shaping individual and family lives, we must remember that individuals are not passive. They are active agents, even as their actions may be constrained or enhanced by broader societal circumstances (Alwin, 2012; Connidis, 2010; Settersten, 2006). There are many examples of individuals following or going against societal norms against history, and how that affected the individuals' lives. For example, in war-torn countries, the decision to leave or stay within that country influences the individual and the family for generations thereafter. The life course perspective will be used in this chapter to foster understanding of families with older adults and the family ties that influence their health. This perspective will be used to think about optimal nursing care for these families, using the nursing process. Furthermore, this approach will be used to explain current social policies influencing older adults and their families.

PROFILE OF AGING FAMILIES

In this section we will explore demographic trends that influence families in mid and later life, including family structures and functions. We will also examine different facets of family relationships, from same-generation and intergenerational relationships to challenges of ambivalence and conflict.

Family structures and many of the functions of family are changing at a rapid pace. Several trends have emerged as our population ages, and many of these trends affect families and nursing care of families. The most dramatic is the increased numbers of adults older than 65 years worldwide (Christensen, Doblehammer, Rau, & Vaupel, 2009; Federal Interagency Forum on Aging-Related Statistics, 2012). Older adults are part of families, offering historical context, developmental perspective, and support for younger adults and children. With greater longevity, families have older members and many family relationships last decades longer than in the past. With advanced age, the assistance of younger family members may be

needed to maintain independent living or care for progressive chronic illnesses. Other trends include greater racial and ethnic diversity in later life; more older adults living with chronic illnesses; delayed marriage and childbirth; changing family structure due to increasing numbers of divorced older adults, more who have never married (but may have intimate partnerships), and greater numbers of grandparents living with and/or raising grandchildren (Cherlin, 2010). These trends contribute to changing family relationships, including increased reliance on support across generations and the challenge of intergenerational conflicts. Caregiving, which includes the unpaid assistance provided by family members for an individual with one or more chronic conditions, is increasingly a normative feature of middle and late life (Family Caregiver Alliance, 2006).

Demographic Profile

The aging of the population worldwide is unprecedented historically and has implications for all aspects of society. The 40.3 million adults older than 65 represent 13% of the population of the United States. In Canada, over 33 million (15.5%) are 65 or older. More than 50 countries have at least 10% of their populations over the age of 65. Japan leads with 22.8%, followed by Germany and Italy with over 20% (Federal Interagency Forum on Aging-Related Statistics, 2012). By 2050, numbers in the United States will more than double, resulting in an aging population comprising over 25% of the population (Vincent & Velkoff, 2010). The fastest growing segment of the population in all developed nations is those older than 85 years (Christensen et al., 2009). The United States will see an increase of 36% in this age group between 2010 and 2020, from 5.5 to 6.6 million (Administration on Aging, 2011).

As a group, older adults are healthier, better educated, and more financially secure than in previous generations. People throughout the world are living longer than ever before. At 65 years, an individual in the United States can expect to live nearly 19 more years; women reaching age 85 can expect to live more than seven more years, whereas men are likely to have about six more years of life (Federal Interagency Forum on Aging-Related Statistics, 2012). Most of these individuals, even those who are very old, live independently and in good health. Three quarters of those older than 65 years report having good, very good, or excellent health (Federal Interagency Forum on Aging-Related Statistics, 2012). This is especially true for whites; over 78% report being in good to excellent health compared to about 62% for both African Americans and Hispanic/Latino elders.

Many people report being in good health in spite of having one or more chronic conditions. Although the prevalence of older adults with chronic disabilities declined steadily between the 1980s and 2004 (Manton, 2008), most older adults continue to experience chronic disease, particularly arthritis, heart disease, uncontrolled hypertension, cancer, and diabetes. More important than having a chronic disease is whether and how it affects an individual's ability to function and engage in desired and meaningful activity. Spillman (2004) reported that about 75% of older adults, including those with chronic conditions, indicated no difficulty or disability related to ADLs (basic self-care tasks such as bathing, eating, or dressing), or in instrumental activities of daily living (IADLs). IADLs include basic functions and activities that allow elderly individuals to continue to live independently, such as using the telephone, managing money, doing laundry, maintaining one's home, and managing transportation. Declines in the need for assistance with IADLs may be explained in part by use of technology, including new mobility devices. Declines in disabilities related to ADLs are due to improved management of chronic disease, particularly cardiovascular disease (Manton, 2008).

Recent data suggest that the favorable trends in both chronic disease and functional abilities may be changing, often due to lifestyle. This can be seen most dramatically with the obesity epidemic, consequences of which can be seen in older as well as younger age groups (Christiansen et al., 2009). More than two-thirds of those over age 60 are overweight or obese; 31% are obese. More women than men are obese. This contributes to decreased physical activity and ultimately to poorer health and physical function (Riebe et al., 2009). This trend has important implications for caregiving within families; for example, obesity increases the strain on both the caregiver and the recipient of care due to increased physical strain.

In the United States, older adults are more diverse ethnically and racially than in previous generations. This includes growing proportions of minority older adults in the population. The older African American population will quadruple between 2000 and 2050, whereas the Hispanic and Asian/Pacific Islander populations will be seven and six-and-a-half times larger, respectively (Dilworth-Anderson, Williams, & Gibson, 2002). Minority older adults have shorter life expectancies and report poorer health throughout the life course (Federal Interagency Forum on Aging-Related Statistics, 2012). In addition, racial and ethnic minority groups tend to receive poorer quality care than whites, even controlling for socioeconomic status and severity of illness or condition (Kronenfeld, 2006).

Although the outlook for a healthy old age is generally positive, older adults have the greatest need for health care and are the major users of health care services, especially those older than 85 years. Approximately 25% of older adults have chronic conditions that interfere with daily activities (Kronenfeld, 2006). This means that close to seven million older adults in the United States have significant chronic disabilities (Manton, 2008; Spillman, 2004). In 2002, about half of hospital patients were older than 65 and accounted for 41% of all hospitalizations (Kleinpell, Fletcher, & Jennings, 2008). Unlike younger adults and children, older adults are more likely to have chronic illnesses, and most of those with chronic illnesses have more than one. In 2004, six of the top seven causes of death were chronic illnesses: heart disease, malignant neoplasms, cerebrovascular diseases, chronic lower respiratory diseases, diabetes mellitus, and Alzheimer's disease (Federal Interagency Forum on Aging-Related Statistics, 2012). Other chronic diseases common in old age include arthritis and hypertension. Older adults also experience sensory impairments with age. Kronenfeld (2006) reported that, in 2002, nearly half of older men and about one third of older women indicated they had trouble hearing. Vision problems, even after correction from glasses or contact lenses, occurred in 16% of men and 19% of women. Between 9% and 21% of those older than 70 years have both hearing and vision loss (Saunders & Echt, 2007). Sensory changes may interfere with abilities to function or to interact socially. Hearing loss can be particularly difficult, leading to social isolation or mistaken perceptions by others that the elder is cognitively impaired. Vision loss can affect or prohibit the ability to drive, which can increase dependency on others. Senses related to smell and taste generally remain stable into old age when one is healthy, but can be negatively affected by disease or medications. This in turn may lead to poor nutritional status, which will adversely affect health status (Maas et al., 2001; Mattes, 2002).

All nurses will work with increasing numbers of older adults simply because the population is aging so rapidly. Even nurses who focus on maternal and child or pediatric nursing are likely to encounter grandparents in the course of their work more often now than in the past, because of increased longevity of grandparents and the increasing numbers of grandparents raising their grandchildren. As discussed later in this chapter, more grandparents are assuming parenting roles because their adult children are unable to function as parents (Dolbin-MacNab, 2006; Uhlenberg & Kirby, 1998).

Family Structure

With increasing life expectancy, family relationships now last for decades. It is common to see newspaper photos of couples celebrating their 60th anniversaries, and to know "children" in their sixties or seventies who have living parents. We now encounter siblings with relationships of 90 years or longer; even grandparent-grandchild relationships increasingly extend five or more decades. These long-lasting relationships with their histories of shared experiences, traditions, and exchanges of help will most often be an asset to the older adult as illnesses or functional declines occur. With declining birth rates, however, older adults in the future will have a smaller pool of family members to draw on for help.

Gender Differences

Differences in life expectancy by sex influence family structures and functions in old age. Women outlive men across all ethnic groups and in all age groups. Women are more likely than men to be widowed throughout the life course, but especially in the oldest age groups: 73% of very old women (those 85 years and older) and 35% of very old men are widowed (Federal Interagency Forum on Aging-Related Statistics, 2012). Living arrangements show a similar pattern, with men more likely to live with their spouses and women more likely to live alone or with other relatives in advanced old age. As a result, men are much more likely to have a spouse caregiver than women (Connidis, 2010). Men are

much more likely than women to be married in old age due to greater longevity for women and somewhat higher rates of remarriage after widowhood or divorce for men. For example, more than 78% of men 65 to 74 years old are married compared with 56% of women. By the time they reach old age, the disparity is even greater; 58% of men 85 years and older are married, whereas only 18% of women in that age group are married (Federal Interagency Forum on Aging-Related Statistics, 2012). Marital status varies by ethnicity, with a greater proportion of African American and Hispanic adults widowed or divorced when compared to whites (Connidis, 2010). In addition, African Americans have greater rates of cohabitation than the general population throughout adulthood. Asian, African American, Hispanic, and Native American elders are more likely to live with nonspouse kin and less likely to live alone than whites.

Financial Disparities

Women's marital status is closely linked to financial status in old age. Women, especially minority women, experience significant losses in income and net worth when their husbands die (Angel, Jimenez, & Angel, 2007). Compared with men, today's oldest women have not had careers or worked in jobs with pension benefits. Those with a history of low-wage jobs, more frequent marital disruption, and fewer opportunities to accumulate assets during their working years are especially vulnerable. More than 10% of older women are poor compared with less than 7% of men (Federal Interagency Forum on Aging-Related Statistics, 2012). On average, Social Security provides 60% of income for older women, and it is the sole source of income for 20% of older women (Herd, 2005). Disparities by race and ethnicity are even greater. For example, older African American women are more than twice as likely to live below the poverty level than are older white women (Herd, 2005).

Marriage, Divorce, and Fertility

Divorce rates increased dramatically during the 20th century, more than doubling between the 1960s and 1980s before stabilizing in the 1990s; most divorces occurred in young or middle adulthood (Faust & McKibben, 1999). As a result, only about 20% of marriages are expected to survive for 50 years because of divorce or widowhood (Wu & Schimmele, 2007). Although many will enter old age as divorced persons, divorce occurring in late life is a growing phenomenon, with many older adults no longer willing to live another 20 or 25 years in an unsatisfying relationship. Reasons for late-life divorce are similar to those found in other age groups, including falling out of love, emotional or physical abuse, substance abuse, or infidelity. Women tend to leave their spouses more frequently than men (Wu & Schimmele, 2007).

This portrait of family structure will continue to change as society changes. Cherlin (2010) described several demographic trends in the first decade of the century that will affect family life in old age in the future. First, age at first marriage continues to rise, particularly for those with college educations. Second, although risk of divorce is beginning to decline, the lifetime probability of divorce remains between 40% and 50%. Like age at marriage, risk of divorce is associated with education; those with more education are less likely to divorce. Thus, we see that experiences with family life will become increasingly divided by educational and economic status. Third, fertility rates in the United States, unlike many developed countries, are at population replacement levels. Fertility varies among ethnic groups, with the highest levels among Hispanic populations with Mexican origins. Over the last several decades, the number of children born outside of marriage has increased significantly, accounting for nearly 40% of all births in 2007. Fourth, cohabitation has become more common in all age groups. We can no longer assume that those who are single are without partners. Furthermore, increasing numbers of children are born to unmarried, and often unpartnered women. Cherlin (2010) reported that partnerships through cohabitation are less stable than those of married couples. This has implications for intergenerational family ties in old age. Other recent trends include the growth of socially and legally recognized same sex unions, increasing numbers of children who have a parent living in a different household, and a growing percentage of foreign born (Cherlin, 2010). These changes mean that older families of the future will be increasingly diverse in terms of ethnicity, economics, structure, and individual experiences with family.

Family Relationships

A prevailing myth in the United States is that older adults, particularly those who are part of the dominant culture, are isolated from and neglected by their younger family members, and ultimately are abandoned in nursing homes. Study after study has demonstrated that most family ties are strong and characterized by affection, caring, and many shared values (Fingerman & Birditt, 2011; Rossi & Rossi, 1990). Furthermore, families have demonstrated remarkable adaptability to social change. Although the family structure has changed in recent decades, much about family life has remained the same, including valuing families. Individuals continue to travel through life in the company of others, which Antonucci and Akiyama (1995) described as "social convoys." Some people come and go in our convoys, but many, especially family members, remain constant social companions for decades. Families value exchanges of emotional and practical support throughout the life course (Sechrist, Suitor, Pillemer, Gilligan, Howard, & Keeton, 2012; Walker, Manoogian-O'Dell, McGraw, & White, 2001).

We now consider family ties in terms of same-generation and intergenerational relationships. Same-generation relationships include intimate partnerships and sibling relationships. Intergenerational relationships examined in this chapter include parent-child and grandparent-grandchild ties.

Same-Generation Relationships

Intimate partnerships: In general, older adults who are married or are in egalitarian relationships have better physical health and psychological well-being when compared to those who are single, widowed, divorced, or separated (Connidis, 2010). This is especially true for men and for couples who report high-quality relationships (Bookwala, 2012). Relationship quality is influenced by retirement status, as well as by health, mental health, and caregiving roles. All of these situations have the potential to influence relationships in negative ways. The way one partner responds to a stressor such as chronic illness influences how the other responds, emphasizing the importance of focusing on family and not just individuals when working with older adults.

As a group, people who have never married tend to have high levels of well-being, though they are second in well-being to those in satisfying partnerships. Because those who have never married often have a history of living alone, they typically have higher levels of life satisfaction than those who are widowed, divorced, and separated. This is because most have created satisfying and robust social networks, typically including close friends, siblings, and other family members. It is important to emphasize that the "never married" group is becoming more diverse. Particularly in future cohorts, we can no longer assume that never married means unpartnered or without children (Cherlin, 2010).

Those who have experienced dissolution of a partnership, whether through divorce or widowhood, must adjust to living alone. This puts them at greater risk of low morale and adverse health. Divorce, particularly for men, can result in strained relationships with adult children placing them at an even greater risk of isolation in old age (Connidis, 2010). Older adults who are widowed or divorced often form new relationships, frequently choosing cohabitation over remarriage. A growing number of older adults are also forming partnerships without sharing a household, termed *living apart together* (LAT). This is often appealing to women who value both autonomy and an intimate relationship (Bookwala, 2012). Until recently, same-sex couples did not have the option of marriage, so formed cohabitating or LAT partnerships. Societal attitudes are shifting, with marriage increasingly an option for same-sex couples in many states and countries.

Sexuality is central to intimate partnerships throughout the life course regardless of gender or partnership status. Women and men continue to desire sexual relationships well into later life, with many reporting increased freedom to explore sexuality because of decreased concern over procreation and decreased family responsibilities. Older adults with partners tend to rate sex as important; most couples who have been sexually active in middle age tend to remain so in old age. Those who are sexually active tend to report greater emotional and physical well-being (Bookwala, 2012). Sexuality continues into later life and is dependent on physical health, quality and availability of relationships, change in role from procreation to pleasure and validation, attitudes toward sexuality, societal influences, and previous sexual experiences (DeLamater & Moorman, 2007). DeLamater and Moorman (2007) emphasized the danger of viewing sexuality from only a biological or medical perspective, noting that attitude is more salient in predicting continued sexual desire and behavior than presence or absence of chronic illness or age. Nevertheless, advancing age

is associated with decline in sexual activity for many people. Declines often result from lack of a partner, typically through widowhood but also through divorce or disability (e.g., Alzheimer's disease). Poor health is another common cause of decline in sexual functioning. Schmall (1994), however, emphasized that sexuality involves more than sexual intercourse, highlighting the importance of intimacy, touch, affection, body image, and one's identity as a sexual being. Sexuality, in intimate, same-generation partnerships, therefore, continues to be an important part of life in spite of increasing frailty and dependence. Loss of a partner through widowhood often means the loss of all these different facets of sexuality, facets that often are unrecognized or unacknowledged. DeLamater's (2002) integrated model of assessing sexuality in later life can aid nurses in understanding the role of sexuality in the lives of older adults. The model includes the following:

- Biological influences: physical health (i.e., presence of chronic conditions that impact sexual function or desire, or both), age, hormonal levels, medical treatments that may impact sexual function
- Psychological: attitudes toward sexuality, role of sexual relationships, knowledge, past experiences, mental health
- Social: availability of partner, including duration and quality of relationship, societal views and influences on sexuality in later life, socioeconomic status

Siblings: Siblings represent important but often overlooked same-generation family relationships (Bedford & Avioli, 2012; Walker, Allen, & Connidis, 2005). They typically are the family tie of the longest duration and, as such, siblings largely experience the same historical and social context. As with all family relationships, identifying siblings can be complex. They may include full biological relationships, siblings through adoptions, half or step siblings, and fictive relationships. With divorce, there can also be relationships of "former siblings." In adulthood, family ties expand through sisters- and brothers-in-law, and nieces and nephews, relationships made possible through sibling ties. Although often intense during childhood, many sibling relationships become inactive in young adulthood as people focus on their partners, children, and career development. During middle and late life, sibling ties are often reactivated as older adults have more time to devote to the relationship and as aging parents require increasing assistance. This illustrates both the voluntary and the obligatory aspects of the sibling tie (Walker et al., 2005). Siblings tend to feel obligations to work together in support of aging parents and also respond to each other in times of need. Conflicts, when they do arise, appear to have roots in family history, and may be related to differential treatment as children. Of course, many siblings remain emotionally close and interact frequently throughout their lives. Siblings are most likely to report being close to a sister. Throughout the life course, those who are unmarried, without children, and live in close proximity retain active ties to siblings. Having sibling relationships is associated with less loneliness in old age (Bedford & Avioli, 2012).

Intergenerational Relationships

Intergenerational relationships may be of growing importance in family life, particularly as divorce has become more common (Sechrist et al., 2012). Most older adults have one grown child who lives within an hour's drive. This has remained relatively constant despite the often-cited geographical mobility of younger generations. At the same time, adult children with college degrees are more likely to live farther away (Uhlenberg, 2004). Contact between generations is common, with the majority of adult children reporting contact with their parents at least once a week. Contact with mothers is more frequent than contact with fathers, and contact between mothers and daughters is the most common intergenerational interaction, reflecting that the strongest intergenerational tie is between mothers and daughters. Contact between grandparents and grandchildren is similar to that between parents and adult children, with 66% of grandparents living within an hour's drive from at least one set of grandchildren. The strongest predictor of grandparent-grandchild relationships is the quality of relationships between parents and grandparents (Monserud, 2008; Thiele & Whelan, 2006). The amount of contact by adult children is influenced by parental marital status, with the lowest contact being with fathers who are widowed, divorced, or remarried, and with remarried mothers.

Relationship quality is as important as contact. Feelings of closeness between generations are the norm, with most adult children reporting feeling very close to parents, especially to mothers. The older generation even more frequently reports feeling very close to their adult children. When adult children report that they are not close to their parents, they are more likely to be describing their relationships with their fathers than their relationships with their mothers (Silverstein & Bengtson, 1997). Exchanges of help and support between generations occur throughout the life course and are motivated by affection, as well as by a sense of obligation. Until late old age, older adults provide more help than they receive in all areas of support, including caring for family members, financial support, and instrumental support (Sechrist et al., 2012). We explore exchanges among generations further in our discussion of caregiving later in the chapter.

Significant intergenerational family relationships include grandparents and grandchildren. Almost all older adults with children are likely to become grandparents, usually around age 50, although the transition can occur both earlier and later in the life course. It is a role that is contingent on the actions of others for timing, number, location, and amount of contact (Hayslip & Page, 2012; Thiele & Whelan, 2006). Sometimes called a "roleless role," grandparents often create their role within the family based on the family's stage in the life course and the family history of grandparenting roles. Grandparents are influenced by experiences with their own grandparents and with their parents as grandparents. Also, relationships with grandchildren are strongly shaped by the quality of relationships with adult children. When the grandparent-parent relationship is strong, grandparents and grandchildren are also likely to enjoy strong connections. If the role is perceived to come too early, as in the case of teenage pregnancy, the transition to grandparenthood may be altered by disappointment, anxiety, and emotional and financial distress.

As in other family relationships, the ways that grandparents relate to grandchildren vary widely among families (Silverstein & Marenco, 2001; Stelle, Fruhauf, Orel, & Landry-Meyer, 2010; Thiele & Whelan, 2006). Most older adults, however, find grandparenting meaningful and experience the role with both satisfaction and pleasure (Roberto, 1990; Szinovacz, 1998). Grandparents are often an important resource for their adult children. For example, they are a major provider of child care when grandchildren are young (Luo, LaPierre, Hughes, & Waite, 2012; Vandell, McCartney, Owen, Booth, & Clarke-Stewart, 2003). With the aging of both grandparents and grandchildren, the nature of relationships will change. Older grandparents, for example, are more likely to provide money and gifts as grandchildren get older rather than direct care (Thiele & Whelan, 2006).

Family Ambivalence and Conflict

Although family relationships are generally strong and characterized by affection and caring, family gerontology researchers have increasingly focused on the complexity of family life. The concept of ambivalence has received increasing attention, recognizing that family members simultaneously hold positive and negative feelings about one another, often as a result of contradictory roles (Connidis & McMullin, 2002; Katz, Lowentstein, Phillips, & Daatland, 2005; Pillemer & Suiter, 2005; Sechrist et al., 2012). Fingerman (2001) found adult daughters tended to express more ambivalence about their mothers than mothers expressed about their daughters. Pillemer and Suitor (2005) report that the majority of parents felt "torn in two directions" about their adult children. They found that ambivalence was frequently related to their adult children's achievements, particularly achievements of their oldest child. More ambivalence was expressed toward those who did not attain normative adult statuses, such as completing college, getting married, or becoming financially independent. Peters, Hooker, and Zvonkovic (2006) conclude that ambivalence is a normal part of family life. In their study, older adults experienced ambivalence surrounding their adult children's busy lives and boundaries related to communication (e.g., holding back on opinions and feelings about being left out). Older adults had uncertainties about the availability of help from children should they need it, though Peters and her colleagues found that those who needed help received it.

Though less common than ambivalence, family conflict, or negative social interactions, can have serious consequences for family relationships. Furthermore, negative aspects of relationships may lead to poorer health, and may decrease the amount and quality of support available when needed (Lachman, 2003; Rook, 2003). Newsom, Rook, Nishishiba, Sorkin, and Mahan (2005) reported on a growing body of research that describes the disproportionate effect of negative social exchanges on psychological health when compared with positive social exchanges. They found that failure of those in one's social network to provide help when it was needed was evaluated most negatively. Umberson, Williams, Powers, Liu, and Needham (2006) examined marriage quality and health over the life course, finding that poor marriage quality was associated with accelerated health declines in old age. They suggested that stress related to marital conflicts undermines immune functioning and has a cumulative effect on health over time. Conflicted families are less likely to provide assistance to each other throughout the life course and may have little contact, share few values, and generally are more detached. As such, they are less likely to be resources to older family members in need (Scharlach, Li, & Dalvi, 2006).

Divorce is often a factor in these situations and has implications for intergenerational relationships throughout the life course. Although not focusing on conflict specifically, Bucx, van Wel, Knijin, and Hagendoorn (2008) reported less contact by adult children with divorced mothers and fathers. Moreover, mothers may be mediating relationships between fathers and adult children, as indicated by increased contact between adult children with widowed mothers, but not with widowed fathers. Less contact was also reported with divorced and remarried fathers, although no differences were found in contact with widowed and remarried mothers (Bucx et al., 2008). Those who are most vulnerable with respect to family relationships, therefore, are divorced men. They may have fewer ties that connect them to informal care and may rely more on formal services, such as nursing homes, than their married counterparts.

An extreme consequence of family conflict is elder abuse or mistreatment. Elder mistreatment includes physical pain or injury, psychological anguish, neglect or abandonment, and financial exploitation. Estimates of prevalence of all types of mistreatment range from 1.3% to 10% of older adults (Fulmer, Guadagno, Bitondo, & Connolly, 2004; Teaster, Wangmo, & Vorsky, 2012). Most perpetrators are adult children, although other family members, paid caregivers, and predatory acquaintances may be abusers. Causes of mistreatment remain poorly understood, but risk factors include unhealthy dependency of the perpetrator on the victim; disturbed psychological state of the perpetrator; frailty, disability, or impairment of the victim; and isolation of the family (Wolf, 1996). Risk of abuse increases with age and women are more likely to be victims. Beach, Schulz, Castle, and Rosen (2010) also found that African American elders were at greater risk for both financial exploitation and psychological mistreatment. Most abuse occurs in domestic settings; those living alone are at greatest risk for financial exploitation (Teaster et al., 2012).

In addition to mistreatment by family members, frail older adults are also at risk for mistreatment by care providers. Nurses and other professionals have a responsibility to screen and assess elders for abuse. Fulmer (2012) reviewed and evaluated several assessment tools. One of the recommended tools is the Elder Assessment Instrument, which can be found on the *Try This* section of the Hartford Institute for Geriatric Nursing (HIGN) Web site (Fulmer, 2012).

As illustrated by the discussions on ambivalence and conflict, it is evident that many family relationships are complex and the strengths of association may vary considerably over time. To add to the complexity, levels of ambivalence and conflict vary within families (Sechrist et al., 2012). An individual may have conflicted feelings about one family member and close, affectionate feelings about another. Both ambivalence and conflict may be apparent for nurses and other health providers when an older adult needs care. Nurses should be aware that the families vary considerably with respect to the quality of relationships and the availability of family resources in times of crisis and health decline. Nurses must be sensitive to underlying tensions and be able to provide support in nonjudgmental ways, remembering that the current family dynamics are embedded in a lifetime of relationships and actions.

FAMILY CAREGIVING

As described previously, family life is characterized by exchanges of help and support throughout the life course. Until very old age, parents are more often givers than receivers in this exchange, regardless of income. They provide financial assistance to younger adults in college or those who are making major purchases such as cars or homes (Bengtson & Harootyan, 1994). Grandparents are a frequent source of childcare for grandchildren, particularly in their first 3 years (Vandell et al., 2003). They provide child care for their grandchildren while

their adult children work or are unable to care for their children because of illness or planned absences (e.g., vacations). Less typical is providing care for dependent adult children with cognitive or physical disabilities. In some cases, caring for dependent children can be a lifelong role (Bilmes, 2008; Pruchno & Meeks, 2004; Seltzer, Greenberg, Floyd, & Hong, 2004; Yeoman, 2008). Grandparents also are often a source of stability when parents divorce. Growing numbers of grandparents are filling parenting roles for grandchildren because their parents are unable or unwilling to fulfill their parental obligations (Hayslip & Kaminski, 2005).

Regardless of the type of care provided, family caregiving grows out of ongoing family relationships and refers to support given to those who are dependent on that support for everyday functioning (Pruchno & Gitlin, 2012; Waldrop, 2003). The transition from the normal and mutual aid to support that is defined as caregiving is often a gradual process. Many wives, for example, do not describe what they do as caregiving, because the work they do in support of their increasingly dependent husbands is part of their ongoing family roles related to meal preparation, housework, and laundry. Walker, Pratt, and Eddy (1995) noted that adult daughters do similar things for dependent mothers as they do for mothers who are more self-sufficient, including running errands, preparing meals, and assisting with housework. Caregiving may simply mean "keeping an eye on" an older adult to monitor well-being (Messecar, 2012). As dependency increases and more time is spent on providing support, the family member and now caregiver recognizes that the care recipient is no longer able to perform these tasks without help.

In contrast to a gradual process, transitions to caregiving can happen suddenly if an otherwise healthy older adult has a traumatic injury, or experiences a stroke or cardiac arrest. For many older adults, a health crisis may signal a sudden end to independence or ability to live alone. In this case, a variety of decisions are made regarding informal and formal care services. Depending on the situation, including the nature of the disability, availability of services, and personal resources, the older person may receive support services in several different settings. About half (51%) receive care in their own home, and about a third live in the caregiver's home (National Alliance for Caregiving & AARP, 2009). Others move into supported living situations, such as assisted living or nursing homes.

Whether the onset of caregiving is sudden or gradual, most caregivers are family members, accounting for 80% to 90% of care received by older adults (Pruchno & Gitlin, 2012). Few older adults who live in their own or in their caregiver's home rely on formal services, with 35% using any type of paid care, such as a housekeeper or aide (National Alliance for Caregiving & AARP, 2009). Those with higher incomes are more likely to use paid help.

Estimates of the prevalence of caregiving range widely depending on how caregiving is defined. Care may support IADLs, which consist of functions related to laundry, housekeeping, transportation, food preparation, shopping, handling finances, using the phone, and medication management (Graf, 2007). Increasing dependency requires care specific to ADLs, which involve intimate, personal care related to bathing, dressing, eating, toileting, transferring, and mobility (Wallace & Shelkey, 2007). Messecar (2012) reported that between 22.4 and 52 million people provide some care to family members every year. The smaller estimates are related to the more intense ADLs care, whereas the larger estimates include those who receive assistance with IADLs only. Combining all levels of care, Reinhard, Given, Petlick, and Bemis (2008) cited the statistic of 44 million caregivers, about 20% of the adult population. The National Alliance for Caregiving and AARP (2009) estimate that nearly a third of U.S. households (36.5 million) have a caregiver present. Indeed, caregiving is now considered an expected role in middle and late life. Clearly, providing care to an older adult is becoming part of the normative life experience in families; most adults will experience caring for another adult family member at least once in their lifetime (Pruchno & Gitlin, 2012).

Most caregivers are middle-aged or older and are most likely to be wives and daughters, although men are increasingly assuming this role. Research has shown consistently that women provide more personal care, more hours of caregiving, and more housekeeping, whereas men provide financial assistance (such as money management), make arrangements for formal care, and do home and yard maintenance work. These historically gendered roles, however, are becoming less distinct. Reinhard et al. (2008) report a 50% increase between 1984 and 1994 in the number of caregiving men who provide physical care. Similarly, Neal and Hammer (2007) reported that men in dual-earner couples were taking on substantially more parent care responsibilities, including ADLs care, although their wives were providing about 2 more hours of caregiving per week than husbands. The trend of increasing involvement by men in all facets of caregiving likely will continue as the number of older adults needing support increases.

Duration of caregiving may last for days or decades, with the average length of time 4.6 years; 15% of caregivers have been providing care for 10 years or longer. About half of caregivers provide 8 hours of care or more each week, with 26% of caregivers providing 21 hours or more (National Alliance for Caregiving & AARP, 2009). As in families described by Neal and Hammer (2007), working couples are often involved in providing parent care for more than one person, such as providing care to both parents or to one's parent and a parent-in-law. The Hooper family case study below illustrates such multiple caregiving demands as Maria provides care to both her father and her mother-in-law.

Estimates of the value of unpaid family care are difficult to determine and are as high as $375 billion annually (Pruchno & Gitlin, 2012). Out-of-pocket medical expenses are 2.5 times greater for caregivers than noncaregivers (Family Caregiver Alliance, 2006). Furthermore, caregiving often results in lost income if spouses and adult children leave the workforce early to care for older family members. Those who maintain their jobs often lose time and, therefore, wages, promotions, or other job opportunities because of parent care responsibilities. As discussed earlier, the loss of income may be particularly difficult for those with low incomes to begin with. Family members are often faced with the difficult decision of having less income due to less time in the workforce versus dealing with the expense of paid care either in the home or at a residential care facility.

Family Caregiving Roles

Family roles, like family structure, have shifted across time. Major changes in mid and late life frequently include an increase in caregiving. This section focuses on caregiving for older adults by spouses and adult children, caring for grandchildren, and care for disabled adult children. It also covers ways in which nurses can support caregivers.

Caring for Older Adults

The experience of caregiving differs by role. Spouses are generally the first line of caregivers. Because women live longer than men, wives are more likely than husbands to become caregivers. Spouse caregivers, in particular, may have their own health concerns that are exacerbated by strains related to caregiving. Messecar (2012) reported that caregiving spouses have a 63% greater mortality rate than others their age who are not caregivers. At times, the spouse who is designated as caregiver is also in need of support services. It is not unusual for husbands and wives to support each other; they are both caregivers and care recipients. These situations are often tenuous but can work for a while. Spouses typically experience greater burden and depression than adult children who provide care (Messecar, 2012). Spouses are more likely to experience chronic illnesses and frailty themselves. Because spouse caregivers typically live with the care recipient, they are at risk for not getting rest, not having time to recuperate from illnesses, and experiencing health declines. This is particularly true if the person they are caring for has Alzheimer's disease or some other kind of dementia (Reinhard et al., 2008). Those who care for someone with dementia are at increased risk for depression, greater levels of stress, and lower levels of subjective well-being, especially wives (Pinquart & Sorensen, 2006).

Adult children, especially daughters, experience the stresses of care in other ways. More than half are working while providing care, and make a range of adjustments at work. This may include going in late or leaving early, cutting down on hours worked, or leaving the labor force entirely (National Alliance for Caregiving & AARP, 2009). Adult children have to balance caregiving and other family obligations. Some are doing substantial caregiving for parents while caring for young children at home (Neal & Hammer, 2007). Grandchildren may also participate in providing care to their grandparents as they age, especially if their mothers are primary caregivers. The ways that grandchildren cope with this caregiving role is influenced by their previous relationships with their grandparents (Stelle et al., 2010).

Caregiving is influenced by culture. It is important to be aware of and sensitive to possible ethnic differences in caregiving experiences and resources. At the same time, it is important not to stereotype and make assumptions based on race or ethnicity. More differences are found within ethnic groups than between them. With that caution, Dilworth-Anderson et al. (2002) argue that "culture affects caregiving experiences. Findings on values and norms provide evidence that individuals and groups use explicit rules and guidelines that influence who provides care to elders as well as interactions between caregivers, family members, and social institutions" (p. 264). From their review of the literature, it appears that minority caregivers often have a more diverse group of extended helpers than do white caregivers. But although more people might be involved in providing care to a dependent family member, minority caregivers are no more likely to feel supported by their social network than are caregivers from the dominant culture. Whites are more likely to care for a spouse, which is related to whites having more married couples in later life and a longer life expectancy for men. African Americans are more likely to include church connections to assist with caregiving tasks. They are also more likely to have a network of kinship relationships that assist with caregiving. African Americans and Hispanics are least likely to use formal services and yet are most likely to express the need for assistance with caregiving responsibilities. Cultural values do influence who takes on the leadership role of caregiving within a family (Dilworth-Anderson et al., 2002). These values are affected by a sense of filial obligation and a sense of responsibility, cultural norms regarding who provides care (i.e., daughter or daughter-in-law), values of giving back, culturally based illness meanings (e.g., a view that disease is normal or that there is a stigma), and larger belief systems such as religion. Because of poorer health status found in most minority populations, caregiving often begins at a younger age, but the duration is shorter.

African American caregivers are more likely to have children younger than 18 years living in the household than other ethnic groups. They are more likely to be working and caring for a family member, and also spending more time and money to support the person they care for. This commitment contributes to the financial burden for the family, increasing their risk for living at a low socioeconomic level. African American caregivers are more likely to say caregiving is a financial hardship. Asian American caregivers are found, as a rule, to have more education and higher incomes when compared with other racial ethnic groups. This group is less likely to report emotional stress and be more able to pay for assistance with caregiving. White caregivers tend to be older and also living in a higher income bracket when compared with other racial groups (Dilworth-Anderson et al., 2002).

Our discussion of providing care to frail older adults reflects research in this area, as well as the population most at need of family caregiving (Riebe et al., 2009). It is important to emphasize, however, that many older adults are primary caregivers of younger members of their families.

Grandparents Caring for Grandchildren

Unlike caregiving for older adults, which often evolves over time, grandparents may suddenly find themselves in the role of raising their grandchildren. This may occur when teenagers have children or as a result of traumatic circumstances surrounding the parent generation, including divorce, substance abuse, incarceration, child abuse or neglect, or death (Hayslip & Page, 2012). The number of grandparents who are raising their grandchildren has risen dramatically, increasing 30% between 1990 and 2000 (Hayslip & Kaminski, 2005). According to census data reported in 2006, about 2.4 million grandparents are in this position (Goodman, 2012). Lumpkin (2008) reported 11% of grandparents in the United States were parenting their grandchildren. The trend continued from 2000 to 2008, with increases of another 8%. Most of that occurred from 2007 to 2008 (Luo et al., 2012). These grandparent-grandchild families are more likely to live below the poverty line and lack health insurance. Some grandparents leave the workforce to care for grandchildren, whereas others feel that they cannot retire for financial reasons. Grandparent caregivers are most often women, are in poorer physical health, and have a greater incidence of depression than other grandparents. Ongoing conflict with adult children (parents of their grandchildren) is common, with accompanying feelings of disappointment, resentment, feeling taken advantage of, and grief. If parents have been substance abusers, grandchildren may have physical and behavioral problems that cause further anxiety for grandparents (Hayslip & Kaminski, 2005; Leder, Grinstead, & Torres, 2007).

Many custodial grandparents are saddened by the loss of the traditional grandparent role that emphasizes indulgence and fun, instead of being responsible for discipline, financial support, and a myriad of activities related to daily care. Caregiving grandparents may be isolated from their age peers who are pursuing more traditional grandparent-, work-, or retirement-related activities. They also may have little in common with the parents of their grandchildren's friends (Landry-Meyer & Newman, 2004). Most grandparents who raise grandchildren are non-Hispanic whites, yet the largest proportion of any ethnic or racial group of grandparents raising grandchildren are African Americans. African American and Latino grandparents are more likely to assume the responsibility because of economic conditions and teen pregnancies, whereas white grandparents are more likely to be parenting because of substance abuse by their adult children. White grandparents are also more likely to report greater levels of burden and more intergenerational conflict than those in other ethnic groups. This may be because of combined circumstances of normative expectations and issues related to substance abuse (Goodman & Silverstein, 2006).

As with caregiving in general, grandparents and their grandchildren experience many benefits from grandparents parenting. Grandparents are often a stabilizing influence, and their grandchildren generally do well in school, are less likely to be on welfare, and have fewer negative behaviors. Grandparents, in spite of their grief and the burdens associated with care, report benefits such as realizing their inner strength, close relationships with their grandchildren, and a sense of accomplishment and purpose (Hayslip & Kaminski, 2005; Waldrop, 2003). Goodman (2012) followed grandmothers raising grandchildren over 9 years. She found that those who had close relationships with their grandchildren did not experience many of the negative consequences described earlier, suggesting that interventions that support these relationships are particularly important.

Older Adults Caring for Adult Children

Much of the literature addresses parents caring for adult children with developmental disabilities or mental illness. Seltzer and her colleagues have followed aging mothers of adults with mental retardation or severe mental illness for many years. Their research indicates many similarities and also some important differences between these mothers (Seltzer et al., 2004; Seltzer, Greenberg, Krause, &

Hong, 1997). The onset of disability occurred at different times in the life course—at birth for those with mental retardation and in young adulthood for those with mental illness. Mothers of those with mental retardation experienced more gratification and less subjective burden than mothers of those with mental illness. They also received more social support and had developed more effective coping skills. Mothers of children with mental illness experienced greater levels of stress and burden. The course of the child's illness was less predictable, sometimes involving repeated crises involving hospitalization or incarceration. As mothers of disabled children aged, they required additional supports, including placement of their children in residential care. Reasons leading to placement varied. For mothers of children with mental retardation, placement often occurred because of poor health and mother's declining abilities. Mothers in both groups maintained a high frequency of contact with their disabled child (Seltzer et al., 1997).

Magana, Seltzer, and Krauss (2002) focused on Latino populations, finding that they had higher service needs than the general population, in part because of lack of knowledge and the difficulty of navigating the system. When programs were culturally sensitive and provided opportunities for peer support, however, Latinos did increase use of services.

The consequences of a lifetime of caring for an adult child with intellectual or developmental disabilities are significant. Although Seltzer, Floyd, Song, Greenberg, and Hong (2011) found similarities to parents of children with no disabilities with respect to health, attainment, and life satisfaction in midlife, they did find parents of those with disabilities differed with respect to lower employment levels for women and lower social participation rates. These patterns continued as parents entered their sixties. This was especially true for those who continued to co-reside with their children. Challenges included higher rates of depression, divorce, widowhood and poorer physical health and functional status when compared to other parents whose children did not have disabilities (Seltzer et al., 2011).

Many parents are finding themselves caring for disabled war veterans as an aftermath of the Iraq and Afghanistan wars (Yeoman, 2008). As of November 2009, over 36,000 servicemen had been wounded and many more are likely to suffer ill

effects from traumatic brain injury, post-traumatic stress disorder, depression, and other conditions that lead to chronic disability. For example, over 106,000 received mental health diagnoses following deployment (Institute of Medicine, 2010). Nearly half of the soldiers in the armed forces are not married, so when they are disabled, their parents are most likely to become caregivers and advocates. Parents of soldiers, who are themselves parents, may also see increased involvement with their grandchildren during deployment and, in the case of disability and death, a greater role in raising grandchildren (Yeoman, 2008).

Nursing Role in Assessing and Supporting Caregivers

Much of the care and support that older adults receive is related to needs associated to chronic illness or disability. Long-term services and supports encompass a wide range of services, both paid and unpaid. Although the term *long-term care* (LTC) is sometimes used interchangeably with *nursing home care*, nursing homes represent only one type of LTC service. A variety of community-based care services are available, including in-home care, supportive housing, adult day care, and a range of residential care settings. Residential care includes assisted living, board and care, and adult foster homes (Stone, 2006). Nurses may work with older adults and their family caregivers in all of these settings. Family caregivers are particularly important during times of transition. This includes transitions from one care setting to another, as well as the transition from good health and independence to increasing disability, frailty, and dependence (Gitlin & Wolff, 2011). Little is known about how these transitions are experienced by family systems, but we do have knowledge regarding caregiver needs and supports.

Eliopoulous (2009) described a continuum of care with three points. On one end are older adults who are able to live independently and receive preventive services provided in communities. In the middle are those who require partial or intermittent assistance to manage health and self-care needs. Examples are older adults receiving home health care or residing in assisted living communities (see Boxes 15-1 and 15-2 for descriptions of these and other services). Intermittent assistance also includes care provided to those who are admitted to a long-term care

BOX 15-1
Home- and Community-Based Services

Home- and community-based services (HCBS) include a range of personal, support, and health services provided in the home or community to help individuals stay at home and live as independently as possible. These services are often provided by family caregivers, but can also be provided by a variety of home- and community-based providers. Home- and community-based services include the following:

Adult Day Service Programs

Adult Day Service (ADS) programs provide social interaction and a safe place for people to go while family caregivers are at work. ADS programs may also provide a variety of health, social, and other support services in a protective setting. Most operate during normal business hours. Some have evening, night, and weekend hours, but these programs do not provide 24-hour care.

ADS programs include health model and social models. The health model provides some health care services onsite. The social model provides social services, such as exercise classes or arts and crafts. Some programs offer both types of services.

Case Managers or Geriatric Care Managers

Case managers or geriatric care managers are typically nurses or social workers who can help individuals and families choose and manage long-term care services, develop a plan of care, and monitor long-term care needs over time.

Emergency Response Systems

Emergency response systems provide a signaling device you can wear at home. If there is a medical or other emergency, the person presses a button to alert an operator who contacts emergency personnel. This can be especially useful for those who live alone.

Friendly Visitor and Companion Services

Friendly visitor and companion services can provide visitors who regularly spend time with individuals who are frail or living alone so that they do not become isolated.

Home Health Care and Home Care

Home health care services typically offer skilled services such as the nursing and physical therapy that your doctor orders. Generally these services are limited to 60 or fewer days. Home care services are often limited to personal care assistance services, such as bathing and dressing, and may include homemaker services, such as meal preparation or household chores.

Homemaker or Chore Services

Homemaker or chore services help with your general household activities, such as meal preparation and routine household care, and sometimes heavier household chores, such as washing floors or shoveling snow.

Home Modifications

Home modifications support continued independent living at home. Some examples include building a wheelchair ramp or installing handrails in a shower or tub, modifications that are typically done by a contractor.

Meals Programs

Meals programs, such as meals-on-wheels, deliver meals directly to a person's home or provide communal meals.

Respite Care

Respite care gives unpaid caregivers time off from their responsibilities. Respite care is offered in the home, adult day centers, and nursing homes.

Senior Centers

Senior centers provide nutritional, recreational, social, and educational services. They provide comprehensive information and referrals to help find needed care and services.

Transportation Services

Transportation services provide transportation to medical appointments and shopping centers. They can transport people to community services and resource centers.

Villages

Villages are private membership programs in communities that provide or arrange assistance with activities, such as basic home health, lawn and garden care, transportation, and grocery shopping.

Source: Adapted from National Clearinghouse for Long-Term Care (Administration on Aging). (2013). Understanding long-term care. Retrieved February 12, 2013, from http://www.longtermcare.gov/LTC/Main_Site/Understanding/Services/Home_Community_Services.aspx

facility for rehabilitation or recovery from an acute illness with the intent to return to their prior living situation. At the other end of the continuum are older adults who need regular and continuous assistance during hospitalization for an acute condition or need to reside permanently in a nursing home due to significant limitations in their ability to manage their health and self-care needs.

Because many family caregivers are unprepared for their role, they are at risk for negative outcomes.

BOX 15-2
Facility-Based Long-Term Care Options

Services provided by long-term care facilities vary by type of facility. All facilities provide housing and related housekeeping services. Some also provide help with managing medications, assistance with personal care, supervision, special programs for people with Alzheimer's disease, or 24-hour nursing care. Typically, the state in which the facility is located will regulate which services are offered. For example, some states do not allow some types of facilities to include residents who are wheelchair bound or who cannot exit the facility on their own if there is an emergency. Facility-based service providers include the following:

Adult Foster Care

Adult foster care programs match people who cannot live safely on their own with a foster family that provides room and board 24 hours a day and helps with personal care activities such as bathing, eating, and medication. Foster families may take one person or a small group of adults. Licensure requirements and the terminology used for this type of facility vary greatly from state to state.

Board and Care Homes

The two main types of board and care homes are residential care facilities and group homes. Residential care facilities usually have 20 or fewer residents. Most group homes have six or fewer residents. Both types provide meals, personal care, and a 24-hour staff. These homes generally do not offer nursing and medical services. Rooms may be private or shared. State licensing requirements and the names for these types of facilities vary greatly.

Assisted Living

Like board and care homes, assisted living is designed for people who want to live in a community setting but need help with personal care, other daily activities, or supervision, but who do not need as much care as that provided by a nursing home. In general, assisted living facilities are larger than board and care homes. Residents often live in their own apartment or room, though this varies by state. Services provided typically include meals, assistance with personal care, help with medications, housekeeping, and laundry, 24-hour security, onsite staff for emergencies, and social programs. Some AL provide ADL support. The cost of assisted living depends on the kinds of services you need and the types of amenities the facility provides. Regulations for assisted living facilities vary greatly among states.

Continuing Care Retirement Communities

Continuing care retirement communities offer several levels of care in one location. They offer a mix of independent housing (for people who need little or no care), assisted living, and nursing facilities for those who need more care and supervision. If you live in the independent housing unit of a CCRC and become unable to live independently, you can either receive help there or move to the assisted living area. If necessary, you can enter the onsite or affiliated nursing home. The fee arrangements for CCRCs vary and include both a monthly fee and an entrance fee.

Nursing Homes

Nursing homes, also called skilled nursing facilities (SNFs), provide a range of services, including nursing care, 24-hour supervision, and assistance with ADLs. They also offer rehabilitation services such as physical, occupational, and speech therapy. Nursing home services may be needed for a short period of time for recovery or rehabilitation after a serious illness or operation. Longer stays are common when chronic physical health problems or cognitive problems (e.g., memory loss) make it necessary for 24-hour care or supervision.

Source: Adapted from National Clearinghouse for Long-Term Care (Administration on Aging). (2008). Understanding long-term care. Retrieved February 12, 2013, from http://www.longtermcare.gov/LTC/Main_Site/Understanding/Services/Facility_Based_Services.aspx

The degree of risk is influenced by the context of caregiving, including family history and dynamics, the nature of impairment (such as physical care needs compared to behavioral problems related to dementia), the level of care recipient dependency, and a wide range of personal and financial resources. Messecar (2012) identified seven categories of nursing care strategies for working with family caregivers (Box 15-3). To be effective, these strategies must be based on a thorough assessment and tailored to the individual caregiving situation. Yet needs of caregivers are not assessed routinely, and caregivers remain at risk for burnout and care recipients at risk for not receiving appropriate care, either at home or in another setting.

When nurses assess family caregiving situations, they tend to focus on ADLs (bathing, dressing, eating, toileting, hygiene, and mobility) and IADLs (shopping, managing finances, meal preparation, driving, and managing medications). ADLs are

BOX 15-3

Nursing Care Strategies to Support Caregivers

1. Identify content and skills needed to increase preparedness for caregiving.
2. Form a partnership with the caregiver before generating strategies to address issues and concerns.
3. Identify the caregiving issues and concerns on which the caregiver wants to work and generate strategies.
4. Assist the caregiver in identifying strengths in the caregiving situation.
5. Assist the caregiver in finding and using resources.
6. Help caregivers identify and manage their physical and emotional responses to caregiving.
7. Use an interdisciplinary approach when working with family caregivers.

Source: Messecar, D. C. (2012). Family caregiving. In M. Boltz, E. Capezuti, T. Fulmer, & D. Zwicker (Eds.), *Evidence-based geriatric nursing protocols for best practice* (4th ed.). New York, NY: Springer.

useful for determining how much physical assistance a care recipient may need from the caregiver. IADLs may determine whether an individual can live independently in the community. For example, a person may have significant mobility problems but if she has the ability to plan and direct care through execution of IADLs, it may be possible to remain at home. In any event, Reinhard et al. (2008, p.2) recommend that assessments be done for families as clients and for families as providers of care, and that assessments go beyond a listing of needs related to ADLs and IADLs for the following reason:

Those concepts do not adequately capture the complexity and stressfulness of caregiving. Assistance with bathing does not capture bathing a person who is resisting a bath. Helping with medications does not adequately capture the hassles of medication administration, especially when the care recipient is receiving multiple medications several times a day, including injections, inhalers, eye drops, and crushed tablets.

Limiting assessment to ADLs and IADLs also neglects to acknowledge the role nurses play in helping family members manage multiple and chronic illnesses.

To address the lack of systematic attention to assessing caregiver needs, the National Center on

Caregiving at the Family Caregiver Alliance identified "Fundamental Principles for Caregiver Assessment" (Box 15-4). Domains to be included in assessments are context; caregiver perception of health and functional status of the care recipient; caregiver values and principles; well-being of the caregiver; consequences of caregiving; skills, abilities, and knowledge to provide care; and potential resources that the caregiver could choose to use (Family Caregiver Alliance, 2006). Examples of assessment tools are presented in Box 15-5. Some of these are specific to nursing and/or specific settings.

Multiple interventions have been developed and tested to address the needs of caregivers, both as clients and as providers. In a meta-analysis, Pinquart and Sorensen (2006) identified six types of interventions: (a) psychoeducational, (b) cognitive-behavioral therapy (CBT), (c) counseling/case management, (d) support—training the care recipient, (e) respite

BOX 15-4

Fundamental Principles for Caregiver Assessment

1. Because family caregivers are a core part of health care and long-term care, it is important to recognize, respect, assess, and address their needs.
2. Caregiver assessment should embrace a family-centered perspective, inclusive of the needs and preferences of both the care recipient and the family caregiver.
3. Caregiver assessment should result in a plan of care (developed collaboratively with the caregiver) that indicates the provision of services and intended measurable outcomes.
4. Caregiver assessment should be multidimensional in approach and periodically updated.
5. Caregiver assessment should reflect culturally competent practice.
6. Effective caregiver assessment requires assessors to have specialized knowledge and skills. Practitioners' and service providers' education and training should equip them with an understanding of the caregiving process and its effects, as well as the benefits and elements of an effective caregiver assessment.
7. Government and other third-party payers should recognize and pay for caregiver assessment as a part of care for older people and adults with disabilities.

Source: Family Caregiver Alliance. (2006). *Caregiver assessment: Principles, guidelines and strategies for change. Report from a National Consensus Development Conference* (vol. I, p. 12). San Francisco, CA: Author.

BOX 15-5

The *Try This: Best Practices in Nursing Care to Older Adults* Series of Assessment Tools Is to Provide Knowledge of Best Practices in the Care of Older Adults

1. SPICES: An Overall Assessment Tool of Older Adults
2. Katz Index of Independence in Activities of Daily Living
3. Mental Status Assessment of Older Adults: The Mini-Cog
4. The Geriatric Depression Scale (GDS)
5. Predicting Pressure Ulcer Risk
6.1. The Pittsburgh Sleep Quality Index
6.2. The Epworth Sleepiness Scale
7. Assessing Pain in Older Adults
8. Fall Risk Assessment
9. Assessing Nutrition in Older Adults
10. Sexuality Assessment for Older Adults
11.1. Urinary Incontinence Assessment in Older Adults: Part I—Transient Urinary Incontinence
11.2. Urinary Incontinence Assessment in Older Adults: Part II—Persistent Urinary Incontinence
12. Hearing Screening in Older Adults
13. Confusion Assessment Method (CAM)
14. The Modified Caregiver Strain Index (CSI)
15. Elder Mistreatment Assessment
16.1. Beers Criteria for Potentially Inappropriate Medication Use in the Elderly. Part I. Criteria Independent of Diagnoses or Conditions
16.2. Part II. Criteria Considering Diagnoses or Conditions
17. Alcohol Use Screening and Assessment
18. The Kayser–Jones Brief Oral Health Status Examination (BOHSE)
19. Horowitz's Impact of Event Scale: An Assessment of Post-Traumatic Stress in Older Adults
20. Preventing Aspiration in Older Adults With Dysphagia
21. Immunizations for the Older Adult

22. Assessing Family Preferences for Participation in Care in Hospitalized Older Adults
23. The Lawton Instrumental Activities of Daily Living (IADL) Scale
24. The Hospital Admission Risk Profile (HARP)
25. Confusion Assessment Method for the Intensive Care Unit (CAM-ICU)
26. Transitional Care Model (TCM) Hospital Discharge Screening Criteria for High Risk Older Adults
27. General Screening Recommendations for Chronic Disease and Risk Factors in Older Adults
28. Preparedness for Caregiving Scale

Specialty Practice Series

Series on Dementia:
D1 Avoiding Restraints in Patients with Dementia
D2 Assessing Pain in Persons with Dementia
D3 Brief Evaluation of Executive Dysfunction
D4 Therapeutic Activity Kits
D5 Recognition of Dementia in Hospitalized Older Adults
D6 Wandering in the Hospitalized Older Adult
D7 Communication Difficulties: Assessment and Interventions
D8 Assessing and Managing Delirium in Persons with Dementia
D9 Decision Making in Older Adults with Dementia
D10 Working With Families of Hospitalized Older Adults With Dementia
D11.1 Eating and Feeding Issues in Older Adults with Dementia. Part I. Assessment
D11.2 Eating and Feeding Issues in Older Adults with Dementia. Part II. Interventions

Source: Hartford Institute for Geriatric Nursing. Try this: And how to try this series assessment tools on the care of older adults. Retrieved February 19, 2013, from http://hartfordign.org/practice/try_this

care, and (f) multicomponent interventions (combinations of more than one type of intervention). Outcomes of interest included reducing burden, depression, care recipient symptoms, and institutionalization of the care recipient, as well as increasing subjective well-being and caregiver knowledge and ability. The largest effects were with CBT, which helped to reduce depression and, to a lesser extent, helped reduce feelings of burden. CBT concentrates on helping caregivers identify and modify beliefs related to the situation, and develop new behaviors to cope with caregiving demands. Psychoeducational

programs contributed to small-to-moderate effects related to decreasing burden, depression, subjective well-being, and care receiver symptoms. Only care receiver education and multicomponent interventions were successful in reducing institutionalization. Other interventions that show some promise in reducing stress include moderate intensity exercise programs, and yoga and meditation activities (Messecar, 2012).

Pinquart and Sorensen (2006) suggest that more effort needs to be given to designing multicomponent interventions that target individual caregiver needs. For example, teaching caregivers to provide care and helping caregivers attend support groups can be powerful interventions that contributes to feelings of mastery. Those with high mastery have more positive experiences with caregiving and more positive health behaviors (Reinhard et al., 2008). They are also more likely to provide safe care and develop critical thinking skills.

CARE SETTINGS

We turn now to the settings in which older adults receive long-term services and supports. This exploration of care settings begins with community-based care, where most older adults receive care. Particular attention is given to the unpaid long-term care system, which occurs mostly in the older adult's or a family member's home. Next is a discussion of long-term care in residential settings, such as assisted living and nursing homes. The focus is on the formal care system, as well as family caregiving roles. This section of the chapter will conclude with a discussion of acute care.

Home- and Community-Based Care

Most older adults live in community settings with no or minimal support to manage their personal and health needs. Recent studies show that 72% of adults from 65 to 85 years of age report being in good health. Further, nursing home residency for this age group is projected to drop from 4.6% in 1985 to 3.4% by 2030 (Administration on Aging, 2011). For those over age 85 years and at the highest risk for needing daily assistance, the trend is similar with 22% needing nursing home care in 1985, but only 16% are projected to need nursing home care by 2030 (Administration on Aging, 2011). Nurses may encounter these older adults where they receive their primary health care or to help them learn to manage chronic health problems. A variety of home- and community-based programs have been developed to support the preference of older adults to remain in their homes (see Box 15-1). Many older adults and their families, however, have limited knowledge about what might be needed to continue living at home, the range of service options available in their communities, and how to access them.

Health care providers also have limited knowledge about services outside of their own agencies.

Aging and Disability Resource Centers (ADRCs) are available in most states and are designed to be a single access point for connecting people to the wide range of LTC services in communities. Nurses in all settings can make referrals to ADRCs and use these organizations to enhance their own knowledge. The goal for ADRCs is to provide people information and assistance regardless of age, income, or disability. "Options counseling" is a core function of ADRCs. Options counselors are knowledgeable about public and private resources and assist older adults, people with disabilities, and their families to access needed services. Services are designed to meet individual values and preferences and options counselors emphasize self-determination. Options counselors assist people in planning for the future to help preserve personal financial resources and to avoid crisis situations.

Options counselors can work with older adults and families to ensure that supports needed are in place if the person is discharged to home. They are an important partner for nurses. Although hospital discharge planners may assist with arranging home health services, older adults may have continuing needs for supports once their qualifications for home health services through Medicare ends. Options counselors can help identify other types of assistance. Thus, they are an important resource to providers and older adults in making a successful transition from hospitals and nursing facilities to a lesser level of care, whether it is back to the person's home, assisted living, or other residential setting. To find the ADRCs in your state, use the interactive map at ADRC Technical Assistance Exchange, http://www.adrc-tae.org.

Not all ADRCs function statewide. Another resource for identifying local long-term services and supports is Eldercare Locater (http://www.eldercare.gov/Eldercare.NET/Public/Index.aspx; 1-800-677-1116), which will provide contact information for a local Area Agency on Aging (AAAs). The AAAs and the organizations that subcontract with them (e.g., Senior Centers, Adult Day Service, Meals Programs) administer the services listed in Box 15-1. Other resources for older adults and their caregivers include organizations associated with a variety of health problems, such as the Alzheimer's Association, the American Heart Association, and the Arthritis Foundation. Such organizations contain a wealth of consumer information on their Web sites, including tools for monitoring chronic health problems, guides for caregivers, and links to local resources.

Nurses may also work with older adults in a several established and emerging programs to maintain or improve their health, reduce hospitalization, and support family caregivers. Examples of these programs are listed in Box 15-6 and Box 15-7. Technology is also increasingly used in home settings, including intravenous therapy, enteral nutrition, telehealth, or devices to monitor chronic health problems. While this technology contributes to early detection and prevention of many health problems and treatment of chronic health needs, learning how to use the equipment can also be a source of stress and anxiety for caregivers (Saunders, 2012).

One of the major reasons older adults prefer to remain in their own homes is to maintain autonomy and control over their lives. Yet family members are often more concerned about safety. Nurses can play an important role in working with families to identify ways to balance safety and risk related to mobility and cognitive problems such as dementia. Nurses can also help caregivers understand the normal aging process, including recognition of changes that should prompt an evaluation for potential problems. For example, Keyser, Buchanan, and Edge (2012) designed a program to teach caregivers about recognizing risk factors and signs of delirium in community-dwelling elders with a goal of early intervention. This intervention, in turn, helps caregivers feel more capable and competent, and keeps care recipients safer by addressing treatable conditions more quickly and successfully.

Residential Long-Term Care

Residential care includes services that are considered community-based (e.g., adult foster care, board and care homes, assisted living) and nursing home settings. Continuing care retirement communities (CCRCs) include elements of both, ranging from apartments for independent living to skilled nursing. CCRCs often provide home care or assisted living services as well. The terms and amount of regulation for community-based residential care and CCRCs vary by state, including minimal educational requirements for the staff, staff-client ratios, and service requirements. General descriptions of residential LTC options were presented in Box 15-2. Families continue to be integrally involved in all of these care settings, and nurses play a vital role in assessment and managing care and supporting older adults and their families. This section focuses on two aspects of residential LTC: assisted living (AL) and nursing homes. Throughout this discussion, we examine the changing role of LTC nurses and the partnership of nurses with LTC consumers, their family members, and other LTC providers.

BOX 15-6
Chronic Care Programs for Older Adults

National PACE Association: http://www. npaonline.org/website/article.asp?id=4

The Program of All-inclusive Care for the Elderly (PACE) model is centered around the belief that it is better for the well-being of seniors with chronic care needs and their families to be served in the community whenever possible.

Guided Care: http://www.guidedcare.org

"Guided Care® is a new solution to the growing challenge of caring for older adults with chronic conditions and complex health needs. A Guided Care nurse, based in a primary care office, works with 2–5 physicians and other members of the care team to provide coordinated, patient-centered, cost-effective health care to 50–60 of their chronically ill patients. The Guided Care nurse conducts in-home assessments, facilitates care planning, promotes patient self-management, monitors conditions monthly, coordinates the efforts of all health care professionals, smooths transitions between sites of care, educates and supports family caregivers, and facilitates access to community resources."

Patient-Centered Primary Care Collaborative: http://www.pcpcc.net

Describes the patient-centered medical home model of chronic illness management.

BOX 15-7
Programs and Models to Improve Quality of Care for Older Adults in Hospitals

Nurses Improving Care to Health System Elders (NICHE): Initiated in 1992, this is a nationwide program of staff education and system evaluation to deliver "sensitive and exemplary nursing care" to older adults (Mezey et al., 2004, p. 452). As of 2008, more than 200 hospitals were participating in this effort.

Geriatric Resource Nurse (GRN) Model: In this unit-based model, staff nurses with an interest in working with older adults are provided with additional knowledge and skills for working with this specialized population. They serve as resources for other nurses on their units by implementing best practices and providing consultation to their peers. The GRN is usually a key component in hospitals that have implemented the NICHE program (Mezey et al., 2004).

Geriatric Syndrome Management Model: This model uses advanced practice nurses, usually gerontological clinical nurse specialists (GCNSs), as consultants to assess and manage problems common to hospitalized older adults, such as delirium, falls, and incontinence. These nurses also provide staff education and evaluate policies, procedures, and other system issues to identify barriers to design strategies to provide optimal care for older adults (Mezey et al., 2004).

Acute Care for the Elderly (ACE) Model: These are hospital units designed specifically to meet the needs of older adults. An interdisciplinary team approach is used, often with a GCNS as the team coordinator. The goal is to prevent loss of function while being hospitalized for an acute health problem.

Hospital Elder Life Program (HELP): This model also uses an interdisciplinary approach with a focus on ongoing assessment to identify and treat problems promptly. Volunteers are also incorporated in this model (Inouye, Bogardus, Baker, Leo-Summers, & Cooney, 2000).

Family-Centered Geriatric Resource Nurse (FCGRN) Model: This combines the GRN role with concepts from the Family-Centered Care (FCC) Model. The FCC Model, previously used for working with chronically ill children, was adapted for care of hospitalized older adults. The focus is on assessment of the family, as well as the individual older adult (Salinas, O'Connor, Weinstein, Lee, & Fitzpatrick, 2002). This model is used in one of the case studies in this chapter.

Older Adults Services Inpatient Strategies (OASIS): This program was developed at a hospital in Atlanta and combined features from other programs based on the local needs and resources. It used an interdisciplinary approach with a GCNS as the team coordinator (Tucker et al., 2006). *Note:* This should not be confused with the OASIS (Outcome Assessment and Information Set), a comprehensive assessment and database used in home health care.

Hospital at Home: Initially a research project, this model focused on community-dwelling older adults requiring hospital admission for exacerbation of chronic obstructive pulmonary disease (COPD), chronic heart failure (CHF), community-acquired pneumonia, or cellulitis. If specific criteria were met, older adults were offered the option of receiving care at home with direct nursing care as well as other services as indicated. Outcomes of care were equal to or better than those of patients cared for in the hospital, especially regarding functional ability (Frick et al., 2009; Leff et al., 2009). The Veterans Administration has continued this model in several locations under the name Program at Home (Mader et al., 2008).

Assisted Living (AL)

AL was developed in part as a response to the institutional environment of nursing homes. Nursing homes were considered to function under a medical model that was unresponsive to the quality-of-life needs of residents. In contrast, the assisted living approach was described as a social model of care that would serve as an extension of "home." Keren Brown Wilson (2007) was a pioneer in this effort in the early 1980s. She was interested in creating housing that would match the needs of frail elders for support while maintaining their autonomy, privacy, and a sense of home. The idea was to provide help to people who required some assistance because of physical or cognitive impairment and could not live safely at home but did not require levels of nursing care found in traditional nursing homes. The key features of this assisted living model included a private living space with locking doors, a kitchenette, and the right of residents to make a wide range of choices about their lives, including visits from friends and family, and their health care.

The state of Oregon, as an example of a state using new model of care, supports the vision of AL proposed by Wilson. Oregon obtained a Medicaid Waiver to support low-income clients in using assisted living and other community-based care settings. Oregon administrative rules identify five values that are necessary for assisted living: independence, choices, dignity, homelike environments, and privacy (Carder, 2002). In contrast, most other states use LTC Medicaid funds predominantly for nursing home care. The Medicaid Waiver allowed Oregon to use Medicaid funds to support individuals in assisted living, adult foster care (homes with five or fewer residents), and a variety of other home care services. Evaluations of these services indicated that these new forms of community-based care were generally viewed positively by consumers, and they were substituting for nursing home care (Wilson, 2007). Costs are also significantly lower compared to nursing home care.

A number of assisted living models developed independently and simultaneously around the United States (Stone & Reinhard, 2007; Wilson, 2007; Zimmerman & Sloan, 2007). By the 1990s, the number of assisted living housing units and those served by them had exploded to become the fastest growing type of LTC service. By 2005, the number of residential or assisted living beds was similar to the number of nursing home beds (Sloane, Zimmerman, & Sheps, 2005). With this growth came increasing divergence in the definitions of assisted living and the services associated with it. Some assisted living facilities no longer emphasized private units, and the types of supportive services varied widely—some offering simple medication reminders to others offering a full range of ADL and dementia care services. Each state has developed its own definitions and regulations that influence how assisted living is implemented. Financing varies greatly; only some states use Medicaid dollars to fund assisted living. In other states, only those with significant personal financial resources have assisted living as a housing option.

Because assisted living is regulated by states, the services may vary but typically include presence of staff 24 hours/day, meals, modified special diets, assistance with personal care, housekeeping and laundry, transportation, and medication management and health monitoring (Mitty et al., 2010; Oregon Department of Human Services, 2011) Depending on the organization, additional services may be available for additional fees. Although staff is available 24 hours per day, a licensed nurse typically is not on duty at all times. In many AL settings,

unlicensed staff may carry out most care activities, including those that might be considered nursing care, such as medication administration. Similarly, training requirements for resident assistants are less standardized and/or demanding as compared to nursing assistants in nursing homes.

Many people who move into assisted living apartments may expect to remain there for the rest of their lives. Because of the gap between needs and services that exist in many facilities, however, individuals may be asked to move to a nursing home or perhaps a foster care placement. Some facilities may have strict admission criteria that residents must meet to remain in the assisted living community and discharge criteria that will require relocation. For example, in a review of research on AL, Stone and Reinhard (2007) found that a sizable number (75% in one study) of AL would not keep residents who required nursing home level care for more than 2 weeks. In contrast, they described another study that suggested that as residents become increasingly frail and dependent, AL can and does become a substitute for nursing home care, providing additional services as the need arises. These different findings demonstrate the difficulties of providing care in the least restrictive environment whenever possible, while at the same time ensuring residents receive the needed care to avoid jeopardizing their health and avoiding unnecessary transitions. This goal is often referred to as "aging in place." When working with older adults and their families, it is critical that they understand the characteristics of assisted living related to staffing and services available so they can make informed decisions. In some cases, AL residents may be eligible to receive additional support from Medicare home health care or hospice care if they meet the requirements for those programs.

Roles and Responsibilities of AL Nursing

The role of nurses in long-term care residential settings is evolving and expanding. It is as variable as are the models of assisted living, in part because residents are generally less disabled and the availability of nursing services is lower than in nursing homes. Some AL communities include full-time or part-time registered nurses (RNs) as part of their staff, some do not employ nurses, and still others contract with nurses to provide assessment of residents' health and self-care needs and other services. As a general matter, important roles and responsibilities of nurses in AL include assessment of resident needs, communication with residents and families to help them understand what services and care are available, and whether there are specific admission and/or discharge criteria. AL nurses may also provide staff education. If nurses function in a consultation role, they are not direct supervisors of staff and need to consider different strategies to encourage staff to adopt their recommendations for care. Additional nursing activities, often initiated at the requests of families who do not live with the older adult, include assisting direct care workers with documentation; teaching paid care workers what to expect in caring for residents; and advocacy, monitoring, and support through long-term trusting relationships.

Nursing Homes

Although a very small proportion of older adults live in nursing homes, about one-third of those over age 65 may spend some time in one (AARP, 2004). Attempts to control health care costs through shortened hospital stays beginning in the 1980s resulted in nursing homes increasingly being the location for rehabilitation and recovery from surgery and acute illness. The number of older adults who permanently reside in nursing homes has declined as more residential care alternatives have become available (Stone, 2006). Costs of care are high and are the responsibility of residents unless they meet the strict requirements for Medicare or qualify for Medicaid. Moving to a nursing home represents considerable losses for an older adult, including loss of health, privacy, independence, choice, quality of life, and autonomy. Due to space limitations, they may not be able to bring many personal possessions with them.

Most older adults and their families consider nursing homes to be undesirable and the option of last resort, largely because nursing homes have a poor image and a reputation for providing poor quality of care. The Nursing Home Reform Act, passed in 1987 as part of the Omnibus Reconciliation Act (OBRA 1987), attempted to address shortcomings by changing practice and systems of care. Practice changes included reducing restraint use (both physical and chemical or medications used to manage behavior symptoms), addressing psychosocial and physical care, and developing a national data system known as the Minimum Data Set

(MDS) (Sloane et al., 2005). Although there have always been nursing homes where excellent, nurturing care is provided, and although extensive federal and state regulations have attempted to address shortcomings, the prevailing public view and experience of nursing homes for many older adults, their families, and nurses has remained negative.

The Pioneer Network (1997), a group of LTC innovators, initiated the culture change movement, which focuses on person-directed care. It is a way of thinking about care that honors and values the person receiving care, with an emphasis on both quality of care and quality of life so that the individual is not lost in the process of providing care. Other terms used include *person-centered care*, *resident-centered care*, *individualized care*, and *person-centered thinking* (White, Newton-Curtis, & Lyons, 2008). Research suggests that nursing home culture is changing, although improvements are still needed (Miller et al., 2010; Rahman & Schnelle, 2008).

Roles and Responsibilities of Nursing Home Nurses

Nurses historically have played major roles in nursing home (NH) care, but like their counter parts in AL, the role of nurses is evolving and expanding in these settings. Care is increasingly complex and residents in skilled and rehabilitation units resemble hospitalized patients of the not too distant past. As in AL, NH nurses must be able to work independently, assume leadership roles, and possess strong assessment and prioritizing skills. They must be able to work effectively and collaboratively on interdisciplinary teams consisting of direct care workers, administrators, other NH staff who support residents (e.g., social services, rehabilitation, dietary), and other providers who may not be on staff but are critical to the well-being of residents, such as hospice teams, physicians, options counselors, and other home- and community-based care providers. Understanding of best practices in care of older adults is constantly evolving. Practices such as those related to pressure ulcer prevention and treatment, pain assessment and management, dementia care, use of restraints (physical, pharmaceutical, or electronic), and mental health care continue to evolve. A key role of NH nursing is to maintain knowledge of and implement best practices. Some useful sources are listed in Box 15-8. The most skilled nurses are needed for these settings.

BOX 15-8
Resources for Best Practices

Medicare: http://www.medicare.gov/index.html

Provides resources for consumers for finding nursing home and home health care agencies, including important questions to ask, information about quality of care, and staffing.

Creating Enriched Learning Environments Through Partnerships in Long-Term Care: http://www.ecleps.org/PRWR.html

Includes peer-reviewed Web sites and learning activities for nurses.

Transitional Care Model: http://www. transitionalcare.info

Interdisciplinary model developed by the University of Pennsylvania School of Nursing for comprehensive discharge planning for high-risk hospitalized older adults.

Pioneer Network: http://www.pioneernetwork. net/Providers/ForNurses

Resources about culture change and other innovative practices in nursing homes.

Geriatric Education Centers: http://bhpr.hrsa. gov/grants/geriatricsalliedhealth/gec.html

These are located in most states and focus on education and training of health professionals. Most centers have Web sites and post educational materials. For a listing of GECs, go to "active grants" at the bottom of the GEC program Web site.

Next Step in Care: http://www.nextstepincare. org/About_the_Campaign

Sponsored by the United Hospital Fund to support partnerships between family caregivers and health care providers, especially during times of transitions between care settings.

Many nurses are participating in efforts to promote culture change in all residential care settings. Person-directed care is consistent with nursing values, in that nursing strives to individualize care and put the individual ahead of the task (Koren, 2010, Robinson & Rosher, 2006; Talerico, O'Brien, & Swafford, 2003). This is also true for family care, where the nurse puts family-centered care before tasks or hospital regulations that exclude family members. Common elements include personhood, knowing the person and their family, autonomy/choice, including family members in decision making, comfort, and valuing relationships (White et al.,

2008). New regulations from the Centers for Medicare and Medicaid Services have made changes in regulations and support culturally and family-directed care practices. The Pioneer Network and leaders in gerontological and long-term care nursing developed "Nurse Competencies for Nursing Home Culture Change" (Box 15-9).

Family Involvement in Residential Care Settings

Contrary to prevailing myths, families typically do not abandon their older members once they move into facility-based care, nor do they cease providing care, although the nature of that care will be different (Keefe & Fancey, 2000). Decades

BOX 15-9
Nurse Competencies for Nursing Home Culture Change

1. Models, teaches, and utilizes effective communication skills such as active listening, giving meaningful feedback, communicating ideas clearly, addressing emotional behaviors, resolving conflict, and understanding the role of diversity in communication
2. Creates systems and adapts daily routines and "person-directed" care practices to accommodate resident preferences
3. Views self as part of team, not always as the leader
4. Evaluates the degree to which person-directed care practices exist in the care team and identifies and addresses barriers to person-directed care
5. Views the care setting as the residents' home and works to create attributes of home
6. Creates a system to maintain consistency of caregivers for residents
7. Exhibits leadership characteristics/abilities to promote person-directed care
8. Role models person-directed care
9. Problem solves complex medical/psychosocial situations related to resident choice and risk
10. Facilitates team members, including residents and families, in shared problem solving, decision making, and planning

These competencies are useful in identifying specific skills needed by nurses working in care settings involved in culture change. It is a first step in creating measurement and other tools useful in educating and supporting nurses in this work.

Developed through a collaboration of Pioneer Network & Hartford Institute for Geriatric Nursing. (2010). Retrieved from http://www.pioneernetwork.net/Providers/ForNurses

of research in nursing homes have revealed that family members continue to visit and provide emotional support, as well as some types of informal care, after transition into a nursing facility. Families typically desire to work in partnership with facility staff to support (Bauer & Nay, 2011; Pillemer et al., 2003). Nurses and other staff members can inadvertently set up barriers that decrease the ability of family members to participate in the life of the resident, such as by limiting visiting hours, limiting family knowledge or involvement in care, or discounting or discouraging family input into care decisions. Developing a successful relationship actually begins before a resident is admitted, when a family member makes an initial visit to the facility. In addition to evaluating the physical environment, families begin to consider the quality of care provided, and whether they can trust the staff to become partners in caring for their family member (Legault & Ducharme, 2009). Nurses and other staff, therefore, can assist to strengthen the staff-family partnership through communication, making family members feel comfortable and welcomed, and providing assurance that the staff is competent and providing good care.

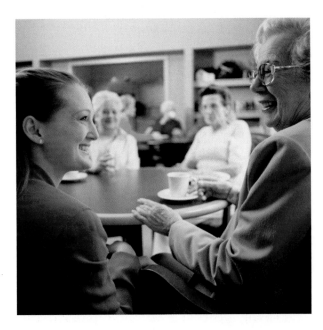

Person-centered, or person-directed, care is consistent with the needs and values of nursing home residents and their families. Family members want staff to gain knowledge about the resident, often striving to be role models in demonstrating how to give care to the individual (Duncan & Morgan, 1994). Partnerships between families and staff help staff members to know residents in meaningful ways. Families are key informants with respect to individuals' history, likes and dislikes, personality, routines, and what is and has been important to them (Austin et al., 2009; Boise & White, 2004; Iwasiw, Goldenberg, Bol, & MacMaster, 2003; Legault & Ducharme, 2009; Logue, 2003; Reuss, Dupuis, & Whitfield, 2005). This knowledge is critical, particularly when residents have dementia and cannot clearly communicate this information themselves. Family members can provide insight into resident actions, which in turn can help the staff respond more quickly to resident needs as conveyed through their behavior.

Families provide considerable psychological support to residents through their visits. Families are key members of the resident's social network, contributing to identity, dignity, and quality of life (Boise & White, 2004; Iwasiw et al., 2003). Another important role of family members is in monitoring the quality of care and advocating for the resident if needed (Friedemann, Montgomery, Maiberger, & Smith, 1997). In addition, family members continue to provide hands-on care, including helping a family member eat, attending activities, and handling personal care. Families help residents to maintain connections with the larger community by taking them to public events such as concerts, parks, shopping, and to family gatherings.

Palliative Care and End-of-Life Care in Residential Care Settings

Currently, about 20% of all deaths occur in nursing homes; this proportion is expected to increase due to the aging population (Davidson, 2011; Kelly, Thrane, Virani, Malloy, & Ferrell, 2011). Still, staff and families of residents generally do not identify nursing homes as a location for providing palliative and end-of-life or hospice care. In contrast, nursing home residents, as well as those in assisted living, view death as a normal occurrence, something to be expected living in a community with a large number of older adults (Munn et al., 2008). As older adults begin to age in place in AL and other community-based care settings, these settings are increasingly the places where death occurs. End-of-life care in these settings has its own challenges in part due to limited staffing, limited staff knowledge, and the emphasis on resident independence and autonomy (Cartwright, Miller, & Volpin, 2009).

As noted in Chapter 10, palliative care and end-of-life or hospice care are often considered synonymous. To clarify for the discussion here, the focus of palliative care is to improve the quality of life for persons with chronic, life-limiting illnesses through careful identification and management of symptoms. These symptoms may include pain, shortness of breath, fatigue, constipation, nausea, loss of appetite, problems with sleep, and side effects of medical treatments (National Institute of Nursing Research, 2011). Palliative care may continue for years; ideally, it begins when the chronic condition is first identified. The focus of end-of-life care, on the other hand, is the immediate time around death.

Most long-stay nursing home residents have multiple chronic illnesses and are ideal candidates for palliative care. Because of the confusion about these terms, however, health team members may not initiate discussion about palliative care until the person is close to the end of life. Several other barriers to providing effective palliative and end-of-life care in nursing homes exist, including lack of education of staff, high turnover, and low reimbursement. Another barrier is the dual mission of nursing homes as organizations that provide rehabilitation and short-term care for persons recovering from acute illness with the goal of returning home, as well as care for people at the end of their lives (Davidson, 2011; Kelly et al., 2011). Another challenge is the high proportion of nursing home residents who have dementia, which is often not recognized as a terminal condition by families or staff, including physicians. Dementia also has a less predictable trajectory or pattern of transition to end of live compared to other chronic conditions, making it more difficult to identify when changes are likely to happen and when additional resources such as hospice may be appropriate.

An important part of palliative care is working with older adults and their families to prepare advance directives, such as a durable power of attorney for health care or a living will. The process of preparing these documents provides an opportunity to discuss and understand values and preferences to guide decisions when the individual is not able to directly communicate. Advance directives are not just about what treatments are not wanted; they can also be used to request treatment (Mitty, 2012).

Although often associated with a location or service, hospice is, most important, a philosophy of care provided at the end of life. Most hospice care is provided at home, although assisted living and nursing home residents may also qualify for hospice as a Medicare benefit. Cartwright et al. (2009) found that quality end-of-life care was greatly influenced by the AL staff commitment to the resident dying in the AL and the respectful collaboration of multiple care providers, including AL nurses, direct care workers, family members, and the hospice team. Hospice also provides continued support to family members after the death. The culture change initiative in nursing homes has the potential to facilitate provision of palliative and end-of-life care in this setting. The cultures of both initiatives focus on person-centered care, understanding behavior as a way of communicating needs, comfort, and honoring values and preferences of older adults and their families (Long, 2009).

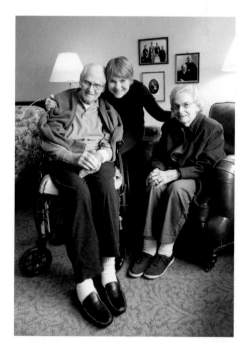

Acute Care

Although most nurses who work in acute care do not consider themselves gerontological nurses, a high proportion of acute care patients are over age 65. This includes both general acute care and critical care units where up to 50% of patients may be older adults (Balas, Casey, & Happ, 2012; Steele, 2010). Older adults are also commonly seen in emergency departments, where they account for up to 25% of trauma admissions (Cutugno, 2011). Older adults are often admitted to the hospital for conditions associated with chronic conditions, such as an exacerbation of heart failure or surgery to replace joints damaged from osteoarthritis. In this section, we discuss two risks for older adults associated with hospitalization: loss of functional ability and development of delirium. We focus on the nurses' crucial role in assessment of risk factors and early intervention to eliminate or reduce these risks.

Comprehensive assessment is essential to identify potential problems and design interventions to prevent complications and maintain function. Four areas are critical to assess in all older adults: (1) ADLs, (2) IADLs, (3) cognitive status, and (4) presence of sensory impairments. Although nurses are always assessing through observations and interactions with clients, the use of standardized tools facilitates consistent data collection over time to be able to evaluate baseline status, detect changes, and evaluate response to interventions. Several tools are available to assess an older adult admitted to acute care (see Box 15-5).

As described previously, ADL assessment includes bathing, dressing, eating, toileting, hygiene, and mobility. This information is important for planning care during hospitalization and for discharge. IADL function often determines a person's ability to continue to live independently; these functions include shopping, managing finances, meal preparation, driving, and managing medications. Persons with visual or hearing impairments will have difficulty participating in assessment of ADLs and IADLs. Failure to recognize hearing and visual impairments risks making erroneous diagnoses. Providing the person's glasses and hearing aides are easy but important interventions.

Hospitalization puts older adults at great risk for functional decline. Kleinpell et al. (2008) report that, after two days of bed rest, 71% of older patients experienced declines in mobility, transferring, toileting, feeding, and grooming. This deconditioning is also responsible for accelerated bone loss, reduced cardiovascular efficiency, and decreased muscle strength. As a result, older adults are at increased risk for falls, delirium, nosocomial infections, adverse drug reactions, and pressure ulcers. Furthermore, after discharge, they continue to experience functional decline and prolonged recovery.

Because persons with pre-existing cognitive impairment are especially at risk during hospitalization, careful assessment helps to distinguish between the presence of any of the "three D's": dementia, delirium, and depression. Although some symptoms are similar, these disorders are distinct and require very different kinds of interventions. Dementia is a group of several progressive cognitive disorders that results in memory loss, confusion, loss of judgment, and loss of various executive functions such as ability to plan or organize activities. Onset is slow and insidious. Alzheimer's disease is the most common form of dementia and risk increases with age; estimates are that 50% or more of those older than 85 years have the disease (Doerflinger, 2007).

Delirium also involves confusion, though onset occurs rapidly. Symptoms include inattention, disorganized thinking, and altered level of consciousness (Waszynski, 2007). Because of their more fragile physiological balance, older adults are more susceptible to delirium, which is usually due to physiological causes such as infection, adverse effects of medications, dehydration, and fluid and electrolyte imbalance. With estimates of 14% to 56% of older patients experiencing delirium in hospitals, it is extremely important to be alert to symptoms. Postoperative patients appear to be especially vulnerable. Family members can provide essential information about baseline cognitive status. Delirium can be prevented by identifying and eliminating or minimizing risk factors, and reversed if detected and the underlying causes treated early. Morbidity and mortality rates are high for older adults who develop delirium. Costs of hospitalization are also higher for persons who develop delirium.

Depression is a mood disorder with affective, cognitive, and physical symptoms (Harvath & McKenzie, 2012). Although common in older adults (up to 30% to 40% in some settings), depression is not a normal result of aging. It is often not recognized and consequently is undertreated, diminishing quality of life. Depression presents a complex picture in this population: it is associated with many chronic conditions, which contributes to its high prevalence for older adults; it may interfere with chronic illness self-management; and some medications to treat chronic conditions may cause symptoms of depression (Byrd & Vito, 2011; Harvath & McKenzie, 2012). Left untreated, however, depression may persist or progress. It is also a major risk factor for suicide; adults over age 65 have the highest rates of suicide (15 to 20 per 100,000) with the rate for white males over age 85 even higher (80 to 113 per 100,000) (Harvath & McKenzie, 2012).

Screening for depression should be part of routine health and nursing assessment. Several brief and easy-to-use tools are available, such as the Geriatric Depression Scale: Short Form (GDS-SF; Greenberg, 2007). The first two items of the Patient Health Questionnaire (PHQ)-9 can also be used as an initial screen; if either is answered positively, the remaining seven items are administered. Once identified, depression can be treated by a variety of methods, including medications, exercise, and psychosocial approaches such as cognitive behavioral therapy, and reminiscence or life review (Harvath & McKenzie, 2012). Most of the newer antidepressant medications are effective for older adults and also have an improved side-effect profile compared to older drugs. Older adults who do not tolerate medications may benefit from electroconvulsive therapy (ECT). Nursing interventions include assessing and providing safety for persons at risk for suicide, supporting health and physical function, enhancing autonomy and control, and providing encouragement and advocacy to obtain optimal treatment (Byrd & Vito; Harvath & McKenzie, 2012). As noted previously, family caregivers are also at risk for depression and should be included in assessment and treatment.

The hospital experience is further complicated for patients, families, and nurses due to the fact that the "three D's" often occur in combination. For example, delirium superimposed on dementia is receiving increasing attention in nursing literature (Steis & Fick, 2012; Steis et al., 2012; Voyer, Richard, Doucet, & Carmichael, 2011). This challenge presents opportunities for nurses and family members to collaborate. For example, hospital nurses are at a disadvantage because they are not familiar with the usual behavior of a person with dementia and are not able to recognize a subtle change due to delirium. Family members may be able to provide valuable information about the person's usual behavior to prompt the nurse to assess for potential delirium. Nursing home staff may also be an important resource for a resident who does not have family available; staff may be an important resource about the person's usual mental status. Family members may be alarmed by behavior changes seen in a hospitalized older adult without prior cognitive impairment who develops delirium and might assume the patient has developed dementia. Nurses can offer reassurance that these changes may be due to a physiological cause and when corrected, the person's usual cognitive abilities will return.

Family Case Study: Hooper Family

Using the life course perspective illustrated by Maria Hooper and her family (see Figure 15-1, which depicts the Hooper family genogram), we explore transitions that families experience as a result of declining health and increasing dependency common in old age. From a wider perspective, we take in the intersection of older families with the health care system.

Maria, age 60, is the oldest of four siblings. She has two brothers, James and Paul, and a sister, Ruth. Maria always counts Jane as her sister, too. Jane is a year younger than Maria and is the daughter of one of her mother's closest friends. When Jane needed a home as a young teenager, Maria's parents, Sarah and Louis, took her in, and Jane lived with them for 5 years. She and Maria became especially close, and now Jane and her family participate in all of Maria's and her extended family's gatherings.

Sarah, age 82, and Louis, age 84, have lived in their community since their marriage 60 years earlier. They enjoy good health, except for Sarah's arthritis and mild

hearing loss, and Louis's diabetes and hypertension, which are well controlled. They experience no limitations in ADLs, although both complain that it takes them longer to get things done. Still, they both volunteer for several different organizations and spend time with their friends. Maria lives 40 miles away from her parents, closer than the rest of her siblings. Maria and her parents talk on the phone about twice a week and they get together for dinner every couple of weeks.

Maria was divorced when her children, Jason and Kyra, were in elementary school. She still maintains connections with her ex-mother-in-law, Carol, who is now 87 years old. Carol has been widowed for 40 years. When Maria and her husband were divorced, Carol was determined that she would not lose contact with her grandchildren, as she had seen that happen with some of her friends. Maria had always been on good terms with Carol and felt it important that her children know their paternal grandmother, so both Maria and Carol made the effort to maintain contact. Carol lived about an hour away, but Maria and her children would spend at least one Saturday a month with her until

(continued)

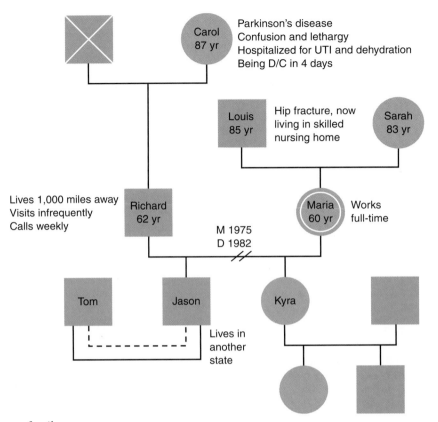

FIGURE 15-1 Hooper family genogram.

the children entered into high school and were involved with multiple activities. Their visits became more sporadic, but Carol would come and watch her grandchildren's games and music concerts whenever she could.

When Carol was diagnosed with Parkinson's disease about 10 years ago, Maria became part of a community support system. Her role was to visit monthly, purchase groceries, and do some housekeeping. In addition to Parkinson's disease, Carol began to have problems with her memory and could no longer live alone. With some reluctance, she moved into an assisted living (AL) residence in her community. Maria has continued to visit her nearly every month. Carol usually knows Maria, but sometimes forgets she is divorced from her son. They mostly reminisce about the grandchildren.

Maria's life is quite busy. She is the office manager of a small business, and in addition to her parents and mother-in-law, Maria is involved in her children's lives. Jason and his partner live several hundred miles away, but Maria talks with him every couple of weeks. Maria often spends her vacations with them. Kyra is married and has two children of her own. Because Kyra lives close, Maria frequently babysits and

delights in having each child spend the night about once a month. Maria enjoys being a grandparent, yet feels badly for her sister, Ruth, who has had sole responsibility for raising her own grandchildren for the past two years.

Discussion:

Maria's family is reflective of many older families. At 60 years, Maria is part of the baby boom, and like many in her generation, she has several siblings who represent potential support systems for both Maria and her parents. This includes Jane, who is fictive kin and has a close and family-like relationship with Maria and her parents. Typical for most families, Maria lives relatively close to her parents and is in regular contact with them. Generally, they have a good relationship, characterized by affection, a history of mutual exchanges of help, and many shared values. Maria and her children are especially close to her parents because they provided considerable support as Maria was going through her divorce. Support included temporary housing, child care, and some financial assistance. Now, Sarah and Louis (Maria's parents) are close to becoming the "old-old" generation, that is, those older than 85 years. Although they are independent, engaged in their community, and consider themselves in good health, both have several chronic illnesses that could cause them problems in the future. Maria's former mother-in-law, Carol, has not been as fortunate. She was widowed "off-time" in her forties and has lived alone since her son grew up and left home. Her activities have been limited for many years because of Parkinson's disease and, more recently, cognitive impairment. She has resided for several years in an AL that accepts Medicaid clients.

Transition 1—Louis Home to Hospital:

Sarah (now age 83) spent most of the day at a friend's house. When she returned home about 4 p.m., she found her husband, Louis (age 85), on the floor in the garage. He told her that he tripped on the stairs while carrying a chair that needed repair; this occurred about 9:30 a.m. He tried to get up or crawl up the three steps from the attached garage to the kitchen, but he could not move because the pain was too great. Sarah called 911, and Louis was taken to the emergency department. Fortunately, it was a relatively uncomplicated fracture of his hip. He was able to have a surgical repair the next morning. Because he experienced some confusion after surgery, the nurses were reluctant to give him pain medication, believing the medication would cause more confusion. He started physical therapy the day after surgery but could participate only to a limited extent because of the pain. He was also started on insulin to control his diabetes (he previously took an oral medication).

Louis's needs are common. As an older adult, Louis was at a greater risk for falls and related injuries even though he did not have other risk factors. Hospital care by those unfamiliar with the needs of older adults can exacerbate rather than prevent negative outcomes. Knowing, for example, that untreated pain can increase confusion and delay successful rehabilitation is important for nurses.

Transition 2—Louis Hospital to Skilled Nursing Facility:

After 4 days in the hospital, Louis was discharged to the skilled care unit of a nursing home for additional rehabilitation, with the goal of returning to his own home. The timing of the discharge came as a surprise to Sarah and Maria, giving them little time to visit and select a skilled nursing facility (SNF) or for other siblings to arrive from out of town to provide support. Fortunately, Sarah and Louis had friends who had had a good experience in one that was located about 30 minutes away. It had space available; Maria stopped by to look at it and thought it would work. At the SNF, Louis' pain was finally controlled and he was

eager to begin physical and occupational therapy so that he could go home. Although attention was focused on Louis, Sarah also needed support to bring Louis home as quickly and successfully as possible. See Figure 15-2, the Hooper family ecomap. One spouse's response to stress will affect the way that the other spouse experiences stress. During this transitional period, it is important to be cognizant of stress levels and needs of both Sarah and Louis. For example, nurses and others can help them consider changing their home environment to prevent future falls and they will need instruction in managing Louis's pain while his hip heals. Louis's diabetes needs to be monitored and assessed to determine whether he will continue to need insulin injections or be able to return to managing through oral medications.

Without including Sarah in the transition planning, Louis is likely to spend a longer time in the SNF or return home without sufficient support. Without support, Sarah is likely to experience greater levels of stress and caregiver burden in her expanded role as caregiver. Because of her hearing loss, Sarah does not always understand what the physician, nurses, and other staff tell her. Maria noticed that providers tend to treat her mother as if she has dementia and often do not include her in conversations. As a result, Maria feels the need to be present as much as possible. She has missed a lot of work, is worried about losing her job, and cannot afford to take more time off. Fortunately, nurses at the SNF are aware of these constraints and are able to arrange a care conference with Louis, Sarah, and Maria after regular business hours to begin planning for Louis's discharge to home. Maria and her parents are aware that Medicare is funding rehabilitation services, but are surprised to learn that these benefits will run out, sooner if Louis does not keep progressing toward independence.

Transition 3—Louis SNF to Home:

Once again, discharge came quickly with little time to locate a home health care agency. The SNF discharge coordinator provided a list of agencies and Maria selected one. The therapists at the SNF gave Sarah and Maria a list of adaptive devices (e.g., raised toilet seat, grabber, elastic shoestrings, a device to help Louis put on his socks, walker) to purchase before Louis's discharge. Because Louis still qualified for Medicare services, he was able to see a physical therapist, an occupational therapist, and a nurse once a week at home. These three providers collaborated to complete a home safety assessment to identify potential risk and strategies to eliminate or reduce the risks. A home health care worker also came to the house to assist with Louis's shower twice a week.

(continued)

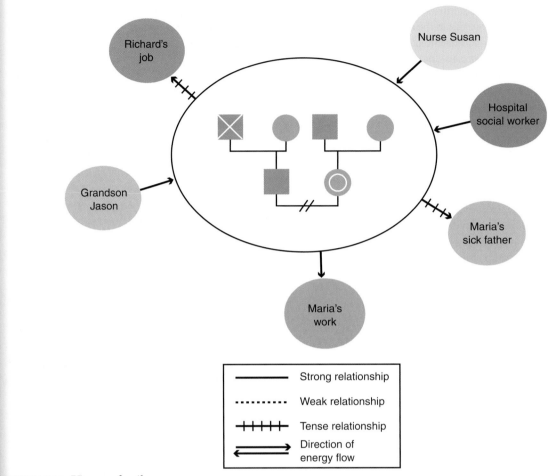

FIGURE 15-2 Hooper family ecomap.

The social worker at the nursing facility had suggested that the family contact the Aging and Disability Resource Center (ADRC) in the community. An Options Counselor (OC) from the ADRC met with the family in the nursing facility and again once Louis was home. She was able to provide information about services beyond those provided by the home health agency. Once Medicare benefits ran out, she provided them information about home care workers. Sarah and Louis hired a worker to continue to help him with showers and to do a little light housekeeping. The OC also identified an organization that put a grab bar in the shower and, if needed in the future, could build a ramp into the house. Because Sarah was exhausted, the options counselor helped arrange for home-delivered meals. With time, Louis recovered and although he now used a cane, he resumed most of his community activities. His diabetes was once again managed through diet and oral medications and Sarah soon decided that they no longer needed the home care worker and meals. They kept the phone number of the options counselor on their refrigerator in case they needed assistance in the future.

Transition 4—Carol Apartment to Assisted Living:

Recall that Carol, Maria's former mother-in-law, had been living in an AL for several years. She moved there because her worsening Parkinson's disease made it impossible to remain at home in her apartment. In the community, Carol's main support system came from friends and neighbors, with Maria and her children helping when they could. Richard, Carol's son and Maria's ex-husband, lived in another state but would visit two or three times a year to fix things around the apartment and to handle Carol's finances. The year before Carol moved into the AL, she began losing weight because she was not able to prepare meals. In response, Maria and some of Carol's friends often prepared meals and froze these meals in individual portions. Maria also did grocery shopping during her monthly visits. A local volunteer organization provided some house cleaning, and friends from Carol's church would take her to lunch or bring her dinner at least once a week. At Maria's urging, Richard arranged for meals-on-wheels from a local community center. Carol often did not eat the food from this service, however (her reasons included "It's not like my own cooking," and "It all tastes the same"). Several times, when the volunteer delivered the meal, she found Carol on the floor because she had fallen. Concern about Carol's safety prompted Richard, her friends, and Maria to convince her to move to the AL, which was also closer to Maria's home. Although Carol had limited income from Social Security, the AL accepted residents receiving housing subsidy as a Medicaid benefit.

Carol was initially reluctant to move to the AL. She was not familiar with AL and thought her family wanted her to move to a nursing home, which she strongly opposed. She changed her mind after visiting a few AL communities and learned that she could still have her own apartment. After moving in, she discovered she enjoyed the opportunities to participate in many of the activities. Her strength also improved; at her apartment, it had been difficult to get regular exercise because of limited space and a short flight of stairs to get outside. At the AL, the long hallways provided a safe walking space, and with the elevator she did not need to worry about stairs. As a result, she was able to go outside more often. Carol developed close friendships with several other residents during the time she lived at the AL. She recognized that she had become somewhat isolated in her apartment because of her increasing difficulty with mobility. As she received three meals daily in the dining room, her weight improved. She also received assistance with bathing twice a week. Bathing had been a challenge in her apartment because she had only a tub and shower combination, and the owner would not allow her to have safety bars installed in the bathroom.

Transition 5—Carol Assisted Living to Hospital:
After living successfully in the AL for 3 years, Carol gradually developed memory problems; her physician was not sure whether it was Alzheimer's disease or dementia secondary to the Parkinson's disease. The AL staff frequently had to go find her at mealtimes. Like many older adults, Carol took several medications, both prescription and over-the-counter drugs. She had been able to take them

safely and accurately once the med-aide had set them up for her in a pill box, but now when Maria visited, she found Carol has not taken about half of the doses. When cleaning her apartment, the staff also noted clothes soiled with urine in her bathroom. One morning, when she did not come to breakfast, the resident assistant found her still in bed. She was very difficult to wake up, she had been incontinent, and could not stand even with the help of the resident assistant. When the AL nurse came on duty, she assessed Carol and suspected she had an infection. She contacted Richard, who lives several hundred miles away. He called Maria, who arranged to take time off work and took Carol to see her physician. The physician determined that Carol was dehydrated and had a urinary tract infection (UTI). He had her admitted to the hospital for treatment.

Note that incontinence is not "normal" for older adults; development of incontinence may indicate a change in health status. For example, it may be a sign of a UTI. Other changes in urinary elimination, such as burning or frequency, may also be signals that further evaluation is warranted. Because of her memory problems, Carol may not have remembered to mention these symptoms to Maria or the AL staff. If identified early, the UTI could probably have been successfully treated with oral antibiotics and hospitalization avoided.

Unlike nursing homes, ALs do not have nurses available 24 hours per day; other staff members may have limited training and experience working with older adults (unlike nursing homes, training requirements for direct care workers are limited). Nurses can provide staff training focusing on normal aging- and health-related changes. Staff should also understand the importance of reporting changes in the resident's usual condition, such as a change in continence, to the nurse, who will then follow up with additional assessments and evaluations. For example, although Carol had memory problems, she was usually awake and alert, so for the resident assistant to find her difficult to awaken represented a significant change.

Transition 6—Carol Hospitalization:
Carol was admitted to a general medical-surgical unit of a community hospital later that afternoon. The hospital recently implemented a program similar to the Family-Centered Geriatric Resource Nurse model that Salinas, O'Connor, Weinstein, Lee, and Fitzpatrick (2002) describe (see Box 15-7). This model incorporates the acronyms SPICES and FAMILY as frameworks for assessing both the older adult and her family. Susan Jones, the admitting nurse, obtained the information from Maria and also from

(continued)

the AL nurse because Carol was still quite lethargic when she first arrived at the hospital:

- **S**leep disorders: No problems.
- **P**oor nutrition: Carol has a history of problems, but over the past year her weight has been stable and within the ideal range for her height.
- **I**ncontinence: As noted earlier, this is a recent development. The bathroom in Carol's apartment has safety bars and is arranged in a manner that makes it easily accessible for persons with mobility problems.
- **C**onfusion: The admitting nurse recognizes that Carol is experiencing the "hypoactive" form of delirium as demonstrated by lethargy (it was difficult for the resident assistant to get her to wake up) and is at risk for it worsening.
- **E**vidence of falling: Carol has a history of falls but none in the past year. She has not sustained any serious injuries from falling.
- **S**kin breakdown: No problems.

The nurse continued to collect information using the FAMILY acronym:

- **F**amily involvement: Carol has regular contact with Maria, who provides assistance with a variety of needs. Carol also has come to consider her close friends at the AL to be part of her family. Her son Richard calls about once a week but visits infrequently. Susan learns that Maria is also involved with her own parent care activities and that her father Louis is recovering from his hip fracture. Maria has used most of her vacation days providing parent care and cannot afford to take many days without pay.
- **A**ssistance needed: Because of her current mental status changes, Carol needs extensive assistance with eating and drinking, changing position, hygiene, and other activities. Because Carol has missed some doses of her anti-Parkinson's medication, her mobility is not as good as usual, and she has lost some function even from this relatively short illness. She may require more assistance than her family or the AL staff can provide.
- **M**embers' needs (what family members need from staff to be able to continue to provide care): Maria needs to be updated regularly about Carol's condition so she can keep other family members informed (particularly Carol's son, Richard). She also needs to know whether Carol will be able to return to the AL, and if not, what options are available. At the same time, Maria expresses some resentment to Susan about Richard's apparent lack of willingness to step up and take more responsibility for the care of his mother. She reports feeling pulled by the needs of her parents, Carol, her grandchildren, and her sister, who is raising her grandchildren.

- **I**ntegration into care plan (inclusion of family in planning and teaching activities): Susan gives Maria a business card for the unit social worker; she also shares Maria's contact information with the social worker. The team will meet the following day to evaluate Carol's situation. She will probably be in the hospital for 2 to 4 days; therefore, it is important to start planning for discharge as soon as possible.
- **L**inks to community support: Before the team meeting, Susan will follow up with the AL nurse to learn what care can be provided after discharge. One option could be for Carol to return to the AL and receive home health care from an outside agency for additional support and follow-up.
- **Y**our intervention: On admission, Susan completed the Confusion Assessment Method (Waszynski, 2007). She knows that Carol has a diagnosis of dementia. Carol is too lethargic to participate in any structured assessments of ADL or IADL function. Susan will reassess her in the morning. By then, Carol should have improved hydration and will have received a few doses of the antibiotic to treat the UTI and may be alert enough for further assessment. This will be important information to gather before the team meeting.

Transition 7—Hospital to Nursing Home:

Carol's condition did improve by the next day, but she was not able to return to the AL because she needed more assistance than could be provided. She was transferred to the rehabilitation unit of a nearby nursing home with the long-term goal to return to AL. She received physical therapy twice daily. Another important aspect of her care was to get her reestablished on her medication regimen to manage the symptoms of her Parkinson's disease to improve her mobility. The nursing staff also used scheduled voiding to help Carol regain continence.

Although Carol experienced some improvements, it was clear that she would not return to the AL. Richard reviewed Medicare's Nursing Home Compare Web site (www.medicare.gov/nursinghomecompare). Maria called the Options Counselor who had helped with her father and was directed to the AARP Web site about choosing a nursing home (http://www.aarp.org/relationships/caregiving/info-2006/embedded_sb.html). Finally, they found a guide to help them select a nursing home that was committed to culture change and person-centered care. At his children's insistence, Richard made several visits and after discussion with the administrator and staff, he selected a facility he thought would best meet his mother's needs. Because of her frailty and dementia he opted not to move her closer to him. Maria and her daughter agreed to continue monthly visits.

Family Case Study: Brown Family

Helen Brown and her family illustrate the family lives of people who have never married and/or have no children in their social networks. Family lives of these individuals are often rich, but many experience challenges in old age, particularly with declining health and abilities, that those with children and spouses may not encounter. The life course perspective also informs our understanding of Helen and her family's resources, although we will focus mostly on the intersection with social services, long-term care financing, and community-based care.

Discussion:

Helen just celebrated her 90th birthday. She enjoyed the gathering of friends and family and felt quite special. Helen never married, caring for her disabled mother when she was young and middle-aged. Her father died when she was 6 and her brother was 3. Her mother supported the family as a seamstress. Later, Helen supported her mother and herself as a school teacher, with her brother occasionally helping out. Helen retired shortly before her 65th birthday but continued teaching piano lessons well into her eighties. Her mother died shortly after Helen's retirement, after a brief illness. Helen then became involved in many volunteer activities, which she found fulfilling. Although she has "retired" from most of her volunteer activities, Helen still enjoys being out of doors and always has had a garden full of vegetables and flowers. She has many close friends and feels very tied to the community through her long involvement as a teacher and community member. She never regretted not getting married and although she wondered what it would have been like to have children of her own, she found satisfaction with her students and nieces and nephews. All in all, Helen feels she has had a full and rich life.

It is only in the past year that Helen has begun to feel somewhat vulnerable. She lives in the two-story home that she shared with her mother. Most of the neighbors she was close to have moved away, although she has made efforts to meet some of the new ones as they move in. She describes herself as in good health, but has had increasing difficulties with balance. This began after a bout with the flu 3 months ago. With great reluctance, she started using a walker when she leaves her home, which she tries to do every day when the weather is good. She also has much less energy than she used to have and finds housework and meal preparation daunting. She is no longer able to go up or down stairs without a lot of effort. Still, she is adamant about remaining in her own home and is determined to get her strength back. She has a modest income, mostly Social Security and a very small pension, totaling about $2,200 per month. She had trouble paying her heating bills last winter. She frets over her garden. When she got sick, she began paying one of her youngest great-nieces to help keep it weeded, but her niece will be moving away to attend college soon.

Helen has two relatives of her generation who live nearby and have been central to her social network (see Figure 15-3, the Brown family genogram). Both have her very worried. Her younger brother Roy, 87, is widowed and is dealing with prostate cancer, now at stage three. His children are attentive, but are debating among themselves about his living situation. Two of his children feel he needs 24-hour care in a nursing home, and the other two feel that he needs to be in familiar surroundings without a lot of strangers around. His physician has suggested that they consider hospice care. His children are all over 60 and only two live close by.

Mostly, Helen is fearful for her cousin and best friend, Alice, who is 88. Like Helen, Alice did not have children of her own. She did marry, however, and her husband, Charles, had several siblings. Charles and Alice doted on their many nieces and nephews and their home was often a fun-filled destination for these children and later for their children. Alice's husband was a successful businessman and Alice had a lot of money after he died. She was glad to help out her nieces and nephews as they went through school, got married, and had children of their own. As Alice's health began to decline, Beth, one of her nieces, offered to move in to help her out. It seemed like a good idea, but now Helen hardly talks to or sees Alice. When she does, Alice's manner has changed: she is no longer upbeat, she is not keeping herself carefully groomed, and seems quite distracted. She has also lost weight. One of Alice's nephews told Helen that many of the family photos have been removed from Alice's walls. Helen noticed that Beth is driving a new car, has very fashionable clothes, and recently went to Europe with her boyfriend and her daughter. Helen hates to think that Beth is stealing from Alice, but she can't come up with an alternative explanation. Because Roy is so sick, she is not sure who she should talk to.

Transition 1—Independence to Supportive Services:

As she has begun to "slow down," as she puts it, Helen is increasingly worried about her ability to maintain her independence (see Figure 15-4, the Brown family ecomap). She tried to save money for "a rainy day" because she has no children to provide support, but knows her funds are limited. Through friends and the local Senior Center, she made a connection with an Options Counselor to help

(continued)

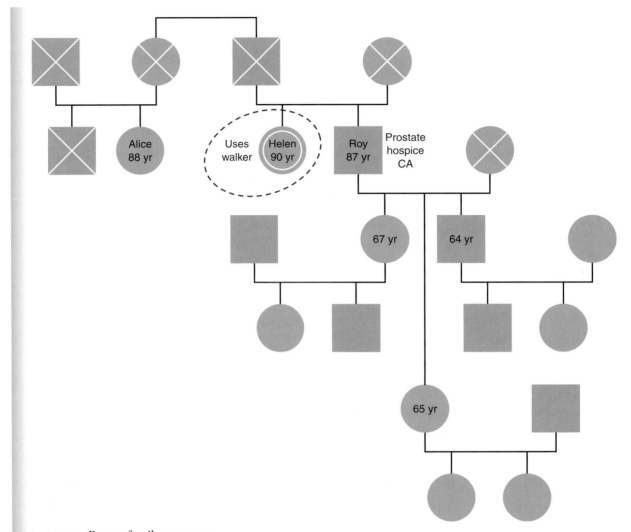

FIGURE 15-3 Brown family genogram.

Helen make a plan for herself. The Options Counselor learned that staying at home and in her neighborhood is very important to Helen. Helen has important strengths that make this possible. She is capable of making decisions for herself and she is successfully managing her health. Importantly, she is determined to get better and stay well and is doing the things that will make that possible. She is engaged in her community and has good relationships with others and at least one great-niece is likely to provide short-term assistance should she need it.

The options counselor helps Helen to come up with strategies that will keep her active. This includes taking advantage of a low-cost transportation service to visit the Senior Center where she can continue volunteer activities

and participate in an exercise group. The van also stops at the grocery store twice a week. She also learned that she can afford to use the services of a small nonprofit gardening organization that teaches children to garden. The staff of this agency will work with children in Helen's garden in exchange for sharing in Helen's harvest. Finally, she learned about an energy assistance program that will reduce her monthly payments.

Transition 2—Transition to Hospice:
Health providers have an important role in communicating with and supporting families as the end of life approaches (see Chapter 10). In this case study, health professionals will have to be sensitive in working with Roy's children.

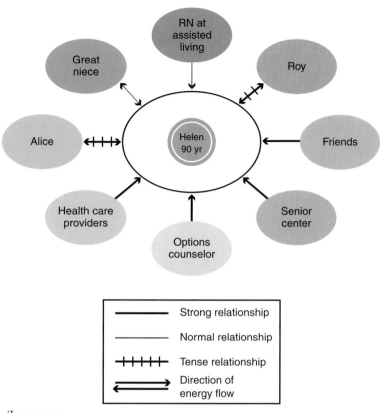

FIGURE 15-4 Brown family ecomap.

Although hospice care is provided in residential care settings, nursing homes, and at home, Roy needs to be involved as much as possible regarding the location of services. Health professionals can help families explore pros and cons, alleviate fears and uncertainties, and help to identify services that will support the family, as well as Roy. By including Roy in discussions with his children, hospice workers helped Roy's children come to agreement that hospice care at home was a feasible and desirable option for Roy. They helped establish a schedule and a list of tasks so that each child and grandchild could be present in a way that was comfortable for them and for Roy. They were able to supplement with paid caregivers to assist family members who were not comfortable being alone with Roy in case he needed help they did not feel comfortable providing. One of his children made sure that Helen was able to visit with Roy during the last days of his life. Roy's symptoms were well managed and he died peacefully at home.

Transition 3—Transition to Assisted Living:
At her most recent visit to her nurse practitioner, Helen began to describe her worries about her cousin. The NP listened carefully and took down Alice's name, address,

and contact information. After Helen left, the NP contacted Adult Protective Services and reported this potential abuse. The agency followed up with Alice and did find evidence of neglect and financial exploitation, and worked with the family to recover some of Alice's funds and to get appropriate help into her home. (Helen could also have alerted her Options Counselor to the possibility of abuse and the Options Counselor would have made the referral to protective services.) As a result of their investigation into Alice's situation, the protective service worker suggested that Alice be evaluated for dementia; older single women with dementia and living alone are at risk for financial exploitation.

The situation with Beth caused considerable tension and conflict within the family. Beth denied that she had taken funds inappropriately and insisted that Alice had, as she had in years past, insisted on giving Beth money. Beth felt she earned those funds because of the increasing difficulty in taking care of Alice as her health and cognitive status declined. Some were supportive of Beth, but other family members blamed Beth for isolating Alice from other family members, keeping her deteriorating cognitive status

(continued)

from other family members, and taking advantage of her previous generosity. Not all family members agreed with the dementia diagnosis.

As the extent of Alice's condition became clear to the extended family, the only area of agreement was that Alice could not remain at home without assistance. As a consequence, Alice was moved into an assisted living residence with a memory care unit. Although Alice did not yet need to live on the memory care unit, no one in her family felt comfortable with any other alternative. Living with another family member was not an option because no one wanted to worry that decisions they made would be second guessed or criticized by other family members. Because Alice still had financial resources, her family felt confident that she had the resources needed to stay in the AL for the rest of her life, and that she could pay out of pocket for additional charges should they arise. Once her nieces and nephews agreed that an assisted living placement was appropriate, they consulted an elder law attorney who helped to manage Alice's assets for her care.

Alice was not happy with the decision and had a difficult adjustment period. Helen visited regularly at first, but she found that Alice was becoming more confused and kept asking to leave and return to her home. Over time, Helen's visits became less frequent because transportation was difficult to arrange and Helen felt distressed by these visits. Helen continued to call Alice at least weekly and often sent notes and cards.

SUMMARY

This chapter has described the aging population in the United States and provided an overview of family ties of older adults.

- Using the life course perspective, we discussed the diversity of family structure in later life and how it has been influenced by societal trends, such as increasing life expectancy, increasing divorce rates, changing fertility patterns, greater ethnic diversity, and changes in economic status and work patterns.
- Most elders are embedded in social networks in which kin are important sources of emotional and instrumental support. Given the diversity of family life, many configurations of "family" exist. In most families, individuals enjoy strong and affectionate relationships,

and can count on family members to provide care and support when needed. Nonetheless, it is also common for families to have both positive and negative feelings toward one another because they are providing support. In some families, negative feelings may predominate, which will have consequences for health, well-being, and availability of support.

- Older adults, especially those of advanced years, have unique health care needs that must be addressed whether in clinics, at home, in hospitals, or through a variety of LTC services.
- Nursing and other professionals in gerontology have developed evidence-based assessment tools and interventions that are the basis for optimal care. Nurses must be familiar with these tools and apply them routinely and appropriately.
- Professionals must also recognize that older adults, including many care recipients, are also providers of care to their spouses, children, grandchildren, or friends. In fact, family members deliver the majority of care.
- As the population ages, it is increasingly important that nurses develop expertise in geriatric care, regardless of setting. Nurses with strong leadership skills are needed, especially in community-based care and nursing home settings.
- In all settings, nurses must partner with elders and their family members in designing and providing care that addresses unique needs and supports relationships.

REFERENCES

AARP. (2004). AARP Public Policy Institute analysis of the 2004 National Nursing Home Survey (NNHS) and U.S. Census Bureau population estimates. Retrieved from http://assets.aarp.org/rgcenter/il/fs10r_homes.pdf

Administration on Aging. (2011). A profile of older Americans: 2011. Retrieved from http://www.aoa.gov/AoARoot/Aging_Statistics/Profile/index.aspx

Alwin, D. F. (2012). Demographic transitions and life-span development. In K. L. Fingerman, C. A. Berg, J. Smith, & T. C. Antonucci (Eds.), Handbook of life-span development (pp. 673–699). New York, NY: Springer.

Angel, J. L., Jimenez, M. A., & Angel, R. J. (2007). The economic consequences of widowhood for older minority women. Gerontologist, 47, 224–234.

Antonucci, T. C., & Akiyama, H. (1995). Convoys of social relations: Family and friendships within a life span context. In

R. Blieszner & V. H. Bedford (Eds.), *Handbook of aging and the family*. Westport, CT: Greenwood Press.

Austin, W., Goble, E., Strang, V., Mitchell, A., Thompson, E., Lantz, H., . . . Vass, K. (2009). Supporting relationships between family and staff in continuing care settings. *Journal of Family Nursing, 15*(3), 360–383.

Balas, M. C., Casey, C. M., & Happ, M. B. (2012). Comprehensive assessment and management of the critically ill. In M. Boltz, E. Capezuti, T. Fulmer, & D. Zwicker (Eds.), *Evidence-based geriatric nursing protocols for best practice* (4th ed., pp. 600–627). New York, NY: Springer.

Bauer, M., & Nay, R. (2011). Improving family-staff relationships in assisted living facilities: The view of family. *Journal of Advanced Nursing, 67*(6), 1232–1241.

Beach, S. R., Schulz, R., Castle, N. G., & Rosen, J. (2010). Financial exploitation and psychological mistreatment among older adults: Differences between African Americans and non–African Americans in a population-based survey. *Gerontologist, 50*, 744–757.

Bedford, V. H., & Avioli, P. S. (2012). Sibling relationships from midlife to old age. In R. Bleizner & V. H. Bedford (Eds.), *Handbook of families and aging* (2nd ed., pp. 125–152). Santa Barbara, CA: Praeger.

Bengtson, V. L., & Allen, K. R. (1993). The life course perspective applied to families over time. In P. G. Boss, W. J. Doherty, R. LaRossa, W. R. Schumm, & S. K. Steinmetz (Eds.), *Sourcebook of family theories and methods: A contextual approach* (pp. 469–498). New York, NY: Plenum Press.

Bengtson V. L., & Harootyan, R. A. (1994). (Eds.). *Intergenerational linkages: Hidden connections in American society*. New York, NY: Springer.

Bianchi, S. M., & Casper, L. M. (2005). Explanations of family change: A family demographic perspective. In V. L. Bengtson, A. C. Acock, K. R. Allen, P. Dilworth-Anderson, & D. M. Klein (Eds.), *Sourcebook of family theory and research* (pp. 93–117). Thousand Oaks, CA: Sage.

Bilmes, L. J. (2008, March/April). Iraq's 100-year mortgage. *Foreign Policy*, pp. 84–85.

Boise, L., & White, D. (2004). The family's role in person-centered care: Practice considerations. [Electronic version.] *Journal of Psychosocial Nursing, 42*, 12–20.

Bookwala, J. (2012). Marriage and other partnered relationships in middle and late life. In R. Bleizner & V. H. Bedford (Eds.), *Handbook of families and aging* (2nd ed., pp. 91–124). Santa Barbara, CA: Praeger.

Bucx, F., Van Wel, F., Knijin, T., & Hagendoorn, L. (2008). Intergenerational contact and the life course status of young adult children. *Journal of Marriage and Family, 70*, 144–156.

Byrd, E. H., & Vito, N. A. (2011). Nursing assessment and treatment of depressive disorders of late life. In K. D. Mililllo & S. C. Houde (Eds.), *Geropsychiatric and mental health nursing* (2nd ed.). Sudbury, MA: Jones & Bartlett Learning.

Carder, P. C. (2002). The social world of assisted living. *Journal of Aging Studies, 16*, 1–18.

Cartwright, J. C., Miller, L., & Volpin, M. (2009). Hospice care in assisted living: Promoting good quality care at end of life. *Gerontologist, 49*, 508–516.

Cherlin, A. J. (2010). Demographic trends in the United States: A review of research in the 2000s. *Journal of Marriage and Family, 72*, 403–419.

Christensen, K., Doblehammer, G., Rau, R., & Vaupel, J. W. (2009). Ageing populations: The challenges ahead. Author manuscript, NIH Public Access. Retrieved from http://www.ncbi.nlm.nih.gov/pmc/articles/PMC2810516

Connidis, I. A. (2010). *Family ties and aging* (2nd ed.). Thousand Oaks, CA: Pine Forge.

Connidis, I. A., & McMullin, J. A. (2002). Sociological ambivalence and family ties: A critical perspective. *Journal of Marriage and Family, 64*, 558–567.

Cutugno, C. L. (2011). The "graying" of trauma care: Addressing traumatic injury in older adults. *American Journal of Nursing, 111*(11), 40–48.

Dannefer, D. (2003). Cumulative advantage/disadvantage and the life course: Cross-fertilizing age and social science theory. *Journals of Gerontology, Series B, Psychological Sciences and Social Sciences, 58*(6) S327–S337.

Davidson, K. M. (2011). Family preparedness and end-of-life support before the death of a nursing home resident. *Journal of Gerontological Nursing, 37*(2), 11–16.

DeLamater, J. (2002). Sexuality across the life course: A biopsychosocial perspective. Paper presented at the Midcontinent and Eastern regions meeting of the Society for the Scientific Study of Sexuality, Big Rapids, MI.

DeLamater, J., & Moorman, S. M. (2007). Sexual behavior in later life. *Journal of Aging and Health, 19*(6), 921–945.

Dilworth-Anderson, P., Williams, I. C., & Gibson, B. E. (2002). Issues of race, ethnicity, and culture in caregiving research: A 20-year review (1980–2000). *Gerontologist, 42*, 237–272.

Doerflinger, D. M. C. (2007). How to try this: The Mini-Cog. *American Journal of Nursing, 107*(12), 62–71.

Dolbin-MacNab, M. L. (2006). Just like raising your own? Grandmothers' perceptions of parenting a second time around. *Family Relations, 55*, 564–575.

Duncan, M. T., & Morgan, D. L. (1994). Sharing the caring: Family caregivers' views of their relationships with nursing home staff. *Gerontologist, 34*, 235–259.

Eliopoulos, C. (2009). *Gerontological nursing* (7th ed.). Philadelphia, PA: Lippincott Williams & Wilkins.

Family Caregiver Alliance. (2006). *Caregiver assessment: Principles, guidelines and strategies for change. Report from a National Consensus Development Conference* (vol. I). San Francisco, CA: Author.

Faust, K. A., & McKibben, J. N. (1999). Marital dissolution: Divorce, separation, annulment, and widowhood. In M. B. Sussman, S. K. Steinmetz, & G. W. Peterson (Eds.), *Handbook of marriage and the family* (2nd ed.). New York, NY: Plenum.

Federal Interagency Forum on Aging-Related Statistics. (2012, June). *Older Americans 2012: Key indicators of well-being.* Federal Interagency Forum on Aging-Related Statistics. Washington, DC: U.S. Government Printing Office. Retrieved from http://www.agingstats.gov/agingstatsdotnet/main_site/default.aspx

Fingerman, K. L. (2001). *Aging mothers and their adult daughters: A study in mixed emotions.* New York, NY: Springer.

Fingerman, K. L., & Birditt, K. S. (2011). Relationships between adults and their aging parents. In K. W. Schaie & S. L. Willis (Eds.), *Handbook of the psychology of aging* (7th ed.). New York, NY: Elsevier.

Frick, K. D., Burton, L. C., Clark, R., Mader, S. I., Naughton, W. B., Burl, J. B., . . . Leff, B. (2009). Substitutive hospital at home for older persons: Effects on costs. *American Journal of Managed Care, 15*(1), 49–56.

Friedemann, M. L., Montgomery, R. J., Maiberger, B., & Smith A. A. (1997). Family involvement in the nursing home: Family-oriented practices and staff-family relationships. *Research in Nursing & Health, 20,* 527–537.

Fulmer, T. (2012). Elder mistreatment assessment. In M. Boltz (Series Ed.), *Try this: Best practices in nursing care to older adults* (Issue No. 15). Retrieved from http://consultgerirn.org/uploads/File/trythis/issue15.pdf

Fulmer, T., Guadagno, L., Bitondo, C., & Connolly, M. T. (2004). Progress in elder abuse screening and assessment instruments. [Electronic version.] *Journal of the American Geriatrics Society, 52,* 297–304.

Gitlin, L. N., & J. Wolff (2011). Family involvement in care transitions of older adults: What do we know and where do we go from here? *Annual Review of Gerontology and Geriatrics, 31,* 31–64.

Goodman, C. C. (2012). Caregiving grandmothers and their grandchildren: Well-being nine years later. *Children and Youth Services Review, 34,* 648–654.

Goodman, C. C., & Silverstein, M. (2006). Grandmothers raising grandchildren: Ethnic and racial differences in well-being among custodial and coparenting families. *Journal of Family Issues, 27,* 1605–1626.

Graf, C. (2007). The Lawton instrumental activities of daily living scale. In M. Boltz (Series Ed.), *Try this: Best practices in nursing care to older adults* (Issue No. 23). Retrieved from http://consultgerirn.org/uploads/File/trythis/issue23.pdf

Greenberg, S. A. (2007). How to try this: The geriatric depression scale: Short form. *American Journal of Nursing, 107*(10), 60–69.

Hanson, B. G. (1995). *General systems theory beginning with wholes.* Washington, DC: Taylor & Francis.

Harvath, T. A., & McKenzie, G. (2012). Depression in older adults. In M. Boltz, E. Capezuti, T. Fulmer, & D. Zwicker (Eds.), *Evidence-based geriatric nursing protocols for best practice* (4th ed., pp. 469–499). New York, NY: Springer.

Hayslip, B., & Kaminski, P. L. (2005). Grandparents raising their grandchildren: A review of the literature and suggestions for practice. *Gerontologist, 45,* 262–269.

Hayslip, B., Jr., & Page, K. S. (2012). Grandparenthood: Grandchild and great-grandchild relationships. In R. Bleizner & V. H. Bedford (Eds.), *Handbook of families and aging* (2nd ed., pp. 183–212). Santa Barbara, CA: Praeger.

Herd, P. (2005). Ensuring a minimum: Social Security reform and women. *Gerontologist, 45,* 12–25.

Hungerford, T. L. (2007). The persistence of hardship over the life course. *Research on Aging, 29,* 491–511. Retrieved from http://psychsocgerontology.oxfordjournals.org/content/65B/3/358.full.pdf+html

Inouye, S. K., Bogardus, S. T., Baker, D. I., Leo-Summers, L., & Cooney, L. M. (2000). The Hospital Elder Life Program: A model of care to prevent cognitive and functional decline in older hospitalized patients. [Electronic version.] *Journal of the American Geriatrics Society, 48,* 1697–1706.

Institute of Medicine. (2010). Returning home from Iraq and Afghanistan: Preliminary Assessment of readjustment needs of veterans, service members, and their families. Retrieved from http://www.nap.edu/catalog/12812.html

Iwasiw, C., Goldenberg, D., Bol, N., & MacMaster, E. (2003). Resident and family perspectives: The first year in a long-term care facility. *Journal of Gerontological Nursing, 29,* 45–54.

Katz, R., Lowenstein, A., Phillips, J., & Daatland, S. O. (2005). Theorizing intergenerational family relations: Solidarity, conflict, and ambivalence, in cross-national contexts. In V. L.

Bengtson, A. C. Acock, K. R. Allen, P. Dilworth-Anderson, & D. M. Klein (Eds.), *Sourcebook of family theory and research* (pp. 393–420). Thousand Oaks, CA: Sage.

Keefe, J., & Fancey, P. (2000). The care continues: Responsibility for elderly relatives before and after admission to a long term care facility. *Family Relations, 49,* 235–244.

Kelly, K., Thrane, S., Virani, R., Malloy, P., & Ferrell, B. (2011). Expanding palliative care nursing education in California: The ELNEC geriatric project. *International Journal of Palliative Nursing, 12*(3), 188–194.

Keyser, S. E., Buchanan, D., & Edge, D. (2012). Providing delirium education for family caregivers of older adults. *Journal of Gerontological Nursing, 38*(2), 24–31.

Kleinpell, R. M., Fletcher K., & Jennings, B. M. (2008). Reducing functional decline in hospitalized elderly. In Hughes, R. G. (Ed.), *Patient safety and quality: An evidence-based handbook for nurses.* Rockford, MD: Agency for Healthcare Research and Quality. Retrieved from http://www.ahrq.gov/qual/nurseshdbk/docs/KleinpellR_RFDHE.pdf

Koren, M.J. (2010). Person-centered care for nursing home residents: The culture-change movement. *Health Affairs, 29*(2), 312-317.

Kronenfeld, J. J. (2006). Changing conceptions of health and life course concepts. [Electronic version.] *Health, 10,* 501–517.

Lachman, M. E. (2003). Negative interactions in close relationships: Introduction to a special section. *Journal of Gerontology: Psychological Sciences, 52B,* P69.

Landry-Meyer, L., & Newman, B. M. (2004). An exploration of the grandparent caregiver role. *Journal of Family Issues, 25,* 1-5-1-25.

Leder, S., Grinstead, L. N., & Torres, E. (2007). Grandparents raising grandchildren: Stressors, social support, and health outcomes. *Journal of Family Nursing, 13,* 333–352.

Leff, B., Burton, S., Mader, S. L., Naughton, B., Burl, J., Greenough, W. B., . . . Stinwachs, D. (2009). Comparison of functional outcomes associated with hospital at home care and traditional acute hospital care. *Journal of the American Geriatrics Society, 57*(2), 273–278.

Legault, A., & Ducharme, F. (2009). Advocating for a parent with dementia in a long-term care facility: The process experienced by daughters. *Journal of Family Nursing, 15*(2), 198–219.

Logue, R. M. (2003). Maintaining family connectedness in long-term care. *Journal of Gerontological Nursing, 29*(6), 24–31.

Long, C. O. (2009). Palliative care for advanced dementia: Approaches that work. *Journal of Gerontological Nursing, 35*(11), 19–24.

Lumpkin, J. R. (2008). Grandparents in a parental or near-parental role: Sources of stress and coping mechanisms. *Journal of Family Issues, 29,* 357–372.

Luo, Y., LaPierre, T. A., Hughes, M. E., & Waite, L. J. (2012). Grandparents providing care to grandchildren: A population-based study of continuity and change. *Journal of Family Issues, 33,* 1143–1167.

Maas, M. L., Buckwalter, K. C., Hardy, M. D., Tripp-Reimer, T., Titler, M. G., & Specht, J. P. (2001). *Nursing care of older adults: Diagnoses, outcomes, and interventions.* St. Louis, MO: Mosby.

Mader, S. L., Medcraft, M. C., Joseph, C., Jenkins, K. L., Benton, N., Chapman, K., . . . Schutzer, W. (2008). Program at home: a Veterans Affairs healthcare program to deliver hospital care in the home. *Journal of the American Geriatrics Society, 56*(12), 2317–2322.

Magana, S., Seltzer, M. M., & Krauss, M. W. (2002). Service utilization patterns of adults with intellectual disabilities: A comparison of Puerto Rican and non-Latino white families. *Journal of Gerontological Social Work, 37*(3/34), 65–86.

Manton, K. G. (2008). Recent declines in chronic disability in the elderly U.S. population: Risk factors and future dynamics. *Annual Review of Public Health, 29*, 91–113. Retrieved from arjournals.annualreviews.org

Mattes, R. D. (2002). The chemical senses and nutrition in aging: Challenging old assumptions. [Electronic version.] *Journal of the American Dietetic Association, 102*, 192–196.

Messecar, D. C. (2012). Family caregiving. In M. Boltz, E. Capezuti, T. Fulmer, & D. Zwicker (Eds.), *Evidence-based geriatric nursing protocols for best practice* (4th ed., pp. 469–499). New York, NY: Springer.

Mezey, M., Kobayashi, M., Grossman, S., Firpo, A., Fulmer, T., & Mitty, E. (2004). Nurses improving care to health system elders (NICHE): Implementation of best practice models. *Journal of Nursing Administration, 34*, 451–457.

Miller, S. C., Miller, E. A., Jung, H.-Y., Sterns, S., Clark, M., & Mor, V. (2010). Nursing home organizational change: The "culture change" movement as viewed by long-term care specialists. *Medical Care Research and Review, 67* (4 Suppl), 65S–81S. Mitty, E. L. (2012). Advance directives. In M. Boltz, E. Capezuti, T. Fulmer, & D. Zwicker (Eds.), *Evidence-based geriatric nursing protocols for best practice* (4th ed., pp. 579–599). New York, NY: Springer.

Mitty, E., Resnick, B., Allen, J., Bakerjian, D., Hertz, J., Gardner, W., . . . Mezy, M. (2010). Nursing delegation and medication administration in assisted living. *Nursing Administration Quarterly, 34*(2), 162–171.

Monserud, M. A. (2008). Intergenerational relationships and affectual solidarity between grandparents and young adults. *Journal of Marriage and Family, 70*, 182–195.

Munn, J. C., Dobbs, D., Meier, A., Williams, C. S., Biiola, H., & Zimmerman, S. (2008). The end-of-life experiences in long-term care: Five themes from focus groups with residents, family members, and staff. *Gerontologist, 48*(4), 485–494.

National Alliance for Caregiving & AARP. (2009). Caregiving in the U.S. Bethesda, MD. Retrieved from http://www.caregiving.org/research/caregiving-research/general-caregiving

National Clearinghouse for Long-Term Care (Administration on Aging). (2013). Understanding LTC services. Retrieved from http://www.longtermcare.gov/LTC/Main_Site/Understanding/Services/Home_Community_Services.aspx

National Institute of Nursing Research. (2011). *Palliative care: The relief you need when you're experiencing the symptoms of serious illness.* Bethesda, MD: Author.

Neal, M. B., & Hammer, L. B. (2007). *Working couples caring for children and aging parents: Effects on work and well-being.* Mahwah, NJ: Lawrence Erlbaum Associates.

Newsom, J. T., Rook, K. S., Nishishiba, M., Sorkin, D. H., & Mahan, T. L. (2005). Understanding the relative importance of positive and negative social exchanges: Examining specific domains and appraisals. *Journal of Gerontology: Psychological Sciences, 60B*, P304–P312.

Oregon Department of Human Services. (2011). *Oregon consumer guide: Assisted living and residential care facilities.* Salem, OR: Author.

Peters, C. L., Hooker, K., & Zvonkovic, A. M. (2006). Older parents' perceptions of ambivalence in relationships with their children. *Family Relations, 55*, 539–551.

Pillemer, K., & Suitor, J. J. (2005). Ambivalence and the study of intergenerational relations. In M. Silverstein (Ed.), Focus on intergenerational relations across time and place [electronic version]. *Annual Review of Gerontology and Geriatrics, 24*, pp. 3–28.

Pillemer, K., Suitor, J. J., Henderson, C. R., Meador, R., Schultz, L., Robison, J., & Hedgman, C. (2003). A cooperative communication intervention for nursing home staff and family members of residents. *Gerontologist, 43*, 96–106.

Pinquart, M., & Sorensen, S. (2006). Helping caregivers of persons with dementia: Which interventions work and how large are their effects? [Electronic version.] *International Psychogeriatrics, 18*, 577–595.

Pioneer Network. (1997). Toward a new culture of aging: Mission, vision and values. Retrieved from http://www.pioneernetwork.net/AboutUs/Values

Pioneer Network & Hartford Institute for Geriatric Nursing. (2010). Nurse competencies for nursing home culture change. Retrieved from http://www.pioneernetwork.net/Providers/ForNurses

Pruchno, R., & Gitlin, L. N. (2012). Family caregiving in later life: Shifting paradigms. In R. Bleizner & V. H. Bedford (Eds.), *Handbook of families and aging* (2nd ed., pp. 515–541). Santa Barbara, CA: Praeger.

Pruchno, R. A., & Meeks, S. (2004). Health-related stress, affect, and depressive symptoms experienced by caregiving mothers of adults with a developmental disability. [Electronic version.] *Psychology and Aging, 19*, 394–401.

Quadagno, J. (2008). *Aging and the life course: An introduction to social gerontology* (4th ed.). New York, NY: McGraw Hill.

Rahman, A. N., & Schnelle, J. F. (2008). The nursing home culture-change movement: Recent past, present, and future directions for research. *Gerontologist, 48*, 142–148.

Reinhard, S. C., Given, B., Petlick, N. H., & Bemis, A. (2008). Supporting family caregivers in providing care. In *Patient safety and quality: An evidence-based handbook for nurses.* Agency for Healthcare Research and Quality. Retrieved from http://www.ahrq.gov/qual/nurseshdbk

Reuss, G. F., Dupuis, S. L., & Whitfield, K. (2005). Understanding the experience of moving a loved one to a long-term care facility. [Electronic version.] *Journal of Gerontological Social Work, 46*, 17–46.

Riebe, D., Blissmer, B. J., Greaney, M. L., Garber, C. E., Lees, F. D., & Clark, P. G. (2009). The relationship between obesity, physical activity, and physical function in older adults. *Journal of Aging and Health, 21*, 1159–1178.

Roberto, K. A. (1990). Grandparent and grandchild relationships. In T. H. Brubaker (Ed.), *Family relationships in later life* (2nd ed., pp. 100–112). Newbury Park, CA: Sage.

Robinson, S. B., & Rosher, R. B. (2006). Tangling with the barriers to culture change: Creating a resident-centered nursing home environment. *Journal of Gerontological Nursing, 32*(10), 19–25.

Rook, K. S. (2003). Exposure and reactivity to negative social exchanges: A preliminary investigation using daily diary data. [Electronic version.] *Journals of Gerontology, Series A, Biological Sciences and Medical Sciences, 58*, P100–P111.

Rossi, A. S., & Rossi, P. H. (1990). *Of human bonding.* New York, NY: Aldine de Gruyter.

Salinas, T. K., O'Connor, L. J., Weinstein, M., Lee, S. Y. V., & Fitzpatrick, J. J. (2002). A family assessment tool for hospitalized elders. *Geriatric Nursing, 23*, 316–319.

Saunders, G. H., & Echt, K. V. (2007). An overview of dual sensory impairment in older adults: Perspectives for rehabilitation. *Trends in Amplification, 11*, 243–258.

Saunders, M. M. (2012). Perspectives from family caregivers receiving home nursing support: Findings from a qualitative study of home care patients with heart failure. *Home Healthcare Nurse, 30*(2), 82–90.

Scharlach, A., Li, W., & Dalvi, T. B. (2006). Family conflict as a mediator of caregiver strain. *Family Relations, 55*, 625–635.

Schmall, V. (1994). *Sexuality in later years. Essentials of aging for health, mental health, and social services provider series.* DVD published by the Oregon Geriatric Education Center. 47 minutes. Call no. SX5.S10.

Sechrist, J., Suitor, J. J., Pillemer, K., Gilligan, M., Howard, A. R., & Keeton, S. A. (2012). Aging parents and adult children: Determinants of relationship quality. In R. Bleizner & V. H. Bedford (Eds.), *Handbook of families and aging* (2nd ed., pp. 153–182). Santa Barbara, CA: Praeger.

Seltzer, M. M., Floyd, F., Song, J., Greenberg, J., & Hong, J. (2011). Midlife and aging parents of adults with intellectual and developmental disabilities: Impacts of lifelong parenting. *American Association on Intellectual and Developmental Disabilities, 116*, 479–499.

Seltzer, M. M., Greenberg, J. S., Floyd, F. J., & Hong, J. (2004). Accommodative coping and well-being of midlife parents of children with mental health problems or developmental disabilities. *American Journal of Orthopsychiatry, 74*, 187–195.

Seltzer, M. M., Greenberg, J. S., Krause, M. W., & Hong, J. (1997). Predictors and outcomes of the end of co-resident caregiving in aging families of adults with mental retardation or mental illness. *Family Relations, 46*, 13–22.

Settersten, R. A. (2006). Aging and the life course. In R. H. Binstock & L. K. George (Eds.), *Handbook of aging and the social sciences* (6th ed., pp. 3–19). New York, NY: Academic Press.

Silverstein, M., & Bengtson, V. L. (1997). Intergenerational solidarity and the structure of adult child-parent relationships in American families. *American Journal of Sociology, 103*, 429–460.

Silverstein, M., & Marenco, A. (2001). How Americans enact the grandparent role across the family life course. [Electronic version.] *Journal of Family Issues, 22*, 493–522.

Sloane, P. D., Zimmerman, S., & Sheps, C. G. (2005). Improvement and innovation in long-term care: A research agenda report and recommendations from a national consensus conference. University of North Carolina at Chapel Hill. Retrieved from http://www.pragmaticinnovations.unc. edu/FinalReport/Pragmatic%20Innovations%20Final %20Report%201-9-05.pdf

Spillman, B. C. (2004). Changes in elderly disability rates and the implications for health care utilization and cost. [Electronic version.] *Milbank Quarterly, 82*, 157–194.

Steele, J. S. (2010). Current evidence regarding models of acute care for hospitalized geriatric patients. *Geriatric Nursing, 31*(5), 331–347.

Steis, M. R., & Fick, D. M. (2012). Delirium superimposed on dementia: Accuracy of nurse documentation. *Journal of Gerontological Nursing, 38*(1), 32–42.

Steis, M. R., Prabhu, V., Kolanowski, A., Kang, Y., Bowles., K. H., Fick, D., & Evans, L. (2012). Detection of delirium in community-dwelling persons with dementia. *Online Journal of Nursing Informatics, 16*(1). Retrieved from http://ojni.org/issues/?p=1274

Stelle, C., Fruhauf, C. A., Orel, N., & Landry-Meyer, L. (2010). Grandparenting in the 21st century: Issues of diversity in grandparent-grandchild relationships. *Journal of Gerontological Social Work, 53*, 682–701.

Stone, R. I. (2006). Emerging issues in long-term care. In R. H. Binstock & L. K. George (Eds.), *Handbook of aging and the social sciences* (6th ed., pp. 397–418). New York, NY: Academic Press.

Stone, R. I., & Reinhard, S. C. (2007). The place of assisted living in long-term care and related service systems. *Gerontologist, 47*(Special Issue III), 23–32.

Szinovacz, M. E. (Ed.). (1998). *Handbook of grandparenthood.* Westport, CT: Greenwood Press.

Talerico, K. A., O'Brien, J. A., & Swafford, K. L. (2003). Person-centered care: An important approach for 21st century health care. *Journal of Psychosocial Nursing, 41*, 12–16.

Teaster, P. B., Wangmo, T., & Vorsky, F. B. (2012). Elder abuse in families. In R. Bleizner & V. H. Bedford (Eds.), *Handbook of families and aging* (2nd ed., pp. 409–429). Santa Barbara, CA: Praeger.

Thiele, D. M., & Whelan, T. A. (2006). The nature and dimensions of the grandparent role. *Marriage & Family Review, 40*, 93–108.

Tucker, D., Bechtel, G., Quartana, C., Badger, N., Werner, D., Ford, I. F. & Connelly, L. (2006). The OASIS Program: Redesigning hospital care for older adults. *Geriatric Nursing, 27*, 112–117.

Uhlenberg, P. (2004). Historical forces shaping grandparent-grandchild relationships: Demography and beyond. In M. Silverstein (Ed.), Focus on intergenerational relations across time and place [electronic version]. *Annual Review of Gerontology and Geriatrics, 24*, pp. 77–97.

Uhlenberg, P., & Kirby, J. P. (1998). Grandparenthood over time: Historical and demographic trends. In M. E. Szinvocz (Ed.), *Handbook of grandparenthood* (pp. 23–39). Westport, CT: Greenwood Press.

Umberson, D., Williams, K., Powers, D. A., Liu, H., & Needham, B. (2006, March). You make me sick: Marital quality and health over the life course. [Electronic version.] *Journal of Health and Social Behavior, 47*, 1–16.

Vandell, D. L., McCartney, K., Owen, M. T., Booth, C., & Clarke-Stewart, A. (2003). Variations in child care by grandparents during the first three years. *Journal of Marriage and Family, 65*, 375–381.

Vincent, G. K., & Velkoff, V. A. (2010, May). The next four decades: The older population in the United States: 2010 to 2050. U.S. Department of Commerce, Economics and Statistics Administration, U.S. Census Bureau. P 25 1138. Retrieved from http://books.google.com/books?id=gALA2 NWAFZ4C&dq=+Vincent,+G.+K.,+%26+Velkoff,+V.+A.+ %282010,+May%29.+The+next+four+decades:+The+older+ population+in+the+United+States:+2010+to+2050.+U.S.+ Department+of+Commerce,+Economics+and+Statistics+ Administration,+U.S.+Census+Bureau.+P+25+1138.+&lr= &source=gbs_navlinks_s

Voyer, P., Richard, S., Doucet, L., & Carmichael, P. (2011). Factors associated with delirium severity among older persons with dementia. *Journal of Neuroscience Nursing, 43*(2), 62–69.

Waldrop, D. P. (2003). Caregiving issues for grandmothers raising their grandchildren. *Journal of Human Behavior in the Social Environment, 7*, 201–223.

Walker, A. J., Allen, K. R., & Connidis, I. A. (2005). Theorizing and studying sibling ties in adulthood. In V. L. Bengtson, A. C. Acock, K. R. Allen, P. Dilworth-Anderson, & D. M. Klein (Eds.), *Sourcebook of family theory and research* (pp. 167–190). Thousand Oaks, CA: Sage.

Walker, A. J., Manoogian-O'Dell, M., McGraw, L. A., & White, D. L. (2001). *Families in later life: Connections and transitions.* Thousand Oaks, CA: Pine Forge Press.

Walker, A. J., Pratt, C. C., & Eddy, L. (1995). Informal caregiving to aging family members: A critical review. *Family Relations, 44,* 402–411.

Wallace, M., & Shelkey, M. (2007). Katz index of independence in activities of daily living (ADL). In M. Boltz (Series Ed.), *Try this: Best practices in nursing care to older adults* (Issue No. 2). Retrieved from http://consultgerirn.org/uploads/File/trythis/issue02.pdf

Waszynski, C. M. (2007). Detecting delirium. *American Journal of Nursing, 107*(12), 50–59.

White, D. L., Newton-Curtis, L., & Lyons, K. S. (2008). Development and initial testing of a measure of person-directed care. *Gerontologist, 48*(Special Issue 1), 114–123.

Wilson, K. B. (2007). Historical evolution of assisted living in the United States, 1979 to the present. *Gerontologist, 47*(Special Issue III), 8–22.

Wolf, R. S. (1996). Understanding elder abuse and neglect. [Electronic version.] *Aging, 367,* 4–9.

Wu, A., & Schimmele, C. M. (2007). Uncoupling in late life. [Electronic version.] *Generations, 31*(3), 41–46.

Yeoman, B. (2008, July/August). When wounded vets come home. *AARP Magazine.* Retrieved from http://www.aarp.org/relationships/caregiving/info-05-2008/iraq-vets-when-wounded-vets-come-home.html

Zimmerman, S., & Sloane, P. D. (2007). Definition and classification of assisted living. *Gerontologist, 47*(Special Issue III), 33–39.

chapter 16

Family Mental Health Nursing

Laura Rodgers, PhD, PMHNP

Critical Concepts

- All parts of the family system are interconnected; therefore, all members are affected when a member has a mental health condition.

- The family of a person with a mental health condition needs to be involved in treatment because it enhances the effectiveness of the health care treatment.

- Comorbidities are frequently present when someone has a mental health condition (e.g., depression often coexists with eating disorders or anxiety disorders; substance abuse and alcohol/drug addictions commonly occur with mood disorders). As a result, mental health conditions typically require integrated and complex treatment.

- Psychoeducation and participating in formal and/or informal support groups are effective interventions for family members who have a member with a mental health condition.

- Nurses must examine their personal attitudes and stigmas toward persons and families who have a member with a mental health condition and seek additional education and training to challenge the negative stigmas so they can then serve as effective advocates for these families in both community and acute care settings.

- Nurses must use nonjudgmental and nonblaming communication interactions with families who have a member with a mental health condition in order to establish a therapeutic professional relationship with the family.

Mental health has been defined as a (1) state of well-being such that (2) an individual is able to perform mental functions that allow her to adapt to change and cope with adversity in order to (3) function well in society while (4) being mostly satisfied with life in general (American Nurses Association [ANA], American Psychiatric Nurses Association [APNA], & International Society of Psychiatric–Mental Health Nurses [ISPN], 2007). In other words, an individual has achieved a state of mental health when she is able to adapt to internal and environmental life stressors, as demonstrated by age and culturally appropriate thoughts, feelings, and behaviors (Robinson, 1983). A person who can

cope with the normal stress of family, work, and friends; can work productively; and is able to make a contribution to her community (World Health Organization [WHO], 2001a) would represent someone in a state of psychological, emotional, and social well-being.

By contrast, a disturbance in thoughts or mood caused by a mental disorder or mental illness can lead to maladaptive behavior, inability to cope with normal stresses of life, and interference with daily functioning (ANA, APNA, & ISPN, 2007). The diagnoses of mental disorders are based on diagnostic criteria from either the American Psychiatric Association's (APA's) (2013) *Diagnostic and Statistical*

Manual of Mental Disorders, Fifth Edition (DSM-5) or the *International Classification of Disease–10* (ICD-10), which is endorsed by the WHO (2010). The DSM-5 was 13 years old before its recent revision and the ICD-10 is currently under revision and due to be released within the next several years. Each describes mental disorders as conditions characterized by alterations in a person's thinking, mood, or behavior that (1) cause an individual distress, (2) impair his occupational or social functioning, and/or (3) place the individual at significant risk for experiencing death, pain, disability, or a loss of freedom (APA, 2013).

Rather than describe an individual who has been diagnosed with a mental disorder as "mentally ill," the term used throughout this chapter will be "an individual with a mental or behavioral health condition," or a person with an MHC. Although mental disorders have discrete diagnostic criteria, there are some mental disorders that consume a larger burden of care in the community and often have the most negative and intrusive effects on an individual's life and on family members' lives. Individuals with these disorders will be noted as persons with a serious mental illness (SMI). Examples of disorders that cause significant impairment to an individual throughout his lifetime are schizophrenia, bipolar disorder, pervasive developmental disorders, and major depressive disorder. The Substance Abuse and Mental Health Services Administration (SAMHSA) (2012a) has defined persons with SMIs as individuals 18 or older who currently or at any time in the past year have had a diagnosable mental, behavioral, or emotional disorder (excluding developmental and substance use disorders) that has met diagnostic criteria specified in the DSM-IV (APA, 2000), has resulted in serious functional impairment, and has substantially interfered with one or more major life activities. On the other hand, examples of disorders that typically do not cause significant social, emotional, or behavioral disability include generalized anxiety disorder, adjustment disorder, and dysthymia.

This chapter covers mental health family nursing. The chapter begins with a brief demographic overview of the pervasiveness of MHCs in both Canada and the United States. The remainder of the chapter focuses on the impact a specific mental health condition can have on the individual with the MHC, individual family members, and the family as a unit. Although the chapter does not go into specific diagnostic criteria for various conditions, it does offer nursing interventions to assist families. Note that the impact and treatment of substance abuse is discussed within the Johnson family case study.

MENTAL HEALTH CONDITIONS IN THE UNITED STATES AND CANADA

The WHO (2001a) estimated that more than 25% of people worldwide will be affected by an MHC at least once in their lifetime and that approximately 10% of the adult population at any given time has an MHC. More specifically, 20% of adult Canadians (those 18 and older) have an MHC (Mental Health Commission of Canada, 2012) and the remaining 80% have a friend, family member, or colleague who has an MHC (Health Canada, 2002). Similarly, 20% of adults in the United States have an MHC in a given year and a subpopulation of about 5.4% have SMIs (U.S. Department of Health and Human Services, 1999). Researchers estimate that, in the United States, the chance of being diagnosed with any MHC during one's lifetime is 46.4% (Kessler, Berglund, et al., 2005), and the overall prevalence of mental disorders is about the same across genders (WHO, 2001a). This section addresses the prevalence of MHCs in the United States and Canada, comorbidities associated with MHCs, general approaches being taken toward those with MHCs, and the stigma associated with having an MHC.

Prevalence of MHCs

Mental disorders are the leading cause of disability in both Canada and the United States (WHO, 2008) and of all diseases, with the exception of heart disease, account for the most years lived with a disability (National Institute of Mental Health [NIMH], 2001). Only one-third of those persons who need mental health services in Canada receive the care (Statistics Canada, 2002) and only 5.5% of these conditions receive health care dollars even though these illnesses constitute more than 15% of the burden of disease in Canada (Institute of Health Economics, 2008); in other words, though 15% of the estimated costs associated with all diseases in Canada are due to mental health conditions, insufficient monetary resources are allocated to mental health services. In the United States, adult outpatient mental health services are paid for by private health insurance (37.9%), self-payment or payment by a family member living in the household (33.7%), Medicare (15.2%), Medicaid (11.9%), or an employer (11.9%) (SAMHSA, 2012b). Only 17.4 million adults in the United States received mental health services in 2001 despite there being 45.6 million adults with mental illness (SAMHSA, 2012b). Financial costs may be a barrier to people accessing care.

In 2001 in the United States, the percentage of persons 18 or older who had any diagnosable mental, behavioral, or emotional disorder (excluding developmental and substance use disorders) of sufficient duration to meet DSM-IV-TR diagnostic criteria within the past year was 15.9% among Hispanics, 16.1% among Asians, 18.8% among blacks, 20.5% among whites, 28.3% among persons reporting two or more races, and 28.9% among American Indians or Alaska Natives (SAMHSA, 2012b). Although MHCs are pervasive across the general population in Canada and the United States, some groups experience a greater impact of poor mental health. In Canada, families in the lowest income group are three to four times more likely to report poor mental health than those in the highest income group (Statistics Canada, 2002). Likewise in the United States, the number of persons with an MHC is highest among low-income families (SAMHSA, 2012b).

Mental Health and Comorbidities

It is common for someone with an MHC to have another condition, either mental or physical; the coexistence of multiple conditions is termed *comorbidity*. For example, depression often coexists with eating disorders such as anorexia nervosa and bulimia nervosa, or anxiety disorders, such as post-traumatic stress disorder (PTSD), obsessive-compulsive disorder, panic disorder, social phobia, and generalized anxiety disorder (Devane, Chiao, Franklin, & Kruep, 2005). Likewise, the coexistence of substance abuse and mood disorders has been documented among the U.S. population (Conway, Compton, Stinson, & Grant, 2006). Women are more prone than men to having a coexisting anxiety disorder at the same time as depression and men are more likely than women to exhibit alcohol and substance abuse or dependence

when depression is present (Kessler et al., 2003). Given the prevalence of comorbidities, it is important that nurses take a holistic view of the person with an MHC and approach interventions from multiple perspectives, rather than simply focusing on a single MHC.

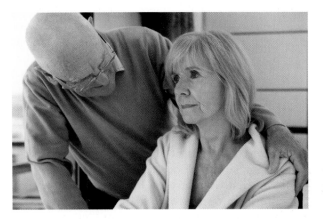

Serious physical medical illnesses may accompany, and even be exacerbated by, a mental health condition. For example, heart disease, stroke, cancer, HIV/AIDS, diabetes, Parkinson's disease, thyroid problems, and multiple sclerosis are some of the conditions that often coexist with depression (Cassano & Fava, 2002). There is evidence that when depression accompanies a serious physical illness, both conditions tend to show more severe symptoms, medical costs increase, and people have more difficulty adapting to the physical condition compared to those without the MHC (Katon & Ciechanowski, 2002). Treating the depression along with the coexisting physical illness may help ease both conditions (Katon & Ciechanowski, 2002).

Mental Health and General Approaches Toward Those With an MHC

Recovery from a mental health disorder is the major goal for mental health care. SAMHSA (2012a) has established a set of principles for recovery and has defined recovery as "a process of change through which individuals improve their health and wellness, live a self-directed life, and strive to reach to their full potential" (p. 3). Health, home, purpose, and community have been identified as the four major areas that contribute to maintaining a life in recovery.

The 10 guiding principles of the Recovery Model are as follows:

- Hope
- Person-driven
- Many pathways (nonlinear)
- Holistic
- Peer support
- Relational (interactions with others, both formally and informally)
- Culture
- Addresses trauma
- Strengths/responsibilities
- Respect

Unlike previous views of MHCs, especially in relation to the more severe conditions, that some MHCs are chronic and very difficult if not impossible to manage, part of the recovery model is the assertion that there are no limits to the potential for an individual to recover from any mental health condition (Till, 2007).

Another recovery model with a similar philosophy has been implemented in Canada. Called the Tidal Model, it also emphasizes a shift in how nurses think about the care provided to people with an MHC. Rather than focusing on disease and illness, this model stresses the importance of the individual with an MHC actively participating in decision making related to care and including family in the overall care (Caldwell, Sclafani, Swarbrick, & Piren, 2010). The Tidal Model was developed by nurses in collaboration with other mental health care providers and has transformed nursing practice in mental health care settings (Brookes, Murata, & Tansey, 2006, 2008). At the center of both of these models, the Recovery Model and the Tidal Model, is the philosophy that nurses recognize the uniqueness of each individual with an MHC and that nurses must collaborate not only with these individuals to provide person-centered care, but also with their families. There are improved outcomes when this collaboration takes place (Kaas, Lee, & Peitzman, 2003), such as reduced morbidity and mortality rates in persons with MHCs and improved preservation of the psychological and physical health of their family members. In line with this philosophy, the President's New Freedom Commission on Mental Health (2003) final report (Box 16-1) recommended six national goals to move mental health care in the United States toward a recovery-oriented system,

---

BOX 16-1

Goals Identified by the New Freedom Commission on Mental Health

- Americans understand that mental health is essential to overall health.
- Mental health care is consumer and family driven.
- Disparities in mental health services are eliminated.
- Early mental health screening, assessment, and referral to services are common practice.
- Excellent mental health care is delivered and research is accelerated.
- Technology is used to access mental health care and information.

Source: New Freedom Commission on Mental Health. (2003). *Achieving the promise: Transforming mental health care in America.* Rockville, MD: U.S. Department of Health and Human Services. Retrieved from http://govinfo.library.unt.edu/mentalhealthcommission/reports/reports.htm

---

with the overall goal of improving mental health care for Americans.

Also in line with this philosophy, there has been an international trend to provide care to persons with an MHC in the community rather than in an institutional setting. Past practice had been to institutionalize persons with an MHC, often for a lengthy period of time; however, the recovery approaches shift both the focus and the locus of care provision. Large inpatient, mental health care institutions have been closed in most areas, but many governments have not provided funding for other resources to deliver the care that persons with an MHC might need. This change has resulted in the transfer of care from the institutional to the family level, a fact that is especially pertinent for families providing care to individuals with SMIs (Doornbos, 2002). The stress and burden of care experienced by these families has been well documented (NIMH, 2001). Families often suffer financial and social deprivations when providing care to family members with an MHC, and they often live in fear that the family member with an MHC will cause disruption to family life due to a recurrence or exacerbation of the MHC (WHO, 2001b). Common needs for families living with a family member with an MHC are support, information, skills and training, advocacy, and referral sources (Yamashita & Forsyth, 1998).

More than ever, families are an integral and instrumental resource for recovery for individuals with an MHC and especially those individuals with an SMI. One qualitative Canadian study examined the role of family in supporting recovery for people with an MHC who lived in structured, community housing (Piat, Sabetti, Fleury, Boyer, & Lesage, 2011). The researchers found that, even though the mental health consumers lived apart from their families and relied heavily on formal services, the residents identified their families—more than mental health professionals, friends, or residential caregivers—as those who most believe in them and in their recovery. These same mental health consumers stated that their recovery was supported by their families' affection, emotional support, and active involvement. Families offered more hope in recovery than professional providers. It is evident that nurses and other health professionals must engage the families of individuals with an MHC in their recovery.

Mental Health and Stigma

Stigma has been defined as labeling, stereotyping, separation, status loss, and discrimination (Link, Yang, Phelan, & Collins, 2004). Our society singles out mental illness as undesirable and devalues the person who possesses an MHC (Brunton, 1997). Society's stigma influences how an individual feels about himself, which can lead to self-stigma and can exacerbate mental health conditions (Link & Phelan, 2001). The media are responsible for perpetuating misconceptions about persons with an MHC (Mental Health America, 2012), often by sensationalizing crimes in which persons with an MHC are involved and using pejorative terms to describe the individual with the MHC.

Stigma affects both the individual with the MHC and the family members. As family members become responsible for providing more and more care to individuals with an MHC, they are reporting their perceptions of caregiving as stressful and stigmatizing (Dalky, 2012). For example, families may perceive that their family reputation has been disgraced because a member has a mental illness; they may be embarrassed at the behavioral outbursts sometimes associated with MHCs (Dalky, 2012). Stigma can cause individuals with an MHC and their families to become isolated and feel ashamed or stigma can make individuals and family members engage in denial or a wish for things to appear normal, which may then discourage them

from talking about their needs and seeking help (Abrams, 2009).

Stigma and discrimination toward persons with an MHC can prevent care and treatment from reaching people with mental illnesses (WHO, 2001a). For example, stigma toward a parent who has an MHC, or who is providing care to a child with an MHC, may prevent the parent from obtaining community support because of her fear that others may assume she is not a fit parent; she may not access care because she fears losing custody of her child (Obadina, 2010). People with MHCs also may fear workplace reprisals if they seek mental health care through work-provided insurance.

In fact, the stigma can be quantified. Just over 50% of Canadians say they would tell a friend or coworker that a family member has an MHC, compared to 72% who would discuss a cancer diagnosis or 68% who would discuss diabetes in the family (Canadian Medical Association, 2008). Only 12% of Canadians would hire a lawyer who has an MHC; just 49% would socialize with a friend who has an SMI; and many Canadians (46%) think that people use mental illness as an excuse for bad behavior (Canadian Medical Association, 2008). The proportion of Americans who believe SMI is associated with violent and dangerous behaviors doubled between 1950 and 1996 (Phelan, Link, Stueve, & Pescosolido, 2000), and 27% of Canadians are fearful of being around people with an SMI (Canadian Medical Association, 2008). Unfortunately, nurses and professionals are not immune to demonstrating stigma toward individuals with an MHC and their families. For example, nurses providing care to a mother parenting a child with attention-deficit hyperactivity disorder (ADHD) may blame poor parenting for the child's behavioral challenges.

But there is some cause to hope for decreasing stigma toward those with an MHC. For instance, in 2006, 67% of the public agreed that depression had a neurobiological cause compared to only 54% in 1996 (Pescosolido et al., 2010). Personal contact with someone with an MHC has been shown to decrease one's stigma toward persons with an MHC (Schafer, Wood, & Williams, 2010). In addition, peer-led interventions have been shown to be effective in reducing family self-stigma (Perlick et al., 2010). Education of health care professionals about specific disorders and their treatments can also help reduce or prevent behaviors or discrimination due to stigma. Increased understanding about the symptoms and behaviors arising from an MHC allows professionals to provide optimal care. For instance, instead of blaming poor parenting, nurses working with a mother whose child has ADHD can focus on identifying those behaviors that are ADHD related and work with the mother to develop targeted interventions that compensate for the executive function deficits and emotional dysregulation issues associated with this condition.

FAMILY MEMBERS OF INDIVIDUALS WITH A MENTAL HEALTH CONDITION

The whole family may be affected by and involved in care of the member who has an MHC, or individual relationships and responsibilities may be more pronounced. For example, a spouse may be providing care to her husband. Parents may be providing care to young or adult children. In some cases, the parent has the MHC and so a child takes care of the parent. Siblings may provide care for siblings, and so on. The "normal" relationships and dynamics within the family may be disrupted. Nurses need to pay attention to family dynamics and to the potential burdens faced by individual members and the family as a whole when a member has an MHC. This section focuses on the general burden of family caregiving, spousal caregiving, role changes within the family, children living with a parent or sibling who has an MHC, and parenting a child who has an MHC.

Burden of Family Caregiving

Family caregivers often take on their role because of a sense of responsibility, as well as a perceived lack of available resources or services (Decima Research Inc., 2004). Families who provide care for a family member with an MHC can find the role demanding and stressful. Research has shown that family members and caregivers of persons with an MHC experience shame, guilt, and sorrow (Sjoblim, Pejlert, & Asplund, 2005), as well as chronic stress, poor health behaviors, and adverse immune and neuroendocrine consequences (Nadkarni & Fristad, 2012). Financial stress related to insufficient resources, educational level, and the age of the care

provider also affects the care provider's burden (Tan et al., 2012). Single, divorced, separated, or widowed caregivers have more depressive symptoms than married care providers (Kamel, Bond, & Froelicher, 2012). Women are typically the providers of care, with estimates ranging from 56.6% to 69% of caregivers (Zauszniewski, Bekhet, & Suresky, 2008). Each year, 54 million Americans are affected by an SMI and though the women who provide care to their family members with an SMI are resourceful, the overall burden causes many of these women to experience depression, poorer quality of life (Zausniewski et al., 2008), and lower levels of subjective well-being and physical health than men who are caregivers (Moller, Gudde, Folden, & Linaker, 2009; Pinquart & Sorensen, 2006). Regardless of the relationship of the caregiver to the person with the MHC, formal (professional therapy) and informal (social, including support groups) support has been shown to buffer the caregiver's symptoms of depression (Chen & Lukens, 2011).

A small qualitative Canadian study (Veltman, Cameron, & Stewart, 2002) confirmed the paradox that family care providers report not only negative impacts of providing care to a relative with an MHC but also beneficial effects, such as feelings of gratification, love, and pride. Most respondents in the study believed that caregiving made them stronger, more patient, and more appreciative of time with their families, as well as less judgmental of others (Veltman et al., 2002). Family caregivers also report being more secure (Foster, 2010) and sensitive (Chen & Lukens, 2011), and having more hope (Tranvag & Kristofferson, 2008). Many family care providers gain a deep respect for their family member's struggle, as portrayed in this mother's comment about providing care to her son who has schizophrenia: "He's always on my mind, I'm always worried about him, it breaks my heart, I wish he had friends, I wish he had a job, but he tries the best he can, the best he knows how, struggling every day, I don't know how he does it, but I'm proud of each of his accomplishments, no matter how small" (Veltman et al., 2002, p. 112).

Caregivers express worries about the deterioration of their family member's general health over time as the care recipient ages (Corsentino, Molinari, Gum, Roscoe, & Mills, 2008). Moreover, care providers frequently mention that their own physical health as they age is a major issue for them. But what caregivers fear the most is what happens to the individual with an MHC if the caregiver is no longer able to provide care (Corsentino et al., 2008).

Spousal Caregiving

Approximately one in four family caregivers caring for someone with a mental illness provide care to a spouse (Decima Research Inc., 2004). Care is typically provided in the family home and the most common tasks performed on a daily basis are providing companionship, providing emotional support during a crisis, and monitoring symptoms (Decima Research Inc., 2004). Other aspects of care include providing or monitoring medications, paying bills, advocating for the person to receive help, arranging and coordinating services and appointments, assisting with personal grooming, looking after household chores, and going to appointments with the person who has an MHC (Decima Research Inc., 2004). These tasks and aspects of care are common to anyone who has an MHC, regardless of whether the person is the spouse, child, sibling, and so on.

Spousal care providers may feel angry about the changes that they see in their spouse due to the onset, exacerbations, and remissions of the MHC (O'Connell, 2006). Spouses may find themselves blaming their spouse for having a character flaw rather than understanding the cause of and treatments for the MHC. Additional financial and parental responsibilities can also increase the stress and negatively affect the relationships between family members. Couple and family therapy and spousal support groups can help these families adapt to the demands of the MHC (O'Connell, 2006).

Family Role Changes

It is not unusual for family caregivers of persons with an MHC to change their relationships or roles within the family (Ali, Ahlstrom, Krevers, & Skarsater, 2012). For example, an adult younger brother may find it challenging to maintain his role as younger brother, while also being caregiver and guardian to his older sister who has an SMI. On the other hand, Aldridge (2006) contended that children as caregivers to parents do not necessarily change their status. Rather, the child may take on some parenting roles—such as providing personal and emotional care to a parent, engaging in household chores, providing care to brothers and sisters,

administering medication to parents, or providing crisis support to a parent during an acute psychotic episode or self-harming—but not others (Aldridge, 2006). Thus, parents may maintain their role as parents, though there might be some interdependence between the child and parents. Being a child (under the age of 18 years) in the caregiver role to a parent can have a positive effect on the child's development, including improved family relationships, but it can also negatively affect the child's development and overall childhood experience (Aldridge, 2006).

Role changes may not be welcomed by the family. For instance, some family caregivers describe feeling obliged to provide care to their relative with an MHC, whether the obligation is willingly accepted or suddenly pushed on them (Rowe, 2012). They may find themselves needing to learn about their legal and moral roles in the new caregiving situation. Family care providers often struggle with unexpected and unfamiliar expectations placed on them in their new roles. Legal and moral rights related to providing care to the family member with an MHC often cause conflict between the family care provider and the professional staff. Frequently, professional staff members neither appreciate nor understand the legal needs and moral rights of the family care provider but, rather, focus on the legal and moral rights of the person with the MHC. For example, professionals may pressure a parent to take his adult child home with him because they believe that the person with the MHC will benefit by being cared for at home. But the parent may not feel that he has the capacity to care for his daughter, or he may have made a decision not to attempt to provide care because of previous negative consequences to the family when the daughter has been at home. This difference in perspectives can cause barriers between health care professionals and family care providers (Rowe, 2012). It is important to note, however, that family care providers and families in general want to be included and supported in the treatment and care decision making for their family member.

Children With a Family Member With a Mental Health Condition

When an adult with an MHC accesses care, it is imperative that nurses ascertain whether there are children in the family because research has shown that children living with a family member with an

MHC are at increased risk for developing psychopathology; developing emotional and behavioral problems (Ahern, 2003; Korhonen, Pietila, & Vehvilainen-Julkunen, 2010), including anxiety or personality disorders (Kendler & Gardner, 1997); suffering abuse and neglect (Mahoney, 2010); and being involved in accidents (Obadina, 2010). Mental health professionals often overlook children who live with a family member with an MHC; they focus their attention solely on the individual who has the MHC. Unless a child shows signs of abuse or neglect, or is in the custody of child protective services, children tend to be invisible to the professionals who are treating the child's parent (Gladstone, Boydell, & McKeever, 2006). Even though one in six Canadian children younger than 12 years of age live with a family member who has an MHC (Bassani, Padoin, Phillip, & Veldhuizen, 2009), nurses who provide care to adults with an MHC inconsistently ask if there are children in the family (Foster, O'Brien, & Korhonen, 2012). One recommendation to avert omission of this important information is to change the hospital assessment forms to include a section that asks about children living in the home (Mordoch & Hall, 2002). Regardless, nurses should make it standard practice to ask the question.

Not only should nurses determine if there is a child in the family of a person with an MHC, but nurses need to understand that children may perceive their own role in a negative way. Strained relationships between family members are not uncommon and can lead to a chaotic family life (Foster, 2010). Appropriate assessment and intervention are important to ameliorate any negative consequences for a child who is living with a person who has an MHC, regardless of whether that person is the child's parent or sibling or has another relationship with the child. At the same time, nurses should remember that, in spite of the associated risks, many of these children remain emotionally and mentally healthy (Ahern, 2003; Place, Reynolds, Cousins, & O'Neill, 2002).

Nurses need to be aware that children living with a family member with an MHC often believe they caused the MHC and may have feelings of guilt, anger, or anxiety (Obadina, 2010). In addition, the children may feel alone (Foster, 2010). Nurses must initiate a conversation with the child and not wait until a child asks for help. It is important for nurses to tell the child that she did not cause the parent's illness or strange behavior nor is she responsible for taking care of the family member; nurses should reinforce that there are professionals who will provide care to the family member (Obadina, 2010). Providing age-appropriate information about the parent's MHC and treatment decreases the child's feelings of guilt and also decreases the child's negative feelings toward the MHC (Obadina, 2010). Developing a relationship with the child ameliorates the feelings of being isolated and alone. If there are several children of different ages in the living situation, the nurse must remember to provide teaching and answers to each child, appropriate to the child's developmental and cognitive ability. Children who are knowledgeable about a parent's illness are able to understand the parent's behaviors better in relation to the specific illness (Mordoch & Hall, 2002). Children need to be provided thoughtful, developmentally appropriate information about their parent's illness and treatment. Children who are not given the whole story are left to formulate unrealistic scenarios, which only adds to their emotional confusion (Mordoch & Hall, 2002). Support for family relationships and other networks must be part of the care that nurses provide to parents in any setting (Korhonen, Vehvilainen-Julkunen, & Pietila, 2008).

While a primary role for a nurse who is providing care to an adult with an MHC is to identify the presence of children living in the family and to offer support and education to those children, the nurse also needs to perform a family-centered assessment of the children's needs (Korhonen et al., 2010), followed by referral to relevant services (Mahoney, 2010). Once needs are identified, nurses can develop a plan for assisting the child. For example, with parental consent and within the limits of confidentiality, nurses can contact a child's school to apprise teachers or administrators of the family situation affecting the child (Mahoney, 2010). Nurses can facilitate access to other professional services and family support, such as family and/or individual therapy. Therapy that teaches children and youth how to communicate easily and have fewer arguments with their parents may be beneficial as those factors have been shown to contribute to improved mental health among adolescents ages 11 to 15 years in a very large cross-national study involving 43 countries, including 26,078 young Canadians (Freeman, King, & Pickett, 2011). In addition, it is important to provide services that can enhance a child's coping skills (Ahern, 2003), because children with effective coping skills are less likely to have behavioral or emotional problems (Gladstone et al., 2006).

Although the majority of professional services for family members with an MHC are in the community, there are times when a family member may be hospitalized. Nurses need to remember to ask the hospitalized family member if there are children. Children whose family members are hospitalized want and need information about the hospitalized family member (Foster et al., 2012) and appreciate having a nurse talk with them about visiting the psychiatric facility and having someone take a genuine interest in explaining what is happening to their family member (O'Brien, Anand, Brady, & Gillies, 2011). Nurses are encouraged to "view children as complex young persons who are competent to express their views and recount their experiences" (Gladstone et al., 2006, p. 2547), rather than as children who are too young to understand what is happening. Simple words and explanations can be used even with very young children and toddlers and may alleviate a lot of the child's anxiety.

Children Living With a Parent With a Mental Health Condition

In addition to the more general areas noted above, nurses also must recognize that specific issues may arise when a child is living with a parent with an MHC. Children growing up with a parent with an MHC may express anger toward the parent with the MHC because their parent is not like other parents and they may experience extreme sadness when they remember a time that the parent was healthy (O'Connell, 2006). These children also frequently worry, often needlessly, that they will inherit and develop the MHC, but they will only share this concern with another person after the person has gained their trust (Foster, 2010). Circumstances such as maternal depression can have a negative impact on the child's normal development and on his likelihood of developing a mental health problem. Therefore, nurses need to pay particular attention to specific risks when the parent is the person with an MHC.

Risks to Normal Development

Several disorders, including depression, schizophrenia, and bipolar disorder, not only affect an adult's ability to parent, but also can have an impact on a child's growth and development. It is estimated that about 8% of women of childbearing age have depression (Smith, 2004). The impact of maternal depression on children from infancy to adolescence has been observed in clinic and community settings. Maternal depression can have negative effects on a child's language development and intelligence, behavior, development of depressive symptoms, sleep patterns, physical health, parent/child relationship, and attachment (Smith, 2004). There is very little information about the effect paternal depression may have on children's growth and development.

Parents with depression may communicate pessimism and sadness to their infants, as well as laugh less and demonstrate less affection, tenderness, and responsiveness. Decreased close and continuous contact with infants can have the most harmful effects on infants (Brockington et al., 2011). A child's mental health and social competence is predicted less by illness variables and categorical diagnosis than by multiple contextual risks (Brockington et al., 2011). In any case, Smith (2004) asserted that effective interventions for the child should occur before negative outcomes are observed in the child. These interventions include teaching parenting skills, assessing the family and children for potential or actual problems, and minimizing parenting disruptions.

Children benefit by consistency in parenting behavior. Similar to children of parents with depression, children of parents with bipolar disorder are at increased risk for parenting disturbances related to the cyclical nature of the disorder. Inconsistent parenting behavior can be related to the parent's depression, manic/hypomanic or mixed state, chronicity of episodes, suicidality/suicide attempts, risky behavior associated with mania, problems with adherence to treatment, withdrawn/irritable behavior during a depressed mood, relapse in spite of treatment, and/or recovery time between episodes (Nadkarni & Fristad, 2012). Parenting difficulties in themselves can be challenging stressors for any parent, but parents who have bipolar disorder may experience exacerbation of the bipolar symptoms with increases in stress (Calam, Jones, Sanders, Dempsey, & Sadhnani, 2012). Nurses can provide assistance to these parents by collaborating with the parent, child, family, and other professionals to address the health needs determined by the family needs assessment.

Nurses, teachers, and family members may not recognize the concerns and issues that children who are living with a parent who has an MHC can face unless the child demonstrates a learning or behavior problem in school or a parent requests specific support for the child (Ahern, 2003; Mordoch & Hall, 2002). Therefore, children of parents with an MHC should be routinely assessed for parent/child relational problems and possible developmental delays so that appropriate interventions can be implemented in a timely manner.

Risks of Developing a Mental Health Condition

It has been estimated that one in five children have a parent with an MHC and that they are more likely than their peers to develop a mental health problem (Mayberry, Goodyear, & Reupert, 2012). In one study, 61% of children who had a parent with depression had developed a mental health disorder by adolescence, with 40% to 70% of those children having a comorbid diagnosis of substance abuse, dysthymia, and/or anxiety (Beardslee, Versage, & Gladstone, 1998). Children's development of depression may be influenced by genetic factors, environmental influences, marital or partner stress or violence, or even disruptions in parenting (Smith, 2004). Not only are children who live with a parent with an MHC at elevated risk for developing a mental health problem, including being developmentally delayed, but they are also at increased risk of being abused and neglected (Aldridge, 2006; Mahoney, 2010). Children of parents with an MHC should be routinely assessed for potential mental health concerns and, where warranted, appropriate interventions should be implemented.

Other Risks

Disruption of relationships within the family and increases in risky behaviors can be an issue, particularly for youth. Adolescents often give up hope of being able to live in a family that does not have a parent with an MHC. They may struggle with the stigma associated with the MHC and may opt out of a relationship with the parent and instead use maladaptive coping mechanisms that can lead to risky behaviors or problems with the justice system (Mordoch & Hall, 2002). Nurses need to be cognizant of this possibility, make sure to assess teenagers for adaptive and maladaptive coping mechanisms, and then intervene as necessary.

Some children have parents with an MHC, such as schizophrenia, major depressive disorder, or bipolar disorder, that is more likely than other MHCs to lead to hospitalization. These children often worry about what will happen to them if a parent is hospitalized. A small-scale Canadian study (Garley, Gallop, Johnson, & Pipitone, 1997) found that the children's biggest fear was parental separation due to a parent's illness. The children worry that they may be removed from their home and placed in foster care or another unknown living situation; they worry about what is happening to their parent who is hospitalized; and they become anxious when their daily rhythms are disrupted by their parent's hospitalization (Mordoch & Hall, 2002). The children become worried and stressed when no one tells them how their parent is doing—often leaving them to their own thoughts and feelings, wondering what is happening to their parent (Ostman, 2008). Nurses can alleviate some of the concern and uncertainty by assisting these families to develop a crisis intervention plan and inviting the entire family to participate (Reupert & Mayberry, 2007). This plan should include a contact person if the parent is ill or in the hospital, someone with whom each child might stay, and who should be told if the child is staying with another friend or family member (Reupert & Mayberry, 2007).

Nurses also must remember to dispel the myth that parents with an MHC are unfit parents. Rather, nurses must emphasize that a parent with an MHC can be a very competent, effective, nurturing, and loving parent. Children and parents will benefit from continuous assessment of the child's needs and ongoing professional support and treatment for the parents. There are many effective psychotherapeutic and psychological interventions available, including family therapies, mother and infant psychotherapies, and brief cognitive therapy appropriate to the age and stage of child development (Brockington et al., 2011). Nurses can provide support to parents who have an MHC by actively listening to the parents' concerns about parenting, providing realistic information about parenting skills, and assessing for the need for interventions to support the children (Mahoney, 2010).

Adult children who grew up living with a parent with an MHC may remember negative experiences caused by their parent's illness and the lack of information and support from mental health services. They may remember worrying about their parent's well-being, wondering if their parent was going to commit suicide, being fearful that the parent was not getting the care needed (Knutson-Medin, Edlund, & Ramklint, 2007), and being anxious about coming home from school because they did not know how their parent was going to respond to them (Foster, 2010). These adult children may remember having to approach either the parent without the health condition or a health professional to get information about their parent's condition, rather than the professional offering them this information. Sadly, some may recall growing up not being able to distinguish between the parent and the MHC (Foster, 2010). Children are not in a place to seek information; rather, nurses must offer and provide this information to children so that they do not grow into adults with negative memories about their experience.

Children Living With a Sibling With a Mental Health Condition

Sibling relationships have a profound impact on the development of a child. The sibling relationship provides the connection for a child to learn how to interact with others, manage quarrels, handle rivalries, share secrets, and try on different roles (Abrams, 2009). Siblings share a common genetic and social background, early life experiences, and a family cultural background that can last a lifetime (Goetting, 1986). Brothers and sisters also share unique private information about their parents and families (Abrams, 2009). Goetting (1986) contended that the common bond siblings experience can be a source of support and companionship for the sisters and brothers. But an MHC in one sibling can interfere negatively with sibling relationships. Some siblings experience guilt for not being the brother or sister with the MHC. Abrams described situations where brothers or sisters would tell friends they were an only child or would refuse to answer questions about the sibling with the MHC because of the shame or guilt they felt toward the sibling with the MHC. Unfortunately, these kinds of actions often lead to more silence and isolation for the unaffected sibling.

Sisters and brothers who have a sibling with a SMI, such as schizophrenia or bipolar disorder, often struggle to understand what has happened to the affected sibling and the impact the condition has on their relationship with their affected sibling, as well as the entire family. For example, siblings who observe an affected sibling experience his first

psychotic episode may feel haunted the rest of their life. Unfortunately, too often siblings of individuals with an SMI have their needs met by mental health professionals at only the lowest level (Ostman, Wallsten, & Kjellin, 2005). Yet, these siblings want more help; for example, they want health professionals to be available to answer their questions and to clarify their role in the future care of their sibling (Friedrich, Lively, & Rubenstein, 2008). When they get older, siblings may also have problems developing and keeping intimate relationships because they are fearful of passing on any genetic deficiencies to their own children (Abrams, 2009).

Sibling participation in a support group specifically for siblings who have a brother or sister with an MHC has been shown to decrease the siblings' feelings of being alone, and helps them gain information about their sibling's MHC and learn ways to support their affected sibling (Ewertzon, Cronqvist, Lutzen, & Andershed, 2012). One study suggested that the top-ranked coping strategies for supporting siblings of persons with schizophrenia are education about the illness, a supportive family, and having their sibling suffer less because the symptoms are controlled (Friedrich et al., 2008). Providing education to siblings can clarify misperceptions about the MHC and its treatment (O'Connell, 2006). Although it is important to address the needs of the brothers' and sisters' current experiences with their affected brother or sister, nurses must also be future oriented and provide education and support to these siblings in preparation for becoming future primary care providers to their sibling.

Nurses also need to be aware of other ways in which the dynamic in the family might be problematic when one sibling has an MHC and the other does not. For example, parents may focus their time and energy on the sibling with the MHC, leaving the unaffected sibling feeling neglected and resentful of the attention given to his sibling. It is important that the needs of healthy siblings are not ignored, no matter how unintentional the neglect by parents may be. Nurses can work with parents to help them shape how the unaffected sibling perceives the affected sibling and the MHC, as well as identify ways in which the parents can provide the needed attention to healthy siblings. Family assessment is critical, followed by appropriate psychoeducation, discussions about how parents might relate to the unaffected sibling, and referral to supports as needed.

Parenting Children With a Mental Health Condition

Parents provide care to children with an MHC on a regular basis in what can often be a long-term, ongoing activity; they frequently are the care providers for their adult child with an MHC. Parents often experience grief, isolation, and stigma when their child has an MHC or blame themselves for their child's MHC. They may face health professionals who are suspicious of parental involvement and do not allow parent participation in the care of the child, especially when the child is hospitalized. In addition, grandparents are assuming a caregiving role for their adult children who have an MHC and also have children.

Grief and chronic sorrow are common experiences that parents encounter after being told their child has an MHC. Parent caregivers tend to experience more grief than sibling caregivers (Chen & Lukens, 2011) and this grief can affect the parent's psychological well-being, health status, and the parent-child relationship (Godress, Ozgul, Owen, & Foley-Evans, 2005). The grief can be prolonged as the parents may experience grief differently across the life course of their child's illness. Chronic sorrow, pervasive sadness that is permanent, periodic, and potentially progressive in nature (Olshansky, 1962), also enhances parental grief. Parents may experience grief for the loss of the child that they can no longer have or may even feel they have a different child from the one they started with (O'Connell, 2006); parents grieve for their future losses, for what their child may not be able to accomplish. Some parents may feel the need to provide regular care for their child well into adulthood and, thus, they grieve not seeing their children grow up into independent individuals. They also may grieve losses in their own lives, such as not becoming empty nesters.

Parents who have a more secure affection bond and a more positive relationship with their child may experience less grief than other parents (Godress et al., 2005). On the other hand, parents who have a more ambivalent and anxious relationship with their child may experience more grief and greater negative relationships with their affected child. In one small study, parents of children diagnosed with either bipolar disorder or schizophrenia reported experiencing chronic sorrow that was often triggered by their unending responsibilities to provide care to their child (Eakes, 1995). Nurses need to recognize and validate the grief and sorrow parents experience and provide interventions that decrease their emotional distress and life disruption (Godress et al., 2005).

Some parents of children with an MHC experience isolation and stigma from family, friends, teachers, and school administrators. Many parents are forced to leave work to meet with teachers or administrators, which may cause them to lose their jobs or change to a less demanding job, thus adding further to the financial strain they may already be experiencing (O'Connell, 2006). Many parents of adult children with an SMI experience significant frustration as they try to navigate a health care system that they perceive as full of obstacles (O'Connell, 2006).

Parents who have a child with bipolar disorder, for instance, often blame themselves for their child's MHC, e.g., because of childhood adversity, bad parenting, or substance misuse (Crowe et al., 2011). Such parents may request family interventions including psychoeducation, communication enhancement, and problem-solving skills training to help the family understand and manage the disorder (Crowe et al., 2011; Nadkarni & Fristad, 2012). Nurses should offer such interventions even if a family does not request them.

Parents want to be involved at an early stage in the treatment of their child with an MHC and it is important to them that their opinions and experiences are heard (Nordby, Kjonsbert, & Hummelvoll, 2010). Yet, many health professionals are suspicious of parental involvement and do not allow parent participation in the care of the child (Jakobsen & Severinsson, 2006). Although trust and honesty are critical elements in relations between professionals and family, trust does not develop naturally (Piippo & Aaltonen, 2004). Collaboration between health professionals, parents, family members, and other disciplines enhances trust among everyone involved.

Many parents experience the hospitalization of their child with an MHC. Parents report that the admission process can be very difficult for them and that they often feel in crisis; they want nurses and other health professionals to understand these challenges (Scharer, 2002). They typically need written and verbal information related to their child's care, such as an up-to-date handbook that tells them who to call for information about their child, what to expect during the hospitalization, hospital costs, what the child can or cannot do, what they should be doing about school, and a list of nearby inexpensive lodging during the hospitalization, as well as easy access to the child and better access to care before, during, and after hospitalization (Scharer, 2002). Parents welcome practical tips and timely, accurate, situation-specific information that is communicated to them in a clear and honest manner (Eakes, 1995). In addition, parents strongly suggest that they be recommended to a parent support group and also be given a list of parents who have undergone a similar experience and are willing to talk with them. Many parents experience guilt and shame related to their child's hospitalization and find it helpful when nurses talk to them about their guilt and shame in a nonjudgmental manner.

Some parents whose child has an SMI and never achieves independence may need to assume the responsibility of caring for their grandchildren (O'Connell, 2006). A small Canadian study (Seeman, 2009) described the role of the grandmother as one with divided loyalties: the toll of providing care to their grandchildren but also the rewards that come with raising their grandchildren. In the United States in 2008, 5.7 million children, 8% of all children, lived with a grandparent. Mental disorders in the parent of the child was one of the 11 reasons why the grandmother was raising the child (U.S. Census Bureau, 2008). Caring for grandchildren involves physical exertion and dedication over time. If the grandparent is also caring for her adult child with MHC, the physical and mental toll can be overwhelming. A particularly vulnerable time for the grandparent is when the grandchild approaches the age at which the child's mother or father began developing symptoms (Seeman, 2009). Nurses should be aware of such dates and offer support to grandparents rather than waiting for the grandparents to request help. Although grandparents often provide the daily care for their grandchildren, nurses must recognize that typically it is the child's parent who is recognized as the legal guardian. This situation can present problems for the grandparent and cause negative caregiving experiences (Seeman, 2009). The grandparents may view the parent's influence as not beneficial to the child's well-being and so they may feel tempted to minimize visitations, though many do try to sustain a relationship between the parent

and child. Grandparent caretakers sometimes are put into adversarial conditions with the parent and may even have to sue for custody of the child (Seeman, 2009).

FAMILIES OF INDIVIDUALS WITH A SPECIFIC MENTAL HEALTH CONDITION

Several mental health conditions warrant specific discussion in this chapter, either due to the stigma associated with these disorders or the serious impact these disorders can have on family function and well-being. The following five disorders will be discussed:

- Schizophrenia
- Bipolar disorder (BD)
- Major depressive disorder (MDD)
- Dementia
- Attention-deficit hyperactivity disorder (ADHD)

The diagnostic criteria for these disorders can be found in the DSM-5 (APA, 2013). This section will discuss the impact these specific disorders can have on families and will include implications for nursing practice. Note that substance abuse is a common comorbidity with these conditions, so it too needs assessment and intervention. The Johnson family case study, later in the chapter, discusses assessment and treatment for substance abuse.

Schizophrenia, BD, and MDD should be considered potentially terminal illnesses for persons with these disorders. It is estimated that around one-third of people with schizophrenia attempt suicide and up to 15% of those are successful (Caldwell & Gottesman, 1990; Hawton, Sutton, Haw, Sinclair, & Deeks, 2005; Lambert & Kinsley, 2005; Meltzer, 2005; Radomsky, Haas, Mann, & Sweeney, 1999). Approximately two-thirds of people with MDD consider suicide and about 10% to 15% of them complete suicide (Sadock & Sadock, 2008). These high rates of attempted and completed suicides are cause for nurses consistently and diligently to assess for suicidality/suicidal ideations in these populations. Several suicide screening tools are available on the Internet (e.g., http://www.integration.samhsa.gov/clinical-practice/screening-tools), and the agencies where nurses work should have an identified suicide assessment screening tool available.

Schizophrenia

Schizophrenia is a chronic condition of disturbed thought processes, perceptions, and affect that can lead to severe social and occupational dysfunction and sometimes hospitalization. It has a life prevalence of 1% in Canada (Health Canada, 2002) and the United States (NIMH, 2001), with equal distribution between women and men (Robins & Regier, 1991) and typically affects someone for the first time in his late teens to early twenties. Schizophrenia is a severe disorder characterized by distorted thinking and perception and inappropriate emotions. False, fixed beliefs not based on reality (delusions), as well as hallucinations, social withdrawal, and amotivation, are additional features of this disorder that can cause significant individual and family dysfunction. A person with schizophrenia may demonstrate disturbed behavior during some phases of the disorder, which can lead to unfavorable social consequences for the individual and family.

There is complete symptomatic and social recovery in about 30% of persons with schizophrenia. Up to 80% of individuals with schizophrenia may have a major depressive disorder at some time in their life, which is conjectured to be linked with the 20-fold increase in suicide over the general public (Sadock & Sadock, 2008). Globally, schizophrenia decreases the person's lifespan by an average of 10 years (WHO, 2001a), with the most frequent causes of premature death other than suicide being heart disease, cerebrovascular disease, and pulmonary disease (Colton & Manderscheid, 2006; Hennekens, Hennekens, Hollar, & Casey, 2005). People with schizophrenia also have a higher mortality rate from accidents and natural causes than the general population (WHO, 2001b).

Inpatient treatment for persons with an SMI such as schizophrenia is more likely to be limited to days rather than weeks or months (Gerson & Rose, 2012). This approach means that treatment and symptom management tend to occur in the community. Some individuals with schizophrenia live with their families, but many do not. Some live on their own, others live with roommates or in a group setting; still others are homeless. Because they are adults who are considered competent when their condition is at least fairly well managed, it can be very challenging for families to help the person obtain the care he or she needs, especially if the person with schizophrenia is not managing well and is refusing care.

Regardless of whether the person with schizophrenia lives with the family or not, families need help with understanding how to manage the situation. Individuals with schizophrenia and their family members state that their greatest need from mental health professionals is to receive more general information about schizophrenia and guidance on how to cope with the symptoms of schizophrenia, including communication and social relationships (Gumus, 2008). Psychological distress is a significant predictor of family functioning (Saunders, 1999), and having a family member with schizophrenia is a major stressor for the family (Saunders & Byrne, 2002). Being informed and knowing what to look for can help family members recognize early signs of changes in the individual's symptoms and behaviors that may need professional involvement (Chen & Lukens, 2011); if changes are addressed early, it is possible to avoid hospitalization and reduce family stress. For example, families need information about how to interact safely with a family member who may be having command hallucinations, especially if the hallucination is commanding the individual to harm herself or others. Nurses need to inform family members that it is not appropriate to argue or disagree with the person who is actively hallucinating or having a delusion. Rather, family members should have a plan already in place to implement. If there are children in the household, the behavior the person is exhibiting may be frightening to them. Children should have a safe, prearranged place to go, such as a nearby neighbor, or have contact information to call a trusted person to come be with the child. Nurses should engage in open discussions with family members about how to interact with their family member who may be hallucinating or having a delusional thought, preferably before the experience.

Families who have a family member with schizophrenia need nurses to understand the frustration and exhaustion they frequently experience; they also want to feel respected by health care professionals (Saunders & Byrne, 2002). On the other hand, nurses need to remind family members to be patient with the affected family member. Family members may be aware of the positive symptoms (i.e., hallucinations and delusions) and negative symptoms (i.e., anergy, amotivation, apathy, avolition) of schizophrenia. Still, many family members complain that the person with schizophrenia is lazy, manipulative, socially inept, or even incompetent, rather than realizing that these are manifestations of the illness (Muhlbauer, 2008). Even though most individuals with schizophrenia do not live with a family member, when the person who has schizophrenia does live at home, the tasks that family caregivers typically provide on a daily basis are similar to those needed when anyone has an MHC: providing companionship, providing emotional support during a crisis, monitoring symptoms, assisting with personal grooming, and so on (Decima Research Inc., 2004). The nature of this condition can make it difficult for families to provide the care they perceive the person needs, especially when the medications are not effective (or the person with schizophrenia has stopped taking them). Nurses need to provide assistance to these families in managing the individual's illness, including living arrangements, job placement, day-to-day activities (Fortinash & Worrett, 2007), and medications. The family's coping ability and family functioning are enhanced when appropriate social support systems are in place, and such supports can even buffer the family from the emotional distress that can occur when providing care to a family member with schizophrenia (Caqueo-Urizar, Gutierrez-Maldonada, & Mirnada-Casatillo, 2009). Nurses need to remind families that there are limits to what they can do for their family member and refer families to appropriate resources and support groups, including the National Alliance on Mental Illness (NAMI).

Medication adherence is a major part of treatment for managing the symptoms and behaviors of schizophrenia, but compliance is variable and frequently less than optimal. The side effects of medications can lead the person with schizophrenia to stop his medication, resulting in exacerbation of the condition. It is important to engage the individual and appropriate family members in administering medications and in monitoring the effects and effectiveness of the medications (Fortinash & Worrett, 2007). Many of the medications have serious adverse effects. Neuroleptic malignant syndrome (NMS) and extrapyramidal symptoms (EPS), including akathisia and tardive dyskinesia (TD),

which affect the muscles, are serious and life-threatening complications that can be caused by typical and atypical antipsychotic medications. The individual and appropriate family members need to know what to do and who to call should they observe a dangerous or life-threatening side effect, such as difficulty in swallowing or breathing, and they should have the emergency information readily available. Selective serotonin reuptake inhibitors (SSRIs; e.g., sertraline and citalopram) can interact with some antipsychotics and cause another significant medical problem, *metabolic syndrome*, a term to describe a group of risk factors (central obesity, insulin resistance, elevated blood pressure, and abnormal lipid profile) (Grundy et al., 2005) that are thought to be highly predictive of risk for heart disease. The atypical antipsychotics, such as olanzapine and risperidone, that are used to treat schizophrenia and other mood disorders, can lead to metabolic syndrome. There is no treatment for metabolic syndrome (Ganguli & Strassnig, 2011). Rather, there are interventions to decrease the risk of coronary heart disease, such as reduction of weight, treatment of high blood pressure, and treatment of elevated lipid levels (Ganguli & Strassnig, 2011). In addition, interventions to prevent metabolic syndrome, such as eating healthy foods and participating in regular exercise, can help to maintain a healthy body and decrease the risk for developing metabolic syndrome.

Hospitalization is not uncommon, partly because of the challenges of noncompliance with medication regimens, and it is a stressful time for the individual and family. Family members often do not understand the use and purpose of physical restraints or seclusion and may need to be taught this information by nurses in a nonjudgmental and positive manner, making sure the family understands the temporary use of these safety measures. Related to issues of hospitalization is the topic of involuntary commitment. Nurses need to be familiar with their state/provincial involuntary commitment statutes and inform families about what is involved in these laws so that families and individuals do not become overwhelmed or frustrated should involuntary commitment occur. Involuntary civil commitment means that an individual is admitted to a mental health unit against her will. The three main reasons for involuntary commitment are mental illness, substance addiction, and developmental disability. Being dangerous to oneself, including being unable to provide for one's basic needs, or to others usually defines the typical commitment standard for mental illness. Most jurisdictions provide for a hearing, the right to counsel, and a periodic judicial review.

Despite the legal possibility of involuntary commitment, many families experience stress because of their frustration with a legal system that they perceive as not taking their concerns seriously (Saunders & Byrne, 2002). Families often feel powerless to protect themselves or the individual with schizophrenia from physical threats or violence at a point early enough in time that no major harm has yet occurred; rather than being able to prevent harm, they feel that the involuntary commitment laws require that they wait until the inevitable happens. Families also report that the legal system, including the police, is not receptive to their input. Further, families are often very concerned that their family member with schizophrenia may not receive treatment even when the individual is demonstrating overt psychotic symptoms (Saunders & Byrne, 2002).

Two final comments about schizophrenia are worthy of consideration for nurses. First, persons with schizophrenia should not be labeled or called "schizophrenics" but rather identified by their names. It is more professional and respectful and less pejorative to identify the person by name and not by illness. Second, the number of children born to parents with schizophrenia has increased due to improved medications and deinstitutionalization; the fertility rate is close to that for the general population (Sadock & Sadock, 2008). First-degree biological relatives of persons with schizophrenia have a greater than 10-fold risk for developing schizophrenia compared with the general population (Sadock & Sadock, 2008). The aforementioned statements have teaching and education implications for nurses working with families who have a family member with schizophrenia.

Major Depressive Disorder

Major depressive disorder (MDD), also called major depression or clinical depression, is a medical condition that causes a persistent feeling of sadness and loss of interest; it affects how someone thinks, feels, and behaves and it can lead to emotional and physical problems. People with MDD often have trouble doing normal day-to-day activities and they may feel as if life is not worth living. MDD, a chronic illness that usually requires long-term treatment, affects 8% of Canadians (Health Canada, 2002) and about 5% to 8% of Americans (Kessler, Chiu, Demler, & Walters, 2005; NIMH, 2012). Worldwide, 6% of men and 10% of women will experience a depressive episode serious enough to receive psychiatric treatment (Smith, 2004). Based on detailed interviews with over 89,000 people from 18 countries, including the United States, Bromet et al. (2011) illustrated that people from high-income countries were more likely than those from low-/middle-income countries to experience depression over their lifetime (15% vs. 11%), with 5.5% having had depression in the last year. Women were twice as likely as men to suffer depression. The number of major depressive episodes was higher in high-income countries (28% vs. 20%) and especially high (over 30%) in France, the Netherlands, and the United States (Bromet et al., 2011). MDD is the leading cause of disability in the United States (WHO, 2008), the fourth leading cause of burden among all diseases (WHO, 2001b), and the 10th leading cause of death in the United States (NIMH, 2012). In Canada, about one-fifth of boys and one-third of girls (ages 11 to 15) feel depressed or low on a weekly basis or more (Freeman et al., 2011).

Sadock and Sadock (2008) asserted that the life event most often associated with development of depression is the loss of a parent before a child is 11 years old, and the environmental stressor most associated with onset of a depressive episode is the loss of a spouse. Nurses should assess for depression using a variety of evidence-based assessment tools, such as the Patient Health Questionnaire–9 (Spitzer, Kroenke, & Williams, 1999), which is in the public domain and available online. Adults with depression experience the following: anhedonia (the inability to experience pleasure from activities normally found to be enjoyable), anxiety (Sadock & Sadock, 2008), decreased energy, feelings of guilt, and changes in appetite or sleep. Depression often coexists with eating disorders or anxiety disorders (Devane et al., 2005), as well as substance abuse and alcohol/drug addictions (Conway et al., 2006) and physical medical conditions (Cassano & Fava, 2002). MDD interferes with social, occupational, and interpersonal functioning. Elderly persons may manifest depression with somatic symptoms. Unfortunately, many health care professionals underdiagnose and undertreat older persons with depression because they assume that MDD is a natural part of aging—which it is not.

MDD can jeopardize marriages and lead to marital discord. Over 50% of spouses report that they would not have married their spouse or had children had they known that their partner was going to develop a mood disorder (Sadock & Sadock, 2008). Family and couples therapy are important strategies to help families and they can be effective in improving the psychological well-being of the whole family.

Psychotherapy and psychopharmacology are common treatments for persons with depression. Selective serotonin reuptake inhibitors (SSRIs) and serotonin-norepinephrine reuptake inhibitors (SNRIs) are two common types of drugs used to treat depression. Individuals who are prescribed these medications and their families need to be aware of a potentially life-threatening drug interaction that can occur if inadvertently taken with other drugs, or in the case of overdose: serotonin syndrome (SS). Serotonin is a chemical produced by the body that allows nerve cells and the brain to function. Too much serotonin may cause mild symptoms such as shivering and diarrhea, but severe SS may led to muscle rigidity, fever, and seizures, which can be fatal if not treated. Herbs such as St. John's wort; stimulants, such as methylphenidate; and opioids, such as hydrocodone, can interact to produce SS. Families need to be educated about the signs and symptoms of SS and receive information on how to contact the health care provider or emergency support services. Nurses should be familiar with the classification of drugs that are prescribed to their clients, such as SSRIs, SNRIs, or norepinephrine-dopamine reuptake inhibitors (NDRIs), as well as the neurotransmitters and parts of the brain these drugs affect. Drugs are used to treat symptoms and behaviors and not to treat diagnoses. There are numerous psychopharmacology textbooks, as well as many excellent online resources, available for nurses to learn more about these drugs.

Children and Depression

Depression is not always easily recognized in children because many everyday stresses, such as the birth of a sibling, can cause changes in a child's behavior. It is important to be able to tell the difference between typical behavior changes and those associated with more serious problems. Symptoms of depression in children may be demonstrated by excessive clinging to parents or by phobias, and adolescents often exhibit poor academic performance, substance abuse, antisocial behavior, sexual promiscuity, or truancy, or they run away (Sadock & Sadock, 2008). Other behaviors to pay special attention to include problems across a variety of settings, such as at school, at home, or with peers; changes in appetite or sleep; social withdrawal; fear of things the child normally is not afraid of; returning to behaviors more common in younger children, such as bed-wetting, for a long time; signs of being upset, such as sadness or tearfulness; signs of self-destructive behavior, such as head-banging, or a tendency to get hurt often; and repeated thoughts of death (NIMH, 2009).

Children who live with a parent who has MDD are often aware of the parent's depression and are both emotionally affected and inappropriately involved in managing everyday life, such as taking over daily living or financial tasks that are normally completed by an adult (Ahlstrom, Skarsater, & Danielson, 2007). Even though children want to help their parent, they do not feel capable, which often can lead to feelings of guilt. Guilt is a feeling that children living with a depressed parent experience more often than other children (Beardslee et al., 1998). Some children worry that their depressed parent may attempt or complete suicide while they are away from home. It promotes children's health when the family as a whole learns about depression and learns how to talk more openly about it (Beardslee, Gladstone, Wright, & Cooper, 2003). It is important for nurses to help children understand that they did not cause the parent's depression and also to help the parents convey this message to their children (Ahlstrom et al., 2007). Nurses also need to include the family in discussions. For example, a mother with MDD who had two children (ages 19 and 11) stated that she herself had received invaluable support and help from her mental health professionals but that this made no difference when the family members were excluded (Ahlstrom et al., 2007). The 19-year-old son thought that finances and untidiness were the cause of his mother's depression, while the 11-year-old daughter linked the depression to family arguments that frightened her. The family members reacted differently to depression. It is important for nurses to develop strategies that assist all members of the family to participate actively in the care of the parent with depression—the child's experience of living with a depressed parent must be included in the overall treatment and management of the depressed parent. In addition, family group cognitive-behavioral interventions that focus on improving positive parenting (e.g., use of praise, scheduling pleasant family activities) contribute to the benefits for the children and the family (Compas et al., 2010).

Bipolar Disorder

Bipolar disorder (BD) affects about 2.6% of adult Americans in any given year (Kessler, Chiu, et al., 2005) and worldwide the prevalence is around 0.4% (WHO, 2011). Bipolar I disorder, a subdiagnosis of BD that is characterized by one or more manic episodes, is more common in divorced and single persons than among married people (Sadock & Sadock, 2008). BD is a recurring, treatable but incurable MHC that causes cycles of mania and depression. Episodes of mania or depression can last from one day to months, with euthymic (normal mood) periods between these mood shifts. It is these dramatic shifts in moods that can disrupt family function and cause damage to relationships, academic problems, financial problems due to loss of jobs, and even legal problems, including confrontations with the police. Family members can find it very difficult to interact with a family member who is demonstrating manic symptoms—euphoria, reduced need for sleep, excessive talking, irritability, overactivity, overconfidence, impaired concentration, increased pleasure-seeking or risk-taking behaviors, and elevated surges of energy (NIMH, 2012; WHO, 2011). Children especially can become disturbed when living with a family member who is manic. The child's safety can be in jeopardy and the child may feel afraid being near someone who is behaving irrationally. On the other hand, it can be equally disconcerting for families to live with or provide care to someone who is depressed and demonstrating hopelessness, extreme sadness, and loss of energy (Kessler, Berglund, et al., 2005).

Families with a member who has BD are consistently challenged by the fickleness and unpredictability that this MHC can have on the family and the individual. They live with uncertainty, not knowing which mood to expect at any given time or when a change will occur. Parents of adult children with BD have more compromised mental and physical health and more difficulties in marriage and work life than comparison families (Aschbrenner, Greenberg, & Seltzer, 2009). Additionally, parents who already have an MHC before the onset of their child's BD are even more vulnerable to problems with mental health issues, psychological well-being, and work life than parents who do not have an existing MHC (Aschbrenner et al., 2009). Consequently, obtaining the history of MHC in parents and the immediate family is important to inform the nurse's interventions in promoting the well-being of each member of the family.

Family history of BD conveys a greater risk for BD disorders in general (Sadock & Sadock, 2008). Nurses need to teach families about the genetic implications of this MHC and educate families on the signs and symptoms so that families can recognize the early signs and symptoms and initiate early professional treatment. BD is a difficult MHC to diagnose accurately, yet it is important that this MHC be differentiated from MDD, personality disorders, substance use, anxiety disorders, and schizophrenia (Sadock & Sadock, 2008) because the treatments can be significantly different. Although BD typically emerges in young adulthood, the range of onset of BD can occur as early as 5 to 6 years of age to 50 years of age or older.

Because children and adolescents can manifest symptoms of mania and depression differently from adults, they are often misdiagnosed as having antisocial personality disorder or schizophrenia rather than BD (Sadock & Sadock, 2008). Child and adolescent symptoms of mania can include substance abuse, irritability that can lead to fights, academic problems, suicide attempts, obsessive-compulsive symptoms, somatic complaints, and antisocial behaviors. Misdiagnosis has tremendous implications in young people. Making differential diagnoses in children and adolescents is difficult, and it is important for nurses to advocate for additional assessments as new signs and symptoms emerge in children and adolescents so that they are treated appropriately and so that they can avoid unnecessary treatments and complications.

Just as misdiagnosis of BD in the younger population is problematic, it is also problematic for the older population. Older adults with BD are more often misdiagnosed as having schizophrenia, with older minority persons being misdiagnosed twice as frequently as white older persons or younger minorities (Luggen, 2005). Elderly persons are also more likely to be diagnosed with depression rather than BD, which can result in antidepressant medications inadvertently placing these older persons at higher risk for having a manic episode (Luggen, 2005). Equally important, many of the medications that are used to treat symptoms of depression and mania can have significant adverse effects on the older person, thus making it even more important for accurate assessment and treatment among this vulnerable population. Some of the medications used to treat these symptoms, such as the second-generation antipsychotic drugs, may place an older person at higher risk for death or cerebrovascular event (Stahl, 2011).

Mental health professionals have typically done a less than adequate job in assessing the needs of spouses who have a family member with BD and in providing information to these spouses (van der Voort, Goossens, & van der Bijl, 2009). Yet, it has been shown that care providers who receive both psychoeducation and health promotion interventions have significantly less depression, improved health, and less subjective burden of care and role dysfunction (Perlick et al., 2010). Not only might the care providers receive benefit from these two interventions, but the family member with BD may demonstrate a decrease in mania and depression, due in part to the improved health of the provider of care (Perlick et al., 2010).

Caregivers of persons with BD often have felt overlooked by health professionals and they report that if professionals would offer support, it would decrease their burden of care (Rusner, Carlsson, Brunt, & Nystrom, 2012; Tranvag & Kristoffersen, 2008). Caregivers who provide care to a family member with BD identified two main themes that would make their caregiving experiences more positive (Maskill, Crowe, Luty, & Joyce, 2010). First, they would feel more supported if the mental health nurses showed understanding of the complexities associated with BD and were nonjudgmental and noncritical of the family. Second, they identified the importance of care providers collaborating with mental health staff. Professionals should recognize the uniqueness of the care provider and the recipient of the care. Care providers also encourage mental health staff to be honest with them about the fact that BD is not curable, but to maintain hope nonetheless (Maskill et al., 2010).

Although BD is treatable, the condition can cause significant social and economic stress for families. Educational interventions for family members living with a person with BD reduce stress for the family members, increase family members' understanding of the condition, and enhance family members' ability to remain socially functional (Jonnson, Wijk, Danielson, & Skarsater, 2011). It is essential that nurses teach family members to observe for early signs of relapse into mania, such as provocative dressing, unrestrained buying sprees, hypersexuality, being more talkative than usual, or grandiosity (APA, 2013); or signs of relapse into depression, such as increased sleeping, problems sleeping, problems with concentration, anhedonia, or recurrent thoughts of suicide. It is important that family members monitor these changes in their family member who has BD (Sorell, 2011) and notify the appropriate health care professional when there are changes.

Dementia

Dementia is a syndrome that affects memory, thinking, behavior, learning capacity, judgment, and the ability to perform daily activities; it is one of the major causes of disability and dependency among older people worldwide (WHO & Alzheimer's Disease International, 2012). Globally, approximately 35.6 million people have dementia and these numbers are expected to double by 2030 and more than triple by 2050 as the population ages (WHO & Alzheimer's Disease International, 2012). In the United States, about 5% of the general population over age 65, and 20% to 40% over age 85, has dementia. Alzheimer's disease is the most common type of dementia (approximately 60% to 70% of dementia cases). People can live for many years with dementia and, thus, with appropriate support many can remain engaged in and contribute to society. There is currently no cure or treatment to alter the progressive nature of the condition.

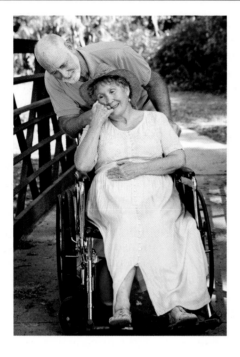

Dementia can dramatically affect the lives of individuals with dementia and their families, not only health-wise, but also economically, socially, and legally. Providing care to a family member with dementia can interrupt the normal family activities. Depending on the severity of the dementia, families may need to take on responsibility for tasks ranging from paying bills to ensuring the individual attends medical appointments to full personal grooming. Discussions about power of attorney and substitute decision making (living wills) need to take place, preferably soon after diagnosis.

The majority of care to persons with dementia is provided by family and informal community support services, though some individuals receive long-term, institutional care. Women typically provide family home-based care to persons with dementia. Emotional and physical stressors are not uncommon among caregivers. The loss of the ability to interact meaningfully with a loved one who no longer, or perhaps intermittently, remembers you is a source of grief and stress for many families. Caregivers have a very high prevalence of depression (Cuijpers, 2005) and may have a compromised immune system (Vitaliano, Zhang, & Scanlan, 2003). Psychoeducation programs have been shown to decrease depression and stress among caregivers (Gallagher-Thompson et al., 2012) and are one source of support that nurses can help families

obtain. These caregivers need strong support from health professionals; assessment and intervention are critical. More detailed information about dementia assessment and intervention is available in Chapter 15.

Despite the commonly held societal belief, dementia is not a normal part of the aging process; dementia is much more than slight memory loss. A family's cultural-based beliefs about dementia can be a barrier to accessing care (Gallagher-Thompson et al., 2012). For instance, families can view dementia as a medical illness, a mental illness, or as part of normal aging. When conducting a family assessment, the nurse should explore each of these views. In addition, it is important that the nurse listen to each member of the family's story. These stories can be used to map the journey of the person with dementia and the family's journey as it lives this experience (Doherty, Benbow, Craig, & Smith, 2009). Other sources, such as extended family members, other informal caregivers, health care records, and formal health care providers should also be used to obtain information. Information collected from a variety of sources can be used to develop effective family-focused interventions.

Although the family member with dementia may have increased confusion and decreased ability to communicate, it is important that nurses not treat this person as a child. The person with dementia is an adult and should still be treated with respect as an adult. Speaking to an adult as if she were a young child is demeaning to the individual and to the family members. There may be some similarities between a young child and an older person with dementia, such as incontinence or inability to dress oneself. Nevertheless, the adult should be treated as an adult who has a cognitive deficit and not as a child. For example, it is important to use normal conversational pitch and words when talking to an older adult, rather than affecting a high-pitched voice or using words that are appropriate to a child's developmental level rather than that of an adult.

New technologies are being used to assist family caregivers who are caring for persons with dementia. Telehealth, for instance, allows family members to communicate with their health care professionals via the Internet, and Smart Phones and new applications provide information to family members about dementia, caring for a person with dementia, and support sources for the family. These technologies can be used to inform families on how to handle daily problems, such as wandering, falling, decreased memory, and eating problems (Gallagher-Thompson et al., 2012). A new multidisciplinary field—gerontechnology—has developed to interface between technology and older people. The mission of the International Society for Gerontechnology (IGS) is to "encourage and promote technological innovations in products and services that address older peoples' ambitions and needs on the basis of scientific knowledge about ageing processes including cultural and individual differences" (http://www.gerontechnology.info/index.php/journal/pages/view/isghome). The IGS values not only meeting the needs of older people, but also supporting the caregivers. Developments such as gerontechnology offer exciting possibilities about how to provide needed support to caregivers of persons with dementia.

Attention-Deficit Hyperactivity Disorder (ADHD)

ADHD is one of the most common MHCs among children and adolescents (Foley, 2010), with more prevalence in boys ranging from 2:1 to as much as 9:1 (Sadock & Sadock, 2008). The underrepresentation of girls may be attributed to underdiagnosis, however, because girls often present with the inattentive rather than hyperactive type of ADHD and are overlooked. In the United States, the presence of ADHD varies from 2% to 20% among grade-school children and the incidence of the symptoms of ADHD persisting into adulthood is about 40% to 50% or 4% of the adult population (Sadock & Sadock, 2008). Children, adolescents, and adults with ADHD typically demonstrate diminished sustained concentration, increased levels of impulsivity, hyperactivity, and problems with social interactions. Other people may view them as lazy, stupid, reckless, or uncaring because of how the symptoms affect the person with ADHD. Some children, especially girls, may be inattentive rather than hyperactive, and the hyperactivity in adults is often internal rather than external. ADHD has a genetic component (Foley, 2010) and so it is not uncommon to have more than one family member with ADHD, including one or both parents (Singh et al., 2010). Diagnosis is complex and requires collaborating with many key adults in the child's life, including teachers, parents, friends, and other community adults with whom the child may interact.

Diagnosis in adults often follows a diagnosis for one of their children.

Young people who are diagnosed with ADHD often endure stigma from their peers, teachers, family, and society. Examples of stigma include teachers and peers thinking that a person with ADHD chooses to be inattentive in class or that the person with ADHD has a character trait flaw rather than an MHC. Many young people struggle with the negative assumptions that others have toward them and that they have toward themselves (Kildea, John, & Davies, 2011). They often experience a lack of empathy and understanding from key adults in their lives (Singh et al., 2010). Young people with ADHD frequently feel that the diagnosis itself gives them a bad reputation, including thinking that others consider them stupid (Singh et al., 2010).

Parents of children with ADHD often report feeling blamed by professionals, their families, and society for their child's behavior (Kildea et al., 2011). Families of children with ADHD have a higher level of dysfunction than other families; thus, earlier identification and intervention with these families can result in healthier family function and child outcomes (Foley, 2010). For instance, families who received eight to twelve 50-minute sessions that included psychoeducation about ADHD, behavioral principles, and specific parenting skills and strategies demonstrated improved parenting behaviors and less parenting stress for mothers (Gerdes, Haack, & Schneider, 2012). Examples of parenting skills and strategies include having regular and consistent daily routines, such as mealtimes (Tamm, Holden, Nakonezny, Swart, & Hughes, 2012), praising positive behavior, ignoring mildly negative behavior, consistently using time out, and giving effective instructions (Gerdes et al., 2012). It is also recommended that families eliminate computer/screen time before bed to decrease sleep problems (Becker, Goobic, & Thomas, 2009). Parenting skills should include supervision and provision of assistance to the child so he can remain organized and focused when doing homework; short movement breaks at regular intervals also are helpful (Becker et al., 2009).

Although it is very beneficial for parents to learn about and use home management skills, it is also important that the parents request appropriate neuropsychological and psychoeducational evaluations for their child to determine if the child might benefit from school-based supports, particularly if their child has academic difficulties, a learning disorder, or executive functioning difficulties (Becker et al., 2009). For example, in the United States some children with ADHD qualify through a federal law, the Individuals with Disabilities Act, to receive an Individual Educational Plan (IEP) that is unique to the child and supports the child's educational needs. Another plan, the 504 Plan, is provided by a civil rights law that protects children with ADHD from being discriminated against because of their MHC and so some children who may not qualify for an IEP may receive additional educational support under the 504 Plan. IEPs are also common in Canada after appropriate assessment and evaluation.

Treatment for ADHD may include medications, psychotherapy such as behavioral therapy, psychoeducation including lifestyle changes, coaching, and other interventions to decrease the number and severity of stressors in the individual's and family's life. Family therapy will help to maintain and promote healthy family functioning. Family therapy is also indicated if the condition jeopardizes the marriage, for example, if a spouse whose partner has ADHD is considering leaving the marriage (Sadock & Sadock, 2008). Family therapy is especially recommended if a child and a parent have ADHD, because it may be difficult for a parent to recognize her own disorganization, inconsistent responses to the child's behaviors, and/or impulsivities and the impact they can have on the family (Singh et al., 2010).

Medications are used to treat ADHD, in conjunction with other interventions, but the decision to use these medications needs to be based on the benefits of taking the medication versus the consequences of not taking the medications. The parent or adult needs to make these decisions without outside pressure from family or media who may be misinformed. Parents of children with ADHD often experience misgivings about administering a stimulant to their child, based on feedback they get from their family, friends, or the media (Jackson & Peters, 2008) even though stimulants are the recommended treatment. Much of the information parents obtain about treating ADHD with medications is secondary and not evidence based. Nurses have a responsibility to provide accurate information to parents so the parents can make a thoughtful and informed decision about whether or not to treat their child with medication. Amphetamine-containing formulations of stimulants are the most

commonly prescribed ADHD medications in Canada and the United States (Berman, Kuczenski, McCracken, & London, 2009). Though stimulants have been used successfully for decades, there has been a link to slower bone growth in children taking amphetamines and to psychosis in adults taking amphetamines (Berman et al., 2009). The child and adult prescribed a stimulant require regular checkups. Just as many clinical settings contact patients for follow-up visits, such as for diabetes management, these settings should likewise designate a nurse to be the point person to provide this service to persons with ADHD and their families (Van Cleave & Leslie, 2008).

Medication adherence and behavior modification can be problematic for individuals with ADHD and their families. It has been suggested that professionals approach ADHD as a chronic health condition, which includes long-term therapy (Van Cleave & Leslie, 2008). Nurses should educate families that medication neither cures ADHD nor necessarily eliminates the impulsive behaviors a child or adult may be exhibiting. Families should be aware of the advantages and disadvantages of taking medication several times during the day versus taking a long-acting stimulant.

ROLE OF THE FAMILY MENTAL HEALTH NURSE

In order to establish a collaborative relationship with the family, nurses must have a nonblaming and accepting attitude toward family members (Doornbos, 2001). Families value interactions with health providers that demonstrate openness, cooperation, confirmation, and continuity (Ewertzon et al., 2012). As family members increasingly have assumed the role of primary caregivers for mentally ill individuals, it is more important than ever to include them as partners in the delivery of mental health care. Care delivery systems that involve family members acknowledge the effect mental disorders have on entire family systems. They seek to prevent the return or exacerbation of a disorder, and they alleviate pain and suffering experienced by family members. To fulfill these goals, researchers (Dixon et al., 2001) have identified 15 evidence-based principles that can be incorporated into family nursing interventions for families of individuals with a mental illness (Box 16-2). This

BOX 16-2

Evidence-Based Principles for Working With Families of Individuals With a Mental Illness

- Organize care so that everyone involved is working toward the same treatment goals within a collaborative, supportive relationship.
- Attend to both the social and clinical needs of the primary patient.
- Provide optimal medication management.
- Listen to family's concerns and involve them in all elements of treatment.
- Examine family's expectations of treatment and expectations of the primary patient.
- Evaluate strengths and limitations of family's ability to provide support.
- Aid in the resolution of family conflict.
- Explore feelings of loss for all parties.
- Provide pertinent information to patients and families at appropriate times.
- Develop a clear crisis plan.
- Help enhance family communication.
- Train families in problem-solving techniques.
- Promote expansion of the family's social support network.
- Be adaptable in meeting the family's needs.
- Provide easy access to another professional if current work with the family ceases.

Adapted from Dixon, L., McFarlane, W., Lefley, H., Lucksted, A., Cohen, M., Falloon, I., . . . Sondheimer, D. (2001). Evidence-based practices for services to families of people with psychiatric disabilities. *Psychiatric Services, 52*(7), 903–910.

section briefly examines a few areas of focus for mental health nurses within care delivery systems: prevention of MHCs, psychoeducation, crisis plans, and providing culturally sensitive care.

Prevention of Mental Health Conditions

Arguably, the most important role for the nurse in mental health care is to engage in professional activities that *prevent* mental health conditions. Stress during childhood, especially before 3 years of age when synapses are still being formed, can trigger the expression of genes that may otherwise have remained unexpressed (Grayson, 2006). Neglect and abuse are negative experiences that can cause serious hormonal and chemical changes in the brain and interrupt normal brain development (Grayson, 2006). The "physical connections between neurons formed in childhood are not 'hard-wired' or

'unchangeable'" (Grayson, 2006, p. 1). It has been suggested that stress can trigger changes to alter a child's brain development (Teicher, 2002). Genetics influence brain development and yet stress, such as physical, emotional, and sexual abuse; famine; and natural disasters profoundly affect the emotional, behavioral, cognitive, social, and physical functioning in children (Perry, Pollard, Blakley, Baker, & Vigilante, 1995). Secure attachments and ample nurturing not only allow for a positive environment for the brain to build neural connections to integrate the brain systems but also strengthen an infant's ability to cope with stress (Grayson, 2006). When babies cry and their needs are taken care of, such as through food or attention and comfort, their neuronal pathways are strengthened and they learn how to get their needs met both physically and emotionally (Grayson, 2006). On the other hand, babies who are abused or neglected learn other lessons that can be damaging and may interfere with a child's ability to self-regulate. For instance, the child whose needs are not met and who endures repeated painful disappointments may abandon crying for help, resulting in problems with hyperarousal or dissociation.

Teicher (2002) conjectured that maltreatment at an early age can have enduring effects on the development and function of a child's brain. Child maltreatment can manifest internally—depression, anxiety, or suicidality—or outwardly, with aggression, impulsiveness, hyperactivity, delinquency, or substance abuse. He further conjectured that there is a strong association between maltreatment in childhood and a person being diagnosed with borderline personality disorder. Borderline personality disorder is characterized by seeing others and situations in black-and-white terms, having unstable relationships, having feelings of abandonment, exhibiting self-harm, having problems with anger, and escaping through substance abuse. The limbic system plays a key role in regulating emotion and memory of one's experiences. Research has shown that abuse in children can cause permanent damage to the neural structure and function of the brain. People with borderline personality disorder often have reduced integration between the left and right brain hemispheres, a smaller corpus callosum, and limbic electrical irritability.

There is also some evidence that a mother smoking and drinking alcohol during pregnancy affects the growth of neural pathways and can contribute to the development of conditions such as ADHD (Nigg, 2006). Healthy lifestyle behaviors, including diet, exercise, stress-reduction strategies, and non-consumption of alcohol, cigarettes, or illegal substances seem to play a role in reducing the risk of developing an MHC. Nurses should put effort into encouraging and supporting healthy lifestyles, whether prenatally or for children, youth, or adults.

Nurses must, of course, advocate for good parenting and must offer parenting support in a non-judgmental way. Nurses should be at the forefront of ensuring that childhood maltreatment does not take place. Nurses can provide resources for caretakers of children so they learn the necessary skills to provide responsible care, support, and nurturing to their child. Moreover, nurses should be active in local, state, and national policies that affect child welfare. "Early assessment and intervention can be prophylactic—helping prevent a prolonged acute neurophysiological, neuroendocrine, and neuropsychological trauma response" (Perry et al., 1995, p. 291).

Psychoeducation

A major role for a professional nurse in working with families who have a member with an MHC is to provide psychoeducation. Psychoeducation includes teaching clients about the cause and treatments of the MHC, while being attuned to each of the family members' unique needs. Family psychoeducation is a term used to describe various family programs that incorporate the following three elements:

- Family education
- Training in coping skills
- Social support (Schock & Gavazzi, 2005)

The time commitment and emphasis on each of these elements is what differs among the diverse psychoeducational models. Currently, these interventions may continue for months or years. Because psychoeducational programs are multifaceted and involve such long-term relationships, they are typically delivered by teams of professionals working together (Marsh & Johnson, 1997). Nurses' training and education make them well suited to participate in such interdisciplinary teams that emphasize client and family education, enhance coping skills, and develop supportive networks.

The educational element of these programs involves providing information to relatives regarding diagnoses, cause of mental illness, prognosis, and treatment. Skills training may include coping skills for family members and social skills training for the family member with the MHC. In addition, the entire family may work on developing communication skills so members can communicate more effectively with one another. Nurses can enhance social support for the family by actively including relatives as members of the treatment team and by helping to establish connections to other families with similar experiences. Through networking with one another, families can find support and share problem-solving strategies. A local chapter of the NAMI is one support and advocacy organization that families may find helpful.

Nurses can teach individuals and family members about no-cost relaxation techniques to reduce stress (e.g., breathing techniques and exercises, guided imagery, yoga, and progressive muscle relaxation) and provide pet and/or music therapy. Nurses have the skills to help families cope with feelings of anger and disappointment as they go through the grief process after learning about the MHC of one of their family members. It is important to realize that it may take time for families to accept the diagnosis and the level of acceptance will vary between members of the family (O'Connell, 2006). A variety of family intervention strategies are outlined in Box 16-3.

Crisis Plans

Nurses are integral in assisting families to develop a crisis plan that is put in place before the need for such a plan; it is more challenging to manage a crisis when you do not have a predetermined plan to follow. Part of this plan may include a visit to the local police precinct to ascertain the best way to deescalate a violent situation (Nadkarni & Fristad, 2012). Nurses should suggest that families have a binder/notebook available with the following information:

- A list of health care providers, emergency professional contact names, and telephone numbers
- Suicide hotline telephone numbers
- Insurance information

BOX 16-3
Family Intervention Strategies

- Coordinate information and treatment plans across settings and with multiple health care providers.
- Ensure that communication is bidirectional from health care providers to families and from families to health care providers.
- Provide validation for commitment and work being done by all family members.
- Create ways for families to manage treatment plans that affect everyday routines.
- Identify realistic ways that the mentally ill family member can participate in and contribute to the family.
- Articulate an action plan to implement during times of crisis.
- Negotiate ways to manage specific problem behaviors.
- Connect with appropriate social resources (individual/group therapy, support groups, extended family, friends, religious organizations).
- Provide diagnostic and treatment-related family psychoeducation.
- Encourage self-care behaviors for all family members.
- Identify effective coping skills for individual family members.
- Advocate for policy changes that benefit individuals with mental health conditions and their family members.
- Challenge detrimental stereotypes and stigma of persons with a mental health condition and their families.

- Details about the best route to the appropriate emergency department or health care facility, including specific directions to get to the sites
- Safe locations where children or other members of the family can go during escalation times

This binder should be readily available to family members and needs to be updated regularly (Nadkarni & Fristad, 2012). Also included in this binder should be advance agreements set up with the person who has an MHC when she was well; these agreements should specify the individual's preferred treatment and note with whom information can be shared during periods of exacerbation of the MHC (Gray, Robinson, Seddon, & Roberts, 2008).

Providing Culturally Competent Care

Nurses must remember that cultural norms and beliefs shape family members' perceptions of coping

and managing care for relatives with an MHC (Dalky, 2012). NAMI's informative Web site (NAMI, n.d.) includes mental health fact sheets for different ethnic groups in the United States (African American, American Indian and Alaska Native, Asian American and Pacific Islander, Latino/Hispanic). Nurses are encouraged to review these fact sheets to become more informed about facts that will help them in practice, and so they can decrease myths and stereotypes about different ethnic groups. For example, American Indian and Alaska Native languages do not include the words "depression" and "anxious," nor does the word "depression" exist in some Chinese languages. Somatization of mental health conditions is more common in African American and Asian cultures than in Caucasian counterparts.

NAMI also has fact sheets about depression among the following groups: veterans, lesbian/gay/bisexual/transgendered, seniors, women, men, and children/adolescents. Misdiagnosis and undertreatment are not uncommon among some cultural groups; improved understanding about various cultural groups will enhance nursing practice. In addition, because psychiatric medications are a significant part of treating MHC, it is important for nurses to know which populations may be fast metabolizers and which might be slow metabolizers in order to avoid overmedicating or undermedicating a specific individual. At the same time, it is important not to stereotype individuals or families based on their cultural identity but rather to use cultural identity as one aspect of the nursing assessment to take into consideration when developing a nursing plan for the entire family.

Family Case Study: Johnson Family

The following case study of the Johnson family demonstrates the assessment, diagnosis, outcome identification, planning, implementation, and evaluation for care of a family with a member who has been diagnosed with bipolar disorder and substance abuse.

Setting: Inpatient acute care hospital, cardiac intensive care unit (ICU).

(continued)

Nursing Goal: Work with the family to assist them in planning for discharge in the next 3 days to a less intensive care facility.

Family Members:
- Steve: father, 55 years old, small business owner
- Mary: mother, 49 years old, stay-at-home mother
- Debbie: stepmother, 54 years old, schoolteacher
- Harold: stepfather, 60 years old, successful building contractor
- Tony: identified patient, 23 years old, oldest child, son, unemployed, sleeping on couches of friends
- Susie: younger daughter, Tony's sister, 14 years old, eighth grader, overachiever and "perfect" child
- Bobby: Tony's half-brother, mother's son, 12 years old
- Rachael: stepmother's daughter from previous marriage, 30 years old
- Thomas: Mary's father, 86 years old, wealthy businessman
- Emma: Mary's mother, 85 years old, abuses alcohol

Johnson Family Story:

Tony Johnson is a 23-year-old man who was admitted to the hospital cardiac ICU through the emergency department in acute cardiac distress from an accidental methamphetamine overdose. He arrived at the emergency department by ambulance from his drug-free friend Doug's single-room occupancy hotel room. Tony is currently homeless. He had been sleeping on his drug dealer's couch for a week until he was arrested for assault. Since his arrest a few days ago, he has been sleeping on Doug's floor.

Tony has been in and out of substance abuse treatment programs since he was 17 years old. He was diagnosed with bipolar disorder at the first treatment program he attended. His father and stepmother convinced him to enter that program just before his 18th birthday and paid for the expensive 3-month program. As with all of the programs he has attended, he left soon after admission to the program.

During a previous emergency department admission, Tony got angry at his family, tore off his electrocardiogram leads and oxygen mask, and left the hospital against medical advice. During the present hospitalization, Tony called his father from the emergency department to ask him to come and help get him admitted to another treatment facility. Tony has agreed to see his sister and stepmother, but not his stepfather or stepsiblings. He also refuses to see his mother because he says she "is the cause of all my problems." His mother and father separated, and later divorced, when Tony was 10 years old and his younger sister was about 1. He and his mother fought constantly when he was a child, and she was overprotective of him. Tony was an obedient child who then began using alcohol and drugs and stealing from family members beginning in his early teens.

Tony's father has maintained Tony on his small business's health insurance policy. Tony is eligible for short-term residential treatment if he can prove to the director of the program that he intends to cooperate this time. His father is again willing to pay for longer-term drug and psychiatric treatment if Tony proves that he is intent on cooperating with his treatment plan.

Tony stopped taking his mood-stabilizing medications approximately 2 weeks ago, when his most recent binge use of methamphetamine started. Currently, the doctors are reluctant to prescribe his mood-stabilizing medications while the methamphetamine is still affecting his major systems.

Family Members:

The admitting nurse and the ICU social worker have gleaned the following familial information from Steve, Mary, and Debbie. The Johnson family genogram is illustrated in Figure 16-1. The Johnson family ecomap is illustrated in Figure 16-2.

Steve is very concerned about his son's health and reminds him that the doctors have said he will not survive another year if he continues to use methamphetamines. Steve recognizes his son's depression and anger and feels guilty that he did not notice sooner that Tony was depressed and "self-medicating" with alcohol and drugs. He blames himself for the divorce, which he believes precipitated Tony's alcohol and drug abuse. He also regrets his workaholism during Tony's early years and for being a co-dependent, allowing Tony to live at Steve's home when Tony was drinking and using drugs to excess, and sleeping round the clock between drug-induced manic episodes. Steve initiated the divorce when he discovered his ex-wife was having affairs and using cocaine. Steve was diagnosed at the time of the divorce as having bipolar disorder, with a manic episode that resulted in his hospitalization. He is maintained on medications and has had no further episodes.

Mary, Tony's mother, became a stay-at-home mom when she gave birth to Tony. She was overprotective with him but secretly resented that he was not a good student. She punished him severely for his learning difficulties, especially when she was drinking. Her closet drinking became cocaine use after Tony's sister Susie was born, when Tony was 9 years old. Tony both resented his sister for taking his mother's attention away from him and was relieved not to be the sole focus of her anger. Mary is currently recovering from drug abuse but drinks wine still, even drinking with Tony when they are speaking to one another.

Debbie, Tony's stepmother, met Tony's father about a year after his divorce. Tony was living with his father at the time and refused to accept his stepmother as a mother figure for him for several years. Debbie is a better limit-setter than Steve and is often more practical about recognizing and

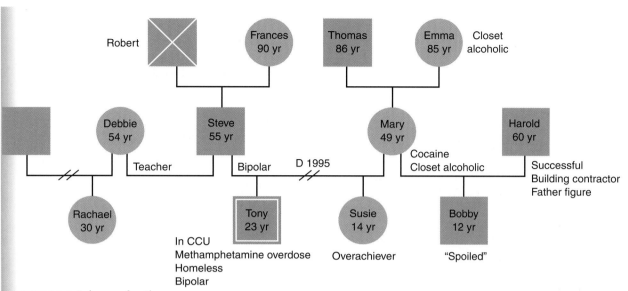

FIGURE 16-1 Johnson family genogram.

addressing Tony's needs. She is influential with both Steve and Mary in making decisions about Tony. She has a daughter from a previous marriage, Rachael, who is 30 years old.

Harold, Tony's stepfather, is 11 years older than Mary and, in many ways, is a father figure for his wife. He dotes on his 12-year-old son and largely ignores his stepson and stepdaughter; he does brag about Susie's successes. He is a successful building contractor and is able to provide a luxurious life for his wife and son.

Susie, 14 years old, is bright and well behaved. Tony calls her the "perfect" child he never was. She is an honor student, talented in music and art, and well liked by her fellow students and by adults. She worries about Tony and has always tried to please him. She can't understand why he gets so mad at his parents and her; she tries to encourage him to enter treatment and tells him she misses him very much. Her parents divorced when she was about a year old, and she has lived most of the time with her mother who remarried and had another son soon after the divorce. Her stepfather is very attached to her half-brother and takes him with him to work and on fishing trips. Susie loves her father very much but sees him only every other weekend and holidays.

Steve's mother, Frances, lives about an hour away, is 90 years old, and is very fond of and sympathetic to Tony. Steve's father died when Tony was young. His parents owned a grocery store that they ran as a family.

Mary's parents, Thomas and Emma, live nearby. Thomas is a wealthy but distant businessman who gave money rather than time to his wife and children. Emma

was a stay-at-home wife and mother; she is a drinking alcoholic who fairly successfully hides her alcoholism except on family occasions when she often makes a scene.

Discharge Plans:

Tony will be discharged from the ICU in 3 days; his insurance does not cover a longer hospital stay once his acute methamphetamine poisoning is treated.

Family Systems Theory in Relation to the Johnson Family:

The health event the Johnson family is managing will be viewed through the lens of a nurse who used Family Systems Theory as the foundational approach to working with this family. A more detailed discussion of this family nursing system can be found in Chapter 3.

Concept 1—All Parts of the System Are Interconnected: In the Johnson case, all members of the family are affected by Tony's dual DSM-5 diagnoses of amphetamine dependence and bipolar disorder, and his dramatic overdoses and near-death experiences. His father feels enormous guilt and is afraid to confront and set limits with his son for fear of sending him to his death. His mother reluctantly verbalizes feeling guilty but lacks sincerity. Her son feels she does not want to change her own behavior; thus, admitting guilt is not possible for her. His stepmother is more realistic because she is not as emotionally attached to Tony, but she worries about the effects of Tony's drug use and the worry it causes Steve, and she fears a relapse of Steve's own bipolar symptoms.

(continued)

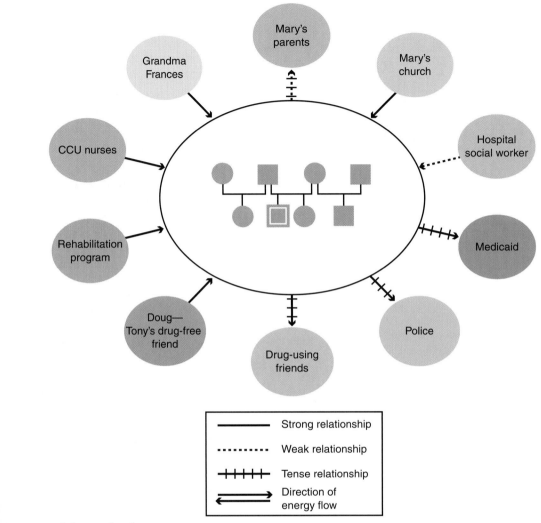

FIGURE 16-2 Johnson family ecomap.

Concept 2—The Whole Is More Than the Sum of Its Parts: In the Johnson family case study, the complexity of the blended family increases the interconnectedness and interdependence of the family members. It is not just parents and children or grandparents and parents, but a complex system involving different permutations of the family relationships that can deteriorate over time as the stress of Tony's illness takes its toll on the entire system.

Concept 3—All Systems Have Some Form of Boundaries or Border Between the System and Its Environment: In the Johnson family, the normal boundaries of self and others, and of family and outsiders, are dysfunctional. Spousal boundaries are violated by infidelity; parent-child boundaries are violated by theft and

parents drinking with substance-abusing children. Some of the boundaries are closed by distant, aloof parents and spouses. Tony demonstrates some flexible boundaries by refusing to allow visits by some family members who can negatively affect his recovery but allowing visits from others who can support his treatment outcome.

Concept 4—Systems Can Be Further Organized Into Subsystems: The Johnson family has many subsystems: parent, parent-stepparent, parent-child, grandparent-parent, sibling, grandparent, and in-law. Each of these subsystems can be mobilized to help with the goals defined for the family. Specifically, the mother-father-stepmother-son subsystem will probably prove most influential in discharge planning.

Family Impact:

In the Johnson family, objective impact includes the financial costs of treatment, physical strain and damage, effects on the health of other family members, and disruption in the daily lives of many of the family members. The subjective impact is the enormous guilt and fear felt by the family members, the damage to Tony's mental and social health, the disruption felt by other children in the family, the strain placed on the marriages, and the disrupted family routines, such as regular mealtimes and leisure time.

Social Support and Stigma:

The Johnson family has been moderately successful in previous generations at hiding the substance abuse and dysfunction. Although more acceptable now than in previous generations, some social stigma is attached to divorce, remarriage, alcoholism, drug addiction, and mental illness—all of which affect the Johnson family. Methamphetamine addiction carries a large social stigma today. Family and professional care providers need information that is evidence based to increase the understanding of the immense physical, mental, and social impact this addiction has on the family. Providing family members with accurate information about the disorder and the treatments can improve the social support family members provide to the individual with the substance use problem, as well as improve family functioning.

Coping and Resiliency:

The Johnson family is in need of intervention to teach it more successful ways of dealing with Tony's and others' behaviors, and with feelings of worry and concern. Most mental health professionals would suggest that they attend 12-step meetings for families of substance abusers, and that they have family counseling with Tony. All subsystems need help learning more effective coping strategies, from those who remain aloof from the problems to those who become overly enmeshed in the lives of other family members.

Assistance From Mental Health Professionals:

The Johnson family needs referral to a treatment facility that focuses on the needs of the family and the enabling behaviors of family members. In addition, the extended family needs counseling concerning the impact of these disorders on the family and the maladaptive coping styles being used. Tony needs treatment for both his substance abuse and his bipolar disorder.

Family psychoeducation for the Johnson family would include education about substance abuse and bipolar disorders, coping skills for Tony and the family members, especially in dealing with grief and anger, and effective communication skills to express feelings constructively.

Mental Health Care Nursing From a Family Systems Perspective:

This section will identify the needs of each member of the Johnson family and address the family as a whole by looking at the family from a Family Systems perspective.

Assessment: The ICU nurse and a social worker conduct the assessment of the Johnson family with Tony, Steve, Mary, and Debbie. It includes the following:

- Perception of and understanding of the illness: The Johnson family has some experience with substance abuse and bipolar disorder. The nurse assesses whether the knowledge is accurate and current.
- The primary complaint, symptoms, or concerns: The Johnson family believes that Tony's illness is the family's "problem." In reality, the dysfunctional family dynamics are more central needs. Since this crisis has arisen, the family's biggest concern is Tony's safety. They now fear that Tony will either end up dead or in prison.
- Physical, developmental, cognitive, mental, and emotional health status: The Johnson family is in a great deal of emotional pain and is in a crisis state at this time. The family's stress level is at an all-time high.
- Health history: The Johnson family has a history of mental health problems but appears to be physically healthy otherwise.
- Treatment history: Tony has a history of unsuccessful treatment attempts, with brief periods of abstinence from alcohol and drugs, and minimal treatment for his bipolar disorder. Tony takes mood-stabilizing medication intermittently but has not had a long-term relationship with a psychiatrist since he was 20.
- Family, social, cultural, racial, ethnic, and community systems: The Johnson family systems have been described and are reflected in the ecomap of the family (see Fig. 15-2). Mary is involved with church activities. Tony is in contact with friends from high school in addition to his friends who use drugs.
- Activities of daily living and health habits: These activities are seriously disrupted for Steve, Debbie, Mary, and Susie. The stress, worry, and concern they have for Tony, and the time and energy they are using to help Tony find a place to live and get into treatment, are affecting their own abilities to spend time focusing on their own health and well-being.
- Substance use: The Johnson family has alcohol, cocaine, and methamphetamine abuse in its history.
- Coping mechanisms used: Although some healthy mechanisms are used by the Johnson family, they also

(continued)

use rationalization, projection, denial, and substance use as ways of coping.

- Spiritual and religious beliefs or values: The Johnson family members state they are Christians, but the only family members to attend services or admit to spiritual practices are Steve, Mary, and Frances. Steve uses meditation to maintain focus in his life but has been unable to do so for many months as a result of his increased time spent on attempting to keep track of Tony.
- Economic, legal, or other environmental factors that affect health: Steve's finances have been strained by Tony's illness. Harold and Mary refuse to accept any of the monetary burden of his care, saying that "he needs to take care of himself," but they remain emotionally involved.
- Health-promoting strengths: There is obvious love between Tony and his father and stepmother, and between Tony and his grandmother, Frances; this can be mobilized to promote healthy family behaviors and communication.
- Complementary therapies used: Tony's friends have recommended acupuncture for his addictions, but he has not been clean long enough to try it. Debbie is trying meditation to ease the stress and is trying to get Steve to join a yoga group with her.
- Family conflicts: Numerous unresolved family conflicts continue in the Johnson family.
- Familial roles and responsibilities: In the Johnson family, Mary alternates between being overprotective and harsh and critical with her children. Steve is an enabler and unable to set appropriate limits. Susie is pseudomature in her relationship with Tony.
- Treatment goals: The treatment goals for the Johnson family are to get Tony into a short-term residential treatment facility and to find a long-term treatment program for families with a member with dual diagnoses. The family desires social support from others with similar experiences, education regarding Tony's ongoing treatment options, and skills training that will help them communicate better with one another and teach them to manage the impact of these disorders on the family in between these intermittent crises.
- The person's ability to remain safe: Without long-term treatment and medication management, Tony is at great risk for harm.

Diagnosis: Tony's dual diagnosis of bipolar disorder with methamphetamine dependence helps determine the best treatment approach for Tony as an individual. His dual disorder probably began when he was an adolescent. For Tony, he describes the feelings of depression and hopelessness preceding his misuse of drugs.

But it is often said that the "mentally ill" patient is just the "delegate to the convention" for the family; most experts advocate for the inclusion of the family in treatment. In addition to the plan of care that staff nurses have established to address Tony's individual nursing diagnoses, family diagnoses for the Johnson family include the following:

- Compromised family coping related to situational crisis as evidenced by Tony's overdose and hospitalization, the family's disruption in their daily activities, and the increased need for support.
- Dysfunctional family process related to drug abuse, as evidenced by familial conflict and ineffective problem solving.
- Ineffective family therapeutic regimen management related to decisional conflict (discharge decision), economic difficulty, and excessive demands on family as evidenced by verbalization of desire to manage Tony's treatment and prevent the negative sequelae of his methamphetamine abuse and untreated bipolar disorder.

Outcome Identification: For the Johnson family and Tony, treatment attempts have failed to date, and it appears that Tony will need to aim for abstinence and control of his mental illness to survive. The desired outcomes for the Johnson family include but are not limited to Tony's recovery from his methamphetamine addiction/abuse and control of his bipolar disorder. Outcomes for the family include identifying familial support systems in the community, exploring financial options for paying for Tony's treatment, making a family decision regarding the best treatment option available for Tony, Tony's acceptance into a residential treatment facility, expressing anger appropriately, discussing openly substance abuse and other "family secrets," setting limits on inappropriate and enabling behavior, and honoring individual and family boundaries and needs.

Planning: For the Johnson family, an integrated program in the community is most appropriate but not easy to find and often quite expensive. Discharge planning for the Johnson family includes the following: the family will be given information about appropriate referrals for residential care, the family (and Tony) will seek out and accept an appropriate referral, and Tony will be discharged to the referral facility. The family will also be given referrals to the Meth Family and Friends Support Group, as well as the NAMI. The family will also be referred for counseling to a therapist/counselor who is available through Steve's insurance plan so family members may work on their communication and coping skills, develop more appropriate boundaries with one another, and address some of their own needs.

Implementation: Tony and his family accepted a referral to a Volunteers of America drug-free facility/ treatment program in which family members participate on a regular basis. This program is free to Tony as long as he continues to work at the facility. He was willing to accept this placement, and it did not burden Steve economically. Other discharge plans were also effectively implemented.

Evaluation: Follow-up is necessary to determine the effectiveness of the referral in assisting the family to function more appropriately, helping Tony to be drug free, and providing treatment for Tony's bipolar disorder.

Benefits of Involving Family: In the Johnson family, Tony is reaching out for help from his family. He has been unsuccessful in receiving and accepting treatment on his own, and he needs the resources of his family (insurance and finances) to get the treatment he needs. The family needs him healthy to improve its self-image and its own successful functioning.

Barriers to Involving Family: Many of the barriers to involving the Johnson family are a result of the family dynamics that the family exhibits. The family has a pattern of rescuing Tony during periods of crisis and has difficulty setting appropriate limits and insisting that Tony take responsibility for his actions. They tend to become overly involved during some periods and remain aloof at others, resulting in inconsistent participation. They are in need of long-term partnership with a treatment team. Tony's lack of commitment to treatment hinders any type of long-term relationship being established with his family. In addition, Steve may experience a sense of guilt that Tony may have inherited the bipolar disorder from him, and he may need counseling to express some of these feelings. The stress of Tony's illness and recent crisis may exacerbate Steve's own disorder.

Family Case Study: Anderson Family

The following brief case study illustrates how a school nurse's interaction with a student led to psychoeducation and support for members of the entire family. The Anderson family consists of a grandmother and the two older children she is raising. See Figure 16-3 for the family genogram.

Karen, age 14, has an older brother, Tom, who is 21 and still lives at home. Tom was diagnosed with paranoid schizophrenia when he was 17. Their grandmother, Emma,

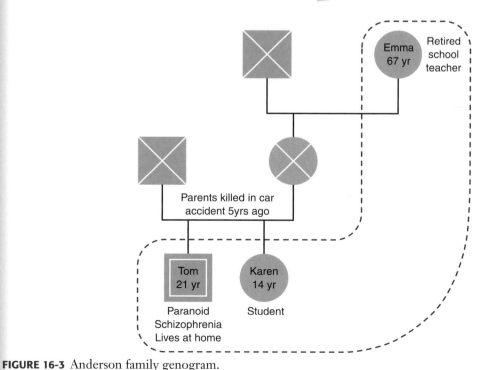

FIGURE 16-3 Anderson family genogram.

(continued)

is raising Karen and Tom because both of their parents were killed in a motor vehicle accident 5 years ago. Emma is 67 and is a retired schoolteacher with a limited income. Karen seldom brings friends over to the house because she does not want to be embarrassed by her brother. Tom has been acting paranoid and frequently mumbles sentences under his breath that don't make any sense to Karen. Karen is aware that the psychiatric mental health nurse practitioner is in the process of regulating his psychiatric medications but she thinks that things will just never get better. Karen is afraid that she's going to become just like her brother when she gets older and worries that her grandmother won't be able to take care of both of them. Karen's grandmother takes Tom to his psychiatric medication appointments and also to individual therapy and is preoccupied with the thought that she is going to have to

take care of Tom for the rest of her life—she loves Tom but had been looking forward to living independently and doing things with her friends.

The school nurse was aware of Karen's living situation and asked Karen to come and see her after school. The nurse did a brief assessment (see Figure 16-4 for the family ecomap) and was able to help Karen voice her fears and concerns about her brother's disorder. She spent some time teaching Karen about schizophrenia and treatments. Karen felt relieved to be able to talk to someone and learn more information that helped her understand why her brother did and said things that did not make sense to her. The nurse was aware of a local NAMI chapter that had a separate parent and sibling support group for families who had a family member with schizophrenia. Reluctantly, Karen went to a meeting where she was relieved to hear

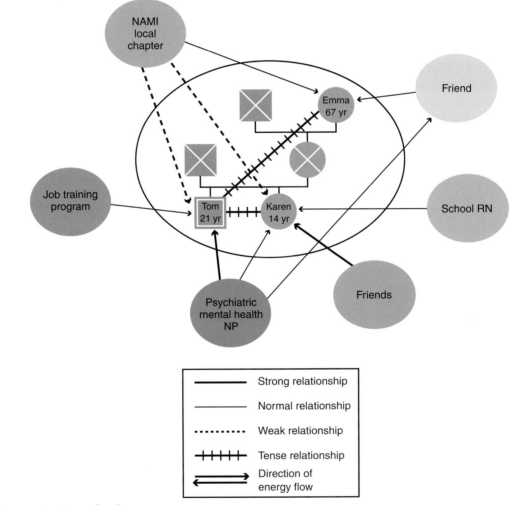

FIGURE 16-4 Anderson family ecomap.

the stories from other kids her age and was surprised to learn that they had similar experiences. Karen's grandmother hesitatingly went to a support group—she had driven Karen to the NAMI meeting and sat in the car and eventually decided to attend a meeting herself. Karen and her grandmother eventually began to talk more openly about their worries and concerns.

Tom's psychiatric mental health nurse practitioner (PMHNP) learned from Tom that his sister and grandmother were attending NAMI support groups. The PMHNP asked Tom if it would be okay if Karen and his grandmother could come to one of his appointments and he agreed. The PMHNP spent time explaining the purpose and adverse effects of the medications Tom was taking and encouraged Karen and Emma to contact her if they noticed changes in his behavior that might suggest his symptoms were increasing or he was having a side effect from the medications.

As Tom became stabilized on his medication he began to be more involved in communicating with his sister and grandmother. Eventually, Karen became more comfortable bringing her friends to the house. Emma was able to learn more about community training programs that Tom could attend during the day to learn a skill that could eventually lead to a job. The job-training program was part of a community grant and so did not add a financial burden to Emma. Emma was now able to do more things during the day with her friends. Psychoeducation decreased not only the family stress as a unit, but also Karen and Emma's stress. The school nurse was instrumental in providing psychoeducation, which led Karen and Emma to peer-led support groups.

SUMMARY

Nurses play an important role in not only helping families manage their lives when a member of the family has an MHC, but also in preventing MHCs from occurring. Providing mental health nursing care may be challenging due to the stigmas associated with MHCs, but it is also a privilege. The nurse-family relationship is very important in effecting positive outcomes: nurses can reduce stigmas; correct myths about MHCs; offer family-centered interventions that promote family health, including referrals to appropriate resources; and provide nursing approaches that change a potentially negative experience into a positive one. The following

points highlight critical concepts that are addressed in this chapter:

- A family-focused approach to providing mental health care to families, that is, viewing the family as a unit, includes supporting families in their natural caregiving roles in ways that encourage family collaboration and choice in treatment decisions.
- There are improved outcomes for the person with an MHC if the health professional collaborates with families when providing treatment to the individual.
- Physical and/or mental comorbidities are frequently present when someone has a mental health condition.
- Common needs for families living with a family member with an MHC are support, information, skills and training, advocacy, and referral sources.
- Families value interactions with health providers that demonstrate openness, cooperation, confirmation, and continuity.
- Nurses must have an attitude toward family members that is perceived as nonblaming and accepting in order to establish a collaborative relationship with the family.
- There are many effective psychotherapeutic and psychological interventions available, including family therapies, mother and infant psychotherapies, and brief cognitive therapy appropriate to the age and stage of child development.

REFERENCES

Abrams, M. S. (2009). The well sibling: Challenges and possibilities. *American Journal of Psychotherapy, 63*(4), 305–317.
Ahern, K. (2003). At-risk children: A demographic analysis of the children of clients attending mental health community clinics. *International Journal of Mental Health Nursing, 12,* 223–228.
Ahlstrom, B. H., Skarsater, I., & Danielson, E. (2007). Major depression in a family: What happens and how to manage—A case study. *Issues in Mental Health Nursing, 28*(7), 691–706.
Aldridge, J. (2006). The experiences of children living with and caring for parents with mental illness. *Child Abuse Review, 15,* 79–88.
Ali, L., Ahlstrom, B. H., Krevers, B., & Skarsater, I. (2012). Daily life for young adults who care for a person with mental illness: A qualitative study. *Journal of Psychiatric and Mental Health Nursing, 19,* 610–617.
American Nurses Association, American Psychiatric Nurses Association, & International Society of Psychiatric–Mental Health Nurses. (2007). *Psychiatric–mental health nursing: Scope and standards of practice.* Silver Spring, MD: Author.

American Psychiatric Association. (2000). *Diagnostic and statistical manual of mental disorders* (DSM-IV-TR) (4th ed., text rev.). Washington, DC: Author.

American Psychiatric Association. (2013). *Diagnostic and statistical manual of mental disorders* (DSM-5(tm)) (5th ed.). Washington, DC: Author.

Aschbrenner, K. A., Greenberg, J. S., & Seltzer, M. M. (2009). Parenting an adult child with bipolar disorder in later life. *Journal of Nervous and Mental Disease, 197*(5), 298–304.

Bassani, D. G., Padoin, D. V., Phillip, D., & Veldhuizen, S. (2009). Estimating the number of children exposed to parental psychiatric disorders through a national health survey. *Child and Adolescent Psychiatry and Mental Health, 3,* 6.

Beardslee, W. R., Gladstone, T. R. G., Wright, E. J., & Cooper, A. B. (2003). A family-based approach to the prevention of depressive symptoms in children at risk: Evidence of parental and child change. *Pediatrics, 112*(2), 119–131.

Beardslee, W. R., Versage, E. M., & Gladstone, T. R. G. (1998). Children of affectively ill parents: A review of the past 10 years. *Journal of the American Academy of Child and Adolescent Psychiatry, 37*(11), 1134–1141.

Becker, L., Goobic, K., & Thomas, S. (2009). Advising families on AD/HD: A multimodal approach. *Pediatric Nursing, 35*(1), 47–52.

Berman, S. M., Kuczenski, S., McCracken, J. T., & London, E. D. (2009). Potential adverse effects of amphetamine treatment on brain and behavior: A review. *Molecular Psychiatry, 14*(2), 123–142.

Brockington, I., Chandra, P., Dubowitz, H., Jones, D., Moussa, S., Nakku, J., & Ferre, I. (2011). WPA guidance on the protection and promotion of mental health in children of persons with severe mental disorders. *World Psychiatry, 10,* 93–102.

Bromet, E., Andrade, L. H., Hwang, I., Sampson, N. A., Alonso, J., de Girolamo, G., . . . Kess, R. C. (2011). Cross-national epidemiology of DSM-IV major depressive episode. *BMC Medicine, 9,* 90.

Brookes, N., Murata, L., & Tansey, M. (2006). Guiding practice development using the Tidal Commitments. *Journal of Psychiatric and Mental Health Nursing, 13,* 460–463.

Brookes, N., Murata, L., & Tansey, M. (2008). Tidal waves: Implementing a new model of mental health recovery and reclamation. *Canadian Nurse, 104*(8), 22–27.

Brunton, K. (1997). Stigma. *Journal of Advanced Nursing, 26,* 891–898.

Calam, R., Jones, S., Sanders, M., Dempsey, R., & Sadhnani, V. (2012). Parenting and the emotional and behavioural adjustment of young children in families with a parent with bipolar disorder. *Behavioral and Cognitive Psychotherapy, 40,* 425–437.

Caldwell, B. A., Sclafani, M., Swarbrick, M., & Piren, K. (2010). Psychiatric nursing practice and the Recovery Model of Care. *Journal of Psychosocial Nursing, 48*(7), 42–48.

Caldwell, C. B., & Gottesman, I. I. (1990). Schizophrenics kill themselves too: A review of risk factors for suicide. *Schizophrenia Bulletin, 16*(4), 571–589.

Canadian Medical Association. (2008). 8th Annual national report card on health. Retrieved from http://www.cma.ca/multimedia/CMA/Content_Images/Inside_cma/Annual_Meeting/2008/GC_Bulletin/National_Report_Card_EN.pdf

Caqueo-Urizar, A., Gutierrez-Maldonada, J., & Mirnada-Castillo, C. (2009). Quality of life in caregivers of patients with schizophrenia: A literature review. *Health and Quality of Life Outcomes, 7,* 84–88.

Cassano, P., & Fava, M. (2002). Depression and public health, an overview. *Journal of Psychosomatic Research, 53*(4), 849–857.

Chen, W., & Lukens, E. (2011). Well being, depressive symptoms, and burden among parent and sibling caregivers of persons with severe and persistent mental illness. *Social Work in Mental Health, 9,* 397–416.

Colton, C. W., & Manderscheid, R. W. (2006). Congruencies in increased mortality rates, years of potential life lost, and causes of death among public mental health clients in eight states. *Prevention of Chronic Disease, 3*(2), 1–13.

Compas, B. E., Champion, J. E., Forehand, R., Cole, D. A., Reeslund, K. L., Fear, J., . . . Roberts, L. (2010). Coping and parenting: Mediators of 12-month outcomes of a family group cognitive-behavioral preventive intervention with families of depressed parents. *Journal of Consulting and Clinical Psychology, 78*(5), 623–634.

Conway, K. P., Compton, W., Stinson, F. S., & Grant, B. F. (2006). Lifetime comorbidity of DSM-IV mood and anxiety disorders and specific drug use disorders: Results from the National Epidemiologic Survey on Alcohol and Related Conditions. *Journal of Clinical Psychiatry, 67*(2), 247–257.

Corsentino, E. A., Molinari, V., Gum, A. M., Roscoe, L. A., & Mills, W. L. (2008). Family caregivers' future planning for younger and older adults with serious mental illness (SMI). *Journal of Applied Gerontology, 27*(4), 466–485.

Crowe, M., Inder, M., Joyce, P., Luty, S., Moor, S., & Carter, J. (2011). Was it something I did wrong? A qualitative analysis of parental perspectives of their child's bipolar disorder. *Journal of Psychiatric and Mental Health Nursing, 18,* 342–348.

Cuijpers, P. (2005). Depressive disorders in caregivers of dementia patients: A systematic review. *Aging & Mental Health, 9*(4), 325–330.

Dalky, H. F. (2012). Perception and coping with stigma of mental illness: Arab families' perspectives. *Issues in Mental Health Nursing, 33,* 486–491.

Decima Research Inc. (2004). *Informal/family caregivers in Canada caring for someone with a mental illness.* POR 03-82. Contract no.: H1011-030149/001/CY. Ottawa, Canada: Health Canada.

Devane, C. L., Chiao, E., Franklin, M., & Kruep, E. J. (2005). Anxiety disorders in the 21st century: Status, challenges, opportunities, and comorbidity with depression. *American Journal of Managed Care, 11*(Suppl 12), S344–S353.

Dixon, L., McFarlane, W., Lefley, H., Lucksted, A., Cohen, M., Falloon, I., . . . Sondheimer, D. (2001). Evidence-based practices for services to families of people with psychiatric disabilities. *Psychiatric Services, 52*(7), 903–910.

Doherty, D., Benbow, S. M., Craig, J., & Smith, C. (2009). Patients' and carers' journeys through older people's mental health services. *Dementia, 8*(4), 501–513.

Doornbos, M. M. (2001). Professional support for family caregivers of people with serious and persistent mental illnesses. *Journal of Psychosocial Nursing, 39*(12), 39–47.

Doornbos, M. M. (2002). Family caregivers and the mental health care of system: Reality and dreams. *Archives of Psychiatric Nursing, 16*(1), 39–46.

Eakes, G. G. (1995). Chronic sorrow: The lived experience of parents of chronically mentally ill individuals. *Archives of Psychiatric Nursing, 9*(2), 77–84.

Ewertzon, M., Cronqvist, A., Lutzen, K., & Andershed, B. (2012). A lonely life journey bordered with struggle: Being a sibling of an individual with psychosis. *Issues in Mental Health Nursing, 33,* 157–164.

Foley, M. (2010). A comparison of family adversity and family dysfunction in families of children with attention deficit hyperactivity disorder (ADHD) and families of children without ADHD. *Journal for Specialists in Pediatric Nursing, 16,* 39–49.

Fortinash, K. M., & Worret P. A. (2007). *Psychiatric nursing care plans* (5th ed.). Philadelphia, PA: Elsevier.

Foster, K. (2010). "You'd think this roller coaster was never going to stop": Experiences of adult children of parents with serious mental illness. *Journal of Clinical Nursing, 19,* 3143–3151.

Foster, K., O'Brien, L., & Korhonen, T. (2012). Developing resilient children and families when parents have mental illness: A family-focused approach. *International Journal of Mental Health Nursing, 21,* 3–11.

Freeman, J. G., King, M., & Pickett, W. (2011). *The health of Canada's young people: A mental health focus.* Ottawa, ON: Public Health Agency of Canada.

Friedrich, R. M., Lively, S., & Rubenstein, L. M. (2008). Siblings' coping strategies and mental health services: A national study of siblings of persons with schizophrenia. *Psychiatric Services, 59*(3), 261–267.

Gallagher-Thompson, D., Tzuang, Y. M., Au, A., Brodaty, H., Charlesworth, G., Gupta, R., . . . Shyu, Y. (2012). International perspectives on nonpharmacological best practices for dementia family caregivers: A review. *Clinical Gerontologist, 35,* 316–355.

Ganguli, R., & Strassnig, M. (2011). Prevention of metabolic syndrome in serious mental illness. *Psychiatric Clinics of North America, 34,* 109–125.

Garley, D., Gallop, R., Johnston, N., & Pipitone, J. (1997). Children of the mentally ill: A qualitative focus group approach. *Journal of Psychiatric and Mental Health Nursing, 4,* 97–103.

Gerdes, A. C., Haack, L. M., & Schneider, B. W. (2012). Parental functioning in families of children with ADHD: Evidence for behavioral parent training and importance of clinically meaningful change. *Journal of Attention Disorders, 16*(2), 147–156.

Gerson, L. D., & Rose, L. E. (2012). Needs of persons with serious mental illness following discharge from inpatient treatment: Patient and family values. *Archives of Psychiatric Nursing, 26*(4), 261–271.

Gladstone, B. M., Boydell, K. M., & McKeever, P. (2006). Recasting research into children's experiences of parental mental illness: Beyond risk and resilience. *Social Science & Medicine, 62,* 2540–2550.

Godress, J., Ozgul, S., Owen, C., & Foley-Evans, L. (2005). Grief experiences of parents whose children suffer mental illness. *Australian and New Zealand Journal of Psychiatry, 39,* 88–94.

Goetting, A. (1986). The developmental task of siblingship over the life cycle. *Journal of Marriage and Family, 48*(4), 703–714.

Gray, B., Robinson, C., Seddon, D., & Roberts, A. (2008). "Confidentiality smokescreens" and carers for people with mental health problems: The perspectives of professionals. *Health and Social Care in the Community, 16*(4), 378–387.

Grayson, J. (Ed.). (2006). Maltreatment and its effects on early brain development. *Virginia Child Protection Newsletter, 77,* 1–16.

Grundy, S. M., Cleeman, J. I., Daniels, S. R., Donato, K. A., Eckel, R. H., Franklin, B. A., . . . Costa, F. (2005). Diagnosis and management of the metabolic syndrome: An American Heart Association/National Heart, Lung and Blood Institute Scientific Statement. *Circulation, 11*(27), 2735–2752.

Gumus, A. B. (2008). Health education needs of patients with schizophrenia and their relatives. *Archives of Psychiatric Nursing, 22*(3), 156–165.

Hawton, K., Sutton, L., Haw, C., Sinclair, J., & Deeks, J. J. (2005). Schizophrenia and suicide: A systematic review of risk factors. *British Journal of Psychiatry, 187*(1), 9–20.

Health Canada. (2002). *A report on mental illness in Canada.* Ottawa, ON: Author.

Hennekens, C. H., Hennekens, A. R., Hollar, D., & Casey, D. E. (2005). Schizophrenia and increased risks of cardiovascular diseases. *American Heart Journal, 150*(3), 1115–1121.

Institute of Health Economics. (2008). How much should we spend on mental health? Edmonton, AB: Author.

Jackson, D., & Peters, K. (2008). Use of drug therapy in children with attention deficit hyperactivity disorder (ADHD): Maternal views and experiences. *Journal of Clinical Nursing, 17,* 2725–2732.

Jakobsen, E. S., & Severinsson, E. (2006). Parents' experiences of collaboration with community healthcare professionals. *Journal of Psychiatry and Mental Health Nursing, 13,* 498–505.

Jonnson, P. D., Wijk, H., Danielson, E., & Skarsater, I. (2011). Outcomes of an educational intervention for the family of a person with bipolar disorder: A 2-year follow-up study. *Journal of Psychiatric and Mental Health Nursing, 18,* 333–341.

Kaas, M. J., Lee, S., & Peitzman, C. (2003). Barriers to collaboration between mental health professionals and families in the care of persons with serious mental illness. *Issues in Mental Health Nursing, 24,* 741–756.

Kamel, A. A., Bond, A. E., & Froelicher, E. S. (2012). Depression and caregiver burden experienced by caregivers of Jordanian patients with stroke. *International Journal of Nursing Practice, 18,* 147–154.

Katon, W., & Ciechanowski, P. (2002). Impact of major depression on chronic medical illness. *Journal of Psychosomatic Research, 53*(4), 859–863.

Kendler, K. S., & Gardner, S. O. (1997). The risk for psychiatric disorders in relatives of schizophrenic and control probands: A comparison of three independent studies. *Psychological Medicine, 27,* 411–419.

Kessler, R. C., Barker, P. R., Colpe, L. J., Epstein, J. F., Gfroerer, J. C., Hiripi, E., . . . Zaslavsky, A. M. (2003). Screening for serious mental illness in the general population. *Archives of General Psychiatry, 60,* 184–189.

Kessler, R. C., Berglund, P., Demler, O., Jin, R., Merikangas, K. R., & Walters, E. E. (2005). Lifetime prevalence and age-of-onset distributions of DSM-IV disorders in the National Comorbidity Survey Replication (NCS-R). *Archives of General Psychiatry, 62,* 593–602.

Kessler, R. C., Chiu, W. T., Demler, O., & Walters, E. E. (2005). Prevalence, severity, and comorbidity of 12-month DSM-IV disorders in the national comorbidity survey replication. *Archives of General Psychiatry, 62,* 617–627.

Kildea, S., John, W., & Davies, J. (2011). Making sense of ADHD in practice: A stakeholder review. *Clinical Child Psychology and Psychiatry, 16*(4), 599–619.

Knutson-Medin, L., Edlund, B., & Ramklint, M. (2007). Experiences in a group of grown-up children of mentally ill parents. *Journal of Psychiatric and Mental Health Nursing, 14,* 744–752.

Korhonen, T., Pietila, A., & Vehvilainen-Julkunen, K. (2010). Are the children of the clients' visible or invisible for nurses in adult psychiatry? A questionnaire survey. *Scandinavian Journal of Caring Sciences, 24,* 65–74.

Korhonen, T., Vehvilainen-Julkunen, K., & Pietila, A. (2008). Do nurses working in adult psychiatry take into consideration the support network of families affected by parental mental disorder? *Journal of Psychiatric and Mental Health Nursing, 15,* 767–776.

Lambert, K., & Kinsley, C. H. (2005). Clinical neuroscience: The neurobiological foundations of mental health. New York, NY: Worth Publishers.

Link, B. G., & Phelan, J. C. (2001). Conceptualizing stigma. *Annual Review of Sociology, 27,* 363–385.

Link, B. G., Yang, L. H., Phelan, J. C., & Collins, P. Y. (2004). Measuring mental illness stigma. *Schizophrenia Bulletin, 30*(3), 511–541.

Luggen, A. S. (2005). Bipolar disorder: An uncommon illness? Recognizing and caring for the elderly person with bipolar disorder. *Geriatric Nursing, 26,* 326–329.

Mahoney, L. (2010). Children living with a mentally ill parent: The role of public health nurses. *Nursing Praxis in New Zealand, 26*(20), 4–13.

Marsh, D., & Johnson, D. (1997). The family experience of mental illness: Implications for intervention. *Professional Psychology: Research and Practice, 28*(3), 229–237.

Maskill, V., Crowe, M., Luty, S., & Joyce, P. (2010). Two sides of the same coin: Caring for a person with bipolar disorder. *Journal of Psychiatric and Mental Health Nursing, 17,* 535–542.

Mayberry, D., Goodyear, M., & Reupert, A. (2012). The Family-Focused Mental Health Practice Questionnaire. *Archives of Psychiatric Nursing, 26*(2), 135–144.

Meltzer, H. Y. (2005). Suicidality in schizophrenia: Pharmacologic treatment. *Clinical Neuropsychiatry: Journal of Treatment Evaluation, 2*(1), 76–83.

Mental Health America. (2012). *Fact sheet: When a parent has a mental illness: Issues and challenges.* Alexandria, VA: Author. Retrieved from http://www.nmha.org/index.cfm?objectid= e3412bb7-1372-4d20-c8f627a57cd3d00f

Mental Health Commission of Canada. (2012). *Changing directions, changing lives: The mental health strategies of Canada.* Calgary, AB: Author. Retrieved from http://www.cpa.ca/docs/ file/Practice/strategy-text-en.pdf

Moller, T., Gudde, C. B., Folden, G. E., & Linaker, O. M (2009). The experience of caring in relatives to patients with serious mental illness: Gender differences, health and functioning. *Scandinavian Journal of Caring, 23,* 153–160.

Mordoch, E., & Hall, W. A. (2002). Children living with a parent who has a mental illness: A critical analysis of the literature and research implications. *Archives of Psychiatric Nursing, 16*(5), 208–216.

Muhlbauer, S. (2008). Caregiver perceptions and needs regarding symptom attenuation in severe and persistent mental illness. *Perspectives in Psychiatric Care, 44*(2), 99–109.

Nadkarni, R. B., & Fristad, M. A. (2012). Stress and support for parents of youth with bipolar disorder. *Israel Journal of Psychiatry and Related Sciences, 49*(2), 104–111.

National Alliance on Mental Illness. (n.d.). What is mental illness? Retrieved from http://www.nami.org

National Institute of Mental Health. (2001). The impact of mental illness on society (NIH Publication No. 01-4586). Retrieved from http://www.nimh.nih.gov/publicat/burden/htm

National Institute of Mental Health. (2009). Treatment of children with mental illness. Frequently asked questions about the treatment of mental illness in children (NIH Publication No. 09-470)

Retrieved from http://www.nimh.nih.gov/health/publications/ treatment-of-children-with-mental-illness-fact-sheet/nimh- treatment-children-mental-illness-faq.pdf

National Institute of Mental Health. (2012). The numbers count: Mental disorders in America [data file]. Retrieved from http://www.nimh.nih.gov/health/publications/the-numbers- count-mental-disorders-in-america/index.shtml

New Freedom Commission on Mental Health. (2003). *Achieving the promise: Transforming mental health care in America.* Rockville, MD: U.S. Department of Health and Human Services. Retrieved from http://www.mentalhealthcommission.gov/ reports/FinalReport/toc.html

Nigg, J. (2006). *What causes ADHD?* New York, NY: Guilford.

Nordby, K., Kjonsberg, K., & Hummelvoll, J. K. (2010). Relatives of persons with recently discovered serious mental illness: In need of support to become resource persons in treatment and recovery. *Journal of Psychiatric and Mental Health Nursing, 17,* 304–311.

Obadina, S. (2010). Parental mental illness: Effects on young carers. *British Journal of School Nursing, 5*(3), 135–139.

O'Brien, L., Anand, M., Brady, P., & Gillies, D. (2011). Children visiting parents in inpatient psychiatric facilities: Perspective of parents, carers and children. *International Journal of Mental Health Nursing, 20,* 137–143.

O'Connell, K. L. (2006). Needs of families affected by mental illness: Through support, information and skill training, advocacy, and referral, nurses can help families put the pieces together. *Journal of Psychosocial Nursing and Mental Health Services, 44*(3), 40–51.

Olshansky, S. (1962). Chronic sorrow: A response to having a mentally defective child. *Social Casework, 43,* 191–193.

Ostman, M. (2008). Interviews with children of persons with a severe mental illness: Investigating their everyday situation. *Nordic Journal of Psychiatry, 62*(5), 354–359.

Ostman, M., Wallsten, T., & Kjellin, L. (2005). Family burden and relatives' participation in psychiatric care: Are the patient's diagnosis and the relation to the patient of importance? *International Journal of Social Psychiatry, 51*(4), 291–301.

Perlick, D. A., Miklowitz, D. J., Chou, N., Kalvin, C., Adzhiashvili, V., & Aronson, A. (2010). Family-focused treatment for caregivers of patients with bipolar disorder. *Bipolar Disorders, 12,* 627–637.

Perlick, D., Nelson, A., Mattias, K., Selzer, J., Kalvin, C., Wilber, C., . . . Corrigan, P. (2011). In our own voice—Family companion: Reducing self-stigma of family members of persons with serious mental illness. *Psychiatric Services, 62*(12), 1456–1462.

Perry, B. D., Pollard, R. A., Blakley, T. L., Baker, W. L., & Vigilante, D. (1995). Childhood trauma, the neurobiology of adaptation, and "use-dependent" development of the brain: How "states" become "traits." *Infant Mental Health Journal, 16*(4), 271–291.

Pescosolido, B. A., Martin, J. K., Long, J. S., Medina, T. R., Phelan, J. C., & Link, B. G. (2010). "A disease like any other"? A decade of change in public reactions to schizophrenia, depression, and alcohol dependence. *American Journal of Psychiatry, 167*(11), 1321–1330.

Phelan, J. C., Link, B. G., Stueve, A., & Pescosolido, B. A. (2000). Public conceptions of mental illness in 1950 and 1996: What is mental illness and is it to be feared? *Journal of Health and Social Behavior, 41*(2), 188–207.

Piat, M., Sabetti, J., Fleury, M., Boyer, R., & Lesage, A. (2011). "Who believes most in me and in my recovery": The importance of families for persons with serious mental illness living in structured community housing. *Journal of Social Work in Disability & Rehabilitation, 10,* 49–65.

Piippo, J., & Aaltonen, J. (2004). Mental health: Integrated network and family-oriented model for co-operation between mental health patients, adult mental health services and social services. *Journal of Clinical Nursing, 13,* 876–885.

Pinquart, M., & Sorensen, S. (2006). Gender differences in caregiver stressors, social resources, and health: An updated meta-analysis. *Journal of Gerontology, 6,* 333–345.

Place, M., Reynolds, J., Cousins, A., & O'Neill, S. (2002). Developing a resilience package for vulnerable children. *Child & Adolescent Mental Health, 7*(4), 162–167.

Radomsky, E. D., Haas, G. L., Mann, J. J., & Sweeney, J. A. (1999). Suicidal behavior in patients with schizophrenia and other psychotic disorders. *American Journal of Psychiatry, 156*(10), 1590–1595.

Reupert, A., & Mayberry, D. (2007). Families affected by parental mental illness: A multiperspective account of issues and interventions. *American Journal of Orthopsychiatry, 77*(3), 362–369.

Robins, L. N., & Regier, D. A. (Eds.). (1991). *Psychiatric disorders in America: The Epidemiologic Catchment Area Study.* New York, NY: Free Press.

Robinson, L. (1983). *Psychiatric nursing as a human experience* (3rd ed.). Philadelphia, PA: W. B. Saunders.

Rowe, J. (2012). Great expectations: A systematic review of the literature on the role of family carers in severe mental illness, and their relationships and engagement with professionals. *Journal of Psychiatric and Mental Health Nursing, 19,* 70–82.

Rusner, M., Carlsson, G., Brunt, D. A., & Nystrom, M. (2012). The paradox of being both needed and rejected: The existential meaning of being closely related to a person with bipolar disorder. *Issues in Mental Health Nursing, 33,* 200–208.

Sadock, B. J., & Sadock, V. A. (2008). *Kaplan and Sadock's concise textbook of clinical psychiatry* (3rd ed.). Philadelphia, PA: Lippincott Williams & Wilkins.

Saunders, J. (1999). Family functioning in families providing care for a family member with schizophrenia. *Issues in Mental Health Nursing, 20,* 95–113.

Saunders, J., & Byrne, M. (2002). A thematic analysis of families living with schizophrenia. *Archives of Psychiatric Nursing, 14*(5), 217–223.

Schafer, T., Wood, S., & Williams, R. (2010). A survey into student nurses' attitudes toward mental illness: Implications for nurse training. *Nurse Education Today, 31,* 328–332.

Scharer, K. (2002). What parents of mentally ill children need and want from mental health professionals. *Issues in Mental Health Nursing, 23,* 617–640.

Schock, A., & Gavazzi, S. (2005). Mental illness and families. In P. McKenry & S. Price (Eds.), *Families and change: Coping with stressful events and transitions* (3rd ed., pp. 179–204). Thousand Oaks, CA: Sage.

Seeman, M. V. (2009). The changing role of mother of the mentally ill: From schizophrenogenic mother to multigenerational caregiver. *Psychiatry, 72*(3), 284–294.

Singh, I., Kendall, T., Taylor, C., Mears, A., Hollis, C., Batty, M., & Keenan S. (2010). Young people's experience of ADHD and stimulant medication: A qualitative study for the NICE guideline. *Child and Adolescent Mental Health, 15*(4), 186–192.

Sjoblom, L., Pejlert, A., & Asplund, K. (2005). Nurses' view of the family in psychiatric care. *Journal of Clinical Nursing, 14*(5), 562–569.

Smith, M. (2004). Parental mental health: Disruptions to parenting and outcomes for children. *Child and Family Social Work, 9,* 3–11.

Sorrell, J. (2011). Caring for older adults with bipolar disorder. *Journal of Psychosocial Nursing, 49*(7), 21–25.

Spitzer, R. L., Kroenke, K., & Williams, J. B. W. (1999). Validation and utility of a self-report version of PRIME-MD: The PHQ primary care study. Primary care evaluation of mental disorders. Patient Health Questionnaire. *Journal of American Medical Association, 282*(18), 1737–1744.

Stahl, S. (2011). *The prescriber's guide* (4th ed.). New York, NY: Cambridge University Press.

Statistics Canada. (2002). Canadian Community Health Survey: Mental health and well-being (Catalogue no. 82-617-X). Retrieved from http://www.statcan.gc.ca/pub/82-617-x/4067678-eng.htm

Substance Abuse and Mental Health Services Administration. (2012a). National consensus statement on mental health recovery. Retrieved from http://store.samhsa.gov/shin/content/PEP12-RECDEF/PEP12-RECDEF.pdf

Substance Abuse and Mental Health Services Administration. (2012b). *Results from the 2011 National Survey on Drug Use and Health: Mental health findings* (NSDUH Series H-45, HHS Publication No. [SMA] 12-4725). Rockville, MD: Author.

Tamm, L., Holden, G. W., Nakonezny, P. A., Swart, S., & Hughes, C. W. (2012). Metaparenting: Associations with parenting stress, child-rearing practices, and retention in parents of children at risk for ADHD. *ADHD Attention Deficit and Hyperactivity Disorders, 4*(1), 1–10.

Tan, S. C., Yeo, A. I., Choo, I. B., Huang, A. P., Ong, S. H., Ismail, H, . . . Chan, Y. H. (2012). Burden and coping strategies experienced by caregivers of persons with schizophrenia in the community. *Journal of Clinical Nursing, 21,* 2410–2418.

Teicher, M. H. (2002). Scars that won't heal: The neurobiology of child abuse. *Scientific American, 286*(3), 68–75.

Till, U. (2007). The values of recovery within mental health nursing. *Mental Health Practice, 11*(3), 32–36.

Tranvag, O., & Kristoffersen, K. (2008). Experience of being the spouse/cohabitant of a person with bipolar affective disorder: A cumulative process over time. *Scandinavian Journal of Caring Science, 22,* 5–18.

U.S. Census Bureau. (2008). Profile America facts for features. Retrieved from http://www.census.gov/Press-Release/www/releases/archives/facts_for_features_special_editions/012095.html

U.S. Department of Health and Human Services. (1999). Mental health: A report of the Surgeon General. Retrieved from http:///www.surgeongeneral.gov/library/mentalhealth/home.html

Van Cleave, J., & Leslie, L. K. (2008). Approaching ADHD as a chronic condition: Implications for long-term adherence. *Journal of Psychosocial Nursing, 46*(8), 28–37.

van der Voort, T., Goossens, P., & van der Bijl, J. (2009). Alone together: A grounded theory study of experienced burden, coping, and support needs of spouses of persons with a bipolar disorder. *International Journal of Mental Health Nursing, 18,* 434–443.

Veltman, A., Cameron, J. I., & Stewart, D. E. (2002). The experience of providing care to relatives with chronic mental illness. *Journal of Nervous and Mental Disease, 190*(2), 108–114.

Vitaliano, P. P., Zhang, J., & Scanlan, J. M. (2003). Is caregiving hazardous to one's physical health? A meta-analysis. *Psychological Bulletin, 129,* 946–972.

World Health Organization. (2001a). *The world health report 2001. Mental health: New understanding, new hope.* Geneva, Switzerland: Author.

World Health Organization. (2001b). *Strengthening mental health promotion* (Fact sheet no. 220). Geneva, Switzerland: Author.

World Health Organization. (2008). *The global burden of disease: 2004 update.* Geneva, Switzerland: Author. Retrieved from http://www.who.int/healthinfo/global_burden_disease/2004_report_update/en/index.html

World Health Organization. (2010). *The international statistical classification of diseases and related health problems.* Chapter V: Mental and behavioural disorders (pp. F00–F99). Geneva, Switzerland: Author. Retrieved from http://apps.who.int/classifications/icd10/browse/2010/en#/F00-F09

World Health Organization. (2011). *World health statistics 2011.* Geneva, Switzerland: Author. Retrieved from http://www.who.int/whosis/whostat/EN_WHS2011_Full.pdf

World Health Organization & Alzheimer's Disease International. (2012). *Dementia: A public health priority.* Geneva, Switzerland: Author.

Yamashita, M., & Forsyth, D. M. (1998). Family coping with mental illness: An aggregate from two studies, Canada and the United States. *Journal of the American Psychiatric Nurses Association, 4*(1), 1–8.

Zauszniewski, J. A., Bekhet, A. K., & Suresky, M. J. (2008). Factors associated with perceived burden, resourcefulness, and quality of life in female family members of adults with serious mental illness. *Journal of American Psychiatric Nurses Association, 142,* 125–135.

Chapter Web Sites

- *Al Anon:* www.al-anon.alateen.org
- *American Psychiatric Association:* www.psych.org
- *American Psychiatric Nurses Association:* www.apna.org
- *American Psychological Association:* www.apa.org
- *Brain and Behavior Research Foundation:* www.bbrfoundation.org
- *Children and Adults With Attention-Deficit/Hyperactivity Disorder:* www.chadd.org
- *Chinese-American Family Alliance for Mental Health:* www.cafamh.org
- *Family Caregiver Alliance:* www.caregiver.org
- *Federation of Families for Children's Mental Health:* www.ffcmh.org
- *International Society of Gerontechnology Free Discussion List:* http://www.jdc.org.il/mailman/listinfo/isg_discussion
- *International Society of Psychiatric–Mental Health Nurses:* www.ispn-psych.org
- *Mental Health America:* www.nmha.org
- *National Alliance on Mental Illness:* www.nami.org
- *National Institute of Mental Health:* www.nimh.nih.gov
- *Tidal Model:* http://www.tidal-model.com
- *Substance Abuse and Mental Health Services:* www.samhsa.gov
- *Veteran's Administration Mental Health:* www.mentalhealth.va.gov
- *World Health Organization:* www.who.int

chapter 17

Families and Community/ Public Health Nursing

Linda L. Eddy, PhD, RN, CPNP

Annette Bailey, PhD, RN

Dawn Doutrich, PhD, RN, CNS

Critical Concepts

- Community is a mindset, not a place.
- Transitioning from individually focused nursing care to care of families and communities is a process.
- Community/public health nurses care for families in a variety of settings.
- Community/public health nurses view families as subunits of the community or as clients in the context of the community.
- Community/public health nurses aim to meet the holistic needs of families and communities while targeting prioritized health needs.
- Healthy families contribute to healthy communities.
- Community/public health family nursing is grounded in social justice and culturally safe, ethical practice.
- Rather than blaming families for their situations, community/public health nurses think upstream to consider how social, political, economic, and environmental conditions affect families' health choices and outcomes.
- Using a combination of relational collaboration and health promotion strategies and principles, community/public health nurses strive to partner with families to assist with all levels of healthy change.
- Nurses foster interconnectedness among families in the community.
- Family interventions in the community are targeted toward primary, secondary, and tertiary prevention.
- The nurse-family relationship is central in interventions at all three levels of prevention.
- Community/public health nursing is evidence based and policy driven.
- Interventions for families are planned, implemented, and evaluated from a health promotion perspective.

What does health mean to you? What are the indicators you use to conclude that you are either healthy or unhealthy? Different people will apply different indicators of health. A definition of health set by the World Health Organization (WHO) in 1948 is that health is "a state of complete physical, mental, and social well-being, and not merely the absence of disease or infirmity" (WHO, 1948, p. 1). This definition implies that achieving health is much more than treating diseases. Health is not just physical, it is emotional and social. Community/public health nurses understand that creating a balance in the various dimensions of people's lives—culture, society, economic, politics, and their physical environment—is crucial in helping them to cultivate health (WHO, 1986). Community/public health nurses recognize that disease patterns are a result of interactions between human beings and their environments and this understanding guides their actions. But how do community/public health nurses transform this understanding of health into health promotion for families?

A broad definition of *family* guides community/public health nurses toward inclusiveness in working with and understanding complex family systems. Family, for purposes of this text, comprises two or more individuals who depend on one another for emotional, physical, and economic support. The members of the family are self-defined.

Along with this broad definition of family, community/public health nurses utilize two prevalent schools of thought. One view sees the family as the unit of care and the community as context. The other view focuses on the community as client with the family as context. The commonality between these views is that family, and thus family health, is indistinguishably linked to community. Therefore, health promotion actions should be concurrent and encompassing for both contexts. Kaiser, Hays, Cho, and Agrawal (2002) have described the complexity of nursing care based on "family as client" in community/public health nursing. Two key issues that contribute to the complexity are (1) labeling family health problems, and (2) identifying the level of need of the family as a whole. Identifying family needs and developing a plan of care for families cannot be done in isolation from the broader context of their surroundings and experiences. When working with families, nurses need to consider environmental, psychological, and behavioral health issues, as well as those of a more

physiological nature. Doing so recognizes that family health problems have contextual roots.

It is important to note that for some individuals, the definition of self is wrapped up in the family (Doutrich, Wros, Valdez, & Ruiz, 2005). For example, *familismo* has been reported as a typical feature of Hispanic families (Vega, 1990). *Familismo*, according to the classic work of Sabogal, Marín, Otero-Sabogal, Marín, and Pérez-Stable (1987), includes three specific types of value orientations: (1) obligations to provide support; (2) perceived high levels of help and support from family; and (3) the perception of relatives as behavioral and attitudinal referents, meaning that one's family determines how one is perceived and perceives the world. Caring for such families will require attention to these values, and to the understanding that family is the unit of care rather than just the individual. For the community/public health family nurse, this definition of self that is inclusive of family will influence the provision of competent and culturally congruent family care.

Healthy communities are comprised of healthy families. Hence, families as units of relationship are important components of communities, and undoubtedly, are heavily affected by their community's state of health. The word *community* means more than just a geographical space; it is a group of people who share similar interests, needs and outcomes, regardless of geographical location (Young & Wharf Higgins, 2012). Community/public health nurses understand the effects that communities can have on individuals and families, and recognize that a community's health is reflected in the health experiences of its members and their families (Canadian Public Health Association [CPHA], 2010; U.S. Department of Health and Human Services [USDHHS], 2001). Issues of violence, unemployment, unclean physical environments, unsupportive relationships, and poor access to needed resources (i.e., food, shelter) are just a few insignia of an unhealthy community. These issues are inextricably linked to the health of families. Promoting and sustaining health for families means helping them to tap into their personal strength, access social and economic resources, and cope with stressors (CPHA, 2010). Community/public health nurses use health promotion strategies, such as facilitating access to resources, to improve the health of families.

Community nursing places an interest in the social, political, and economic aspects of health to help individuals, families, and communities gain a higher degree of harmony within the mind, body, and soul. A public health nurse who visits a new mother in her home and realizes that a bed used for the newborn baby is infested with bedbugs cannot simply focus on the physical health of the mom and baby. Paying attention to lack of proper resources caused by poverty becomes an essential aspect of the nurse's role in promoting health for this family. In fact, the degree to which nurses can contribute positively to the well-being of vulnerable families in communities depends on their convictions and commitments to modify these factors, as well as society's support and recognition of the importance of their work. This chapter offers a description of community health nursing in promoting the health of families in communities. It begins with a definition of community health nursing, and follows with a discussion of concepts and principles that guide the work of these nurses, the roles they enact in working with families and communities, and the various settings where they work. This discussion is organized around a visual representation of community health nursing. The chapter ends with a discussion of current trends in community/public health nursing.

WHAT IS COMMUNITY/PUBLIC HEALTH NURSING?

According to the CPHA (2010), community/public health nursing involves a synthesis of nursing theory and public health science that focuses on population health promotion and primary health care with the intention of maintaining and promoting health, preventing illnesses and injuries, and developing communities. Congruently, the American Public Health Association (2008) states that "public health nurses integrate community involvement and knowledge about the entire population with personal, clinical understandings of the health and illness experiences of individuals and families within the population" (p. 1). These descriptions communicate the critical role of community/public health nurses in fostering care for families beyond a clinical perspective. In their process of work, community and public health nurses rely on various concepts/principles to promote health for individuals, families, and communities. Drawing from various health promotion

frameworks and set standards of practice, these nurses enact these concepts/principles in various settings, with modifications based on families and communities' needs. This is done through a process of empowerment, with the aim of achieving improved health and empowered families. Empowerment enables families to express aspirations and develop their capacity to lead a fulfilling life. This work could include developing personal skills, and facilitating access to economic resources, housing, and decision-making institutions (Sen, 2000, as cited in William, 2008). The model in Figure 17-1 helps to contextualize community/public health nursing.

HEALTH PROMOTION FRAMEWORKS, STANDARDS, AND PRINCIPLES

Health promotion and disease prevention is foundational to community/public health nurses' work (see Chapter 8 for more in-depth information on family health promotion). Interventions for families are planned, implemented, and evaluated from a health promotion perspective. From this perspective, nurses help to reduce health inequities by engaging families in processes that promote their control over their own health. This includes developing families' skills, increasing participation in their care process, and improving access to resources. To prevent illness and injuries, nurses employ health education to help families modify lifestyles/behaviors (e.g., healthy eating, wearing bicycle helmets/seat belts, tobacco use prevention, and physical activity). Nurses know that for families to modify their behaviors, they must address specific barriers beyond their control, such as lack of money, lack of time, and stress. Rather than blaming families for their situations, community/public health nurses shift their thinking and focus on population health, which is concerned with changing the social, economic, political, and environmental conditions that affect families' health choices and outcomes.

The nurse can intervene in public policy at the community, organizational, and/or the individual level to help improve outcomes for individuals and families. For the most sustainable outcomes, nurses rely on the socio-environmental/socio-ecological approach pictured in Figure 17-1 to guide their actions in addressing factors that impede on families' choices to improve their health. The socio-environmental/socio-ecological model is based on systems theory

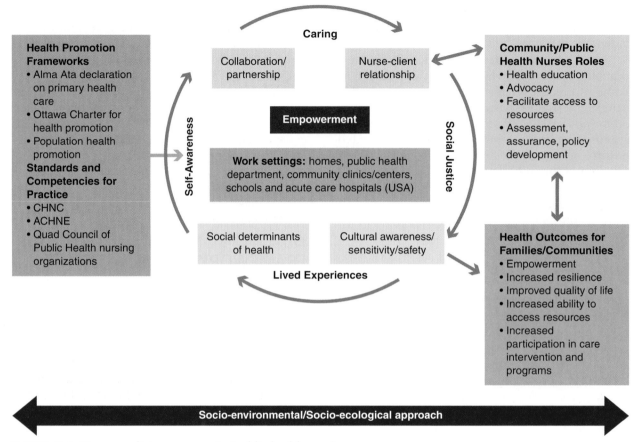

FIGURE 17-1 Contextualizing community/public health nursing.

and is grounded in an understanding of health as influenced by interrelationships between personal and environmental factors (Townsend & Foster, 2011; Young & Wharf Higgins, 2012).

The health of vulnerable families in various settings in society (e.g., homeless families, refugees, victims of intimate partner violence, and families in poverty) is affected negatively by many outside circumstances. An understanding of the factors that negatively affect family health, and strategies to modify these factors, is a priority for the role of community/public health nurses. The use of health promotion strategies is crucial to helping nurses to fulfill this priority. For example, the Breastfeeding Coalition of Oregon (2012) used the socio-ecological framework to outline who/what influences a mother's breastfeeding success and how public health providers can influence these influencers. Using the socio-ecological model, nurses are able to identify and address influences at the individual level (e.g., culture, lack of personal breastfeeding skills), interpersonal level (e.g., lack of support from family

and friends, lack of encouragement from health care providers), community/environmental level (e.g., neighborhood stress, lack of community breastfeeding accommodations, workplaces, and hospitals), and organizational level (e.g., public health organizations, pediatric groups, and the formula industry). Community/public health nurses can target these influencers using various health promotion strategies. At the individual level, nurses need to learn about cultural-specific barriers and needs and build mothers' skills in breastfeeding. At the interpersonal level, nurses can provide education and facilitate access to support services to key influencers to support mothers' breastfeeding efforts. At the community/environment level, community/public health nurses can get involved in advocacy activities such as organizing community activities during World Breastfeeding Week, disseminating breastfeeding materials at workplaces, and helping employers understand and initiate breastfeeding-friendly practices. Finally, at the organizational level, nurses can employ advocacy, coalition building, lobbying, and program evaluation skills targeting public health organizations, pediatric groups, and the formula industry.

Health Promotion Frameworks

Whether working with individuals, families, or a community, nurses use key health promotion (HP) frameworks to guide their work. While various health promotion documents exist, the following three frameworks remain central to health promotion interventions with families and communities:

1. The *Alma Ata Declaration on Primary Health Care* (WHO, 1978) laid the foundation for subsequent HP frameworks. It proposed five interconnected primary health care principles: health promotion, accessibility, public participation, appropriate technology, and intersectoral collaboration. The principles are based on access to health and health care, equity, and empowerment. Because families' social determinants (see Chapter 5) influence how they access resources, manage chronic conditions, and engage in healthy behaviors, addressing the social determinants of health for families by integrating primary health care principles is an integral component of nurses' work. For example, community health nurses who work with families to increase access to needed resources that are cost- or distance-prohibitive are practicing the primary health care principle of accessibility.

2. The *Ottawa Charter for Health Promotion* (WHO, 1986) proposed five overarching strategies: develop personal skills, create supportive environments, build healthy public policy, strengthen community action, and reorient health services. The strategies are intended to enable families and communities to increase control over and improve their health. Using these strategies, nurses work with families to address their physical, mental, and social needs, and attain prerequisites of health, such as shelter, food, sustainable resources, social justice, and equity. For example, to allow newcomers to acquire and sustain needed resources, nurses may facilitate personal skill development in resume writing, job seeking, and interviews for them to acquire employment.

3. The *Population Health Promotion Model* (Hamilton & Bhatti, 1996) draws on two decades of health promotion knowledge to guide practical actions. Key assumptions of this model include the recognition of determinants of health, the use of knowledge gained from research and practice, collaboration with families about the most appropriate actions to care for them, and building relationships with families based on mutual respect and caring, rather than on professional power. In addition to incorporating these assumptions into their work, nurses applying this model are able to focus on the concerns of at-risk groups, such as youth and women in at-risk families. The population health model focuses on the specific issues that put populations at risk. Interventions to modify these issues are targeted at a broad social, political, and economic level, and tailored to meet the needs of groups at the community and family level. For example, the elderly population is victim to ageist assumptions and treatment in society that may infringe on their social engagement and integration. Knowing this, nurses can educate communities and families about ways to prevent age discrimination and promote the health of the elderly.

Health Promotion Standards of Practice

To be effective in their roles, community/public health nurses integrate a broad range of competencies and interrelated standards of practice in their work. In Canada, community health nurses (CHNs) work within the Canadian Community Health Nursing Professional Practice Model outlined by the Community Health Nurses of Canada (CHNC). Seven standards are set by CHNC:

- Health Promotion, Prevention, and Health Protection
- Health Maintenance
- Restoration and Palliation
- Professional Relationships
- Capacity Building
- Access and Equity
- Professional Responsibility and Accountability (CHNC, 2011)

In addition, Core Competencies for Public Health in Canada (CPHA, 2010) provide a baseline for nurses to fulfill effective public health functions These standards/competencies guide community/

public health nurses in delivering acceptable, safe, and ethical care in an effort to protect, preserve, and promote the health of families (CHNC, 2011).

Standards/competencies are also an integral part of U.S. community/public health nursing practice. In the United States, community/public health nursing practice at the generalist and advanced or specialist level is competency based, and is divided into three tiers of practice: the public health nursing (PHN) generalist, the PHN specialist or manager, and the PHN organization leader or administrator (Quad Council of Public Health Nursing Organizations, 2011). The competencies that define these tiers of practice facilitate participatory health promotion in the community (Kulbok, Thatcher, & Meszaros, 2012). Community collaboration is essential to evolving community/public health nursing roles in the context of national initiatives, including *Healthy People 2020* (USDHHS, 2010), the Patient Protection and Affordable Care Act (ACA) (U.S. House of Representatives, 2010), the Family Leave Act HR 1723- 111th Congress, 2009), and the National Prevention, Health Promotion, and Public Health Council: Executive Order 13544 (Obama, 2010). In the United States, the Association of Community Health Nursing Educators (ACHNE) regularly updates the essential documents that guide baccalaureate and graduate nursing practice to delineate core knowledge and competencies related to community nursing practice. Core competencies include the following:

- Communication
- Epidemiology and biostatistics
- Community/population assessment and planning
- Policy development, assurance
- Health promotion and risk reduction
- Illness and disease management
- Information and health care technology
- Environmental health
- Global health
- Human diversity
- Ethics and social justice
- Coordination and management
- Emergency preparedness (ACHNE Education Committee, 2009)

Principles in the Process of Community/ Public Health Nurses' Work

Underlying the role of the community health/public health nurse in any context is a focus on maintenance

and promotion of health and prevention of illnesses and injuries. These concepts and principles include, but are not limited to, the social determinants of health, cultural awareness/sensitivity/safety, collaboration/partnership, nurse-client relationship, and empowerment. These principles are rooted in the values of caring, social justice, self-awareness, and honoring of families' and communities' lived experiences.

Social Determinants of Health

When working with families and communities, one of the most important concepts that influence community/public health nurses' thinking and action is social determinants of health. WHO (2012) defines social determinants of health as "the conditions in which people are born, grow, live, work and age, including the health system. These circumstances are shaped by the distribution of money, power and resources at global, national and local levels" (paragraph 1).

These social determinants of health, or conditions necessary for living, can include factors such as education, income and unemployment, social support and status, culture, housing, childhood development, and access to health services (Mikkonen & Raphael, 2010; Stamler & Gabriel, 2012). These and other determinants shape peoples' vulnerability, put them at risk for illnesses, and influence their social status and the level of respect they gain in society. The resulting health inequities are a substantial social justice issue, with a potentially life-threatening influence on the lives and health of people (WHO, 2009). Social injustice occurs when the health outcomes of individuals, groups, or communities are disproportionally affected because of differences in access and exposure to opportunities (e.g., education, employment).

The effects of the social determinants of health have been found to have a greater impact on health than behavioral factors, such as smoking and dietary habits (Mikkonen & Raphael, 2010). As a result of this significant influence on health equity, it is critical that community/public health nurses recognize and address the social determinants of health as the root cause of many issues faced by families and communities. For instance, community/public health nurses in Toronto, Ontario, working in the Investing in Families program (Table 17-1) provide resources, mental health care, and other support to sole-parent families with children between the ages of 6 and 18 years who are receiving social assistance. For families in this program, determinants of health can be many and interrelated. So, community/public health nurses target prioritized health needs, while trying to meet the holistic needs of families. Key determinants of health needs assessed by nurses would include emotional, economic, employment, educational, housing, and mental health needs. Often, nurses work to facilitate improved access to community mental health services and age-appropriate skill development programs for these family members (Browne et al., 2009).

Table 17-1	Examples of Community/Public Health Nursing			
Name of the Program	**Program Description**	**Role of the Community/ Public Health Nurse**	**Specific Example of Programming**	**Interprofessional Collaboration**
Healthy Baby Healthy Children	To enable all children to attain and sustain optimal health and developmental potential in the areas of • Positive parenting • Breastfeeding • Healthy family dynamics • Healthy eating, healthy weights, and physical activity • Growth and development	Assessments Referrals and recommendations Service coordination Supportive counseling Health promotion Health teaching Advocacy	Supports families with children from 0–4 years old Assesses growth and development, mother-child attachment Links and refers to various community agencies	Family home visitors Registered dietitians Nutrition promotion consultants Community nutrition educators High-risk consultants Health promotion consultants Mental health nurse consultants Infant hearing screeners Family support worker/ social workers Speech-language pathologist Program evaluators
Mental Health Promotion	To promote mental health in Toronto's diverse communities through competent clinical and consultative practice along with education, both internally to Toronto Public Health programs and externally to relevant community agencies	The mental health nurse consultant provides consultation to a variety of internal and external programs Education and training	Using a narrative approach, the mental health promotion team focuses on suicide prevention, violence prevention, and mental health promotion	Examples of internal consultations Healthy communities Chronic disease prevention Healthy families Communicable disease control Healthy environments Examples of external consultations Children's Aid Society Parks, Forestry, and Recreation Shelter, support, and housing Toronto social services Toronto community housing cooperation

(continued)

Table 17-1	Examples of Community/Public Health Nursing—cont'd			
Name of the Program	**Program Description**	**Role of the Community/ Public Health Nurse**	**Specific Example of Programming**	**Interprofessional Collaboration**
Investing in Families	To improve the economic, health, and social status of select families receiving social assistance in Toronto Overall goal of investing in family public health nursing service is to meet the health needs of select, vulnerable families receiving social assistance in Toronto To promote healthy lifestyles To increase personal resilience To improve physical and mental health To enhance social and community supports To improve the family's circumstances through greater access to employment training and supports	Assessments Referrals and recommendations Service coordination Supportive counseling Health promotion Health teaching Advocacy	Supports families with children from 6–18 years Receives referrals from Toronto Social Services Conducts detailed assessments Uses a strengths-based approach assessing the positive assets of the client	Toronto Social Services caseworker Public health nurse Health promotion consultant Mental health nurse consultant Recreationist
School Health	To enhance the physical, mental, social, and spiritual well-being of all the members of the school community To strengthen the capacity of school communities to achieve optimal health To enhance resilience in all school-age children and youth in the city of Toronto	Develop working relationships with all members of the school community to promote healthy schools Work with school communities to increase their capacity to identify health issues, develop and implement a plan of action, evaluate, and build on their successes Participate in existing health committees and advocate for the establishment of new school health committees Engage students and parents in healthy school initiatives Identify and consult with school communities on emerging health issues and trends Link between schools and Toronto Public Health (TPH) services and programs Partner with community organizations that support healthy schools	Liaison public nurse establishes a healthy school committee that assesses the needs of the school in a comprehensive manner The work of the school health committee includes • Creating a shared vision for a healthy school • Assessing strengths and needs of the school community • Prioritizing the issues • Developing a plan • Implementing the plan • Monitoring and evaluating the plan • Celebrating success	School administration School boards Teachers Students Parent council Internal programs in Toronto Public Health Community agencies

Cultural Awareness, Sensitivity, and Safety

Community/public health nurses will often find themselves working with a culturally diverse community. Within this diversity, often there are also inequalities between different groups. To illustrate, a report by the Institute of Medicine (IOM) found that ethnic and racial minority populations "tend to receive a lower quality of health care" (Smedley, Stith, & Nelson, 2003, p. 1) than majority populations even when access and income were controlled. The reasons for this finding are complex but include bias, time pressures, and lack of language and cultural understanding (Smedley et al., 2003). Rectifying these inequalities is not as simple as the nurse developing cultural competencies, because each individual, family, and community will have variations in values and practices based on their unique experiences (Browne et al., 2009). That is, minority populations and diverse communities are heterogeneous. There is wide variation within groups as well as between them.

It is important for nurses working with diverse populations to reflect on similarities and differences, and to undertake nurse-client relationships from that place of understanding. Because community/public health nurses work with people of diverse cultural backgrounds in various settings, it is crucial for them to engage in continuous reflective practice that explores their values and beliefs, as well as those of the groups/families they serve. This reflection can lead to sensitive, client-centered care.

Many families that community/public health nurses care for may not speak English well. This language barrier can create challenges to provision of care. Increasing the numbers of bilingual, bicultural, underrepresented providers is identified as one of the IOM solutions aimed at improving health disparities, and a way for institutions/organizations providing care to demonstrate cultural sensitivity. Refugee families may comprise a subset of those with limited or no English abilities that community/public health family nurses will serve. It is the professional responsibility of nurses to plan ahead for visits with such families and ensure that families understand what is going on in meetings, either through an interpreter or other means.

Added to this context, refugee families, in particular, may have survived war, disaster, and devastating trauma such as torture, rape, and/or watching family members or others die. Often, these families are enduring post-traumatic stress disorder, depression, or both, which may intensify the life challenges they face. In understanding the family's context, nurses need to be aware of not only how to satisfy language deficits, but understand how both theirs and the families' cultural backgrounds and perspectives influence the caring process.

Community/public health nurses can care for culturally diverse populations through the practice of cultural safety. Originally developed in New Zealand, cultural safety goes beyond cultural sensitivity and competence to address the attitudes of health care professionals, with an emphasis on discrimination, power, and the effects of colonization (National Aboriginal Health Organization [NAHO], 2006). Culturally safe care involves the nurse's reflection and self-awareness of his attitudes and beliefs with regard to "nationality, culture, age, sex, political and religious beliefs" (NAHO, 2006). This approach shifts the focus from the nurses' expertise to the expertise of the community, which defines whether the care has been safe or not (Brascoupé & Waters, 2009). Culturally safe care is provided to all within their cultural norms and values, and in a manner that garners their trust and promotes their empowerment. For example, in promoting health for Aboriginal families hurt by colonization processes, community/public health nurses would invite the families to partner with them. This process helps to build their capacity and facilitate trust (Brascoupé & Waters, 2009). Whereas culturally safe care can yield trust, open communication, and empowerment, culturally unsafe care can foster humiliation and disempowerment (Browne et al., 2009; NAHO, 2006). Promoting culturally safe care requires that nurses are sensitive to cultural differences, aware of their own cultural values, and knowledgeable enough to engage in culturally safe practices as defined by the clients.

Collaboration and Partnership

Community/public health nurses are usually one member of a team promoting health and well-being for families and communities. They work in collaboration with other key members of a community/family team. These collaborative relationships are crucial to reaching "a common vision to deliver care" (Betker & Bewick, 2012, p. 30). Nurses' participation in such collaborations depends on the type and purpose for which they were formed. For example, nurses working on a school health team collaborate with various stakeholders—teachers, parents, school board, government officials, and others—to promote health in schools. On such teams nurses may share specialized public health knowledge, share needed resources, interface with external partners, and/or contribute to decision-making processes. The essence of these collaborations is to share knowledge and power among key stakeholders to produce solutions that no one partner could achieve independently. Collaborations are ways in which nurses honor families and community members' lived experience. They realize that health solutions are like large puzzles. The lived experiences, knowledge, and expertise that other members bring to the team represent an important piece of the puzzle toward better health outcomes for families/communities.

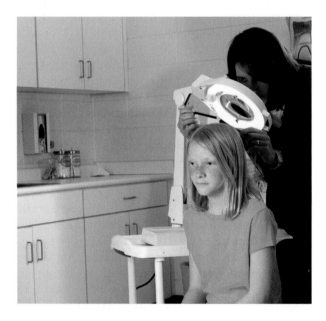

Interprofessional collaboration (IPC) refers to a collaborative partnership between two or more "different health and social care professions who regularly come together to solve problems or provide services" (Reeves, Lewin, Espin, & Zwarenstein, 2010, p. xiii). One example of IPC can be found in Ontario, Canada's, Family Health Teams. These primary care teams feature different professionals working in collaboration with each other and the families. These teams are in existence to address the shortage of family physicians in Ontario, increase access to and quality of care, and decrease the number of individuals visiting the emergency department for minor issues. Rather than going to see a family physician, residents of Ontario are able to receive primary care services from an entire team of health care professionals in the community. A Family Health Team might include a physician, registered nurse, nurse practitioner, pharmacist, social worker, and dietitian. Instead of being referred elsewhere, patients of the Family Health Team are able to acquire services from this team, which collaborates on the provision of their care. As another example, the Investing in Families program involves collaboration between various divisions across the city of Toronto—Parks, Forestry and Recreation, Toronto Social Services, Children Services, and Public Health. At any point, public health nurses can collaborate with any of these partners in the provision of care for families in the program.

Supporting families in their journey toward healthy change within their lives and health requires the development of collaborative partnerships between nurses and individuals, families, and communities (CHNC, 2011). Due to the complex nature of the social determinants of health, community/public health nurses will find themselves engaging in interdisciplinary teamwork. These interdisciplinary teams feature collaboration between individuals from a broad variety of disciplines, such as sociology, economics, and health sciences (Reeves et al., 2010). The collaborative relationships and partnerships with other professionals, disciplines, clients, families, and communities are critical to addressing the complexity of modern health care, because no single profession can accomplish this alone (Reeves et al., 2010).

Nurse-Client Relationship With Families and Communities

Community/public health nurses caring for families in the community rely on the nurse-client relationship as the foundation of their care (McNaughton, 2000, 2005). This relationship allows the nurse to maximize client involvement, recognize strengths and available resources, and ultimately facilitate empowerment at the individual, family, and community level (CHNC, 2011). Within these professional nurse-client relationships, the development of trust is critical. For example, the early phase of home visiting programs is based on the development of trust through helping clients identify problems, engage in mutual problem solving, make decisions about necessary health services, and adopt health-promoting behaviors. This trust-building phase is crucial to the success of a program such as this, for instance, because the efficacy of home visiting programs seems to be greater in longer-term, relationship-based programs than in shorter-term interventions (Koniak-Griffin et al., 2003; McNaughton, 2004). In addition to developing trust, the nurse-client relationship is established for the nurse and the client/families to work as partners toward accomplishing a mutual goal in health. As partners, the expertise of both is valuable to an interactive and therapeutic process.

The nurse-client relationship makes the difference in the success of intervention programs. McNaughton (2005) tested Peplau's Theory of Interpersonal Relations in Nursing as the framework for successful home visits. Using this theoretical framework, she underscored the development of successful nurse-client relationships between public health nurses and pregnant women at risk. The study focused on aspects of the nurse-client relationship, such as amount of nurse-client contact, time spent on assessment versus intervention, and communication skills. The results of this study suggested that the greater number of interactions over time contributes to more effective home visiting programs. Recommendations included strengthening the nurse-client relationship by increasing the number and frequency of visits, making assessments more concise, focusing on interventions, and providing education for nurses on meeting clients' emotional needs.

Doane and Varcoe (2007) state that in the current health care context, nurses' attention to relationships and implementing nursing values and goals is "becoming increasingly challenging" because nurses are managing increased patient acuity, higher nurse/patient ratios, and large workloads (p. 192). Still, relational practice continues to be intensely necessary for holistic, family-oriented care (Tuffrey, Finlay, & Lewis, 2007). Nurses working in the Healthy Baby Healthy Children (HBHC) (see Table 17-1) program, for instance, are trained in implementing principles of home visiting, which includes establishing therapeutic relationships with

families. According to a mental health nurse with the city of Toronto's Public Health Department, "one of the key approaches to building relationships with families in home visiting is for nurses to stay present in the visit, and relinquish the pressing need to fill out paper work" (A. Reid, personal communication, December 29, 2012).

In an example of relational practice, Doutrich and Marvin (2004) paired students enrolled in a community health nursing course with local public health nurses in their clinical rotations. The students reported that they learned to value relationship building with community clients as critical to practice. They described this relationship as the key to "finding the door," getting through it, and establishing a trust relationship with clients. Other important skills these students identified included becoming aware of their own biases, getting the client's story, and not blaming or judging the clients. This ability to remain nonjudgmental usually occurred when the students were truly engaged with families and understood the family's context.

Empowerment

Empowerment can be viewed as a process, a nurse-facilitated, strength-based process in which nurses and families work actively to share knowledge that promotes families capacity to find and sustain solutions for improved health outcomes (Malone, 2012). Most important, although nurses can facilitate empowerment, they cannot "give" it; it is a process as well as an outcome. Although hierarchical relationships still characterize the power dynamics within many provider-client relationships in health care, it should be the goal of all nurses to facilitate empowerment within their community/public health practice.

Facilitating healthy change can be difficult because of the complex and fluctuating nature of the family in its unique environment, and requires considerable skill in various empowerment strategies. Nurses must have the skills to build trusting, nonjudgmental relationships that allow/encourage families to tell their stories so they can jointly uncover the family's needs. For example, in care planning, nurses begin with the client's knowledge of his situation first because this approach recognizes and validates that clients have extensive knowledge about their own health (Anderson, Capuzzi, & Hatton, 2001). In a study by Falk-Rafael

(2001), the author revealed that active participation enabled individuals to increase control over their own health. Additionally, community/public health nurses must have skills that facilitate empowering families to make decisions about their health (Aston, Meagher-Stewart, Vukic, Sheppard-LeMoine, & Chircop, 2006; CHNC, 2011). For example, nurses can adopt the role of mediator or coach rather than director or decision maker. The Community Health Nurses of Canada (CHNC, 2011) suggests a client- or family-centered approach to helping clients problem-solve by building on their strengths and resources available to them. Rather than thinking of clients and families as "powerless" or the nurse as having "power over" them, Falk-Rafael (2001) conceptualizes power as coming from within the person and depending on the situation. Families who have hindrances to participating actively in empowering processes need an advocate. Community family nurses must learn to speak out and are obligated to be actively involved in issues and policies that affect their family clients. By doing so, nurses give voice to the policy and environmental factors that affect families, while also providing support for the "individual, family, group, community, and population to advocate for themselves" (CHNC, 2011, p. 19). These actions are important in transforming families and communities from a state of powerlessness to recognition of their own strengths.

SETTINGS WHERE COMMUNITY/ PUBLIC HEALTH NURSES WORK

Community/public health nurses care for families in a variety of settings, such as the following:

- In their homes
- Community settings, such as schools, clinics, adult day care or retirement centers, and correctional facilities
- Outside for homeless families
- Temporary housing, such as shelters or transitional or recovery programs

Although diversity exists in settings and families specific to socio-demographics (i.e., ethnicity, age, gender, sexual orientation, socioeconomic status, and family type), geographical location, attitudes, values, and subjective well-being, nurses use health promotion concepts/principles to go between people and their interactions with their environment in order to prevent illnesses and promote health (WHO, 2012). Knowing what strategies to use with different families requires an understanding of their diverse needs. This section covers three common settings where community/public health nurses work: family homes, community nursing centers, and public health departments.

Family Homes

Community/public health nurses working with families make home visits to assess family health status, needs, and their environment in order to develop specific interventions and identify available resources. For example, community/public health nurses conduct visits with their client, usually in the client's home, after a baby is born. They visit the home to determine safety, nutrition status, emotional needs, and relationship support needs. They then provide education, counseling, and referral as needed. Nurses help new mothers set goals for making healthy lifestyle choices and fostering personal growth. In some cases, nurses meet with families and their infant to conduct genetic counseling and inform them about the different tests that are possible. In other situations, nurses work with the elderly in their homes to help them remain in their home through case management, home care, and telehealth services. Assessment of the social, emotional, and physical development of families across the age span is a key role of the nurses in home visiting programs. Nurses assess the physical environment of the home, including safety hazards, such as availability of smoke detectors and fire extinguishers, any dangerous equipment, and the adequacy of running water and indoor plumbing.

In the HBHC program (see Table 17-1), for example, nurses promote the health of mothers and children in their homes. The HBHC program is a free public health initiative implemented in Ontario, Canada, to foster social, emotional, and physical health for vulnerable children. Families with anticipated poor birth outcomes, children with challenges to thrive, family stress, little social support, and low income are often referred to the program. In this program, public health nurses and family home visitors work together to assess families' situations (breastfeeding, nutrition, literacy, and social development, such as mother-child bonding), help them to access services and supports, and facilitate skill development of parents (Ontario Ministry of Children and Youth Services [OMCYS], 2011). Community nurses working with the Victorian Order of Nurses (VON) in Canada provide home care services to families recovering from an illness. These nurses conduct assessments, provide personal support, and facilitate links to community services (VON Canada, 2009).

Research has demonstrated the effectiveness of home visiting programs in the United States as well. The work of David Olds and his colleagues in the development and evaluation of the Nurse-Family Partnership program (Olds, 2002; Olds, Kitzman, Cole, & Robinson, 1997) illustrates the effectiveness of family-centered care and community/public health nursing home visitation. Nurses visited low-income, unmarried mothers and their children. The families with home visitation had significantly improved health outcomes. The home visitation was found to contribute to reductions in the following: number of the mothers' subsequent pregnancies, use of welfare, child abuse and neglect, and criminal behaviors for up to 15 years after the first child's birth. The home visit nursing program was found to reduce serious antisocial behavior and substance use as the high-risk children in the study entered adolescence (Olds et al., 1998). As adolescents, they ran away less often, were arrested and convicted less frequently, were less promiscuous, and smoked and drank alcohol less than comparable adolescents who did not receive home visits. The results of this work, which has been rigorously evaluated in controlled trials, demonstrate how community/public health nurse home visits in the community are beneficial for high-risk families.

More recently, Olds et al. (2004) reported on the outcomes of a longitudinal study of prenatal and infancy home visits by nurses, using a primarily African American urban sample. Their results indicate that, compared with the control group, women involved in the nurse home visiting program had fewer subsequent pregnancies and births, longer relationships with partners, and less use of welfare. Eckenrode et al. (2010) found that prenatal and infancy home visits reduced the rate of entrance into the criminal justice system and had other positive program effects that were more noticeable for girls than for boys. Moreover, McNaughton (2004) reviewed 13 home visiting interventions by registered nurses with maternal-child clients from 1980 to 2000 and found that about half of the interventions reported were effective in achieving the desired outcomes.

Empirical evidence for the efficacy of home visit programs reveals that further research is necessary, however. A recent search of the Cochrane Database of Systematic Reviews uncovered two reviews specific to nursing. Hodnett & Fredericks (2003) found that, although the evidence did not support the effectiveness of programs of nurse home visits during pregnancy in reducing the number of babies born too early or with low birth weight, the interventions probably resulted in reduced maternal anxiety and lower cesarean birth rates. Doggett, Burrett, and Osborn (2005) developed programs for postpartum women with drug and alcohol issues. They found evidence that home visits after the birth increased the engagement of these women in drug treatment services, but insufficient data were reported to confirm whether this improved the health of the baby or the mother. Further research is needed, with visits starting during pregnancy. It is important to note that both reviews also involved interventions by a variety of health care professionals, as well as trained lay health workers. In both of these situations, therefore, it is difficult to determine the individual effect of nursing interventions on families. More research is needed tying theory to interventions with regard to nursing home visits and to specify the types of interventions and quantity that are most effective.

Community Nursing Centers

Community/public health nurses also practice within community nursing centers. These unique centers, found in both rural and urban communities in the United States, offer the public access to a wide array of nursing services in a single setting. These programs typically provide services that are not available elsewhere and are likely to focus on the needs of underserved populations (Glick, 1999; Newman, 2005). Within these centers, nurses focus on promoting health and preventing disease; they offer health screening, education, and well-child care. In addition, such centers may offer secondary and tertiary prevention services, such as management of acute and chronic health conditions, and mental health counseling.

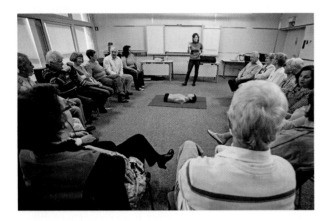

The model for these centers is usually multidisciplinary and strives to provide affordable, accessible, acceptable care that serves to empower individuals across the life span to meet their own health care goals. The focus on social justice in many of these centers is realized by attempts to reach out to marginalized populations and to provide comprehensive, quality, nonjudgmental health care. In keeping with the community-as-mindset concept, community nursing centers may be either physical places or they may be embedded in more traditional health care settings. Some community nursing centers provide educational experiences for nursing students and students from other disciplines, making these centers a place where nursing practice, theory, and research can blend in a model that serves those who need health care the most.

The Ontario Early Years Centers (OEYCs) is a similar model in Canada. OEYCs are government-funded, early learning drop-in programs for parents/caregivers and children that are located in communities across the province of Ontario. Public health nurses and other early years professionals and experts from the community assist parents and caregivers to get the help they need to promote long-term learning, positive behavior, and health among children within the first 6 years of their lives. Parents, caregivers, and children participate actively in educational activities together, while public health nurses provide guidance and support for new parenting skills and linkages to other services in the community, such as prenatal nutrition programs (OMCYS, 2010).

Public Health Departments

Probably the most widely known and accepted model for center-based services for families is that used by county and state departments of health services. Public health departments serve the needs of individuals and families across the life span in both center- and home-based models and, more recently, in acute care settings in the United States. These departments include services to vulnerable groups, such as pregnant and childbearing families (women, infants, and children programs [WIC]), children with special health care needs, individuals at risk for or diagnosed with infectious diseases, and those with chronic conditions. Lahr, Rosenberg, and Lapidus (2005) document an example of effective public health nursing practice with families. These investigators found that, compared with parents receiving newborn care and education from private clinics, those receiving care and education in public health departments were less likely to choose prone sleeping positions for their infant, a major public health initiative to reduce sudden infant death syndrome.

Public health departments care for high-risk clients and are in a unique position to address issues of intimate partner violence, for instance. Shattuck (2002) reports positive outcomes from an intervention program targeted toward preparing family planning nurses who work in a public health department to recognize domestic violence. The intervention, which consisted of a formal curriculum offered to nursing staff, increased intimate partner violence screening from 0% before the program to 16% in a 4-week period, and resulted in approximately 12% of women who screened positive for violence. With respect to reducing intimate partner violence, a goal for *Healthy People 2020* (USDHHS, 2010), a role clearly exists for family-focused community nurses to make a difference.

Although many public health department services are aimed at childbearing and childrearing families, there are programs for older adults with chronic illness. One example is a public health nursing program aimed at educating older adults about their high blood cholesterol levels, implementing better dietary practices, and reducing cholesterol levels. This nursing intervention consisted of three individual diet counseling sessions given by public health nurses. The nurses used a structured dietary intervention (Food for Heart Program), referred elders to a nutritionist if they did not reach lipid goals at 3-month follow-up, made reinforcement phone calls, and sent newsletters. Cholesterol reduction was similar between the groups who received the special interventions and those who received a minimal intervention, but the special intervention group had significantly lower dietary risk assessment scores (Ammerman et al., 2003).

Chronic pain management in older adults living in the community is a pervasive public health problem that can be amenable to public health nursing interventions aimed at individuals and families. Dewar (2006) has reviewed the literature about chronic pain management by nurses in the community. Dewar found that most studies focused on pain assessment tools, and that less focus was on how older adults managed pain and what community resources were available to help these families with pain-management issues. An effective nurse-patient relationship is important in comprehensive assessment and management of pain in the older adult population.

The relationship between community nurses and families of older adults was also found to be important in a study of community nurses working with older clients in Sweden (Weman & Fagerberg, 2006). Caring for older families in the community requires nurses to be alert for signs of elder abuse. Potter (2004) notes that community nurses were often the only professionals invited into peoples' homes, so they must be alert to the many forms abuse takes: physical, psychological, financial, sexual, and verbal. Nurses also must be aware of omission of needed support and attention as a type of abuse. Nurses need to know how to report elder abuse in their communities and be willing to take quick action to prevent further abuse. In many U.S. states, nurses are mandatory reporters of elder abuse. For example, in the states of Oregon and Washington, nurses must report abuse of older adults who sustain physical harm, financial exploitation, verbal or emotional abuse, lack of basic care, involuntary seclusion, wrongful restraint, unwanted sexual contact, or abandonment by the caregiver. Each state has an individual policy for reporting to protective services. More information about reporting elder abuse in the United States can be found at the National Clearinghouse on Abuse in Later Life (NCALL) Web site (http://www.ncall.us).

COMMUNITY/PUBLIC HEALTH NURSING ROLES WITH FAMILIES AND COMMUNITY

In their capacities, community/public health nurses play several roles. These include, but are not limited to, health education, advocacy, facilitation of access to health resources, assessment, assurance, policy development, referrals, building capacity, and consultation. Table 17-1 illustrates some of the diverse roles assumed by these nurses. In this section we discuss community/public health nursing roles in health education, facilitation of resources, assessment, assurance, and policy development.

Health Education

Health education is essential to the promotion of health and the prevention of disease in families. Using information gained through family health appraisals/assessments, community health nurses reinforce health-promoting behaviors, and provide health information and teaching in identified at-risk areas. The Centers for Disease Control and Prevention (CDC) lists five major determinants of health: (1) genes and biology, (2) health behaviors, (3) social environment or social characteristics, (4) physical environment or total ecology, and (5) health services or medical care (CDC, 2012; WHO, 2012). Community/public health nurses have a role in facilitating high-level wellness for their clients by advocating for positive changes in health determinants, including health behaviors, social environment and characteristics, physical environment and ecology, and health services.

Community health nurses use a variety of strategies to modify behaviors, characteristics, or care limitations identified in the health appraisal. Teaching and health information can be used to discuss immunizations, nutrition, rest, exercise, use of seat belts, and abuse of harmful substances, such as alcohol and drugs. Community health nurses may refer families to programs and resources that assist in their lifestyle modifications (e.g., smoking cessation classes, exercise programs). One example of this is the "Biggest Loser" intervention program that was designed to assist clients in a West Virginia county to lose weight. This intervention was developed in response to high obesity rates and included a program based loosely on the television show of the same name. Nurses provided specific education, social supports, weigh-ins, exercise, and dietary help to the participants, though in the public health intervention, no one was voted off.

Health teaching, based on appraisal of the physical environment, might also include information on child safety and prevention of falls for older adults. Other teaching might focus on psychological or social environmental problems, such as family communications or dealing with peer pressure. In some situations, community health nurses promote a healthy and safe environment by meeting with the school board to provide evidence about playground hazards or poor food-handling practices.

Facilitate Access to Resources

A major health-promotion strategy is to ensure access to health promotion and prevention services, including immunizations, family planning, prenatal care, well-child care, nutrition, exercise classes, and dental hygiene. These services may be provided directly by community health nurses, or community health nurses facilitate access to these services through referrals, case management, discharge planning, advocacy, coordination, and collaboration.

Nurses must consider access to resources within a context of what choices families realistically have. For example, eating healthy meals requires that healthy foods be available in locations that families can access easily and without expensive transportation. Also, accessing health providers and facilities requires that, in the United States, families have some type of health insurance or other means to pay. According to the 2010 U.S. census report, almost 50 million Americans (16%) do not have health insurance (DeNavas-Walt, Proctor, & Smith, 2012). This number is scheduled to improve with the implementation of the Affordable Care Act (ACA).

Facilitating access to resources for families who are deprived due to race, social class, and gender requires understanding of how social injustice operates on a social level to cause such depravity. Paul Farmer, a physician and author best known for his medical work in Haiti and worldwide with tuberculosis and AIDS, wrote about structural violence in his book, *Pathologies of Power: Health, Human Rights and the New War on the Poor* (Farmer, 2003). Structural violence refers to historical, economic, and political roots of generational oppression. It is about unequal treatment, racism, classism, and discrimination. In short, it refers to systematized, unequal access to resources. Working toward social justice requires a partnership between families and professionals. The community/public health nurses' responses to the structural violence perpetuated by policy, the myth of meritocracy (that anyone who is hard working and deserving can succeed), and our biases make it an ethical obligation to engage in deep relational practice with the families we serve.

Assessment, Assurance, and Policy Development

Community/public health nurses are engaged in the core public health functions of assessment, assurance, and policy development. These core functions include assessing and monitoring the health of communities and populations at risk to identify health problems and priorities; ensuring that all populations have access to appropriate and cost-effective care (assurance); and formulating policies designed to solve identified local and national health problems and priorities. Assessment is facilitated by the trust that public health nurses have earned from their clients, agencies, and private providers, trust that provides ready access to populations that are otherwise difficult to access and engage in health care. In addition, these nurses have knowledge of current and emerging health issues through their daily contact with high-risk and vulnerable populations. This trust and knowledge provides the foundation for ways nurses work with communities (populations) and families and individuals in the community. Table 17-2 lists the different assessment approaches nurses can use in the community, based on the focus of the health care.

Assurance activities are the direct individual-focused services that public health nurses provide. Measuring health department performance is another example of assurance (Novick, 2003; Zahner & Vandermause, 2003). Although the current shift in emphasis is toward assessment and policy development, critical assurance activities remain for the public health nurse. Assurance activities at the community, family, and individual levels are outlined in Table 17-3.

In 1988 the Institute of Medicine (IOM) compiled a report called *The Future of Public Health*. At that time the IOM articulated the Core Functions

Table 17-2	Comparison of Assessment Approaches	
Community	**Family**	**Individual**
Analyze data on and needs of specific populations or geographical area.	Evaluate a specific family's strengths and areas of concern. This involves a comprehensive assessment of the physical, social, and mental health needs of the family.	Identify individuals within the family who are in need of services.
Identify and interact with key community leaders, both formally and informally.		Evaluate the functional capacity of the individual through the use of specific assessment measures, including physical, social, and mental health screening tools.
Identify target populations that may be at risk. These populations may include families living in high-density low-income areas, preschool children, primary and secondary school children, and elderly adults.	Evaluate the family's living environment, looking specifically at support, relationships, and other factors that might have a significant impact on family health outcomes.	Develop a nursing diagnosis for the individual that describes a problem or potential problem, causative factors, and contributing factors.
Participate in data collection on a target population.		Develop a nursing care plan for the individual.
Conduct surveys or observe targeted populations, such as preschools, jails, and detention centers, to gain a better understanding of needs.	Assess the larger environment in which the family lives (their block or specific community) for safety, access, and other related issues.	

Table 17-3	Assurance Activities in Community, Family, and Individual Care	
Community	**Family**	**Individual**
Provide service to target populations, such as child care centers, preschools, worksites, minority communities, jails, juvenile detention facilities, and homeless shelters. Interventions may include health screening, education, health promotion, and injury prevention programs.	Provide services to a cluster of families within a geographical setting. Services may be provided in a variety of settings, including homes, child care centers, preschools, and schools. Services may include physical assessment, health education and counseling, and health and developmental screening.	Provide nursing services based on standards of nursing practice to individuals across the age continuum. These services may encompass a variety of programs including, specifically, First Steps and Children With Special Health Care Needs, and more generally, child abuse prevention, immunizations, well-child care, and HIV/AIDS programs.
Improve quality assurance activities with various health care providers in the community. Examples include education on new immunization policies, educational programs for communicable disease control, assistance in developing effective approaches, and support techniques for high-risk populations.	Provide care in a nursing clinic to a specific group of families in a geographical location.	Assess and support the individual's progress toward meeting outcome goals.
Maintain safe levels of communicable disease surveillance and outbreak control.		Consult with other health care providers and team members regarding the individual's plan of care.
Participate in research or demonstration projects.		Prioritize individual's needs on an ongoing basis.
Provide expert public health consultation in the community.		Participate on quality-assurance teams to measure the quality of care provided.
Ensure that standards of care are met within the community (assurance).		

of Public Health and the Ten Essential Services of Public Health in the United States. The Core Functions identified in this report were Assessment, Policy Development, and Assurance (IOM, 1988). These remain the guiding framework for U.S. Public Health (CDC, 2011). In some areas over time this changed the focus of public health from delivering primary health care or providing safety-net services to individuals to a more population, upstream, data-driven, policy-focused organization. See Table 17-4 to review ways that policy comes about relative to public health. Though many local health departments still provide some level of health care to individuals or families, comprised mainly of mothers and children, this movement toward the core functions has meant changes in what it means to be a public health nurse or provider. For example, the growing number of new cases of pertussis in the United States requires us to consider all health as public health. With most serious morbidity and mortality from pertussis occurring in infants who are too young to mount an immune response to active

vaccines, community/public health nurses are actively working in acute care and long-term care facilities to vaccinate all adults to provide "herd" immunity that shields our youngest and most vulnerable family members.

In response to the guiding framework of the core functions and the research identifying built environment and the social determinants of health, one local public health department decided to develop a lens for public health planning and policy. Called the Growing Healthier Report, it was developed to inform the process of updating the comprehensive growth management plan. The Growing Healthier Report is comprised of eight chapters, each having to do with one of the social determinants of health. The chapters are (1) Access to Healthy Food; (2) Active Transportation and Land Use; (3) Parks and Open Spaces; (4) Economic Opportunity; (5) Affordable, Quality Housing; (6) Climate Change and Human Health; (7) Environmental Quality; and (8) Safety and Social Connections. Each chapter contains the up-to-date research evidence, the current conditions locally (local data from the assessment

Table 17-4   Activities That Influence Policy Development

Community	Family	Individual
Provide leadership in convening and facilitating community groups to evaluate health concerns and develop a plan to address the concerns.	Recommend new or increased services to families based on identified needs.	Recommend or assist in the development of standards for individual client care.
Recommend specific training and programs to meet identified health needs.	Recommend programs to meet specific families' needs within a geographical area.	Recommend or adopt risk classification systems to assist with prioritizing individual client care.
Raise awareness of key policymakers about health regulations, budget decisions, and other factors that may negatively affect the health of communities.	Facilitate networking with families with similar needs or issues. Guide policymakers on specific issues that affect clusters of families.	Participate in establishing criteria for opening, closing, or referring individual cases.
Recommend programs to target populations such as child care centers, retirement centers, jails, juvenile detention facilities, homeless shelters, worksites, and minority communities.	Request additional data and analyze information to identify trends in a group or cluster of families.	Participate in the development of job descriptions to establish roles for various team members who will provide service to individuals.
Act as an advocate for the community and individuals who are not willing or able to speak to policymakers about issues and programs of concern.	Identify key families in a community who may either oppose or support specific policies or programs, and develop appropriate and effective intervention strategies to use with these families.	
Work with business and industry to develop employee health programs.		

function), conditions research identified as "needed to thrive," and policy/planning recommendations (the policy development function). The goals and timelines are measurable and there are strategies that can provide benchmarks (the assurance function) to help public health and community members understand how well the strategies are working. See Box 17-1 for an example of health policy.

TRENDS IN PUBLIC HEALTH

Community/public health nursing positions in the United States, rather than growing with population needs, have declined. In the past two decades, fewer nurses are public health nurses and these nurses make up a lower proportion of the public health workforce (Baldwin, Lyons, & Issel, 2011). Like nurses in many contexts, those community/public health nurses with positions in public health are being asked to do more with less. Responding to workforce and economic constraints, some public health services have switched to a focus on the core functions and community/neighborhood interventions. Skills in connecting planning to social determinants of health, understanding the multi-perspective views of all stakeholders, and being able to translate (almost in a multilingual way) the contextual realities of clients are among the skills required (SmithBattle, Diekemper, & Leander, 2004). Community/public health nurses today must become comfortable with geographical information system (GIS) (Box 17-2) mapping and epidemiology, and should know and be able to connect with the communities these representations depict.

Nurse Practitioner Roles in Community/Public Health Nursing

In April 2013, the National Organization of Nurse Practitioner Faculties (NONPF) released the following six nurse practitioner population-foci competencies: Family/Across the Lifespan, Neonatal, Acute Care Pediatric, Primary Care Pediatric, Psychiatric–Mental Health, and Women's Health/Gender Related. NONPF incorporated population health into nursing education programs for nurse practitioners, and into its accreditation for these programs, with the intent that all nurse practitioners be educated and competent in population health.

One example of a program employing nurse practitioners in population health takes place in Oregon. Oregon has a comprehensive network of child abuse assessment and intervention centers designed to minimize trauma to child abuse victims

---

BOX 17-1
Example of Public Health Policy

The *Growing Healthier Report* (Clark County Public Health, 2012) is considered a living document and it will change over time. One of the chapters, "Access to Healthy Food," is of high concern to Clark County, Washington, where two-thirds of the adults and one-third of 10th-graders are overweight or obese. Research supports the idea that people's eating choices are strongly affected by the options available. So having convenient healthy choices increases the likelihood of making healthy choices. Likewise, being surrounded by sources of unhealthy food leads to an increased risk for obesity and chronic diseases. One goal related to the "Access to Healthy Food" chapter is "protect resources that enhance community food security" with a measurable objective that says, "By 2015, the County will adopt a local agricultural protection plan" (p. 10). Policies and strategies to meet this objective include the following: "3.1 Implement measures to increase the consumption and/or sale of locally-produced food. 3.1.1 Support and promote current farmers markets and development of new markets. 3.1.2 Work with farmers to develop a measure of healthy food distribution. 3.1.3 Require or incentivize community gardens or urban agriculture space to accompany new development through dedications, easements, or impact fees. 3.1.4 Establish community gardens in existing parks and open spaces" (p. 10).

BOX 17-2
Geographical Information Systems

Geographical information systems (GISs) visually display, analyze, and manipulate spatial data to locate geographical areas, potential hazards, water sources, and other important information. This digital technology helps the user to understand trends and issues of concern by rendering data visually, in the forms of maps, charts, histograms, and a variety of reports. Having access to this type of detailed data in visual format allows community/public health nurses to intervene more quickly and accurately to enhance public health and safety.

by coordinating the local community's response to reports of suspected child abuse. This community-based, interprofessional child maltreatment intervention model offers population-focused nurse practitioners the opportunity to prevent, recognize early, and treat families that have experienced dysfunction and/or child maltreatment in order to prevent some of the negative life impacts of these early experiences. Services include interviews of suspected victims of child abuse, medical evaluations, mental health treatment and/or referrals, provision or coordination of other victim services, and individual- and community-specific needs. This important work grew, in part, out of findings from the Adverse Childhood Events (ACES) study (Felitti et al., 1998). This study revealed the following: (1) more than half of study participants had experienced at least one of the adverse events studied (psychological, physical, or sexual abuse; violence against mother; or living with household members who were substance abusers, mentally ill or suicidal, or ever imprisoned); (2) persons who had experienced four or more categories of childhood exposure, compared to those who had experienced none, had a 4- to 12-fold increased health risk for alcoholism, drug abuse, depression, and suicide; (3) persons who had experienced four or more categories of childhood exposure had a 2- to 4-fold increase in smoking, poor self-rated health, greater than 50 sexual intercourse partners, and sexually transmitted disease; and (4) persons who had experienced four or more categories of childhood exposure had a 1.4- to 1.6-fold increase in physical inactivity and severe obesity. Quality care for families in the community can be enhanced when rigid understandings of place and/or position of nursing care are rethought and flexed according to family and community needs.

Population-focused nurse practitioners often fill positions in inpatient and outpatient settings that focus on the care of groups of clients with particular chronic illnesses, such as diabetes or heart disease. These nurse practitioners provide primary care to these clients, as well as offer individual and group health education and other health promotion activities. Their interest and expertise in a particular health condition lends itself well to advocating for necessary resources for their population of interest, and to becoming active in health policy change on behalf of their clients.

Family Case Study: Jamison-Jensen Family

We visited the Jamison-Jensen family in their home. Stacie Jensen is a 21-year-old high-school graduate, sometimes girlfriend of Griff Jamison, and a first-time mom. Her daughter Danni was born at 27 weeks' gestation with a birth weight of 2½ pounds. Danni remained in the neonatal intensive care unit (NICU) for 10 weeks and encountered many complications, including infection, respiratory compromise, and vision difficulties. The local public health nurse assigned to care for the family visited them briefly 1 week before Danni's hospital discharge to establish a relationship, and to describe available in-home and clinic-based services. One week after Danni's arrival home the nurse visited again. Stacie and Danni seemed to be settling into their new routines at home fairly well, but concern about Danni's well-being had relegated Stacie to being a captive in her own home. She was so worried about Danni getting sick that she had asked friends not to visit at a time when she needed all the support she could get. When asked about supportive people in her life, she reported that Griff was not around much. Because Stacie was unable to work, she moved into a small house with her stepfather, mother, and brother, but Stacie's relationships with them were tenuous and she yearned for a home of her own. Figure 17-2 presents the Jamison-Jensen family genogram. The home environment was clean but very crowded with the oxygen and monitoring equipment required for Danni's care. Stacie was overwhelmed by the physical care of Danni, and worried that she would do something wrong. With these issues so all-consuming, the idea of filling out the many forms required for financial support and medical insurance to which Danni was entitled was too much. Stacie had tears in her eyes when she told the community health nurse, "I don't think I can do this anymore!" A plan of care for the family utilized a family-as-client perspective in helping them to develop much-needed community. Initial health appraisal found an infant whose growth and development was on target for her prematurity-corrected age, and who was receiving appropriate preventive well-child care and immunizations from a local nurse practitioner. This provider-family microsystem was stable and just required maintenance: refer to Figure 17-3, the Jamison-Jenson family ecomap. During the 13 weeks of Danni's hospitalization, the NICU become a supportive community for Stacie, and she missed it. Because Stacie derived comfort from this health care community, the nurse connected her to a support group for parents of children with special needs. The nurse also assessed the health of Griff and Stacie's relationship.

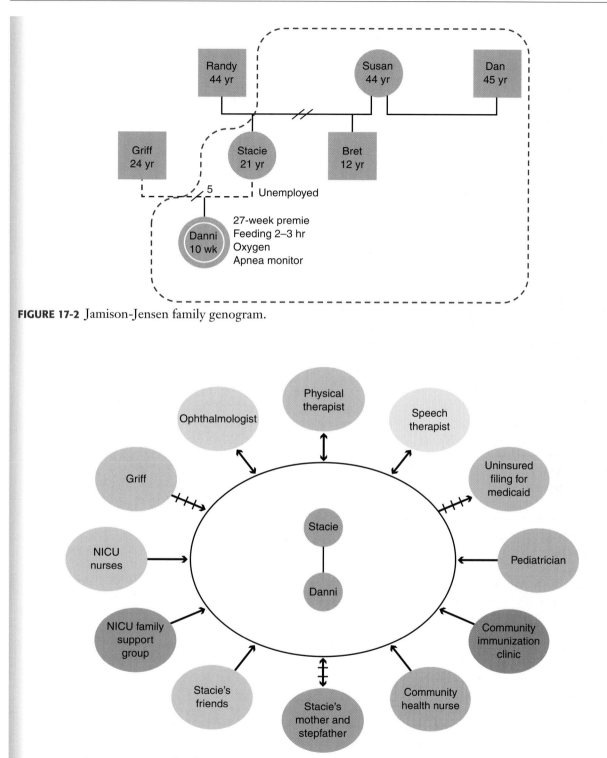

FIGURE 17-2 Jamison-Jensen family genogram.

FIGURE 17-3 Jamison-Jensen family ecomap.

(continued)

With Danni's health and development progressing nicely at 6 months of age, Griff felt more comfortable with supporting Stacie and caring for Danni. The relationship seemed to be a nurturing one, so the nurse helped the parents arrange respite care so that they had some time alone as a couple. Stacie knew that their family needed to move from her parents' home and start life on their own, but she felt hopeless about opportunities for work. The nurse answered questions about social and financial services that were available to help the family, and supported and encouraged Stacie and Griff as they completed the necessary paperwork and interviews. Helping this family move into their own home required creativity. Ultimately, they chose to move in with another family with a young infant so that child care issues could be shared. The family, with the help of the nurse, entered this new extended-family microsystem with a better understanding of the importance of communication in building stable relationships. With Danni's health much improved at year's end, the nurse and the family began the process of terminating the nurse-client relationship.

Setting: Home.

Health Promotion/Standard:
- Create supportive environment.

Concepts/Principles Used By Nurse:
- Access to resources
- Determinant of health (employment, housing)
- Nurse-client relationship

Role Played By Nurse:
- Advocate
- Support
- Facilitate access to support and resource

SUMMARY

Community health nurses forge strong nurse-client partnerships as they maneuver through the maze of interventions and resources in providing family-centered nursing. They are concerned with the health of families and the ways in which family health influences the health of communities.

- Nurses foster interconnectedness among families in the community.
- The settings in which community/public health nurses work with families vary and include, but are not limited to, public and private health agencies, schools, and occupational sites.
- Community/public health nursing roles vary according to whether the nurse is focusing on the family as the unit of care in the context of the community, or focusing on the health of the community with families being a subunit.
- Community/public health nurses aim to meet the holistic needs of families and communities while targeting prioritized health needs.
- Rather than blaming families for their situations, community/public health nurses consider how social, political, economic, and environmental conditions affect families' health choices and outcomes.
- Family interventions in the community are targeted toward primary, secondary, and tertiary prevention. The nurse-family relationship is central in interventions at all three levels of prevention.
- Interventions for families are planned, implemented, and evaluated from a health promotion perspective.
- Using a combination of relational collaboration and health promotion strategies and principles, community/public health nurses strive to partner with families to assist with all levels of healthy change.

REFERENCES

ACHNE Education Committee. (2009). Essentials of baccalaureate nursing education for entry level community/public health nursing. Retrieved from http://www.achne.org/files/Essentials OfBaccalaureate_Fall_2009.pdf

American Public Health Association. (2008). Public health nursing section. Retrieved from http://www.apha.org/membergroups/sections/aphasections/phn

Ammerman, A. S., Keyserling, T. C., Atwood, J. R., Hosking, J. D., Zayed, H., & Krasny, C. (2003). A randomized controlled trial of a public health nurse directed treatment program for rural patients with high blood cholesterol. *Preventive Medicine, 36*(3), 340–351.

Anderson, D. G., Capuzzi, C., & Hatton, D. C. (2001). Families and public health nursing in the community. In S. M. Harmon Hanson (Ed.), *Family health care nursing* (2nd ed., pp. 345–361). Philadelphia, PA: F. A. Davis.

Aston, M., Meagher-Stewart, D., Vukic, A., Sheppard-LeMoine, D., & Chircop, A. (2006). Family nursing and empowering relationships. *Pediatric Nursing, 32*(1), 61–67.

Baldwin, K. A., Lyons, R. L., & Issel, M. (2011). Creating a brand image for public health nursing. *Public Health Nursing, 28*(1), 57–67.

Bender, K., Benjamin, G., Fallon, M., Jarris, P. E., & Libbey, P. M. (2007). Commentary: Exploring accreditation: Striving for a consensus model. *Journal of Public Health Management Practice, 13*(4), 334–336.

Berkman, L. F., & Kawachi, I. (2000). *Social epidemiology.* New York, NY: Oxford University Press.

Betker, C., & Bewick, D. (2012). Financing, policy, and politics of healthcare delivery. In L. L. Stamler & L. Yiu (Eds.), *Community health nursing: A Canadian perspective* (3rd ed., pp. 21–41). Toronto, ON: Pearson Prentice Hall.

Brascoupé, S., & Waters, C. (2009). Cultural safety—Exploring the applicability of the concept of cultural safety to Aboriginal health and community wellness. *Journal of Aboriginal Health, 5*(2), 6–41. Retrieved from http://www.naho.ca/jah/english/archives.php

Breastfeeding Coalition of Oregon. (2012). Brochure. Retrieved from http://www.breastfeedingor.org/communities/social-ecological-model

Browne, A. J., Varcoe, C., Smye, V., Reimer-Kirkham, S., Lynam, M. J., & Wong, S. (2009). Cultural safety and challenges of translating critically oriented knowledge in practice. *Nursing Philosophy, 10*, 167–179.

Canadian Public Health Association. (2010). Public health–Community health nursing practice in Canada. Retrieved from http://www.cpha.ca/uploads/pubs/3-1bk04214.pdf

Centers for Disease Control and Prevention. (2011). Updated recommendations for use of tetanus toxoid, reduced diphtheria toxoid and acellular pertussis (Tdap) vaccine in pregnant women and persons who have or anticipate having close contact with an infant aged less than 12 months—Advisory Committee on Immunization Practices (ACIP). *MMWR Morbidity and Mortality Weekly Report, 60*(41), 1424–1426.

Centers for Disease Control and Prevention. (2012). Social determinants of health. Retrieved from http://www.cdc.gov/socialdeterminants/FAQ.htm

Clark County Public Health. (2012). Growing healthier report. Retrieved from http://www.clark.wa.gov/public-health/community/growing_healthy/documents.html

Community Health Nurses of Canada. (2011). *Canadian community health nursing: Professional practice models and standards of practice, revised.* Toronto, ON: Author. Retrieved from http://www.chnc.ca/documents/CHNC-Professional-PracticeModel- EN/index.html

DeNavas-Walt, C., Proctor, B. D., & Smith, J. C. (2012). Income, poverty, and health insurance coverage in the United States: 2011. Retrieved from http://www.census.gov/prod/2012pubs/p60-243.pdf

Dewar, A. (2006). Assessment and management of chronic pain in the older person living in the community. *American Journal of Advanced Nursing, 24*(1), 33–38.

Doane, G. H., & Varcoe, C. (2007). Relational practice and nursing obligations. *Advances in Nursing Science, 30*(3), 192–205.

Doggett, C., Burrett, S., & Osborn, D. A. (2005). Home visits during pregnancy and after birth for women with an alcohol or drug problem. *Cochrane Database of Systematic Reviews, 4*, CD004456.

Doutrich, D., & Marvin, M. (2004). Education and practice: Dynamic partners in improving cultural competence in public health. *Family and Community Health, 27*(4), 298–307.

Doutrich, D., Wros, P., Valdez, R., & Ruiz, M. E. (2005). Professional values of Hispanic nurses: The educational experience. *International Hispanic Health Care, 3*(3), 161–170.

Eckenrode, J., Campa, M., Luckey, D. W., Henerson, M. A., Cole, R., Kitzman, H., . . . Olds, D. (2010). Long-term effects of prenatal and infancy nurse home visitation on the life course of youths: 19 year follow-up of a randomized trial. *JAMA Pediatrics, 164*(1), 9–15.

Falk-Rafael, A. (2001). Empowerment as a process of evolving consciousness: A model of empowered caring. *Advances in Nursing Science, 24*(1), 1–16.

Farmer, P. (2003). *Pathologies of power: Health, human rights and the new war on the poor.* Berkeley, CA: California University Press.

Felitti, V. J., Anda, R. F., Nordenberg, D., Williamson, D. F., Spitz, A. M., Edwards, V., . . . Marks, J. S. (1998). Relationship of childhood abuse and household dysfunction to many of the leading causes of death in adults. The Adverse Childhood Experiences (ACE) study. *American Journal of Preventive Medicine, 14*, 245–258.

Glick, D. F. (1999). Advanced practice community health nursing in community nursing centers: A holistic approach to the community as client. *Holistic Nursing Practice, 13*(4), 19–27.

Hamilton, N., & Bhatti, T. (1996). *Population health promotion: An integrated model of population health and health promotion.* Ottawa, ON: Health Promotion Development Division, Health Canada.

Hodnett, E. D., & Fredericks, S. (2003). Support during pregnancy for women at increased risk of low birth weight babies. *Cochrane Database of Systematic Reviews, 3*, CD000198.

H.R. 1723—111th Congress: *Family Leave Insurance Act of 2009.* (2009). Retrieved from http://www.govtrack.us/congress/bills/111/hr1723

H.R. 3590-111th Congress of the United States of America: *Patient Protection and Affordable Care Act.* (2010). Retrieved from http://democrats.senate.gov/pdfs/reform/patient-protection-affordable-care-act-as-passed.pdf

Institute of Medicine. (1988). *The future of public health.* Washington, DC: National Academy Press.

Kaiser, K. L., Hays, B. J. Cho, W., & Agrawal, W. (2002). Examining health problems and intensity of need for care in family-focused community and public health nursing. *Journal of Community Health Nursing, 19*(1), 17–32.

Koniak-Griffin, D., Verzemnieks, I. L., Anderson, N. L. R., Brecht, M., Lesser, J., & Kim, S. (2003). Nurse visitation for adolescent mothers: Two year infant health and maternal outcomes. *Nursing Research, 52*(2), 127–136.

Kulbok, P. A., Thatcher, E., Park, E., & Meszaros, P. S. (2012). Evolving public health nursing roles: Focus on community participatory health promotion and prevention. *Online Journal of Issues in Nursing, 17*(2), manuscript 1.

Lahr, M. B., Rosenberg, K. D., & Lapidus, J. A. (2005). Health departments do it better: Prenatal care site and prone infant sleep position. *Maternal and Child Health Journal, 9*(2), 165–172.

Malone, M. (2012). Violence in societies. In L. L. Stamler & L. Yiu (Eds.), *Community health nursing: A Canadian perspective* (3rd ed., pp. 405–419). Toronto, ON: Pearson Prentice Hall.

McNaughton, D. (2000). A synthesis of qualitative home visiting research. *Public Health Nursing, 17*(6), 405–414.

McNaughton, D. B. (2004). Nurse home visits to maternal-child clients: A research review. *Public Health Nursing, 21*(3), 207–219.

McNaughton, D. B. (2005). A naturalistic test of Peplau's theory in home visiting. *Public Health Nursing, 22*(5), 429–438.

Mikkonen, J., & Raphael, D. (2010). Social determinants of health: The Canadian facts. Retrieved from http://www.thecanadianfacts.org/The_Canadian_Facts.pdf

National Aboriginal Health Organization. (2006). Fact sheet: Cultural safety. Retrieved from http://www.naho.ca/english/documents/Culturalsafetyfactsheet.pdf

Newman, D. M. (2005). A community nursing center for the health promotion of senior citizens based on the Neuman systems model. *Nursing Education Perspectives, 26*(4), 221–223.

Novick, L. F. (2003). Core public health functions: 15 year update. *Public Health Management Practice, 9*(1), 5.

Obama, B. (2010). *Executive Order 13544: Establishing the national prevention, health promotion, and public health council.* Retrieved from http://www.whitehouse.gov/the-press-office/executive-order-establishing-national-prevention-health-promotion-and-public-health

Olds, D. L. (2002). Prenatal and infancy home visiting by nurses: From randomized trials to community replication. *Prevention Science, 3*(3), 153–172.

Olds, D., Kitzman, H., Cole, R., & Robinson, J. (1997). Theoretical foundations of a program of home visitation for pregnant women and parents of young children. *Journal of Community Psychology, 25*(1), 9–25.

Olds, D. L., Kitzman, H., Cole, R., Robinson, J., Sidora, K., Luckey, D. W., . . . Holmberg, J. (2004). Effects of nurse home-visiting on maternal life course and child development: Age 6 follow-up results of a randomized trial. *Pediatrics, 114*(6), 1550–1559.

Olds, D., Pettitt, L., Robinson, J., Henderson, C., Jr., Eckenrode, J., Kitzman, H., . . . Powers, J. (1998). Reducing risks for antisocial behavior with a program of prenatal and early childhood home visitation. *Journal of Community Psychology, 26*(1), 65–83.

Ontario Ministry of Children and Youth Services. (2011). Healthy babies healthy children. Retrieved from http://www.children.gov.on.ca/htdocs/English/topics/earlychildhood/health/index.aspx

Potter, J. (2004). The importance of recognizing abuse of older people. *British Journal of Community Nursing, 10*(4), 185–187.

Quad Council of Public Health Nursing Organizations. (2011). Quad Council competencies for public health nurses. Summer 2011. Retrieved from http://www.achne.org/files/Quad%20Council/QuadCouncilCompetenciesforPublicHealthNurses.pdf

Reeves, S., Lewin, S., Espin, S., & Zwarenstein, M. (2010). *Interprofessional teamwork for health and social care.* Oxford, UK: Wiley-Blackwell.

Sabogal, F., Marín, G., Otero-Sabogal, R., Marín, B. V., & Pérez-Stable, E. J. (1987). Hispanic familism and acculturation: What changes and what doesn't? *Hispanic Journal of Behavioral Sciences, 9*, 397–412.

Shattuck, S. R. (2002). A domestic violence screening program in a public health department. *Journal of Community Health Nursing, 19*(3), 121–132.

Smedley, B. D., Stith, A. Y., & Nelson, A. R. (Eds.). (2003). *Unequal treatment: Confronting racial and ethnic disparities in healthcare.* Washington, DC: National Academies Press.

SmithBattle, L., Diekemper, M., & Leander, S. (2004). Moving upstream: Becoming a public health nurse, part 2. *Public Health Nursing, 21*(2), 95–102.

Stamler, L. L., & Gabriel, A. (2012). Poverty and homelessness. In L. L. Stamler, & L. Yiu (Eds.), *Community health nursing: A Canadian perspective* (3rd ed., pp. 420–433). Toronto, ON: Pearson Prentice Hall.

Townsend, N., & Foster, C. (2011). Developing and applying a socio-ecological model to the promotion of healthy eating in the school. *Public Health Nutrition, 10*, 1–8.

Tuffrey, C., Finlay, F., & Lewis, M. (2007). The needs of children and their families at end of life: An analysis of community nursing practice. *International Journal of Palliative Nursing, 13*(1), 64–71.

U.S. Department of Health and Human Services. (2001). Healthy people in healthy communities [brochure]. Retrieved from http://www.odphp.osophs.dhhs.gov/pubs/healthycommunities/creating.html

U.S. Department of Health and Human Services. (2010). *Healthy people 2020.* Washington, DC: Office of Disease Prevention and Health Promotion. Retrieved from http://www.healthypeople.gov/2020

Vega, W. A. (1990). Hispanic families in the 1980's: A decade of research. *Journal of Marriage and the Family, 52*, 1015–1024.

Victorian Order of Nurses (VON) Canada. (2009). About VON. Retrieved from http://www.von.ca/en/about/default.aspx

Weman, K., & Fagerberg, I. (2006). Registered nurses working together with family members of older people. *Journal of Clinical Nursing, 15*, 281–289.

William, L. (2008). Developing personal skills: Empowerment. In A. R. Vollman, E. T. Anderson, & J. McFarlane (Eds.), *Canadian community as partner: Theory and multidisciplinary practice* (pp. 94–112). Philadelphia, PA: Wolters Kluwer/Lippincott Williams & Wilkins.

World Health Organization. (1948). *Constitution of the World Health Organization.* Geneva, Switzerland: Author.

World Health Organization. (1978). *Declaration of Alma-Ata.* International Conference on Primary Health Care, Alma-Ata, USSR, September 6–12. Geneva, Switzerland: Author.

World Health Organization. (1986). *Ottawa charter of health promotion.* Geneva, Switzerland: Author.

World Health Organization. (2009). Social determinants of health. Retrieved from http://www.who.int/social_determinatns/en

World Health Organization. (2012). World conference on social determinants of health. Retrieved from http://www.who.int/sdhconference/en

Young, L. E., & Wharf Higgins, J. (2012). Concepts of health. In L. L. Stamler & L. Yiu (Eds.), *Community health nursing: A Canadian perspective* (3rd ed., pp. 76–88). Toronto, ON: Pearson Prentice Hall.

Zahner, S. J., & Vandermause, R. (2003). Local health department performance: Compliance with state statutes and rules. *Public Health Management Practice, 9*(1), 25–34.

Family Systems Stressor-Strength Inventory (FS³I)

Shirley May Harmon Hanson

Karen B. Mischke

INSTRUCTIONS FOR ADMINISTRATION

The Family Systems Stressor-Strength Inventory (FS³I) is an assessment and measurement instrument intended for use with families (see Chapter 3 for theory behind the approach and Chapter 13 for an example of a nurse using it with a family). It focuses on identifying stressful situations occurring in families and the strengths families use to maintain healthy family functioning. Each family member is asked to complete the instrument on an individual form before an interview with the clinician. Questions can be read to members unable to read.

After completion of the instrument, the clinician evaluates the family on each of the stressful situations (general and specific) and the strengths they possess. This evaluation is recorded on the family member form.

The clinician records the individual family member's score and the clinician perception score on the Quantitative Summary. A different color code is used for each family member. The clinician also completes the Qualitative Summary, synthesizing the information gleaned from all participants. Clinicians can use the Family Care Plan to prioritize diagnoses, set goals, develop prevention and intervention activities, and evaluate outcomes.

Family Name _____   Date _____

Family Member(s) Completing Assessment _____

Ethnic Background(s) _____

Religious Background(s) _____

Referral Source _____

Interviewer _____

(continued)

Family Members	Relationship in Family	Age	Marital Status	Education (highest degree)	Occupation
1.					
2.					
3.					
4.					
5.					
6.					

Family's current reasons for seeking assistance:

Part I: Family Systems Stressors (General)

DIRECTIONS: Each of 25 situations/stressors listed here deals with some aspect of normal family life. They have the potential for creating stress within families or between families and the world in which they live. We are interested in your overall impression of how these situations affect your family life. Please circle a number (0 through 5) that best describes the amount of stress or tension they create for you.

STRESSORS	FAMILY PERCEPTION SCORE						CLINICIAN PERCEPTION
	DOES NOT APPLY	LITTLE STRESS		MEDIUM STRESS		HIGH STRESS	SCORE
1. Family member(s) feel unappreciated	0	1	2	3	4	5	_____
2. Guilt for not accomplishing more	0	1	2	3	4	5	_____
3. Insufficient "me" time	0	1	2	3	4	5	_____
4. Self-image/self-esteem/ feelings of unattractiveness	0	1	2	3	4	5	_____
5. Perfectionism	0	1	2	3	4	5	_____
6. Dieting	0	1	2	3	4	5	_____
7. Health/illness	0	1	2	3	4	5	_____
8. Communication with children	0	1	2	3	4	5	_____
9. Housekeeping standards	0	1	2	3	4	5	_____
10. Insufficient couple time	0	1	2	3	4	5	_____
11. Insufficient family playtime	0	1	2	3	4	5	_____

STRESSORS	DOES NOT APPLY	FAMILY PERCEPTION SCORE						CLINICIAN PERCEPTION SCORE
		LITTLE STRESS		MEDIUM STRESS		HIGH STRESS		
12. Children's behavior/ discipline/sibling fighting	0	1	2	3	4	5		_____
13. Television	0	1	2	3	4	5		_____
14. Overscheduled family calendar	0	1	2	3	4	5		_____
15. Lack of shared responsibility in the family	0	1	2	3	4	5		_____
16. Moving	0	1	2	3	4	5		_____
17. Spousal relationship (communication, friendship, sex)	0	1	2	3	4	5		_____
18. Holidays	0	1	2	3	4	5		_____
19. In-laws	0	1	2	3	4	5		_____
20. Teen behaviors (communication, music, friends, school)	0	1	2	3	4	5		_____
21. New baby	0	1	2	3	4	5		_____
22. Economics/finances/ budgets	0	1	2	3	4	5		_____
23. Unhappiness with work situation	0	1	2	3	4	5		_____
24. Overvolunteerism	0	1	2	3	4	5		_____
25. Neighbors	0	1	2	3	4	5		_____

Additional Stressors: _____

_____

_____

Family Remarks: _____

_____

_____

Clinician: Clarification of stressful situations/concerns with family members.

Prioritize in order of importance to family members: _____

_____

Part II: Family Systems Stressors (Specific)

DIRECTIONS: The following 12 questions are designed to provide information about your specific stress-producing situation/problem or area of concern influencing your family's health. Please circle a number (1 through 5) that best describes the influence this situation has on your family's life and how well you perceive your family's overall functioning.

The specific stress-producing situation/problem or area of concern at this time is: _____

_____

_____

STRESSORS	FAMILY PERCEPTION SCORE			CLINICIAN PERCEPTION SCORE
	LITTLE	MEDIUM	HIGH	
1. To what extent is your family bothered by this problem or stressful situation? (e.g., effects on family interactions, communication among members, emotional and social relationships)	1 2	3 4	5	_____

Family Remarks: _____

_____

Clinician Remarks: _____

_____

2. How much of an effect does this stressful situation have on your family's usual pattern of living? (e.g., effects on lifestyle patterns and family developmental task)	1 2	3 4	5	_____

Family Remarks: _____

_____

Clinician Remarks: _____

_____

3. How much has this situation affected your family's ability to work together as a family unit? (e.g., alteration in family roles, completion of family tasks, following through with responsibilities)	1 2	3 4	5	_____

Family Remarks: _____

_____

Clinician Remarks: _____

_____

STRESSORS	FAMILY PERCEPTION SCORE			CLINICIAN PERCEPTION SCORE
	LITTLE	MEDIUM	HIGH	

Has your family ever experienced a similar concern in the past?

1. YES   If YES, complete question 4

2. NO   If NO, complete question 5

4. How successful was your family in dealing with this situation/problem/concern in the past? (e.g., workable coping strategies developed, adaptive measures useful, situation improved)   1   2   3   4   5   _____

Family Remarks: _____

_____

Clinician Remarks: _____

_____

5. How strongly do you feel this current situation/problem/concern will affect your family's future? (e.g., anticipated consequences)   1   2   3   4   5   _____

Family Remarks: _____

_____

Clinician Remarks: _____

_____

6. To what extent are family members able to help themselves in this present situation/problem/concern? (e.g., self-assistive efforts, family expectations, spiritual influence, family resources)   1   2   3   4   5   _____

Family Remarks: _____

_____

Clinician Remarks: _____

_____

7. To what extent do you expect others to help your family with this situation/problem/concern? (e.g., what roles would helpers play; how available are extra-family resources)   1   2   3   4   5   _____

Family Remarks: _____

_____

Clinician Remarks: _____

_____

(continued)

STRESSORS	POOR	SATISFACTORY	EXCELLENT	SCORE

8. How would you rate the way your family functions overall? (e.g., how your family members relate to each other and to larger family and community) 1 2 3 4 5 _____

Family Remarks: _____

_____

Clinician Remarks: _____

_____

9. How would you rate the overall physical health status of each family member by name? (Include yourself as a family member; record additional names on back.)
   a. _____ 1 2 3 4 5 _____
   b. _____ 1 2 3 4 5 _____
   c. _____ 1 2 3 4 5 _____
   d. _____ 1 2 3 4 5 _____
   e. _____ 1 2 3 4 5 _____

10. How would you rate the overall physical health status of your family as a whole? 1 2 3 4 5 _____

Family Remarks: _____

_____

Clinician Remarks: _____

_____

11. How would you rate the overall mental health status of each family member by name? (Include yourself as a family member; record additional names on back.)
   a. _____ 1 2 3 4 5 _____
   b. _____ 1 2 3 4 5 _____
   c. _____ 1 2 3 4 5 _____
   d. _____ 1 2 3 4 5 _____
   e. _____ 1 2 3 4 5 _____

12. How would you rate the overall mental health status of your family as a whole? 1 2 3 4 5 _____

Family Remarks: _____

_____

Clinician Remarks: _____

_____

Part III: Family Systems Strengths

DIRECTIONS: Each of the 16 traits/attributes listed below deals with some aspect of family life and its overall functioning. Each one contributes to the health and well-being of family members as individuals and to the family as a whole. Please circle a number (0 through 5) that best describes the extent to which the trait applies to your family.

MY FAMILY	DOES NOT APPLY	FAMILY PERCEPTION SCORE				CLINICIAN PERCEPTION SCORE
		SELDOM	USUALLY	ALWAYS		
1. Communicates and listens to one another	0	1	2	3	4 5	_____

Family Remarks: _____

Clinician Remarks: _____

2. Affirms and supports one another	0	1	2	3	4 5	_____

Family Remarks: _____

Clinician Remarks: _____

3. Teaches respect for others	0	1	2	3	4 5	_____

Family Remarks: _____

Clinician Remarks: _____

4. Develops a sense of trust in members	0	1	2	3	4 5	_____

Family Remarks: _____

Clinician Remarks: _____

5. Displays a sense of play and humor	0	1	2	3	4 5	_____

Family Remarks: _____

Clinician Remarks: _____

(continued)

MY FAMILY	DOES NOT APPLY	FAMILY PERCEPTION SCORE				CLINICIAN PERCEPTION SCORE
		SELDOM	USUALLY		ALWAYS	
6. Exhibits a sense of shared responsibility	0	1 2	3	4	5	_____

Family Remarks: _____

Clinician Remarks: _____

| 7. Teaches a sense of right and wrong | 0 | 1   2 | 3 | 4 | 5 | _____ |

Family Remarks: _____

Clinician Remarks: _____

| 8. Has a strong sense of family in which rituals and traditions abound | 0 | 1   2 | 3 | 4 | 5 | _____ |

Family Remarks: _____

Clinician Remarks: _____

| 9. Has a balance of interaction among members | 0 | 1   2 | 3 | 4 | 5 | _____ |

Family Remarks: _____

Clinician Remarks: _____

| 10. Has a shared religious core | 0 | 1   2 | 3 | 4 | 5 | _____ |

Family Remarks: _____

Clinician Remarks: _____

| 11. Respects the privacy of one another | 0 | 1   2 | 3 | 4 | 5 | _____ |

Family Remarks: _____

Clinician Remarks: _____

| MY FAMILY | DOES NOT APPLY | FAMILY PERCEPTION SCORE | | | | CLINICIAN PERCEPTION |
		SELDOM	USUALLY	ALWAYS		SCORE
12. Values service to others	0	1 2	3 4	5		_____

Family Remarks: _____

Clinician Remarks: _____

| 13. Fosters family table time and conversation | 0 | 1 2 | 3 4 | 5 | | _____ |

Family Remarks: _____

Clinician Remarks: _____

| 14. Shares leisure time | 0 | 1 2 | 3 4 | 5 | | _____ |

Family Remarks: _____

Clinician Remarks: _____

| 15. Admits to and seeks help with problems | 0 | 1 2 | 3 4 | 5 | | _____ |

Family Remarks: _____

Clinician Remarks: _____

| 16a. How would you rate the overall strengths that exist in your family? | 0 | 1 2 | 3 4 | 5 | | _____ |

Family Remarks: _____

Clinician Remarks: _____

16b. Additional family strengths: _____

_____

16c. Clinician: Clarification of family strengths with individual members: _____

_____

Source: Hanson, S. M. H. (2001). *Family health care nursing: Theory, practice, and research* (2nd ed., pp. 425–437). Philadelphia, PA: F. A. Davis.

FAMILY SYSTEMS STRESSOR-STRENGTH INVENTORY (FS³I) SCORING SUMMARY

Section 1: Family Perception Scores

Instructions For Administration

The Family Systems Stressor-Strength Inventory (FS³I) Scoring Summary is divided into two sections: Section 1, Family Perception Scores, and Section 2, Clinician Perception Scores. These two sections are further divided into three parts: Part I, Family Systems Stressors (General); Part II, Family Systems Stressors (Specific); and Part III, Family Systems Strengths. Each part contains a Quantitative Summary and a Qualitative Summary.

Quantifiable family and clinician perception scores are both graphed on the Quantitative Summary. Each family member has a designated color code. Family and clinician remarks are both recorded on the Quantitative Summary. Quantitative Summary scores, when graphed, suggest a level for initiation of prevention/intervention modes: Primary, Secondary, and Tertiary. Qualitative Summary information, when synthesized, contributes to the development and channeling of the Family Care Plan.

Part I: Family Systems Stressors (General)

Add scores from questions 1 to 25 and calculate an overall numerical score for Family Systems Stressors (General). Ratings are from 1 (most positive) to 5 (most negative). The Does Not Apply (0) responses are omitted from the calculations. Total scores range from 25 to 125.

Family Systems Stressor Score (General)

$$(25) \times 1 =$$

Graph score on Quantitative Summary, Family Systems Stressors (General), Family Member Perception Score. Color-code to differentiate family members. Record additional stressors and family remarks in Part I, Qualitative Summary: Family and Clinician Remarks.

Part II: Family Systems Stressors (Specific)

Add scores from questions 1 through 8, 10, and 12 and calculate a numerical score for Family Systems Stressors (Specific). Ratings are from 1 (most positive) to 5 (most negative). Questions 4, 6, 7, 8, 10 and 12 are reverse scored.* Total scores range from 10 through 50.

Family Systems Stressor Score (Specific)

$$(10) \times 1 =$$

Graph score on Quantitative Summary, Family Systems Stressors (Specific) Family Member Perception Score. Color-code to differentiate family members.

Summarize data from questions 9 and 11 (reverse scored) and record family remarks in Part II, Qualitative Summary: Family and Clinician Remarks.

Part III: Family Systems Strengths

Add scores from questions 1 through 16 and calculate a numerical score for Family Systems Strengths. Ratings are from 1 (seldom) to 5 (always). The Does Not Apply (0) responses are omitted from the calculations. Total Scores range from 16 to 80.

Family Systems Strengths Score

$$(16) \times 1 =$$

Graph score on Quantitative Summary: Family Systems Strengths, Family Member Perception Score. Record additional family strengths and family remarks in Part III, Qualitative Summary: Family and Clinician Remarks.

---

*Reverse scoring:
Question answered as (1) is scored 5 points.
Question answered as (2) is scored 4 points.
Question answered as (3) is scored 3 points.
Question answered as (4) is scored 2 points.
Question answered as (5) is scored 1 point.

Section 2: Clinician Perception Scores

Part I: Family Systems Stressors (General)*

Add scores from questions 1 through 25 and calculate an overall numerical score for Family Systems Stressors (General). Ratings are from 1 (most positive) to 5 (most negative). The Does Not Apply (0) responses are omitted from the calculations. Total scores range from 25 to 125.

Family systems Stressor Score (General)

$$(_{25}) \times 1 =$$

Graph score on Quantitative Summary, Family Systems Stressors (General) Clinician Perception Score. Record clinicians' clarification of general stressors in Part I, Qualitative Summary: Family and Clinician Remarks.

Part II: Family Systems Stressors (Specific)

Add scores from questions 1 through 8, 10, 12 and calculate a numerical score for Family Systems Stressors (Specific). Ratings are from 1 (most positive) to 5 (most negative). Questions 4, 6, 7, 8, 10, and 12 are reverse scored.* Total scores range from 10 to 50.

Family Systems Stressor Score (Specific)

$$(_{10}) \times 1 =$$

Graph score on Quantitative Summary, Family Systems Stressors (Specific), Clinician Perception Score. Summarize data from questions 9 and 11 (reverse order) and record clinician remarks in Part II, Qualitative Summary: Family and Clinician Remarks.

Part III: Family Systems Strengths

Add scores from questions 1 through 16 and calculate a numerical score for Family Systems Strengths. Ratings are from 1 (seldom) to 5 (always). The Does Not Apply (0) responses are omitted from the calculations. Total scores range from 16 to 80.

Family Systems Strengths Score

$$(_{16}) \times 1 =$$

Graph score on Quantitative Summary, Family Systems Strengths, Clinician Perception Score. Record clinicians' clarification of family strengths in Part III, Qualitative Summary: Family and Clinician Remarks.

Source: Mischke-Berkey, K., & Hanson, S. M. H. (1991). *Pocket guide to family assessment and intervention.* St. Louis, MO: Mosby.
*Reverse scoring:
Question answered as (1) is scored 5 points.
Question answered as (2) is scored 4 points.
Question answered as (3) is scored 3 points.
Question answered as (4) is scored 2 points.
Question answered as (5) is scored 1 point.

Quantitative Summary of Family Systems Stressors: General and Specific Family and Clinician Perception Scores

DIRECTIONS: Graph the scores from each family member inventory by placing an "X" at the appropriate location. (Use first name initial for each different entry and different color code for each family member.)

SCORES FOR WELLNESS AND STABILITY	FAMILY SYSTEMS STRESSORS (GENERAL)		SCORES FOR WELLNESS AND STABILITY	FAMILY SYSTEMS STRESSORS (SPECIFIC)	
	FAMILY MEMBER PERCEPTION SCORE	CLINICIAN PERCEPTION SCORE		FAMILY MEMBER PERCEPTION SCORE	CLINICIAN PERCEPTION SCORE
5.0‡			5.0		
4.8			4.8		
4.6			4.6		
4.4			4.4		
4.2			4.2		
4.0			4.0		
3.8			3.8		
3.6			3.6		
3.4			3.4		
3.2			3.2		
3.0			3.0		
2.8			2.8		
2.6			2.6		
2.4†			2.4		
2.2			2.2		
2.0			2.0		
1.8			1.8		
1.6			1.6		
1.4			1.4		
1.2			1.2		
1.0*			1.0		

*PRIMARY Prevention/Intervention Mode: Flexible Line   1.0–2.3
†SECONDARY Prevention/Intervention Mode: Normal Line   2.4–3.6
‡TERTIARY Prevention/Intervention Mode: Resistance Lines   3.7–5.0
Breakdowns of numerical scores for stressor penetration are suggested values.

Family Systems Strengths Family and Clinician Perception Scores

DIRECTIONS: Graph the scores from the inventory by placing an "X" at the appropriate location and connect with a line. (Use first name initial for each different entry and different color code for each family member.)

SUM OF STRENGTHS AVAILABLE FOR PREVENTION/ INTERVENTION MODE	FAMILY SYSTEMS STRENGTHS	
	FAMILY MEMBER PERCEPTION SCORE	CLINICIAN PERCEPTION SCORE
5.0‡		
4.8		
4.6		
4.4		
4.2		
4.0		
3.8		
3.6		
3.4		
3.2		
3.0		
2.8		
2.6		
2.4†		
2.2		
2.0		
1.8		
1.6		
1.4		
1.2		
1.0*		

*PRIMARY Prevention/Intervention Mode: Flexible Line   1.0–2.3
†SECONDARY Prevention/Intervention Mode: Normal Line   2.4–3.6
‡TERTIARY Prevention/Intervention Mode: Resistance Lines   3.7–5.0
Breakdowns of numerical scores for stressor penetration are suggested values.

QUALITATIVE SUMMARY FAMILY AND CLINICIAN REMARKS

Part I: Family Systems Stressors (General)

Summarize general stressors and remarks of family and clinician. Prioritize stressors according to importance to family members.

_____

_____

_____

Part II: Family Systems Stressors (Specific)

A. Summarize specific stressors and remarks of family and clinician.

_____

_____

B. Summarize differences (if discrepancies exist) between how family members and clinicians view effects of stressful situation on family.

_____

_____

C. Summarize overall family functioning.

_____

_____

D. Summarize overall significant physical health status for family members.

_____

_____

E. Summarize overall significant mental health status for family members.

_____

_____

Part III: Family Systems Strengths

Summarize family systems strengths and family and clinician remarks that facilitate family health and stability.

_____

_____

_____

Family Care Plan*

DIAGNOSIS AND GENERAL AND SPECIFIC FAMILY SYSTEM STRESSORS	FAMILY SYSTEMS STRENGTHS SUPPORTING FAMILY CARE PLAN	GOALS FOR FAMILY AND CLINICIAN	PREVENTION/INTERVENTION MODE		
			PRIMARY, SECONDARY, OR TERTIARY	PREVENTION/ INTERVENTION ACTIVITIES	OUTCOMES, EVALUATION, AND REPLANNING

*Prioritize the three most significant diagnoses.

The Friedman Family Assessment Model (Short Form)

The following Friedman Family Assessment Short Form is useful as a quick instrument to help highlight areas of family function that will need more exploration. Before using the following guidelines in completing family assessments, two words of caution are noted: First, not all areas included below will be germane for each of the families visited. The guidelines are comprehensive and allow depth when probing is necessary. The student should not feel that every subarea needs be covered when the broad area of inquiry poses no problems to the family or concern to the health worker. Second, by virtue of the interdependence of the family system, one will find unavoidable redundancy. For the sake of efficiency, the assessor should try not to repeat data, but to refer the reader back to sections where this information has already been described.

IDENTIFYING DATA

1. **Family Name**
2. **Address and Phone**
3. **Family Composition: The Family Genogram**
4. **Type of Family Form**
5. **Cultural (Ethnic) Background**
6. **Religious Identification**
7. **Social Class Status**
8. **Social Class Mobility**

DEVELOPMENTAL STAGE AND HISTORY OF FAMILY

9. **Family's Present Developmental Stage**
10. **Extent of Family Developmental Tasks Fulfillment**
11. **Nuclear Family History**
12. **History of Family of Origin of Both Parents**

ENVIRONMENTAL DATA

13. **Characteristics of Home**
14. **Characteristics of Neighborhood and Larger Community**
15. **Family's Geographical Mobility**
16. **Family's Associations and Transactions With Community**

FAMILY STRUCTURE

17. **Communication Patterns**
    Extent of Functional and Dysfunctional Communication (types of recurring patterns)
    Extent of Emotional (Affective) Messages and How Expressed
    Characteristics of Communication Within Family Subsystems

Extent of Congruent and Incongruent Messages
Types of Dysfunctional Communication Processes Seen in Family
Areas of Closed Communication
Familial and Contextual Variables Affecting Communication

18. **Power Structure**
Power Outcomes
Decision-making Process
Power Bases
Variables Affecting Family Power
Overall Family System and Subsystem Power (Family Power Continuum Placement)

19. **Role Structure**
Formal Role Structure
Informal Role Structure
Analysis of Role Models (optional)
Variables Affecting Role Structure

20. **Family Values**
Compare the family to American core values or family's reference group values and/or identify important family values and their importance (priority) in family.

Congruence Between the Family's Values and the Family's Reference Group or Wider Community
Disparity in Value Systems
Presence of Value Conflicts in Family
Effect of the Above Values and Value Conflicts on Health Status of Family

FAMILY FUNCTIONS

21. **Affective Function**
Mutual Nurturance, Closeness, and Identification
Separateness and Connectedness
Family's Need-Response Patterns

22. **Socialization Function**
Family Child-rearing Practices
Adaptability of Child-rearing Practices for Family Form and Family's Situation
Who Is (Are) Socializing Agent(s) for Child(ren)?
Value of Children in Family
Cultural Beliefs That Influence Family's Child-rearing Patterns

Social Class Influence on Child-rearing Patterns
Estimation About Whether Family Is at Risk for Child-rearing Problems and If So, Indication of High-Risk Factors
Adequacy of Home Environment for Children's Needs to Play

23. **Health Care Function**
Family's Health Beliefs, Values, and Behavior
Family's Definitions of Health-Illness and Its Level of Knowledge
Family's Perceived Health Status and Illness Susceptibility
Family's Dietary Practices
   ■ Adequacy of family diet (recommended 3-day food history record)
   ■ Function of mealtimes and attitudes toward food and mealtimes
   ■ Shopping (and its planning) practices
   ■ Person(s) responsible for planning, shopping, and preparation of meals
Sleep and Rest Habits
Physical Activity and Recreation Practices
Family's Therapeutic and Recreational Drug, Alcohol, and Tobacco Practices
Family's Role in Self-care Practice
Medically Based Preventive Measures (physicals, eye and hearing tests, immunizations, dental care)
Complementary and Alternative Therapies
Family Health History (both general and specific diseases—environmentally and genetically related)
Health Care Services Received
Feelings and Perceptions Regarding Health Services
Emergency Health Services
Source of Payments for Health and Other Services
Logistics of Receiving Care

FAMILY STRESS, COPING, AND ADAPTATION

24. **Family Stressors, Strengths, and Perceptions**
Stressors Family Is Experiencing
Strengths That Counterbalance Stressors
Family's Definition of the Situation

25. Family Coping Strategies
How the Family Is Reacting to the Stressors
*Extent of Family's Use of Internal Coping
    Strategies (past/present)*
*Extent of Family's Use of External Coping
    Strategies (past/present)*
*Dysfunctional Coping Strategies Utilized
    (past/present; extent of use)*

26. Family Adaptation
Overall Family Adaptation
Estimation of Whether Family Is in Crisis
**27. Tracking Stressors, Coping, and
Adaptation Over Time**

Source: Friedman, M. M., Bowden, V. R., & Jones, E. G. (2003). *Family
nursing: Research, theory, and practice* (5th ed., pp. 593–594). Upper Saddle
River, NJ: Prentice Hall.

PHOTO CREDITS

INDEX

A

AARP, 488
Aboriginal people, 171
  linguistic diversity, 172
  in poverty, 170
Abortion, 22, 38
  social policy and, 155
Abuse, 175–177, 335, 363
  child, 406–408
Access to health care, 154, 177–178
Accidents, automobile, 150
Accommodating management style,
  243–244
Activities of daily living (ADLs), 42, 478,
  481, 488, 493–494
  assessment, 504
Acute Care for the Elderly (ACE) Model,
  498
Acute care settings, 434
  advance directives in, 448–449
  assessments in, 109–110
  brief therapeutic conversations in, 126
  cardiopulmonary resuscitation in,
  449–450
  case study, 453–471
  communication with families in,
  443–444
  Do Not Resuscitate (DNR) orders in,
  448, 450
  elder care, 503–505
  end-of-life family care in, 446–453
  families in, 434–441
  family interventions at discharge from,
  445–446
  family needs during discharge from,
  444–445
  intensive care unit (ICU), 300, 304,
  434–441
  life-sustaining therapies withdrawal or
  withholding in, 450–453
  medical-surgical units, 441–446
  organ donation and, 453
  visiting policy, 437–438, 442–443
Acute illness
  acute onset of chronic illness and,
  87–88
  during childbearing, 371
Adaptation Model, 72
Adaptation to chronic illness, family,
  251–252
Adaptive model of family health, 208
Ad hoc family interpreters, 110
ADLs. *See* Activities of daily living (ADLs)
Administration on Aging, 155
Adolescents, 150
  with chronic illness transition to adult
  services, 256–258
  as emancipated minors, 417
  family meals and, 223
  genetic testing in, 194
  risks, 408–409
  sexual activity among, 408–409
Adoption, 48–51, 367–369
Adult foster care, 493
Advance care planning, 295–296
Advance directives, 448–449
Adverse Childhood Experiences Study,
  329, 578
Advocate, nurse as, 14, 146
  in palliative and end-of-life care,
  295–297
  social policy and, 156–159
Affective functions of the family, 23–24
Affordable Care Act (ACA), 139, 157, 409,
  574
After-school activities, 403–404
Aging. *See also* Elder care; Elderly, the
  case study, 505–514
  demographic changes, 38–39, 480–482
  diversity of experiences in, 477–478
  families, profile of, 480–487
  family ambivalence and conflict in,
  486–487
  family caregiving and, 487–496
  family relationships and, 483–487
  family structure and, 482–483
  intergenerational relationships and,
  485–486
  life course perspective, 478–480,
  505–514
  population policy, 154
  same-generation relationships and,
  483–485
  siblings and, 484–485
  social-emotional, cognitive, and physical
  dimensions of individual development
  and, 392–396
Aging and Disability Resource Centers
  (ADRCs), 496
AHRC. *See* Assisted Human Reproduction
  Canada (AHRC)
Akathisia, 535
Alcohol use, 149–150, 176–177, 543–544
  by adolescents, 150
  binge drinking, 149, 239
*Alma Ata Declaration on Primary Health
  Care*, 563
Alzheimer's disease, 189, 493, 539
American Academy of Pediatrics (AAP),
  152, 216, 408
American Association of Caregiving
  Youth, 253
American Association of Critical Care
  Nurses (AACN), 437–438
American College of Critical Care
  Medicine, 434, 438
American Community Survey, 35, 39
American Lung Association, 145
American Medical Association (AMA), 406
American Nurses Association (ANA), 4,
  157–158, 438, 449
American Psychiatric Association (APA),
  521
American Psychological Association (APA),
  322
Americans with Disabilities Act, 151
America's Promise Alliance, 409
ANA. *See* American Nurses Association
  (ANA)
Anticipatory guidance, 222
Appraisal support for families with
  chronically ill member, 260
Area Agency on Aging (AAAs), 496
Arthritis Foundation, 497
ARTs. *See* Assisted reproductive
  technologies (ARTs)
Ashkenazi Jews, 200
Assessments. *See also* Interventions;
  specific assessment models
  activities of daily living (ADLs), 504
  in acute care settings, 109–110
  caregiving, 491–496
  characteristics and selection, 115–116
  community-based appointments for,
  108–109
  community/public health nursing,
  574–577
  depression, 505
  engaging families in care, 107–111
  evaluation and, 127–128
  family-centered meetings and care
  conferences in, 110–111
  family functions and, 22–25
  family health literacy, 120
  Family Health Model, 248
  family nursing, 106–111
  family processes and, 25–30
  family structure and, 20–22
  genetic family history, 197–199
  genograms and ecomaps, 116–120
  interpreters used in, 110
  models and instruments, 111–120
  nurse and family reflection in, 129–133
  palliative and end-of-life care, 286–305
  preconception, 199–200
  PTSD, 336–337
  shared decision making and, 123–125
Assisted Human Reproduction Canada
  (AHRC), 48
Assisted living facilities, 493, 498–500
Assisted reproductive technologies
  (ARTs), 47–48, 367
Association of Community Health
  Nursing Educators (ACHNE), 564
Asthma, 145
  policy, 153
Attachment, 325–326, 362, 374
Attention-deficit hyperactivity disorder
  (ADHD), 413, 533, 541–542
Authoritarian parenting style, 401–402
Authoritative parenting style, 401, 406
Automobile accidents, 150

Autosomal recessive conditions, 198
Avoiders, 6

B

Baby boomers, 37
Balanced families, 7
Behavioral Risk Factor Surveillance
  System (BRFSS), 239
Behavioral Systems Model for Nursing,
  70, 72
Beliefs and Illness Model, 123
Bereavement care, 285, 302–303
  when death is sudden or traumatic,
    304–305
Bidirectional interactions, 85
Binge drinking, 149, 239
Bioecological Systems Theory, 83–87,
  100–101, 213–219
  aging and, 478–480
Bipolar disorder, 532, 533, 538–539
  case study, 545–551
Birth control, 46
Blended families, 56
Board and care homes, 493
Body mass index (BMI), 148
Boomerang children, 43
Boundaries, Family Systems Theory on,
  77–78
Brain development and early trauma,
  328–329
Breast cancer, 188–189, 194
Breastfeeding, 360–361, 373–374
Breckinridge, Mary, 16, 157
Bronfenbrenner, Urie, 83–85, 323

C

Calgary Family Assessment Model
  (CFAM), 111, 113–115
Calgary Family Intervention Model
  (CFIM), 111
Canada
  aging population in, 38–39
  alcohol use in, 150
  cohabitation in, 44, 55
  in context, 169–173
  definition of family in, 147
  economic burden of chronic disease in,
    240
  economic changes in, 36–37
  economic diversity, 170–171
  ethnocultural diversity, 171–172
  family as safe and nurturing in,
    175–177
  fathering in, 54
  fertility rate, 45–47
  geographical diversity, 169–170
  health care context, 177–178
  health care policy in, 140–141
  health resources in, 147
  heterosexual nuclear families as norm
    in, 173–174
  how family is understood in, 173–177

  ideas of motherhood and women in,
    174–175
  illegal drug use in, 150
  immigration to, 39–40
  income gap in, 143
  life expectancy in, 38–39
  linguistic diversity, 172
  living arrangements in, 40–45
  multigenerational households in,
    41–42
  obesity in, 148, 149
  parental leave policies, 376–377
  poverty in, 143, 170
  religious diversity, 172–173
  same-sex couple families in, 55
  school nursing in, 152–153
  single mothers in, 54
  stepfamilies in, 56
  tobacco use in, 149
Canadian Addiction Survey, 176
Canadian Centre for Policy Alternatives
  (CCPA), 153
Canadian Child Welfare Research
  Portal, 170–171
Canadian Community Health Nursing
  Professional Practice Model, 563
Canadian Community Health Survey,
  170, 176, 217
Canadian Council on Learning, 146
Canadian Hospice Palliative Care
  Association, 295–296
Canadian Incidence Study (CIS), 176
Canadian Nurses Association (CNA),
  158
Canadian Tobacco Use Monitoring
  Survey (CTUMS), 239
Cancer, 146
  deaths from, 239
  genetics and, 188–189, 194
Cardiopulmonary resuscitation, 449–450
Cardiovascular disease, 146, 239
Career, family, 390, 398
Caregiving
  chronic illness and family, 252–256
  family, 487–496
  grandparents caring for grandchildren,
    490
  for individuals with mental health
    conditions, 526–533
  nursing role in assessing and
    supporting, 491–496
  palliative and end-of-life care and,
    282–284
  roles, 488–491
  self-care talk for family, 126–127
Care Model, 141–142
Carrier genetic tests, 190
Case-finder, nurse as, 14
Case manager, nurse as, 15
CDC. *See* Centers for Disease Control
  and Prevention (CDC)
Cell phones in the ICU, 438
Centers for Disease Control and Prevention
  (CDC), 214, 239, 329, 573

Centers for Medicare and Medicaid
  Services, 139–140
CFAM. *See* Calgary Family Assessment
  Model (CFAM)
CFIM. *See* Calgary Family Intervention
  Model (CFIM)
Change Theory, 71
Childbearing. *See also* Parenting
  adjusting to changed communication
    patterns after, 362–363
  adoption and, 367–369
  arranging space for a child and,
    358–359
  assisted reproductive technologies
    (ARTs) and, 47–48
  assuming mutual responsibility for child
    care and nurturing after, 360–362
  complications, 48
  establishing family rituals and routines
    after, 365
  facilitating role learning of family
    members during and after, 362
  family case studies, 377–381
  Family Developmental and Life Cycle
    Theory and, 358–366
  family nursing, 355–356
  family nursing of postpartum families,
    372–376
  family stressors, 366–371
  family systems theory and, 357–358
  family transitions and, 365–366
  feeding management and, 373–374
  fertility rate and, 22, 45–47
  financing child rearing and, 359–360
  high-risk, 371–372
  historical perspective, 354–355
  infertility and, 366–367
  maintaining family members' motivation
    and morale through, 364–365
  perinatal loss and, 369–370
  planning for subsequent children and,
    363
  policy implications for family nursing
    in, 376–377
  postpartum depression and, 375–376
  preconception assessment and education
    prior to, 199–200
  realigning intergenerational patterns
    and, 363–364
  single mothers and, 34, 46, 51–54
  social policy and, 155–156
  theory-guided, evidence-based
    nursing, 356–366
  threats to health during, 371–372
Child care, 403–404
Child care Resource and Referral
  Services, 404
Child health nursing
  care of children with chronic illness and
    their families in, 410–415
  case study, 420–426
  child care, after-school activities, and
    children's health promotion and,
    403–404

concepts of, 390–398
consent in, 415–418
elements of family-centered care and, 388–390
family career and, 390
family stages and, 390–391
family tasks and, 391
in the hospital, 418–420
identifying health risks and teaching prevention strategies in, 404–410
nursing interventions to support care of well children and families, 398–410
parenting a child with chronic illness and, 412–415
transitions and, 391, 396–398
understanding and working with family routines in, 403
web sites of interest in, 426
Child Poverty Report Card, 2011, 170
Children. *See also* Parents
  abuse of, 176, 335, 363, 406–408
  adoption of, 48–51
  attachment of, 325–326, 362, 374
  boomerang, 43
  brain development and early trauma in, 328–329
  caregiving for adult, 252–253
  with chronic illness, 410–415
  of cohabiting couples, 44, 55
  communication with families with, 399–400
  costs associated with special health care needs, 241–242
  death of, 302, 306–309
  depression and, 537–538
  developmental trauma theory and, 326–329
  families caring for chronically ill, 253–256
  fathering and, 54–55
  grandparents caring for grand-, 490
  health promotion, 403–404
  hospital care of, 418–420
  identifying health risks and teaching prevention strategies for, 404–410
  mutual responsibility for care and nurturing of, 360–362
  nursing interventions to support care of well, 398–410
  obesity and overweight among, 148–149, 405–406
  older adults caring for adult, 490–491
  in poverty, 409–410
  preparation for surgery using hospital play, 400
  risks associated with PTSD in, 337–338
  of same-sex couples, 48, 55–56, 174
  siblings of chronically ill, 258–259
  social-emotional, cognitive, and physical dimensions of individual development in, 392–396

stages, tasks, and situational needs of families of disabled and chronically ill, 416–417
in stepfamilies, 56–57
systems of care for chronically ill, 259
trauma in, 326–330
unintentional and intentional injuries in, 405
when family member is critically ill, facilitating connections for, 303–304
of working mothers, 27, 36, 175
Children's Health Insurance Program (CHIP), 409
Children's Health Insurance Program Reauthorization Act (CHIPRA), 140
Child Welfare Information Gateway, 407
Chronic illness, 237–238
  bioecological systems theory applied to, 86–87
  care programs for older adults, 497
  case study, 74–76, 262–272
  during childbearing, 371
  in children, 241–242
  children with, 410–415
  chronic illness framework applied to, 90–91
  core family processes and, 247–248
  course of, 88–89
  defined in families with sick children, 410–412
  developmental and family life cycle theory applied to, 82–83
  economic burden of, 240–242
  families caring for children living with, 253–256
  family adaptation to, 251–252
  family assessment and intervention model applied to, 94–95
  family caregiving and, 252–256
  family functioning in, 90
  Family Health Model and, 244–249
  Family Management Style Framework (FMSF), 242–244
  family nursing intervention during, 261–262
  family systems theory applied to, 78–79
  framework, 87–91, 101
  as a global concern, 238–242
  gradual or acute onset of, 87–88
  as health determinant, 144–146
  health promotion for prevention of, 249
  helping families live with, 249–261
  maintaining family life with child having, 413–414
  normalization and family management styles in childhood, 415
  nurturing a child with, 413
  parenting a child with, 412–415
  parents taking care of self and child with, 414–415
  policy related to, 153–154

Rolland's Chronic Illness Framework, 242
self-management and, 250–251
siblings of children with, 258–259, 413–414
social support for, 259–261
stages, tasks, and situational needs of families of children with disabilities and, 416–417
surveillance of, 239–240
systems of care for children with, 259
theoretical perspectives on, 242–249
time phases, 89–90
trajectory of, 89
transition of adolescents to adult services for, 256–258
Chronic Illness Framework, 242
Chronic obstructive pulmonary disease (COPD), 145
Chronosystems, 84, 85
Cigarette smoking, 149, 543–544
  by adolescents, 150
Circumplex Model of Marital and Family Systems, 6
Clarification and interpretation by nurses, 14
Client, family as, 10, 11
Clinical model of family health, 208
Closed boundaries, 77
Cochrane Database of Systematic Reviews, 571
Cohabitation, 38, 43, 44
  parenting and, 55
Cohesion, family, 7
Collaboration and partnership in community/public health nursing, 567–568
Collaborator, nurse as, 14
Commonwealth Care, 140
Communication
  childbearing and adjusting to changed patterns of, 362–363
  cybernetics and, 114
  with families with children, 399–400
  family, 29
  of genetic information, 192–195
  in the medical-surgical unit, 443–444
  in palliative and end-of-life care, 287–289
  at time of actively dying, 301
Community and trauma, 334–335
Community-based appointments, 108–109
Community Care Access Centre (CCAC), 152
Community Health Nurses of Canada, 570
Community nursing centers, 571–572
Community/public health nursing, 560–561
  assessment, assurance, and policy development in, 574–577
  case study, 578–580

collaboration and partnership in, 567–568
in community nursing centers, 571–572
cultural awareness, sensitivity, and safety, 567
defined, 561
empowerment through, 569–570
examples of, 565–566
facilitating access to resources, 574
health education in, 573–574
health promotion frameworks, 563
health promotion standards of practice, 563–564
nurse-client relationship with families and communities in, 568–569
principles in process of, 564
public health departments and, 572–573
roles with families and community, 573–577
settings for, 570–573
social determinants of health and, 564–565
trends in public health and, 577–578
Comorbidities and mental health, 523
Component of society, family as, 11, 12
Concepts, 69
Conceptual models
chronic illness, 242–249
defined, 69
foundations for, 70–76
nursing, 69–70
theory-guided, evidence-based childbearing nursing, 356–366
Conflict, family, 6
aging and, 486–487
role strain and, 28–29
Connections with families, establishing and sustaining, 289–290
Consent in family child health nursing, 415–418
Constant illness, 88–89
Consultant, nurse as, 14
Contempt, 6
Context
Canada in, 169–173
Canadian health care, 177–178
domain, 246
embedded, 209
family as, 10, 11
Family Health Model, 245–246
family nursing practice attending to, 178–184
integral to family nursing, 169
Continuing care retirement communities (CCRCs), 493, 497
Contract, family self-care, 220
Coordinator, nurse as, 14
Coping, family, 25–26
Core Competencies for Public Health in Canada, 563
Counselor, nurse as, 14
Course of chronic illness, 88–89

Creating Enriched Learning Environments Through Partnerships in Long-Term Care, 501
Crisis plans, mental health, 544–545
Critical Care Family Needs Inventory (CCFNI), 435
Critical care units. *See* Intensive care unit (ICU)
Criticism, 6
Cultural awareness, 197
community/public health nursing and, 567
mental health conditions and, 545
Cultural values, 197
about death and dying, 281–282
Culture, family, 217–218
Current Population Surveys, 35
Cybernetics, 114
Cystic fibrosis, 189

D

Death. *See also* End-of-life care; Palliative care
adolescent, 150
awareness of possibility of, 297
bereavement care after, 285, 302–303
from cancer, 239
care at time of, 300–302
of children, 302
from chronic illness, 239
finding meaning and, 299–300
at home, 305
perinatal, 369–370
personal assumptions and biases about, 280–281
personal assumptions and biases about people and their backgrounds and, 281–282
settings, 279
signs of imminent, 301
sudden or traumatic, 304–305
Decision making
family, 29–30
in the ICU, 440
in palliative and end-of-life care, 296–297
shared, 123–125, 440
Deductive reasoning, 68
Defensiveness, 6
Delirium, 504
Deliverer and supervisor of care and technical expert, nurse as, 14
Dementia, 189, 493, 533, 539–541
Demographics
adoption, 48–51
aging, 38–39
aging families, 480–482
assisted reproductive technologies, 47–48
changing family norms and, 37–38
cohabitation, 55
economic, 36–37
fathering, 54–55

fertility rate, 22, 45–47
gender roles, 36–38
geographical diversity and, 169–170
grandparenting, 57–58
immigration and ethnic diversity, 39–40
implications for health care providers, 40
information sources, 35
living arrangements, 40–45
overview, 34–35
parenting, 45–59
same-sex couple families, 55–56
single mothers, 51–54
stepfamilies, 56
Denham's Family Health Model, 73
Department of Health and Human Services, U. S. (USDHHS), 147
Depression
children and, 537–538
in the elderly, 504–505
major depressive disorder (MDD), 533, 536–538
postpartum, 375–376
Determinants of health, 138, 142–147
Development
childbearing and individual, 398
individual, 398
nuclear families, 19
social-emotional, cognitive, and physical dimensions of individual, 392–396
theory (*See* Family Developmental and Life Cycle Theory)
Developmental Model of Health and Nursing (DMHN), 211–212
Developmental trauma theory, 326–329
Diabetes, 145, 149, 189, 239
case study, 262–266
self-management, 250
Diagnostic and Statistical Manual of Mental Disorders, Fifth Edition (DSM-V), 122, 322, 521–522
Diagnostic genetic tests, 190
Dietary Guidelines for Americans 2010, 218
Direct-to-consumer genetic tests, 190–191
Disabled veterans, 491
Disasters, families affected by, 333
Disaster syndrome, 327
Discrimination and genetic testing, 196
Disparities. *See* Health disparities
Diversity
economic, 170–171
ethnocultural, 171–172
geographic, 169–170
linguistic, 172
religious, 172–173
Divorce, 6, 26, 34, 38
aging and, 482–484
family life cycle for families of, 81
stepfamilies and, 56–57
DNA (deoxyribonucleic acid), 188
Domestic violence, 175–177, 332–333
Dominant conditions, 198

Donation, organ, 453
Do not resuscitate (DNR) orders, 448, 450
Down syndrome, 189, 256
DSM-V. *See Diagnostic and Statistical Manual of Mental Disorders, Fifth Edition (DSM-V)*
Durable power of attorney for health care, 448

E

Early trauma, 325–330
Ecological Systems Theory, 83
    trauma and, 323–325, 338–339
Ecomaps, family, 116–120
Economics. *See also* Poverty
    aging and, 482
    at-risk pregnancy and, 372, 373
    burden of chronic illness, 240–242
    changes, 36–37
    children in poverty and, 409–410
    diversity, 170–171
    elder care and, 42
    fertility rate and, 46
    financing childbearing and child rearing and, 359–360
    functions of the family, 24
    housing and poverty reduction policies and, 153
    resources influences on family health, 213–214
    single mothers and, 52
Education
    of children with special needs, 412–413
    health, 573–574
    as health determinant, 147
    nursing, 159
    in palliative and end-of-life care, 281
    policy, 151–153
    preconception assessment and, 199–200
    school nursing and, 152
Elder care, 155, 489–490
    acute care, 503–505
    assisted living, 493, 498–500
    caring for, 489–490
    case study, 505–514
    chronic care programs, 497
    demographic diversity of, 481–482
    family caregiving, 487–496
    home- and community-based services (HCBS), 492, 496–497
    hospice care, 511–514
    nursing homes, 493, 500–503
    palliative and end-of-life care in, 502–503
    residential long-term care, 493, 497
    settings, 496–505
Elderly, the. *See also* Aging
    abuse of, 176
    caring for adult children, 490–491
    chronic care programs for, 497
    living arrangements of, 41–42

programs and models to improve hospital quality of care for, 498
    public health departments and, 573
    social policy and, 155
Elementary and Secondary Education Act, 151
Emancipated minors, 417
Embedded context, 209
Emotional health and decision to have genetic testing, 195–196
Emotional support for families with chronically ill member, 260
Empowerment, family, 221
    community/public health nursing and, 569–570
    in palliative and end-of-life care, 291–293
End-of-life care. *See also* Death
    advance care planning in, 295–296
    awareness of possibility of death and, 297
    balancing hope and preparation, 294–295
    barriers to optimal, 285–286
    bereavement care, 285, 302–303
    building on strengths, 297
    cardiopulmonary resuscitation, 449–450
    care at time of actively dying and, 300–302
    case studies, 305–314
    connections between families and nurses in, 286–289
    decision making in, 296–297
    defined, 278–280
    empowering families, 291–293
    encouraging patients and families through, 298
    facilitating choices, 295–297
    facilitating healing between family members, 298–299
    family meetings in, 299
    family nursing practice assessment and intervention, 286–305
    finding meaning through, 299–300
    in the hospital, 446–453
    involvement of interprofessional team in, 284–285
    involvement of the family in illness and, 282–284
    key areas of focus for education in, 281
    life-sustaining therapies (LSTs), 450–453
    managing negative feelings through, 298
    offering resources, 297–298
    organ donation and, 453
    personal assumptions and biases about death and dying and, 280–281
    providing information in, 293–294
    relevant literature, 279–280
    relieving the patient's suffering in, 289–291
    in residential care settings, 502–503
    special situations in, 303–305

Enduring management style, 243–244
Energized family, 6
Engagement in care, family, 107–111
Environmental influences on family health, 214
Environmental specialist, nurse as, 14
Epidemiologist, nurse as, 14
Equal Rights Amendment (ERA), 38
Essential Nursing Competencies and Curricula Guidelines for Genetics and Genomics, 187
Ethnicity
    adolescence and, 150, 409
    alcohol use and, 149–150
    caregiving and, 489–490
    cigarette smoking and, 149
    demographic changes, 39–40
    diversity, 39–40, 171–172
    as health determinant, 144
    mental health conditions care and, 545
    obesity and, 148–149
    poverty and, 409
    social determinants and resulting health disparities, 142
Ethnicity Diversity Survey, 171
Ethnocultural diversity, 171–172
Eudaimonistic model of family health, 208
European history and families, 19
Evaluation, 127–128
Exosystems, 84, 85, 213–216
    trauma and, 325
Extrapyramidal symptoms (EPS), 535

F

Facility-based long-term care, 493
Familial hypercholesterolemia, 189
Families
    adaptation, 251–252
    affected by disasters, 333
    affected by war, 331–332
    affective functions of, 23–24
    assumptions and expectations about, 173–177
    balanced, 7
    caregivers, 126–127
    caring for children living with chronic illness, 253–256
    Circumplex Model of Marital and Family Systems, 6
    as client, 10, 11
    communication, 29
    as component of society, 11, 12
    conflict within, 6
    as context, 10, 11
    coping, 25–26
    culture, 217–218
    decision making, 29–30
    defined, 4–5, 146–147, 560
    development, 79–83
    economic functions of, 24
    empowerment of, 221, 291–293
    encouragement for, 298

energized, 6
engaged in care, 107–111
European history, 19
facilitating healing within, 298–299
family career and, 390, 398
functioning in chronic illness, 90
functions, 22–25
genograms and ecomaps, 116–120
health care functions of, 24–25
health literacy, 120
healthy, 5–8
history of, 18–20
housekeeper and child care role in, 27
industrialization and, 19
involvement in one family member's illness, 282–284
lifestyle patterns, 218
marriage health and, 6
meals, 223–224
meetings, 299
norms, changing, 37–38
North American, 19
and nurse reflections, 129–133
prehistoric, 18–19
processes, 25–30, 217
provider role in, 27
reproductive functions of, 22–23
rituals and routines, 30, 222–223, 365
roles, 26–29
as safe and nurturing, 175–177
same-sex couple, 55–56, 174
secrets, 194
sick role in, 27–28
single-parent, 34, 46, 170
socialization functions of, 23
social policy, 138–139
sources of information on demography of, 35
stages, 390–391, 416–417
story analysis, 120–125
structure, 20–22, 34–35, 40–41, 217, 246, 482–483
as system, 10–12, 11
tasks, 391
today, 20
transitions, 365–366, 391, 396–398
trauma, 330–334
as unit of care, 16
violence and PTSD, 332–333
Families With Young Adults: Launching Phase, 82
Familismo, 560
Family advocate, nurse as, 14
Family and Medical Leave Act, 155, 241, 376
Family Assessment and Intervention Model (FS3I), 91–99, 101–102, 111, 112
Family Assessment Device (FAD), 209
Family-centered care
   elements of, 388–390
   meetings and care conferences, 110–111

Family-Centered Geriatric Resource Nurse (FCGRN), 498
Family child health nursing
   care of children with chronic illness and their families in, 410–415
   case study, 420–426
   child care, after-school activities, and children's health promotion and, 403–404
   concepts of, 390–398
   consent in, 415–418
   elements of family-centered care and, 388–390
   family career and, 390
   family stages and, 390–391
   family tasks and, 391
   in the hospital, 418–420
   identifying health risks and teaching prevention strategies in, 404–410
   nursing interventions to support care of well children and families, 398–410
   parenting a child with chronic illness and, 412–415
   transitions and, 391, 396–398
   understanding and working with family routines in, 403
   web sites of interest in, 426
Family Developmental and Life Cycle Theory, 71, 79–83, 100
   childbearing and, 358–366
Family health. *See also* Family health promotion
   adaptive model, 208
   clinical model, 208
   definition of, 5, 206–207
   economic influences on, 213–214
   environmental influences on, 214
   eudaimonistic model, 208
   exosystem and macrosystem influences on, 213–216
   family nursing interventions for, 219–224
   governmental health and families policies influences on, 214
   media influences on, 214–216
   microsystem and mesosystem influences on, 216–219
   model, 208–209
   models of, 207–209
   potential, 212
   role-performance model, 208
   routines, 209, 210, 262
Family health care nursing, 3–4
   approaches to, 10–12
   context integral to, 169, 178–184
   defined, 8
   historical perspectives, 15–20
   levels of, 8, 9
   nature of interventions in, 9–10
   obstacles to, 15
   of postpartum families, 372–376
   roles, 12–15

theoretical and conceptual foundations, 70–76
   variables that influence, 12
Family Health Model, 73, 244–249
   chronic illness and, 261
Family health promotion, 205–206. *See also* Family health
   case studies, 224–231
   common theoretical perspectives, 207–213
   defined, 205
   ecosystem influences on, 213–219
   historical perspectives of, 215
   models for, 209–213
   policies, 154–155
   prevention of chronic illness through, 249
Family history, genetic, 197–199
Family life cycle theory, 478
Family Management Style Framework (FMSF), 242–244
Family nursing assessment. *See* Assessments
Family Reasoning Web, 121
Family self-care contract, 220
Family social policy, 138–139
Family social science, 16
   theories, 70, 73
Family Systems Stressor-Strength Inventory, 457–471
Family Systems Theory, 68, 69, 71, 76–79, 100
   aging and, 478
   childbearing family nursing and, 357–358
   trauma and, 325
Family Systems Therapy Theory, 72
Family therapy theories, 70, 73
Fast food, 218
Fathering, 54–55
   childbirth and, 354
Feeding management of infants, 373–374
Fertility rate, 22, 45–47, 482–483
Fight-or-flight response, 326
First Nations people, 147
Five Core Needs, 326
Flexibility, family, 7
Flexible boundaries, 77
Floundering management style, 243–244
Foster care adoption, 49
Framework of Systemic Organization, 73
Frameworks, 69
Friedemann's Framework of Systemic Organization, 73
Friedman Family Assessment Model, 111, 112–113
Frontier Nursing Service (FNS), 16, 157
FS³I. *See* Family Assessment and Intervention Model

Functional domain, 246
Functions, family, 22–25
"Fundamental Principles for Caregiver Assessment," 494
Future of Nursing: Leading Change, Advancing Health, The, 157
Future of Public Health, The, 574

G

Gender differences. *See also* Men; Women
  aging, 482
  economic role, 27, 36
  elder care, 41–42
  financial disparities, 482
  as health determinant, 144
  life expectancy, 38, 41
  marriage age, 36
Genes, 188
Genetic Information Nondiscrimination Act (GINA), 196
Genetics
  cultural values and, 197
  decision to test, 195–196
  evaluation of interventions with genomics and, 201–202
  family history, conducting, 197–199
  genomics and, 188–189
  information, family disclosure of, 192–195
  information and nurses' role, 196–202
  preconception assessment and education, 199–200
  providing information and resources with testing of, 201
  risk assessment in adult-onset diseases and, 200–201
  testing, 189–192
Genograms, family, 116–120
Genomics, 188–189, 201–202
Geographical diversity of Canada, 169–170
Geographical information systems (GIS), 577
Geriatric Education Centers, 501
Geriatric Resource Nurse (GRN) Model, 498
Geriatric Syndrome Management Model, 498
Gestalt, 206
Global Economic Burden of Non-communicable Diseases, The, 240
Goal Attainment Theory, 72
Goals, family, 209
Gradual onset of chronic illness, 87–88
Grandchildren, 490
Grandparents, 57–58, 364
  caring for grandchildren, 490
Growing Healthier Report, 577
Guided Care, 497
Guttmacher Institute, 155

H

Hague Convention on Protection of Children and Co-operation in Respect of Intercountry Adoption, 50
Hartford Institute for Geriatric Nursing (HIGN), 487
Head Start, 147
Health, social determinants of, 141, 142–147, 564–565
Health care
  access to, 154, 177–178
  decisions and genetic testing, 196
  deliverers, 14
  family role in, 27
  home, 155
Health care functions of the family, 24–25
Health care reform
  social policy and, 156–159
  United States, 139–140, 157
Health determinants, 138
Health disparities, 155
  areas in need of additional social policy to avoid growing, 155–156
  in Canada, 140–141
  defined, 138
  elder care and, 155
  LGBT, 156
  risks and behaviors that contribute to, 148–151
  social determinants and resulting, 142–147
  in the United States, 139–140
Health education, 573–574
Health insurance in the United States, 139–140, 409, 574
Health Insurance Portability and Accountability Act (HIPAA), 140, 257
Health literacy, 146
  family, 120
Health missionaries, 16
Health policy. *See* Social policy
  influence on family health, 214
Health potential, 212
Health promotion. *See* Family health promotion
  child care, after-school activities, and children's, 403–404
  frameworks, standards, and principles in community/public health nursing, 561–570
  strategies for families with children, 410
Health resources as health determinant, 147
Health teacher, nurse as, 13–14
Health work, 212
Healthy Baby Healthy Children, 565
Healthy Marriage Initiative, 147
Healthy People 2000, 154, 215
Healthy People 2010, 146
Healthy People 2020, 152, 156, 214, 215, 216, 564, 572

Heart disease, 189
Henry Street Settlement, 157
Heterosexual nuclear families, 173–174
High-risk pregnancies, 371–372
Historical perspectives of family health care nursing, 15–20
HIV/AIDS, 145–146
  policy, 153
Home- and community-based services (HCBS), 492, 496–497
Home health care, 155
  death at home and, 305
  nursing role in assessing and supporting caregivers in, 491–496
Homelessness, 146
Homeostasis, 91, 328
Home visits, 108–109, 126
  in community/public health nursing, 569, 570–571
Homicide, 150
Homosexuality and LGBT health disparities, 156
Hospice care, 511–514
Hospital at Home, 498
Hospital care. *See also* Acute care settings
  of children, 418–420
  end-of-life care in, 446–453
  programs and models to improve quality of care for older adults in, 498
Hospital Elder Life Program (HELP), 498
Household, family, 246
  tasks assumed during childbearing, 371–372, 373
Housekeeper and child care roles in families, 27
Housing and poverty reduction policies, 153
Housing First program, 153–154
Human Becoming Theory, 73
Human Ecology Theory, 83
Huntington's disease, 189, 192, 195
Hurricane Katrina, 325
Hypotheses, 69

I

ICD-10, 522
ICD-9-CM. *See International Classification of Diseases: Clinical Modifications, Ninth Edition (ICD-9-CM)*
Identity, 23–24
IFNA. *See* International Family Nursing Association (IFNA)
IFNC. *See* International Family Nursing Conference (IFNC)
Illegal drug use, 150
Immigration and ethnic diversity, 39–40, 171–172
  interpreters and, 110
  religious diversity and, 172–173
Incapacitation due to chronic illness, 89
Individual development, 398. *See also* Development
Individual family service plan (IFSP), 413

Individualized educational program (IEP), 256
Individuals with Disabilities Education Act (IDEA), 412–413
Inductive reasoning, 68
Industrialization and families, 19
Infertility, 366–367
Informational support for families with chronically ill member, 260
Initial/crisis time phase, chronic illness, 89
Injuries, unintentional and intentional child, 405
Institute for Patient and Family Centered Care (IPFCC), 110
Institute of Medicine (IOM), 142, 146, 157, 249, 250, 567, 574, 576
Instrumental activities of daily living (IADLs), 481, 488, 493–494
Instrumental support for families with chronically ill member, 260
Instruments, family assessment, 111–120
Intensive care unit (ICU), 300, 304, 434–435
  cell phones in, 438
  family interventions, 439–441
  family needs in, 435–436
  family relocation stress and transfer anxiety, 441
  nursing role ambiguity and conflict, 436–437
  visiting policy, 437–438
  waiting rooms, 438
Intergenerational relationships, 485–486
International adoption, 49–50, 368
International Classification of Diseases: Clinical Modifications, Ninth Ediction (ICD-9-CM), 122
International Family Nursing Association (IFNA), 16
International Family Nursing Conference (IFNC), 16
International Family Therapy Theory, 72
International Red Cross, 333
International Society for Gerontechnology (IGS), 541
Interpreters, 110
Interprofessional collaboration (IPC), 568
Interprofessional team in palliative care, 284–285
Interventions, 9–10, 125–127. *See also* Assessments
  adopting families, 369
  brief therapeutic conversations in acute care, 126
  childbearing and child care, 361–365
  for childbearing families experiencing chronic threats to health, 373
  during chronic illness, 261–262
  at discharge from medical-surgical unit, 445–446
  evaluation of genomics and genetics nursing, 201–202

family health promotion, 219–224
Family Systems Theory and, 78–79
home visits and telephone support, 126
ICU, 439–441
infertility and nursing, 367
mental health crisis plans, 544–545
palliative and end-of-life care, 286–305
postpartum depression, 376
prevention of mental health conditions, 543–544
psychoeducation, 544
PTSD, 336–337
self-care talk for family caregivers, 126–127
to support care of well children and families, 398–410
Intimate partner violence (IPV), 332–333
Investing in Families, 566
IOM. *See* Institute of Medicine (IOM)
IPFCC. *See* Institute for Patient and Family Centered Care (IPFCC)

J

Johnson's Behavioral Systems Model for Nursing, 70, 72
Justice, social, 139

K

King's Goal Attainment Theory, 72
Knowledge, acquisition of, 28

L

Letter, therapeutic family, 128
LGBT persons
  adoption by, 367
  health disparities, 156
Liaison, nurse as, 14
Life course perspective, 478–480
  case study, 505–514
Life expectancy, 38–39, 41
Lifespan Respite Care Act, 241
Lifestyle patterns, family, 218
Life-sustaining therapies (LSTs), 450–453
Linguistic diversity, 172
Literacy, health, 120, 146
Living apart together (LAT), 484
Living arrangements, 40–45
  elderly, 41–42
  young adults, 42–44
Living wills, 448
Longitudinal Survey of Immigrants to Canada (LSIC), 174
Long-term care (LTC), 491, 500
  facility-based, 493
  residential, 493, 497
Low birth weight, 48
Lung diseases, 145

M

Macrosystems, 84, 85, 213–216
  trauma and, 325
Major depressive disorder (MDD), 533, 536–538
Maltreatment, child, 406–408
Marriage, 6, 34. *See also* Families
  age, 36, 37, 43
  aging and, 482–484
  cohabitation outside of, 38, 43, 44
  family roles and, 26–29
  same-sex, 45
  stepfamilies and, 56–57
McMaster Clinical Rating Scale (MCRS), 209
McMaster Model of Family Functioning (MMFF), 209
Meals, family, 223–224
Meaning, finding, 299–300
Media influences on family health, 214–216
Medicaid, 139–140, 155, 409–410, 498–499, 500
Medical Care Act, 140
Medical decisions and genetic testing, 196
Medical-surgical units, 441–446
Medicare, 39, 139–140, 155, 500
  best practices, 501
Meetings, family, 299
Men. *See also* Gender differences
  child care by, 27
  elderly, 41–42
  family roles and, 26–29
  as fathers, 54–55
  life expectancy, 38–39
  marriage age, 36, 37, 43
Mental health conditions, 146
  attention-deficit hyperactivity disorder (ADHD), 413, 533, 541–542
  bipolar disorder, 532, 533, 538–539, 545–551
  burden of family caregiving for, 526–527
  case studies, 545–552
  children living with a parent with, 529–531
  children living with a sibling with, 531
  children with family member with, 527–531
  comorbidities, 523
  crisis plans, 544–545
  defined, 521
  dementia, 533, 539–541
  diagnosis, 521–522
  families of individuals with specific, 533–542
  family members of individuals with, 526–533
  family role changes and, 527
  general approaches toward those with, 523–525
  major depressive disorder (MDD), 533, 536–538

older adults caring for adult children with, 490–491
parenting children with, 532–533
policy, 153–154
postpartum depression, 375–376
prevalence of, 522–523
prevention of, 543–544
providing culturally competent care for, 545
psychoeducation, 544, 551–553
Recovery Model, 524
role of family mental health nurse and, 542–545
schizophrenia, 533, 534–536
spousal caregiving for, 527
stigma of, 525–526
in the United States and Canada, 522–526
Mental health promotion, 565
Mesosystems, 84, 85, 216–219
trauma and, 323–325
Metabolic syndrome, 535
Microsystems, 84, 85, 216–219
trauma and, 323
Mid-time phase, chronic illness, 89–90
Military OneSource, 331
Model of Health-Promoting Family, 212–213
Models
conceptual, 69
family assessment, 111–120
nursing process, 106
social policy, 141–142
Moderation, 209
Moral distress and palliative care, 286
Multiple sclerosis (MS), 306–309
Mutual responsibility for child care and nurturing, 360–362

N

NANDA. *See* North American Nurses Diagnosis Association (NANDA)
National Advance Care Planning Task Group, 296
National Alliance for Caregiving, 488
National Alliance on Mental Illness (NAMI), 535
National Association of School Nurses (NASN), 152
National Cardiovascular Data Registry, 239
National Center for PTSD, 330
National Clearinghouse on Abuse in Later Life (NCALL), 573
National Comprehensive Cancer Network, 189
National Congress of Men, 19
National Council of Family Relations, 16
National Family Caregiver Program, 241
National Health and Nutrition Examination Survey (NHANES), 35, 239
National Health Interview Survey, 35

National Organization for Women (NOW), 19
National Organization of Nurse Practitioner Faculties (NONPF), 577
National PACE Association, 497
National Study of Adolescent Health, 150
National Survey of Children with Special Health Care Needs, 2009-2010, 253
National Survey of Family Growth, 35, 55
Native Americans
automobile accidents among, 150
binge drinking among, 149–150
Neglect, child, 406–408
Neuman Systems Model, 70, 73, 91
Neuroaffective Relational Model, 326
Neuroleptic malignant syndrome (NMS), 535
New England Journal of Medicine, 445
Next Step in Care, 501
NIC. *See* Nursing Intervention Classification (NIC)
Nightingale, Florence, 16
Nightingale nursing theory and model, 72
No Child Left Behind (NCLB), 151
Nonnormative changes in families, 82
Normalcy in families with childhood chronic illness, 415
Normative changes in families, 82
Norms, changing family, 37–38
North American families, 19
North American Nurses Diagnosis Association (NANDA), 121, 122
Nuclear families, 19
as the norm, 173–174
Nurse practitioners, 577–578
Nurses Improving Care to Health System Elders (NICHE), 498
Nursing. *See also* Family health care nursing
anticipatory guidance and information offered through, 222
assisted living, 499–500
conceptual frameworks, 70–76
contract, 220
cultural awareness in, 197
education, 159
family mental health, 542–545
nurse navigator and, 446
nursing home, 500–501
process model, 106
research, 159
school, 152
theories, 69–70, 73
Nursing: Scope and Standards of Practice, 4
Nursing Home Reform Act, 500
Nursing homes, 493, 500–503
Nursing Intervention Classification (NIC), 121
Nursing's Social Policy Statement, 4

O

Obesity, 148–149, 335–336
in families with children, 405–406
Obstacles of family health care nursing, 15

Older adults. *See* Aging; Elderly, the
Older Adults Services Inpatient Strategies (OASIS), 498
Omaha System-Community Health Classification System, 122
Ontario Early Years Centers (OEYCs), 572
Open boundaries, 77–78
Orem's Self-Care Deficit Theory, 73
Organ donation, 453
Ottawa Charter for Health Promotion, 563
Overnutrition, 218

P

Palliative care. *See also* Death
advance care planning in, 295–296
awareness of possibility of death and, 297
balancing hope and preparation, 294–295
barriers to optimal, 285–286
bereavement care, 285, 302–303
building on strengths, 297
care at time of actively dying and, 300–302
case studies, 305–314
connections between families and nurses in, 286–289
decision making in, 296–297
defined, 278–280
empowering families, 291–293
encouraging patients and families through, 298
facilitating choices, 295–297
facilitating healing between family members, 298–299
family meetings in, 299
family nursing practice assessment and intervention, 286–305
finding meaning through, 299–300
involvement of interprofessional team in, 284–285
involvement of the family in illness and, 282–284
key areas of focus for education in, 281
managing negative feelings through, 298
offering resources, 297–298
personal assumptions and biases about death and dying and, 280–281
personal assumptions and biases about people and their backgrounds and, 281–282
providing information in, 293–294
relevant literature, 279–280
relieving the patient's suffering in, 289–291
in residential care settings, 502–503
special situations in, 303–305
Parenting. *See also* Childbearing; Children
adoption and, 48–51
arranging space for a child and, 358–359
assisted reproductive technologies (ARTs) and, 47–48

a child with chronic illness, 412–415
cohabitation and, 55
communication patterns and, 362–363
demographics, 45–59
establishing family rituals and routines
during, 365
Family Management Style Framework
and, 242–244
family transitions during, 365–366
fertility rate and, 22, 45–47
financing and, 359–360
grand-, 57–58, 364
maintaining family members' motivation
and morale during, 364–365
by men, 54–55
mutual responsibility for, 360–362
planning for subsequent children and,
363
realigning intergenerational patterns,
363–364
role learning of family members and,
362
by same-sex couples, 55–56
single-parent, 34, 46, 81
in stepfamilies, 56–57
styles, 401–402
Parent Resource for Information Development and Education (PRIDE),
368
Parents. *See also* Children
of boomerang children, 43
communication of genetic information
to, 193–194
same-sex couples as, 45
single, 34
taking care of self with child suffering
from chronic illness, 414–415
Parkinson's disease, 238, 240,
266–272
Parse's Human Becoming Theory, 73
Patient-Centered Primary Care
Collaborative, 497
Patient/Parent Information and
Involvement Assessment Tool
(PINT), 115, 123–124
Patients
encouraging, 298
family meetings with, 299
finding meaning, 299–300
making choices in palliative and
end-of-life care, 295–297
managing negative feelings, 298
Patient Self-Determination Act, 448
Patriarchy, 19
Peplau's Theory of Interpersonal Relations
in Nursing, 569
Perinatal loss, 369–370
pregnancy following, 370–371
Permissive parenting, 402
Personal Responsibility and Work
Opportunity Reconciliation Act
(PRWORA), 52, 53
Person-centered care, 502
Pharmacogenetic testing genetic tests, 190

Physician orders for life-sustaining
treatment (POLST), 448
PINT. *See* Patient/Parent Information
and Involvement Assessment Tool
(PINT)
Pioneer Network, 500, 501
Policy. *See* Social policy
childbearing family nursing, 376–377
public health, 577
Population Health Promotion Model, 563
Postpartum depression, 375–376
Postpartum families, family nursing of,
372–376
Post-traumatic stress disorder (PTSD),
322–323
community and, 334–335
developmental trauma theory and,
326–329
family functioning and, 333–334
family trauma and, 330–334
family violence and, 332–333
nursing assessment and intervention,
336–337
risks associated with, 337–338
secondary traumatization and, 334, 338
systemic trauma and, 335–336
theory applied to, 323–325
Potential, health, 212
Poverty. *See also* Economics
in Canada, 170
children in, 409–410
education and, 147
health care insurance and, 139
as health determinant, 143–144
reduction policies, 153
single parents living in, 46
welfare reform and, 52
Preconception assessment and education,
199–200
Predictive and presymptomatic genetic
tests, 190, 191–192, 195
Pregnancy. *See also* Childbearing
family nursing of postpartum families
and, 372–376
following perinatal loss, 370
postpartum depression after, 375–376
preterm birth and, 48, 377–381
threats to health during, 371–372
Prehistoric family life, 18–19
Prenatal Care Assistance Program
(PCAP), 140
Prenatal diagnosis genetic tests, 190
Preselection, 195
Preterm delivery, 48
case study, 377–381
Private adoption, 368
Private domestic adoption, 49
Processes, family, 25–30, 217
chronic illness and, 247–248
Program of All-inclusive Care for the
Elderly (PACE), 497
Progressive chronic illness, 88–89
Project F-EAT, 223
Propositions, 69

Provider role in families, 27
Psychoeducation, 544, 551–553
Public health
departments, 572–573
nursing (*See* Community/public health
nursing)
nursing (PHN) generalists, 564
policy, 577

R

Race. *See* Ethnicity
Ray's Adaptation Model, 72
Reasoning, inductive and deductive, 68
Recovery Model, 524
Reflections, nurse and family, 129–133
Registered Nurses Association of Ontario
(RNAO), 158
Relapsing/episodic illness, 88–89
Relational inquiry, 168
Relational nursing
Canada in context and, 169–173
Canadian health care context and,
177–178
in community/public health nursing,
568–569
context integral to, 169
facilitating healing between family
members, 298–299
family nursing practice attending to
context and, 178–184
in palliative and end-of-life care,
286–289
Relationships
ambivalence and conflict in, 486–487
family, 483–487
intergenerational, 485–486
same-generation, 483–485
in theories, 69
Religion
diversity, 172–173
influence on family health, 218–219
Relocation stress, 441
Reproductive functions of the family,
22–23. *See also* Childbearing
Researcher, nurse as, 14–15, 159
Residential care facilities, 493, 497
family involvement in, 501–502
nursing home, 493, 500–503
palliative care and end-of-life care in,
502–503
Resilience, 24, 329–330
Responsiveness, 401
Restlessness, terminal, 301
Resuscitation, child, 420
Retirement, 37
Risks
adolescent, 408–409
assessment in adult-onset diseases,
200–201
and behaviors that contribute to health
disparities, 148–151
child health nursing and identifying,
404–410

Rituals and routines, 30, 222–223, 365
    establishment of, 365
    family health, 209, 210, 246–247, 262
    perinatal loss, 371
    understanding and working with family, 403
Roe v. Wade, 155
Roger's Science of Unitary Human Beings, 72
Role model, nurse as, 15
Role-performance model of family health, 208
Roles, family, 26–29
    caregiving, 488–491
    mental health conditions and, 527
Rolland's Chronic Illness Framework, 242

S

Same-generation relationships, 483–485
Same-sex couples, 35, 45, 174
    adoption by, 367
    assisted reproductive technologies and, 48
    families, 48, 55–56
    LGBT health disparities and, 156
"Sandwich" generation, 58
Sanger, Margaret, 16
Scared Sick: The Roles of Childhood Trauma in Adult Disease, 336
Schizophrenia, 533, 534–536
School health, 566
School nursing, 152
Science and technology influences on family health, 216
Science of Unitary Human Beings, 72
Secondary traumatization, 334, 338
Selective serotonin reuptake inhibitors (SSRIs), 537
Self-care contract, family, 220
Self-Care Deficit Theory, 73
Self-care talk for family caregivers, 126–127
Self-identity, 23–24
Self-management, 250–251
Selye, Hans, 328
Sexuality
    adolescents and, 408–409
    throughout the life course, 484
Shaken baby syndrome, 363
Shared decision making, 123–125
    in the ICU, 440
Siblings, 374
    aging and, 484–485
    of children with chronic illness, 258–259, 413–414
    of hospitalized children, 419
    of individuals with mental health conditions, 531
    realigning intergenerational patterns and, 364
Sickle cell anemia, 189
Sick role in families, 27–28
Single mothers, 34, 46, 51–54

Single-parent families, 34, 46
    family life cycle, 81
    poverty and, 170
Skilled nursing facilities (SNFs), 493
Smoking. *See* Cigarette smoking
Social Determinants of Health Model, 141, 142–147, 564–565
Social-emotional, cognitive, and physical dimensions of individual development, 392–396
Socialization functions of the family, 23
Social justice, 139
Social policy
    aging population, 154
    areas in need of additional social policy to avoid growing disparities, 155–156
    defining, 138–141
    determinants of health and, 138, 142–147
    educational policy, 151–153
    elder care, 155
    family, 138–139
    health promotion, 154–155
    historical involvement of nurses in, 156–157
    housing and poverty reduction policies, 153
    LGBT health disparities and, 156
    models, 141–142
    nurse's role in advocacy for, 156–159
    nursing policy, research, and education influencing, 158–159
    nursing today and, 157–158
    related to chronic illness, 153–154
    in the United States, 139–140
    women's reproduction and, 155–156
Social science, 16
Social Security benefits, 37
Social support for chronic illness, 259–261
Society
    aging, 38–39
    families as component of, 11, 12
Society for Adolescent Medicine, 258
Special health care needs (SHCN) children, 253–256, 410–415
Spirituality. *See* Religion
Spousal caregiving, 527
Stages, family, 390–391
    tasks, and situational needs of families of children with disabilities and chronic illness, 416–417
State Child Health Insurance Program (SCHIP), 139–140
Stepfamilies, 56–57
Stigma and mental health, 525–526
Stonewalling, 6
Story analysis, family, 120–125
Strain, role, 28–29
Strengths-based nursing care, 221
Stress
    chronic, 145
    family relocation, 441
    toxic, 336

Stressors, family
    adoption, 367–369
    childbearing, 366–371
    family structure and, 217
    in family systems, 93–99
    Family Systems Stressor-Strength Inventory, 457–471
    infertility, 366–367
    perinatal loss, 369–370
    pregnancy following perinatal loss, 370–371
    when raising a child with chronic health conditions, 255–256
Structural domain, 246
Structural Family Therapy Theory, 72
Structural Functional Theory, 71
Structure, family, 20–22, 34–35, 40–41, 217, 482–483
    Family Health Model and, 246
Struggling management style, 243–244
Substance abuse, 150, 176–177, 336
Substance Abuse and Mental Health Services Administration (SAMHSA), 522, 523
Subsystems, 78
Sudden or traumatic death, 304–305
Surgery, preparing children for, 400
Surrogate, nurse as, 14
Surveillance of chronic illness, 239–240
Symbolic Interaction Theory, 71
System, family as, 10–12, 11
Systemic trauma, 335–336
Systems Model, 70, 73, 91

T

TANF. *See* Temporary Assistance to Needy Families (TANF)
Tardive dyskinesia (TD), 535
Tasks, family, 391
Tay-Sachs disease, 200
Technical expert, nurse as, 14
Teenage mothers, 47
Telehealth, 540
Telephone support, 126
Temporary Assistance to Needy Families (TANF)
    creation of, 53
    legal definition of family and, 147
Terminal restlessness, 301
Terminal time phase, chronic illness, 90
Theoretical frameworks. *See* Conceptual models
Theories, 67–68. *See also* specific theories
    concepts in, 69
    defined, 68–69
    hypotheses in, 69
    nursing conceptual frameworks, 70–76
    perspectives and applications to families, 76–99
    propositions in, 69
    relationship between practice, research, and, 68–70
Therapeutic family letter, 128
Thriving management style, 243–244

Tidal Model, 524
Time phases, chronic illness, 89–90
Tobacco use, 149
    by adolescents, 150
    surveillance, 239
Toxic stress, 336
Trajectory of illness, 89
Transfer anxiety, 441
Transitional Care Model, 501
Transition of care, 256–258
Transitions, family, 365–366, 391, 396–398
    during hospital care, 419–420
Transition Theory, 71
Transmission of family patterns, 116
Transracial adoption, 50, 368
Trauma, 321–323
    assessment and intervention, 336–337
    attachment and, 325–326
    brain development and early,
        328–329
    cases studies, 339–347
    community and, 334–335
    death due to, 304–305
    developmental trauma theory and,
        326–329
    disasters and, 333
    early, 325–330
    ecological theory applied to, 323–325,
        338–339
    family, 330–334
    family functioning and, 333–334
    Family Systems Theory applied to, 325
    nurses and, 336–339
    post-traumatic stress disorder (PTSD)
        and, 322–325
    risks associated with PTSD and,
        337–338
    secondary, 334, 338
    systemic, 335–336
    understanding of adult trauma through
        early childhood, 329–330
    war and, 331–332
Type 1 diabetes, 262–266
Type 2 diabetes, 145, 149, 239
    self-management, 250

U

Unemployment, 359–360
*Unequal Treatment: Confronting Racial
    and Ethnic Disparities in Health Care,*
    142
Unified Parkinson's Disease rating scale,
    270–272
Uninvolved parenting, 402
United States, the

adoption in, 48–51
aging population in, 38–39
alcohol use in, 149–150
American family in, 19
cohabitation in, 44, 55
definition of family in, 147
economic changes in, 36–37
Family and Medical Leave Act, 155,
    241, 376
fathering in, 54
fertility rate, 45–47
grandparenting in, 57–58
health care policy in, 139–140, 157, 574
illegal drug use in, 150
immigration to, 39–40
income gap in, 143
life expectancy in, 38–39
living arrangements in, 40–45
multigenerational households in,
    41–42
obesity in, 148–149
poverty in, 143–144
same-sex couple families in, 55
stepfamilies in, 56
tobacco use in, 149
welfare reform in, 52, 53

V

Validators, 6
Veterans, disabled, 491
Victorian Order of Nurses (VON), 571
Violence
    adolescents and, 408
    against children, 405, 406–408
    domestic, 175–177, 332–333
    PTSD and, 332–333
    screening questions, 407
Visiting policy
    ICU, 437–438
    medical-surgical units, 442–443
Volatiles, 6

W

Waiting rooms, ICU, 438
Wald, Lillian, 157
War. *See also* Post-traumatic stress
    disorder (PTSD)
    developmental trauma theory and,
        327
    disabled veterans of, 491
    families affected by, 331–332
    toxic stress and, 336
Warfarin, 189–190
Welfare reform, 52, 53

Welfare-to-Work program, 139
Well-being, 247, 249
WHO. *See* World Health Organization
    (WHO)
WIC. *See* Women, Infants, and Children
    Program (WIC)
Widowhood, 483–484
Wills, living, 448
Women. *See also* Childbearing; Gender
    differences
    changing economy and society effects
        on, 36
    elderly, 41–42
    family roles and, 26–29
    financial disparities, 482
    historical roles, 15–16
    life expectancy, 38–39, 41
    marriage age, 36, 37, 43
    postpartum depression in, 375–376
    as single mothers, 34, 46, 51–54
    violence against, 176
    women's movement and, 19, 38
    women's reproduction social policy
        and, 155–156
    as working mothers, 27, 36, 175, 359
Women, Infants, and Children Program
    (WIC), 140, 148, 361
Work, health, 212
World Health Organization (WHO), 5,
    122, 522, 560
    on determinants of health, 138
    on health disparities, 138
World War II
    economic changes after, 36
    public health nursing during, 16
    women's roles after, 37

X

X-linked recessive condition, 198

Y

Young adults
    bioecological model of aging and, 479
    living arrangements of, 42–44
    mortality risk in, 150
    social-emotional, cognitive, and
        physical dimensions of individual
        development in, 392–396
Youth Risk Behavior Surveillance System
    (YRBS), 408